ACSM'S RESOURCE MANUAL

for

GUIDELINES FOR EXERCISE TESTING AND PRESCRIPTION

Third Edition

AMERICAN COLLEGE OF SPORTS MEDICINE

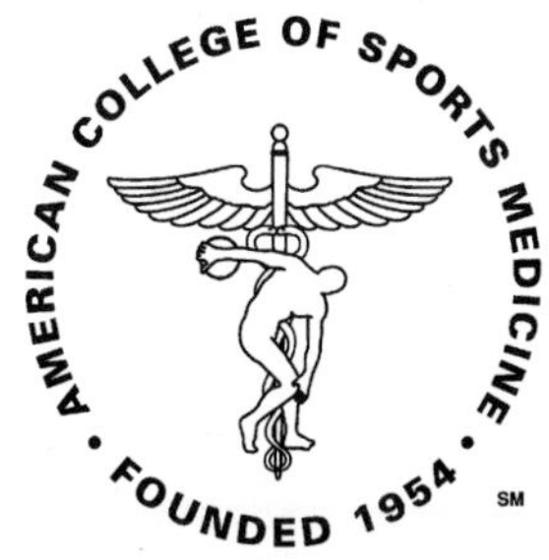

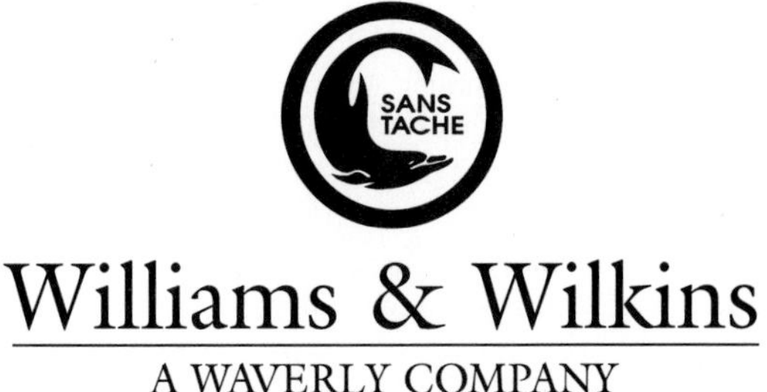

Williams & Wilkins
A WAVERLY COMPANY

BALTIMORE • PHILADELPHIA • LONDON • PARIS • BANGKOK
BUENOS AIRES • HONG KONG • MUNICH • SYDNEY • TOKYO • WROCLAW

Editor: Eric P. Johnson
Managing Editor: Jennifer Schmidt
Marketing Manager: Christine Kushner
Production Coordinator: Danielle Hagan
Project Editor: Jeffrey S. Myers
Text/Cover Designer: Graphic World, Inc.
Coverphoto: John Riley/Tony Stone Images

3511 West Camden Street
Baltimore, Maryland 21201–2436 USA

Rose Tree Corporate Center
1400 North Providence Road
Building II, Suite 5025
Media, Pennsylvania 19063–2043 USA

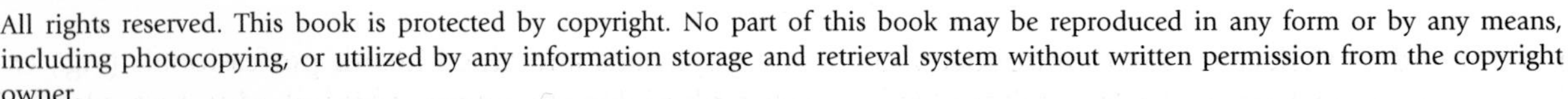

Accurate indications, adverse reactions and dosage schedules for drugs are provided in this book, but it is possible that they may change. The reader is urged to review the package information data of the manufacturers of the medications mentioned.

Printed in the United States of America

First Edition, 1988
Second Edition, 1993
Third Edition, 1998

Library of Congress Cataloging-in-Publication Data

American College of Sports Medicine.
ACSM's resource manual for Guidelines for exercise testing and prescription / American College of Sports Medicine.—3rd ed. / senior editor, Jeffrey L. Roitman : section editors, Moira Kelsey . . . [et al.]
p. cm.
Companion v. to: Guidelines for exercise testing and prescription. 4th ed. 1991.
Includes bibliographical references and index.
ISBN 0-683-00026-8
1. Exercise therapy. 2. Exercise tests. I. Roitman, Jeffrey L. II. Kelsey, Moira. III. Title.
[DNLM: 1. Exercise Test. 2. Exercise Therapy. 3. Exertion. 4. Exercise—physiology. WE 103 A5125g 1991 Suppl. 1998]
RM725.R42 1998
615.8′2—dc21
DNLM/DLC
for Library of Congress 97–50181
CIP

The publishers have made every effort to trace the copyright holders for borrowed material. If they have inadvertently overlooked any, they will be pleased to make the necessary arrangements at the first opportunity.

Call our customer service department at **(800) 638–0672** for catalog information or fax orders to **(800) 447–8438.** For other book services, including chapter reprints and large quantity sales, ask for the Special Sales department.

To purchase additional copies of this book or for information concerning American College of Sports Medicine certification and suggested preparatory materials, call the ACSM Certification Resource Center at **(800) 486–5643** or visit **www.wwilkins.com/acsmcrc.**

Canadian customers should call **(800) 665–1148,** or fax **(800) 665–0103.** For all other calls originating outside of the United States, please call **(410) 528–4223** or fax us at **(410) 528–8550.**

Visit Williams & Wilkins on the Internet: **http://www.wwilkins.com** or contact our customer service department at **custserv@wwilkins.com.** Williams & Wilkins customer service representatives are available from 8:30 am to 6:00 pm, EST, Monday through Friday, for telephone access.

98 99 00 01 02
1 2 3 4 5 6 7 8 9 10

ACSM's RESOURCE MANUAL

for

GUIDELINES FOR EXERCISE TESTING AND PRESCRIPTION

Third Edition

SENIOR EDITOR

JEFFREY L. ROITMAN, EdD, FACSM
DIRECTOR, CARDIAC REHABILITATION
RESEARCH MEDICAL CENTER
KANSAS CITY, MISSOURI

SECTION EDITORS

MOIRA KELSEY, RN, M.S.
Clinical Coordinator
Division of Thoracic and Cardiovascular Surgery
Ohio State University Medical Center
Columbus, Ohio

THOMAS P. LAFONTAINE, PhD, FACSM
Manager
WELLAWARE Disease Prevention and Community Wellness Program
Boone Hospital Center
Columbia, Missouri

DOUGLAS R. SOUTHARD, PhD
Director, Physician Assistant Program
College of Health Sciences
Roanoke, Virginia

MARK A. WILLIAMS, PhD, FACSM
Professor of Medicine
Division of Cardiology
Director, Cardiovascular Disease Prevention and Rehabilitation
Cardiac Center of Creighton University
Omaha, Nebraska

TRACY YORK, MS
Director of Operations
Lake Austin Spa Resort
Austin, Texas

Foreword

It is an honor and a privilege for me to introduce you to the Third Edition of the *American College of Sports Medicine's Resource Manual for Guidelines for Exercise Testing and Prescription*. This textual compendium of 80 individual chapters and accompanying appendices largely represents the fundamental knowledge that must be mastered by candidates applying for ACSM's certifications in preventive and rehabilitative exercise programming. Accordingly, the editors have recruited a prestigious group of scientists, clinicians, and researchers who have painstakingly worked to summarize, in a clear and concise manner, the core material and latest research findings in their respective areas of expertise, with specific reference to lifestyle modifications, anatomy and biomechanics, exercise physiology, cardiopulmonary and other chronic diseases, electrocardiography, exercise programming, human development, behavior change, and program implementation.

An impressive gain in the management of persons with and without chronic disease has been the establishment of the benefits of regular physical activity and its progressive incorporation into the mainstream of contemporary medical care. Exercise is now accepted as a bona fide preventive and therapeutic measure. However, special deficits or defects resulting from congenital deformities, injury, or disease, and the needs and limitations imposed by these conditions must be considered in formulating safe and effective exercise prescription. To this end, we have come to recognize the usefulness of exercise testing in evaluating the cardiorespiratory, hemodynamic, and electrocardiographic responses to physical exertion, both before and after various therapeutic interventions.

In the era of managed, capitated health care, primary care physicians and allied health professionals (e.g., exercise physiologists, nurses, physical educators, physical therapists, registered dietitians) will assume an increasingly important role in implementing exercise-based primary and secondary prevention programs. Although hypertension, hyperlipidemia, obesity, and diabetes mellitus may be favorably affected by regular physical activity, optimal health-related outcomes will only be achieved by complementing exercise with education and counseling, medical surveillance and emergency support (when appropriate), pharmacotherapy (if necessary), and interventions to enhance psychosocial functioning and long-term adherence to lifestyle changes. The latter include assessing the client's/patient's "readiness" for change, providing services that are designed to circumvent or attenuate common barriers to enrollment and adherence (e.g., offering group and home-based programs), keeping goals short-term and attainable, using motivational incentives accruing to periodic exercise testing and risk factor assessment, recruiting spouse and family support of the intervention, and archiving goal achievements.

As we approach the next millennium, our changing medical environment will dictate that there will be greater individual responsibility to maintain health and prevent disease. This text provides substantial reinforcement for the adoption of exercise as part of the armamentarium of interventions necessary to achieve this objective. Those who master the material in this volume will be especially well-prepared to "help others help themselves." The challenge is yours!

Barry A. Franklin, PhD, FACSM

Preface

The American College of Sports Medicine certification program for exercise professionals began in 1975 with the publication of the First Edition of *ACSM's Guidelines for Exercise Testing and Prescription* ("*The Guidelines*") and the subsequent examination of candidates for certification. The First Edition of the *Resource Manual for Guidelines for Exercise Testing and Prescription* was published in 1988. The original purpose of this book was as a companion to *The Guidelines.* This book continues to serve that purpose for fitness professionals who are candidates for certification as well as for those professionals requiring the resources behind *The Guidelines.*

The objectives for certification, originally called "behavioral objectives" and subsequently re-named "Knowledges, Skills and Abilities" or "KSAs," are written to describe a set of minimum competencies that various levels of exercise professional should possess to function professionally. They are, therefore, required "Knowledges, Skills and Abilities" for successful certification. The KSAs are divided into those associated with the Health/Fitness Track and the Clinical Track.

The Third Edition of *The Resource Manual,* presents background information for the KSAs to assist both professionals in the field and candidates for certification. This edition has changed significantly from the previous edition. Material similar to that found in previous editions has been updated, information has been added in the form of whole sections and chapters to present information to assist exercise professionals in staying abreast of current trends and concepts. Most chapters have been shortened to concentrate material in order to make it easier to find and study.

One of the most significant changes is the indexing of KSAs to chapters at the front of the book. In addition, numbered KSAs, matched by icon to the level of certification can be found at the beginning of each chapter. In this way, the book becomes more "user friendly" to the professional wishing to find information referring to specific KSAs. This type of format also enables the reverse indexing of the KSAs, thus the list in the front also contains references to chapters where the KSA may be found.

No single reference can provide all of the answers for professionals or candidates for certification, but The *Resource Manual* is an authoritative source. The contributors are among the best in their specialty, each a well known researcher or practitioner. The information is current and presents what is presently known about the topic, we hope in a way that will make it useful to the exercise professional and candidate for certification.

The Resource Manual continues to be a primary reference source for KSAs as well as for information relative to the practice of the fitness professional (both health/fitness and clinical professionals). More broadly, *The Resource Manual* is a reference work for those working in either the clinical or the health/fitness environment for topics relative to exercise physiology disease management, wellness, prevention of disease, behavioral psychology, program administration and the wide array of topics that exercise professionals encounter on a daily basis.

How to Use This Book

HOW TO USE THIS BOOK

In the section of the front material entitled "KSA Listing," the KSAs are printed exactly as they are in *The Guidelines,* but are numbered in consecutive order. A second column shows the chapter number where material relative to that KSA can be found. Note that in many instances, more than one chapter is listed because information relative to KSA is found in more than one chapter. Similarly, at the beginning of each chapter you will find an icon with a number. The icon illustrates the level of certification and the number can be matched back to the individual KSA in the front of the book. This index is not exhaustive, in that every single piece of information about a KSA has been indexed. Candidates for certification are encouraged to look through the Table of Contents and the index seeking additional sources for material which interests them.

This system allows candidates studying for certification to locate information pertinent to a KSA quickly and easily. By simply using the table of KSAs at the front and referring to the specific chapter(s) indexed, individual KSAs can be located. Likewise, when reading and studying individual chapters, information concerning the KSAs covered in that chapter can be found at the beginning of the chapter.

Icon Key

Health/Fitness Track

Health Fitness Director

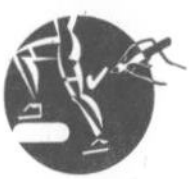

Health Fitness Instructor

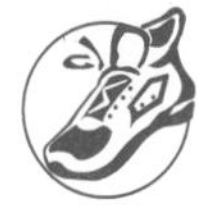

Exercise Leader

Clinical Track

Clinical Program Director

Exercise Specialist

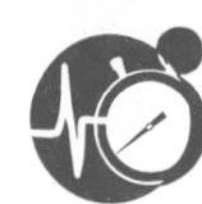

Exercise Test Technologist

KSA Listing

KSA: Health/Fitness Track

KSA: FUNCTIONAL ANATOMY AND BIOMECHANICS

	KSA Number	Chapter
Exercise Leader		
1. Describe the basic structures of bone, skeletal muscle, and connective tissues.	1	9, 54
2. Describe the basic anatomy of the heart, cardiovascular system, and respiratory system.	2	7, 8
3. Identify the major bones and muscles and their actions. Major muscles include, but are not limited to, trapezius, pectoralis major, latissimus dorsi, biceps, triceps, abdominal, erector spinae, gluteus maximus, quadriceps, hamstrings, and gastrocnemius.	3	9
4. Define the following terms: supination, pronation, flexion, extension, adduction, abduction hyperextension, rotation, and circumduction.	4	9, 10, 44
5. List and describe the types of joints in the body.	5	9
6. Identify the interrelationships among center of gravity, base of support, balance, and stability.	6	11, 12
7. Describe the following abnormal curvatures of the spine: lordosis, scoliosis, kyphosis.	7	13
8. Describe low back pain syndrome and describe exercises used to prevent this problem.	8	13
9. Describe the biomechanical effects and potential risks of using hand/ankle weights.	9	
10. Describe and demonstrate exercises designed to enhance muscular strength and/or endurance of specific major muscle groups.	10	
11. Describe and demonstrate exercises for enhancing musculoskeletal flexibility	11	
Health/Fitness Instructor		
12. Describe the structure and nature of movement in the major joints of the body.	12	9, 44
13. Describe the factors that determine range of motion in the major joints of the body.	13	9, 44
14. Describe the biomechanical principles that underlie performance of the following activities: walking, jogging, running, swimming, cycling, weight lifting, and carrying or moving objects.	14	12
15. Locate the common sites for measurement of skinfold thickness, skeletal diameter, girth measurements for estimation of body composition; the anatomic landmarks for palpation of peripheral pulses; locate the brachial artery and correctly place the cuff and stethoscope in position of blood pressure measurement.	15	10
Health/Fitness Director		
16. Discuss the relationship among biomechanical efficiency, oxygen cost of activity (economy), and performance of physical activity.	16	11, 12
17. Discuss the application of biomechanical principles (e.g., Newton's Laws of Motion) to human movement.	17	11, 12

KSA: EXERCISE PHYSIOLOGY

	KSA Number	Chapter
Exercise Leader		
1. Define aerobic and anaerobic metabolism.	18	14, 15
2. Identify the role of aerobic, anaerobic and ATP-PC systems in the performance of various physical activities.	19	14, 15
3. Define the following terms: ischemia, angina pectoris, tachycardia, bradycardia, myocardial infarction, cardiac output, stroke volume, lactic acid, oxygen consumption, hyperventilation, systolic blood pressure, diastolic blood pressure.	20	14
4. Describe the role of carbohydrates, fats, proteins as fuels for aerobic and anaerobic metabolism.	21	14
5. Demonstrate an understanding of the components of fitness: cardiorespiratory fitness, muscular strength, muscular endurance, flexibility, body composition.	22	17, 18, 19, 53, 54
6. Define the major components of motor fitness: agility, speed, balance, coordination, power.	23	
7. Describe the normal cardiorespiratory responses to static and dynamic exercise in terms of heart rate, blood pressure, and oxygen consumption.	24	15, 17
8. Describe how heart rate, blood pressure, and oxygen consumption responses change with adaptation to chronic exercise training and how men and women may differ in response.	25	15, 17, 19
9. List the physiological adaptations associated with strength training in men and women.	26	18, 19
10. Define and describe the relationship of METs and kilocalories to physical activity.	27	Appendix A
11. Identify the common sites for pulse and palpation and describe how heart rate is determined by pulse palpation. List precautions in the application of these techniques.	28	10
12. Identify the physiological principles related to warm-up and cool-down.	29	52
13. List the effects of temperature, humidity, altitude, and pollution on the physiological response to exercise.	30	24, 25
14. Identify the physical and physiological signs of over-exercising, over-training, overuse.	31	52, 57
15. Describe the common theories of muscle fatigue and delayed onset muscle soreness (DOMS).	32	18, 19, 20
Health/Fitness Instructor		
16. Describe the primary anaerobic and aerobic energy systems and their role during exercise.	33	14, 15
17. Describe the basic properties of cardiac muscle and the normal pathways of conduction in the heart.	34	7, 48
18. Calculate the energy cost in METs and kilocalories for given exercise intensities in stepping exercise, bicycle ergometry, and during horizontal and graded walking and running.	35	Guidelines
19. Identify approximate MET equivalents for various sport, recreational, and work tasks.	36	Appendix A
20. Discuss the physiological basis of the major components of physical fitness: flexibility, cardiovascular fitness, muscular strength, muscular endurance, and body composition.	37	15, 18, 19, 44, 53, 54
21. Explain the differences in the cardiorespiratory responses to static exercise compared with dynamic exercise, including possible hazards of static exercise.	38	16
22. Explain how the principle of specificity relates to the components of fitness.	39	17, 19, 53, 56
23. Define and describe the implications of ventilatory anaerobic threshold ("anaerobic threshold") as it relates to physical conditioning programs and cardiovascular assessment.	40	
24. Explain the concept of detraining or reversibility of conditioning and its implications in fitness programs.	41	21, 22, 23
25. Discuss the physical and psychological signs of over-training and provide recommendations to deal with these problems.	42	
26. Describe the structure of the skeletal muscle fiber and the basic mechanism of contraction.	43	9
27. Describe the functional characteristics of fast and slow twitch fibers.	44	9, 14, 18

28. Explain contraction of muscle in terms of the sliding filament theory.	45	9
29. Explain twitch, summation, and tetanus in terms of muscle contraction.	46	9
30. Discuss the physiological principles involved in promoting gains in muscular strength and endurance.	47	18, 19, 53
31. Demonstrate an understanding of the relationship between number of repetitions, intensity, number of sets, and rest with regard to strength training.	48	19, 53
32. Describe how each of the following differ from the normal condition: dyspnea, hypoxia, hypoventilation, orthostatic hypotension, premature atrial contractions, and premature ventricular contractions.	49	36
33. Describe blood pressure responses associated with exercise and changes in body position.	50	15, 16
34. Define hypotension and hypertension and explain why blood pressure should be monitored during exercise testing.	51	15, 16
35. List the physiologic adaptations to the muscular system, metabolism, and the cardiorespiratory system that occur at rest, during submaximal and maximal exercise following chronic anaerobic and aerobic training.	52	15, 17, 21
36. Describe the response of the following variables to steady state submaximal exercise and maximal exercise: heart rate, stroke volume, cardiac output, pulmonary ventilation, tidal volume, respiratory rate, arteriovenous oxygen difference.	53	15, 16, 17
37. Describe the physiologic and metabolic responses to exercise associated with chronic disease (e.g., heart disease, hypertension, diabetes mellitus, and pulmonary disease).	54	32
Health/Fitness Director		
38. Discuss the physiological and biochemical characteristics of fast and slow twitch muscle fibers.	55	9, 14, 18, 19
39. Explain the concept of muscular fatigue during specific conditions of task intensity, duration, and the accumulative effects of exercise.	56	20
40. Contrast the cardiorespiratory responses to acute graded exercise in conditioned and unconditioned subjects.	57	15, 17
41. Compare the relative and absolute cardiorespiratory responses to levels of exercise intensity in conditioned and unconditioned subjects.	58	15, 17

KSA: HUMAN DEVELOPMENT AND AGING

	KSA Number	Chapter
Exercise Leader		
1. Describe the changes that occur in maturation from childhood to older adulthood for the following areas: skeletal muscle, bone structure, reaction and movement time, coordination, tolerance to hot and cold environments, maximal oxygen consumption, strength, flexibility, body composition, resting and maximal heart rate, resting and maximal blood pressure.	59	59, 60, 61
2. List the benefits and risks associated with exercise training in pre- and post-pubescent youth.	60	60
3. Identify benefits and precautions associated with resistance and endurance training in the older adult.	61	19, 61
4. Describe special leadership techniques which might be used for children, adolescents, and older participants.	62	60, 61
Health/Fitness Instructor		
5. Demonstrate and understand the effect of the aging process on the structure and function of the human organism at rest, during exercise, and during recovery.	63	59
6. Characterize the differences in the development of an exercise prescription for children, adolescents, and older participants.	64	60, 61

7. Describe the unique adaptations to exercise training in children, adolescents, and older participants with regard to strength, functional capacity, and motor skills.	65	60, 61
8. Describe common orthopedic and cardiovascular considerations of older participants and what modifications in exercise prescription are indicated.	66	61
HEALTH/FITNESS DIRECTOR		
9. Demonstrate a knowledge and a practical understanding of programming techniques as they relate to markets of all ages.	67	61
10. Identify the various components involved with implementing successful programs for children, adolescents, adults, and older participants.	68	60, 61

KSA: PATHOPHYSIOLOGY/RISK FACTORS

	KSA NUMBER	CHAPTER
EXERCISE LEADER		
1. Identify risk factors for coronary artery disease (CAD) and designate those that may be favorably modified by regular and appropriate physical activity habits.	69	1, 5, 30
2. Define the following terms: total cholesterol, high density lipoprotein cholesterol (HDL-C), low density lipoprotein cholesterol (LDL-C), total cholesterol/high density lipoprotein cholesterol ratio anemia, and hypertension.	70	
3. Be familiar with the plasma cholesterol levels for various ages as recommended by the National Cholesterol Education Program.	71	
4. Identify the following cardiovascular risk factors or conditions that may require consultation with medical or allied health professionals prior to participation in physical activity or prior to a major increase in physical activity intensities and habits; inappropriate resting, exercise, and recovery HR's and BP's; new discomfort or changes in the pattern of discomfort in the chest area, neck, shoulder or arm with exercise or at rest; heart murmurs; myocardial infarction; fainting or dizzy spells, claudication, ischemia, cigarette or other tobacco use, lipoprotein profile.	72	4, Guidelines
5. Identify the following respiratory risk factors that may require consultation with medical professionals prior to participation in physical activity or prior to major increases in physical activities or habits; extreme breathlessness after mild exertion or during sleep, asthma, exercise-induced asthma, bronchitis, emphysema.	73	36, Guidelines
6. Identify the following metabolic risk factors that may require consultation with medical professionals prior to participation in physical activity or prior to major increases in physical activity intensities and habits: body weight more than 20% above optimal, thyroid disease, diabetes or glucose intolerance, McArdle's syndrome, hypoglycemia.	74	31, Guidelines
7. Identify the following musculoskeletal risk factors that may require consultation with medical professionals prior to physical activity or prior to major increases in physical activity intensities and habits: osteoarthritis, rheumatoid arthritis, acute or chronic back pain, prosthesis-artificial joints.	75	13, 57
8. Demonstrate an understanding of muscle atrophy and the loss of strength and endurance with disuse/sedentary behavior.	76	23
9. Define shin splints, sprains, strains, tennis elbow, bursitis, stress fracture, tendinitis, contusions, osteoporosis, arthritis, overweight, chondromalacia, blisters, skin irritations, and low back discomfort.	77	57
HEALTH/FITNESS INSTRUCTOR		
10. Demonstrate an understanding of the pathophysiology of atherosclerosis and how this process is influenced by physical activity.	78	1, 26, 30

11. Identify common drugs from each of the following classes of medications and describe the principal action and the effects on exercise testing and prescription: A. Antianginal (nitrates, beta blockers, calcium channel blockers, etc.) B. Antihypertensive C. Antiarrhythmic D. Bronchodilators E. Hypoglycemics F. Psychotropics G. Vasodilators	79	Appendix C
12. Identify the effects of the following substances on exercise response: antihistamines, tranquilizers, alcohol, diet pills, cold tablets, caffeine, and nicotine.	80	4
HEALTH/FITNESS DIRECTOR		
13. Explain the risk factor concept of coronary artery disease (CAD) and the influence of heredity and lifestyle upon the development of CAD.	81	1, 3, 4, 5, 6, 30
14. Explain the process of atherosclerosis, the factors involved in its genesis, and the methods which may potentially reverse the process.	82	1, 4, 5, 6, 26, 30
15. Discuss in detail how lifestyle factors and heredity influence lipid and lipoprotein profiles.	83	1, 3, 30, 35
16. Explain the genesis of myocardial ischemia and infarction.	84	26, 27
17. Explain the causes of hypertension, obesity, hyperlipidemia, diabetes, chronic obstructive and restrictive pulmonary diseases, arthritis, and gout.	85	31, 32, 35, 37
18. Identify and explain the effects of the above diseases or conditions on cardiorespiratory and metabolic function at rest and during exercise.	86	15, 16, 31, 32, 36, 37, 38, 39
19. Describe muscular, cardiorespiratory, and metabolic responses to exercise following a decrease in physical activity, bed rest, or casting of a limb for a period of one month.	87	22, 23
20. Identify and discuss the causes and mechanisms of chronic obstructive pulmonary disease (COPD), exercise-induced asthma, chronic asthma, chronic diseases, and immunosuppressive disease.	88	31, 37
21. Identify current drugs from each of the following classes of medications. Explain the principal action, mechanism of action, and major side-effects. A. Antianginal B. Antihypertensive C. Antiarrhythmic D. Bronchodilators E. Hypoglycemics F. Psychotropics G. Vasodilators	89	Appendix C

KSA: HUMAN BEHAVIOR/PSYCHOLOGY

	KSA NUMBER	CHAPTER
EXERCISE LEADER		
1. List several techniques to deal with disruptive individuals in group programs (e.g., non-complier, comedian, chronic complainer, and the over-exerciser)	90	67
2. Define the psychological principles which are critical to health behavior change (i.e., behavior modification, reinforcement, goal-setting, social support and peer pressure).	91	4, 65, 67, 68, 69, 70, 71
3. Describe the personal communication skills necessary to develop rapport in order to motivate individuals to begin exercise, enhance adherence, and return to exercise.	92	62, 65, 68, 69
4. Identify several techniques that can be used in an exercise program to facilitate skill development in muscular relaxation.	93	
5. List specific techniques to enhance motivation: posters, recognition, bulletin boards, games, competitions, etc.	94	69

	KSA Number	Chapter
Health/Fitness Instructor		
6. Describe the specific strategies (e.g., operant conditioning) aimed at encouraging the initiation, adherence, and return to participation in an exercise program or any other healthy lifestyle behaviors.	95	4, 65, 67, 68, 69
7. Describe effective counseling communication skills in order to bring about behavioral change.	96	4, 62
8. Describe how each of the following terms may impact the successful management of an exercise program; anxiety, depression, fear, denial, rejection, rationalization, aggression, anger, hostility, empathy, arousal, euphoria, and relaxation.	97	*64*, 65, 66
9. Discuss the potential manifestation of test anxiety (i.e., performance, appraisal, threat) during exercise testing and how it may disrupt accurate physiological responses to testing.	98	63
10. Describe the differential effects of exercise and progressive relaxation as stress management techniques for modifying anxiety, depression, anger, and for generating relaxation.	99	5, 66
11. Discuss the behavioral change strategies that are appropriate or inappropriate for modifying body composition.	100	70
Health/Fitness Director		
12. Describe basic cognitive-behavioral intervention, such as shaping, goal-setting, motivation, cueing, problem solving, reinforcement strategies, and relaxation management.	101	65, 68, 69
13. Describe the selection of appropriate behavioral and outcome goals, and the suggested method and frequency of outcome evaluation.	102	65, 70

KSA: HEALTH APPRAISAL AND FITNESS TESTING

	KSA Number	Chapter
Exercise Leader		
1. Describe and demonstrate the use of health history appraisal to obtain information on past and present medical history, orthopedic limitations, prescribed medications, activity patterns, nutritional habits, stress and anxiety levels, family history of heart disease, smoking history, and use of alcohol and illicit drugs and know when to recommend medical clearance.	103	40, 41, 42, 46 Guidelines
2. Describe the use of informed consent forms and medical clearances prior to exercise participation.	104	75
3. Demonstrate the ability to conduct group field assessment, such as Cooper 12-minute test, step test, strength, muscular endurance, and flexibility assessment.	105	44
4. State the rationale for determining body composition.	106	45, 46
5. Describe the types of tests for cardiorespiratory fitness, evaluation of strength and flexibility, and techniques used to determine body composition, and the purposes for which each may be used (i.e., base-line, comparison, motivation, etc.).	107	41, 42, 43, 44, 45
6. Describe the difference between maximal and submaximal cardiorespiratory exercise tests.	108	41
7. Demonstrate the ability to measure pulse rate accurately both at rest and during exercise.	109	
8. Demonstrate the ability to measure blood pressure accurately at rest.	110	
Health/Fitness Instructor		
9. Demonstrate or identify appropriate techniques for health appraisal and use of fitness evaluations.	111	40, 41
10. State the purpose and demonstrate basic principles of exercise testing.	112	41, 42
11. Describe the categories of participants who should receive medical clearance prior to administration of an exercise test or participation in an exercise program.	113	40, 42 Guidelines
12. Identify relative and absolute contraindications to exercise testing or participation.	114	58 Guidelines
13. Demonstrate the ability to obtain appropriate medical history, informed consent, and other pertinent information prior to exercise testing.	115	40, 41, 42, 75

14. Discuss the limitations of informed consent and medical clearances prior to exercise testing.	116	75
15. Demonstrate the ability to instruct participants in the use of equipment and test procedures.	117	
16. Demonstrate the ability to assess muscular strength, muscular endurance, and flexibility.	118	43, 44
17. Demonstrate various techniques of assessing body composition and discuss the advantages/disadvantages and limitations of the various techniques.	119	45
18. Discuss and demonstrate various submaximal and maximal cardiorespiratory fitness tests using various modes of exercise and interpret and critique the information obtained from the various tests.	120	41, 42
19. Discuss modification of protocols and procedures for cardiorespiratory fitness tests in children, adolescents, and older adults.	121	
20. Explain the purpose and procedures for monitoring clients prior to, during, and after cardiorespiratory fitness testing.	122	41, 42
21. Demonstrate the ability to accurately measure heart rate, blood pressure, and rating of perceived exertion at rest and during exercise according to established guidelines.	123	
22. Demonstrate the ability to interpret results of fitness evaluations on apparently healthy individuals and those with stable disease.	124	41, 42
23. Describe and demonstrate techniques for calibration of a cycle ergometer and a motor-driven treadmill.	125	
24. Identify appropriate criteria for discontinuing a fitness evaluation and demonstrate proper procedures to be followed after discontinuing such a test.	126	41, 42 Guidelines
Health/Fitness Director		
25. Explain the use and value of the results of the exercise test and fitness evaluation for various populations.	127	
26. Demonstrate the ability to design and implement a health appraisal/fitness assessment programming; including but not limited to staffing needs, physician interaction, documents, equipment, marketing, ongoing evaluations.	128	72
27. Demonstrate the ability to recruit, train, and evaluate appropriate staff personnel for performing exercise tests and fitness evaluations.	129	73

KSA: EMERGENCY PROCEDURES AND SAFETY

	KSA Number	Chapter
Exercise Leader		
1. Demonstrate skills necessary to obtain basic life support and cardiopulmonary resuscitation certification.	130	
2. Describe appropriate emergency procedures (i.e., telephone procedures, written emergency procedures, personnel responsibilities, etc.) in a variety of exercise settings.	131	Guidelines
3. Describe basic first aid procedures for exercise-related injuries such as: bleeding skin wounds, contusions, strains/sprains, fractures, dizziness, syncope, and metabolic abnormalities including hypo/hypertension, hypo/hyperglycemia, hypo/hyperthermia.	132	57, 58, 79
4. Demonstrate an understanding of the risks associated with exercise participation.	133	57, 58
5. Describe the signs/symptoms for participants (including special populations) to defer, delay, or terminate the exercise session.	134	Guidelines
6. Demonstrate the basic precautions taken in a weight room area to ensure participant safety (e.g., spotting, buddy system, control speed of movement, weights returned to rack, safe passageways, check loose parts on equipment, etc.)	135	79
Health/Fitness Instructor		
7. Demonstrate knowledge of safety plans, emergency procedures, and first aid techniques needed during fitness evaluations, exercise testing, and exercise training.	136	79
8. Identify the components that create and maintain a safe environment.	137	77

9. Identify the content and discuss the use of informed consent and exercise waivers.	138	75
10. Discuss the instructors responsibilities, limitations, and the legal implications of carrying out emergency procedures.	139	75 Guidelines
11. Describe potential musculoskeletal injuries (e.g., contusions, strains/sprains, fractures), cardiovascular/pulmonary complications (e.g., tachycardia, bradycardia, hypo/hypertension, tachypnea), and metabolic abnormalities (e.g., fainting/syncope, hypo/hyperglycemia, hypo/hyperthermia).	140	57, 58
12. Explain the initial management and first aid techniques associated with open wounds, musculoskeletal injuries, cardiovascular/pulmonary complications, and metabolic abnormalities.	141	57, 79
13. Describe the components of an equipment maintenance/repair program and how it may be used to evaluate the condition of exercise equipment in order to reduce potential risk of injury.	142	77
Health/Fitness Director		
14. Provide instruction in the principles and techniques used in cardiopulmonary resuscitation.	143	10
15. Design and update emergency procedures for a preventive exercise program and an exercise testing facility.	144	79
16. List emergency drugs that should be available during exercise testing.	145	Guidelines
17. Train staff in safety procedures, the epidemiology of risk of injury and cardiovascular complications, risk reduction techniques, and emergency techniques.	146	79
18. Demonstrate an understanding of the legal implications of documented safety procedures, the use of incident documents, ongoing training, and drills.	147	75

KSA: EXERCISE PROGRAMMING

	KSA Number	Chapter
Exercise Leader		
1. State the recommended intensity, duration, frequency, and type of physical activity necessary for development of cardiorespiratory fitness in an apparently healthy population.	148	52
2. Differentiate between the dose of exercise required for various health benefits and the dose required for fitness development.	149	52, 70
3. Describe the differences between improvement and maintenance exercise training programs.	150	52
4. Describe the principles of overload, specificity, and progression and how they relate to exercise programming.	151	52, 53, 56
5. Describe and demonstrate appropriate exercises used in warm-up and cool-down for: cardiorespiratory conditioning classes, weight training, and sport participation (racquet sports, volleyball, basketball, etc.).	152	52
6. Demonstrate an understanding of the components incorporated into an exercise session and their proper sequence (i.e., warm-up, aerobic stimulus phase, cool-down, muscular endurance, and flexibility).	153	52
7. Define overload, specificity of exercise conditioning, use-disuse, progressive resistance, isotonic, isometric, isokinetic, concentric, eccentric, atrophy, hypertrophy, sets, repetitions, plyometrics, Valsalva maneuver.	154	52, 53
8. Define RPE and describe the relationship to the physiological responses to exercise and its role in exercise programming.	155	52
9. Demonstrate an understanding of calculation of predicted maximal and training heart rate ranges.	156	52 Guidelines
10. Demonstrate various methods for monitoring exercise intensity such as heart rate and perceived exertion.	157	52
11. Describe the signs and symptoms of excessive effort that would indicate a change in intensity, duration, or frequency of exercise.	158	52

12. Describe and demonstrate appropriate modifications in exercise programs that may be recommended by a physician for the following: older adults, acute illness, controlled conditions such as exercise-induced asthma, allergies, hypertension, pregnancy and postpartum, obesity, and low back pain.	159	13, 32, 70
13. Demonstrate the ability to recognize proper technique and use of all exercise equipment (i.e., proper body mechanics, proper positioning on apparatus, appropriate settings for cardiovascular and resistance training, proper monitoring techniques, safety considerations, etc.).	160	
14. Describe the importance of flexibilty and recommend proper exercises for improving range of motion of all major joints.	161	13, 54
15. Demonstrate the ability to modify exercises in the group setting for apparently healthy persons of various fitness levels.	162	
16. Describe and demonstrate exercises for the improvement and maintenance of muscular endurance and muscular strength.	163	19, 53
17. Describe how the following weight training methods may be used in resistance programming: progressive resistance exercise, super sets, pyramiding, split routines, plyometrics, isokinetic, isotonic, isometric.	164	19, 53
18. Identify various types of isometric, isotonic, and isokinetic equipment.	165	77
19. List advantages and disadvantages of various aerobic exercise equipment such as stair climbers, rowing machines, treadmills, bicycles, etc.	166	77
20. Describe the hypothetical concerns and potential risks that may be associated with the use of exercises, such as straight leg sit-ups, double leg raises, full squats, hurdler's stretch, plough, forceful back hyperextension, and standing straight-leg, toe-touch.	167	13, 79
21. Describe the differences between interval, continuous, and circuit training programs.	168	52
22. Demonstrate appropriate and effective group exercise management and teaching techniques.	169	
23. Describe various locations a leader may take within a group to enhance visibility, participant interactions, and communication.	170	
24. Demonstrate the ability to communicate effectively with exercise participant in the group and one-on-one setting.	171	
25. Describe an exercise regimen for a water exercise class.	172	
26. Describe partner resistance exercises that can be employed in a class setting.	173	
27. Demonstrate a knowledge of techniques for a accommodating various fitness levels within the same class.	174	
28. Identify the differences between high impact and low impact exercise classes and which class is appropriate for various participants.	175	
29. Identify the short-term and long-range advantages/benefits associated with fitness participation.	176	2, 15, 19
Health/Fitness Instructor		
30. Design, implement, and evaluate individualized and group exercise programs based on health history and physical fitness assessments.	177	72
31. Define exercise prescription guidelines for apparently healthy, higher risk, and clients with controlled disease.	178	52
32. Demonstrate the use of the variables of mode, intensity, duration, frequency, and progression in designing cardiorespiratory and resistive training.	179	18, 52, 53
33. Design exercise programs to improve or maintain cardiorespiratory endurance.	180	52
34. Demonstrate the use of various methods for establishing and monitoring levels of exercise intensity including heart rate, RPE, and METs.	181	52
35. Design resistive exercise programs to increase or maintain muscular strength and/or endurance for the purpose of general fitness, hypertrophy, injury prevention, and sports conditioning.	182	19
36. Demonstrate the proper techniques for performing resistive exercises for all major muscle groups using calisthenics, free weights, resistive equipment, and machines.	183	
37. Demonstrate an ability to establish appropriate resistance levels on circuit weight training equipment and various free weight exercises.	184	53

38. Design flexibility programs to improve or maintain range of motion at all major joints.	185	54
39. Demonstrate proper techniques for performing flexibility exercises for all major muscle groups.	186	54
40. Discuss the advantages and disadvantages of implementation of interval, continuous, and circuit training programs, and design programs for each.	187	52
41. Discuss the advantages and disadvantages of various commercial exercise equipment in developing cardiorespiratory fitness, muscular strength, and muscular endurance.	188	53, 77
42. Describe special precautions and modifications of exercise programming for participation at altitude, different ambient temperatures, humidities, and environmental pollution.	189	25
43. Describe modifications in type, duration, frequency, progression, level of supervision, and monitoring techniques in exercise programs for patients with heart disease, diabetes mellitus, obesity, hypertension, musculoskeletal problems pregnancy/postpartum, and exercise-induced asthma.	190	70
44. Demonstrate an understanding for the components incorporated into an exercise session and their proper sequence (i.e., pre-exercise evaluation, warm-up, aerobic stimulus phase, cool-down, muscular endurance, and flexibility).	191	52, 54
45. Describe the types of exercise programs available in the community and how these programs are appropriate for various populations.	192	72
46. Demonstrate an understanding of the importance of recording exercise sessions and performing periodic evaluations to assess changes in fitness status.	193	52

KSA: NUTRITION AND WEIGHT MANAGEMENT

	KSA Number	Chapter
Exercise Leader		
1. Define the following terms: obesity, overweight, percent fat, lean body mass, anorexia nervosa, bulimia, and body fat distribution.	194	70
2. Discuss the relationship between body composition and health.	195	45, 55
3. Compare the effects of diet plus exercise, diet alone, and exercise alone as methods for modifying body composition.	196	55, 70
4. Describe misconceptions about spot reductions and rapid weight loss programs.	197	55, 70
5. Explain the concept of energy balance as it relates to weight control.	198	55, 70
6. Identify the functions of fat and water soluble vitamins and contrast their potential risk of toxicity with over-supplementation.	199	3
7. Discuss the ramifications of the use of salt tablets, diet pills, protein powder, and other nutritional supplements.	200	3
8. Describe the importance of and procedures for maintaining normal hydration at times of heavy sweating, and describe appropriate beverages for fluid replacement during and after exercise.	201	24
9. Demonstrate familiarity with the USDA Food Pyramid and US Dietary Guidelines.	202	3, 55
10. Demonstrate an understanding of the importance of calcium and iron in women's health.	203	3
11. Describe the effects of diet and exercise on the blood lipid profile.	204	1, 3, 35
12. Describe the myths and consequences associated with inappropriate weight loss methods: saunas, vibrating belts, body wraps, electric simulators and sweat suits.	205	
13. List the number of kilocalories in 1 gram of the following: fat, carbohydrate, protein, and alcohol. List the number of kilocalories in 1 pound of fat.	206	3, 55, 70
14. Describe appropriate weekly weight loss goals.	207	55, 70
Health/Fitness Instructor		
15. List the six essential nutrients and describe their nutritional role.	208	3
16. Discuss the recommended distribution of calories from fat, carbohydrate, and protein.	209	3, 55

17. Describe the health implications of variation in body fat distribution patterns and the significance of waist/hip ratios.	210	45, 70
18. Discuss guidelines for caloric intake for an individual desiring to lose or gain weight.	211	55, 70
19. Discuss common nutritional ergogenic aids, their purported mechanism of action and any risks and/or benefits (e.g., carbohydrates, protein/amino acids, vitamins, minerals, sodium bicarbonate, bee pollen, etc.).	212	3
20. Describe nutritional factors related to the female athlete triad syndrome (i.e., eating disorders, menstrual cycle abnormalities, and osteoporosis).	213	
21. Demonstrate familiarity with the NIH Consensus statement on health risks of obesity, Nutrition for Physical Fitness Position Paper of the American Dietetic Association (endorsed by ACSM), and the ACSM Position Stand on proper and improper weight loss programs.	214	

KSA: PROGRAM AND ADMINISTRATION/MANAGEMENT

	KSA Number	Chapter
Health/Fitness Instructor		
1. Understand the health fitness instructor's supportive role in administration and program management within a health/fitness facility.	215	76
2. Demonstrate an ability to administer fitness-related programs within established budgetary guidelines.	216	74
3. Demonstrate an ability to develop marketing materials for the purpose of promoting fitness-related programs.	217	80
4. Describe various sales techniques for prospective program clients/participants.	218	80
5. Describe the documentation required when a client shows signs or symptoms during an exercise session and should be referred to a physician.	219	
6. Demonstrate the ability to create and maintain records pertaining to participant exercise adherence, retention, and goal setting.	220	
7. Demonstrate the ability to develop and administer educational programs (i.e., lectures, workshops, etc.) and educational materials (i.e., participant handouts).	221	72
8. Demonstrate an understanding of management of a fitness department (e.g., working with a budget, training exercise leaders, scheduling, running staff meetings, etc.).	222	76
9. Discuss the importance of tracking and evaluating member retention.	223	
Health/Fitness Director		
10. Describe a management plan for the development of staff, materials for education, marketing, client records, billing, facilities management, and financial planning.	224	76
11. Discuss how each of the following affect the decision-making process: budget, market analysis, program evaluation, facilities, staff allocation, and community development.	225	72, 74, 76, 80
12. Discuss the development, evaluation, and revision of policies and procedures for programming, and elements of a program evaluation report.	226	78
13. Discuss the use of the outside consultation: establishing contacts, contracting for services and follow-up procedures.	227	73
14. Discuss how the computer can assist in data analysis, spreadsheet development, and daily tracking of customer service and utilization.	228	72
15. Describe and discuss the management-by-objective decision-making approach.	229	
16. Interpret applied research in the areas of testing, exercise, and educational programs in order to maintain a comprehensive and current state-of-the-art program.	230	
17. Compare and contrast the various evaluation design models such as cross-sectional, longitudinal, case control, and randomized clinical trials.	231	

18. Discuss the establishment of a database, including type of data to be collected, data management, and analysis.	232	
19. Discuss the organization of a risk factor screening program; describe procedures, staff training, feedback, and follow-up.	233	72
Health/Fitness Director: Personnel		
20. Demonstrate an understanding of personnel management.	234	73
21. Describe effective interviewing, hiring, and employee termination procedures.	235	73
22. Diagram and explain an organizational chart and show the staff relationships between a health fitness director, governing body, medical advisor, and staff.	236	73
23. Discuss various staff training techniques.	237	73
24. Describe performance reviews and their role in evaluating staff.	238	73
25. Discuss legal obligations and problems involved in personnel management.	239	
26. Discuss incentive-based compensation management.	240	73
27. Describe effective methods of implementing a sales commission system.	241	
28. Discuss the significance of a benefits program for staff.	242	73
29. Describe the process of establishing a wage-based scale.	243	73
30. Identify the procedures of writing and implementing job descriptions.	244	73
31. Describe personnel time management techniques.	245	73
Health/Fitness Director: Budget/Finance		
32. Demonstrate an understanding of the principles of financial management.	246	74
33. Demonstrate an understanding of basic accounting principles, such as accounts payable, accounts receivable, liabilities, assets, and return on investment.	247	74
34. Identify the various forms of a business enterprise such as sole proprietorship, partnership, corporation, and S-corporation.	248	74
35. Identify the procedures involved with developing, evaluating, revising, and updating capital and operating budgets.	249	74
36. Describe recommended expense management techniques.	250	74
37. Develop an understanding of taxes and how they impact various health/fitness organizations.	251	74
38. Develop an understanding of financial statement analysis.	252	74
39. Demonstrate an understanding of the current financial industry trends.	253	74
40. Demonstrate an understanding of program-related break-even analysis.	254	74
41. Discuss the importance of return on investment.	255	74
43. Demonstrate an understanding of the principles of operational costs versus revenue generated in regard to membership programs and profit centers.	256	74
Health/Fitness Director: Marketing/Sales		
43. Demonstrate an understanding of sales and marketing.	257	80
44. Identify the steps in the development, implementation, and evaluation of a marketing plan.	258	80
45. Discuss the components of a needs assessment/market analysis.	259	80
46. Describe the various sales techniques for prospective members.	260	80
47. Discuss techniques for advertising, marketing, sales promotion, and public relations.	261	80
48. Discuss the principles of evaluating product and established pricing.	262	80
49. Describe various membership tracking techniques and the steps of implementation and evaluation of a plan.	263	80
Health/Fitness Director: Operations		
50. Demonstrate an understanding for implementing capital improvements.	264	

51. Discuss the principles of pricing and purchasing equipment and supplies.	265	77
52. Demonstrate an understanding of facility layout and design.	266	
53. Demonstrate the ability to establish and evaluate an equipment preventive maintenance and repair program.	267	77
54. Describe a plan for implementing a daytime and nighttime housekeeping program.	268	
55. Describe the importance of short-term and long-term planning.	269	72
56. Identify and explain operating policies for preventive exercise programs including data analysis and reporting, reimbursement of service fees, confidentiality of records, relationships between program and referring physicians, continuing education of participants and family, legal liability, and accident or injury reporting.	270	78
57. Explain the legal concepts of tort, negligence, contributory negligence, liability, indemnification, standards of care, consent, contract, confidentiality, malpractice, and the legal concerns regarding emergency procedures and informed consent.	271	75
Health/Fitness Director: Member Service/Communications		
58. Demonstrate effective skills and techniques for communication and public speaking.	272	
59. Discuss various techniques for obtaining customer feedback.	273	72
60. Describe an understanding of developing surveys for the purpose of customer communication.	274	72
61. Discuss the strategies for managing conflict.	275	73
62. Identify the recommended techniques of effective front desk management.	276	76
Health/Fitness Director: Health Promotion		
63. Demonstrate an understanding of health promotion programs, such as nutrition and weight management, smoking cessation, stress management, healthy back, substance abuse, and dependent care.	277	5, 6 70, 71
63. Discuss appropriate content within specific health promotion programs.	278	5, 6
64. Discuss different methods used in implementing health promotion programs (e.g., health communications, referral programs, sponsored intervention programs, etc.).	279	72
65. Discuss resources available for various programs and delivery systems.	280	6, 72
66. Discuss appropriate selection criteria for programs and providers.	281	72
67. Demonstrate an understanding of the role of evaluating health promotion programs in reducing health care costs and improving profitability in the workplace.	282	72
68. Describe the concepts of cost-effectiveness and cost-benefit as it relates to the evaluation of health promotion programming in the workplace.	283	72
69. Discuss the means and amounts by which health promotion programs might reduce care costs and improve profitability in the workplace.	284	72
70. Demonstrate an understanding of how health promotion programs may interrelate with Employee Assistance Programs (EAPs).	285	73

KSA: Clinical Track Certification

KSA: FUNCTIONAL ANATOMY/BIOMECHANICS

	KSA Number	Chapter
Exercise Test Technologist		
1. Demonstrate a knowledge of surface anatomy as related to exercise testing and fitness evaluation.	286	10, 47
2. Locate the appropriate sites for the limb and chest leads for standard and bipolar resting and exercise ECGs.	287	10, 47

3. Locate the brachial artery and describe the cuff and stethoscope positions for blood pressure measurement.	288	10
4. Locate anatomic landmarks for palpation of radial, brachial, and carotid pulses.	289	10
5. Locate the anatomic landmarks used during cardiopulmonary resuscitation and emergency defibrillation.	290	10
EXERCISE SPECIALIST		
6. Demonstrate an understanding of the biomechanical factors associated with various disease states, neuromuscular disorders, and orthopedic problems.	291	11, 12, 13
7. Discuss common gait abnormalities.	292	
8. Discuss abnormal curvatures of the spin and their effects on the biomechanics of movement.	293	13
9. Discuss how muscular weakness and/or neurologic disorder affect the biomechanics of movement.	294	
10. Locate common sites for measurement of skinfold thicknesses, widths, and girths.	295	10

KSA: EXERCISE PHYSIOLOGY

	KSA NUMBER	CHAPTER
EXERCISE TEST TECHNOLOGIST		
1. Demonstrate a knowledge of exercise physiology as it relates to exercise testing.	296	15, 16
2. List the cardiorespiratory responses associated with postural changes.	297	15
3. List the differences in the physiological responses to various modes of ergometry (i.e., treadmill, cycle, or arm ergometer) as they relate to exercise testing.	298	15, 16
4. Describe the principle of specificity of training as it relates to the mode of exercise testing.	299	56
5. Explain the meaning of maximal oxygen ($\dot{V}O_2$) consumption and how it is measured.	300	15
6. Describe the normal cardiorespiratory responses to graded exercise.	301	15, 36
7. Explain the common variables measured during cardiopulmonary exercise testing including heart rate slope, anaerobic threshold, ventilatory slope, maximum ventilation, breathing pattern, wasted ventilation, and wasted pulmonary circulation and their relationship to various diseases.	302	36, 37
EXERCISE SPECIALIST		
8. Demonstrate an understanding of clinical applications of exercise physiology.	303	16, 42
9. Describe the aerobic and anaerobic metabolic demands of various exercises for patients with cardiovascular, pulmonary, and/or metabolic diseases undergoing rehabilitation and their implications.	304	Appendix A
10. Describe how each of the following varies for the healthy individual vs. the patient with coronary artery disease (CAD): function of the myocardium, the generation of the action potential, repolarization, and major variants in pathways of electrical activity.	305	
11. Describe the cardiovascular responses to postural change before and after exercise testing.	306	42
12. List and be able to plot the normal resting and exercise values associated with increasing exercise intensity (and how they may differ from the CAD and/or COPD patient) for: heart rate, stroke volume, cardiac output, double product, arteriovenous O_2 difference, O_2 consumption, systolic and diastolic blood pressure, minute ventilation, tidal volume, and breathing frequency.	307	15, 36
13. Discuss the potential hazards of isometric exercise for subjects with low functional capacity or patients with cardiovascular disease.	308	
14. Describe the physiological effects of bed rest and discuss the appropriate physical activities which might be used to counteract these changes.	309	21, 22, 23
15. Compare the unique hemodynamic responses of arm vs. leg exercise and of static vs. dynamic exercise.	310	15, 16
16. Identify activities which are primarily aerobic or anaerobic.	311	15

17. Describe the determinants of myocardial O_2 consumption and the effects of exercise training on those determinants.	312	17
Program Director		
18. Discuss the mechanisms by which functional capacity and cardiovascular, respiratory metabolic, endocrine, and neuromuscular adaptations occur in response to physical conditioning programs.	313	14, 15, 17, 18, 56

KSA: HUMAN DEVELOPMENT AND AGING

	KSA Number	Chapter
Exercise Test Technologist		
1. Demonstrate competence in selecting an appropriate test protocol according to the age of the patient.	314	60, 61
2. Describe adjustments that may be necessary for testing younger and older patients; specifically, instructions to the patient and modification of the testing protocol and equipment.	315	60, 61
3. Explain differences in overall policy and procedures for the inclusion of different age groups in an exercise program.	316	60, 61
4. Discuss facility and equipment adaptations necessary for different age groups.	317	60, 61

KSA: HUMAN BEHAVIOR AND PSYCHOLOGY

	KSA Number	Chapter
Exercise Test Technologist		
1. Demonstrate knowledge of psychological factors that may affect exercise test patients.	318	5, 63
2. Identify factors that may increase anxiety in the patient undergoing exercise testing and describe how anxiety in a patient may be reduced.	319	5, 62, 63, 64
3. Identify specific psychological and physiological manifestations of test anxiety that can influence the response to an exercise test.	320	5, 63
Exercise Specialist		
4. Demonstrate an understanding of basic behavioral psychology and group dynamics as they apply to crisis management, coping, and lifestyle modifications.	321	64, 66
5. Describe signs and symptoms of maladjustment/failure to cope during an illness crisis and/or personal adjustment crisis (e.g., job loss) that might prompt a psychological consult or referral to other professional services.	322	62, 63, 64,
6. Describe the general principles of crisis management and factors influencing coping and learning in illness states.	323	64
7. Describe the psychological issues to be confronted by the patient and by family members of patients who have cardiorespiratory disease, and/or who have had an acute myocardial infarction or cardiac surgery.	324	66
8. Contrast the psychological issues associated with an acute cardiac event vs. those associated with chronic cardiac conditions.	325	
9. Describe the psychological stages involved with the acceptance of death and dying and recognize when it is necessary for a psychological consult or referral to a professional resource available in the community.	326	64
Program Director		
10. Demonstrate an understanding of the need for psychosocial consultation and referral of individuals who exhibit signs of psychological distress.	327	62, 64, 66
11. Describe community resources for psychosocial support and behavior modification and outline an example of a referral system.	328	64, 65, 67

12. Describe the observable signs and symptoms of psychological distress secondary to cardiopulmonary disorders.	329	5, 63, 66

KSA: PATHOPHYSIOLOGY AND RISK FACTORS

	KSA Number	Chapter
Exercise Test Technologist		
1. Demonstrate knowledge of the basic pathophysiology of coronary artery and pulmonary diseases.	330	26, 37
2. Define myocardial ischemia and list the methods that are used to measure ischemic responses.	331	16, 26, 27, 28
3. List the effects of CAD (including myocardial infarction) upon performance and safety during an exercise test.	332	
4. List primary and secondary risk factors for CAD.	333	1
5. Describe abnormal chronotropic and inotropic response to exercise testing.	334	16
6. Explain indications for combining exercise testing with radionuclide imaging.	335	28, 42
7. Describe common procedures used for radionuclide imaging (such as thallium, technetium, sestamibi, SPECT, RVG, MUGA, etc.).	336	28
8. Name the drugs commonly encountered during exercise testing and describe how they may affect the ECG, heart rate, or blood pressure at rest or during exercise. A. Cardiovascular agents (beta adrenergic blockers, nitrates, calcium channel antagonists, antiarrhythmics, ACE-inhibitors) B. Anticoagulant and antiplatelet drugs (dipyridamole, aspirin, etc.) C. Digitalis glycosides D. Decongestants and antihistamines E. Diabetes agents (oral and injection) F. Electrolytes (potassium, etc.) G. Hormones (estrogen, thyroid preparations, etc.) H. Lipid-lowering agents I. Psychotropic agents (antianxiety, antidepressants, antipsychotic agents, etc.) J. Respiratory therapy agents (bronchial dilators) K. Seizure disorders L. Smoking cessation aids (nicotine gum, nicotine patches, etc.)	337	Appendix C
9. Define reversible airway (obstructive) and restrictive lung diseases and how they may affect exercise testing.	338	37, 38, 39
Exercise Specialist		
10. Demonstrate an understanding of the cariorespiratory and metabolic responses to increasing intensities of exercise in certain diseases and conditions.	339	15, 16
11. Describe the cardiorespiratory and metabolic responses in myocardial dysfunction and ischemia at rest and during exercise.	340	16
12. Describe the cardiorespiratory and metabolic responses which accompany or result from pulmonary diseases at rest and during exercise.	341	36, 37, 38
13. Describe the signs and symptoms of peripheral vascular diseases and the effects different types of exercise may have on each.	342	33
14. Describe the metabolic responses and possible complications of a diabetic patient at rest and during exercise.	343	31
15. Describe the influence of exercise on weight reduction, hyperlipidemia, and diabetes.	344	31, 35
16. Describe the effects of variation in ambient temperature, humidity, carbon dioxide, and altitude on functional capacity and the exercise prescription. Explain required adaptations to the exercise prescription when environmental extremes exist.	345	24, 25
17. Describe the etiology of atherosclerosis.	346	26
18. Describe the implications, symptoms, and mechanisms of classical and vasospastic angina.	347	27
19. Describe the methods used to measure ischemic responses.	348	28, 42

20. Discuss the pathophysiology of the healing myocardium and the potential complications that may occur after an acute myocardial infarction (extension, expansion, rupture, etc.)	349	26, 27
21. Discuss Risk Stratification of patients after MI. What materials are used and what are the prognostic indicators for high risk patients post MI?	350	42 Guidelines
22. Describe the effects of the following classifications of drugs on the ECG, heart rate, and blood pressure. Also, list the common major symptoms of drug intolerance or toxicity in the following classes of medications (see Appendix C). A. Antianginal (nitrates, beta adrenergic blockers, calcium channel antagonists, etc.) B. Antiarrhythmic C. Anticoagulant and antiplatelet D. Lipid-lowering drugs E. Antihypertensive (diuretics, vasodilators, etc.) F. Digitalis glycosides G. Bronchodilators H. Tranquilizers, antidepressants, and antianxiety drugs I. Hypoglycemics	351	29, Appendix C
23. List the major effects of the above nine classes of drugs on physiological responses and symptomatology, including ECG changes, at rest and during exercise testing and training.	352	
24. Demonstrate an understanding of various modalities applied in the medical diagnosis and therapeutic management of certain diseases.	353	28, 29, 37, 38
25. Describe the purpose and utility of coronary angiography and radionuclide imaging.	354	28
26. Describe percutaneous transluminal coronary angioplasty (PTCA).	355	29
27. Describe the use of streptokinase and other thrombolytic agents.	356	29
PROGRAM DIRECTOR		
28. Demonstrate an understanding of the relationship between different disease states and rehabilitative therapy.	357	31, 32, 33, 36, 37, 39
29. Explain the process of atherosclerosis including current hypotheses regarding onset and rate of progression and/or regression.	358	26
30. Demonstrate an understanding of lipoprotein classifications and their relationship to atherosclerosis or other diseases.	359	1, 35
31. Contrast the signs and symptoms in the pulmonary vs. cardiac patient during exercise testing and exercise training.	360	27, 36, 37
32. Explain the diagnostic and prognostic value of the results of the graded exercise test for various populations.	361	28, 42
33. Explain the diagnostic and prognostic value of the low level predischarge exercise test vs. the symptom-limited test and the indications for use with CAD patients.	362	28, 42
34. Identify and explain the mechanisms by which exercise may contribute to preventing or rehabilitating individuals with cardiovascular, respiratory, or metabolic diseases.	363	30, 31, 32, 33, 35
35. Demonstrate an understanding of the following drug classifications, explain the mechanisms of principle actions, and list the major side effects, including ECG changes at rest and during exercise (see Appendix C). A. Antianginal (nitrates, beta adrenergic blockers, calcium channel antagonists, etc.) B. Antiarrhythmic C. Anticoagulant and antiplatelet D. Lipid-lowering drugs E. Antihypertensive F. Digitalis glycosides G. Bronchodilators H. Hypoglycemics I. Psychotropics J. Emergency medications	364	Appendix C
36. Demonstrate an understanding of the various diagnostic and treatment modalities currently used in the management of cardiovascular disease.	365	28, 29, 33, 42

37. Describe coronary angiography, radionuclide imaging, echocardiography imaging, and pharmacologic stress studies, including the type of information obtained, sensitivity, specificity, and associated risks and indications for use.	366	28, 29, 42
38. Describe PTCA as an alternative to medical management or coronary artery bypass surgery (CABS) in CAD. Demonstrate an understanding of the indications and limitations for PTCA in different subsets of CAD patients vs. CABS or management with medications.	367	29
39. Describe the use of thrombolytic therapy in acute MI.	368	29

KSA: HEALTH APPRAISAL AND FITNESS TESTING

	KSA NUMBER	CHAPTER
EXERCISE TEST TECHNOLOGIST		
1. Demonstrate the skills and knowledge for administering an exercise test.	369	41, 42
2. Recognize inappropriate calibration of testing equipment and explain procedures for calibration (i.e., a motor-driven treadmill, cycle ergometer (mechanical), arm ergometer, electrocardiograph, aneroid and mercury sphygmomanometer, and spirometers).	370	
3. Obtain a routine medical history prior to exercise testing, ensure informed consent is obtained, explain procedures and protocol for the exercise test, recognize the contraindications to an exercise test, and summarize and present screening information to the physician.	371	40, 42 Guidelines
4. Recognize the significance of patient medical history and physical exam findings as they relate to exercise testing.	372	28, 40, 41
5. Identify patients for whom physician supervision is recommended during maximal and submaximal exercise testing.	373	Guidelines
6. Perform routine tasks prior to exercise testing including: taking a standard and exercise 12-lead ECG on a participant in the supine, upright, and post-hyperventilation conditions; accurately recording right and left arm blood pressure in different body positions; demonstrating the ability to instruct the test participant in the use of rating of perceived exertion (RPE) scale and other appropriate subjective scales, such as dyspnea and angina scales.	374	10, 42
7. Discuss the techniques used to minimze ECG artifact and the value of a single-lead and multiple electrocardiographic lead systems in exercise testing.	375	10
8. Discuss the selection of the exercise test protocol in terms of modes of exercise, starting levels, increments of work length of stages, and frequency of physiological measures.	376	42
9. Discuss how age, weight, level of fitness, and health status are considered in the selection of an exercise test protocol.	377	41
10. Contrast exercise testing procedures for pulmonary patients with that of cardiac patients in terms of exercise modality, protocol, physiological measurements, and expected outcomes.	378	38, 42
11. Demonstrate appropriate techniques of measurement of physiological and subjective responses (i.e, symptoms, ECG, blood pressure, heart rate, RPE, and O_2 consumption measures) at appropriate intervals during the test.	379	42
12. Identify appropriate endpoints for exercise testing for various populations.	380	38, 42 Guidelines
13. Discuss technical factors that may indicate test termination (e.g., loss of ECG signal, loss of power, etc.).	381	41, 42 Guidelines
14. Discuss immediate post-exercise procedures and list various approaches to cool-down.	382	41, 42
15. Record, organize, and perform necessary calculations of test data for summary presentation to test interpreter.	383	
16. Describe differences in test protocol and procedures when the exercise involves radionuclide imaging procedures.	384	28
17. Demonstrate the ability to administer basic resting spirometric test including FEV_1, FVC, and MVV.	385	
18. Describe basic equipment and facility requirements for exercise testing.	386	41, 42
19. Describe the responsibilities of the exercise test technologist on a typical testing day.	387	
20. Demonstrate competence in the interpretation of the exercise test for a rehabilitation program.	388	28

21. Describe the techniques used to calibrate a motor-driven treadmill, cycle ergometer (mechanical), arm ergometer, electrocardiograph, aneroid and mercury column sphygmomanometer, spirometers, and respiratory gas analyzers.	389	
22. Demonstrate appropriate techniques for measurement of O_2 consumption at appropriate intervals during an exercise test.	390	
23. Modify testing procedures and protocol for children with clinical conditions.	391	
24. Demonstrate the ability to provide objective recommendations to a patient following a cardiovascular event regarding physical conditioning, return to work, and performance of selected activities for daily living (such as driving, stair climbing, sexual activity) based on exercise test results and clinical status.	392	Guidelines
25. Understand the prognostic implications of the exercise ECG and hemodynamic responses, radionuclide imaging, and Holter monitoring in post infarction risk stratification. Use this information in determining the appropriate setting for exercise, level of supervision, and level of monitoring.	393	42 Guidelines

KSA: ELECTROCARDIOGRAPHY

	KSA Number	Chapter
Exercise Test Technologist		
1. Demonstrate knowledge of normal and abnormal resting ECGs and be able to recognize commonly encountered abnormalities during exercise testing.	394	48
2. Describe the resting ECG by identifying waveforms (P, QRS, T) segments (ST), intervals (PR, QRS, QT), and axis (QRS) which comprise the normal resting ECG.	395	47, 48
3. Recognize changes in the ST segment, the presence of abnormal T waves, and significant Q waves as well as their importance in resting and exercise ECGs.	396	49
4. Define the ECG criteria for terminating an exercise test due to ischemic changes.	397	Guidelines
5. Identify ECG patterns of common conduction defects and arrhythmias and their importance at rest and during exercise. A. Identify ECG changes associated with the following abnormalities: 1. Bundle branch blocks 2. Atrioventricular blocks 3. Sinus bradycardia (< 60 beats/min) and tachycardia (> 100 beats/min) 4. Sinus arrest 5. Supraventricular premature depolarizations and tachycardia 6. Ventricular premature depolarizations (including frequency, form, couplets, salvos, tachycadia) 7. Atrial fibrillation 8. Ventricular fibrillation B. Define the limits or considerations for initiating and terminating an exercise test based on the ECG abnormalities listed above.	398	48, 50
Exercise Specialist		
6. Demonstrate an understanding of the important ECG patterns at rest and during exercise in healthy persons and in patients with CAD, pulmonary diseases, and metabolic diseases.	399	49, 50, 51
7. Describe the electrophysiological events involved in the cyclic depolarization and repolarization of the heart.	400	47
8. Describe the ECG changes which are associated with myocardial ischemia, injury, and infarction. A. Identify ECG complexes typically seen in acute subendocardial ischemia, epicardial injury, and acute and chronic transmural and non Q-wave infarction. B. Identify ECG changes which correspond to ischemia in various myocardial regions (inferior, posterior, anteroseptal, anterior, anterolateral, lateral). C. Differentiate between Q-wave and non-Q-wave infarction.	401	49
9. Identify ECG changes which typically occur due to hyperventilation, electrolyte abnormalities, and drug therapy.	402	51
10. Identify resting ECG changes associated with diseases other than CAD (such as hypertensive heart disease, cardiac chamber enlargement, pericarditis, pulmonary disease, metabolic disorders).	403	50, 51

11. Explain possible causes of ischemic ECG changes and various cardiac dysrhythmias. Explain the significance of their occurrence during rest, exercise, and recovery.	404	50
12. Identify potentially hazardous dysrhythmias or conduction defects that may be observed on the ECG at rest, during exercise, and recovery. Explain what procedures would be followed in the event of such dysrhythmias or conduction defects.	405	50
13. Identify the significance of important ECG abnormalities in the designation of the exercise prescription and in activity selection.	406	
14. Discuss the indications and methods for ECG monitoring during exercise testing and during exercise sessions.	407	Guidelines
15. Identify ECG patterns with the following conduction defects and dysrhythmias: fascicular blocks and atrial flutter.	408	50
Program Director		
16. Demonstrate the ability to identify ECG patterns and to discuss implications for exercise testing, exercise programming, prognosis, and risk stratification.	409	28, 42, 49
17. Explain the diagnosis and prognostic significance of ischemic ECG responses or arrhythmias at rest, during exercise, or recovery.	410	49
18. Explain the causes and means of reducing false positive and false negative exercise ECG responses.	411	
19. Understand Baye's theorem as it relates to pretest likelihood of CAD and the predictive value of positive or negative diagnostic exercise ECG results.	412	
20. Discuss the role of ECG exercise testing as it relates to radionuclide imaging and echocardiography imaging.	413	28, 42

KSA: EMERGENCY PROCEDURES AND SAFETY

	KSA Number	Chapter
Exercise Test Technologist		
1. Demonstrate competency in responding with appropriate emergency procedures to situations that might arise prior to, during, and after administration of an exercise test.	414	58
2. List and describe the use of emergency equipment that should be present in an exercise testing laboratory.	415	10
3. Demonstrate competency in verifying operating status of and maintaining emergency equipment.	416	
4. Describe emergency procedures for a preventive and rehabilitative exercise testing program.	417	
5. Possess current Basic Cardiac Life Support certification or equivalent credentials, including the use of a pocket airway mask.	418	
Exercise Specialist		
6. Demonstrate competence in responding with the appropriate emergency procedures to situations in rehabilitative settings which might arise prior to, during, and after exercise.	419	
7. Describe the emergency response(s) to cardiac arrest, hypoglycemia, bronchospasm, and sudden onset hypotension.	420	
8. Identify the emergency drugs that should be available in exercise testing and participation situations and describe the mechanisms of action.	421	
Program Director		
9. Demonstrate knowledge about appropriate emergency procedures for situations in rehabilitative settings that might arise prior to, during, and after exercise.	422	
10. Diagram an emergency response system and discuss minimum standards for equipment and personnel required in setting for rehabilitative exercise program.	423	

KSA: EXERCISE PROGRAMMING

	KSA NUMBER	CHAPTER
EXERCISE SPECIALIST		
1. Demonstrate an understanding of the implications of exercise for persons with CAD risk factors and for patients with established cardiovascular, respiratory, metabolic, or orthopedic disorders and demonstrate competence in executing individualized exercise prescription.	424	30, 32, 33, 34
2. Discuss the level of supervision and level of monitoring recommended for various patient populations in exercise programs.	425	Guidelines
3. Prescribe appropriate exercise based on medical information and exercise test data including intensity, duration, frequency, progression, precautions, and type of physical activity.	426	Guidelines
4. Modify a patient's exercise program (type of physical activity, intensity, duration, progression) according to the current health status of the patient with the following conditions: immediate post-CABS, MI, PTCA, heart transplantation, COPD, diabetes, obesity, renal disease, and common orthopedic and neuromuscular conditions.	427	34, 39, 70
5. Discuss basic mechanism of action of medications that may affect the exercise prescription: beta adrenergic blockers, diuretics, calcium channel antagonists, antihypertensives, antihistamines, hypoglycemics, tranquilizers, alcohol, diet pills, cold tablets, caffeine, and nicotine.	428	
6. Discuss warm-up and cool-down phenomena with specific reference to angina and ischemic ECG changes, dysrhythmias, and blood pressure changes.	429	
7. Discuss the differences in the physiological response to arm and leg exercise in cardiac patients.	430	15
8. Discuss the appropriate use of static and dynamic exercise by cardiac patients.	431	15, 53
9. Design a program of strength training for cardiac patients.	432	53
10. Discuss modifications in monitoring of exercise intensity for various patient groups.	433	39
11. Discuss possible adverse responses to exercise in various patient groups and what precautions may be taken to prevent them.	434	
12. Discuss contraindications to exercise as related to the current health status of the participant.	435	Guidelines
13. Given a clinical case study, devise supervised exercise programs for the first 6 weeks after hospitalization for MI, PTCA, CABS, and angina and for the 3 months following.	436	
14. Identify characteristics which correlate or predict poor compliance to exercise programs.	437	
15. Identify and describe the role of various allied health professionals and the indications and procedures for referral necessary in a multidisciplinary rehabilitation program.	438	

KSA: PROGRAM ADMINISTRATION

	KSA NUMBER	CHAPTER
PROGRAM DIRECTOR		
1. Demonstrate the ability to administer a clinical program including personnel, finance, program development, and continuous quality improvement.	440	
2. Diagram and explain an organizational chart and show the staff relationships between and exercise program director, governing body, exercise specialist, exercise test technologist, fitness instructor, medical director or advisor, and a participant's personal physician.	441	73
3. Identify and explain operating policies for preventive and rehabilitative exercise programs.	442	78
4. Describe the role of the medical director and referring physician in the program design and implementation; and describe the responsibility of the program director to these individuals.	443	73
5. Describe and explain strategies for enhancing the understanding of the role of rehabilitation on the part of the public, health care policy-makers, health care providers, and the medical community.	444	
6. Discuss the development and implementation of the comprehensive patient care plan.	445	

7. Discuss the role of the rehabilitative staff in the development and implementation of the comprehensive patient care plan.	446	
8. Demonstrate the ability to justify the inclusion of a comprehensive rehabilitation program in the health care setting.	447	
9. Describe the concept of risk stratification and its application to program administration.	448	Guidelines
10. Identify and explain operating policies for clinical exercise programs including data analysis and reporting, reimbursement of service fees, confidentiality of records, relationships between program and referring physicians, continuing education of participants and family, legal liability, and accident or injury reporting.	449	78
11. Demonstrate the ability to assume fiscal (financial) responsibility for clinical programs.	450	
12. Demonstrate the ability to implement and monitor a comprehensive continuous quality improvement process.	451	

Acknowledgments

The editors thank these individuals who contributed to this book by reviewing manuscripts and providing editorial assistance:

Paul A. Becker, MD
Dale R. Bergren, PhD
Jeffrey J. Betts, PhD
Elaine Filusch Betts, PhD, PT
Gordon Blackburn, PhD
Susan A. Bloomfield, PhD
Michael S. Bolander, PT
Charles J. Brooks, MD
William N. Brodine, MD
Ellsworth R. Buskirk, PhD
Brian W. Carlin, MD
Tom Clanton, PhD
Diane Cullen, PhD
Bill Day, PhD
Robert Doroghazi, MD
Ami M. Drimmer, PhD
Barbara L. Drinkwater, PhD
J. Larry Durstine, PhD
Marigold A. Edwards, PhD
JoAnne M. Eickhoff-Shemek, PhD
Paul S. Fardy, PhD
Andrew W. Gardner, PhD
Richard Gevirtz, PhD
Terry Glenn, PhD, PT
James Hagberg, PhD
Susan J. Hall, PhD
Larry F. Hamm, PhD
Steven H. Herman, PhD
Elizabeth Holford, PhD
Kady Hommel Anderson, MBA
Reed Humphrey, PhD, PT
Dianne R. Jewell, MS, PT
W. Larry Kenney, PhD
Steven J. Keteyian, PhD
Joy A. Kistler, MS
Kennneth L. Knight, PhD
Harold W. Kohl, III, PhD
David Lombard, PhD
Ben Londeree, EdD
Terry Marble, PhD, PT
Carol Mayberry, PhD
David A. Mays, PharmD, BCPS
Timothy R. McConnell, PhD
Diane McCullen, PhD
Henry S. Miller, Jr, MD
Byron Nelson, PG
Richard B. Parr, EdD
Robert W. Patton, PhD
Jody Payne, BS
Claire Peel, PhD, PT
Linda S. Pescatello, PhD
George B. Pierson, MD
Robin B. Purdie, MS
Janet Walberg Rankin, PhD
Scott O. Roberts, PhD
Eric Samaniego, MS
Albert B. Schultz, PhD
Wayne E. Sinning, PhD
L. Kent Smith, MD
Wayne Sotile, PhD
Catherine J. Spangler Perry, RN, MSN
Kerry Stewart, PhD
Michael H. Stone, PhD
James Stray-Gundersen, MD
Tom Thomas, PhD
Janet P. Wallace, PhD
Mary Watson, MS, RD
Michael J. Waxman, MD
Mary Ellen Wewers, PhD, RN, ANP
Mark A. Williams, PhD
Richard Winett, PhD
Nancy C. Zambraski, MS

It would be remiss of me not to acknowledge those who supported the time and effort that went into this revision. First, to my wife and partner for almost 20 years, thank you for your patience and support. Allowing me the time to do this was not easy on either of us and I love you. To the Section Editors whose creativity have made this revision an excellent update of the Second Edition. Thanks to our two editors at Williams & Wilkins, Jennifer Schmidt and Jeff Myers, who have been amazingly patient with me and have been remarkedly helpful in making the book a work of high quality. Finally, I want to thank the present and former staff of the Cardiac Rehabilitation program of Research Medical Center for carrying a heavy load and allowing me to complete my work on this book.

JEFFREY L. ROITMAN

Contributors

Frank Ancharski, MS
The Fitness Company
Iselin, New Jersey

Tony G. Babb, PhD
Division of Pulmonary and Critical Care Medicine
University of Texas Southwestern Medical Center
Dallas, Texas

Kenneth C. Beck, PhD
Division of Pulmonary and Critical Care Medicine
Mayo Clinic
Rochester, Minnesota

Sue Beckham, PhD
Exercise, Sport and Health Studies
University of Texas at Arlington
Arlington, Texas

Thomas E. Bernard, PhD
College of Public Health
University of South Florida
Tampa, Florida

Susan A. Bloomfield, PhD
Department of Health and Kinesiology
Texas A&M University
College Station, Texas

Sorin J. Brener, MD
Interventional Cardiology
Cleveland Clinic Foundation
Cleveland, Ohio

Kelly D. Brownell, PhD
Department of Psychology
Yale University
New Haven, Connecticut

Peter H. Brubaker, PhD
Cardiac Rehabilitation
Wake Forest University
Winston-Salem, North Carolina

Cedric X. Bryant, PhD
Randall Sportsmedicine
StairMaster
Kirkland, Washington

Jill A. Bush, MS
Noll Laboratory
The Pennsylvania State University
University Park, Pennsylvania

Gayle Butterfield, PhD, RD
Nutrition Studies
Palo Alto VA Healthcare System
Palo Alto, California

Barbara N. Campaigne, PhD
ACSM National Center
American College of Sportsmedicine
Indianapolis, Indiana

Richard Casaburi, MD, PhD
Division of Respiratory and Critical Care Physiology
Harbor-UCLA Medical Center
Torrance, California

Michael Caton, MEd
FitLinxx
Stamford, Connecticut

Chris Cole, MD
Department of Cardiology
Cleveland Clinic Foundation
Cleveland, Ohio

Edward F. Coyle, PhD
Human Performance Laboratory
University of Texas
Austin, Texas

Brent Darden, MS
Cooper Aerobics Center
Dallas, Texas

Mark Davis, PhD
Department of Exercise Science
University of South Carolina
Columbia, South Carolina

Paul G. Davis, MS
Department of Exercise Science
University of South Carolina
Columbia, South Carolina

Rebecca Davis, PhD
Department of Physiology
The University of Arizona
Tucson, Arizona

Gary A. Dudley, PhD
Department of Exercise Science
University of Georgia
Athens, Georgia

J. Larry Durstine, PhD
Department of Exercise Science
University of South Carolina
Columbia, South Carolina

Robert S. Eliot, MD
(recently deceased)
Paradise Valley, AZ
(1929–1997)

Nestor Fernandez, II, MBA
Western Athletic Clubs
University of San Francisco
San Francisco, California

Robert Fitts, PhD
Department of Biology
University of Wisconsin-Milwaukee
Milwaukee, Wisconsin

Steven J. Fleck, PhD
Department of Sport Science
Colorado College
Colorado Springs, Colorado

Barry A. Franklin, PhD
Cardiac Rehabilitation and Exercise Testing Laboratory
William Beaumont Hospital
Royal Oak, Michigan

Denise M. Fredette, MS, PT
School of Physical Therapy
Texas Women's University
Houston, Texas

Scott Going, PhD
Department of Physiology
The University of Arizona
Tucson, Arizona

Neil F. Gordon, MD, PhD, MPH
Center for Heart Disease Prevention
Savannah, Georgia

Andrew M. Gottlieb, PhD
The Health Psychology Center
Palo Alto, California

Mark D. Grabiner, PhD
Department of Biomedical Engineering
Cleveland Clinic Foundation
Cleveland, Ohio

James E. Graves, PhD
Department of Exercise Science
Syracuse University
Syracuse, New York

Carlos Grilo, PhD
Yale Psychiatric Institute
Yale University School of Medicine
New Haven, Connecticut

Larry R. Gurchiek, DA, ATC
Department of Health and Physical Education
University of South Alabama
Mobile, Alabama

Linda K. Hall, PhD
Health and Disease Management
Baptist Memorial Hospital
Memphis, Tennessee

Joseph Hamill, PhD
Department of Exercise Science
University of Massachusetts
Amherst, Massachusetts

Sharon A. Harvey, MA
EKG and Stress Laboratories
Cleveland Clinic Foundation
Cleveland, Ohio

George Havenith, PhD
Department of Human Sciences
Loughborough University
Loughborough, United Kingdom

Gregory W. Heath, DHSc, MPH
Division of Adult and Community Health
National Center for Chronic Disease Prevention and Health Promotion
Atlanta, Georgia

Kathryn Hellweg, PhD
Department of Teaching and Learning
Rochester Public Schools
Rochester, Minnesota

David L. Herbert, JD
Herbert, Benson and Scott
Canton, Ohio

William G. Herbert, PhD
Department of Exercise Science
Virginia Technological University
Blacksburg, Virginia

William G. Hiatt, MD
Department of General Internal Medicine
University of Colorado Medical Center
Denver, Colorado

Michael Holewijn, PhD
Research and Development Department
Netherlands Aerospace Medical Laboratory
Soesterberg, The Netherlands

Robert G. Holly, PhD
Department of Exercise Science
University of California
Davis, California

Connie C. Hsia, MD
Department of Internal Medicine
University of Texas Southwestern Medical Center
Dallas, Texas

Reed Humphrey, PhD, PT
School of Physical Therapy
Medical College of Virginia
Richmond, Virginia

Donna Israel, RD, PhD
Fitness Formula Inc.
Richardson, Texas

Bruce D. Johnson, PhD
Division of Pulmonary and Critical Care Medicine
Mayo Clinic
Rochester, Minnesota

Leonard A. Kaminsky, PhD
Human Performance Laboratory
Ball State University
Muncie, Indiana

Michaela Kiernan, PhD
Department of Medicine
Stanford University School of Medicine
Palo Alto, California

Abbey C. King, PhD
Department of Medicine
Stanford University School of Medicine
Palo Alto, California

John E. Kovaleski, PhD, ATC
Department of Health and Physical Education
University of South Alabama
Mobile, Alabama

William J. Kraemer, PhD
Noll Laboratory
The Pennsylvania State University
University Park, Pennsylvania

Tom P. LaFontaine, PhD
Wellaware Disease Prevention and Community Wellness
Boone Hospital Center
Columbia, Missouri

John A. Larry, MD
Division of Cardiology
The Ohio State University Medical Center
Columbus, Ohio

Richard W. Latin, PhD
School of HPER
University of Nebraska–Omaha
Omaha, Nebraska

John M. Lawler, PhD
Human Performance Laboratory
Texas A&M University
College Station, Texas

Ben Levine, MD
Department of Cardiology
University of Texas Southwestern Medical School
Dallas, Texas

Donald A. Mahler, MD
Section of Pulmonary and Critical Care Medicine
Dartmouth Hitchcock Medical Center
Lebanon, New Hampshire

Tina M. Manos, EdD
Department of Exercise Science and Sports Studies
Springfield College
Springfield, Massachusetts

John E. Martin, PhD
Department of Psychology
San Diego State University
San Diego, California

Phillip E. Martin, PhD
Department of Exercise Science and Physical Education
Arizona State University
Tempe, Arizona

Timothy R. McConnell, PhD
Cardiac Rehabilitation
Geisinger Medical Center
Danville, Pennsylvania

Stuart M. McGill, PhD
Department of Kinesiology
University of Waterloo
Waterloo, Ontario, Canada

Jonathan Meyers, MS
Cardiac Rehabilitation
Wake Forest University
Winston-Salem, North Carolina

Nancy Houston Miller, RN, BS
Stanford Cardiac Rehabilitation Program
Stanford University School of Medicine
Palo Alto, California

Sandy Minor, MS
Health Studies
Texas Women's University
Denton, Texas

Julie M. Murray, PhD, PT
Department of Physical Therapy
Guadalupe Valley Hospital
Seguin, Texas

Tinker D. Murray, PhD
Department of HPER
Southwest Texas State University
San Marcos, Texas

Fredric J. Pashkow, MD
Cardiac Health Improvement and Rehabilitation
Cleveland Clinic Foundation
Cleveland, Ohio

James A. Peterson, PhD
Monterey, CA

Michael L. Pollock, PhD
Center for Exercise Science
University of Florida
Gainesville, Florida

Scott R. Powers, PhD
Center for Exercise Science
University of Florida
Gainesville, Florida

Elizabeth J. Protas, PhD, PT
School of Physical Therapy
Texas Women's University
Houston, Texas

Judith G. Regensteiner, PhD
Department of General Internal Medicine
University of Colorado Medical Center
Denver, Colorado

Paul M. Ribisl, PhD
Department of Health and Exercise Science
Wake Forest University
Winston-Salem, North Carolina

Rosemary Riley, PhD, RD
Ross Products Division
Abbott Laboratories
Columbus, Ohio

Jeffrey L. Roitman, EdD
Cardiac Rehabilitation
Research Medical Center
Kansas City, MO

Mark A. Russell, MS
Interior Fitness Design
Dallas, Texas

Stephen F. Schaal, MD
Division of Cardiology
The Ohio State University Medical Center
Columbus, Ohio

James D. Shaffrath, PhD
Department of Exercise Science
University of California
Davis, California

Janet M. Shaw, PhD
Department of Exercise and Sport Science
University of Utah
Salt Lake City, Utah

Sally A. Shumaker, PhD
Bowman Gray School of Medicine
Wake Forest University
Winston-Salem, North Carolina

Wesley E. Sime, PhD
Health and Human Performance
University of Nebraska-Lincoln
Lincoln, Nebraska

Patricia M. Smith, PhD
Department of Health Studies and Gerontology
University of Waterloo
Waterloo, Ontario, Canada

Lori L. Ploutz Snyder, PhD
Department of Physical Education
Syracuse University
Syracuse, New York

Erik E. Solberg, MD
Department of Cardiology
Ulleval University Hospital
Oslo, Norway

Wayne M. Sotile, PhD
Sotile Psychological Associates
Winston-Salem, North Carolina

Barbara H. Southard, MS, RN
Merck and Company, Inc.
Floyd, Virginia

Douglas R. Southard, PhD, MPH, PA-C
Physician Assistant Program
College of Health Sciences
Roanoke, Virginia

Daniel H. Spriggs, MD
Department of Family Practice
University of South Alabama Medical Center
Mobile, Alabama

Ray W. Squires, PhD
Cardiovascular Health Clinic
Mayo Clinic
Rochester, Minnesota

Suzanne Nelson Steen, PhDSc, RD
Graduate Department of Nutrition Education
Immaculata College
Immaculata, Pennsylvania

Kerry J. Stewart, EdD
Cardiac Rehabilitation
Francis Scott Key Medical Center
Baltimore, MD

C. Barr Taylor, MD
Department of Psychiatry and Behavioral Sciences
Stanford Medical Center
Palo Alto, California

Tom R. Thomas, PhD
Human and Environmental Science
University of Missouri
Columbia, Missouri

Jeff S. Volek, PhD, RD
Noll Laboratory
The Pennsylvania State Univeristy
University Park, Pennsylvania

Mitchell A. Whaley, PhD
Human Performance Laboratory
Ball State University
Muncie, Indiana

Mark A. Williams, PhD
Division of Cardiology
Creighton University School of Medicine
Omaha, Nebraska

Kara A. Witzke, PhD
Bone Research Laboratory
Oregon State University
Corvalis, Oregon

Julie Zuckerman, RN
University of Texas Southwestern Medical School
Dallas, Texas

Linda D. Zwiren, EdD
Department of HPER
Hofstra University
Hempstead, New York

Table of Contents

SECTION ONE

Lifestyle and Health

SECTION EDITOR: *Mark Williams, PhD, FACSM*

69, 204 81, 82, 83 333 359, 363

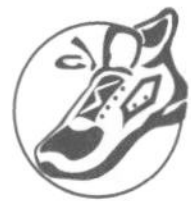
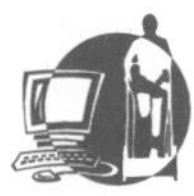
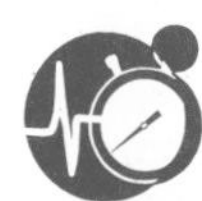
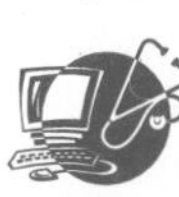

CHAPTER 1

Conceptual Basis for Coronary Artery Disease Risk Factor Assessment

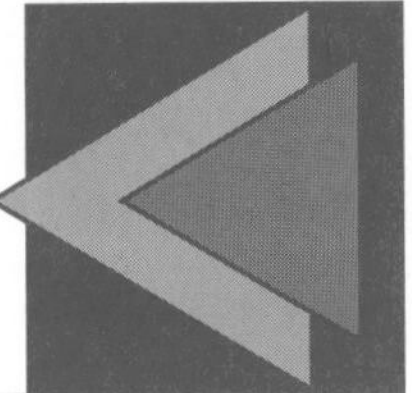

Neil F. Gordon

Understanding the concept of risk factors is central to both the primary and secondary prevention of coronary artery disease (CAD). From a practical standpoint, primary prevention involves intervention before the onset of CAD, whereas secondary prevention involves intervention after the onset of CAD (1). Although the risk for a recurrent cardiac event is affected by indicators of disease severity, such as left ventricular dysfunction and residual myocardial ischemia, all factors associated with the first episode or manifestation of CAD are also predictive of the risk for recurrent events.

PREVENTIVE PATHOPHYSIOLOGY: MODIFIABLE RISK FACTORS

The risk factor concept for CAD is now well evolved. A risk factor may be defined as "an aspect of personal behavior or lifestyle, an environmental exposure or inherited characteristic, which, on the basis of epidemiologic evidence, is known to be associated with health-related conditions considered to be important to prevent (2). It must be emphasized that the term "associated" does not necessarily imply causation. Causation is best evaluated on the basis of evidence generated from randomized clinical trials. Certain risk factors are nonmodifiable and, as in the case of some modifiable risk factors, it may be unethical to expose people to substances (cigarettes, for example) that are potentially harmful. Therefore, most risk factors are never evaluated in randomized clinical trials. Rather, they are identified using observational studies from which the likelihood of causation is implied based on the strength of the association, exposure antedating disease onset, dose-dependency, consistency of the relationship under diverse circumstances, specificity of the association, and biological plausibility.

CAD risk factors are typically classified as shown in Table 1.1. For clinical purposes, however, the importance of a specific risk factor in the primary and secondary prevention of CAD is best judged by the extent to which changes in the factor have been proven to influence the future clinical course (3). In view of this, Table 1.2 illustrates proposed risk factor categories for use in a clinical setting (4). For the purposes of this chapter, risk factors having to do with lifestyle and health will be discussed.

Cigarette Smoking

Tobacco use has been cited as the chief avoidable cause of illness and death. It is responsible for over 400,000 deaths in the United States each year. Despite this fact, cigarette smoking is surprisingly prevalent. Recent estimates are that 25% of Americans smoke cigarettes (5). Moreover, smoking prevalence among adolescents appears to be increasing, with more than 3,000 children and adolescents becoming addicted to tobacco each day (5).

There is overwhelming evidence from observational studies that incriminate cigarette smoking as a major risk factor for CAD (6). A linear relation has been shown to exist between the risk for cardiovascular disease and the number of cigarettes smoked (Fig. 1.1) (7). The risk also increases in accordance with the number of years of smoking and the depth of inhalation (8). Acutely, cigarette smoking accentuates risk by elevating the myocardial oxygen demand (due to increases in heart rate and blood pressure), reducing oxygen transport, increasing susceptibility to malignant ventricular arrhythmias, predisposing to coronary artery spasm, and increasing platelet adhesiveness. Chronically, cigarette smoking lowers high-density lipoprotein (HDL) cholesterol levels, promotes oxidation of low-density lipoprotein (LDL) cholesterol, elevates blood fibrinogen concentration, increases blood viscosity by inducing secondary polycythemia, and damages the arterial endothelium. Smoking also amplifies the effect of other CAD risk factors, thereby accelerating the atherosclerotic process. Patients who continue to smoke cigarettes after an acute myocar-

Table 1.1. Coronary Artery Disease Risk Factors

Positive Risk Factors	Defining Criteria
1. Age	Men > 45 years; women > 55 or premature menopause without estrogen replacement therapy
2. Family history	MI or sudden death before 55 years of age in father or other male first-degree relative, or before 65 years of age in mother or other female first-degree relative
3. Current cigarette smoking	
4. Hypertension	Blood pressure ≥ 140/90 mm Hg, confirmed by measurements on at least 2 separate occasions, or on antihypertensive medication
5. Hypercholesterolemia	Total serum cholesterol > 200 mg/dL (5.2 mmol/L) (if lipoprotein profile is unavailable) or HDL < 35 mg/dL (0.9 mmol/L)
6. Diabetes mellitus	Persons with insulin dependent diabetes mellitus (IDDM) who are > 30 years of age, or have had IDDM for > 15 years, and persons with noninsulin dependent diabetes mellitus (NIDDM) who are > 35 years of age should be classified as patients with disease
7. Sedentary lifestyle/physical inactivity	Persons comprising the least active 25% of the population, as defined by the combination of sedentary jobs involving sitting for a large part of the day and no regular exercise or active recreational pursuits
Negative Risk Factor	**Comments**
1. High serum HDL cholesterol	> 60 mg/dL (1.6 mmol/L)

Notes: (1) It is common to sum risk factors in making clinical judgments. If HDL is high, subtract one risk factor from the sum of positive risk factors, since high HDL decreases CAD risk; (2) Obesity is not listed as an independent positive risk factor because its effects are exerted through other risk factors (e.g., hypertension, hyperlipidemia, diabetes). Obesity should be considered as an independent target for intervention.

(With permission from ACSM. ACSM's Guidelines for Exercise Testing and Prescription. 5th ed. Baltimore: Williams & Wilkins, 1995.)

dial infarction have a 22% to 47% greater subsequent risk of death and reinfarction (3). After bypass surgery, continued cigarette smoking results in a two-fold increase in the relative risk of death (3).

Regardless of the dose or duration of cigarette smoking, cessation reduces the risk of CAD (9). In particular, the risk of acute myocardial infarction declines more rapidly with cigarette smoking cessation than does the overall risk of death from cardiovascular disease. The greatest proportion of reducing the risk of acute myocardial infarction and of reducing overall cardiovascular mortality occurs in the first several months of cessation. The risk continues to decline over the ensuing several years, but at a more gradual rate. The early decline in risk is thought to be derived from improvements in endothelial function and the prothrombotic state, whereas the late benefit is thought to result from a delay in progression or reversal of the underlying atherosclerotic process (10).

In addition, environmental exposure to second-hand smoke (passive smoking) is estimated to cause 53,000 heart disease deaths each year in the United States (6). It constitutes one of the leading causes of preventable death in this country. Paradoxically, the risk may be greater in non-smokers than in smokers due to a degree of "conditioning" of habitual smokers to the adverse effects of exposure to cigarette smoke (11).

LDL Cholesterol

A large body of epidemiologic evidence supports a direct relationship between serum total cholesterol concentration and CAD risk (Fig. 1.2). Of the various lipopro-

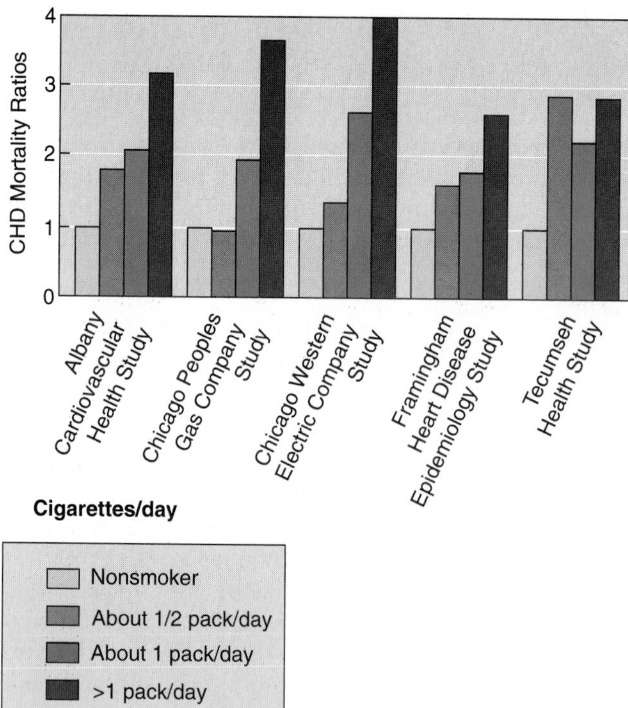

Figure 1.1. Coronary heart disease mortality ratios according to the amount of ciagarettes smoked in five populations. (Reprinted with permission from The Pooling Project Research Group. Relationship of blood pressure, serum cholesterol, smoking habit, relative weight, and ECG abnormalities to incidence of major coronary events: Final report of the Pooling Project. J Chron Dis 1978;31:202.)

Table 1.2. Cardiovascular Risk Factors: The Evidence Supporting Their Association With Disease, the Usefulness of Measuring Them and Their Responsiveness to Intervention

	Evidence for Association With CVD		Clinical Measurement	Response to	
Risk Factor	Epidemiologic	Clinical Trials	Useful?	Nonpharmacologic Therapy	Pharmacologic Therapy
Category I (risk factors for which interventions have been proved to lower CVD risk)					
Cigarette smoking	+ + +	+ +	+ + +	+ + +	+ +
LDL cholesterol	+ + +	+ + +	+ + +	+ +	+ + +
High fat/cholesterol diet	+ + +	+ +	+ +	+ +	—
Hypertension	+ + +	+ + + (stroke)	+ + +	+	+ + +
Left ventricular hypertrophy	+ + +	+	+ +	—	+ +
Thrombogenic factors	+ + + (fibrinogen)	+ + + (aspirin, warfarin)	+ (fibrinogen)	+	+ + + (aspirin, warfarin)
Category II (risk factors for which interventions are likely to lower CVD risk)					
Diabetes mellitus	+ + +	+	+ + +	+ +	+ + +
Physical inactivity	+ + +	+ +	+ +	+ +	—
HDL cholesterol	+ + +	+	+ + +	+ +	+
Triglycerides; small, dense LDL	+ +	+ +	+ + +	+ +	+ + +
Obesity	+ + +	—	+ + +	+ +	+
Postmenopausal status (women)	+ + +	—	+ + +	—	+ + +
Category III (risk factors associated with increased CVD risk that, if modified, might lower risk)					
Psychosocial factors	+ +	+	+ + +	+	—
Lipoprotein(a)	+	—	+	—	+
Homocysteine	+ +	—	+	+ +	+ +
Oxidative stress	+	—	—	+	+ +
No alcohol consumption	+ + +	—	+ +	+ +	—
Category IV (risk factors associated with increased CVD risk, but which cannot be modified)					
Age	+ + +	—	+ + +	—	—
Male gender	+ + +	—	+ + +	—	—
Low socioeconomic status	+ + +	—	+ + +	—	—
Family history of early-onset CVD	+ + +	—	+ + +	—	—

CVD = cardiovascular disease; HDL = high density lipoprotein; LDL = low density lipoprotein; + = weak, somewhat consistent evidence; + + = moderately strong, rather consistent evidence; + + + = very strong, consistent evidence; — = evidence poor or nonexistent.
(With permission from Fuster V, Pearson TA. 27th Bethesda Conference: Matching the intensity of risk factor management with hazard for coronary disease events. *J Am Coll Cardiol* 27:957–1047, 1996.)

teins, LDL cholesterol is most strongly associated with the risk for CAD and accounts for most of the risk resulting from elevated total cholesterol concentrations. Indeed, evidence from epidemiologic, genetic, animal, and clinical investigations strongly supports a causal link between elevated LDL cholesterol and CAD risk (12).

In a primary prevention setting, lowering LDL cholesterol levels 1 mg/dl results in approximately a 1% to 2% reduction in the relative risk for CAD (3). In the West of Scotland Coronary Prevention Study, a 26% reduction in LDL cholesterol resulted in a 31% reduction in coronary events and a 22% reduction in the risk of death from any cause (13). Likewise, lowering LDL cholesterol via lifestyle intervention and/or drug therapy is highly effective in a secondary prevention setting (14). Thus, there is a strong rationale for the long-term aggressive control of LDL cholesterol as an essential strategy to normalize coronary artery endothelial function, halt or reverse the progression of coronary atherosclerosis, prevent the instability, rupture, and thrombosis of atherosclerotic plaques, and reduce mortality, recurrent hospitalization, and the ongoing cost of medical care in persons with established CAD.

Initiation and goal LDL cholesterol levels for dietary intervention and drug therapy in adults are summarized in Table 1.3. Dietary intervention is primarily aimed at reducing the intake of saturated fat and cholesterol. Overweight patients can further lower LDL cholesterol level by eliminating excess total calories and increasing physical activity.

High Fat/Cholesterol Diet

Over 50 years of research demonstrates that diet is one of the, if not the, major environmental causes of

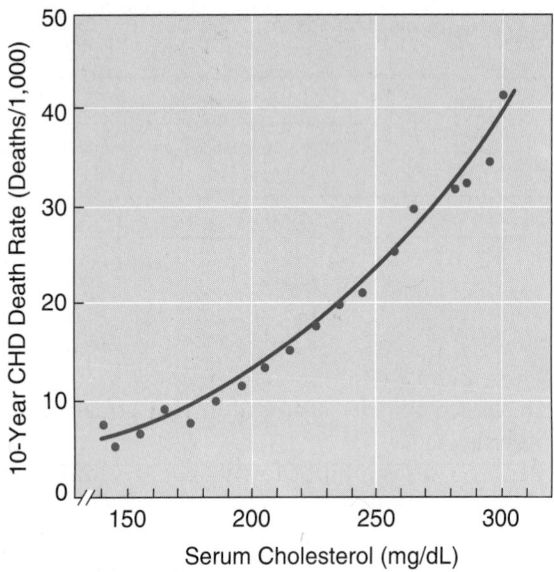

Figure 1.2. Relationship between serum cholesterol level and CHD death rate. (With permission from Expert Panel on Detection, Evaluation, and Treatment of High Blood Cholesterol in Adults (Adult Treatment Panel II). Second report of the National Cholesterol Education Program (NCEP) Men Screened for MRFIT Program. *NIH Publication* No. 93, 1993;361, 662.)

CAD. Within populations, serum total cholesterol and LDL cholesterol concentrations are strongly associated with dietary intake of fat, saturated fat and cholesterol (15). As mentioned above, dietary modification is universally recommended as the first step in managing individuals with hypercholesterolemia. Diet further predisposes to CAD by contributing to obesity, hypertension, and diabetes mellitus. Dietary saturated fat intake is also associated with increased thrombogenicity (10). More recently, ingestion of foods high in antioxidants, folate, vitamins B_6 and B_{12}, and soluble fiber have been suggested to lower CAD risk.

Hypertension

Nonfatal and fatal cardiovascular diseases, including CAD and all-cause mortality, increase progressively with higher levels of both systolic and diastolic blood pressure. In the general population, risks are lowest for adults with systolic blood pressure below 120 mmHg and diastolic blood pressure below 80 mmHg. At every level of diastolic blood pressure, the risk for CAD is greater with higher levels of systolic blood pressure (16).

Blood pressure may be classified as outlined in Table 1.4 and persons with values above normal should be followed-up as outlined in Table 1.5. The goal of treating patients with hypertension is to prevent morbidity and mortality associated with high blood pressure and to control blood pressure by the least intrusive means possible (16). To accomplish this, systolic and diastolic blood pressure should be reduced and maintained below 140 mmHg and 90 mmHg, respectively, while simultaneously optimizing the control of other modifiable risk factors for CAD (16).

Hypertension is believed to predispose patients to CAD by both the direct vascular injury caused by high blood pressure and its adverse effects on the myocardium, which include increased wall stress and myocardial oxygen demand. Although there is substantial evidence attesting to the health benefits of reducing blood pressure, the reduction in CAD events with antihypertensive therapy has been less than anticipated in most studies. This finding should not detract from the importance of lowering blood pressure, but has raised concern about the potentially proatherogenic effects of certain antihypertensive treatments (such as the unfavorable effect of beta-blockers and thiazide diuretics on serum lipids and lipoproteins) (17).

Lifestyle modification, including weight reduction, increased physical activity, and moderation of dietary sodium and alcohol intake, are recommended both as definitive or adjunctive therapy for hypertension (16). If blood pressure remains > 140/90 mm Hg despite 3 to 6 months of lifestyle modification, drug therapy should

Table 1.3. Treatment Decisions Based on LDL-Cholesterol

Dietary Therapy		
	Initiation Level	LDL Goal
Without CHD and with fewer than 2 risk factors	≥ 160 mg/dL	<160 mg/dL
Without CHD and with 2 or more risk factors	≥ 130 mg/dL	< 130 mg/dL
With CHD	> 100 mg/dL	≤ 100 mg/dL
Drug Treatment		
	Consideration Level	LDL Goal
Without CHD and with fewer than 2 risk factors	≥ 190 mg/dL*	< 160 mg/dL
Without CHD and with 2 or more risk factors	≥ 160 mg/dL	< 130 mg/dL
With CHD	≥ 130 mg/dL**	≤ 100 mg/dL

* In men under 35 years of age and premenopausal women with LDL-cholesterol levels 190–219 mg/dL, drug therapy should be delayed except in high-risk patients such as those with diabetes.

** In CHD patients with LDL-cholesterol levels 100–129 mg/dL, the physician should exercise clinical judgment in deciding whether to initiate drug treatment.

(With permission from Second Report of the National Expert Panel on Detection, Evaluation, and Treatment of High Blood Cholesterol in Adults (Adult Treatment Panel II). NIH Publication No. 93, 1993.)

Table 1.4. Classification of Blood Pressure for Adults Age 18 Years and Older*

CATEGORY	SYSTOLIC (MM HG)	DIASTOLIC (MM HG)
Normal†	< 130	< 85
High normal	130–139	85–89
Hypertension**		
STAGE 1 (Mild)	140–159	90–99
STAGE 2 (Moderate)	160–179	100–109
STAGE 3 (Severe)	180–209	110–119
STAGE 4 (Very Severe)	≥ 210	≥ 120

* Not taking antihypertensive drugs and not acutely ill. When systolic and diastolic pressures fall into different categories, the higher category should be selected to classify the individual's blood pressure status. For instance, 160/92 mm Hg should be classified as stage 2, and 180/120 mm Hg should be classified as stage 4. Isolated systolic hypertension (ISH) is defined as SBP ≥ 140 mm Hg and DBP < 90 mm Hg and staged appropriately (e.g., 170/85 mm Hg is defined as stage 2 ISH).
† Optimal blood pressure with respect to cardiovascular risk is SBP < 120 mm Hg and DBP < 80 mm Hg. However, unusually low readings should be evaluated for clinical significance.
** Based on the average of two or more readings taken at each of two or more visits following an initial screening.
Note: In addition to classifying stages of hypertension based on average blood pressure levels, the clinician should specify presence or absence of target-organ disease and additional risk factors. For example, a patient with diabetes and a blood pressure of 142/94 mm Hg plus left ventricular hypertrophy should be classified as "stage 1 hypertension with target-organ disease (left ventricular hypertrophy) and with another major risk factor (diabetes)." This specificity is important for risk classification and management.

be initiated. This is especially important in individuals with target organ disease and/or other known CAD risk factors (16). A variety of factors, including concomitant disease, demographic characteristics, the use of accompanying drugs that may lead to drug interactions, cost of medication, and metabolic and subjective side effects should be considered in the selection of initial and subsequent antihypertensive drug therapy (16).

Physical Inactivity

Despite the absence of adequately powered randomized clinical trials, physical inactivity is recognized as a risk factor for CAD (18). Epidemiologic criteria used to establish causal relationships can be applied to the association between physical activity and CAD, with the following principles of causality having been met:

1. Consistency—the association has been documented in a variety of settings and populations, with the better-designed studies showing the strongest associations;
2. Strength—the relative risk of CAD associated with physical inactivity is comparable to that observed for cigarette smoking, hypercholesterolemia, and hypertension;
3. Temporal sequencing—physical inactivity has been observed to predate the diagnosis of CAD;
4. Dose response—the risk of CAD increases as physical activity decreases; and
5. Biologic plausibility (19).

The precise mechanism by which physical inactivity predisposes patients to CAD has yet to be fully elucidated. Postulated mechanisms include:

1. Improvement of the balance between myocardial oxygen supply and demand at a given submaximal exercise intensity,
2. Decreased platelet aggregation and enhanced fibrinolysis,
3. Reduced susceptibility to malignant ventricular arrhythmias,
4. Improved endothelial-mediated vasomotor tone, and
5. Beneficial effect on other CAD risk factors.

Regarding the beneficial effect on other CAD risk factors, regular physical activity has been shown to lower resting systolic and diastolic blood pressure, reduce serum triglyceride levels, increase serum HDL cholesterol levels, and enhance glucose tolerance and insulin sensitivity (18, 19).

Studies of physical activity in both animals and humans with established CAD have demonstrated slowing of atherosclerotic progression and, in some instances, regression of atherosclerosis (20). Meta-analyses of ran-

Table 1.5. Recommendations for Follow-up Based on Initial Set of Blood Pressure Measurements for Adults Age 18 and Older

INITIAL SCREENING BLOOD PRESSURE (MM HG)*		
SYSTOLIC	DIASTOLIC	FOLLOWUP RECOMMENDED†
< 130	< 85	Recheck in 2 years
130–139	85–89	Recheck in 1 year**
140–159	90–99	Confirm within 2 months
160–179	100–109	Evaluate or refer to source of care within 1 month
180–209	110–119	Evaluate or refer to source of care within 1 week
≥ 210	≥ 120	Evaluate or refer to source of care immediately

* If the systolic and diastolic categories are different, follow recommendation for the shorter time followup (e.g., 160/85 mm Hg should be evaluated or referred to source of care within 1 month).
† The scheduling of follow-up should be modified by reliable information about past blood pressure measurements, other cardiovascular risk factors, or target-organ disease.
** Consider providing advice about lifestyle modifications (see Chapter 3).

domized clinical trials of aerobic exercise training in post myocardial infarction patients have documented a powerful (20% to 30%) reduction in coronary deaths (21, 22). Interestingly, no reduction in nonfatal myocardial infarction was observed.

Despite the above evidence, millions of U.S. adults remain essentially sedentary. Indeed, the number of individuals who are inactive is substantially greater than the number who smoke cigarettes, have hypercholesterolemia, or have hypertension. Thus, it has been hypothesized that the overall impact of stimulating Americans to lead a more physically active lifestyle could effectively lower CAD rates more than by reducing any other single risk factor (8).

Diabetes Mellitus

The prevalence of CAD is increased two- to fourfold in persons with diabetes mellitus. Atherosclerosis accounts for 80% of all diabetic mortality, with CAD accounting for 75% of these deaths. It is estimated that 25% of all myocardial infarctions in the United States occur in patients with diabetes mellitus. In patients with established CAD, diabetes remains a risk factor for adverse prognosis even after consideration of angiographic and other clinical characteristics (3, 8).

Multiple mechanisms have been implicated in the pathogenesis of atherosclerosis in diabetes (1, 3, 8). However, in the Diabetes Control and Complications Trial, improved glucose control in patients with insulin dependent diabetes mellitus was shown to convincingly reduce the risk for microvascular complications (23). Whether optimization of blood glucose control reduces CAD in persons with insulin dependent or non-insulin dependent diabetes mellitus remains to be seen. Control of hyperglycemia and the aggressive management of other CAD risk factors remains the most logical approach to cardiovascular disease risk reduction in persons with diabetes mellitus.

Obesity

The prevalence of obesity in the U.S. appears to have increased substantially during the past decade and 1 of 3 adults is now considered overweight (24). Obesity contributes to many adverse health outcomes and obesity-related conditions are estimated to contribute to 300,000 deaths annually in the United States (25). Obesity is associated with an accentuated risk for cardiovascular disease (Fig. 1.3). Analysis of the relationship between obesity and CAD is difficult because of its association with other risk factors, in particular, physical inactivity, hypertension, hyperlipidemia, and diabetes. However, recent reports from the Framingham Heart Study support the independence of obesity as a risk factor for CAD (26).

In the syndrome referred to as syndrome X, visceral or central abdominal obesity, high triglyceride levels, low HDL cholesterol levels, insulin resistance, and hypertension are metabolically linked. This form of obesity is relatively common and associated with a markedly increased risk for CAD.

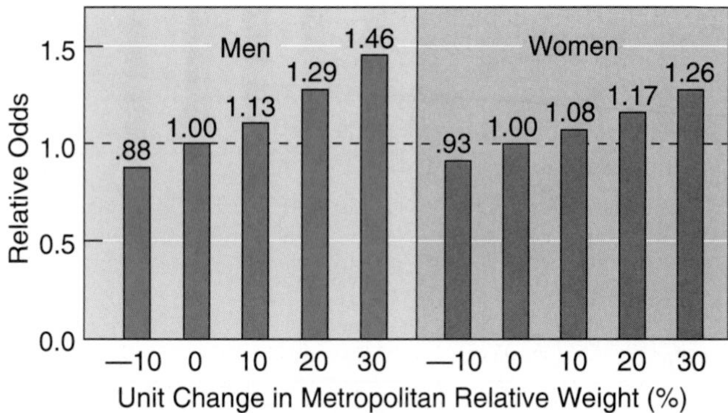

Figure 1.3. The relative odds of developing cardiovascular disease corresponding to degrees of change in metropolitan relative weight between age 25 years and entry into the Framingham Study. The odds ratios reflect adjustments for the effects of relative weight at age 25 years and risk factor levels at exam 1. (With permission from Hubert HB, et al. Obesity as an independent risk factor for cardiovascular disease: a 26-year follow-up of participants in the Framingham Heart Study. *Circulation* 1983;67:968.)

No studies have specifically evaluated the impact of weight loss on CAD events. Thus, obesity is classified as a Category II risk factor on the basis that weight management alters CAD risk by virtue of a favorable impact on other risk factors. Comprehensive programs that incorporate behavioral modalities to increase physical activity and improve diet have been shown to induce weight loss sufficient to produce significant cardiovascular health benefits in many obese individuals. In this respect, even modest weight loss of 5% to 10% of initial body weight has positive benefits on CAD risk factors, and weight loss of this magnitude may be realistic for many individuals (27).

Unfortunately, improvements in CAD risk factors are not maintained if weight is regained, and the vast majority of individuals who lose a significant amount of weight regain the lost weight within a relatively short period of time. Recognition of the need for long-term, and perhaps even lifelong, treatment has led certain experts to embrace the concept of long-term drug therapy, as is used in other chronic diseases. A national task force on the prevention and treatment of obesity, however, recently concluded that until more long-term data are available, pharmacotherapy cannot be recommended for routine use in obese individuals, although it may be helpful in carefully selected patients (28). Physicians who choose to administer anorexiant medications should do so only in the context of a comprehensive program that includes behavioral strategies targeted at nutrition and physical activity.

Triglycerides

Elevated serum triglyceride levels are positively correlated with CAD risk in univariate analyses. However, triglyceride levels lose some or most of their ability to predict CAD in multivariate analyses (29). The link between triglycerides and CAD is complex and may be related to the association between high triglycerides and low HDL cholesterol, increased thrombogenicity, insulin resistance, or high concentrations of LDL subclass pattern B (10). Regarding high concentrations of LDL subclass pattern B, small, dense LDL are more susceptible to oxidation and are believed to accentuate the risk for CAD (30). The Helsinki Heart Study and the Prospective Cardiovascular Munster Study have demonstrated that the combination of elevated LDL cholesterol and triglyceride levels and low HDL cholesterol constitutes a particularly atherogenic lipoprotein profile (31, 32).

The National Cholesterol Education Program classifies triglyceride levels as normal (< 200 mg/dl), borderline-high (200–399 mg/dl), high (400–999 mg/dl), and very high (> 1,000 mg/dl) (12). Triglyceride levels can be lowered by lifestyle interventions, including weight loss, exercise, dietary changes, decrease in alcohol consumption, and cigarette smoking cessation. Fibric acids and niacin are the most potent triglyceride lowering agents.

HDL Cholesterol

Existing animal and human studies support the concept that HDL cholesterol may prevent the entry of cholesterol into the atherogenesis process or even remove cholesterol from atherosclerotic lesions (so-called "reverse cholesterol transport") (29). As is the case for most lipoproteins, HDL cholesterol is a heterogeneous collection of particles of differing size and composition. In this respect, HDL cholesterol containing apo A-I but not apo A-II appears to be protective against CAD, whereas HDL cholesterol with both apolipoproteins appears to be neutral. Apo A-I has been identified as a prostacyclin-stabilizing factor, an attribute which may contribute to its cardioprotective benefit (3).

In the Framingham Heart Study, the Lipid Research Clinic Mortality Follow-up Study and Coronary Primary Prevention Trial, and the Multiple Risk Factor Intervention Trial data were consistent with a 2% to 3% decrease in CAD risk for each 1 mg/dl increase in HDL cholesterol after adjustment to control for other risk factors (29). Interventions that increase HDL cholesterol have been shown to favorably impact the underlying atherosclerosis process in secondary prevention, angiographic regression studies. The relationship between HDL cholesterol and CAD appears to be equally strong among asymptomatic individuals as well as in patients with established CAD and in men and women (29).

In the Helsinki Heart Study, the reduction in CAD with gemfibrozil exceeded that expected from the magnitude of reduction in LDL cholesterol alone (31). This observation has been interpreted to indicate a therapeutic benefit from raising HDL cholesterol. However, because gemfibrozil and other lipid-active agents and lifestyle interventions studied to date affect multiple lipid and lipoprotein fractions simultaneously, it has been difficult to convincingly demonstrate that an increase in HDL cholesterol independently lowered CAD risk.

The National Cholesterol Education Program has recommended the addition of HDL cholesterol to initial cholesterol testing, designating a high HDL cholesterol (> 60 mg/dl) as a negative risk factor and a low HDL cholesterol (< 35 mg/dl) as a positive risk factor for CAD, and considering HDL cholesterol levels in the choice of drug therapy (12). Recommended lifestyle interventions include diet, weight control, and exercise. Because of inherent problems, alcohol is not recommended for the purpose of raising HDL cholesterol.

OTHER RISK FACTORS FOR CAD

A number of factors have received attention because of their potential for increasing the risk of CAD. Unfortunately, in most cases, the impact of lifestyle modification on these factors has either little recognized relevance to reducing risk for CAD or has yet to be scientifically substantiated. Nonetheless, a brief discussion of each is warranted in order to provide a more complete understanding of the risk factor concept.

Left Ventricular Hypertrophy

Left ventricular hypertrophy occurs in response to chronic pressure and/or volume overload and constitutes a risk factor for cardiovascular disease (32, 33). Small studies of lifestyle interventions, such as weight loss and reduction of dietary sodium intake, that reduce left ventricular mass and wall thickness in patients with high blood pressure have been documented to result in regression of left ventricular hypertrophy (15). Additionally, a recent report from the Framingham Heart Study shows that persons with documented electrocardiographic evidence of regression of left ventricular hypertrophy are at substantially reduced risk for a cardiovascular event compared to persons without such evidence of regression (35). The presence of left ventricular hypertrophy should, at the very least, be regarded as an indication for effective blood pressure control (16).

Fibrinogen

Of the various hemostatic determinants, the association of fibrinogen with an increased risk of CAD is the most consistent and powerful (36). A recent meta-analysis has further indicated that the positive relation between plasma fibrinogen and CAD is independent of other risk factors (37). However, smoking, physical inactivity, and elevated triglycerides all are associated with increased fibrinogen levels.

Postmenopausal Status

CAD manifests itself approximately a decade later in women than in men. Nevertheless, CAD remains the leading cause of death among women in the U.S. (38). The concept that endogenous estrogen protects women against CAD is supported by the observation that the protection conferred upon women against CAD diminishes after natural or surgical menopause (39). Increasing evidence concerning the benefits of postmenopausal estrogen replacement has been derived from observational studies, but suggest that estrogen replacement may reduce the risk of developing CAD by as much as 50% (40). Among women with pre-existing CAD, data suggest an even greater reduction in risk with estrogen replacement therapy (40). However, definitive proof of the protective effect of estrogen replacement in females and potential risk of such therapy awaits the results of prospective clinical trials which are currently in progress.

Psychosocial Factors

According to several prospective studies, a variety of psychosocial factors are associated with CAD risk. These include the so-called "Type A" personality, hostility, depression, chronic stress produced by situations with "high demand and low control," and social isolation (Fig. 1.4) (3, 7). Psychosocial factors are postulated to accentuate CAD risk via two major mechanisms. First, they may exert their detrimental influence by direct mechanisms which include primarily neuroendocrine effects such as changes in catecholamine and serotonin levels. Second, they may indirectly accentuate risk by influencing adherence to lifestyle recommendations and compliance with drug therapy. Interventions of potential benefit include behavior modification, biofeedback, meditation, exercise, and when indicated, pharmacotherapy (3, 7).

Lipoprotein(a)

There is evidence from observational studies that lipoprotein(a) is associated with an accentuated risk for CAD, particularly in the presence of other risk factors (30, 41). Lifestyle interventions do not appear to lower lipoprotein(a) levels and niacin is the only conventional lipid agent known to lower lipoprotein(a). Estrogen replacement may also be beneficial.

Homocysteine

Homocysteine is postulated to predispose patients to CAD by virtue of procoagulant effects or direct injury of vascular endothelium. Among patients with vascular disease, 25% to 45% have been found to have increased levels of homocysteine (42). Serum homocysteine levels can be reduced by vitamin B_6, vitamin B_{12}, or folate supplements.

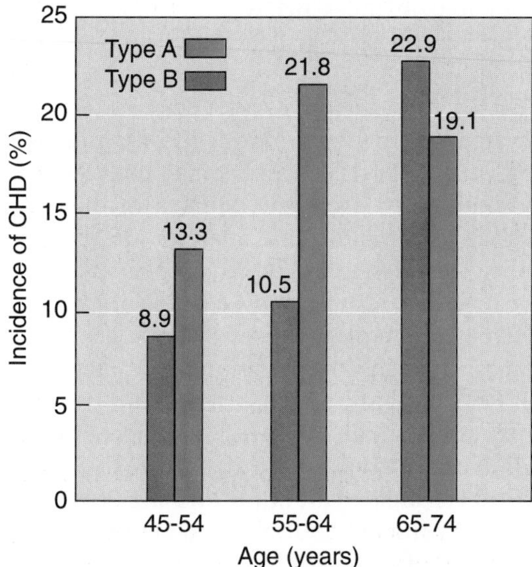

Figure 1.4. Eight-year incidence of coronary heart disease among men by the Framingham Type A and B behavior patterns. (With permission from Haynes SG, Feinleib M, Kannel WB. The relationship of psychosocial factors to coronary heart disease in the Framingham Study. III. Eight-year incidence of coronary heart disease. *Am J Epidemiol* 1980;111:37.)

Oxidative Stress

In the very early stages of atherogenesis, endothelial cells are responsible for mild oxidation of LDL cholesterol, which plays a role in monocyte recruitment. Monocytes differentiate into macrophages after entering the vessel wall and are believed to convert mildly oxidized LDL into highly oxidized LDL. Highly oxidized LDL binds to the scavenger receptors of macrophages and enters the cells, converting them into foam cells. When saturated with lipid, foam cells rupture and liberate products which further damage the endothelium and accelerate the atherosclerosis process (10). Antioxidants increase LDL resistance to oxidation and have been associated with a reduction in CAD risk. Specifically, there is the suggestion that diets high in vitamin C and, in particular, vitamin E are cardioprotective (3). In the recent Cambridge Heart Antioxidant Study of 2,002 patients with CAD, 400 or 800 IU of vitamin E was associated with a 47% reduction in the risk for acute myocardial infarction as compared to placebo (43).

Alcohol Consumption

Excessive alcohol consumption is associated with an increased risk for cardiovascular disease mortality, possibly as a result of alcoholic cardiomyopathy, cardiac arrhythmias, or hypertension. Regarding the hypertension,

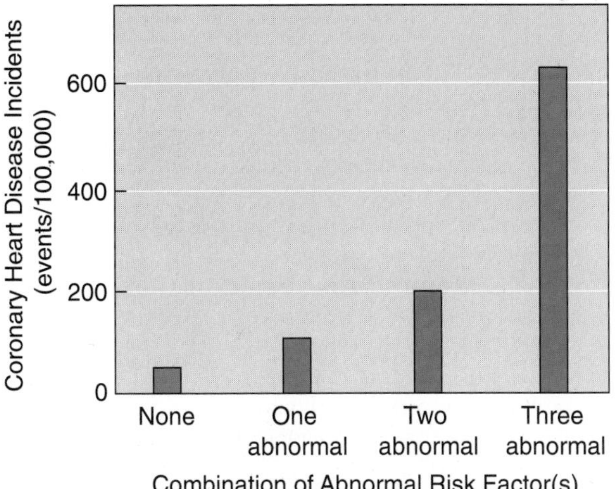

Figure 1.5. Relationship between a combination of abnormal risk factors (cholesterol ≥ 250 mg/dL; systolic blood pressure ≥ 160 mm Hg; smoking ≥ 1 pack of cigarettes/day) and incidence of coronary heart disease. (With permission from Kannel WB, Gordon T. The Framingham Study: an epidemiological investigation of cardiovascular disease. Section 30. Washington, Public Health Service, NIH, DHEW Publication (NIH) 1974;74-599.)

almost all of the more than 30 cross-sectional studies performed to date have identified an association between alcohol intake (three drinks or more, or approximately 40 g of ethanol per day) and blood pressure (16). In contrast, moderate alcohol consumption of one to three drinks daily has been reported to reduce CAD risk by 40% to 50% (3). Postulated mechanisms include an increase in HDL cholesterol, beneficial effect on vascular reactivity, and an improvement in hemostatic factors. Specifically regarding the improvement in hemostatic factors, both red wine and grape juice inhibit platelet activity in vivo, raising the possibility that the alcohol containing beverage itself may also impact CAD risk. The potential risks of excessive alcohol intake undoubtedly outweigh the potential benefits of moderate alcohol consumption. Therefore, persons who do not drink alcohol should not be encouraged to do so.

NON-MODIFIABLE RISK FACTORS

Age, male gender, family history of premature CAD (Table 1.1), and, to a certain degree, low socioeconomic status are risk factors for CAD which are not amenable to intervention. Recognition of the above risk factors is of importance in helping to reduce the risk for future cardiac events. Although they cannot be modified, they should be considered when attempting to match the level of management with the level of risk (4, 8). In particular, individuals with multiple CAD risk factors are at greatest risk (Fig. 1.5).

SUMMARY

Risk factors for CAD are characteristics which imply association with, but not causation of the disease. The risk factors can be divided into classifications including those that are modifiable and those that are not modifiable. Lifestyle modification may significantly reduce the morbidity and/or mortality associated with certain risk factors while change in others may not influence prognosis. Both primary and secondary prevention of CAD through modification of risk factors is efficacious.

References

1. Furberg CD, Hennekens CH, Hulley SB, et al. Task Force 2. Clinical epidemiology. The conceptual basis for interpreting risk factors. *J Am Coll Cardiol* 27:976–978, 1996.
2. Last JM. *A Dictionary of Epidemiology*. 2nd ed. New York: Oxford University Press, 1988.
3. Pasternak RC, Grundy SM, Levy D, et al. Task Force 3. Spectrum of risk factors for coronary heart disease. *J Am Coll Cardiol* 27:978–990, 1996.
4. Fuster V, Pearson TA. 27th Bethesda Conference. Matching the intensity of risk factor management with the hazard for coronary disease events. *J Am Coll Cardiol* 27:957–1047, 1996.
5. Fiore M, Bailey WC, Choen SJ, et al. Smoking Cessation. Clinical Practice Guideline No.18. Rockville, MD. U.S. Department of Health and Human Services, Public Health Service, Agency for Health Care Policy and Research. *AHCPR Publication* No. 96–0692, 1996.
6. Glantz SA, Parmley WW. Passive and active smoking. A problem for adults. *Circulation* 94:596–598, 1996.
7. Doll R, Peto R. Mortality in relation to smoking: 20 years' observations on male British doctors. *Br Med J* 2:1525–1536, 1976.
8. Caspersen CJ, Heath GW. The risk factor concept of coronary heart disease. In: ACSM's Resource Manual for Guidelines for Exercise Testing and Prescription. 2nd ed, Lea & Febiger, Philadelphia. 151–167, 1993.
9. The Health Benefits of Smoking Cessation. A report of the Surgeon General. Washington (D.C.): *U.S. Department of Health and Human Services*, 1990.
10. Fuster V, Gotto AM, Libby P, et al. Task Force 1. Pathogenesis of coronary disease: the biologic role of risk factors. *J Am Coll Cardiol* 27:964–976, 1996.
11. Glantz SA, Parmley WW. Passive smoking and heart disease. Mechanisms and risk. *JAMA* 273:1047–1053, 1995.
12. Second Report of the National Cholesterol Education Program (NCEP) Expert Panel on Detection, Evaluation, and Treatment of High Blood Cholesterol in Adults (Adult Treatment Panel II). *NIH Publication* No. 93, 1993.
13. Shepherd J, Cobbe SM, Ford I, et al. Prevention of coronary heart disease with pravastatin in men with hypercholesterolemia. *N Engl J Med* 333:1301–1307, 1995.
14. Smith SC Jr, Blair SN, Criqui MH, et al. AHA Medical/Scientific Statement. Consensus panel statement: preventing heart attack and death in patients with coronary disease. *Circulation* 92:2–4, 1995.
15. Committee on Diet and Health Food and Nutrition Board Co. *Diet and Health* 7:1989.

16. Joint National Committee on Detection, Evaluation, and Treatment of High Blood Pressure. The Fifth Report of the Joint National Committee on Detection, Evaluation, and Treatment of High Blood Pressure (JNC V). *Arch Intern Med* 153:154–183, 1993.
17. Roberts WC. Blood lipid levels and antihypertensive therapy. *Am J Cardiol* 60:33E–35E, 1987.
18. Fletcher GF, Balady G, Blair SN, et al. Statement on Exercise: benefits and recommendations for physical activity programs for all Americans: a statement for health professionals by the Committee on Exercise and Cardiac Rehabilitation of the Council on Clinical Cardiology, American Heart Association. *Circulation* 94:857–862, 1996.
19. Pate RR, Pratt M, Blair SN, et al. Physical activity and public health: a recommendation from the Centers for Disease Control and Prevention and the American College of Sports Medicine. *JAMA* 273:402–407, 1995.
20. Schuler G, Hambrecht R, Schlierf G, et al. Regular physical exercise and low-fat diet: effects on progression of coronary artery disease. *Circulation* 86:1–11, 1992.
21. Oldridge NB, Guyatt GH, Fischer ME, et al. Cardiac rehabilitation after myocardial infarction: Combined experience of randomized clinical trials. *JAMA* 260:945–950, 1988.
22. O'Connor GT, Buring JE, Yusuf S, et al. An overview of randomized trials of rehabilitation with exercise after myocardial infarction. *Circulation* 80:234–244, 1989.
23. The effect of intensive treatment of diabetes on the development and progression of long-term complications in insulin-dependent diabetes mellitus: The Diabetes Control and Complications Trial Research Group. *N Engl J Med* 329:977–986, 1993.
24. Kuezmarski RJ, Flegal KM, Campbell SM, et al. Increasing prevalence of overweight among US adults. *JAMA* 272: 205–211, 1994.
25. Pi-Sunyer FX. Medical hazards of obesity. *Ann Intern Med* 110:655–660, 1993.
26. Hubert HB, Feineib M, McNamara PM, et al. Obesity as an independent risk factor for cardiovascular disease: a 26-year follow-up of participants in the Framingham Heart Study. *Circulation* 67:968–77, 1983.
27. Blackburn GL, Rosofsky W. Making the connection between weight loss, dieting, and health: the 10% solution. *Weight Control Dig* 2:121–127,1992.
28. National Task Force on the Prevention and Treatment of Obesity. Long-term pharmacotherapy in the management of obesity. *JAMA* 276:1907–1915, 1996.
29. NIH Consensus Development Panel on Triglyceride, High-Density Lipoprotein, and Coronary Heart Disease. Triglyceride, high-density lipoprotein, and coronary heart disease. *JAMA* 269:505–510, 1993.
30. Superko HR. Beyond LDL cholesterol reduction. *Circulation* 94:2351–2354, 1996.
31. Frick MH, Elo O, Haapa K, et al. Helsinki Heart Study: primary-prevention trial with gemfibrozil in middle-aged men with dyslipidemia: safety of treatment, changes in risk factors, and incidence of coronary heart disease. *N Engl J Med* 317:1237–1245, 1987.
32. Assmann G, Schulte H. Relation of high-density lipoprotein cholesterol and triglycerides to incidence of atherosclerotic coronary artery disease (the PROCAM experience). Prospective Cardiovascular Munster study. *Am J Cardiol* 70:733–737, 1992.
33. Kannel WB, Gordon T, Castelli WP, et al. Electrocardiographic left ventricular hypertrophy and risk of coronary heart disease. The Framingham Study. *Ann Intern Med* 72: 813–822, 1970.
34. Kannel WB, Gordon T, Offutt D. Left ventricular hypertrophy by electrocardiogram. Prevalence, incidence, and mortality in the Framingham Study. *Ann Intern Med* 71:89–105, 1969.
35. Levy D, Salomon M, D'Agostino RB, et al. Prognostic implications of baseline electrocardiographic features and their serial change in subjects with left ventricular hypertrophy. *Circulation* 90:1786–1793, 1994.
36. Fuster V. Mechanisms leading to myocardial infarction: Insights from studies of vascular biology. *Circulation* 90: 2126–2146, 1994.
37. Yang XC, Jing TY, Resnick LM, et al. Relation of hemostatic risk factors to other risk factors for coronary heart disease and to sex hormones in men. *Arterioscler Thromb Vasc Biol* 13(4):467–471, 1993.
38. Fetters JK, Peterson ED, Shaw IJ, et al. Sex-specific differences in coronary artery disease risk factors, evaluation, and treatment: Have they been adequately evaluated? *Am Heart J* 131:796–813, 1996.
39. Grodstein F, Stampfer M. The epidemiology of coronary heart disease and estrogen replacement in postmenopausal women. *Prog Cardiovasc Dis* 38:199–210, 1995.
40. Sullivan JM. Estrogen replacement therapy. *Am J Med* 101(Suppl 4A):56S–60S, 1996.
41. Bostom AG, Cuppies LA, Jenner JL, et al. Elevated plasma lipoprotein(a) and coronary heart disease in men aged 55 years and younger. A prospective study. *JAMA* 276:544–548, 1996.
42. Clarke R, Daly L, Robinson K, et al. Hyperhomocysteinemia: An independent risk factor for vascular disease. *N Engl J Med* 324:1149–1155, 1991.
43. Stephens NG, Parsons A, Schofield PM, et al. Randomised controlled trial of vitamin E in patients with coronary disease: Cambridge Heart Antioxidant Study. *Lancet* 347:781–786, 1996.

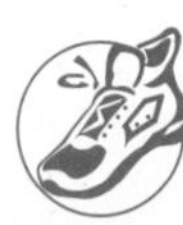

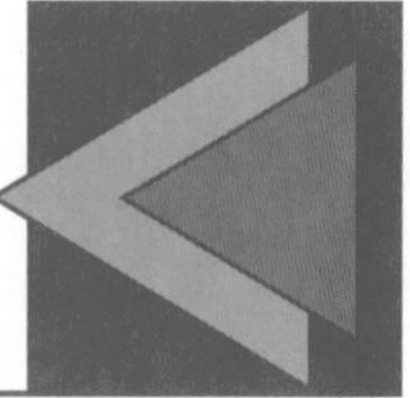

CHAPTER **2**

Epidemiology of Physical Activity, Physical Fitness, and Selected Chronic Diseases

Mitchell A. Whaley and Leonard A. Kaminsky

Based on the observed health-related benefits associated with increased physical activity, several health organizations have published position papers calling for efforts to increase public awareness and to establish recommendations for the appropriate quantity and quality of physical activity for adults (1–3). These position statements were based on the continually increasing volume of scientific literature that demonstrates the inverse association between sedentary lifestyle and morbidity or mortality from a number of chronic diseases. The purpose of this chapter is to review the association between sedentary habits and the risk for chronic disease and to review the most recent physical activity recommendations in light of this evidence.

MEASUREMENT OF LEISURE TIME PHYSICAL ACTIVITY/CARDIORESPIRATORY FITNESS

Most studies that assess the association between physical activity habits or fitness levels and the risk of disease include a measure of leisure time physical activity (LTPA) and/or cardiorespiratory fitness (CRF). Studies that have assessed LTPA commonly use a single self-reported measure of LTPA at baseline, although some more recent studies included measures of LTPA at both baseline and during the follow-up period (4–7). This study design allows the opportunity to assess the impact of changes in physical activity habits across time on disease/mortality risk. The considerable variability in assessment instruments for quantifying LTPA should be considered when comparing results among the studies (8–10). Physical activity habits are usually converted to either an estimate of total energy expenditure (e.g., kilocalories per day or week) or a physical activity index where individuals are assigned to LTPA categories based on a combination of type, amount, and intensity of self-reported physical activity.

In contrast to the studies that focused on LTPA habits among their cohort, a number of studies have used a measure of cardiorespiratory fitness as the variable within their analyses. Based on the weaker associations found in studies that employed less precise measures of CRF, only studies that included a maximal exercise test will be discussed in this review (9, 11–18). Further, it should be recognized that there is a genetic component associated with such a measure of CRF, probably ranging between 10% and 50% (19). Therefore, measures of CRF should appropriately be viewed as a consequence of both hereditary factors and habitual physical activity patterns.

Finally, although LTPA and CRF are of particular interest, it is well established that risk for many chronic diseases is multifactorial. Thus, numerous factors besides LTPA or CRF contribute to the risk of developing a chronic disease. To better understand the association between either LTPA or CRF and a specific disease risk, other risk factors for that disease, often referred to as *confounders,* should be controlled within the analysis. Each of the studies reviewed herein adjusted for most of the important confounders in the analysis and were able to assess the independent association between LTPA or CRF and disease outcome. Therefore, in addition to the specific measure of LTPA or CRF employed within the study, the type of confounders adjusted for within the study should be considered when comparing risk estimates among the available studies.

LTPA/CRF AND CARDIOVASCULAR DISEASE/CORONARY HEART DISEASE

Numerous population-based observational studies have linked a sedentary lifestyle or low fitness to greater risk for cardiovascular disease (CVD) or more specifically, coronary heart disease (CHD) morbidity and mortality. Reviews of early research concluded that CHD risk for sedentary individuals was approximately double that of more physically active individuals and the better quality studies reported stronger inverse relationships between physical activity or fitness and CHD (20, 21). More recent reviews have called for further information regarding the dose-response relationship between physical activity or fitness and premature morbidity/mortality from CHD, and whether adoption of a more active lifestyle or improvements in cardiorespiratory fitness would confer the protection from CHD inferred by earlier studies (22–25). Recent studies provide new insight regarding these topics, and a summary of the study designs and important findings from these papers are presented in Table 2.1. Several of these recent papers are follow-up reports to earlier analyses within the same cohort (6, 7, 10, 26–32).

With few exceptions, the results from the studies of LTPA and CVD/CHD listed in Table 2.1 are consistent with the finding of Powell et al. of a twofold greater risk for CHD when comparing the most inactive to more active men (21, 27, 29). However, several recent studies compared CVD/CHD rates among multiple ordinal categories of LTPA and they provide new information about the dose-response relationship between physical activity and CVD (9, 10, 26, 28, 33–35). Results from two of the cohorts suggest that moderate amounts and intensities of physical activity are adequate for protection from CHD while others reported more vigorous physical activity was necessary to reduce risk for CHD or all-cause death (9, 10, 26, 28, 33, 34).

In summary, although recent studies are consistent in the finding of an inverse and graded relationship between LTPA and CHD, the issue of an intensity threshold has not been clearly resolved. Based on results from the available studies, high-risk men who engage in mostly light to moderate intensity physical activities and accumulate an average of 1500 kilocalories per week of total energy expenditure are likely to experience a 25% to 50% lower CHD risk (7, 10, 34, 35). However, men who engage in more intense physical activities (e.g., >6 metabolic equivalents [METS]) on a regular basis may experience a 60% to 70% lower CHD risk and greater longevity (9, 26, 33).

An additional interesting finding within these data was an upswing in CHD risk for the most active men (those who reported very frequent sporting exercise) (34). This trend was also apparent in an earlier report from the Harvard Alumni cohort (36). Based on subsequent analysis however, it was concluded that the higher CHD risk observed for the most active men was confined primarily to those with hypertension (28). Whether hypertension could also explain the higher mortality risk observed for the most physically active men (>3500 kcal/week) within the Harvard Alumni cohort is unknown.

Several recent studies of physical fitness and CHD are also summarized in Table 2.1. Each of the studies reported an independent, inverse relationship between fitness and CHD/CVD (9, 13, 16). These results, derived from studies that included strong, objective measures of CRF, strengthen the findings from earlier studies of men and extend the findings to women (13, 22). Comparisons among multiple ordinal fitness categories have also been made to evaluate the question of optimal level of CRF for protection from CHD (9, 13, 37). Based on the available studies of fitness and CHD/CVD, it appears that a fitness level below 8 or 9 METS represents a threshold for middle-aged men that is associated with significantly greater risk. Because only one study provides fitness data for women, the thresholds presented in Table 2.2 are reasonable until more data on women become available (13).

Changes in Physical Activity or Fitness

Results from recent reports that used measures of LTPA or CRF during the follow-up period to assess **change** in physical activity habits or fitness level strengthen findings from the numerous studies where physical activity habits or physical fitness was defined only at the time of entry into the study. Two reports from the Harvard Alumni Study indicate similar associations between change in physical activity habits and mortality risk; a 41% lower risk of CHD mortality during the follow-up period was seen in subjects who took up moderately vigorous physical activity (≥4.5 METS intensity) compared to those who never engaged in such activity. In addition, the studies indicated a 28% decrease in all-cause mortality risk in men who increased their total energy expenditure during leisure time to more than 1500 kcal/week (6, 7). It is also worth noting that those men who became less active during the follow-up period had a small but statistically greater mortality risk (13%) compared to those who were inactive at both assessments (7). Additionally, research has demonstrated that men considered fit at two different exams had a 67% and 78% lower risk of all-cause and CVD mortality, respectively, compared to those who were unfit at both exams (12).

LTPA/CRF AND CANCER

Cancer is the second leading cause of death for adult men and women in the United States. Several recent review papers have discussed the available epidemiological studies related to physical activity and/or fitness and risk of cancer. Based on the available data at that time, these review articles concluded that there was significant evidence to support an inverse association between physical activity and colon cancer although no consistent relationships were demonstrated between physical activity and cancers of the rectum, lung, breast, pancreas, or other sites (38–40). Two other recent studies also reported inconsistent results in describing associations between mortality from combined-sites cancer and either physical activity or fitness. One study suggested no association and the other a strong association (8, 13). In the latter study, the lowest fit men were two to three

Table 2.1. Recent Prospective Studies of LTPA/CRF and All-Cause, CVD and CHD Mortality

Study (Ref)	Design	Cohort	CHD Endpoint	Major Findings
Blair *et al.* 1989 (15)	Mean 8 yrs follow-up CRF - maximal treadmill test CRF - total treadmill time CRF Quintiles	ACLS men (10,224) and women (3,120)	Fatal CVD n = 66 men n = 7 women	RR = 7.9[a] (−8.8, −3.3)[b] for men; RR = 9.3[b] (−5.1, 0.5)[b] for women, for low vs. two highest quintiles of fitness.
Morris *et al.* 1990 (33)	9 yrs follow-up week recall of LTPA Vig Aerobic Ex (VAE) Frequency VAE = > 7.5 kcals/min; > 6 METs; > 65% VO_{2max} PA categories	British Civil Servants cohort 9,376 men Age 45–64 yrs @ baseline reported frequent VAE	Fatal & Non-Fatal CHD n = 287 fatal n = 459 non-fatal	Ages 45–54 Yrs: RR[c] Fatal = 0.25 (0.07, 0.93) & Non-Fatal = 0.37 (0.15, 0.77) for Freq VAE vs. No VAE Ages 55–64 Yrs: RR[c] Fatal = 0.53 (0.21, 1.32) & Non-Fatal = 0.43 (0.19, 1.01) for Freq VAE vs. No VAE Data taken from Table 7.
Leon *et al.* 1991 (10)	10.5 yrs follow-up Minnesota LTPA Q PA Tertiles (T1-T3)	MRFIT cohort 12,138 men Age 35–57 yrs @ baseline	Fatal CHD n = 518	RR[d] Fatal CHD = 0.75 (0.59, 0.96) for middle group vs. least active; 0.82 (0.65, 1.03) for most active vs. least active. No Dose-response for quantity of LTPA for Fatal CHD.
Lindsted *et al.* 1991 (8)	26 yrs follow-up Single PA Question 2 PA Categories	Seventh Day Adventist cohort 9,484 men Age > 30 yrs @ baseline Mixture of health status	Fatal CHD n = 1351	RR[e] = 0.55 (0.38, 0.78) for moderately active men compared to less active at age 50, and remained significant up to age 70 years. Association was not statistically significant for higher levels of activity.
Shaper & Wannamethee 1991 (34)	8 yrs follow-up Unique PAI PA Categories	British Regional Heart Study 7,735 men Age 40–59 yrs @ baseline Mixture of health status Included HTNs	Fatal & Non-Fatal CHD n = 217 (fatal) n = 271 (non-fatal)	RR[d] = 0.5 (0.2, 0.8) for moderate active groups compared to least active. RR[d] = 0.9 (0.5, 1.8) for most active vs. least active men. Data taken from Table 4.
Arraiz *et al.* 1992 (11)	7 yrs follow-up LTPA CHS-PAI PA categories	Canadian Men & women combined Age 30–64 yrs @ baseline	Fatal CVD n = 256	RR[f] = 0.8 (0.4, 1.4), 0.3 (0.1, 0.9), 0.8 (0.4, 1.4) for inactive, moderate & active groups compared to the very active group. Data from Table 4.
Hein *et al.* 1992 (12)	17 yrs follow-up Single PA Question PA Categories	4,999 men Age 40–59 yrs @ baseline engaged in "conditioning" activities	Fatal CHD n = 266 (171 MIs)	RR[g] = 1.6 (1.14, 2.21) Low vs. High groups. No difference in CHD among upper 3 or 4 PA groups.
Sandvik *et al.*, 1993 (18)	Mean 15.9 yrs follow-up CRF - maximal leg cycle test CRF - difference in PWC[h]	Norwegian 1,960 men Age 40–59 yrs @ baseline	Fatal CVD n = 143 (127 MIs or SD)	RR[a] = 0.41 (0.20, 0.84) for high vs. low quartile. Dose-response (Q2-3 vs. Q4) was most clear after the first 7 yrs of follow-up. PA was not independently related to CVD.

(continued)

Table 2.1. *(continued)*

Study (Ref)	Design	Cohort	CHD Endpoint	Major Findings
Lakka *et al.* 1994 (9)	4.9 yrs follow-up Modified Minnesota LTPA Q PA Tertiles CRF - maximal leg cycle test CRF - VO_{2max}	Eastern Finnish 1,453 men Age 42–60 yrs @ baseline Mixture of health status	Fatal & Non-Fatal MIs n = 41	LTPA: RR^d = 0.34 (0.12, 0.94) for those with > 2.2 hr/wk of "conditioning" activities vs. those with lesser amounts. LTPA: Non-conditioning activities were not protective. CRF: RR^d = 0.35 (0.13, 0.92) High vs. low fit third; > 2.7 (1 min^{-1}).
Rodriguez *et al.* 1994 (27)	23 yrs follow-up Framingham PAI PA Tertiles	Honolulu Heart Program 7,074 men Age 45–68 yrs @ baseline Free of CHD	Fatal & Non-Fatal CHD n = 340 (fatal) n = 789 (combined)	RR $Fatal^d$ = 0.85 (0.65, 1.13) for High vs. Low PA tertile. RR Combined Fatal & $Non\text{-}Fatal^d$ = 0.95 (0.80, 1.14) for High vs. Low active tertile. No protective effect for middle tertile for either endpoint.
Sherman *et al.* 1994 (29)	16 yrs follow-up Framingham PAI PA Quartiles	Framingham 1,404 women Age 50–74 yrs @ baseline Free of CVD	Fatal CVD n = 106	No relationship between PA and CVD morbidity/mortality.
Shaper *et al.* 1994 (28)	9 yrs follow-up Unique PAI 6 PA Categories	British Regional Heart Study 5,695 men Age 40–59 yrs @ baseline Mixture of health status Normotensive/1806 Hypertensive	Fatal & Non-Fatal CHD n = 125 (fatal) n = 186 (non-fatal)	Normotensive Men RR^d = 0.5 (0.2, 0.9) for moderate/moderately vigorous vs. inactive; RR = 0.5 (0.2, 1.1) for vigorous vs. inactive. Hypertensive Men RR^d = 0.5 (0.2, 0.9) for moderate/moderately vigorous vs. inactive; RR = 1.2 (0.5, 2.7) for vigorous vs. inactive. Data are from Table 3.
Lee *et al.* 1995 (26)	24 yrs follow-up Harvard PAI PA Quintiles Vigorous vs. Non-vigorous PA	Harvard Alumni 17,321 men Free of CVD, cancer and COPD Mean age 46 yrs @ baseline	3728 all-cause deaths	Graded inverse relation between total PA and mortality. RR^i for quintiles of increasing PA were 1.00, 0.94, 0.95, 0.91, and 0.91 (P [trend] < 0.05). RR^i for quintiles of increasing vigorous PA were 1.00, 0.88, 0.92, 0.87, and 0.87, (P [trend] = 0.007). Vigorous PA, but not non-vigorous PA associated with lor.gevity.

Paffenbarger *et al.* 1993, 1994 (6,7)	9 yrs follow-up from 2nd assessment Harvard PAI Change in moderately vigorous LTPA Change in total PAI	Harvard Alumni 10,269 healthy men (1993 paper); 14,786 healthy men (1994 paper) Age 45–84	n = 130 fatal CHD n = 2,343 deaths thru 1988	RR of CHD[i] = 0.77 (0.58, 0.96) and 0.71 (0.55, 0.96) for those who maintained or took up moderately vigorous sports (≥ 4.5 METs). RR of death[i] = 0.72 (0.64, 0.82) and 0.77 (0.69, 0.85) for men who increased to or maintained ≥ 1500 kcals/wk of LTPA across assessments.
Blair *et al.* 1995 (14)	Mean 4.9 yrs follow-up CRF - maximal treadmill change in CRF	ACLS 9,777 men Age 20–82 @ baseline Health & unhealthy	Fatal CVD n = 87	RR[a] = 0.48 (0.31, 0.74) for Unfit-Fit; and 0.22 (0.12, 0.39) for Fit-Fit compared to Unfit-Unfit.

CHD–coronary heart disease, CHS–Canadian Health Survey, CRF–cardiorespiratory fitness, CVD–cardiovascular disease, GXT–graded exercise test, HTN–hypertension, HTNs–hypertensives, LTPA–leisure time physical activity, METs–metabolic equivalents, MI–myocardial infarction, PA–physical activity, PAI–Physical Activity Index, PWC–physical work capacity, RR–relative risk, SD–sudden death (Values in parentheses represent the 95% confidence intervals for the risk ratio)

[a] RR adjusted for age only, although additional adjustments for other factors had little effect.

[b] 95% confidence intervals for linear trend slope.

[c] RR adjusted for age, family history of CVD, height, BMI, smoking, hypertension, diabetes, and angina.

[d] RR adjusted for age and other major CHD risk factors.

[e] RR adjusted for age, sex, BMI, and smoking.

[f] RR adjusted for race, smoking, education, medical illness, BMI, marital status and dietary pattern.

[g] RR adjusted for age, social class, and smoking.

[h] Difference in PWC: PWC was calculated as the sum of all workloads completed, and the difference between the observed and expected PWC was used as the measure of fitness in the analyses.

[i] RR adjusted for age, cigarette smoking, hypertension, and BMI.

Table 2.2. MET Values[a] for Low and High Cardiorespiratory Fitness (CRF) for Adult Men and Women

Age-Category	Men (Low–High Fitness)	Women (Low–High Fitness)
20–39 years	10.1–13.4	7.1–11.1
40–49 years	9.1–12.5	6.6–9.7
50–59 years	8.4–11.7	6.0–8.9
60+ years	7.0–10.5	5.4–8.0

[a] Based on fitness categories as described by Blair SN, Kohl HW, Paffenbarger RS, Clark DG, Cooper KH, Gibbons LW. Physical fitness and all-cause mortality: a prospective study of healthy men and women. *JAMA* 262:2395–2402, 1989.

With permission from Whaley MH, Blair SN. Epidemiology of physical activity, physical fitness and coronary heart disease. *J Cardiovasc Risk* 2:289–295, 1995.

times more likely to die from cancer compared to their more fit counterparts, but due to the low number of cancer deaths within the female cohort, relative comparisons among the fitness categories in women were limited.

A number of recent prospective studies have assessed the association between leisure time physical activity or fitness and cancers from specific sites and are summarized in Table 2.3 (4, 5, 17, 41–45). Results from four of five studies support an inverse association between leisure time physical activity and colon cancer risk which confirm the findings from earlier reports reviewed elsewhere (4, 38–42, 44, 45). Despite the dissimilar physical activity assessment instruments among these recent studies, the average relative risk for colon cancer among the most sedentary men was approximately double that of the most active men. However, based on the results from two of the studies, the association between physical activity and colon cancer is less clear in women (41, 42).

The results from prospective studies assessing the association between other site-specific cancers and LTPA or fitness have been mixed. Three of the four studies reported an inverse association between physical activity or fitness and risk of prostatic cancer in men, while the other reported null results (5, 17, 41, 45). Three of the studies listed in Table 2.3 did not indicate an association between LTPA and rectal cancer, while two of the studies found no association between LTPA and cancer of the breast (4, 41, 43, 45). In addition, no association was observed between leisure time activity and cancers of the lung, cervix, stomach, and urinary bladder (41, 45).

In conclusion, the results from the most recent studies of LTPA/CRF and cancer provide further support for an inverse association for risk of cancers of the colon in men (not women). When combined with results from studies reviewed previously, the recent evidence would also confirm a lack of an association between LTPA and rectal cancer (39). At present, the associations between LTPA/CRF and other site-specific cancers remain unclear and should continue to be a focus of future prospective studies, particularly in women.

LTPA/CRF AND NON-INSULIN DEPENDENT DIABETES MELLITUS

Non-insulin dependent diabetes mellitus (NIDDM) affects some 12 million people in the United States and is a major risk factor for cardiovascular disease morbidity and mortality. Several recent prospective epidemiological studies have assessed the association between physical activity or fitness and risk of developing NIDDM. A brief summary of each study is presented in Table 2.4. Each of these studies included results from multivariate analyses where other variables that might confound the relationship between activity or fitness and NIDDM (e.g., body mass index, traditional CHD risk factors) were taken into consideration. Four of the available studies included male cohorts, while two included women (16, 46–49). In addition, four of the studies used self-report physical activity habits as the variable (46–49), while one assessed the risk of NIDDM as a function of physical fitness (16).

Although the available studies differed significantly in the way they quantified LTPA or physical fitness, collectively, the reports support the finding of an inverse relationship between LTPA and risk for development of NIDDM for both men and women. In addition, the studies that included more elaborate measures of LTPA or a measure of physical fitness also reported stronger associations between inactivity/low fitness and the risk for NIDDM (16, 46, 47). As is the case with several other chronic diseases, future studies should focus on further defining the relationship between the quantity and quality of physical activity and risk of NIDDM.

LTPA/CRF AND STROKE

Stroke is the third leading cause of death in the United States. In a recent review of physical activity and stroke, the authors concluded that the available data were "equivocal concerning the role that physical activity and physical fitness may play in the risk of stroke" (50). Five recent prospective epidemiological studies assessed the association between self-reported LPTA and risk of stroke. A brief summary of each study is presented in Table 2.5 (8, 51–54). Of the five studies reviewed here, all included a cohort of men, while one also included a cohort of women (53).

In summary, although two of the three studies that compared multiple categories of LTPA reported a graded relationship with significantly lower stroke rates for the most active men within the cohort, the existing data are not conclusive regarding a relationship between physical activity and stroke in men or women (53, 54). Future

Table 2.3. **Recent Prospective Studies of LTPA/Physical Fitness and Cancer**

Study (Ref)	Design	Cohort	Cancer Endpoint	Major Findings
Albanes *et al.*, 1989 (41)	10 yrs follow-up 2 questions PA recall (Recreational & Non-recreational PA) 3 PA categories	NHANES I 5,138 men; 7,407 women Age 25–74 yrs @ baseline	Colorectum, lung, prostate, breast, cervix n = 460 combined male cases n = 399 combined female cases	*Non-recreational activity*: RR 1.8[a] (1.4, 2.4) for least active vs. most active men for combined-sites; strongest relationship seen for lung cancer with RR 2.0 (1.2, 3.5) for least active vs. most active men. *Recreational activity*: RR 1.8 (1.0, 3.3) for prostate for most active vs. least active men. No significant associations for women.
Severson *et al.*, 1989 (45)	11 yrs follow-up Framingham PAI PA tertiles	7,858 Japanese men in Hawaii Age 46–68 yrs @ baseline	Colon, rectum, stomach, lung, prostate, urinary bladder n = 929 combined cases	RR[b] = 0.56 (0.39, 0.80) and 0.71 (0.51, 0.99) for the middle and most active tertiles compared to the lowest active for colon cancer. Incidence of cancer at other sites was not associated with PAI.
Ballard-Barbash *et al.*, 1990 (42)	Up to 28 yrs follow-up Framingham PAI PA tertiles	Framingham 1,906 men; 2,308 women Mean age 50 ± 9 yrs @ baseline	Large bowel cancer n = 152 cases	RR[c] = 1.4 (0.8–2.6) and 1.8 (1.0–3.2) for men in the middle and lowest PAI tertiles (compared to the most active tertile), respectively. No significant associations for women.
Lee *et al.*, 1991 (4)	23 yrs of follow-up in Harvard PAI 3 PAI categories (< 1000, 1000–2500, > 2500 kcals/wk of LTPA)	Harvard Alumni 17,719 men Age 30–79 yrs @ baseline	Colon, rectal n = 225 cases n = 44 cases	Increased activity taken at either assessment alone was not related to incidence of cancer. RR[d] for colon cancer = 0.50 (0.27, 0.93) and 0.52 (0.28, 0.94) for men in highest and middle PAI categories at both assessments compared to least active men. No association between PAI and rectal cancer.
Lee *et al.*, 1992 (5)	23 yrs of follow-up Harvard PAI (analysis 2/change in PAI (analysis 1) 3 or 4 PAI categories	Harvard Alumni 17,719 men Age 30–79 yrs @ baseline	Prostate n = 221 cases (analysis 1) n = 419 cases (analysis 2)	RR[e] = 0.12 (0.02, 0.89) for those expending > 4000 kcals/wk vs < 1000 kcals/wk at both assessment points (1962–66 & 1977). RR[e] = 0.53 (0.29, 0.95) for those men age > 70 yrs who expending > 4000 kcals/wk at either assessment (1962–66 or 1977). No evidence of dose-response relationship

(continued)

Table 2.3. *(continued)*

Study (Ref)	Design	Cohort	Cancer Endpoint	Major Findings
Dorgan *et al.*, 1994 (43)	Up to 27 yrs of follow-up Framingham PAI PA quartiles	Framingham 2,307 women	Breast n = 117 cases	No association found between PA and breast cancer.
Giovannucci *et al.*, 1995 (44)	> 5 yrs of follow-up Unique PA index (MET Hrs/wk) PA quintiles	Health Professionals Follow-up 47,723 men Age 40–75 yrs @ baseline	Colon cancer/adenomas n = 203 colon cancer cases n = 586 adenoma cases	RR[f] = 0.53 (0.32, 0.88) for the most active quintile vs. least active quintile. P for Trend across quintiles = 0.03
Oliveria *et al.*, 1996 (17)	Followed to 1990 questionnaire CRF quartiles PA quartiles (< 1000 with 1000 kcal/wk increases)	ACLS 12,975 men Age 20–80 yrs @ baseline	Prostate n = 94 cases	RR[g] = 0.26 (0.10, 0.63) for the most fit quintile vs. least fit quintile. P for Trend across CRF quartiles = 0.004 P for Trend across LTPA quartiles = 0.826

CRF–cardiorespiratory fitness, LTPA–leisure time physical activity, PA–physical activity, PAI–Physical Activity Index, RR–relative risk, SD–sudden death

[a] RR adjusted for age, but additional adjustment for confounders did not alter the findings.

[b] RR adjusted for age and BMI.

[c] Results were unchanged after adjustment for BMI, serum total cholesterol, alcohol, and other potentially confounding variables.

[d] RR adjusted for age.

[e] RR adjusted for age; based on only 1 case in Alumni who were highly active (> 4000 kcals/wk) at both assessments.

[f] RR adjusted for age, BMI, history of polyp diagnosis, parental history of colorectal cancer, pack-yrs smoking, aspirin use, intake of folate, methione, alcohol, dietary fiber, red meat, and total energy.

[g] RR adjusted for age, BMI and smoking status.

Table 2.4. Recent Prospective Studies of LTPA and Non-Insulin Dependent Diabetes Mellitus (NIDDM)

Study (Ref)	Design	Cohort	NIDDM Endpoint	Major Findings
Manson *et al.*, 1991 (49)	8 yrs of follow-up 2 PA questions; Frequency of VIG EX 2 PA categories	Nurses Health Study 87,253 women Age 34–59 yrs @ baseline	Survey; physician-diagnosed n = 1303 cases	RR = 0.83[a] (0.74, 0.93) for women who reported VIG EX at least 1× week vs. those who reported no VIG EX. 56% reported no VIG EX.
Helmrich *et al.*, 1991 (47)	14 yrs of follow-up Harvard PAI Kcal/wk Deciles	Univ Penn Health Study 5,990 men Age 39–68 yrs @ baseline	Survey n = 202 cases	Inverse gradient across PA deciles with 50% drop in risk comparing the low (< 500) to high (> 3500 kcals/wk) decile RR = 0.94[b] (0.90, 0.98) for each increase in 500 kcals/wk in PAI.
Manson *et al.*, 1992 (48)	5 yrs of follow-up 2 PA questions; Frequency of VIG EX 2 PA categories	Physicians Health Study 21,271 men Age 40–84 yrs @ baseline	Survey of physicians n = 285 cases	RR = 0.71[c] (0.54, 0.94) for men who reported VIG EX at least 1× week vs. those who reported no VIG EX. 27% reported no VIG EX.
Jackson *et al.*, 1992 (16)	Ave 4.5 yrs follow-up Max TM Time (CRF) 3 PF categories	ACLS 13,636 men; 4,828 women	Survey; physician-diagnosed n = 67 male cases n = 22 female cases	RR = 4.0 (1.53, 10.4) for low vs. high fit men RR = 1.4 (0.51, 3.71) for low vs. high fit women
Burchfiel *et al.*, 1995 (46)	6 yr incidence rate Framingham PAI PA Quintiles that were a combination of quality and quantity of PA	Honolulu Heart Program 6,815 men Age 45–80 yrs @ baseline	Diabetic medication use during follow-up exam n = 391	Inverse gradient across Quintiles ($p < 0.001$) RR = 0.49[d] (0.34, 0.72) for high vs. low Quintile of PA

CRF–cardiorespiratory fitness, LTPA-Leisure time physical acticity, PA–physical activity, PAI–Physical Activity Index, RR–relative risk, VIG EX–vigorous exercise

[a] Adjusted for age, BMI, family history of NIDDM and follow-up interval

[b] Adjusted for age, BMI, history of HPT, parental history of NIDDM

[c] Adjusted for age, BMI, total cholesterol, smoking, blood pressure, history of hypertension, alcohol consumption, aspirin & beta carotene assignment

[d] Age, BMI, other CHD risk factors

Table 2.5. Recent Prospective Studies of LTPA and Stroke

Study (Ref)	Design	Cohort	Stroke Endpoint	Major Findings
Harmsen *et al.*, 1990 (52)	Mean 11.8 yrs follow-up Occupational & LTPA 4 point scale reduced to 2 groups for analysis	Swedish 9,998 men Age 47–55 yrs @ baseline	Fatal & non-fatal stroke n = 230 cases	No association for combined and type specific stroke.
Lindsted *et al.*, 1991 (8)	26 yrs follow-up Single multiple choice question (4 possible responses) 3 PA categories	Seventh Day Adventist 9,484 men Age > 30 yrs @ baseline	Fatal cerebrovascular disease n = 410 cases	RR[a] = 0.78 (0.61, 1.00) and 0.94 (0.65, 1.36) for the moderate and high activity groups compared to the low active group.
Wannamethee *et al.*, 1992 (54)	9.5 yrs follow-up Unique PAI 6 PA Categories	British Regional Heart Study 7,735 men Age 40–59 yrs @ baseline	Fatal & non-fatal stroke n = 128 cases	RR[b] = 0.50 and 0.20 for moderately and vigorously active compared to inactive men (P trend = 0.008). Association remained after excluding men reporting regular vigorous sporting activity.
Abbott *et al.*, 1994 (51)	22 yrs follow-up Framingham PAI 3 PA categories Age stratified analysis	Honolulu Heart Program 7,530 men Age 45–68 yrs @ baseline Analyses at left excluding men with hypertension, diabetes & left ventricular hypertrophy	Hemorrhagic (Hem) & thromboembolic (TE) Annual exam, hospital records, death cert. n = 537 cases (373 TE; 129 Hem; 35 unknown)	Age-adjusted association between PA & Hem. stroke for older men (32.1, 37.6 & 10.1 incidence rates × 1000) (P trend = 0.001). In Nonsmokers: RR = 2.8[c] (1.2, 6.7) Least vs. Most; RR = 2.4 (1.0, 5.7) Middle vs. Most for TE stroke. RR[c] = 3.7 (1.3, 10.4) Least vs. Most; RR = 2.2 (0.8, 6.4) Middle vs. Most for Hem Stroke. No significant trends for younger men or those who smoked.
Kiely *et al.*, 1994 (53)	18 yrs follow-up Framingham PAI PA tertiles from exam 11–12.	Framingham 1,228 men; 1,676 women in 2nd analysis (mean age = 63 yrs)	Biennial exam diagnoses n = 107 male cases; n = 127 female cases	RR[d] = 0.41 (0.24, 0.69) and 0.53 (0.34, 0.84) for middle and high PA tertiles relative to the low PA tertile for men. No significant associations in women in multivariate model.

HTN–Hypertension, LTPA–leisure time physical activity, LVH–Left ventricular hypertrophy, PA–Physical activity, PAI–Physical Activity Index, RR–Relative risk

[a] Adjusted for age, smoking, education, medical illness, BMI, marital status and dietary patterns.

[b] Adjusted for age, CHD risk factors, heavy drinking and pre-existing Ischemic Heart Disease or stroke.

[c] Adjusted for age, Systolic Blood Pressure and Total Cholesterol, alcohol intake, serum glucose, serum uric acid, and hematocrit.

[d] Age, BMI, other CHD risk factors.

studies should reassess the relationship between physical activity and stroke risk in women, as well as further define the relationship within subtypes of stroke (e.g., hemorrhagic versus thromboembolic).

CURRENT PHYSICAL ACTIVITY RECOMMENDATIONS

The 5th edition of the American College of Sports Medicine's (ACSMs) *Guidelines for Exercise Testing and Prescription* and the 1990 ACSM Position Stand on the quality and quantity of exercise are well accepted as primary sources of recommendations for exercise training programs to develop and maintain physical fitness (55, 56). The scientific basis for these exercise recommendations is well developed and reviewed extensively in the ACSM Position Stand (56). It has been estimated that approximately 250,000 deaths per year can be attributed to sedentary living habits and that only 22% of adults are sufficiently active to derive the health benefits associated with participation in regular physical activity (3, 57, 58).

Based on the high prevalence of sedentary living habits and the numerous observational studies showing reductions in chronic disease associated with increased LTPA/CRF, the Centers for Disease Control and Prevention (CDC) and the ACSM developed new physical activity recommendations for adults that are intended to complement the exercise prescription guidelines from the ACSM (55, 56). The essence of the new recommendations is captured in the following excerpt from the report:

> *"Every US adult should accumulate 30 minutes or more of moderate-intensity physical activity on most, preferably all, days of the week. This recommendation emphasizes the benefits of moderate-intensity physical activity and of physical activity that can be accumulated in relatively short bouts. Adults who engage in moderate-intensity–i.e., enough to expend approximately 200 calories per day–can expect many of the health benefits, described herein" (2).*

A discussion of the above recommendations must begin by reviewing the operational definitions for several important terms found within the statements (59). First, the term **physical activity** refers to "any bodily movement produced by skeletal muscles that results in energy expenditure." Whereas, **exercise** is considered a subclass of physical activity defined as "planned, structured, and repetitive bodily movement done to improve or maintain one or more components of physical fitness." Considering the above definitions, the recent recommendations from the CDC/ACSM should be examined in light of the scientific evidence related to physical activity and risk for chronic disease presented earlier in this chapter.

The recent CDC/ACSM physical activity recommendations represent a paradigm shift from the more traditional exercise prescription model to a model aimed at increasing general physical activity patterns. The new recommendations have several unique aspects related to the new emphasis on moderate intensity and accumulated bouts of physical activity. These issues will be explored in the following section.

Intensity of Physical Activity

One of the major features of the CDC/ACSM physical activity recommendations is the new emphasis on participating in activities that are of **moderate** intensity (e.g., 3 to 6 METS). The recommendations equate the 3 to 6 MET intensity range with walking at 3 to 4 mph. Light activities are described as requiring >3 METS. Heavy or vigorous activities are those requiring >6 METS. Surprisingly, there are few published standards for placing level of activity into categories (60, 61). However, as indicated in Table 2.6, the use of **moderate** intensity has been assigned to a wide range of intensities.

The observational studies reviewed earlier in the chapter are also not consistent in their use of the term intensity. Some studies used the term **moderate** physical activity when referring to the middle of a distribution of quantity of activity (i.e., kcal/week), where others used the term **moderate** in the context of intensity (e.g., light, moderate or vigorous intensity). Based on the measure of LTPA used within a study, many were unable to distinguish between moderate **intensity** and moderate

Table 2.6. Comparison of Physical Activity Intensity Classification Schemes

Reference	Classification	Intensity	
Durnin and Passmore (60)	moderate	Men	~ 4.0–5.9 METs
		Women	~ 2.8–4.3 METs
Bouchard *et al.* (61)	moderate	Young	< 9.0 METs
		Middle-aged	< 7.0 METs
		Old	< 5.0 METs
		Very old	< 2.8 METs
Taylor *et al.* (64)	heavy	> 50% $\dot{V}O_{2max}$	
Paffenbarger *et al.* (36)	light	5 kcal/min	
	mixed	7.5 kcal/min	
	vigorous	10 kcal/min	
Leon *et al.* (35)	moderate	4.5–5.5 kcal/min	
Paffenbarger *et al.* (6) and Helmrich *et al.* (47)	moderately vigorous	≥ 4.5 METs	
Kohl *et al.* (65)	moderate	4 METs	
Morris *et al.* (33)	vigorous	> 7.5 kcal/min or > 65% $\dot{V}O_{2max}$	
Lee *et al.* (26)	non-vigorous (light-moderate)	< 6 METs	
	vigorous	≥ 6 METs	

METs–metabolic equivalents.

amounts of LTPA. Many of the studies that focused more on moderate **amounts** (a middle group within the analysis) showed a lower risk (for the study endpoint) in the intermediate group. However, in those studies that provided a clear analysis of the intensity question, most reported that vigorous LTPA was more protective against the chronic disease endpoint or was associated with lower mortality risk (36, 37, 47).

Another concern about using fixed MET ranges is the issue of the **relative** exercise intensity. A "moderate" range can be quite broad given the large range of functional capacity across genders and age groups. For example, in one study, a 3 MET activity spanned a relative intensity range of 29% to 50% for men and women ages 20 to 79 years in the lowest quintile of physical fitness and a 6 MET activity spanned 57% to 102% (56). This suggests that some adults could actually be exercising **vigorously** (defined as >60% of $\dot{V}O_{2max}$) rather than **moderately** in an attempt to be active (55).

Accumulation of Physical Activity

Another major feature of the physical activity recommendations from the CDC/ACSM is the value of discontinuous physical activities. The CDC/ACSM statement suggests that intermittent physical activity is an appropriate means to attain the recommended quantity of daily activity. Support for the beneficial effects of intermittent physical activity comes from the body of studies reviewed earlier in the chapter. It is likely that many of these studies used physical activity assessment instruments that probably captured a considerable amount of intermittent physical activity for the study participants (4, 5, 9, 10, 26, 34, 42–47, 51, 53, 54). However, most of the studies analyzed a given amount of total physical activity (kcal/week), and thus, could not directly contrast the health benefits of intermittent versus continuous physical activity. The CDC/ACSM statement also cited two experimental studies that support the benefit of intermittent exercise (46, 62). However, whether the results from these studies which employed intermittent **vigorous** exercise bouts (e.g., running) support the notion of health benefits associated with accumulated bouts of **moderate** intensity physical activity is debatable.

The authors of the CDC/ACSM conclude that the **amount** of activity (kilocalories expended) is more important than the manner in which the activity is performed and recommend the accumulation of approximately 200 kcal/day of moderate physical activity on a daily basis (2). The support for this caloric expenditure goal is derived from a number of the epidemiological studies that suggest 1500 kcal/week as the threshold level for benefit. Among the common activities that are recommended to obtain this goal are brisk walking (3 to 4 mph), cycling for pleasure or transportation (≤10 mph), swimming (moderate effort), conditioning exercises (general calisthenics), racket sports, table tennis, golf (pulling cart or carrying clubs), fishing (standing, casting), canoeing leisurely (2.0 to 3.9 mph), mowing lawn (power mower), and home repair (painting).

A question worthy of consideration is how many minutes of this level of activity would be required to achieve the 200 kcal/day goal? The CDC/ACSM statement provides a conversion factor estimate of 4 to 7 kcal/min for the 3 to 6 MET intensity range. Using the midpoint of this range would suggest that 36.5 minutes (200 kcal/5.5 kcal/min) of this level of activity would be required 7 days a week or 42.5 minutes per day would be required if activity was performed 6 days per week. However, the least fit individuals are more likely to be at the lower end of this range (3 METS or 4 kcal/min) and thus would require 50 minutes a day if they were active every day or 58.5 minutes per day if they were active 6 days per week. Although it is beyond the scope of this chapter to discuss behavioral issues, it warrants consideration as to how likely it is that individuals can incorporate 45 to 60 minutes per day of activity into their lifestyle when the most common barrier to participation in physical activity is lack of time (63).

Finally, the authors of the CDC/ACSM report suggest that the expected health benefits derived by increasing physical activity to the recommended level are likely to be greatest for the most sedentary individuals (this concept is presented in Figure 2.1 of the report). It should be emphasized that the dose-response curve presented in the figure is theoretical. The dose-response curve might also be interpreted to suggest that the **majority** of health benefits associated with regular physical activity (≥50%) are available to sedentary individuals who increase their habitual physical activity to the level recommended within the report (30 minutes of moderate activity on most days of the week). However, whether this amount of benefit is truly available for those who invest in mainly moderate intensity activity is not entirely clear based on the varying results among the recent studies regarding the optimal quality and/or quantity of physical activity. The need to define the optimal dose of physical activity (both quality and quantity) remains.

SUMMARY

It is well established that sedentary lifestyle or low cardiorespiratory fitness independently increases morbidity and mortality from several of the most prevalent chronic diseases. Based on the available evidence, it may also be concluded that there is an inverse dose-response gradient of risk across categories of either LTPA or cardiorespiratory fitness. The physical activity gradient, and perhaps the CRF gradient, in most of the studies is the result of a combination of varying levels of both quality and quantity of habitual physical activity. Thus, it is not possible at the present time to definitively describe the dose-response association of physical activity intensity to disease risk and it may well be that there is no single optimal dose of physical activity which yields protection from each of the chronic diseases reviewed within the chapter.

References

1. American Heart Association. Statement on Exercise. Benefits and recommendations for physical activity programs for all Americans. *Circulation* 86:340–344, 1992.
2. Pate RR, Pratt M, Blair SN, Haskell WL, Macera CA, Bouchard C, Buchner D, Ettinger W, Heath GW, King AC. Physical activity and public health: a recommendation from the Centers for Disease Control and Prevention and the American College of Sports Medicine. *JAMA* 273:402–407, 1995.
3. Public Health Service, U.S.Department of Health & Human Services. Healthy People 2000: National Health Promotion & Disease Prevention Objectives. *U.S. Government Printing Office, Washington D.C.* DHHS Publication No. (PHS) 91-50212, 1991.
4. Lee I-M, Paffenbarger RS, Hsieh CC. Physical activity and risk of developing colorectal cancer among college alumni. *J Natl Cancer Inst* 83:1324–1329, 1991.
5. Lee I-M, Paffenbarger RS, Hsieh CC. Physical activity and risk of prostatic cancer among college alumni. *Am J Epidemiol* 135:169–179, 1992.
6. Paffenbarger RS, Hyde RT, Wing AL, Lee IM, Jung DL, Kampert JB. The association of changes in physical-activity level and other lifestyle characteristics with mortality among men. *N Engl J Med* 328:538–545, 1993.
7. Paffenbarger RS, Kampert JB, Lee IM, Hyde RT, Leung RW, Wing AL. Changes in physical activity and other lifeway patterns influencing longevity. *Med Sci Sports Exerc* 26:857–865, 1994.
8. Lindsted KD, Tonstad S, Kuzma JW. Self-report of physical activity and patterns of mortality in Seventh-Day Adventist men. *J Clin Epidemiol* 44:355–364, 1991.
9. Lakka TA, Venalainen JM, Rauramaa R, Salonen R, Tuomilehto J, Salonen JT. Relation of leisure-time physical activity and cardiorespiratory fitness to the risk of acute myocardial infarction. *N Engl J Med* 330:1549–1554, 1994.
10. Leon AS, Connett J. Physical activity and 10.5 year mortality in the Multiple Risk Factor Intervention Trial (MRFIT). *Int J Epidemiol* 20:690–697, 1991.
11. Arraiz GA, Wigle DT, Mao Y. Risk assessment of physical activity and physical fitness in the Canadian Health Survey Mortality Follow-up Study. *J Clin Epidemiol* 45:419–428, 1992.
12. Hein HO, Suadicani P, Gyntelberg F. Physical fitness or physical activity as a predictor of ischaemic heart disease? A 17-year follow-up in the Copenhagen Male Study. *J Intern Med* 232:471–479, 1992.
13. Slattery ML, Jacobs DR. Physical fitness and cardiovascular disease mortality: The US Railroad Study. *Am J Epidemiol* 127:571–580, 1988.
14. Blair SN, Kohl HW, Barlow CE, Paffenbarger RS, Gibbons LW, Macera CA. Changes in physical fitness and all-cause mortality: a prospective study of healthy and unhealthy men. *JAMA* 273:1093–1098, 1995.
15. Blair SN, Kohl HW, Paffenbarger RS, Clark DG, Cooper KH, Gibbons LW. Physical fitness and all-cause mortality: a prospective study of healthy men and women. *JAMA* 262:2395–2401, 1989.
16. Jackson S, Barlow C, Brill P, Blair S. The association between physical fitness and non-insulin dependent diabetes in men and women. *Med Sci Sports Exerc* 24:S61, 1992.
17. Oliveria SA, Kohl HW, Trichopoulos D, Blair SN. The association between cardiorespiratory fitness and prostate cancer. *Med Sci Sports Exerc* 28:97–104, 1996.
18. Sandvik L, Erikssen J, Thaulow E, Erikssen G, Mundal R, Rodahl K. Physical fitness as a predictor of mortality among healthy, middle-aged Norwegian men. *N Engl J Med* 328:533–537, 1993.
19. Bouchard C, Dionne FT, Simoneau J, Boulay MR. Genetics of aerobic and anaerobic performances. *Exer Sport Sci Rev* 1992:27–58.
20. Berlin JA, Colditz A. A meta-analysis of physical activity in the prevention of coronary heart disease. *Am J Epidemiol* 132:612–627, 1990.
21. Powell KE, Thompson PD, Caspersen CJ, Kendrick JS. Physical activity and the incidence of coronary heart disease. *Ann Rev Public Health* 8:253–287, 1987.
22. Blair SN. Physical activity, fitness, and coronary heart disease. In: Bouchard C, Shepard RJ, Stephens T, eds. *Physical Activity, Fitness, and Health.* Champaign, IL: Human Kinetics Publishers, 1994:579–590.
23. Haskell WL. Health consequences of physical activity: understanding and challenges regarding dose-response. *Med Sci Sports Exerc* 26:649–660, 1994.
24. Morris JN. Exercise in the prevention of coronary heart disease: today's best buy in public health. *Med Sci Sports Exerc* 26:807–814, 1994.
25. Whaley MH, Blair SN. Physical activity, physical fitness and coronary heart disease. *J Cardiovasc Risk* 2:289–295, 1995.
26. Lee IM, Hsieh CC, Paffenbarger RS. Exercise intensity and longevity in men: the Harvard Alumni Health Study. *JAMA* 273:1179–1184, 1995.
27. Rodriguez BL, Curb JD, Burchfiel CM, Abbott RD, Petrovitch H, Masaki K, Chiu D. Physical activity and 23-year incidence of coronary heart disease morbidity and mortality among middle-aged men. *Circulation* 89:2540–2544, 1994.
28. Shaper AG, Wannamethee G, Walker M. Physical activity, hypertension and risk of heart attack in men without evidence of ischaemic heart disease. *J Hum Hypertens* 8:3–10, 1994.
29. Sherman SE, D'Agostino RB, Cobb JL, Kannel WB. Physical activity and mortality in women in the Framingham Heart Study. *Am Health J* 128:879–884, 1994.
30. Donahue RP, Abbott RD, Reed DM, Yano K. Physical activity and coronary heart disease in middle-aged and elderly men: The Honolulu Heart Program. *Am J Public Health* 78:683–885, 1988.
31. Kannel WB, Sorlie P. Some health benefits of physical activity: The Framingham Study. *Arch Intern Med* 139:857–861, 1979.
32. Blair SN, Kohl HW, Barlow CE. Physical activity, physical fitness, and mortality in women: Do women need to be active? *J Am Coll Nutr* 12:368–371, 1993.

33. Morris JN, Clayton DG, Everitt MG, Semmence AM, Burgess EH. Exercise in leisure time: coronary attack and death rates. *Br Heart J* 63:325–334, 1990.
34. Shaper AG, Wannamethee G. Physical activity and ischaemic heart disease in middle-aged British men. *Br Heart J* 66:384–394, 1991.
35. Leon AS, Connett J, Jacobs DR, Rauramaa R. Leisure-time physical activity levels and risk of coronary heart disease and death. The Multiple Risk Factor Intervention Trial. *JAMA* 258:2388–2395, 1987.
36. Paffenbarger RS, Hyde RT, Wing AL, Hsieh CC. Physical activity, all-cause mortality, and longevity of college alumni. *N Engl J Med* 314:605–613, 1986.
37. Ekelund LG, Haskell WL, Johnson JL, Whaley FS, Criqui MH. Physical fitness as a predictor of cardiovascular mortality in asymptomatic North American men: The Lipid Research Clinics Mortality Follow-up Study. *N Engl J Med* 319:1379–1384, 1988.
38. Kohl HW, LaPorte RE, Blair SN. Physical activity and cancer: an epidemiological perspective. *Sports Med* 6:222–237, 1988.
39. Lee IM. Physical activity, Fitness and Cancer In: Bouchard C, Shepard RJ, and Stephens T, eds. *Physical activity, fitness, and health.* Champaign, IL: Human Kinetics, 1994:814–831.
40. Shepard RJ. Exercise in the prevention and treatment of cancer: an update. *Sports Med* 15:258–280, 1993.
41. Albanes D, Blair A, Taylor PR. Physical activity and risk of cancer in the NHANES I population. *Am J Public Health* 79: 744–750, 1989.
42. Ballard-Barbash B, Schatzkin A, Albanes D, Schiffman MH, Kreger BE, Kannal WB, Anderson KM, Helsel WE. Physical activity and risk of large bowel cancer in the Framingham Study. *Cancer Res* 50:3610–3613, 1990.
43. Dorgan JF, Brown C, Barrett M, Splansky GL, Kreger BE, D'Agostino RB, et al. Physical activity and risk of breast cancer in the Framingham Heart Study. *Am J Epidemiol* 139:662–669, 1994.
44. Giovannucci E, Ascherio A, Rimm EB, Colditz GA, Stampfer MJ, Willett WC. Physical activity, obesity, and risk for colon cancer and adenoma in men. *Ann Intern Med* 122: 327–334, 1995.
45. Severson RK, Nomura AMY, Grove JS, Stemmermann GN. A prospective analysis of physical activity and cancer. *Am J Epidemiol* 130:522–529, 1989.
46. Burchfiel CM, Sharp DS, Curb JD, Rodriguez BL, Hwang L, Marcus EB, Yano K. Physical activity and incidence of diabetes: the Honolulu Heart Program. *Am J Epidemiol* 141: 360–368, 1995.
47. Helmrich SP, Ragland DR, Leung RW, Paffenbarger RS. Physical activity and reduced occurrence of non-insulin-dependent diabetes mellitus. *N Engl J Med* 325:147–152, 1991.
48. Manson JE, Nathan DM, Krolewski AS, Stampfer MJ, Willett WC, Hennekens CH. A prospective study of exercise and incidence of diabetes among US male physicians. *JAMA* 268:63–67, 1992.
49. Manson JE, Rimm EB, Stampfer MJ, Colditz GA, Willett WC, Krolewski AS, Rosner, B, Hennekens CH, Speizer FE. Physical activity and incidence of non-insulin-dependent diabetes mellitus in women. *Lancet* 338:774–778, 1991.
50. Kohl HW, McKenzie JD. Physical activity, fitness and stroke. In: Bouchard C, Shepard RJ, Stephens T, eds. *Physical activity, fitness, and health.* Champaign, IL: Human Kinetics, 1994:609–621.
51. Abbott RD, Rodriquez BL, Burchfiel CM, Curb JD. Physical activity in older middle-aged men and reduced risk of stroke: the Honolulu Heart Program. *Am J Epidemiol* 139: 881–893, 1994.
52. Harmsen P, Rosengren A, Tsipogianni A, Wilhelmsen L. Risk factors and stroke in middle-aged men in Goteborg, Sweden. *Stroke* 21:223–229, 1990.
53. Kiely DK, Wolf PA, Cupples LA, Beiser AS, Kannel WB. Physical activity and stroke risk: The Framingham Study. *Am J Epidemiol* 140:608–620, 1994.
54. Wannamethee G, Shaper AG. Physical activity and stroke in British middle-aged men. *Br Med J* 304:597–601, 1992.
55. American College of Sports Medicine. *Guidelines for Exercise Testing and Prescription.* 5th ed. Baltimore: Williams & Wilkins, 1995:373.
56. American College of Sports Medicine. The recommended quantity and quality of exercise for developing and maintaining cardiorespiratory and muscular fitness in healthy adults. *Med Sci Sports Exerc* 22:265–274, 1990.
57. Hahn RA, Teutsch SM, Rothenberg RB, Marks JS. Excess deaths from nine chronic diseases in the United States. *JAMA* 264:2654–2659, 1986.
58. McGinnis JM, Forge WH. Actual causes of death in the United States. *JAMA* 270:2207–2212, 1993.
59. Casperson CJ, Powell KE, Christenson GM. Physical activity, exercise and physical fitness. *Pub Health Rep* 100:125–131, 1985.
60. Durnin JVGA, Passmore R. *Energy, work and leisure.* London: Heinmann, 1967.
61. Bouchard C, Shepard RJ. Physical activity and health: the model and key concepts In: Bouchard C, Shepard RJ, Stephens T, eds. *Physical activity, fitness, and health.* Champaign, IL: Human Kinetics, 1994:77–88.
62. Ebisu T. Splitting the distance of endurance running: on cardiovascular endurance and blood lipids. *Japan J Phys Ed* 30:37–43, 1985.
63. Martin JE, Dubbert PM. Exercise applications and promotion in behavioral medicine. *J Consult Clin Psych* 50:1004–1017, 1982.
64. Taylor HL, Jacobs DR, Schucker B, Knudsen J, Leon AS, Debacker G. A questionnaire for the assessment of leisure time physical activities. *J Chron Dis* 31:741–755, 1978.
65. Kohl HW, Blair SN, Paffenbarger RS, Macera CA, Kronefeld JJ. A mail survey of physical activity habits as related to measured physical fitness. *Am J Epidemiol* 127:1228–1238, 1988.

83 208, 209, 212 199, 200, 202, 203, 204, 206

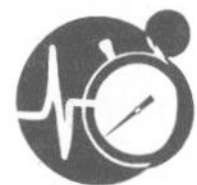

CHAPTER 3

Diet and Nutrition

Suzanne Nelson Steen and Gayle Butterfield

An adequate and balanced diet is essential for optimal functioning and performance. What we eat influences our work, play, psychological status, and health. In industrialized societies, with the abundance of food available, nutrient deficiencies are rare if individuals select a well-balanced diet, but overconsumption is linked to disease. The excessive consumption of calories and fat has been linked to cardiovascular disease, certain forms of cancer, obesity, hypertension and diabetes mellitus.

BASIC FOODS AND FUNCTIONS

More than 50 nutrients are essential (required for life). These nutrients are divided into six classes: fat, carbohydrate, protein, vitamins, minerals, and water. This section discusses each basic nutrient, including function and food sources. Energy (measured in calories) is the potential to do work and is a "nutrient" of concern. The major food components, carbohydrate, fat and protein, each provides energy at a rate of 4, 9, and 4 kcal/gm, respectively. Alcohol, which is metabolized similarly to fat, is thought to contribute 7 kcal/gm. One pound of fat contributes approximately 3,500 kcal.

Fats and Cholesterol

Fat is stored in large quantities in adipose tissue and represents a potential energy store. It also insulates and protects vital organs. In addition to providing energy, dietary fat transports fat-soluble vitamins A, D, E, and K.

The primary fats in food (and in the body) are triglycerides and cholesterol. Triglycerides are composed of three fatty acids (a chain of carbons with a carboxylic acid group on the end) and a glycerol molecule. Fatty acids are categorized as either saturated or unsaturated (including polyunsaturated and mono-unsaturated), depending upon chemical structure.

Saturated fatty acids come primarily from animal products (exceptions are palm oil, coconut oil and cocoa butter) and form triglycerides that are solid at room temperature. Unsaturated fatty acids form triglycerides, liquid at room temperature, and are found in vegetable oils such as soy, sunflower, corn and olive oils.

Dietary fat provides essential fatty acids (EFAs), linoleic and linolenic acids. Arachidonic acid becomes essential if there is insufficient linoleic acid in the diet, from which it is synthesized. These EFAs are required for growth, healthy skin, and for producing elements of the immune system. A deficiency is characterized by scaly dermatitis, hair loss, and poor wound healing. Although the body requires only small amounts of EFA (~ 2% to 3% of total energy), obtaining sufficient amounts may require consuming a diet containing at least 10% of total energy from fat because the proportion of fatty acids in the diet is small (1).

Cholesterol is a waxy, fat-like substance found in foods of animal origin. It is found in the membranes of all cells and performs a number of essential anatomical and physiological functions. It is not found in plants or plant products. The liver produces sufficient amounts of cholesterol to meet requirements, therefore, dietary consumption is unnecessary. Although monitoring cholesterol intake is important, dietary saturated fats have the greatest impact on total blood cholesterol, a risk factor for coronary artery disease (CAD) (2). Cholesterol is not cleared properly from the blood if saturated fat is overconsumed (3). Blood cholesterol is also affected by heredity (4). The National Cholesterol Education Program considers a blood cholesterol level of less than 200 mg/dl desirable, 200 to 239 mg/dl is considered borderline high, and levels of 240 mg/dl or greater are considered high and are associated with increased risk of CAD (5).

Lipoproteins, produced by the liver and intestinal mucosa, transport insoluble fat-like substances, such as cholesterol and triglycerides, through the blood. Very low-density lipoproteins (VLDL) are a major carrier of triglycerides. Low-density lipoproteins (LDL) are principally composed of cholesterol. The cholesterol transported by LDL may be deposited in the arterial walls, contributing to atherosclerosis. The smallest group of lipoproteins, the high-density lipoproteins (HDLs), appear to be protective by carrying cholesterol away from the arterial walls to the liver for catabolism and excretion and by interfering with binding of LDL to cell membranes (6). Therefore, high levels of HDL (> 45 mg/dl for men, > 55 mg/dl for women), low levels of LDL (< 130 mg/dl), low total cholesterol (< 200 mg/dl), and low total cholesterol/HDL cholesterol ratio (< 4:9 for men, < 4:4 for women), carry the lowest risk of CAD (5). The impact of the type of fat consumed (saturated or unsaturated) on blood lipid levels occurs through changes in the metabolism of these lipoproteins. Exercise has been shown to favorably increase HDL levels (7).

Carbohydrates and Fiber

There are two types of carbohydrate, simple and complex. Simple carbohydrates (sugars) include glucose, fructose, sucrose (table sugar), and lactose (milk sugar) are found in foods such as candy, soft drinks, milk and fruits. Complex carbohydrates (starches) are composed of chains of simple sugars and are found in foods such as pasta, bread, cereal, rice, fruits, and vegetables. These food sources also contain B-vitamins, minerals, fiber, and protein, which contribute to a balanced diet.

Dietary fiber is the non-digestible portion of carbohydrate. It is found only in plant foods and may play a role in the prevention and treatment of diabetes, cardiovascular disease, and cancer. It may also benefit those on weight loss regimens by creating a feeling of fullness without a high intake of energy.

There are two types of fiber: soluble and insoluble. Soluble fiber dissolves in water, and is found in citrus fruits, apples, grains, legumes and peas. Soluble fiber has been linked to decreasing cholesterol and offering protection against CAD. Insoluble fiber absorbs water in the large intestine and produces soft stools that pass quickly through the intestinal tract. It is theorized that insoluble fiber protects against colon cancer by reducing the time that potential carcinogens are in contact with the cells of the intestinal tract (8). Insoluble fiber is contained in whole-grain products and vegetables. Recommended fiber intake is 25 to 35 g/day, compared with the current average intake of 10 to 20 g/day (9). Fiber intake can be increased by substituting whole foods for processed foods (Table 3.1).

Protein

Proteins are composed of amino acids and are found in both plant and animal products. Eight of the 20 amino acids (9/20 in children) found in proteins are essential; that is, they cannot be synthesized in adequate amounts by the body and must be supplied in the diet. Proteins from animal sources generally contain the essential amino acids in sufficient amounts for protein synthesis and are considered to be high quality. Proteins from plant sources are lower quality because one or more of essential amino acids may be present in small amounts. Vegetarians must consume a variety of plant proteins to ensure adequate consumption of all essential amino acids to build complete proteins.

Table 3.1. Fiber in Processed and Whole Foods[a]

INSTEAD OF	USE
Apple juice (0.4 g)	Fresh apple (3.5 g)
Orange juice (0.5 g)	Fresh orange (2.6 g)
Polished rice (0.2 g)	Brown rice (1 g)
Pasta (1.1 g)	Whole wheat pasta (4 g)
White bread (0.4 g)	Whole wheat bread (1.4 g)
Potato, no skin (1.4 g)	Potato with skin (2.5 g)

[a] From United States Department of Agriculture. Composition of foods. In: *Agricultural handbook, No. 8-8*, Revised July 1982.

Vitamins

Vitamins are essential for life and cannot be manufactured by the body. They are therefore required in the diet, but in small amounts. The **fat-soluble** vitamins, A, D, E, and K, are stored in fatty tissues and need not be supplied in the diet on a daily basis. On the other hand, they are also potentially toxic (especially vitamins A and D) because they are stored and can accumulate. **Water-soluble** vitamins are not stored and regular consumption is important. **Water-soluble** vitamins include vitamin C, thiamin, riboflavin, niacin, vitamin B_6, folacin, vitamin B_{12}, biotin, and pantothenic acid.

Vitamins have many functions, including facilitating metabolic reactions in which energy is released (thiamin, riboflavin, niacin, vitamin B_6, biotin, pantothenic acid). Others are required for blood coagulation (vitamin K), visual processes (vitamin A), and cellular protection (antioxidants, vitamin E and vitamin C). Table 3.2 summarizes the primary functions, dietary sources, and gives adult recommendations for vitamins.

Vitamin supplementation has not been shown to prevent or cure illness (including the common cold) except when specific deficiencies exist. Some vitamins assist energy metabolism, but do not **provide** energy. With the exception of synthetic vitamin B_6, which is less active due to synthesis of inactive forms, there are no essential differences between a synthetic vitamin and a "natural" vitamin (10). Complications have been reported from large doses of vitamin C, niacin, and vitamin B_6 (10). Vitamin supplements should not be used to compensate for poor dietary habits. However supplementation is advisable during certain phases of the life cycle, such as pregnancy and lactation or when food intake is erratic (10).

Minerals

Although minerals are found in minute amounts in tissue, they are essential to life. Fifteen essential minerals

Table 3.2. Function, Source and Recommended Dietary Allowances (RDA) for Vitamins[a]

VITAMIN	MAIN FUNCTION	GOOD SOURCES	RDA (ADULT)
A	Maintenance of skin, bone, growth, vision, and teeth	Eggs, cheese, margarine, milk, carrots, broccoli, squash, and spinach	m: 1000 μg f: 800 μg
D	Bone growth and maintenance of bones	Milk, egg yolk, tuna, and salmon (sunlight)	m: 5 μg f: 5 μg
E	Antioxidant	Vegetable oils, whole-grain cereal, bread, dried beans, & green leafy vegetables	m: 10 mg f: 8 mg
K	Blood clotting	Cabbage, green leafy vegetables, milk	m: 80 μg f: 65 μg
Thiamine (B1)	Energy-releasing reactions	Pork, ham, oysters, breads, cereals, pasta, green peas	m: 1.5 mg f: 1.1 mg
Riboflavin (B2)	Energy-releasing reactions	Milk, meat, cereals, pasta, mushrooms, dark green vegetables	m: 1.7 mg f: 1.3 mg
Niacin	Energy-releasing reactions	Poultry, meat, tuna, cereal, pasta, bread, nuts, legumes	m: 19 mg f: 15 mg
Pyridoxine (B6)	Metabolism of fats & proteins & formation of red blood cells	Cereals, bread, spinach, avocados, green beans, bananas	m: 2.0 mg f: 1.6 mg
Cobalamin (B12)	Formation of red blood cells & functioning of nervous system	Meat, fish, eggs, milk	m: 2.0 μg f: 2.0 μg
Folacin	Assists in forming proteins & in formation of red blood cells	Dark green leafy vegetables, wheat germ, oranges, bananas	m: 200 μg f: 180 μg
Pantothenic acid	Metabolism of proteins, CHO, & fats, formation of hormones	Bread, cereals, nuts, eggs & dark green vegetables	ESADDI = 7–9 mg
Biotin	Formation of fatty acids & energy-releasing reactions	Egg yolk, leafy green vegetables,	ESADDI = 30–100 μg
C	Maintenance of bones, teeth, blood vessels, & collagen: antioxidant	Citrus fruits, tomatoes, strawberries, melons, green peppers, potatoes	m: 60 mg f: 60 mg

m–male; f–female; ESADDI–Estimated Safe and Adequate Daily Dietary Intake

[a] With permission from the National Resource Council. *Recommended Dietary Allowances,* 10th ed. Washington DC: National Academy of Sciences, 1989.

have been identified, but there are specific recommended allowances for only seven (calcium, phosphorus, magnesium, iron, zinc, selenium, and iodine). The major or macrominerals include calcium, potassium, magnesium, sulfur, sodium, and chloride. The trace minerals (microminerals) are iron, iodine, copper, zinc, flourine, selenium, manganese, molybdenum, and chromium. Table 3.3 lists main functions, food sources, and adult recommendations of minerals.

Supplementation of minerals is generally not necessary. Exceptions, however include women of childbearing age, infants, young children, adolescents, and athletes who are iron-deficient. Good sources of iron include red meat, organ meats, shellfish, eggs, beans, peas, green leafy vegetables, whole and fortified grains. Iron absorption is tripled if it is consumed with vitamin C. Vegetarians should pay special attention to food sources of iron and ensure vitamin C accompanies iron intake.

Chronically low calcium intake in women may contribute to osteoporosis, a disease in which bones become porous, thin and susceptible to fracture. The average calcium intake in adult women is reported to be 550 to 600 mg/day but should be at least 800 mg/day (see Table 3.3). In women under 25 and postmenopausal women, this should be increased to 1200 mg/day (10). Non-dairy calcium sources are difficult to find (see Table 3.4). If insufficient dietary calcium is consumed, supplementation may be necessary. Many supplements are available and absorption varies widely. The best supplement supplies a high concentration of calcium, is inexpensive, and free from toxins found in dolomite and bone meal. Calcium carbonate or calcium citrate are appropriate choices.

Fluids

Water is an essential nutrient that is often neglected. It is the solvent for chemical reactions, it enables the transportation of nutrients to cells, provides a medium for excretion of waste products, and acts as a lubricant between cells; it assists in temperature regulation through evaporation of sweat from skin and by conducting heat from the core to the surface. Although an individual can live without food for up to 30 days, the absence of water limits survival to a few days. Fluid requirement is approximately 2 liters/day.

DIETARY GOALS AND RECOMMENDATIONS

Dietary Goals

Federal agencies have made a variety of recommendations for assessment of dietary habits and evaluating the need for change. The 1995 Dietary Guidelines for Americans set by the Food and Nutrition Board of the

Table 3.3. Function, Source and Recommended Dietary Allowances (RDA) for Minerals[a]

Mineral	Main Function	Good Sources	RDA (adult)
Calcium	Formation of bones, teeth, maintenance of nerve impulses, blood clotting	Cheese, sardines, dark green vegetables, vegetables, clams, milk	m: 800 mg f: 800 mg
Phosphorus	Formation of bones & teeth, acid-base balance	Milk, cheese, meat, fish, poultry, nuts, grains	m: 800 mg f: 800 mg
Magnesium	Activation of enzymes and protein synthesis	Nuts, meat, milk, whole-grain cereal, green leafy vegetables	m: 350 mg f: 280 mg
Sodium	Acid-base balance, body water balance, nerve function	Most foods	min. = 500 mg
Potassium	Acid-base balance, body water balance, nerve function	Meat, milk, many fruits, cereals, vegetables, legumes	min. = 2000 mg
Chloride	Gastric juice formation & acid-base balance	Table salt, seafood, milk, meat, eggs	
Iron	Component of hemoglobin & enzymes	Meats, legumes, eggs, grains, dark green vegetables	m: 10 mg f: 15 mg
Zinc	Component of many enzymes	Milk, shellfish, & wheat bran	m: 15 mg f: 12 mg
Iodine	Component of thyroid hormone	Fish, dairy products, vegetables, iodized salt	m: 150 mg f: 150 mg
Copper	Component of enzymes, delivers iron from storage	Shellfish, grains, cherries, legumes, poultry, oysters, nuts	ESADDI = 1.5–3 mg
Manganese	Component of enzymes, fat synthesis	Greens, blueberries, grains, legumes, fruit	ESADDI = 2–5 mg
Fluoride	Maintenance of bones and teeth	Water, seafood, rice, soybeans, spinach, onions, and lettuce	ESADDI = 1.5–4 mg
Chromium	Glucose and energy metabolism	Fats, meats, clams, cereals	ESADDI = 50–200 μg
Selenium	Functions with vitamin E antioxidant	Fish, poultry, meats, grains, milk, vegetables	m: 70 μg f: 55 μg
Molybdenum	Component of enzymes	Legumes, cereals, dark green leafy vegetables	ESADDI = 70–250 μg

m = male; f = female; ESADDI = Estimated Safe and Adequate Daily Dietary Intake

[a] With permission from the National Resource Council. *Recommended Dietary Allowances*, 10th ed. Washington DC: National Academy of Sciences, 1989.

National Research Council represent general guidelines for improving health (see Table 3.5) (11). These recommendations suggest limiting fat intake to less than 30% of total calories and saturated fat to 10%. Cholesterol intake should be limited to 300 mg/day and protein consumption should be approximately 15% of total calories. Therefore carbohydrate intake should be approximately 55% of total calories with about 15% from simple carbohydrates (preferably from natural sources) (12).

The food industry has addressed the need for reduced fat intake by producing fat substitutes that mimic the taste and feel of fat. However, as fat intake decreases and intake of these substitutes increases, the average waistline has increased, perhaps due to an increase in consumption of calories as "lite" foods. The fear that individuals compensate for reduced fat intake by eating more less-nutrient dense foods seems to be borne out.

Recommended Dietary Allowances

The National Research Council of the National Academy of Sciences has determined a Recommended Dietary Allowance (RDA) that represents the levels of essential nutrients considered to be adequate to meet the needs of most healthy people (10). RDA is applied to population groups and should not be confused with requirements for any specific individual. Because there is a margin of safety built into each RDA, they exceed the requirements of most people. Of approximately 50 known nutrients, an RDA has been established only for those nutrients where adequate data are available. A range of intake, considered safe and adequate, has been identified for those where insufficient data are available to set specific recommendations (see Tables 3.2 and 3.3).

The RDA for caloric intake is set at the mean intake of the normal weight population, and should be adjusted for activity level (10). No RDA has been established for carbohydrate and fat, since these nutrients can be synthesized and are not considered essential. The RDA for protein is based on body weight, with increased amounts required during growth, pregnancy and lactation, and in exercising populations (13). For the average person, the recommended intake is 0.8 g/kg body weight. This requirement can be met by consuming a variety of protein containing foods, such as 5 ounces of meat, fish or poultry, and a cup of milk and a serving of pasta. The RDA for some vitamins and minerals has been determined (see Tables 3.2 and 3.3).

Table 3.4. **Non-dairy Sources of Calcium**[a]

VEGETABLES	AMOUNT	CALCIUM (MG)
Collard greens, fresh, cooked	1 cup	360
Turnip greens, fresh, cooked	1 cup	250
Spinach, fresh, cooked	1 cup	240
Kale, fresh, cooked	1 cup	200
Mustard greens, fresh, cooked	1 cup	150
Dandelion greens, fresh cooked	1 cup	150
Swiss chard, fresh, cooked	1 cup	100
Broccoli, fresh or frozen, ckd	1 cup	100
Butternut squash, boiled	1/2 cup	40
Brussel sprouts	1/2 cup or 4 sprouts	30
Green or red cabbage, ckd	1/2 cup	25
Potato w/skin, baked	1 medium	20
Carrot, raw	1 medium	20
Celery, raw	1 medium stalk	20
Parsley	1 Tbs	10
NUTS AND SEEDS		
Sesame seeds, whole	1 Tbs	90
Almonds	1 oz	80
Filberts/Hazelnuts	1 oz	55
Brazil nuts	1 oz	50
Sunflower seeds	1 oz	35
Pistachios	1 oz	35
Sesame butter (tahini)	1 Tbs	65
Almond butter	1 Tbs	45
BEANS		
Tofu, firm	1/2 cup	250
White beans, cooked	1 cup	175
Navy beans, cooked	1 cup	120
Pinto beans, cooked	1 cup	85
Kidney beans, cooked	1 cup	60
Black beans, cooked	1 cup	50
Lentils, cooked	1 cup	40
FRUITS		
Figs, dried	5	135
Papaya	1 medium	70
Orange	1 medium	50
Prunes	10	40
Raisins	1/3 cup	25
Apricots, dried	1/3 cup	20
Orange juice with calcium added	1 cup	300
OTHER FOODS		
Instant Oatmeal	1 packet	150
Cream of Wheat, ckd	3/4 cup	40
Molasses, blackstrap	1 Tbs	170
Sardines, oil pack	3.75 oz	400
Mackerel, Pacific	4 oz	300
Salmon, red, with bones	4 oz	290
Anchovies, canned	1 oz	70
Clams	3 oz	80
Shrimps, canned or raw	3 oz	50
Oysters, canned	3 oz	40

[a] From United States Department of Agriculture. Composition of foods. In: *Agriculture Handbook, No. 8-8,* Revised July 1982.

Table 3.5. **The Dietary Guidelines for Americans**[a]

- Eat a variety of foods
- Balance the food you eat with physical activity. Maintain or improve your weight.
- Choose a diet with plenty of grain products, vegetables and fruits.
- Choose a diet low in fat, saturated fat and cholesterol.
- Choose a diet moderate in sugars.
- Choose a diet moderate in salt and sodium.
- If you drink alcoholic beverages, do so in moderation.

[a] From U.S. Dept. of Agriculture, U.S. Dept. of Health and Human Services. *Dietary Guidelines for Americans,* 1995.

FOOD GUIDE PYRAMID

A basic principle of nutrition is to consume a variety of foods containing a wide range of nutrients. This strategy is illustrated by the Food Guide Pyramid (Fig. 3.1) devised by the United States Department of Agriculture in which foods are classified on the basis of nutrient content (14). The base of the pyramid consists of complex carbohydrate-containing foods that should comprise the base of a balanced diet. Fruits and vegetables compose a second tier of foods, and meats and dairy products are recommended in moderate amounts. At the top of the pyramid are fats and pure sugar, which should be consumed in small amounts.

NUTRITIONAL CONSIDERATIONS FOR THE ATHLETE

Athletes should adjust their diet to meet the energy demands of their sport. Energy and nutrient requirements vary depending on weight, height, age, sex, metabolic rate, and on the type, intensity, frequency, and duration of training. At least 50% of total calories should come from carbohydrate. The remainder should be obtained from protein (10% to 15%) and fat (20% to 30%). Male athletes may consume up to 70% of calories as carbohydrate, but female athletes should be cognizant of consumption of protein and fat as well and may find it difficult to exceed 60% of energy from carbohydrate, due to a generally lower total energy intake (15).

Carbohydrate

The major source of energy for working muscles is glucose, stored as glycogen in both the muscle and the liver. Adequate glycogen stores for training are ensured by both adequate daily caloric intake and carbohydrate consumption (16). Fasting or crash dieting, a very high-protein diet (30% of total calories), or limiting or omitting high-carbohydrate foods can reduce carbohydrate stores to inadequate levels (16). Symptoms of carbohydrate underconsumption include fatigue, weakness, inability to maintain normal exercise intensity and deterioration of performance.

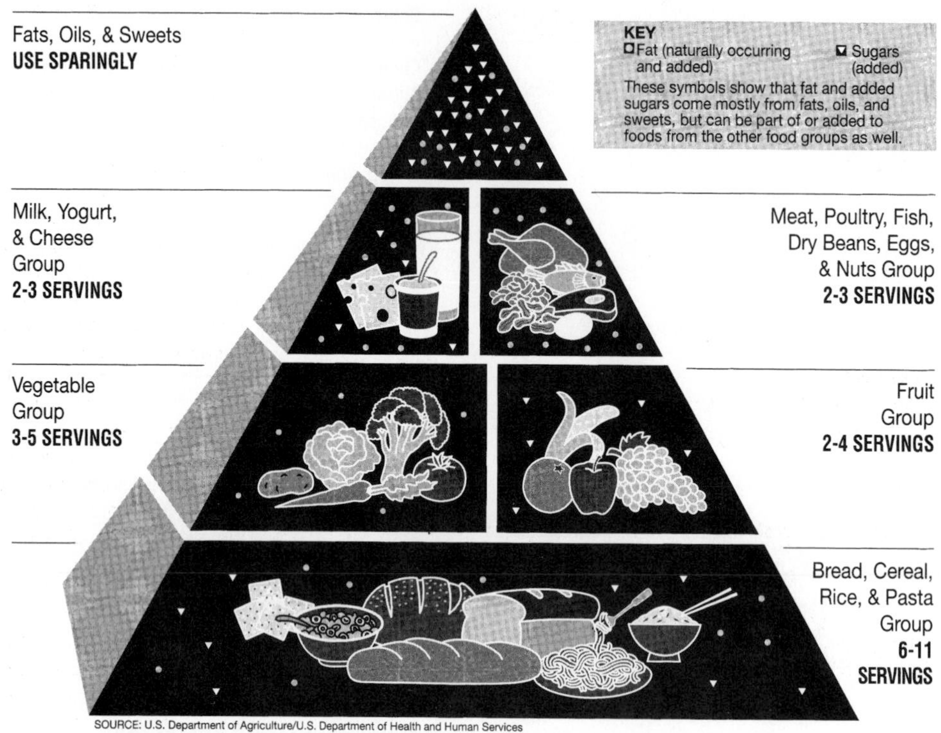

Figure 3.1. Food guide pyramid.

The amount of carbohydrate required depends on body mass. Generally, male athletes should eat 6 to 8 g/kg of carbohydrates. Consuming more than 600 grams of carbohydrate per day does not result in proportionately greater stores of muscle glycogen. Athletes requiring a lower calorie diet (e.g., females on low energy intakes) may have difficulty attaining this level if protein and fat intake are adequate; intakes of 4 to 6 g/kg must suffice for these individuals (15).

Skeletal muscle stores glycogen at the highest rate during the first 2 hours after exercise (17). Practically, an athlete should consume 100 g of carbohydrate (400 kcal) within 15 to 30 minutes after exercise, followed by an additional 100 g every 2 to 4 hours (18). Those with smaller body mass should decrease carbohydrate intake proportionately. See Table 3.6 for foods high in carbohydrate.

A pre-event meal may be instrumental in maintaining blood glucose levels during exercise (19). Such a meal may be consumed 1 to 4 hours before competition and should include readily digestible foods and fluids that enter the blood slowly and are familiar. These require-

Table 3.6. Carbohydrate-rich Foods[a]

Food Group	Food	Grams of Carbohydrate
Milk Group		
	Chocolate milkshake (10 oz)	58
	Blueberry yogurt (1 cup)	42
	Ice milk (1/2 cup)	14
	Low-fat milk	12
Protein Group		
	Pinto beans (1/2 cup)	23
	Refried beans (1/2 cup)	23
	Meatloaf (3 oz)	13
Fruit & Vegetable Group		
	Baked potato	51
	Cranberry juice cocktail (1 cup)	37
	Raisins (1/4 cup)	29
	Grapes (1 cup)	28
	Banana	27
	Orange juice (1 cup)	26
	Applesauce (1/2 cup)	25
	Pear	25
	French Fries (10)	20
	Corn (1/2 cup)	20
	Fruit Roll-ups (1 roll)	12
	Watermelon (1 cup)	12
Grain Group		
	Bagel	38
	Rice	28
	English muffin	28
	Corn flakes (1 oz)	24
	Raisin bran (1 oz)	21
	Hot dog bun	21
Commercial High Carbohydrate Drinks		
	Exceed High Carbohydrate Source (12 oz)	89
	Carboplex (12 oz)	81
	Gatorade (12 oz)	70

[a] From United States Department of Agriculture. Composition of foods. In: *Agricultural Handbook* No. 8-8, Revised July 1982.

Table 3.7. Pre-event Meals

Burrito:	1/2 cup black beans or kidney beans (cooked whole) and 1/2 cup rice (preferably long-grain and definitely not instant) in large flour tortilla
Soup and Bread:	Large bowl of split pea and barley, lentil or mixed-bean soup with a couple of pieces of mixed grain bread (soups not pureed and not instant)
Sandwich:	2 pieces of oat bran or pumpernickel bread with 1 tablespoon of peanut butter and 1 tablespoon of low-sugar or diabetic fruit preserves along with 1/4 cup of dried apricots
Pasta:	1 1/2 cups spaghetti or linguine tossed in *small* amount of olive oil or small amount of marinara sauce (sauce made without sugar), sprinkled *lightly* with parmesan
Salads:	Large sweet potato or yam along with 2 cups green salad topped only with green peas and variety of beans, such as chickpeas (garbanzo), kidney, red, lima, pinto, and black (1/2 cup total). Salad dressing should be low in sugar.
Cereals:	1/2 cup all-bran with 1 cup skim milk or low fat yogurt with an apple-oatmeal muffin (can substitute Bran Buds, Bran Chex, or Muesli for All-Bran)
Hot Cereal:	1 1/2 cups porridge with chopped apples (porridge made with whole oats—the less rolled and processed the better! Cook oats for minimal time. Does not include "instant" oatmeal)
Snack:	3 oatmeal cookies with 1 cup low-fat chocolate milk and peach, pear, or plum

ments can be met by including foods high in complex carbohydrates and low in fat and protein (20). A list of meals that meet the above qualifications is found in Table 3.7. Ingestion of high sodium, high-fiber, or gas producing foods should be avoided. Liberal intake of fluid is recommended.

Fat

Fat is a valuable metabolic fuel for muscle activity during long duration, moderate intensity endurance exercise; however, for health reasons, fat intake should not exceed 30% of daily calories (12). In addition, consumption of a high-fat diet typically decreases calories consumed from carbohydrates. Avoiding a very low fat diet is important to maintain intramuscular triglyceride stores, necessary for prolonged training (21). A balance between fat and carbohydrate intake is required to optimize performance.

Protein

Increased strength can improve performance. However, consumption of large amounts of protein does not appreciably increase muscle size or strength. The most important factors in increasing strength are adequate energy intake and strength training. Daily protein requirements vary slightly according to the type of sport (strength/power sports may have increased protein requirements), intensity of training, stage of training, and most important, energy balance. If caloric intake is sufficient, 0.8 to 1.5 g/kg protein intake is adequate (15).

Claims that amino acids have an anabolic effect, stimulate growth, and reduce body fat are unfounded (22). Although arginine and ornithine are sold as "natural steroids," and arginine and lysine are touted to promote weight loss, these and other such claims for amino acids are not based on any controlled research data.

Fluids

Water is a most important nutrient during any phase of training or competition. Water comprises approximately 60% to 70% of body weight and as little as a 6% decrease in body weight from fluid loss can lead to a significant decrease in muscular strength and endurance. Consumption of fluids should be done before (8 to 12 ounces, 15 minutes before), during (3 to 4 ounces every 10 to 15 minutes), and after exercise (16 ounces for every 0.5 kg weight loss) (24).

For exercise bouts lasting less than 60 minutes, water is recommended for fluid replacement. However, when the exercise exceeds 60 minutes, or in the heat, sports drinks can be beneficial, which supply energy and electrolytes and promote maximum fluid absorption through maintenance of the thirst mechanism, thus promoting fluid consumption can be beneficial (25). The best fluid replacement beverage is one that tastes good and works well in the training regimen, does not cause gastrointestinal distress, promotes rapid fluid absorption and maintenance of extracellular fluid volume, and provides energy (8 ounces of sports drink should provide 14 to 19 g of carbohydrate) (24).

Salt tablets can irritate the lining of the stomach, cause nausea, and increase the requirement for water, therefore they should not be consumed. Sweat contains proportionately more water and less sodium and potassium, than blood plasma. Therefore, it is important to replace fluid loss before replacing electrolytes.

Supplementation

Although it has been shown that inadequate intake of some vitamins can impair performance, it is unusual for an athlete to experience such deficiencies. Even marginal vitamin deficiencies do not appear to significantly affect the ability to exercise and the use of supplements does not guarantee a high level of performance (26). Overconsumption of vitamins and minerals can lead to toxicity as well as a false sense of security and may, in fact, alter use of other nutrients. "Crash diets" that supplement vitamins and minerals without consuming foods result in an inadequate energy supply and lower performance. Megadoses of supplements do not compensate for a lack of training or talent, nor do they give any athlete an edge.

For athletes who maintain a low body weight or repeatedly lose weight, consumption of a one-a-day multivitamin/mineral supplement is prudent. Iron-deficiency anemia can be a problem, particularly for female athletes and endurance athletes, and supplementation under medical supervision may be indicated if a problem is identified. For the female athlete, adequate calcium consumption is important because low levels, in conjunction with amenorrhea, may result in stress fractures and, later in life, osteoporosis (27).

FACILITATING CHANGES IN DIETARY BEHAVIOR

There is clear evidence of dietary change occurring because of large-scale educational efforts that confirm some professional opinion (5). Millions of people are concerned about dietary habits, they read food labels, and seek restaurants with "lighter" menus, salad bars, etc. The climate is right for encouraging even broader changes, but the process of changing eating behavior is complex.

General Principles of Behavior Change

Specific steps can aid in changing general dietary practice or in altering specific nutrient intake (e.g., salt, fat). Assessment of motivation and readiness for change is the first step. Some individuals are ready to change and can be guided through certain steps, while others may not be ready and, in spite of encouragement, will not change.

Analyzing Eating Patterns

Dietary change can be facilitated through analysis of eating patterns using a food diary. This information can identify how the food intake compares to the recommended diet. Other patterns, such as time of eating, association of eating with certain moods, and problems with specific foods can be highlighted in a diet diary. Patterns typically emerge from keeping such a record over several weeks. The information can be individualized, used for motivational purposes and provide targets for change.

Instruction

Relevant information about healthy dietary practice is provided either generally or specifically. For those with no special dietary needs, general information can be provided; however, for those with known health problems or nutritional deficiencies, more detailed information may be required (14). Special meal plans, focused cookbooks, and food preparation classes may be helpful.

Goal Setting

The establishment of reasonable goals is important. A person suddenly motivated by pressure from family, physician, or even social pressure may begin with a burst of motivation, but radical changes tend to be transient.

Altering the Eating Environment

Structuring eating environment can take several forms. Keeping healthy foods available and problem foods out of the house may reduce temptation and curb automatic or compulsive eating. Individuals can benefit from instruction about shopping for food in a careful and planned manner as well as storage, preparation, and serving in ways that promote healthier eating.

▶ SUMMARY

Adequate nutrition is essential for health, well-being, and optimal performance. Much is known about specific types and amounts of food needed for optimal health, but eating behavior does not change easily. Applying current knowledge, assessing and modifying dietary behavior, and combining this with principles of nutrition education, can be instrumental in changing eating habits and, hence, improving public health.

ACKNOWLEDGMENT

We would like to thank Jane Borchers, Helen DeMarco and Stefanie Jensen for their significant contributions to this work.

References

1. Whitney EN, Rolfes SR. *Understanding Nutrition.* 7th ed. St Paul, MN: West Publishing Co, 1996:161–162.
2. Grundy SM, Denke MA. Dietary influences on serum lipids and lipoproteins. *J Lipid Res* 31:1149–1172, 1990.
3. Connor WE, Connor SL. The Dietary Therapy of Hyperlipidemia. In: Schettler G, ed. *Handbook of Experimental Pharmacology,* Vol. 109. New York: Springer-Verlag, 1994.
4. Genest JJ, Martin-Munley SS, McNamara JR, Ordovas JM, Jenner J, Myers RH, Silberman SR, Wilson PW, Salem DN, Schaefer EJ. Familial lipoprotein disorders in patients with premature CAD. *Circulation* 85:2025–2033, 1992.
5. Summary of the Second Report of the National Cholesterol Education Program (NCEP) Expert Panel on Detection, Evaluation and Treatment of High Blood Cholesterol in Adults (Adult Treatment Panel II). *JAMA* 269:3015–3023.
6. Principles and treatment of lipoprotein disorders. In: Schettler G, ed. *Handbook of Experimental Pharmacology,* Vol. 109. New York: Springer-Verlag, 1994.
7. Wood PD, Haskell W, Klein H, Lewis S, Stern MP, Farquhar JW. The distribution of plasma lipoproteins in middle-aged male runners. *Metabolism* 25:1249–1257, 1976.
8. Burkitt DP. Epidemiology of cancer of the colon and rectum. *Nutrition* 4:201–214, 1988.
9. Butrum RR, Clifford CK, Lanza E. NCI Dietary Guidelines: Rationales. *Am J Clin Nutr* 48:888–895, 1988.
10. National Research Council. *Recommended Dietary Allowances,* 10th ed. Washington DC: National Academy of Sciences Press, 1989.
11. U.S. Dept. of Agriculture, U.S. Dept. of Health and Human Services. *Dietary Guidelines for Americans.* 1995.
12. National Research Council. *Diet and Health.* Washington DC: National Academy Press, 1989.
13. Butterfield GE. Protein and Amino Acids. In: Lamb D, Williams M, eds. *Perspectives in Exercise Science and Sports Medicine: Vol. 4: Ergogenics: The Enhancement of Sport Performance.* Carmel, IN: Benchmark Press, 1991.
14. United States Department of Agriculture, Human Nutrition Information Service. USDA's Food Guide Pyramid. *Home and Garden Bulletin* #249. US Government Printing Office, April, 1992.
15. Butterfield GE. Dietary requirements of the athlete. In: Shepard R, ed. *Current Therapy in Sports Medicine.* Philadelphia: Mosby, 1995.
16. Sherman WM. Recovery from endurance exercise. *Med Sci Sports Exerc* 24:S336–S339, 1992.
17. Ivy JL, Katz AL, Cutler CL, Sherman WM, Coyle EF. Muscle glycogen synthesis after exercise: effect of time of carbohydrate ingestion. *J Appl Physiol* 64:1480–1485, 1988.
18. Robergs RA. Nutrition and exercise determinants of postexercise glycogen synthesis. *Intl J Sports Nutr* 1:307–337, 1991.
19. Coyle EF, Coggan AR, Hemmert MK, Ivy JL. Muscle glycogen utilization during prolonged strenuous exercise when fed carbohydrate. *J Appl Physiol* 61:165–172, 1986.
20. Thomas DE, Brotherhood JR, Brand JC. Carbohydrate feeding before exercise: effect of glycemic index. *Intl J Sports Med* 12:180–186, 1991.
21. Hellerstein MK, Christiansen M, Kaempfer S, Kletke C, Wu K, Reid JS, Mulligan K, Hellerstein NS, Shackleton CHL. Measurement of de novo hepatic lipogenesis in humans using stable isotopes. *J Clin Invest* 87:1841–1852, 1991.
22. Williams MH. The use of nutritional ergogenic aids in sports: is it an ethical issue? *Intl J Sports Nutr* 4:120–131, 1994.
23. Greenleaf JE. The body's need for fluids. In: Haskell W, ed. *Nutrition and Athletic Performance.* Palo Alto, CA: Bull Publishing Co., 1982:34–50.
24. American College of Sports Medicine. Position stand on exercise and fluid replacement. *Med Sci Sports Exerc* 28:i–vii, 1996.
25. Nose H, Mack GW, Shi X, Nadel ER. Role of osmolality and plasma volume during rehydration in humans. *J Appl Physiol* 65:325–331, 1988.
26. Telfor RD, Catchpole EA, Deakin V, Hahn AG, Plank AW. The effect of 7 to 8 months of vitamin/mineral supplementation on athletic performance. *Intl J Sports Nutr* 2: 135–153, 1992.
27. Loucks AB, Horvath SH. Athletic amenorrhea: a review. *Med Sci Sports Exerc* 17:56–72, 1985.
28. Gersovitz M, Madded JP, Smicikias-Wright H. Validity of the 24-hour dietary recall and seven day record for group comparisons. *J Am Dietetics Assoc* 73:48–52, 1978.

Suggested Readings

Berning JR, Steen SN, eds. *Sports Nutrition for the 90's; the Health Professional's Handbook.* Gaithersburg, MD: Aspen, 1991.

Clark N. *Nancy Clark's Sports Nutrition Guidebook: Eating to Fuel Your Active Lifestyle.* Champaign, IL: Leisure Press, 1990.

Coleman E. *Eating for Endurance.* Palo Alto, CA: Bull Publishing, 1995.

Coleman E, Steen SN. *The Ultimate Sports Nutrition Handbook.* Palo Alto, CA: Bull Publishing, 1996.

72, 91 80, 81, 82, 95, 96 278

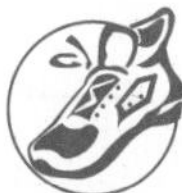

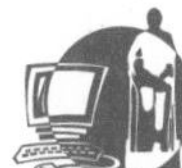

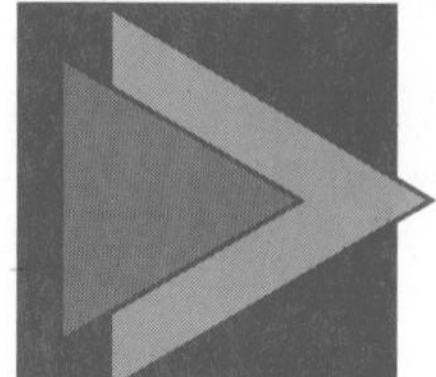

CHAPTER 4
SMOKING CESSATION

Nancy Houston Miller and Patricia M. Smith

Tobacco use is an important public health issue and it is essential that all health care professionals accept their responsibility to intervene with smoking. According to the Centers for Disease Control, tobacco use is the number one preventable cause of premature mortality, and is responsible for more than 470,000 deaths annually (1). More people die from tobacco-related deaths each year than from AIDS, alcoholism, cocaine, heroin, traffic accidents, fire, homicides, and suicides combined (2). Although adult smoking prevalence is at the lowest level in more than 50 years, at least 1 in 4 adults continues to smoke (1). Teen smoking has not decreased since 1980 and approximately 3,000 minors begin to smoke each day. As much as $68 billion annually has been attributed to smoking due to increased health care costs, lost productivity and missed work, higher insurance costs, and higher maintenance costs in the workplace where employees smoke. This chapter is designed to provide the facts on smoking and what health care professionals can do to impact smoking prevalence.

HEALTH RISKS OF SMOKING

All organs and tissues can be damaged by the toxic compounds present in tobacco smoke. Research now suggests that one-third to one-half of all regular cigarette smokers will eventually be killed by their habit (1, 3). Lung cancer, of which approximately 85% of cases are directly attributable to cigarette smoking, is the most common cause of cancer death in both men and women. The prevalence of lung cancer in the United States has increased by 250% since 1950 (4). Although most commonly associated with the risk of lung cancer, smoking is also responsible for cancer of the trachea, larynx, lip, oral cavity, pharynx, esophagus, bladder, kidney, cervix, pancreas, stomach, and leukemia (4). Smoking is also a major cause of atherosclerosis and is one of the four major risk factors for cardiovascular disease including coronary heart disease, cerebrovascular disease (stroke), abdominal aortic aneurysm, and peripheral vascular disease (5). Compared to nonsmokers, women who smoke and use oral contraceptives have a tenfold increased risk of death from coronary heart disease (6). Approximately 50,000 additional fatalities from burns, pediatric diseases, and second hand smoke are attributed to cigarette smoking (1).

Smokers also have a higher prevalence of peptic ulcer disease, chronic bronchitis, asthma, respiratory infections, emphysema, and other chronic obstructive pulmonary disease (6). In women, smoking is associated with earlier menopause and increased risk of osteoporosis due to lower estrogen levels. Smoking during pregnancy can result in fetal hypoxia, increased risk of neonatal death, spontaneous abortion, premature and/or lower birth weight babies, and may adversely affect the child's long-term growth and intellectual development.

The physiological alterations and systems affected by smoking are complex and multidimensional. In the cardiovascular system, for example, nicotine from cigarette smoking releases catecholamines, increasing heart rate and blood pressure, which in turn leads to increased work of the heart. It also lowers high-density lipoprotein levels and increases platelet adhesiveness. Carbon monoxide, another byproduct of smoking, may cause damage by injuring vascular endothelium and interfering with the ability of red blood cells to carry oxygen, thus reducing the amount of oxygen received by the heart muscle (7).

HEALTH BENEFITS OF QUITTING SMOKING

The health benefits of smoking cessation are immediate and substantial for all smokers regardless of age, gender, disease state, and smoking history—the sooner smoking cessation occurs, the lower the risk for disease. The decline in risk with smoking cessation has been reviewed (8). For example, reduced risk with cessation is well-documented for lung and laryngeal cancers, although the extent of reduction over time remains uncertain due to the dose-response relationship between smoking and disease (i.e., lung cancer is related to the number of cigarettes smoked daily and the total number of years smoked). The risks for cancers of the oral cavity, esophagus, pancreas, and bladder drop quickly after cessation and within 10 years of abstinence, reach levels similar to those who have never smoked.

Of the conditions most associated with heart disease (atherosclerosis, promotion of thrombosis, increased risk of coronary artery spasm, production of arrhythmias, and reduced oxygen delivery), all but atherosclerosis are believed to reverse within a short time after smoking cessation. Cessation leads to a rapid reduction in risk for myocardial infarction (MI) in healthy persons and, after periods of 5 to 20 years of abstinence, risks of former smokers have been found to equal to those who have never smoked. Cessation is also related to substantial improvement in patient outcome after MI. In one study, the overall reduction in risk of death was found to be as high as 40%, with 5-year survival rates of quitters and never smokers being comparable. The risk of reinfarction drops by 50% within the first year for patients who quit smoking after MI and within 10 years, the risk is only slightly higher than a nonsmoker (9).

In another study of patients 55 years of age or older following coronary artery bypass surgery, continuing smokers had a higher risk of both MI and death compared to those who did not smoke for > 6 years postoperatively (10). **Although research shows that the risk of cancer and heart disease is much lower in former smokers compared to current smokers, the heterogeneity of former smokers and the degree of existing disease at the time of cessation precludes applying the evidence on cessation to all individual smokers** (8).

FACTS ABOUT SMOKING BEHAVIOR

Smoking is an Addictive Behavior

Smoking causes both physiological and psychological dependence. The drug leading to addiction is nicotine. Smokers regulate their nicotine levels or "fine-tune" the amount of nicotine delivered to the brain by varying the intensity, frequency, and depth of each puff (11). Nicotine also appears to have both stimulating and tranquilizing effects, depending on the dosage; therefore, many smokers may use nicotine to regulate mood (11). All addictive behaviors share common characteristics, which include physical dependence and tolerance for the substance, an immediate sense of gratification, use of the drug despite social and/or medical disapproval and harm to physical, social, psychological or economic well-being; use of the drug to restore physical and psychological comfort, and predictable withdrawal symptoms when attempts to quit are made (12).

Smoking Is a Habit

Smoking is an "over-learned" habit; that is, events such as drinking coffee, driving a car, eating a meal, or talking on the telephone can stimulate the need for a cigarette. Success in getting smokers to quit and remain nonsmokers is partially dependent upon identifying what triggers the person to smoke (13). Smoking cigarettes and the associated nicotine effects are intertwined with many aspects of life.

Initiation and Maintenance of Smoking

The majority of people begin smoking as teenagers (14). Smoking initiation in younger years is, in large part, due to the social environment. Teenagers often feel social pressure from peers, siblings, and parents, or respond to the intrigue and pressure created by advertising. Curiosity, rebelliousness, and lack of social confidence can also play a part in smoking initiation. Young people frequently experiment with cigarettes to make them feel mature, "cool," and sophisticated (14). The majority of teens believe they will not become addicted and will be able to stop smoking whenever they wish. The continuation of a smoking behavior into adulthood, however, is maintained by a variety of mechanisms including nicotine addiction, habit, and psychological effects. Some smokers also continue to smoke to maintain their self-image. As strong as the anti-smoking messages are in society, the tobacco industry spends over 3.9 billion dollars annually on cigarette advertising to create a positive image of smoking (15).

Why People Quit Smoking

The reasons people quit smoking are varied and personal. Concerns about health, however, are the most frequently cited reasons for quitting smoking (16). Moreover, people with smoking-related diseases tend to have the highest cessation rates. Age is also related to smoking cessation with older people being more likely to quit smoking than younger people. It is believed that age is related to cessation because of fear of, or saliency of, smoking-related diseases that tend to occur later in life (17). One group of researchers showed that knowing someone whose health was affected by smoking was related to cessation and that this effect was greater for individuals over 65 years of age (18). Since older individuals have more friends and relatives whose health has been adversely affected by smoking, perceived susceptibility may increase with increasing age. Expense and social pressure from family, children, and friends are other reasons people quit smoking.

Why People Don't Quit Smoking

Most smokers know that smoking is unhealthy, yet many continue smoking. At least 60% to 70% of smokers report they would like to quit (up to 50% attempt to quit each year) (19, 20). Reasons for not quitting include inconvenience, stress, relatives who smoked and lived to be 95 years of age, weight gain, and people simply like to smoke. Smokers also have difficulty quitting due to the effects of nicotine. They experience positive psychological effects such as improved concentration and fear withdrawal symptoms such as headache, irritability, and restlessness. Excuses are difficult to counteract because smokers are good at defending their desire and right to smoke. The approach to smoking cessation intervention suggested by most health care professionals is not to counteract excuses directly but to have the smoker search for meaningful reasons that will make them want to quit.

MAINTENANCE OF ABSTINENCE FROM SMOKING: UNDERSTANDING THE PROCESS OF RELAPSE

Researchers and clinicians working to change addictive behaviors agree there are at least three basic stages of health behavior change: motivation and commitment to change, initial change, and maintaining the change (13). Therefore, even when people successfully quit smoking, it is not necessarily the end of the problem. Relapses are common; up to 80% of smokers who try to quit, fail on their first attempt and many require numerous attempts before they are successful. In the early stages of cessation, relapse often occurs because of withdrawal symptoms. Withdrawal symptoms are strongest during the first week after quitting and usually resolve by 1 month. Relapse after prolonged abstinence may occur due to stressful situations or the memory of the reinforcing properties of cigarettes since urges to smoke may continue over a number of months and even years.

SMOKING CESSATION INTERVENTIONS

Quit Rates

Since the 1960s, major public health initiatives such as the media advertising ban, local ordinances to limit smoking in public places, and tobacco tax initiatives have had a major impact on the decline in smoking prevalence. Per capita consumption is at its lowest since World War II, and among men today, there are more former smokers than current smokers (1). Smoking cessation interventions have played an important role in the decline in smoking prevalence over the last three decades. Interventions result in average quit rates of 15% to 25% in the general population of smokers. Quit rates increase substantially for people with smoking related diseases, with up to 70% of patients quitting one year after MI when provided with an intensive intervention (21). These rates are higher than self-quit rates which have been estimated to be less than 3% in the general population of smokers (22).

What Works?

Based on a meta-analysis of 39 clinical trials from the late 1970s and early-to-mid 1980s, quitting smoking is not necessarily achieved with a specific intervention or delivery system such as nicotine replacement therapy, hypnosis, counseling, or written materials. Rather, it is achieved by increasing reinforcement—that is, increasing the number of contacts made with the smoker who is trying to quit or to abstain after quitting, the types of contacts, and the number of people making the contacts (23). Providing multiple components (e.g., information on the risk of smoking, the benefits of quitting, support, skills and problem solving to deal with difficult situations associated with smoking, and nicotine replacement therapy) and multiple media for delivery (e.g., videotapes, audiotapes, workbooks, telephone calls) rather than any single intervention strategy provides a greater degree of success because people have different needs and may respond differently to each component.

Settings for Smoking Cessation Interventions

Smoking cessation programs can be implemented in any number of settings—the worksite, hospital, outpatient clinic, physician office, rehabilitation center, or a commercial fitness center. A program, however, must be visible, accessible, and capable of reaching large numbers of smokers. Even though 70% of smokers indicate that they would like to quit smoking, very few ever seek out treatment (24). Therefore, the more frequent a message or program is offered, the greater the likelihood that an individual will respond to help with smoking cessation.

Given that over 33 million Americans are hospitalized each year, and at least 25% are smokers, the hospital setting has recently been identified as an important setting to reach large numbers of smokers (25). By offering smoking cessation programs to all hospitalized patients at the bedside, hospitalization provides an especially important opportunity for success due to enforced smoking bans. Moreover, hospitalized patients are often more motivated to quit smoking because they are ill, their daily cues to smoke are removed, and numerous health professionals such as doctors, nurses, and therapists can provide multiple non-smoking messages.

APPROACHING SMOKING BEHAVIOR

Health care professionals and exercise leaders are often asked to help people stop smoking. The Agency for Health Care Policy and Research has identified guidelines for clinicians to help people with the process of quitting (26). Similar to what is offered by many organizations in attempting to help individuals, they suggest a stepped approach to the problem. This suggested approach includes the following:

Step 1: Identify Smokers at Every Encounter

The identification of smokers can be facilitated by the addition of a smoking question to an intake questionnaire or interview. Once a smoker is identified, follow-up at every encounter and asking about smoking status, should be implemented. Stickers on charts or notation on exercise logs provide convenient ways of prompting the smoking status question.

Step 2: Advise Smokers to Quit

A 1 to 2 minute, strong and personalized message to quit may have substantial impact on smokers. Advice should be clear, succinct, and should specify the impact of diseases caused by smoking or the risk associated with continuing to smoke. The message should be personalized to current health or illness, economic costs, motivational level, or impact on others. If additional time permits, reflecting on symptoms an individual is experiencing, such as cough, shortness of breath or chest discomfort (angina), may also be appropriate. Focusing on the benefits of quitting may provide reinforcement for an individual about the value of quitting. Lack of a clear message may only allow smokers to deny or minimize the need for smoking cessation. The more messages the smoker receives from varied health care professionals, the greater the likelihood of impact.

Step 3: Ask Smokers If They Are Willing to Make a Quit Attempt

Asking an individual if they are willing to quit smoking is simply done by a straightforward question such as "*What is your willingness to quit smoking now*?" Individuals who are not willing to quit should receive a "motivational" interview that defines the personal short- and long-term risks associated with continued smoking. Individuals should be asked to identify the potential benefits of quitting and the interview should be repeated at all encounters.

For those who are willing to quit, it is necessary to determine whether the smoker might perceive benefit from a more formal program in the community. Many programs are offered through local hospitals, community colleges, medical groups, and organizations such as the American Lung Association, American Cancer Society, and the American Heart Association. A list of smoking cessation programs offered in the community including the cost, intervention methods, and contact people should be made available to those individuals needing this type of support. Follow-up is important for those individuals to determine whether contact has been made and if individuals have been successful with smoking cessation.

Step 4: Aid Smokers in Quitting

Many smokers may be ready to quit without the aid of a group program. If so, they should be helped to set a quit date within 1 to 2 weeks so their commitment to quitting does not wane. Once the decision to quit has been made, they must decide if they want to quit "cold turkey" or use other methods such as cutting down on the number of cigarettes smoked in the days preceding the quit day. Health care professionals can help in this process by reviewing previous quit attempts with smokers, focusing on what was useful in the past, and helping the smoker identify problems that hindered successful cessation in the past (Table 4.1). Smokers must also be told to prepare for their quit day by getting rid of all ashtrays, matches and tobacco products, and formally acknowledging to family members and friends of the intention to quit and asking for their support.

Nicotine replacement therapy to aid with the physical withdrawal symptoms can be obtained prior to the quit date for use on that day. Specific guidelines for the proper use of nicotine gum or the patch are important if the smoker is to be successful in using pharmacologic therapy. Now that nicotine gum is available over-the-counter without a prescription, it is extremely important to success for the patient to learn how to properly use the gum through appropriate chewing techniques such as using the "chew and park" method, avoidance of acidic beverages before and during chewing, and using gum on a fixed schedule. Appropriate use of the nicotine patch includes rotating patch sites daily and watching for local skin reaction. In addition, the use of low-cost self-help materials such as videotapes, audiotapes and CD ROM programs also offer inexpensive alternatives to

Table 4.1. Counseling a Smoker to Quit: What Can Be Done in 5–15 Minutes?

- Ask about smoking status and offer a firm unequivocal "quit smoking message."
- Determine whether the smoker is willing to quit and set a quit date within 1 to 2 weeks if possible.
- Find out whether there has been an attempt to quit in the past and what was helpful. Use this information to determine the best approach to quitting.
- Assist with preparation to quit by recommending that the smoker:
  - + Prepare the environment for quitting by removing all cues to smoke (ashtrays, matches, and tobacco products).
  - + Inform family members and friends of the intention to quit, asking for their support in not offering cigarettes or not smoking in front of the "ex-smoker."
  - + Plan for withdrawal and consider nicotine replacement therapy.
  - + Identify situations that will pose difficulty in abstaining from tobacco products (e.g., social functions, under stress) and how these situations can be handled. (See Table 4.2)
- Follow-up to determine progress, problem solve, and offer support.

more complex interventions. Many of these materials are available from non-profit organizations.

Step 5: Arrange for Follow-up

If possible, individuals who attempt to quit smoking should be offered at least two contacts in the early stages (first month) of quitting. Telephone calls are a convenient, effective, and inexpensive method of follow-up. They can be used to provide support and reinforcement to those who quit, and to problem-solve difficulties which may be encountered with giving up tobacco products. For those who have relapsed, a quick telephone contact may serve as a method to get them to seriously think about setting another quit date.

IMPORTANT AREAS TO COVER IN COUNSELING SMOKERS ABOUT A QUIT ATTEMPT

Withdrawal

In the early stages of quitting, people will experience withdrawal symptoms similar to withdrawal from other stimulants such as cocaine or heroin. Symptoms include difficulty concentrating, decreased performance on memory tasks or attention tasks, restlessness, irritability, depression, decreased heart rate and blood pressure, increased hunger, sleep disturbance, and weight gain. The strongest symptoms occur during the first 48 to 72 hours and then reach a second peak approximately 1 to 2 weeks after quitting. Most withdrawal symptoms resolve by one month. Nicotine replacement therapy (gum or patch) can be helpful in the initial stages of withdrawal but there is little benefit to continuing nicotine therapy past 8 weeks (26). Nicotine replacement therapy can be especially helpful for highly addicted smokers who have had problems with smoking withdrawal or who smoke at least one pack per day. Little research, however, is available on the use of nicotine replacement therapy in individuals considered to be light smokers (i.e., those smoking ≤ 10 to 15 cigarettes per day). Whether using the gum or the patch, all individuals must refrain from smoking while using these agents. Smokers can be prepared to deal with withdrawal by:

1. Acknowledging that smokers may experience some withdrawal although the symptoms vary.
2. Emphasizing that the worst withdrawal will be within the first 48 to 72 hours. People who successfully endure the first 3 weeks smoke-free have an increased chance of remaining a nonsmoker.
3. Recommending that heavier smokers (> 1 pack/day) consider nicotine replacement therapy to assist with withdrawal symptoms.

Psychological Craving

Psychological craving, urges, and desire to have a cigarette should not be confused with withdrawal symptoms—cravings may persist in some ex-smokers over a prolonged period of time. Cravings are often associated with other behaviors such as driving a car, talking on the telephone, or socializing, especially when alcohol is involved. Various emotional states such as boredom, anger, depression, and stress can also trigger the urge to smoke. Developing behavioral strategies in advance is an important part of the maintenance process. Smokers can be prepared to deal with cravings and urges by:

1. Acknowledging that smokers may experience cravings or urges which may persist over prolonged periods of time or may reappear after a long period of abstinence.
2. Emphasizing that urges can be overcome.
3. Recommending that smokers identify those situations that are most likely to trigger the smoking urge.

For each situation identified, recommend creating one cognitive and one behavioral strategy that can be used to help resist the smoking urge. A list of cognitive and behavioral strategies are shown in Table 4.2.

Relapse

Slips or lapses to smoking are common. They may occur when an individual has a strong smoking urge. Many researchers studying addictive behaviors believe that the method of addressing slips may determine whether a person returns to abstinence or relapses totally (13). It is important to help individuals identify high risk situations which may result in smoking. The riskiest situations for slips and potential total relapse include negative emotional states in which the ex-smoker experiences an unpleasant emotional feeling such as frustration, anger, depression, or boredom; interpersonal conflict during which the ex-smoker experiences conflict with interpersonal relationships at home, work, or socially; and, social pressure situations whereby the ex-smoker is influenced or pressured to smoke by other people or situations. Situations involving alcohol are also difficult for many ex-smokers. If high risk situations are identified ahead of time, the ex-smoker can develop strategies to help them cope with the situation and remain smoke-free. This increases their confidence or "self-efficacy" for coping with these situations. Smokers can be prepared to deal with slips by:

1. Acknowledging that slips or near slips may occur.
2. Emphasizing that slips do not represent failure and do not have to result in a full-blown relapse.
3. Recommending identification of the situation that resulted in smoking; considering location, circumstances, and recommending review of cognitive and

Table 4.2. Cognitive-Behavioral Strategies to Cope with High Risk Situations

Cognitive Strategies	
Focus on the negative effects from smoking such as:	Focus on the personal benefits from not smoking such as:
the physical harm to oneself and others	a reward of a trip or new clothes
suffering from smoking-related diseases	improved sense of smell and taste
lungs turning black	improved respiratory function
a symptom such as chest discomfort	being free of a cough
the negative role-model for children and grandchildren	increased stamina for physical activity
the dangers of second-hand smoke for family and friends	improved self-image and respect
inhaling the more than 4,000 chemicals in cigarettes	
esthetics (yellow teeth, bad breath, yellow fingers, smelly clothes)	
Behavioral Strategies	
Suggested strategies for coping with two high risk situations	
Smoking after a meal:	Smoking while driving:
chew gum or mints after eating	remove your car ashtray
brush your teeth	keep gum and snacks in the car
use a mouthwash	put a photo of your children or grandchildren in the ashtray
get up from the table and work on a hobby	use a straw as something to hold in your hand
play a card game	keep an air freshener in your car

behavioral strategies to deal with high-risk situations (Table 4.2).

Weight Gain

Weight gain is an especially important issue to address for the smoker who is considering quitting because many smokers are fearful of gaining weight and many believe that returning to smoking is the only answer for controlling weight gain (26). The fact is the majority of smokers will gain weight with cessation although the precise mechanisms underlying weight gain are not well understood. However, the weight gained is generally less than 10 pounds. Weight gain tends to be slightly greater for women, and is more often associated with heavier smokers (>25 cigarettes per day), restrained eaters, and those who have a history of weight problems (27). African-Americans and people under the age of 55 years are also at increased risk for weight gain (26). Smokers must realize that the weight gain associated with cessation is minor compared with the risks of continued smoking. Smokers can be prepared to deal with the weight gain by:

1. Acknowledging that most smokers will gain weight.
2. Emphasizing that the first priority should be to manage cessation and then address the weight gain.
3. Recommending that individuals may avoid excessive weight gain through increasing physical activity, limiting alcohol intake, and consuming less fat in the diet.

Social Environment

Being in the presence of other smokers is associated with a return to smoking and partner support is associated with lower rates of relapse (28). Therefore, identification of other smokers within the household is important in aiding the smoker with quitting. While it may not be feasible to get family members to quit smoking together, there are a number of things a smoker can request from family and friends in preparation for quitting. Smokers can be prepared to deal with other smokers in their environment by:

1. Acknowledging that being around other smokers may be difficult.
2. Emphasizing that they may need to restrict socializing with other smokers in the early days of quitting.
3. Recommending that the home environment be more conducive to quitting by asking family members to refrain from smoking in the presence of the quitter, avoid leaving tobacco products around the house, refrain from offering cigarettes to the quitter, and restrict smoking in the home.

SMOKING CESSATION IS A MAJOR LIFESTYLE CHANGE

Smokers can benefit from acknowledgment that quitting can be quite difficult and, in fact, for many it can be associated with significant loss. Incorporating positive changes in lifestyles such as picking up new hobbies, developing reward systems for not smoking, and increasing exercise and relaxation have been shown to help individuals gain better sense of self-control and thus decrease the probability of relapse (13). Exercise can also be an important way to foster long-term abstinence. Previous work with post-MI patients, suggests that those who participated in an exercise training program combined with smoking cessation had greater cessation rates and smoked significantly fewer cigarettes than did smokers not participating in such a program (29). Exercise can bring psychological benefits, help reduce post-cessation weight gain, and minimize withdrawal.

▶ SUMMARY

While adult smoking prevalence is at its lowest level in more than 50 years, a large proportion of Americans (25%) are smokers (1). All health care professionals must realize their responsibility in helping smokers understand the health risks associated with continued smoking and the benefits of quitting. They must also know how to apply appropriate strategies to counsel smokers and do so at every encounter. Developing a planned approach in helping smokers will ensure that a larger proportion of such individuals will succeed with smoking cessation.

References

1. Centers for Disease Control. Cigarette smoking among adults: United States, 1993. *MMWR* 43:925–930, 1994.
2. Warner KE. Health and economic implications of a tobacco-free society. *JAMA* 258:2080–2086, 1987.
3. Doll R, Peto R, Wheatley K, Gray R, Sutherland I. Mortality in relation to smoking: 40 years' observations on male British doctors. *Br Med J* 309:901–911, 1994.
4. Newcomb PA, Carbone PP. The health consequences of smoking: cancer. *Med Clin North Am* 76:305–331, 1992.
5. McBride PE. The health consequences of smoking: cardiovascular diseases. *Med Clin North Am* 76:333–353, 1992.
6. Fielding J. Smoking: health effects and control. *N Engl J Med* 313:491–497, 1985.
7. McGill HC. The cardiovascular pathology of smoking. *Am Heart J* 115:250–252, 1988.
8. Samet JM. The health benefits of smoking cessation. *Med Clin North Am* 76:399–415, 1992.
9. Sparrow D, Dawber T, Colton T. The influence of cigarette smoking on prognosis after a first myocardial infarction. *J Chron Dis* 31:425–432, 1978.
10. Hermanson B, Omenn GS, Kronmal RA, Gersh BJ. Beneficial six-year outcome of smoking cessation in older men and women with coronary artery disease. *N Engl J Med* 319:1365–1369, 1988
11. Pomerleau OF, Pomerleau CS. Neuroregulators and the reinforcement of smoking: towards a biobehavioral explanation. *Neurosci Biobehav Rev* 8:503–513, 1984.
12. American Psychiatric Association. *Diagnostic and Statistical Manual of Mental Disorders.* 3rd ed, Revised. Washington DC: American Psychiatric Association, 1987.
13. Marlatt GA, Gordon JR, eds. *Relapse Prevention: Maintenance Strategies in the Treatment of Addiction.* New York: Guilford Press, 1985.
14. Hooked on tobacco: the teen epidemic. *Consumer Rep* Mar 1995:142–147.
15. MacKenzie TD, Bartecchi CE, Schrier RW. The human costs of tobacco use. *N Engl J Med* 330:975–980, 1994.
16. McWhorter WP, Boyd GM, Mattson ME. Predictors of quitting smoking: the NHANES I followup experience. *J Clin Epidemiol* 43:1399–1405, 1990.
17. Salive ME, Cornoni-Huntley J, LaCroix AZ, Ostfield AM, Wallace RB, Hennekens CH. Predictors of smoking cessation and relapse in older adults. *Am J Public Health* 82: 1268–1271, 1992.
18. Bosse R, Rose CL. Age and interpersonal factors in smoking cessation. *J Health Soc Behav* 14:381–387, 1973.
19. Mason JO, Lindsay GB. A positive approach to smoking prevention and cessation. *Western J Med* 139:721–722, 1983.
20. Kottke TE, Brekke ML, Solberg, Hughes JR. A randomized trial to increase smoking intervention by physicians: doctors helping smokers, round 1. *JAMA* 261:2101–2106, 1989.
21. DeBusk RF, Houston Miller N, Superko R, Dennis CA, Lew HT, Berger WE, 3rd, Heller RS, Rompf J, Gee D, Kraemer HC, Bandura A, Ghandour G, Clark M, Shah RV, Fisher L, Taylor CB. A case management system for coronary risk factor modification following acute myocardial infarction. *Ann Intern Med* 120:721–729, 1994.
22. Cohen S, Lichtenstein E, Prochaska JO, Rossi JS, Gritz CR, Orleans CT, Schoenbach VJ, Biener L, Abrams D, DiClemente C, Curry S, Marlatt GA, Cummings M, Emont SJ, Giovino G, Osspi-Klein D. Debunking myths about self-quitting. Evidence from 10 prospective studies of persons who attempt to quit smoking by themselves. *Am Psychol* 44:1355–1365, 1989.
23. Kottke TE, Battissta RN, DeFriese GH, Brekke ML. Attributes of successful smoking cessation interventions in medical practice. A meta-analysis of 39 controlled trials. *JAMA* 259:2883–2889, 1988.
24. Sherin K. Smoking cessation: the physician's role. *Postgrad Med* 71:99–106, 1982.
25. Houston Miller N, Smith PM, DeBusk RF, Sobel DS, Taylor CB. Smoking cessation in hospitalized patients: Results of a randomized trial. *Arch Intern Med* 157:409–415, 1997.
26. Fiore MC, Wetter DW, Bailey WC, et al. Smoking cessation clinical practice guideline. Rockville, MD: Agency for Health Care Policy and Research, Public Health Service, US Dept of Health and Human Services, 1996.
27. Williamson DF, Madans J, Anda RF, Kleinman JC, Giorino GA, Beyers T. Smoking cessation and severity of weight gain in a national cohort. *N Engl J Med* 324:739–745, 1991.
28. Mermelstein R, Lichtenstein E, McIntyre K. Partner support and relapse in smoking-cessation programs. *J Consult Clin Psychol* 51:6555–6566, 1983.
29. Taylor CB, Houston Miller N, Haskell WL, Debusk RF. Smoking cessation after acute myocardial infarction: the effects of exercise training. *Addict Behav* 13:331–335, 1988.

Suggested Reading

Taylor CB, Killen JD. *The Facts about Smoking.* New York: Consumer Reports Books, 1991.

69 78, 99 81, 82, 277, 278 318, 819, 320 329

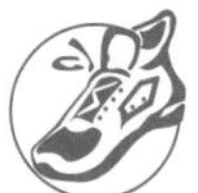
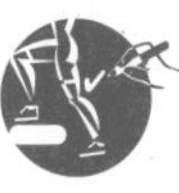
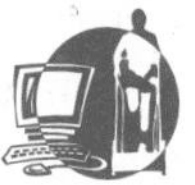
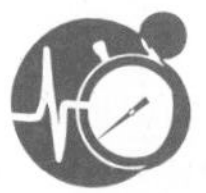

CHAPTER 5
STRESS AND HEART DISEASE

Wesley E. Sime, Robert S. Eliot, and Erik E. Solberg*

One way to assist individuals in understanding how emotional stress affects them personally is to think of stress as any disturbing physical event (ranging from spilled milk to a life threatening personal assault) or any cognitive thought process (ranging from mild stage fright to anticipated financial ruin) that is of sufficient magnitude and duration to elicit an emotional (psychophysiological) reaction, such as nervous sweating, heart pounding, panic, or depression. Ironically, the situation that precipitates an emotional reaction can be either negative (embarrassing, ego-threatening) or positive (excitement). These and other examples of challenges and hassles in daily living are known to cause potent psychophysiological reactions that potentially result in substantial homeostatic disruption as well as significant cardiovascular risk. When this disruption is either excessive or prolonged, the effect on the cardiovascular system is referred to as "strain." Since strain is an outcome of overload, it should be apparent that while some stress can be stimulating, interesting, and perhaps productive, excessive exposure to strain (experienced with great intensity or high frequency over time) can have deleterious pathophysiological consequences. Individual vulnerability to stressful stimulation is determined by many individual personality traits and environmental conditions called "psychosocial" factors.

When combining all possible personality traits together with a multitude of socioeconomic conditions (ranging from low demand, low income jobs to high challenge, high reward professions) and with either supportive or non-supportive family and friends, a complicated risk profile is presented that is unique for every individual predisposition to a variety of stress-related illnesses. One discerning element in this equation is the critical role of cognitive appraisal. That is, the way an individual evaluates the degree of threat, challenge, or opportunity in light of goals and expectations (1). Thus, cognitive appraisal serves to modulate or amplify the severity of the reaction so that a stressor, such as the death of a parent at age 65, can be viewed either as a natural course of events or devastating. Similarly, the cumulative effect of numerous low-grade hassles over a long period of time may be viewed as "no big deal" by one person, while another may find it to be overwhelming and exhausting. The essential question is whether individuals tend to make "mountains out of molehills" or whether they have learned the strong admonition, "Don't sweat the small stuff"(2).

The difficulty in ascribing health risks to specific emotional stress markers is related to the lack of objectivity, validity, and reliability in assessing the level of exposure to stress and to the complexity involved in measuring the level of physiological and psychological responses to real-life stressful experiences. It is important to acknowledge that a certain degree of interesting, yet provocative and challenging stress is both healthy and appropriate for natural growth and development throughout life. Some individuals seem to thrive on higher levels of stress, while others seem to be much more sensitive and reactive to modest stress exposures, manifesting a variety of signs and symptoms of stress that often precede a serious stress-related disorder. The purpose of this chapter is to describe the various aspects of stress responses, present an overview of the apparent heart disease and other health risks associated with stress, and discuss the assessment of stress using psychophysiological stress testing.

STRESS RESPONSES

Every individual exhibits a unique profile of response to stress that includes some combination of physiologi-

* Dr. Eliot died recently at his home in Scottsdale, AZ, during the writing of this chapter. He was a pioneer in stress-related cardiology research and author of numerous scientific articles focusing on sudden cardiac death and the "hot reactor" syndrome which served to stimulate important theories regarding stress and coronary heart disease. He was the author of two popular books of interest to the readers of this volume (ACSM Guidelines). The first was a 1984 publication, "Is It Worth Dying For?" and the more recent (1994) is "From Stress to Strength: How to Lighten Your Load and Save Your Life." We dedicate this chapter to his memory.

cal, cognitive, emotional and behavioral factors. Some of the more prominent and generally accepted examples for each of these four categories are listed in Table 5.1. Since it is difficult to assess stress indicators directly using clinical measures, paying attention to observable signs and symptoms of stress is very important for all staff, especially those close to clients or patients. Initially, one might have a vague sense that an individual is simply nervous or "ill at ease." This could be "situational" if the individual overreacts to a strange environment with some manifestations of anxiety or it could be a reflection of a more significant problem. In the case of a cardiac patient, the anxiety could also be "reactive" to stresses, such as that of an ischemic event or some other psychosomatic factor (e.g., fear of dying). Thus, it is important to discern whether the observed stress response is an inherent personality factor, or simply a reaction to the strange environment and/or to pathological symptoms.

Some of the most obvious behavioral indicators of stress include difficulty speaking, nervous laughter, or other outward appearances (e.g., restlessness, fidgeting, impatience, hypervigilance, despondence, etc.). One of the most interesting and relevant physical signs of stress reaction is cold and sweaty hands as observed in a social situation as when meeting someone for the first time. To amplify this, it is important to pay close attention to the "handshake" at the beginning and the end of an exercise session. Individuals who exhibit a warm, dry handshake are usually comfortable, at ease, and relaxed in that setting. Those with either cool and/or damp hands are exhibiting some degree of arousal while those with cold and/or sweaty hands are highly aroused or stressed. When these and other common signs of stress are exaggerated or persistent, it is important to question the individual cautiously about his/her feelings at the moment and to initiate the steps for coping with the stress. Because the cognitive and emotional symptoms are not obvious or observable, it is necessary to include questions in the conversation to elicit immediate reflections or their recollection of circumstances that might account for existing physical, emotional or behavioral stress reactions.

Table 5.1. Common Physiological, Cognitive, Emotional & Behavioral Stress Reactions

EMOTIONAL STRESS RESPONSES	PHYSIOLOGICAL STRESS RESPONSES
• Withdrawal • Feeling despondent • Frequent nightmares • Feeling of inferiority • Lack of empathy • Increased dependency • Feeling hopelessness • Mistrusting others • Crying easily for no reason	• Cold hands and feet • Heart pounding • Muscle tension (neck, back, jaws) • Nausea or vomiting • Nervous stomach • Diarrhea or constipation • Hyperventilation or breath holding • Dry mouth or stuttering • Restless sleep or insomnia
BEHAVIORAL STRESS RESPONSES	**COGNITIVE STRESS RESPONSES**
• Irritable for no good reason • Increased use of substances • Aggressive actions (driving) • Careless or dangerous actions • Hostile actions • Nervous laughter • Impatience, time urgency • Compulsive behaviors • Increased food intake	• Mental disorganization • Being obsessive about work • Inability to concentrate • Forgetting important tasks • Frequently frustrated • Procrastination • Persistent indecision • Mind goes blank • Increased fantasies

With permission from Raymer KF. Stress management education: Defining the knowledge base. Dissert Abstr Intl, 1991.

STRESS AND HEART DISEASE

Epidemiological evidence that demonstrates that stress is an important risk factor for heart disease is becoming stronger and more consistent. Among several large population studies conducted over extended periods, some as long as 35 years, there is ample evidence linking one of several manifestations of stress with the increased incidence of heart disease. In the 20-year follow-up of the Framingham Study, the incidence of angina was two times greater among those who exhibited higher levels of worry, dissatisfaction with work, feeling undue time pressure/urgency, and competitive drive (3).

In another study using meta-analyisis of five different populations numbering over 12,000 individuals and covering an 18 to 30-year time period, work stress (e.g., lack of control) was associated with higher levels of cholesterol, systolic blood pressure and smoking behavior (4). The Harvard Mastery of Stress Study, one of the longest prospective studies ever conducted in this field, revealed that severe anxiety and conflict with hostility were accurate predictors of not only coronary heart disease, but also of risk of overall future illness (5). Lastly, in two large studies of patients with documented coronary artery disease (13,000 and 2,000 patients, respectively), the high risk group in both studies had significantly more socioeconomic difficulties while simultaneously lacking social support or social connections to deal with stress (6, 7).

More recent studies (shorter duration and smaller populations) document specific markers of emotional stress that are related to heart disease. For example, patients who frequently exhibit outbursts of anger are known to have higher levels of cardiac reactivity (characterized by increased heart rate, systolic blood pressure and peripheral resistance) and greater cardiac dysfunction as well as increased risk of vasospasm and sudden death (8–10). Conversely, those who are angry but repress their feelings are also at increased risk of other noncardiac health complications. Those with a diagnosis of depression are clearly at greater risk for mortality at 6 month follow-up after diagnosis (11, 12). In addition, among the various occupational stress factors that exist, it has been shown that monotonous work, high-paced work, and job burnout are correlated with an increased incidence of heart disease (13, 14).

The mechanism by which stress may influence atherogenesis involves a complex interaction of sympathetic arousal, hypothalamic stimulation, and adrenergic and neurohormonal responses that lead to increased blood pressure, increased circulating catecholamine levels, and increased platelet activity (15–20). The resulting increased shearing forces of blood on the arterial wall, lead to endothelial injury and arterial wall damage. Thus, chronic exposure to emotional stress promotes the development of atherosclerosis that may result in coronary artery occlusion, vasospasm, myocardial ischemia, myocardial infarction, and increased incidence of ventricular arrhythmia, a known risk factor for sudden coronary death (21–23). Furthermore, the most serious impact of chronic stress is observed when hypercholesterolemia is also present (24).

Specific vascular changes resulting from emotional outbursts have also been demonstrated. There is a long history of research showing that emotional stress is clearly associated with angina, which may ultimately lead to sudden death (25–27). However, more recent evidence demonstrates that specific mechanisms of fatality, including silent ischemia, autonomic and adrenergic excesses leading to ventricular arrhythmias, or other electrocardiogram abnormalities, may occur without prior history or warning, and all of which may be provoked by a single dramatic emotional event (15, 16, 21, 28–32). The arbitrary expression of anger and fear, for example, has been shown to result in myocardial ischemia. Theoretically, myocardial ischemia could occur in "normal" coronary arteries (the result of spasm) or in arteries with fixed atherosclerotic lesions; either may result in a higher incidence of cardiac arrhythmias and sudden death (15). Cardiac events may also be triggered by sudden exertion, particularly in untrained persons (33). These findings suggest that both acute and chronic stress increases the risk of sudden events as well as the development of heart disease.

Cardiac Reactivity and Heart Disease

Evidence shows that high levels of cardiac reactivity to a moderate stress load is associated with the development of atherosclerosis, particularly in the presence of a high fat diet (34, 35). In addition, systolic blood pressure reactivity to stress is greatest in patients with severe ischemic heart disease, lowest in those without heart disease, and in-between in patients with mild to moderate ischemic heart disease. Systolic blood pressure reaction is thought to indicate a proportional disease-reactivity relationship (36, 37). Several other studies show that blood pressure reactivity in the presence of mild provocative stress is one element of the equation that links stress to heart disease risk, especially among black males and especially when the expression of anger is manifested (38–41).

The Interaction of Exercise and Stress

Independently, both exercise and stress have been associated with myocardial ischemia. However, the performance of exercise testing or training at times of emotional distress may disproportionately increase the risk of the occurrence of myocardial ischemia, although there is some controversy. In cardiac patients specifically, some emotions, such as depression or competitiveness, and sensitivity levels to discomfort have been predictive of ischemia and angina during exercise while several other responses, including anger and hostility, have not (42). Other investigators examining the relationship between exercise and stress in cardiac patients have suggested that, in patients where cardiac reactivity can be increased by a simple bout of exertion (talking, standing, etc.) compounded by a modest emotional trauma (fear, embarrassment, etc.), the risk of reinfarction is significantly increased (43, 44).

Exercise Training

Numerous studies have been conducted to examine the impact of exercise training on emotional stress responses (45–48). Considerable evidence spanning decades now documents the fact the exercise can enhance emotional well-being and attenuate stress responses (49). In general, exercise training tends to decrease beta-adrenergic myocardial responses to physical and behavioral challenges and has an acute prophylactic effect in reducing blood pressure response to a psychological stressor (39, 50). Furthermore, exercise is a very potent antidote for emotional stress as seen by the reductions in anxiety and depression associated with regular exercise training (51).

Exercise training of moderate intensity and duration is also very effective in reducing acute skeletal muscle tension (52–54). Thus, exercise is an excellent facilitating prelude for relaxation training in individuals who are particularly tense. In many exercise programs, relaxation training is conducted immediately after each exercise session, in part because relaxation effects occur more expeditiously following a moderate bout of exertion. The added advantage of post-exercise relaxation training lies in the safety factor. Because a large proportion of exercise-related cardiac complications occur in the post-exercise period (during the shower or on the way home), the longer the staff can monitor patients after exercise, the more protection is available.

In addition, the potential "cross-training" benefit of exercise training is reported to produce some protective insulation to the effects of stress; that is, both physiological and stress response benefit from exercise training.

Specifically, it has been shown that, along with the physiological benefits of exercise training, the tolerance to stress (level of sympathoadrenal reactivity and catecholamine response to psychological stressors) can be enhanced by the combination of moderate exercise and the specific exposure to the psychological stress of exercising (55, 56). This has been described as the "physiological toughness" model and further serves to support the rationale for the role of exercise training in a program of stress modification.

PSYCHOPHYSIOLOGICAL (EMOTIONAL) STRESS TESTING

Exercise testing procedures are intended to objectively and exclusively measure the metabolic and cardiovascular responses to standardized workloads. Unfortunately however, there are numerous emotional factors that can potentially override or inflate the true cardiovascular response. Some of these confounding emotional factors include exposure to a novel environment, performance anxiety, fear of failure, and apprehension about being observed by medical personnel (57). These factors have been shown to cause inflationary reactions during a first encounter with an exercise test situation, but ordinarily will subside among individuals who are not unduly anxious. As such, exercise testing has been shown to be more reliable and valid especially by the second or third administration for both heart rate and blood pressure (58, 59). Ideally, it would be desirable to conduct a traditional exercise stress test on the first visit together with a repeat exercise test on the second visit followed by an emotional stress test to factor out the physiological and psychological dimensions of stress.

In consideration of the complicated and confounding effect of emotions on exercise performance and response, it is interesting to note that vagal parasympathetic nervous system activity plays a role in the emotional responses to stress, fear and depression (60, 61). Decreased vagal activity often contributes to exaggerated diastolic blood pressure reactivity to mental stress, especially among individuals without a history of exercise training. In addition low vagal tone is associated with faster progression of the atherosclerotic disease process. Apparently these parasympathetic influences are associated with higher risk of myocardial ischemia and ventricular ectopy in the recovery phase following either emotional or exertional challenge. Thus, extreme caution is needed during the recovery period following either exertional and emotional strain.

Mental or emotional stress has been measured based upon non-invasive recording of cardiac output and blood pressure in both the laboratory and the clinical setting (62, 63). One of the most relevant measures uses impedance cardiography to continuously record stroke volume and is valid at rest and during exercise (64). Psychophysiological stress testing (Table 5.2) in this manner has been predictive of mean daily blood pressure as recorded by 24-hour ambulatory monitoring in accordance with the "hot reactor" model (65). In this procedure, individual differences in stress tolerance can be observed during the presentation of simple tasks such as quizzes, mental arithmetic tasks, and cold pressor tests that result in dramatic changes in the cardiovascular function of some individuals (66–70). Abnormal cardiovascular reactivity has been found in borderline hypertensive patients and in post-myocardial infarction patients (71, 72). Based on these findings, emotional stress testing in addition to standard exercise testing has been suggested in order to provide the most comprehensive diagnostic information.

Table 5.2. Psychophysiological (emotional) Stress Testing for Assessing Coronary Risk

PSYCHOPHYSIOLOGICAL STRESSORS

Cognitive Stressors
- Mental Arithmetic
- Competitive Contest
- Vigilance Task
- Word/Color Conflict Task
- Shock-Avoidance Task
- Ego-threatening IQ Test
- Viewing Traumatic Disaster Films
- Interview of Emotionally-charged Events
- Structured Interview for Type A Behavior

Somatic Stressors
- Cold Pressor Test
- Isometric Handgrip

} Both conducted with high challenge to endure

SOME PHYSIOLOGICAL MEASURES OF EMOTIONAL STRESS

Cardiovascular and Pulmonary
- Heart Rate Variability
- Electrocardiograph Changes
- Cardiac Output
- Stroke Volume (by impedance cardiography)
- Blood Pressure (systolic, diastolic, and mean)
- Peripheral Resistance (computed from pressure and cardiac output)
- Respiration Rate and Respiratory Sinus Arrhythmia
- Peripheral Blood Flow (pulse volume or skin temperature)

Autonomic and Skeletal Muscle
- Electrodermal Skin Response (palmar sweating)
- Electromyography (muscle tension)

With permission from Sime WE, Buell JC, Eliot RS. Cardiovascular responses to emotional stress (quiz interview) in post-myocardial infarction patients and matched control subjects. *J Human Stress* 6:39–46, 1980.

Comparing Exercise Testing and Psychophysiological Testing

Previous efforts to compare the efficacy of psychological and exertional testing revealed that exercise was more effective than emotional stimuli in elevating heart rate and blood pressure to a sufficient level to observe ischemic abnormalities (73). More recently however, psychophysiology specialists have improved the techniques for emotional stress testing using more sophisticated stress stimuli and more advanced measures of sympathetic nervous system arousal (skin conductance, pulse amplitude and respiration rate) as well as impedance cardiography and nuclear ventriculography (74–79). Table 5.2 describes detailed procedures for administering cognitive or somatic stressors while monitoring several cardiovascular, pulmonary, autonomic, and skeletal muscle measures.

Finally, it should be noted that heart rate and oxygen consumption responses during exercise are accurate predictors of heart rate responses during psychological testing (80). Using that information, measuring the "additive" heart rate responses during psychological tasks is possible, thus separating the exertional and emotional components of stress (81). Clearly there is a clinical efficacy for including some form of psychophysiological (emotional) stress testing, and though it is not a common practice in most clinical programs, it certainly should be considered in the future.

SUMMARY

The importance of stress in the development of heart disease and the incidence of various cardiovascular events of morbidity and mortality make stress reduction an important component of risk management in cardiovascular disease. Understanding methods that identify the common signs and symptoms of stress overload, including standard exercise testing and psychophysiological testing, are important knowledge for the exercise practitioner.

References

1. Lazarus R. Progress on a cognitive-motivational-relational theory of emotion. *Am Psych* 46:819–834, 1991.
2. Eliot RS. *Is It Worth Dying for?* New York: Bantam, 1984.
3. Eaker ED, Abbott RD, de Knell WB. Frequency of uncomplicated angina pectoris in type A compared with type B persons (the Framingham Study). *Am J Cardiol* 63:1042–1045, 1989.
4. Pieper C, LaCroix A, Karasek R. The relation of psychosocial dimensions on work with coronary heart disease risk factors: a meta-analysis of five United States databases. *Am J Epidemiol* 129:483–494, 1989.
5. Russek LG, King SH, Russek SJ, Russek HI. The Harvard Mastery of Stress Study—35-year follow-up: prognostic significance of patterns of psychophysiological arousal and adaptation. *Psych Med* 52:271–285, 1990.
6. Kaplan GA, Salonsen JT, Cohen RD, Brand RJ, Syme SL, Puska P. Social connections and mortality from all causes and from cardiovascular disease: prospective evidence from eastern Finland. *Am J Epidemiol* 128:370–380, 1988.
7. Williams RB, Barefoot JC, Califf RM, Haney TL, Saunders WB, Pryor DB, Hlatky MA, Siegler IC, Mark DB. Prognostic importance of social and economic resources among medically treated patients with angiographically documented coronary artery disease. *JAMA* 267:520–524, 1992.
8. Burns J, Katkin E. Psychological, situational, and gender predictors of cardiovascular reactivity to stress: a multi-variate approach. *J Behav Med* 16:445–466, 1993.
9. Burg MM, Jain D, Soufer R, Kerns RD, Zaret BL. Role of behavioral and psychological factors in mental stress-induced silent left ventricular dysfunction in coronary artery disease. *J Am Coll Cardiol* 22:440–448, 1993.
10. Boltwood MD, Taylor CB, Burke MB, Grogin H, Giacomini J. Anger report predicts coronary artery basal motor response to mental stress in atherosclerotic segments. *Am J Cardiol* 72:1361–1365, 1993.
11. Siegman AW. Cardiovascular consequences of expressing, experiencing, and repressing anger. *J Behav Med* 16:539–570, 1993.
12. Frasure-Smith N, Lesperance F, Talajic M. Depression following myocardial infarction: impact of six-month survival. *JAMA* 270:1819–1825, 1993.
13. Oleson O, Kristensen T. Impact of work environment on cardiovascular diseases in Denmark. *J Epidemiol Commun Health* 45:4–10, 1991.
14. Appels A, Schouten E. Burnout as a risk factor for coronary heart disease. *Behav Med* 17:53–59, 1991.
15. Verrier RL, Dickerson LW. Autonomic nervous system and coronary blood flow changes related to emotional activation and sleep. *Circulation* 83(Suppl 2):81–89, 1991.
16. Coumel P, Leenhardt A. Mental activity, adrenergic modulation, and cardiac arrhythmias in patients with heart disease. *Circulation* 83(Suppl 2):58–70, 1991.
17. Raab W, Stark E, MacMillan WH, Gigee WR. Sympathetic origin and anti-adrenergic prevention of stress-induced myocardial lesions. *Am J Cardiol* 8:203–211, 1961.
18. Light KC, Koepke JP, Obrist PA, Willis PW 4th. Psychological stress induces sodium and fluid retention in men at high risk for hypertension. *Science* 220:429–431, 1983.
19. Naesh O, Haedersdal C, Hindberg I, Trap-Jensen J. Platelet activation in mental stress. *Clin Physiol* 13:299–307, 1993.
20. Grignani G, Soffiantino F, Zucchella M, Pacchiarini L, Tacconi F, Bonomi E, Pastoris A, Sbaffi A, Fratino P, Tavazzi L. Platelet activation by emotional stress in patients with coronary artery disease. *Circulation* 83(Suppl 2):128–136, 1991.
21. Rozanski A, Krantz DS, Bairey CN. Ventricular responses to mental stress testing in patients with coronary artery disease. *Circulation* 83(Suppl 2):37–44, 1991.
22. Davis A, Natelson B. Brain-heart interactions: neurocardiology of arrhythmia and sudden death. *Tex Heart Inst J* 20:158–169, 1993.
23. Eliot RS, Buell JC, Dembroski TM. Biobehavioral perspectives on coronary heart disease, hypertension and sudden cardiac death. *Acta Med Scand* 660 (Suppl):203–213, 1982.
24. Dimsdale LE, Herd JA. Variability of plasma lipids in response to emotional arousal. *Psych Med* 44:413–430, 1982.
25. Osler W. Angina pectoris. *Lancet* :697–702, 1910.
26. Engel G. Psychologic stress, vasodepressor (vasovagal) syncope, and sudden death. *Ann Intern Med* 89:403–412, 1978.
27. Lown B, Verrier R, Rabinowitz S. Neuro and psychologic mechanisms and the problem of sudden cardiac death. *Am J Cardiol* 39:890–902, 1977.
28. Trauner M, Giang W, Blumenthal J. Prognostic significance of silent myocardial ischemia. *Ann Behav Med* 16:24–34, 1994.

29. Miller P, Light K, Bragdon E. Beta-endorphin response to exercise and mental stress in patients with ischemic heart disease. *J Psych Res* 37:455–465, 1993.
30. Schwartz PJ, Zaza A, Locati E, Moss AJ. Stress and sudden death: the case of the long QT syndrome. *Circulation* 83(Suppl 2):71–80, 1991.
31. Yeung AC, Vekshtein VI, Krantz DS, Vita JA, Ryan TJ Jr, Ganz P, Selwyn AP. The effect of atherosclerosis on the vasomotor response of coronary arteries in mental stress. *N Engl J Med* 325:1551–1556, 1991.
32. Lambert CR, Pepine CJ. Coronary artery spasm. *Hosp Med* 28:29–42, 1992.
33. Tofler GH, Stone PH, Maclure M, Edelman E, Davis VG, Robertson T, Antman EM, Muller JE. Analysis of possible triggers of acute myocardial infarction (the Milis study). *Am J Cardiol* 6:22–27, 1990.
34. Clarkson TB. Personality, gender, and coronary artery atherosclerosis of monkeys. *Arteriosclerosis* 7:1–8, 1987.
35. Burker EJ, Fredrikson M, Rifai N, Siegel W, Blumenthal JA. Serum lipids, neuroendocrine, and cardiovascular responses to stress in men and women with mild hypertension. *Behav Med* 19:155–161, 1994.
36. Krantz DS, Helmers KF, Bariey CM. Cardiovascular reactivity and mental stress-induced myocardial ischemia in patients with coronary artery disease. *Psych Med* 53:1–12, 1991.
37. Williams RB, Jr, Suarez EC, Kuehn DM, Zimmerman EA, Schanberg SM. Behavioral basis of coronary prone behavior in middle-aged men. Part I: evidence for chronic SNS activation in type A's. *Psych Med* 53:517–527, 1991.
38. Cardillo C, De Felice F, Campia U, Folli G. Psychophysiological reactivity and cardiac end-organ changes in whitecoat hypertension. *Hypertension* 21:836–844, 1993.
39. Boone JB, Probst MM, Rogers MW, Berger R. Postexercise hypotension reduces cardiovascular responses to stress. *J Hypertens* 11:449–453, 1993.
40. Calhoun DA, Mutinga ML, Collins AS, Wyss JM, Oparil S. Normotensive blacks have heightened sympathetic response to cold pressor test. *Hypertension* 22:801–805, 1993.
41. Ballard M, Cummings E, Larkin K. Emotional and cardiovascular responses to adults' angry behavior and to challenging tasks in children of hypertensive and normal tensive parents. *Child Devel* 64:500–515, 1993.
42. Davies R, Linden W, Habibi H. Relative importance of psychologic traits and severity of ischemia in causing angina during treadmill exercise. *J Am Coll Cardiol* 21:331–336, 1993.
43. Eliot RS. Detection and management of brain-heart interrelations. *J Am Coll Cardiol* 4:1101–1105, 1988.
44. Pagani M, Mazzuero G, Ferrari A, Liberati D, Cerutti S, Vaitl D, Tavazzi L, Malliani A. Sympathovagal interaction during mental stress. *Circulation* 83(Suppl 2):43–51, 1991.
45. Clayter R. Stress reactivity: Hemodynamic adjustments in trained and untrained humans. *Med Sci Sports Exerc* 23: 873–881, 1991.
46. Sothmann M, Hart B, Horn T. Plasma catecholamine response to acute psychological stress in humans: Relation to aerobic fitness and exercise testing. *Med Sci Sports Exerc* 23:860–867, 1991.
47. De Geus E, Van Doonen L, Orlebeke J. Regular exercise and aerobic fitness in relation to psychological make-up and physiological stress reactivity. *Psych Med* 55:347–363, 1993.
48. Hull E, Young S, Ziegler M. Aerobic fitness affects cardiovascular and catecholamine responses to stressors. *Psychophysiology* 21:353–362, 1984.
49. Sime W. Psychological benefits of exercise. *Adv Inst Adv Health* 1:15–29, 1984.
50. Light KC, Obrist PA, James SA, Strogatz DS. Cardiovascular responses to stress: II relationships to aerobic exercise patterns. *Psychophysiology* 24:79–85, 1987.
51. Sime, W. Guidelines for Exercise Therapy. In: Van Raalts J, Brewer B, eds. *Exploring Sport and Exercise Psychology.* American Washington, DC: Psychological Association, 1996: 257–274.
52. DeVries H, Hams G. Electromyographic comparison of single dose of exercise and meprobamate as to effects on muscular relaxation. *Am J Phys Med* 51:130–141, 1972.
53. Sime W. Acute relief of emotional stress. *Proceedings of the American Association for the Advancement Q Tension Control.* Blacksburg, VA: University Publications, 1978.
54. Sime WE. Discussion: Exercise, fitness, and mental health. In: *Exercise Fitness and Health.* Bouchard C, Shephard RJ, Stephens T, Sutton JR, McPherson BD, eds. Champaign, IL: Human Kinetics, 1990:627–633.
55. Dienstbier RA. Behavioral correlates of sympathoadrenal reactivity: the toughness model. *Med Sci Sports Exerc* 23: 846–852, 1991.
56. Sothman MS, Hart BA, Horn TS. Plasma catecholamine response to acute psychological stress in humans: Relation to aerobic fitness and exercise training. *Med Sci Sports Exerc* 23:860–867, 1991.
57. Cacioppo JT, Rourke PA, Marshall-Goodell BS, Tassinary LG, Baron RS. Rudimentary physiological effects of mere observation. *Psychophysiology* 27:177–185, 1990.
58. Sime WE, Whipple IT, Berkson DM, MacIntyre WC, Stamler J. Reproducibility of heart rate at rest and in response to submaximal treadmill and bicycle ergometric test in middle-aged men. *Med Sci Sports Exerc* 4:14–17, 1972.
59. Sime WE, Whipple IT, Berkson DM, MacIntyre WC, Stamler J. Reproducibility of heart rate at rest and in response to submaximal bicycle ergometic test in middle-aged men. *Human Biol* 47:483–492, 1975.
60. Jiang W, Hayano J, Coleman E. Relation of cardiovascular responses to mental stress and cardiac vagal activity in coronary artery disease. *Am J Cardiol* 72:551–554, 1993.
61. Vingerhoets AJ. Role of the parasympathetic division of the autonomic neurons system in stress and the emotions. *Int J Psych* 32:28–32, 1985.
62. Sime WE, Buell JC, Eliot RS. Psychophysiological (emotional) stress testing for assessing coronary risk. *J Cardiovasc Pulmon Tech* Aug-Sept:27–31, 1980.
63. Eliot RS. *From Stress to Strength: How to Lighten Your Load and Save Your Life.* New York: Bantam, 1994.
64. Wilson MF, Sung BH, Pincomb GA, Lovallo WR. Simultaneous measurement of stroke volume by impedance cardiography and nuclear ventriculography: comparisons at rest and exercise. *Ann Biomed Eng* 17:475–82, 1989.
65. Morales-Balljo H, Eliot R, Boone JL. Psychophysiological stress testing as a predictor of mean daily blood pressure. *Am Heart J* 116:673–681, 1988.
66. Shiffer F, Hartley LH, Schulman CL, Abelmann WH. The quiz electrocardiogram: a new diagnostic and research

technique for evaluating the relation between emotional stress and ischemic heart disease. *Am J Cardiol* 37:41–47, 1976.

67. Brod J, Fencl V, Hejl Z, Jirka J. Circulatory changes underlying blood pressure elevation during acute emotional stress (mental arithmetic) in normotensive and hypertensive subjects. *Clin Sci* 18:269–279, 1959.
68. Williams RB, Jr, Lane JD, Kuhn CM, Melosh W, White AD, Schanberg SM. Type A behavior and elevated physiological and neuroendocrine responses to cognitive tasks. *Science* 218:483–484, 1982.
69. Hines EA, Brown GE. The cold pressor test for measuring the reactibility of blood pressure: data concerning 571 normal and hypertensive subjects. *Am Heart J* 11:1–9, 1936.
70. Lovallo W. The cold pressor test and autonomic function: a review and integration. *Psychophysiology* 12:268–282, 1975.
71. de Champlain J, Petrovich M, Gonzalez M, Lebeau R, Nadeau R. Abnormal cardiovascular reactivity in borderline and mild essential hypertension. *Circulation* 18(Suppl 2): 22–28, 1991.
72. Sime WE, Buell JC, Eliot RS. Cardiovascular responses to emotional stress (quiz interview) in post-myocardial infarction patients and matched control subjects. *J Human Stress* 6:39–46, 1980.
73. DeBusk R, Taylor C, Agras W. Comparison of treadmill exercise testing and psychologic stress testing soon after myocardial infarction. *Am J Cardiol* 43:907–912, 1979.
74. Berman P, Johnson H. A psychophysiological assessment battery. *Biofeedback Self Regul* 10:203–221, 1985.
75. Jacobs SC, Friedman R, Parker JD, Tofler GH, Jimenez AH, Muller JE, Benson H, Stone PH. Use of skin conductance change during mental stress testing as an index of autonomic arousal in cardiovascular research. *Am Heart J* 128: 1170–1177, 1994.
76. Wilson MF, Sung BH, Pincomb GA, Lovallo WR. Simultaneous measurement of stroke volume by impedance cardiography and nuclear ventriculography: comparisons at rest and exercise. *Ann Biomed Eng* 17:475–482, 1989.
77. Zotti AM, Bettinardi O, Soffiantino F, Tavazzi L, Steptoe A. Psychophysiological stress testing in post infarction patients: psychological correlates of cardiovascular arousal and abnormal cardiac responses. *Circulation* 81(Suppl 2): 25–35, 1991.
78. Steptoe A, Vögele C. Methodology of mental stress testing in cardiovascular research. *Circulation* 83(Suppl 2):14–24, 1991.
79. Speccia G, Falcone C, Traversi E, La-Rovere MT, Guasti L, De Micheli G, Ardissino D, De-Servi S. Mental stress as a provocative test in patients with various clinical syndromes of coronary heart disease. *Circulation* 83(Suppl 2):108–114, 1991.
80. Carrol D, Turner JR, Rogers S. Heart rate and oxygen consumption during mental arithmetic, video game, and graded static exercise. *J Psychophysiol* 24:112–121, 1987.
81. Sims J, Carrol D. Cardiovascular and metabolic activity at rest and during and physical challenge in normal tenses and subjects with mildly elevated blood pressure. *Psychophysiology* 27:149–160, 1990.
82. Raymer KF. Stress management education: defining the knowledge base. *Dissert Abstr Int* 1991.

81, 82, 230
277, 278, 280

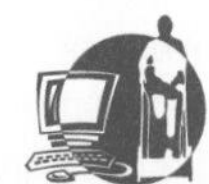

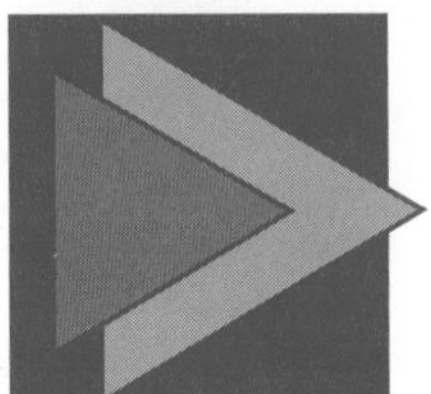

CHAPTER 6

Integration of Lifestyle Behaviors

Patricia M. Smith and C. Barr Taylor

The focus of this chapter is to describe the findings of large multifactor risk reduction trials that integrate two or more interventions for risk reduction in one trial (i.e., sedentary lifestyle, smoking, hypertension, hyperlipidemia, and obesity). Multiple risk factor reduction is important because the adverse effect of several risk factors is cumulative and many of the risk factors are interrelated.

MULTIFACTOR RISK REDUCTION: PRIMARY PREVENTION

Multifactor risk factor reduction for primary prevention originated in the 1970s with the Multiple Risk Factor Intervention Trial (MRFIT). MRFIT was a multi-site study that focused on the simultaneous reduction of smoking, blood pressure, and blood cholesterol levels (1). Until MRFIT, interventions designed to improve risk factors tended to focus on a single risk factor (i.e., smoking cessation or hypertension or lowering blood cholesterol). The premise behind MRFIT was that simultaneous reduction of several risk factors would result in maximum risk factor change and significant reduction in cardiovascular disease (CVD) mortality, nonfatal myocardial infarction (MI), coronary heart disease (CHD) mortality, and all-cause mortality over a 6-year period (1).

MRFIT included over 12,000 men identified as high risk for CHD. The men were randomized to either special intervention or to usual sources of health care. The intervention in MRFIT was multi-component in design, delivered by a multi-disciplinary team, and featured multiple follow-up contact. The overriding theoretical model of MRFIT followed a social learning theory model (2). The intervention was group-based and included various behavior modification techniques (e.g., self-monitoring, goal setting, stimulus control of the environment, systematic desensitization and relaxation, support systems, feedback). The intervention components were interactive and included role-playing, group discussions, food preparation demonstrations, and potluck dinners. Delivery of the intervention was enhanced by generous use of media materials such as films, cassettes, advertising displays, shopping guides, pamphlets, and cookbooks. Family participation was encouraged. Hypertensive medications were prescribed as required.

The historical perspectives, development of the intervention model and protocol, and a summary of the 4-year results of MRFIT have been presented (3). After 4 years, MRFIT evidenced significant changes in the three risk factors, although the changes fell substantially short of the goals (3). MRFIT also demonstrated that multifactor risk reduction could reduce CHD mortality in patients free of CHD at baseline. By the 10.5 year follow-up, mortality rates were 10.6% lower for the intervention group compared to usual care (4).

Since MRFIT was completed, a number of other primary prevention trials, some occurring in worksites, others at the community level, have focused on primary prevention of CVD. The implications of some of these more well-known trials are reviewed by Miettinen and Strandberg (5). These authors remain optimistic about the usefulness of multiple risk factor reduction for CVD prevention although the results of primary prevention trials have been inconsistent. Most notably, prevention has not been consistently obtained even when risk factors have been significantly improved, and differences in risk factor levels between intervention and control group are often diminished after varying periods of follow-up.

MULTIFACTOR RISK REDUCTION: SECONDARY PREVENTION

The remainder of this chapter focuses on multifactor risk reduction trials for secondary prevention, that is, in patients with established CVD. Six clinic-based, randomized controlled trials that targeted at least two risk factors with behavioral interventions (e.g., exercise, diet, smoking cessation) were selected for discussion (5–10). Because the details of multifactor trials are not presented in a consistent format across studies, it can be difficult to ascertain the components and procedures of the interventions in a way that allows for critical examination and replication of methods, and to determine what knowledge, skills, and abilities are required to carry them out. Thus, a series of tables are presented within the chapter that summarize the information. The discussion is divided into the various components of multifactor lifestyle risk reduction.

Investigational Designs

The studies included for discussion were randomized, controlled trials of patients with CVD (Table 6.1). Although most of these studies were multi-disciplinary, the trials originated in medical centers and, in most cases, were led by physicians. Half of the trials offered drug therapy as one of the main intervention components (6, 10, 11). Behavioral interventions for diet and exercise were offered in all studies, and smoking cessation, stress management, and psychosocial interventions were offered in some but not all of the trials (6, 8–11). With one exception, the trials were clinic-based (8). The one program that was not clinic-based involved only an educational mail-out program. The most stringent behavioral intervention featured a strict vegetarian diet, stress management, exercise, psychosocial intervention, and no lipid-lowering drugs (9). Usual care patients in all of the trials received medical care under the direction of their primary care physician. Usual care did allow for medication for hypertension and hyperlipidemia, lifestyle risk factor modification advice, and psychosocial intervention for conditions such as depression. For the purpose of data collection, usual care patients in all but one study were also offered annual medical examinations at which time various tests and evaluations regarding risk factor reduction were administered and feedback of results were provided to the patients and their physicians (8).

The primary outcomes measured varied across the multifactor trials. They included self-reported adherence to the behavioral regimes, changes in depression or psychosocial functioning, physiological changes including functional capacity, biochemically-confirmed smoking status, serum lipid levels, blood pressure, angiograms to determine regression and progression of atherosclerosis, and morbidity and mortality. Across studies, intervention patients had significantly greater changes in most physiological measures than did usual care patients, providing support for the efficacy of the various interventions. The information provided in the tables summarizes the assessment of the behavioral components of the trials. The original articles provide information on other primary outcomes.

Behavioral Prescriptions

The prescriptions of diet, exercise, and psychosocial interventions varied across the studies. In all but one trial, exercise prescription was based on the results of a treadmill test (8). The range of intensity prescribed was 50% to 85% of age-adjusted maximum heart rate, duration was 30 to 60 minutes a session for a total of 2 to 3 hr/week, and frequency was 2 to 5 days/week.

The prescription for the dietary component was based on low fat (< 20% calories/day), low cholesterol (< 5 to 200 mg/day), and high complex carbohydrates (65% to 75%). Protein intake, when specified, was 15% to 20% of calories/day. Alcohol and caffeine restrictions and dietary supplements were the exception rather than the rule (6, 9). Whereas some studies did not identify the underlying premise of the diet component, other studies specified the use of diet plans such as the one in the National Cholesterol Education Program and American Heart Association (6, 7, 9–11). The most stringent study prescribed a strict low fat, vegetarian diet (no animal products except egg white and one cup per day of non-fat milk or yogurt) (9).

Complete abstinence was the prescription for the smoking interventions. Counseling ranged from educational information only to individualized stop-smoking and relapse prevention programs provided by psychologists and specially trained nurses (6, 8, 11). The most detailed program described offered multiple telephone follow-up calls to augment the counseling session and provided a good variety of take-home materials (videotape, workbook, audiotape). Nicotine therapy was reserved for highly addicted patients (11).

Only two studies specified the psychosocial prescription. In one study, patients attended group sessions for social support with a clinical psychologist twice per week for 4 hours, but the length of continued contact was not specified (9). The patients in this study were also prescribed stress management techniques for 1 hour per day. The other study offered five group therapy sessions over the one year study (7). Considering that participants in CVD risk reduction programs were not specifically seeking psychosocial interventions for their physical conditions, factors that need to be considered include the motivation, comfort level and philosophy of the participant regarding psychotherapy and ability to get to a therapy session. Dropout from psychotherapy may be a problem and ways to enhance compliance should be considered when developing an intervention program (12).

Study Length and Follow-up

The length of the intervention and follow-up are important aspects of any program because measurable changes in risk factors take time. Although the interven-

Table 6.1. General Design of Multifactor Risk Reduction Trials

Trial	Population	Selection Criteria and Primary Target	Intervention Length and Follow-up	Provider	Theoretical Model
WHO 10-year Follow-up Hämäläinen *et al.*, 1989 Finland	*N* = 375 (SI = 188, UC = 187) *Males:* 80% *Average age* = 54 yr	*Criteria:* Consecutive non-selected patients treated in-hospital for acute MI *Target:* Secondary prevention post-AMI	*Length:* Intensive contact for 3 months, close contact for 3 years *Follow-up:* 1,2,3,6 & 10 years	Multidisciplinary–internist, social worker, psychologist, dietitian, physiotherapist	Medical model of optimal medical care & medication as needed. Education for smoking, diet, & psychosocial.
Schuler *et al.*, 1992 Germany	*N* = 113 (SI=56 UC=57) *Males:* 100% *Average age* = 53.5 yr	*Criteria:* Stable angina pectoris *Target:* Stop progression of CAD	*Length:* 3 weeks on a hospital metabolic ward, 1 year home-based *Follow-up*: 1 year	Multidisciplinary (not specified)	Educational & psychotherapeutic. Medication as indicated. No lipid-lowering drugs.
Heller *et al.*, 1993 Australia	*N* = 450 (SI=213 UC=237) *Males:* 76% *Average age* = 58.5 yr	*Criteria:* Suspected AMI *Target:* Secondary prevention; increase quality of life	*Length:* 6 months *Follow-up:* 6 months	Not specified	Educational mail-out program
The Lifestyle Heart Trial, Ornish *et al.*, 1990 United States	*N* = 48 (SI=28 UC=20) *Males:* 88% *Average age* = 56–60 yr	*Criteria:* Angiographically documented CAD *Target:* Stop progression of CAD	*Length:* 1 wk residential retreat, 1 yr home-based program *Follow-up:* 1 year	Multidisciplinary–stress management & exercise instructor, counsellors, nurses, chefs, physicians	Non-medical adjuncts to conventional treatment (vegetarian diet, exercise, meditation, stretching, relaxation & breathing) No lipid-lowering drugs.
The Stanford Coronary Risk Intervention Project (SCRIP), Haskell *et al.*, 1994 United States	*N* = 300 (SI=145 UC=155) *Males:* 86% *Average age* = 56 yr	*Criteria:* Angiographically defined coronary atherosclerosis *Target:* Reduce rate of progression of coronary atherosclerosis	*Length:* 4 years *Follow-up:* 4 years	Multidisciplinary–nurse, dietitian, psychologist, physician. Managed by SCRIP staff in co-op with private physician	Physician-supervised nurse case manager, medication as indicated. Combined social learning theory & medical model
MULTIFIT (see Table 3) DeBusk *et al.*, 1994 United States	*N* = 585 (SI=293 UC=292) *Males:* 79% *Average age* = 57 yr	*Criteria:* Hospitalized for AMI *Target:* Secondary prevention and disease management	*Length:* 6–12 months *Follow-up:* 6 months	Multidisciplinary–nurse, psychiatrist, cardiologist, lipid specialist, and nutritionist	Physician-supervised, nurse case manager, lipid-lowering medication. Social learning theory, relapse prevention, & education.

CAD–Coronary artery disease, MI–myocardial infarction, AMI–acute MI, SI–special intervention, UC–usual care.

tions often last for one year, the trend is to front-end load the intervention for the first few months after recruitment, often with multiple follow-up and clinic visits. The patient is then expected to continue the behavioral regimes at home with lessened supervision during the remainder of the study.

The WHO trial offered the most extended program–the intervention itself lasted for 3 years (5, 13). All but one of the trials had a minimum of a 1-year follow-up to the intervention (8). One of the studies extended the follow-up to 4 years with annual follow-up and another followed participants for 10 years (6, 10). The paradox is that, although time is needed to evidence change in risk factors, the rate of risk factor change seems to slow with time and attenuation of many of the early differences between the intervention and usual care groups occurs. Although this slowing of risk factor change could be due to regression to the mean, it is most likely due to lack of continued maintenance to the behavioral regimes. The pattern of behavior change is believed to cycle and result in relapse many times before the habit is successfully integrated.

The success of any program depends on long-term adherence and efforts need to be made to build adherence interventions into the programs (14). The lesson to be gained from these studies is that, although the length of intervention was probably determined more from clinical experience and other goals unique to the project (funding), intensive multifactor risk reduction cannot be achieved without frequent visits, spread over at least a year.

Provider

All but one study, involved a multi-disciplinary team which included a nutritionist/dietitian for the diet component, a clinical psychologist or nurse for the stress reduction and smoking cessation components, and a physician for medications and treadmill testing (8). Physical therapists and exercise physiologists were used for exercise testing, prescription, and supervision. Nurses (or unspecified staff members of the research team) who worked in cooperation with the primary care physician were employed to monitor or manage patients, track medication requirements and symptoms and refer to other medical personnel as necessary (10, 11). The use of multiple health care providers with a broad base of skills and knowledge is critical for success. A multi-disciplinary, multi-component system also requires an infrastructure to ensure that patient needs are met, that patients are moved smoothly through the various components of the program, and that they are not lost to follow-up.

Theory

The importance of psychological theory lies in its ability to elucidate the underlying biopsychosocial mechanisms involved in change and that it can be used to determine what components of the intervention are most effective in bringing about change (15). Only two studies clearly stated that they followed social-learning theory (2, 10, 11). Interventions based on social learning theory strive to build self-efficacy in order to effectively change behavior. The medical model involving optimal medical care, physician activation, and medication dominated in most studies.

Many of the behavioral interventions themselves, however, have antecedents in psychological theory of behavior modification, although these were not specified. One study used non-medical adjuncts to conventional treatment as the guiding principle (e.g., strict vegetarian diet and relaxation) (9). This program was based on literature that indicates the relaxation response and a vegetarian diet may reduce CVD risk factors such as hypertension and hypercholesterolemia. Health education appeared to be an unspecified underlying theoretical approach to a number of interventions. Although health education is important to decrease knowledge deficits, research to substantiate the relationship between health knowledge and health behavior change and maintenance is lacking.

In general, it is evident that multifactor risk reduction programs should follow a theoretical model. This model allows not only for replication across trials, but also provides insight as to the underlying mechanisms of behavior change and provides information that can be used to fine-tune interventions. Social learning theory remains the most comprehensive model.

Behavioral Interventions

Exercise and diet were the two behavior interventions that all studies used. The programs for diet and exercise are found in Tables 6.2 and 6.3. Interventions for smoking cessation were included in most studies, although the interventions were only well-specified for two studies (6, 8–11). Interventions for psychosocial problems involved either group or individual psychotherapy and focused on adaptation to life after a cardiac event (5–8). Topics discussed in therapy included return to work, perceptions of physical ability, anxiety and depression, communication skills, home and work relationships, and strategies for maintaining adherence to risk factor changes. Stress was treated as a separate entity in one study and treatment involved stretching exercises, breathing techniques, meditation, progressive relaxation, and imagery (9). Unfortunately, these studies do not provide sufficient information about the best sequencing or combinations of behaviors to be intervened upon. A variety of different sequencing strategies appear to be effective.

Components of the Behavioral Interventions

The major components included in the interventions were evaluation and assessment, health education, individual or group counseling, relapse prevention and maintenance strategies, optimal medical care, prescribed behavioral goals and regimes, antihypertensive, antiarrhythmic, and lipid-lowering medication, frequent contact with multiple health care providers, and medical examinations. Multiple component interventions featuring multiple follow-up contacts by multiple health care providers were generally found to be the most effective in changing health behaviors such as smoking cessation (16). Because different people change in different ways, the provision of different opportunities and techniques of change should be considered for programs. Thus, there is evidence that multi-component programs are generally more effective than single component programs. The studies presented here, however, do not elucidate the most effective components for changing targeted behaviors and outcomes.

Setting

A number of different settings were used in these trials (outpatient clinics, home-based, hospital metabolic ward, and a residential retreat at a hotel), but all in-

Table 6.2. **Exercise**

TRIAL	COMPONENTS	SETTING	PRESCRIPTION	MEDIA/DELIVERY	EVALUATION
WHO 10-year Follow-up Hämäläinen *et al.*, 1989 Finland	Individually tailored, light exercise. Exercise supervised in Turku, advised only in Helsinki.	Clinic & home	Intensity determined by cycle ergometer test. Details not specified.		Adherence & physical working capacity measured at 1,2,3,6, & 10 yr. post-AMI
Schuler *et al.*, 1992 Germany	Intensive group training. Daily home exercise on cycle ergometer. Group information sessions 5×/yr for patients & spouses.	Initial 3 wks in a hospital metabolic ward. Clinic for group exercise. Home-based for daily exercise.	60 min. 2×/wk (group) with 30 min./day (individual) at 75% MHR	Information & training in-hospital, group sessions for exercise & information, exercise log book	Exercise testing at baseline & 1 year; attendance at group, & daily adherence (log book) at baseline, 3 wk, 3, 6, & 12 mo.
Heller *et al.*, 1993 Australia	Walking program advised by mailout, monthly newsletter reinforcing benefits of exercise	Home-based		4 monthly newsletters, information on "Walking for Pleasure" groups, magnetic reminder sticker, calls	6 mo. self-report questionnaire on exercise performance
The Lifestyle Heart Trial, Ornish *et al.*, 1990 United States	Treadmill testing, moderate aerobic exercise, choice of exercise	Initial 1 wk residential retreat then home-based	50–80% HR, minimum 30 min./session, total 3 hr/wk for 1 year		Questionnaire on type, frequency & duration at baseline & 1 year.
The Stanford Coronary Risk Intervention Project (SCRIP), Haskell *et al.*, 1994 United States	Verbal & written goals and instructions to increase daily activity and exercise endurance	Clinic-based Home-based		Verbal & written goals and instructions. Progress tracked by mail & phone	7-day physical activity recall; progress tracked by phone & mail; progress reports by mail; clinic visits 2–3 mo.
MULTIFIT (see Table 3) DeBusk *et al.*, 1994 United States	Treadmill testing, aerobic exercise (choice of brisk walking, jogging, bicycling, & swimming)	Clinic for treadmill Home-based exercise	60–85% PHR 30 min/day, 5 days/wk; after 4 wks, 100% PHR or 85% age-predicted MHR	Portable HR monitor to regulate training intensity during first 8 wks	Treadmill in-hospital & 3–6 wk post-MI; phone follow/up at 2 wks & monthly; functional capacity at 6 mo.

HR–heart rate, MHR–maximum HR, PHR–peak HR during treadmill, MI–myocardial infarction, AMI–acute MI. Some studies differentiate prescription by patient's heart condition.

volved some clinic involvement (6–11). Most settings for the interventions encompassed a combination of clinic and home-based programs. Treadmill testing and educational, nutritional, psychosocial, and smoking cessation counseling at a clinic were common and patients carried out the exercise and diet regimen at home.

The relative benefit of using only mail and telephone contact that was used in one study is not clear given the lack of significant findings across endpoints in this study (8). The advantage of mail and telephone contact is that the patient does not have to visit the clinic, which enhances the convenience of the intervention and lowers the cost of delivery. The relative benefits of a more intensive residential program used in two studies also remains unclear (7, 8). The advantage of a residential program is control over diet and exercise without contamination of non-compliance with prescribed regimens. Such information may help elucidate more precisely the impact of lifestyle modification on risk factor profile. Adherence to behavior change after the initial residential component, however, remains a problem (as it does in all other approaches) and providing meals to patients is not equivalent to prescribing diets to individuals who must do their own food shopping and preparation. Moreover, residential programs are potentially more costly and perhaps not as feasible as outpatient

Table 6.3. Diet

TRIAL	COMPONENTS	SETTING	PRESCRIPTION	MEDIA	EVALUATION
WHO 10-year Follow-up Hämäläinen *et al.*, 1989 Finland	Health education, nutrition classes, and individual counseling	Clinic	Reduce total fat, sat. fat, salt, coffee, & energy level if needed. Avoid dietary cholesterol, sugar, big meals & alcohol. Increase polyunsaturated fat, fiber vitamins & minerals.		
Schuler *et al.*, 1992 Germany	AHA diet Phase 3. In-hospital teaching. Group info sessions 5×/yr for pts & spouses.	Initial 3 wks in a hospital metabolic ward, then home-based	< 20% fat, < 200 mg chol, 15% protein, 65% carbs, polyunsaturated: saturated fat > 1.0	AHA diet Phase 3 guidelines	24 hr. dietary protocol at baseline, 3 wks, 3,6,9, & 12 mo.
Heller *et al.*, 1993 Australia	3 mailouts, fat reduction targets, behavioral contracts, letters of encouragement, low fat products info & recipes, knowledge quiz phoneline	Home-based		Phone calls, handouts, letters of encouragement, behavioral contracts, monthly newsletters	6 mo. self-report questionnaire on fat intake
The Lifestyle Heart Trial, Ornish *et al.*, 1990 United States	Strict low-fat vegetarian	Initial 1 wk residential retreat then home-based	10% fat, 15–20% protein, 70–75% complex carbs, alcohol limited to 2 units/day, no caffeine, B_{12} suppl		3-day diet diary at baseline & 1 year.
The Stanford Coronary Risk Intervention Project (SCRIP), Haskell *et al.*, 1994 United States	Individualized low-fat & low cholesterol diet. Instruction & record review at clinic. Verbal & written goals.	Clinic and home-based	< 20% fat, < 6% saturated fats, < 75 mg cholesterol/day	Verbal & written goals and instructions. Progress tracked by mail and phone	4-day food records; progress tracked by phone & mail; progress reports by mail; clinic visits every 2–3 mo.
MULTIFIT (Multifactorial Intervention Trial) DeBusk *et al.*, 1994 United States	Low cholesterol & saturated fat, nutritional counseling, progress reports, prioritized dietary goals, relapse prevention, strategies for dietary maintenance	Home-based	National Cholesterol Education Project Step 2 diet	Nutrition workbook; computer-generated progress reports based on a food frequency questionnaire (FFQ). Progress tracked by phone & mail.	FFQ in-hospital, 6, 11, 26 wks after admission; reports mailed to pt. within 48–72 hr after FFQ received; questionnaire-6 & 12 mo.

programs in terms of dissemination, although that has yet to be determined. It is clear that multifactor risk reduction can be done in a variety of settings. However, no studies have been conducted which compare one setting to another relative to efficacy, dissemination, and cost-effectiveness.

Multimedia Approaches for Intervention Delivery

Unfortunately, the type and extent of multimedia approaches were not well specified in most studies. Multimedia presentations are most effective if used in a proactive, interactive fashion (17). Many well-designed multimedia materials are available from agencies such as the National Cancer Institute, National Heart, Lung, and Blood Institute, and the American Heart Association. Multimedia approaches may include information/educational pamphlets, workbooks, video and audiotapes, telephone follow-up, and a personalized, computer-generated series of nutrition guidelines. The most innovative multimedia approach was the use of a personalized, computer-generated series of nutrition guidelines (11). Telephone follow-up contact, which is effective, cost-effective, and convenient for patients because they do not have to make multiple clinic visits, was under-used in most studies. One study focused all of its effort on a mailing and telephone program and had no face-to-face contact except at baseline and 6-month follow-up (8). The authors in that study were very explicit as to the multimedia approach used and included information on the source of their materials and the stepped procedure used for delivery. It is important to carefully consider how media can be used most effectively. Multimedia presentations should be used in an interactive, on-going fashion rather than in a one-time, non-interactive manner.

Evaluation

Evaluation refers to the behavioral component of the intervention only and does not apply to other endpoints such as change in lipid profiles. The method of evaluation was primarily self-report for exercise, diet, smoking adherence, exercise diaries, biochemical verification of smoking status, food frequency questionnaires, and psychosocial questionnaires. The most inconsistent type of assessments were dietary questionnaires ranging from 24 hour recall to 6 month recall. Psychosocial evaluation was not common and follow-up measurement was only specified in two studies (7, 8). The evaluation of compliance remains an important issue in health behavior change. Standardized measurement should be carefully considered not only for internal validity but also to permit comparisons of results across studies.

LIMITATIONS AND FUTURE DIRECTIONS OF MULTIFACTOR RISK REDUCTION

Cost-effectiveness

With the advent of managed care, the cost-effectiveness of multifactor risk reduction has become an important consideration. However, none of these studies provide that data. The cost-effectiveness of individual risk factor reduction (e.g., smoking cessation) has been established and is especially impressive when compared to more invasive and costly medical procedures (18). Using a health care provider, such as a nurse, for managing patients can be a cost-effective method for preventing dropout and enhancing adherence (11, 14). Cost-effectiveness and resource allocation have become important concerns today at worksites and in health care systems and will gain increasing attention in the future (19).

Generalization

Other questions remain regarding multifactor risk reduction programs. For example, to whom do they apply? The majority of trials have focused on white males with little known about the efficacy and effectiveness of such trials with females and other ethnic groups.

Acceptance

The acceptance of multifactor risk reduction programs both in terms of the program components, as well as the convenience of participation in an intensive program is another issue in question. For example, one study prescribed a strict vegetarian diet and another required multiple clinic visits and blood draws. What is the feasibility of residential programs that take people away from family, friends, and work? Other questions relate to the use of group versus individual intervention. The group approach may be too general and time consuming and not specific enough to meet the needs of the individual. Certainly individual intervention tailoring was a strength of the SCRIP and MULTIFIT trials, yet the Lifestyle Heart Trial, which achieved equally favorable results, involved a group format for the initial residential component of the program (9–11).

Compliance and Maintenance

Compliance and long-term adherence to program components are major concerns in multifactor risk reduction programs. A major consideration of multifactor programs is not simply that the participants adopt the desired behaviors, but that they also maintain the behaviors over time. It is therefore imperative that continued attention be focused on enhancing patient compliance in multiple risk factor reduction.

Dissemination

The feasibility and practicality of multifactor risk reduction for the general population has yet to be determined. The questions of how transferable multifactor risk reduction programs are to the community and whether comprehensive lifestyle changes can be sustained in the general population of people with and without CVD remain unanswered. Although we have come a long way in understanding multifactor risk reduction and its implementation, many questions regarding dissemination still remain.

▶ SUMMARY

Many lessons have been learned since the inception of multifactor risk reduction in the 1970s, and researchers continue to refine their methods and interventions. The trials reviewed in this chapter provide some insight to the complexity of the behavioral components of multifactor risk reduction. Even though the mechanisms are unknown, studies have demonstrated that comprehensive risk factor intervention can lead to significant reduction in risk factor profiles, can reverse coronary atherosclerosis, and may impact long-term, all-cause as well as coronary morbidity and mortality. Researchers should continue to improve upon design, methods, and implementation and to expand dissemination from the research model to clinical practice and community settings. At the same time, practitioners have adequate models to allow multifactor lifestyle programs to be integrated with existing exercise programs.

References

1. Zukel WJ, Paul O, Schnaper HW. The multiple risk factor intervention trial (MRFIT): I. Historical perspectives. *Prev Med* 10:387–401, 1981.
2. Bandura A. *Social Foundations of Thought and Action: A Social Cognitive Theory.* Englewood Cliffs, NJ: Prentice-Hall, Inc., 1986.
3. Benfari RC, Sherwin R. Forum: the multiple risk factor intervention trial (MRFIT): The methods and impact of intervention over four years. *Prev Med* 10:387–553, 1981.
4. The Multiple Risk Factor Intervention Trial Research Group. Mortality rates after 10.5 years for participants in the Multiple Risk Factor Intervention Trial. *JAMA* 263: 1795–1801, 1990.
5. Miettinen TA, Strandberg TE. Implications of recent results of long-term multifactorial primary prevention of cardiovascular diseases. *Ann Intern Med* 24:85–89, 1992.
6. Hämäläinen H, Luurila OJ, Kallio V, Arstila M, Hakkila J. Long-term reduction in sudden deaths after a multifactor intervention programme in patients with myocardial infarction: 10-year results of a controlled investigation. *Eur Heart J* 10:55–62, 1989.
7. Schuler G, Hambrecht R, Schlierf G, Niebauer J, Hauer K, Neumann J, Hoberg E, Drinkman A, Bacher F, Grunze M. Regular physical exercise and low-fat diet: effects on progression of coronary artery disease. *Circulation* 86:1–11, 1992.
8. Heller RF, Knapp JC, Valenti LA, Dobson AJ. Secondary prevention after acute myocardial infarction. *Am J Cardiol* 72:759–762, 1993.
9. Ornish D, Brown SE, Scherwitz LW, Billings LW, Armstrong WT, Ports TA, McLanahan SM, Kirkeeide RL, Braud RJ, Gould KL. Can lifestyle changes reverse coronary heart disease? *Lancet* 336:129–133, 1990.
10. Haskell WL, Alderman EL, Fair JM, Maron DJ, Mackey SF, Superko HR, Williams PT, Johnstone IM, Champagne ME, Krauss RM, et al. Effects of intensive multiple risk factor reduction on coronary atherosclerosis and clinical cardiac events in men and women with coronary artery disease. *Circulation* 89:975–990, 1994.
11. DeBusk RF, Houston-Miller N, Superko HR, Dennis CA, Thomas RJ, Lew HT, Berger WE 3rd, Heller RS, Gee D, et al. A case-management system for coronary risk factor modification after acute myocardial infarction. *Ann Intern Med* 120:721–729, 1994.
12. Meichenbaum D, Turk DC. *Facilitating Treatment Adherence: A Practitioner's Guidebook.* New York: Plenum, 1987.
13. Kallio V, Hämäläinen H, Hakkila J, Luurila OJ. Reduction in sudden deaths by a multifactor intervention programme after acute myocardial infarction. *Lancet* 2(8152):1091–1094, 1979.
14. Hill MN, Houston Miller N. Compliance enhancement: a call for multidisciplinary team approaches. *Circulation* 93: 4–6, 1996.
15. Brawley LR. The practicality of using social psychological theories for exercise and health research and intervention. *J Appl Sport Psychol* 5:99–115, 1993.
16. Kottke, TE, Battista RN, DeFriese GH, Brekke ML. Attributes of successful smoking cessation interventions in medical practice: a meta-analysis of 39 controlled trials. *JAMA* 259:2882–2889, 1988.
17. Adler EW. *Print That Works: The First Step-by-step Guide That Integrates Writing, Design, and Marketing.* Palo Alto, CA: Bull Publishing Co, 1991.
18. Goldman L, Garber AM, Grover SA, Hlatky MA. Task force 6. Cost effectiveness of assessment and management of risk factors. *J Am Coll Cardiol* 27:1020–1030, 1996.
19. Jönsson B. Cost-effectiveness: a new criterion for selecting therapy. *J Intern Med* 237:1–3, 1995.

Suggested Readings

Miller NH, Taylor CB. *Lifestyle Management in Patients with Coronary Heart Disease.* Champaign, IL: Human Kinetics Publishers, 1995.

Ornish D. *Dr. Dean Ornish's Program for Reversing Heart Disease.* New York: Ballantine Books, 1990.

Watson DL, Tharp RC. *Self-directed Behavior Change.* Monterey: Brooks/Cole, 1981.

SECTION TWO

Anatomy

SECTION EDITOR: *Mark Williams, PhD, FACSM*

2 34

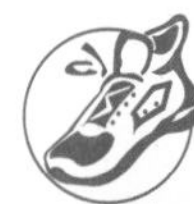

CHAPTER 7
CARDIOVASCULAR ANATOMY

Tinker D. Murray and Julie M. Murray

The cardiovascular system is a continuous, closed arrangement including a pump (the heart) and over 60,000 miles of conduits (blood vessels) (1). The primary function of the cardiovascular system is to provide an environment for the transport of nutrients and removal of waste products. The cardiovascular system assists with maintenance of homeostasis at rest and during exercise.

The cardiovascular system performs the following specific functions (2–4):

1. Transports oxygenated blood from the lungs to tissues and deoxygenated blood from the tissues to the lungs
2. Distributes nutrients (glucose, free fatty acids, amino acids, etc.) to the body's cells
3. Removes metabolic wastes (carbon dioxide, urea, lactate, etc.) from the periphery for elimination or reuse
4. Regulates pH to control acidosis and alkalosis
5. Transports hormones and enzymes to regulate physiological function
6. Maintains fluid volume to prevent dehydration
7. Maintains body temperature by absorbing and redistributing heat

The following sections provide an overview of the basic structures and functions of the heart and blood vessels.

THE HEART

The adult heart is approximately the size of a fist and weighs between 250 and 350 g (5). The heart is positioned obliquely in a space known as the mediastinum (Fig. 7.1). It is anterior to the vertebral column and posterior to the sternum. The lungs flank the heart bilaterally and slightly overlap it.

The heart has four chambers. The two superior chambers are the atria and the two inferior chambers are the ventricles. The external deep grooves of the heart (called sulci) define the boundaries of the four chambers of the heart (4, 6). The coronary sulcus separates the atria from the ventricles while the interventricular sulcus separates the left and right ventricles (LV, RV). The sulci also contain the major arteries and veins that provide circulation to the heart.

The heart has a base and an apex. The base consists mainly of the left atrium (LA), part of the right atrium (RA), and parts of the proximal portion of the large veins that enter the heart posteriorly. It is located superiorly and near the right sternal border at the level of second and third ribs. The apex of the heart is located inferiorly and to the left of the base at the level of the fifth intercostal space. Approximately two-thirds of the mass of the heart is to the left of the midsternal border. As the heart is palpated at the apex (between the fifth and sixth ribs), the contraction can be easily felt. This is referred to as the point of maximal intensity (PMI) (3).

The heart also has borders. The superior border consists of both atria and the bases of the major blood vessels. The right border is formed by the RA. The left border consists of the LV and a small part of the LA. The inferior border is formed primarily by the RV and a portion of the LV at the apex.

The heart is rotated to the left in the chest so that the anterior portion of the heart forms the sternocostal surface which consists mainly of the RA and RV. The diaphragmatic surface consists mainly of the LV where it slopes and rests on the diaphragm.

Tissue Coverings and Layers of the Heart

The heart is covered by a double-walled, loose-fitting membranous sac called the pericardium (Fig. 7.2). The outer wall of the pericardium is referred to as the parietal pericardium and has both a fibrous (tough) layer and a serous (smooth) layer. The interior wall is called the visceral pericardium or epicardium. Between the parietal and visceral layers is the pericardial cavity. The pericar-

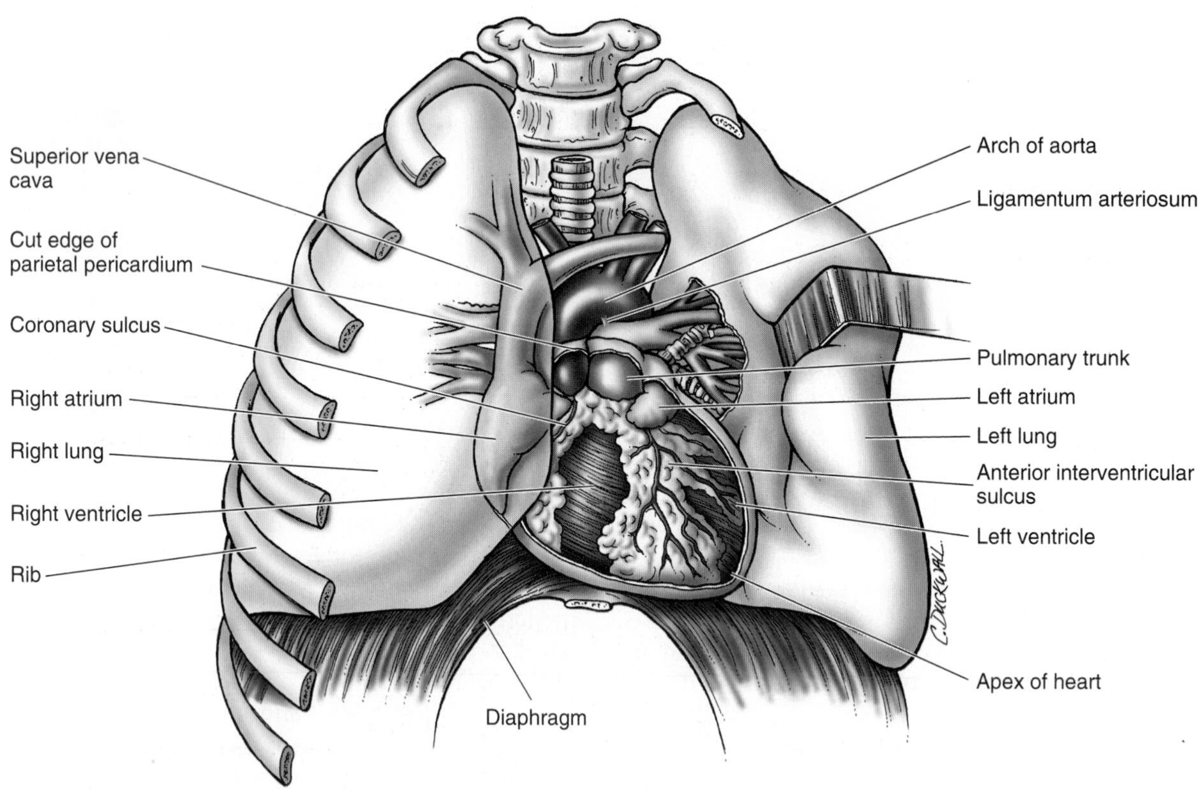

Figure 7.1. Anterior view of the thorax showing the position of the heart in the mediastinum. (With permission from Spence AP, Mason EB, eds. *Human Anatomy and Physiology.* 4th ed. St Paul, MN: West Publishing Co, 1992:595.)

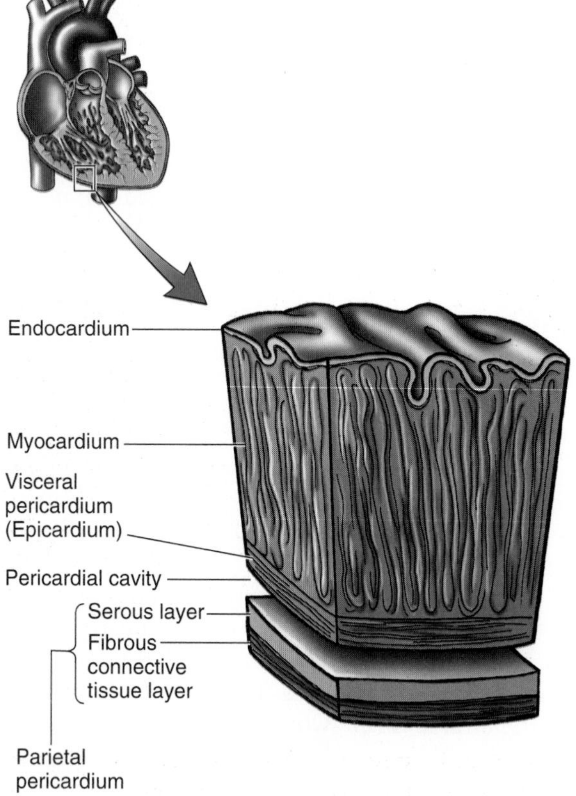

Figure 7.2. The endocardium, myocardium, and pericardium. (With permission from Spence AP, Mason EB, eds. *Human Anatomy and Physiology.* 4th ed. St Paul, MN: West Publishing Co, 1992:596.)

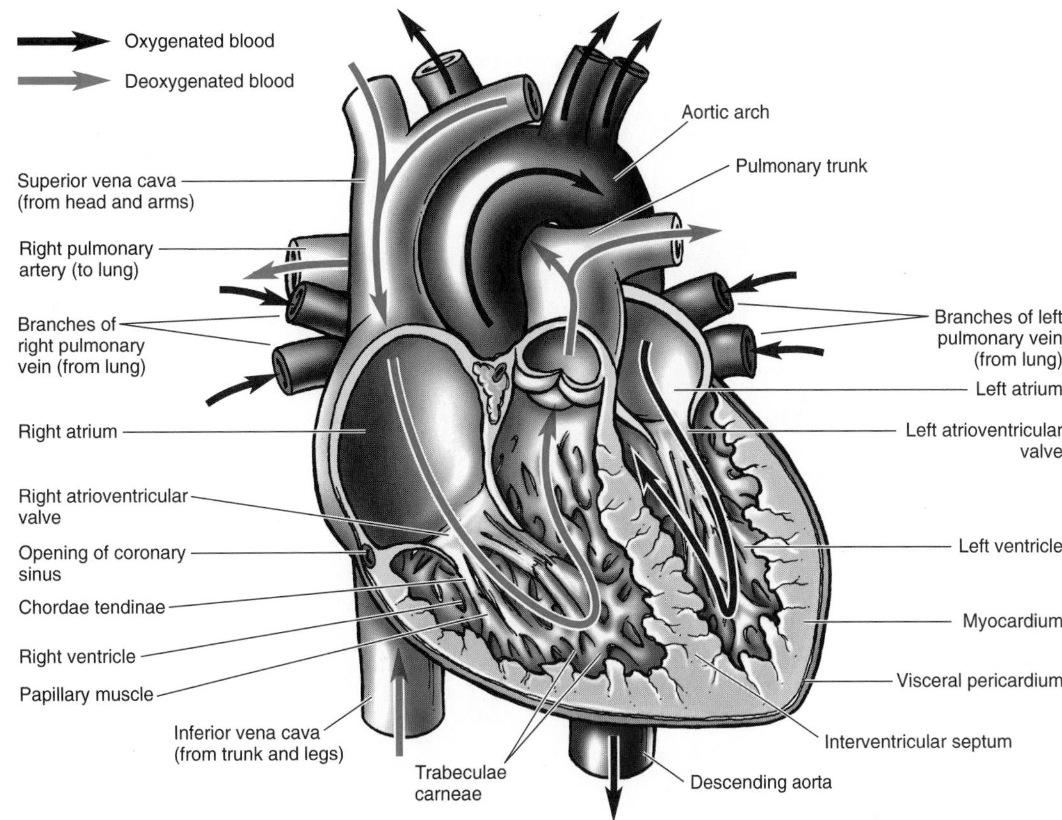

Figure 7.3. Frontal section of the heart. The *arrows* indicate the path of blood flow through the heart. (With permission from Spence AP, Mason EB, eds. *Human Anatomy and Physiology*. 4th ed. St Paul, MN: West Publishing Co, 1992:600.)

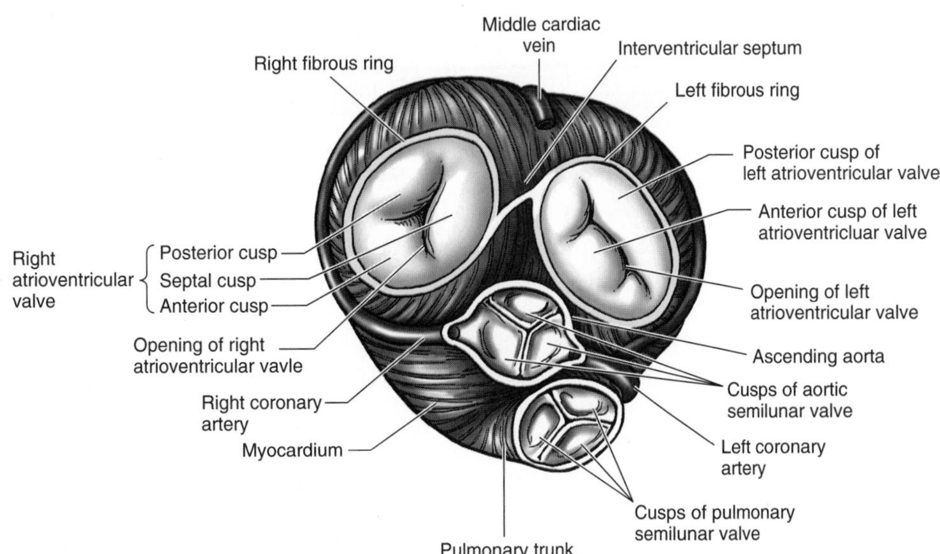

Figure 7.4. Superior view of the heart showing valve openings. (With permission from Spence AP, Mason EB, eds. *Human Anatomy and Physiology*. 4th ed. St Paul, MN: West Publishing Co, 1992:601.)

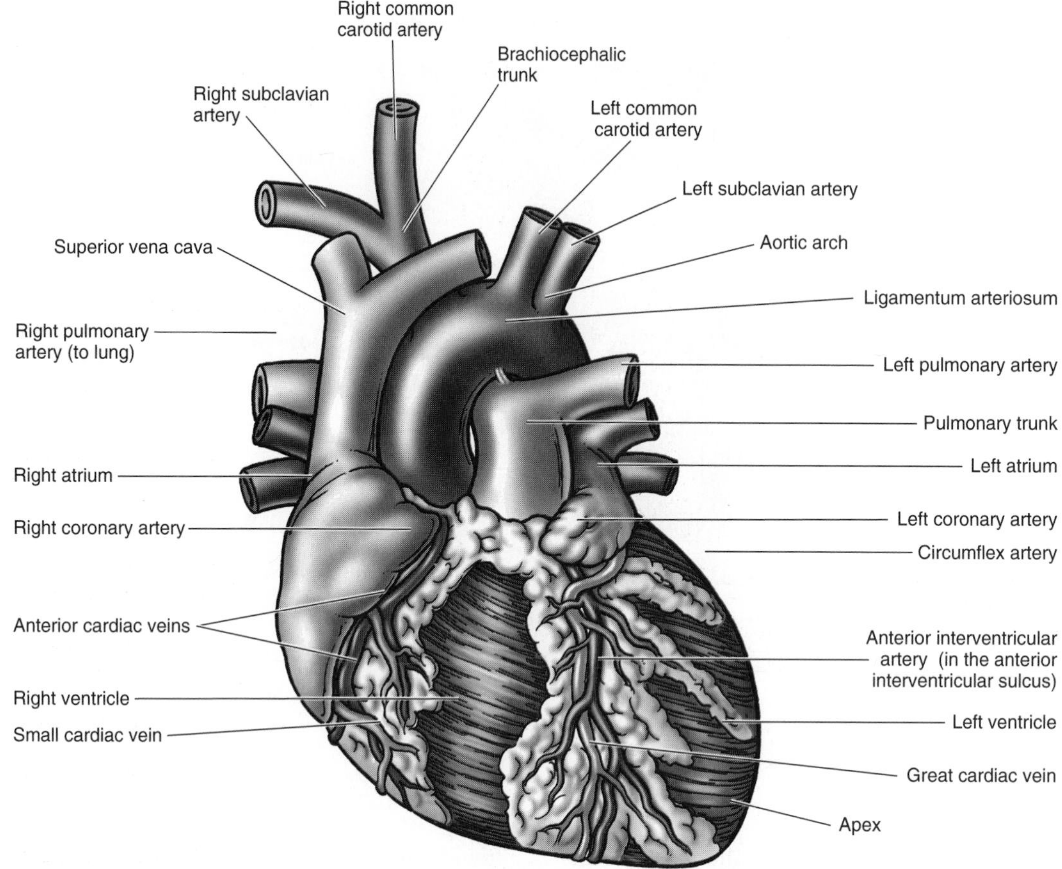

Figure 7.5. Anterior view of the heart. (With permission from Spence AP, Mason EB, eds. *Human Anatomy and Physiology.* 4th ed. St Paul, MN: West Publishing Co, 1992:598.)

dial cavity contains pericardial fluid which acts as a lubricant reducing friction between the membranes during contractions of the heart. If the pericardium becomes inflamed a condition called pericarditis can result in painful adhesions.

The thickest layer of tissue located in the heart is the myocardium or heart muscle. The myocardium is contracting, cardiac muscle. Within the myocardium is a network of crisscrossing connective tissue fibers called the fibrous skeleton. This skeleton provides support for the myocardium and the valves of the heart and provides some separation between the atria and the ventricles.

The inner layer of the myocardium is lined with a thin layer of endothelium called the endocardium. The endocardium forms the inner-most lining of the walls of the various heart chambers as well as the heart valves. The endocardium joins with the endothelial linings of the blood vessels as they leave and enter the heart (7).

Chambers, Valves, and Blood Flow of the Heart

The heart is two pumps in a single unit with four chambers or cavities (Fig. 7.3). The right heart (RA and RV) and the left heart (LA and LV) make up the two pumps. The right side of the heart collects blood from the periphery and pumps it through the lungs (pulmonary circuit). The left side of the heart collects blood from the lungs and pumps it throughout the body (systemic circuit) (8–12).

The atria of the heart are separated by the interatrial septum and the ventricles by the interventricular septum. The LV walls and interventricular septum are two to three times thicker than the RV walls. The atria are smaller in size and have thinner walls than the ventricles. The thicker myocardium of the ventricles allows the ventricles to pump blood against greater resistance to meet the demand of pumping blood through the systemic circuit. Conversely, the RV has only to pump blood a relatively short distance through the pulmonary circuit.

The heart has four valves which function to maintain unidirectional blood flow. The atrioventricular (AV) valves separate the atria from the ventricles. The semilunar valves separate the ventricles from the aorta and pulmonary artery trunk. The AV valves are named for the number of leaflets or cusps formed by the endocardium

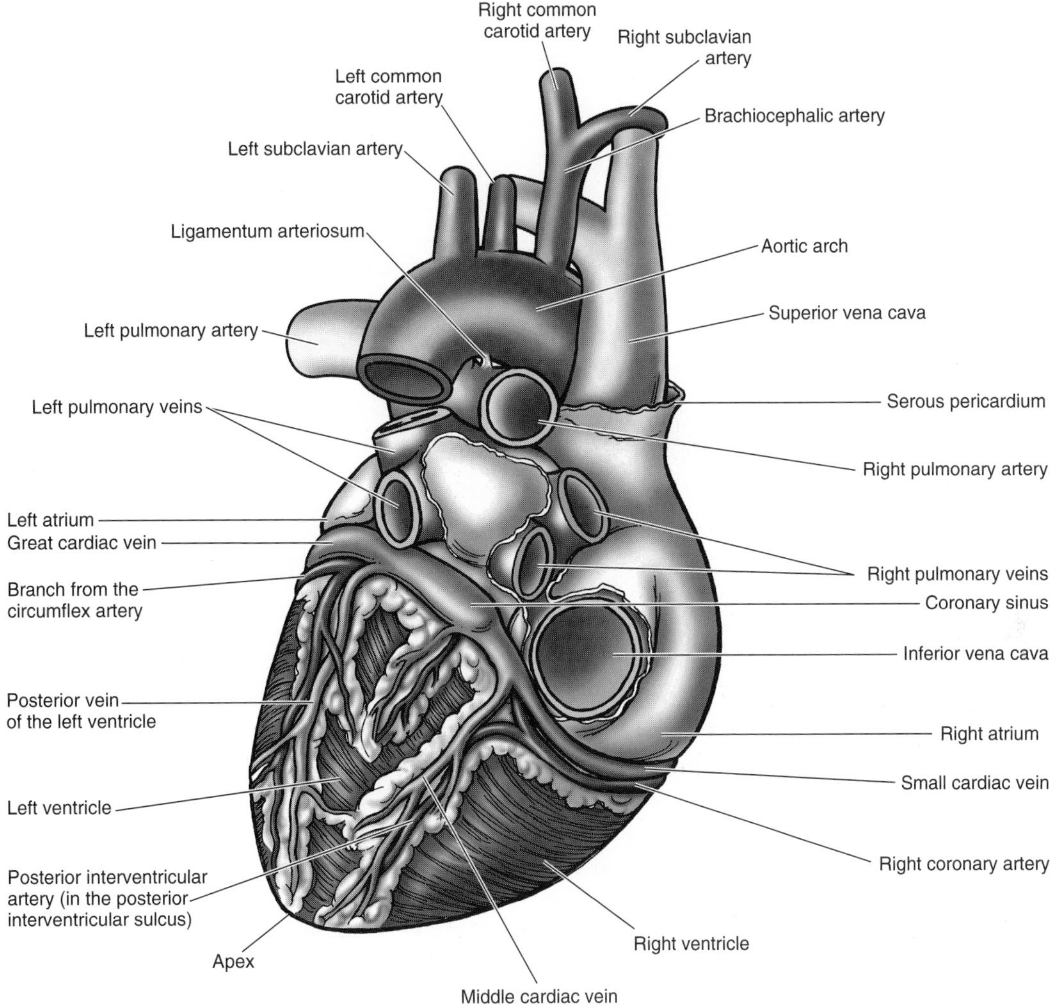

Figure 7.6. Posterior view of the heart. (With permission from Spence AP, Mason EB, eds. *Human Anatomy and Physiology*. 4th ed. St Paul, MN: West Publishing Co, 1992:599.)

(Fig. 7.4). The right AV valve has three cusps and is called the tricuspid valve, while the left AV valve has only two cusps and is called the bicuspid (or mitral) valve. The tricuspid valve controls the flow of blood from the RA to the RV, while the mitral valve controls blood between the LA and LV. The AV valves are attached to chordae tendineae (strong fibrous bands) and papillary muscles which arise from folds and ridges of the myocardium within the ventricles. The chordae tendineae and papillary muscles help open the AV valves and also prevent them from swinging back into the atria which would result in retrograde blood flow (13).

There are two semilunar valves in the heart, each with three cusps. The pulmonic valve lies between the RV and the pulmonary artery. The aortic valve is located between the LV and the aorta. The cusps of the semilunar valves prevent the flow of blood from the atria to the ventricles.

Blood flow through the heart is accomplished by the following sequence of events beginning with the return of systemic blood to the RA:

1. Deoxygenated blood flows into the RA via the superior and inferior vena cava, the coronary sinus, and anterior cardiac veins.
2. The RA free wall contracts and blood moves through the tricuspid valve into the RV.
3. The RV free wall contracts, the tricuspid valve closes, and blood flows through the pulmonic valve into the pulmonary arteries and the branches of that system.
4. Blood enters the alveolar capillaries from the pulmonary trunk where gas exchange occurs.
5. Blood flows back to the LA via the pulmonary veins.

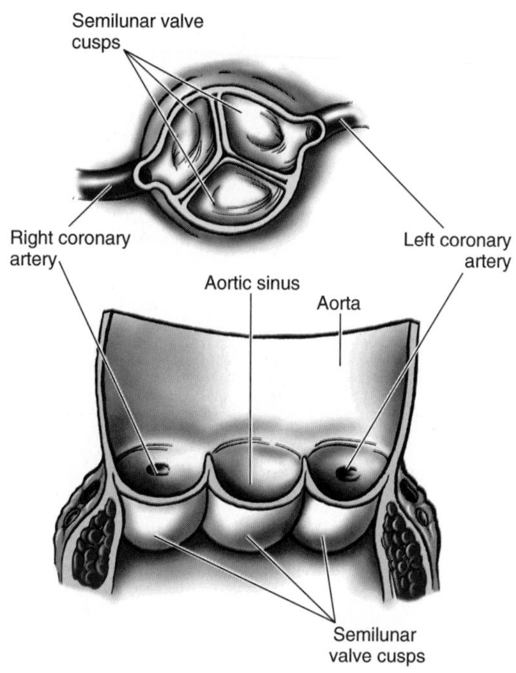

Figure 7.7. The origin of the coronary arteries. (With permission from Spence AP, Mason EB, eds. *Human Anatomy and Physiology.* 4th ed. St Paul, MN: West Publishing Co, 1992:601.)

6. The LA free wall contracts and blood flows through the mitral valve and into the LV.
7. The LV free wall contracts, the mitral valve closes and blood flows through the aortic valve into the aorta and its branches where it is distributed to the coronary circulation and the systemic circulation (13–16).

The Myocardial Blood Supply

Although the interior of the heart chambers are continuously bathed with blood, only the endocardium is nourished directly, because the myocardium is too thick for diffusion to the epicardium to occur. The functional supply of blood for the heart is provided by the coronary circulation via the left and right coronary arteries (LCA, RCA) (Figs. 7.5 and 7.6). The coronary arteries arise from the Sinus of Valsalva which is located at the base of the aorta just above the semilunar valve cusps of the aortic valve (Fig. 7.7).

The LCA angles towards the left side of the heart for about 1 to 2 centimeters before branching into the left anterior descending (LAD) coronary artery and the circumflex artery (CxA) (17). The LAD artery supplies blood to the interventricular septum and anterior walls of both ventricles. The CxA branches towards the left margin of the heart in the coronary sulcus and supplies blood to the laterodorsal walls of the LA and LV. Both the LAD artery and CxA curve around the left ventricular wall and supply small branches that interconnect (anastomose) with the RCA.

The RCA supplies blood to the right side of the heart as it follows the atrioventricular groove before curving to the back of the heart giving off a posterior interventricular artery (posterior descending artery, PDA). The RCA and PDA have numerous branches which supply blood to the anterior, posterior, and lateral surfaces of the right ventricle as well as to the right atrium.

After blood circuits the coronary artery system, which ends with myocardial capillaries, it is collected by the cardiac veins and travels a path similar to the coronary arteries, but in the opposite direction. The cardiac veins form an enlarged vessel called the coronary sinus (on the posterior aspect of the heart) which empties the blood into the RA. Some smaller anterior cardiac veins empty directly into the RA.

Electrical Activity of the Heart

Cardiac muscle has intrinsic properties that allow it to depolarize and contract without neural stimulation. Cardiac cells interconnect end to end and form intercalated discs (2). These intercalated discs allow electrical impulses to spread cell to cell and cause the myocardium to act as a single unit or functional syncytium. The components of the heart's conduction system include the sinoatrial (SA) node, the atrioventricular (AV) node, atrioventricular bundle (bundle of His), right and left bundle branches, and the Purkinje fibers (Fig. 7.8).

The electrical impulse which initiates cardiac contraction begins at the SA node or "intrinsic pacemaker" of the heart. The cells of the SA node located in the posterior wall of the right atrium depolarize spontaneously

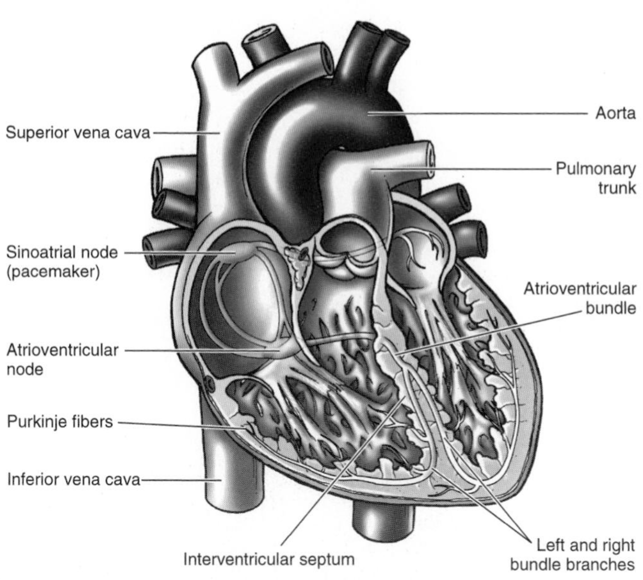

Figure 7.8. The electrical conduction system of the heart. (With permission from Spence AP, Mason EB, eds. *Human Anatomy and Physiology.* 4th ed. St Paul, MN: West Publishing Co, 1992:608.)

about 60 to 80 times per minute (18). From the SA node the electrical impulse spreads via internodal gaps through both atria until it reaches the AV node located in the inferior part of the interatrial septum. The electrical impulse is delayed at the AV node for approximately 0.13 seconds to allow the atria to contract and fill the ventricles (18). The impulse then moves rapidly through the bundle of His, through the right and left bundle branches and through the network of Purkinje fibers in the myocardium of both ventricles. This rapid conduction allows both ventricles to contract approximately at the same time.

The rate and forcefulness of heart contraction does not depend on extrinsic nerve stimulation, but rather, are influenced by extrinsic factors such as autonomic nerve control and hormone activity. Sympathetic nerves stimulate the atria and ventricles of the heart to beat faster (chronotropic effect) and more forcefully (inotropic effect). Parasympathetic nerves (vagi) control the atria and slow heart rate. Hormones like norepinephrine and epinephrine stimulate increases in heart rate and force of contraction.

THE BLOOD VESSELS

After blood flows from the heart, it enters the vascular system which is composed of numerous blood vessels. The blood vessels form a closed system to deliver blood to the tissues; to help promote the exchange of nutrients, metabolic wastes, hormones, and other substances with cells; then to return blood to the heart.

Arteries carry blood away from the heart (Fig. 7.9). Large arteries branch into smaller arteries and eventually to smaller arterioles. Arterioles branch into capillaries which allow the exchange of blood with various tissues (digestive system, liver, kidneys, etc.). On the venous side of the circulation, capillaries converge into small venules, which converge to form larger vessels called veins. The larger veins return blood to the heart.

The walls of blood vessel vary in thickness and size due to the presence or absence of one or more layers of tissues (Fig. 7.10). The tunica intima consists of the endothelium and a thin connective-tissue basement membrane. The tunica intima is the only layer common to all the blood vessels. The internal elastic lamina separates the tunica intima from the middle layer of smooth muscle fibers and elastic fibers called the tunica media. The smooth muscle fibers of the tunica media can be influenced by neural control (parasympathetic and sympathetic nerves), hormones (acetylcholine, norepineph-

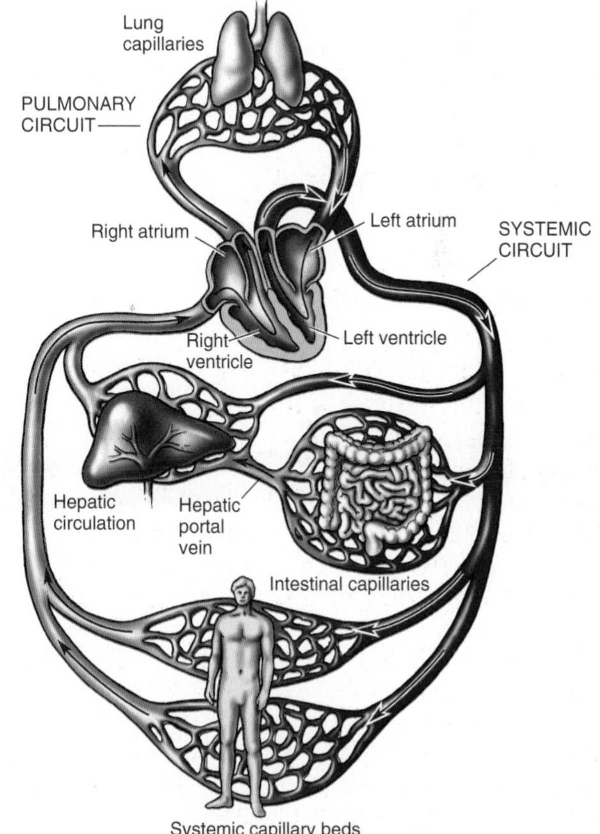

Figure 7.9. Schematic diagram of blood circulation. (With permission from Spence AP, Mason EB, eds. *Human Anatomy and Physiology.* 4th ed. St Paul, MN: West Publishing Co, 1992:604.)

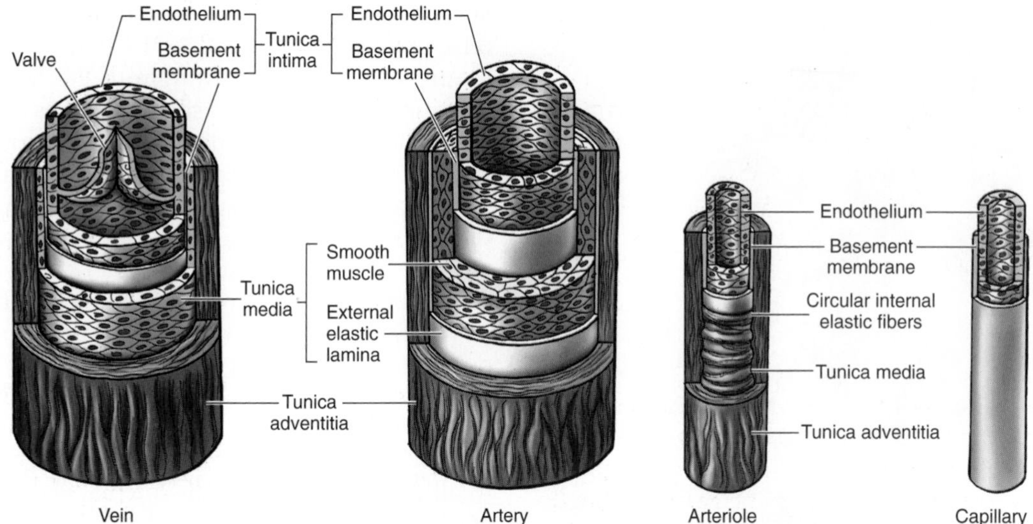

Figure 7.10. Comparison of the structure of blood vessels. (With permission from Spence AP, Mason EB, eds. *Human Anatomy and Physiology*. 4th ed. St Paul, MN: West Publishing Co, 1992:629.)

rine, epinephrine, etc.), or local factors (ph, O_2 levels, CO_2 levels, etc.) which can cause them to vasoconstrict or vasodilate. The external elastic lamina separates the tunica media from the outermost layer of connective tissue called the tunica adventitia. The adventitia helps attach vessels to surrounding tissues (4).

Arteries can be classified as elastic arteries, muscular arteries, or arterioles based on their relative size and function. Large arteries like the aorta and those of the pulmonary trunk are called elastic arteries. The tunica media of these vessels is thick and contains many elastic fibers. The elastic nature of these arteries helps maintain pressure within the vessels. Other arteries are smaller and distribute blood throughout the body. These arteries are called muscular arteries and the tunica media contains primarily smooth muscle fibers. Muscular arteries are less distensible than elastic arteries. Arterioles have lumens smaller than 0.5 mm and the tunica media is largely composed of smooth muscle with scattered elastic fibers (4). Arterioles play a major role in regulating blood flow to the capillaries due to the ability to vasoconstrict or vasodilate.

Capillaries form dense networks that branch throughout all tissues. The average capillary is 1.0 mm in length and 0.01 mm in diameter. This is just large enough for single red blood cells to pass through (3). Capillaries have extremely thin walls and are the site where the exchange of materials between blood and the interstitial fluid takes place.

Venules form from capillaries and consist mainly of tunica intima and tunica adventitia. Veins receive blood from the venules and have the same three tissue layers as arteries. However, the tunica media of the veins is

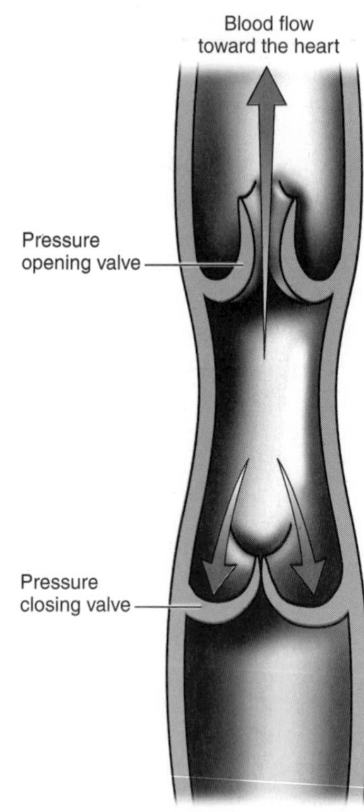

Figure 7.11. Valves of a vein. (With permission from Spence AP, Mason EB, eds. *Human Anatomy and Physiology*. 4th ed. St Paul, MN: West Publishing Co, 1992:632.)

thinner than that found in the arteries. Overall the veins are thinner and more compliant than arteries and act as blood reservoirs. The walls of some veins, such as those in the legs, contain one way valves that help maintain venous return to the heart by preventing retrograde blood flow, even under relatively low pressures (Fig. 7.11). The valves in the veins are made up of folds of tunica intima and are similar in nature to the semilunar valves of the heart.

▶ SUMMARY

In summary, the cardiovascular system is a closed system of pumps, valves and conduits which is coordinated to function both anatomically and physiologically to maintain homeostasis. In times of increased cardiovascular demands, the system functions in an even more sophisticated manner to meet those demands while it continues to attempt to maintain a homeostatic environment.

References

1. McArdle WD, Katch FI, Katch VL. *Essentials of Exercise Physiology.* Philadelphia: Lea & Febiger, 1994.
2. Martini F. *Fundamentals of Anatomy and Physiology.* Englewood Cliffs, NJ: Prentice Hall, 1989.
3. Marieb EN. *Human Anatomy and Physiology.* Redwood City, CA: Benjamin/Cummings, 1989.
4. Spence AP, Mason EB. *Human Anatomy and Physiology.* 4th ed. St Paul, MN: West Publishing, 1992.
5. Anthony CP, Thibodeau GA. *Textbook of Anatomy and Physiology.* 11th ed. St Louis, MO: C.V. Mosby, 1983.
6. Williams PL, Warwick R, Dyson M, Bannister LH, eds. *Grays Anatomy.* 37th ed. London: Churchill Livingstone, 1989.
7. Hole JW. *Essentials of Human Anatomy and Physiology.* 2nd ed. Dubuque, IA: W.C. Brown, 1986.
8. Brooks GA, Fahey TD, White TP. *Human Bioenergetics and its Applications.* 2nd ed. Mountain View, CA: Mayfield, 1996.
9. deVries HA. *Physiology of Exercise.* 4th ed. Dubuque, IA: W.C. Brown, 1986.
10. Fox EL, Bowers RW, Foss ML. *The Physiological Basis of Physical Education and Athletics.* 5th ed. Dubuque, IA: W.C. Brown, 1993.
11. McArdle WD, Katch FI, Katch VL. *Exercise Physiology, Energy, Nutrition, and Human Performance.* 3rd ed. Philadelphia: Lea & Febiger, 1991.
12. Powers SK, Howley ET. *Exercise Physiology: Theory and Application to Fitness and Performance.* 2nd ed. Madison, WI: Brown & Benchmark, 1994.
13. Hall-Craggs ECB. *Anatomy as a Basis for Clinical Medicine.* Baltimore: Williams & Wilkins, 1995.
14. Williams MA. Cardiovascular and respiratory anatomy and physiology: responses to exercise. In: Baechle TR, ed. *Essentials of Strength Training and Conditioning.* Champaign, IL: Human Kinetics, 1994.
15. Montgomery RL. *Basic Anatomy for the Health Professions.* Baltimore: Urban & Schwarzenberg, 1980.
16. Thibodeau GA. *Anatomy and Physiology.* St Louis, MO: Times Mirror/Mosby, 1987.
17. Sokolow M, McIlroy MB. *Clinical Cardiology.* 2nd ed. Los Altos, CA: Lange Medical Publishing, 1979.
18. Wilmore JH, Costill DL. *Physiology of Sport and Exercise.* Champaign, IL: Human Kinetics, 1994.

Suggested Readings

Kapit W, Elson LM. *The Anatomy Coloring Book.* 2nd ed. New York: Harper Collins, 1993.

Moore KL. *Clinically Oriented Anatomy.* 2nd ed. Baltimore: Williams & Wilkins, 1985.

Snell RS. *Clinical Anatomy for Medical Students.* 4th ed. Boston, MA: Appleton & Lange, 1992.

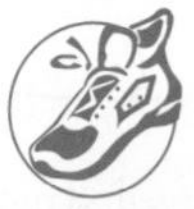

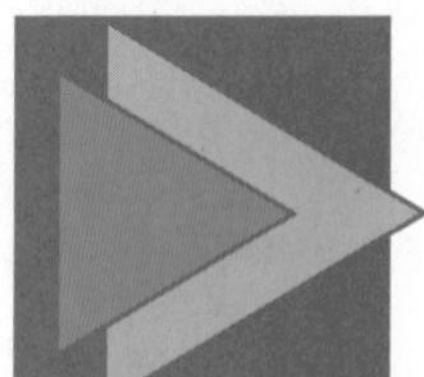

CHAPTER 8

RESPIRATORY ANATOMY

Donald A. Mahler

The objective of this chapter is to describe the basic anatomy of the respiratory system as it relates to function. Clearly, the anatomy of the respiratory system supports the basic function of exchanging carbon dioxide (CO_2), a by-product of cellular metabolism, and oxygen (O_2), which is necessary for cellular activity (1). Other important functions include production and metabolism of vasoactive substances and filtering systemic venous blood prior to entry into the left ventricle. The structural components of the respiratory system (Fig. 8.1) are the framework for the corresponding functions of the system (Table 8.1) (2, 3).

CONTROL OF BREATHING

Because respiratory muscles have no intrinsic automaticity, the control of breathing in an awake person results from the interplay of brainstem and cortical respiratory pathways (4). Automatic control structures are located in the brainstem while voluntary control structures are located in the cerebral cortex.

Automatic Control

The major regions of automatic control are the medullary center and groups of rostral pontine respiratory nuclei. The respiratory neurons in the medulla aggregate into the dorsal respiratory groups (DRG) and ventral respiratory groups (VRG). The DRG contains different types of neurons that initiate inspiration, and the phrenic nerve (which innervates the diaphragm) originates from the DRG. The VRG has various functions, including a forced expiration. The pontine respiratory nuclei act to "fine tune" breathing.

Cortical Modulation

Voluntary pathways in the cerebral cortex originate in cortical neurons with efferent projections via spinal pathways to respiratory muscles. Voluntary respiratory activities, such as breath holding, hyperventilation, coughing, singing, or speaking, can override the automatic brainstem respiratory centers. Integration between voluntary (cortical) and automatic (brainstem) respiration occurs by interconnections in the spinal cord (spinal pathways). During sleep and loss of consciousness, automatic control and feedback become dominant for respiration.

Chemoreceptors

The central chemoreceptors in the medulla are activated by changes in arterial CO_2 tension ($PaCO_2$) and pH. These receptors are normally responsible for most of the input to the DRG. At low to moderate altitude, CO_2 is the major stimulus that determines ventilation in healthy individuals. The peripheral chemoreceptors located at the bifurcation of the carotid arteries are activated by low arterial oxygen tension (PaO_2) and by increased $PaCO_2$. The peripheral chemoreceptors are important in increasing ventilation when PaO_2 decreases (i.e., at high altitudes).

Mechanoreceptors

Various sensory receptors are located in the tracheobronchial tree and transmit information via the vagal nerve to the DRG and higher respiratory centers. Pulmonary stretch receptors that are slow to adapt are located among smooth muscle cells in both intra- and extra-thoracic airways. Their predominant stimulus is lung inflation. Rapidly adapting pulmonary stretch receptors are located among airway epithelial cells primarily near the region of the carina and in the large bronchi. The major stimuli for rapidly adapting receptors are the rate of lung inflation and various types of endogenous and exogenous agents including cigarette smoke, chemicals, and noxious chemicals. Accordingly, these receptors are also known as irritant receptors. C-fiber endings are located in the pulmonary interstitial space and respond to large hyperinflation and various endogenous agents that may be produced with pulmonary congestion or inflammation. In addition, the chest wall (including dia-

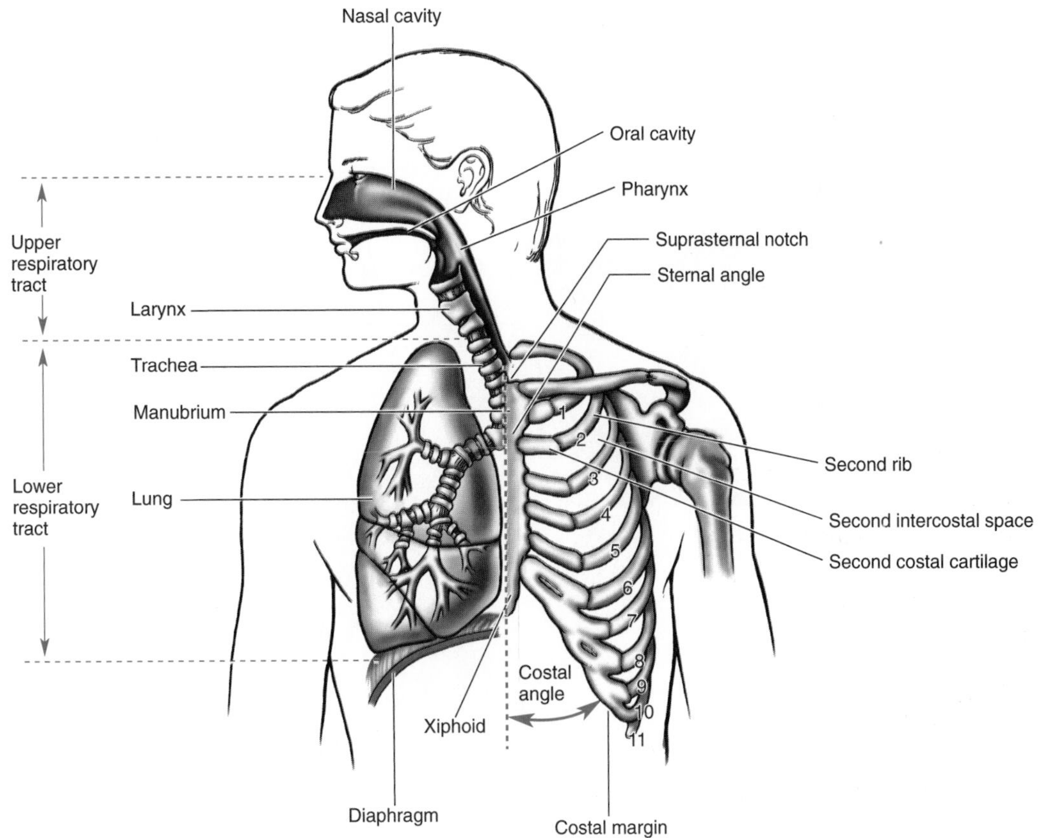

Figure 8.1. The respiratory system consists of an upper respiratory tract (nose, pharynx, and larynx) and a lower respiratory tract (tracheobronchial tree and lungs).

phragm, intercostal muscles, and ribs) contains muscle spindle receptors that detect muscle stretch and Golgi tendon organs that respond to muscle tension.

DISTRIBUTION OF VENTILATION

Ventilation of the pulmonary system is accomplished in two major divisions, the upper and lower respiratory tracts.

Upper Respiratory Tract

The upper respiratory tract includes the nose, paranasal sinuses, pharynx, and larynx (Fig. 8.2), and acts as a conduction pathway for the movement of air into the respiratory tract. The purpose of these structures is to purify, warm, and humidify ambient air before it reaches the gas exchange units. During normal, quiet breathing inspired air is heated to body temperature and the relative humidity is increased to over 90% during passage through the nose. The pharynx is divided by the soft palate into the nasopharynx and the oropharynx. The epiglottis, located at the base of the tongue, protects the laryngeal opening during swallowing. The larynx contains the vocal cords, which contribute to speech and participate in coughing.

Table 8.1. Structural Components of the Respiratory Tract and Their Corresponding Function

Structural Components	Function
Respiratory center Peripheral chemoreceptors Afferent and efferent nerves	Control of breathing
Upper respiratory tract Conducting airways Respiratory bronchioles	Distribution of ventilation
Chest wall, respiratory muscles, and pleura	Ventilatory pump
Pulmonary arteries, capillaries, and veins	Distribution of blood flow
Functional respiratory unit	Gas exchange
Mucociliary escalator	Bronchial clearance
Alveolar macrophages Lymphatic drainage	Lung clearance and defense

Receptors throughout the upper respiratory tract may initiate a cough response. Coughing is produced by closure of the vocal cords along with contraction of the expiratory muscles to create increased intrathoracic pressures. With sudden opening of the vocal cords the positive airway pressure forces air carrying possible mu-

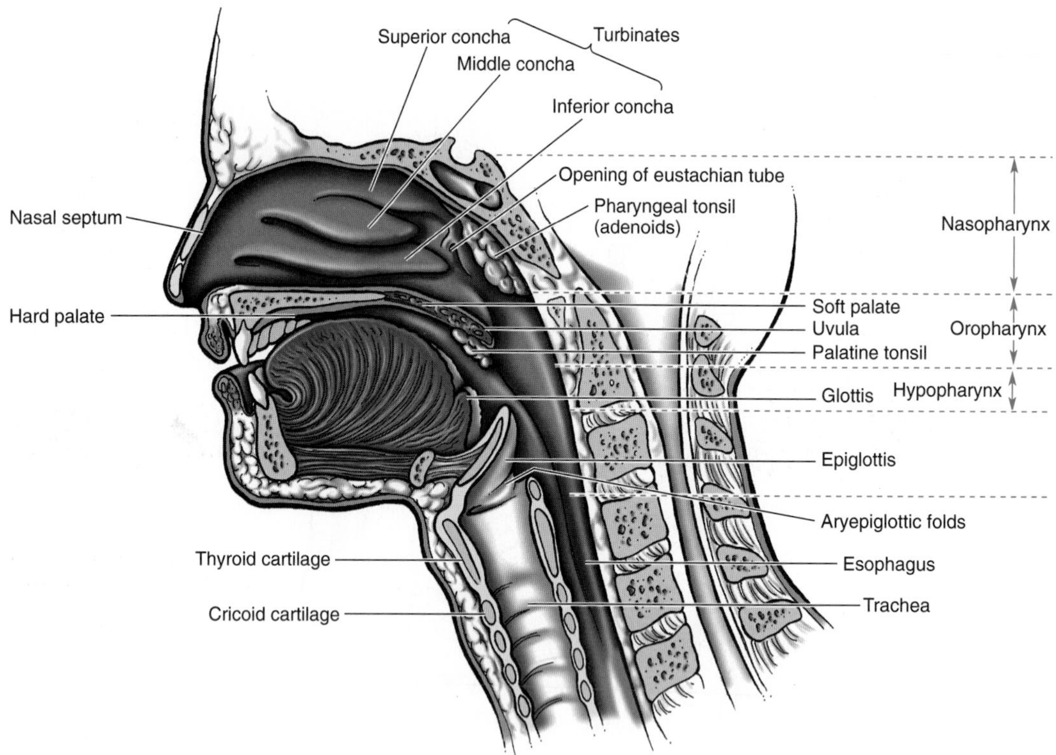

Figure 8.2. Structures of the upper respiratory tract.

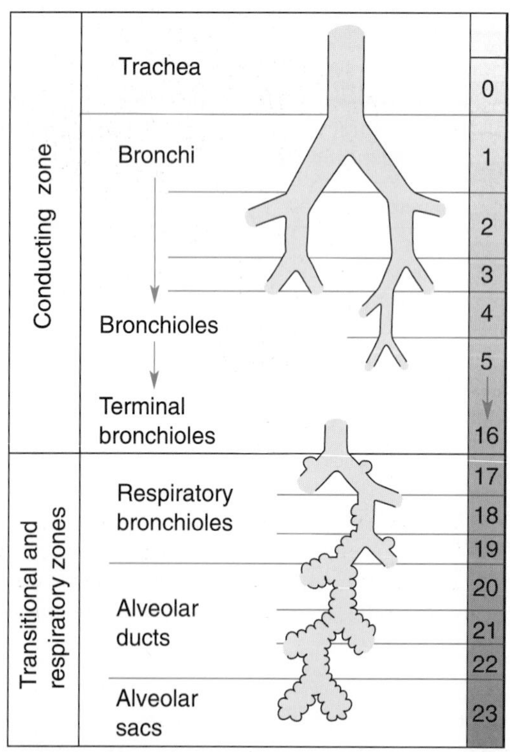

Figure 8.3. Branching of the airways starting from the trachea to the alveolar sacs. There are approximately 23 generations of branching in the tracheobronchial tree.

cus or particles from the tracheobronchial tree into the atmosphere. A cough can move gas from the lung at a rate of 10 L/sec during the expulsion phase.

Lower Respiratory Tract

The lower respiratory tract begins in the trachea just below the larynx and includes bronchi, bronchioles, and alveoli (Fig. 8.3). There are approximately 23 generations of airways; the first 16 are conducting airways and the last 7 are respiratory airways ending blindly in approximately 300 million alveoli which form the gas exchange surface. The structural components of the airways coincide with their functional properties. For example, the volume of the conducting zone is approximately 1 ml of air per pound of body weight and does not contribute to gas exchange; whereas those areas where gas exchange occurs occupy a proportionately greater volume in the lungs.

The **trachea** begins at the base of the neck and extends about 10 to 12 cm to the main carina where it divides into right and left main bronchi. It is located anterior to the esophagus. The trachea consists of a series of anterior horseshoe-shaped cartilaginous rings and a posterior longitudinal muscle bundle.

The major **bronchi** contain cartilage that maintains airway patency as well as large numbers of mucus glands that produce secretions in response to irritation, infection, and/or inflammation. Irritant receptors, which probably have C-fiber endings, are located in large air-

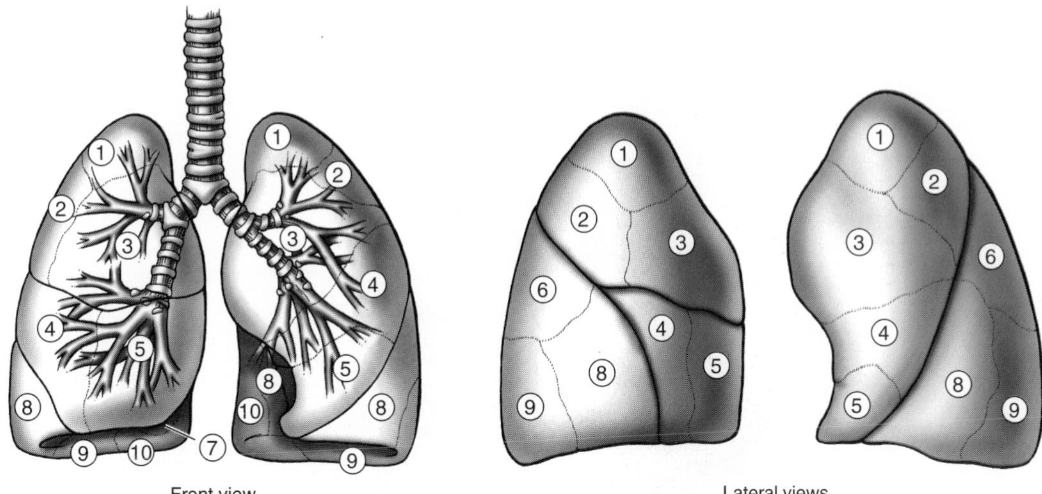

Figure 8.4. Structure of the tracheobronchial tree with corresponding lung segments which originate from segmental bronchi. The right upper lobe contains segments 1–3, the right middle lobe contains segments 4 and 5, and the right lower lobe contains segments 6–10. The left upper lobe contains segments 1–5, and the left lower lobe contains segments 6–10.

way and initiate the cough reflex. The right main bronchus divides into three lobar bronchi (upper, middle, and lower). The left main bronchus divides into two lobar bronchi (upper and lower) (Fig. 8.4). The lobes are separated by fissures (two layers of visceral pleura). The lobar bronchi divide into segmental bronchi and segments, 10 on the right and 10 on the left. Columnar cells line the epithelium (inner lining) of the bronchi and consist predominantly of ciliated cells that contain motile cilia which move or beat in a coordinated manner to move the mucus layer toward the mouth ("mucociliary escalator") (Fig. 8.5). The columnar epithelium is an important barrier for lung defense. Goblet cells are interspersed among the ciliated cells and secrete mucus.

Segmental bronchi bifurcate further until the terminal bronchiole, which has a diameter of about 1 mm. Beyond the terminal bronchiole are respiratory bronchioles, alveolar ducts, and the alveoli (Fig. 8.3). Air flows through the conducting airways and, at the level of the alveolar ducts and alveoli, movement of air or gas is by diffusion. Transition of the epithelium to squamous cells in alveoli is important to facilitate gas exchange.

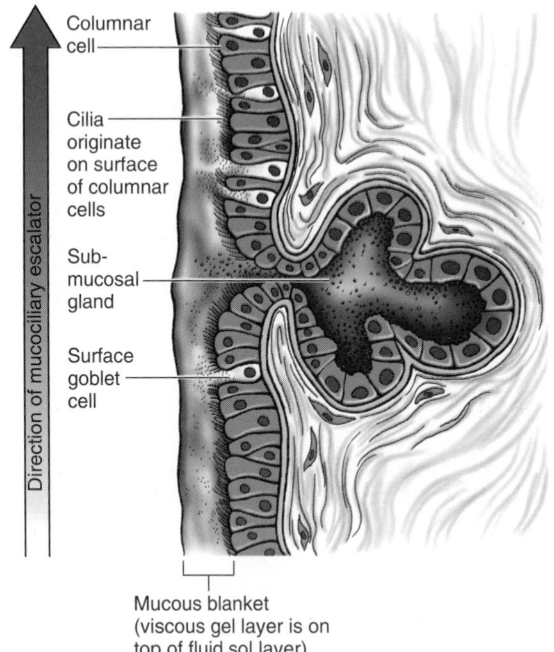

Figure 8.5. Epithelial surface of the bronchial wall contain cilia (fine hair structures which beat in a coordinated manner), columnar cells, goblet cells (which secrete mucus), and mucus (which consists of a viscous gel layer and a fluid sol layer).

VENTILATORY PUMP

The ventilatory pump consists of the chest wall, the respiratory muscles, and the pleural space (Figs. 8.6 and 8.7).

Chest Wall

The chest wall includes muscles of respiration (primarily intercostal muscles) and bones (primarily the spine, ribs, and sternum). The ribs are hinged on the spine by ligaments and cartilage so that the ribs move upward and outward during inspiration, and downward and inward during expiration. The hinging movement results in a change in thoracic volume. At rest and at the end of a normal expiration the elastic properties of the

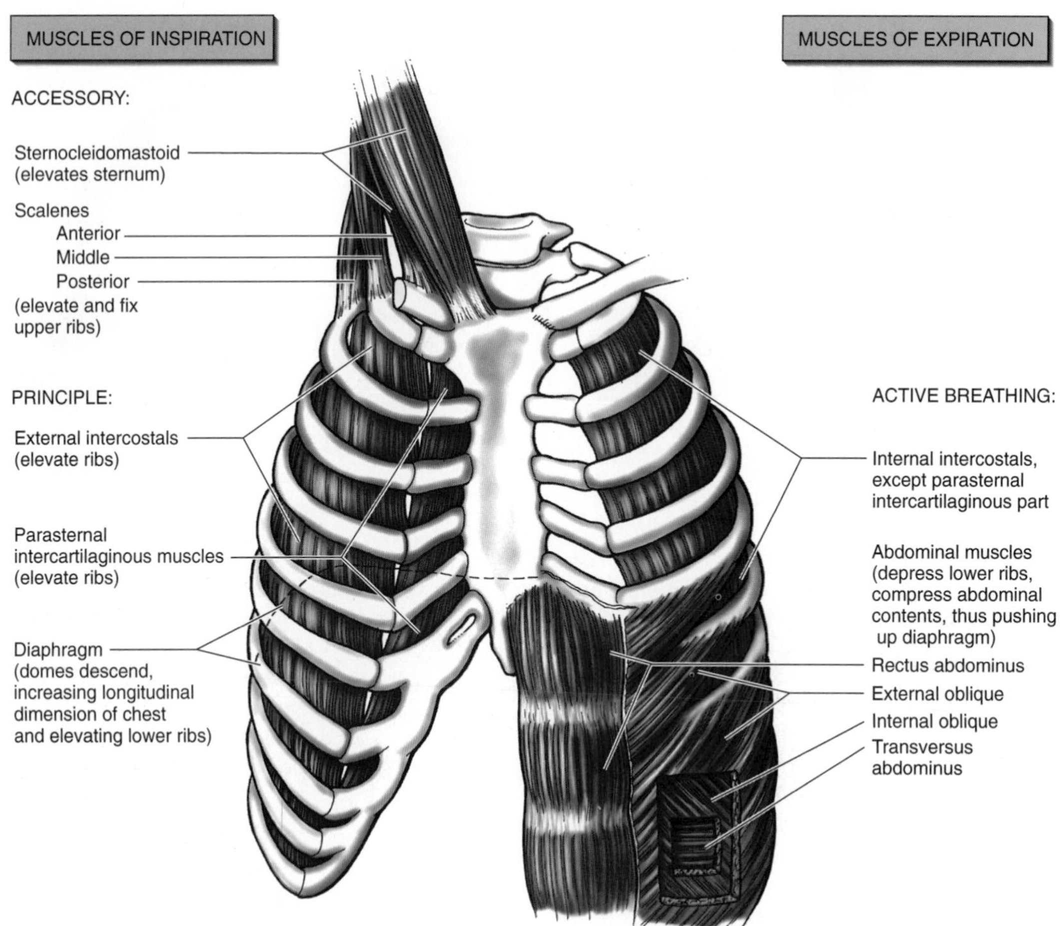

Figure 8.6. Diagram of the major muscles of respiration. The principal inspiratory muscles are illustrated on the left and include the diaphragm, external intercostals, and the parasternal muscles. The principal expiratory muscles are shown on the right and include the internal intercostals and the abdominal muscles (rectus, transversus, and internal/external obliques).

chest wall exert an outward (expansion) force, whereas the elastic properties of the lung parenchyma exert an inward (recoil) force. Inspiration (air flow into the lungs) occurs by activation of the respiratory muscles, particularly the diaphragm, which creates a more negative pressure in the pleural space and the lungs. Air enters the lung until the intrapulmonary gas pressure equals atmospheric pressure. During expiration, when the respiratory muscles relax, air flows from the lung into the atmosphere because of the positive pressure generated by the elastic recoil of the lungs.

Respiratory Muscles

The muscles of respiration are the only skeletal muscles essential to life. The muscles of inspiration and expiration are illustrated in Figure 8.6. The diaphragm, the major muscle of inspiration, is innervated by the phrenic nerve, which originates from the third to fifth cervical spinal segments. Spinal cord transection due to injury at or above this level compromises respiratory muscle function and consequently ventilation.

The diaphragm consists of a flat crural portion and vertical-oriented muscles called the costal portion. The diaphragm functions as a piston with contraction/relaxation of the vertical muscle fibers. With contraction, the crural portion (or dome) moves downward and displaces the abdominal contents so that the abdomen moves outward as does the chest wall. Expiration is normally passive under quiet breathing due to elastic recoil of the lung and requires no work. However, during active breathing when ventilatory requirements are increased (e.g., exercise) the muscles of expiration are recruited. The major muscles of expiration are the internal intercostals and the abdominal muscles (rectus abdominus, external and internal oblique, and transverse abdominus).

In patients with airflow obstruction (e.g., acute bronchoconstriction in asthma or emphysema), there is hyperinflation of the lungs which stretches the lung tissue (and leads to additional elastic recoil) and forces the crural portion of the diaphragm downward, thus shortening the vertically-oriented muscle fibers. This result places the diaphragm at a mechanical disadvantage because of the altered length-tension relationship.

Pleura

The visceral (inner layer) and parietal (outer layer) pleura are each a thin membrane located between the lung and the chest wall and converge at the lung hila (Fig. 8.7) (5). The intrapleural space is located between the visceral and parietal pleura and contains a small amount of fluid. As the pleural space is airtight, and the chest wall and lung tissue pull against each other across the pleural space, a negative pressure is produced at rest. During inspiration both the visceral and parietal pleura expand outward while more negative pressure develops in the pleural space.

Air can enter the pleural space (i.e., pneumothorax) by spontaneous rupture of a subpleural bleb or by trauma to the chest wall (e.g., a fractured rib with penetration of the parietal pleura). With a pneumothorax the lungs collapse while the chest wall expands due to intrinsic elastic properties. The parietal pleura contains abundant pain fibers and irritation of this membrane by a pneumothorax or inflammation produces localized chest pain exacerbated by motion of the pleura (e.g., a deep inspiration).

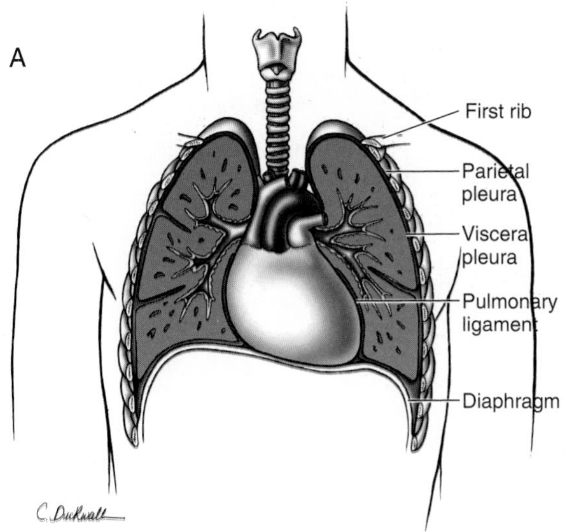

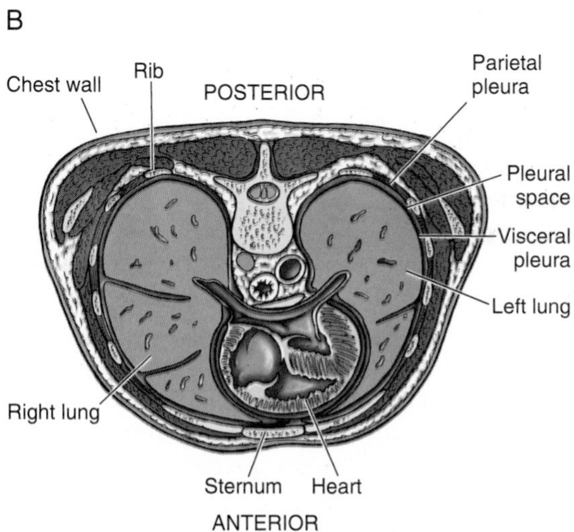

Figure 8.7. Frontal and cross section views of the chest and lungs shows the pleural layers (visceral and parietal) and the pleural space. With inspiration, negative pressure develops in the pleural space. This allows air to move from the atmosphere into the tracheobronchial tree for gas exchange. The negative intrathoracic pressure also facilitates return of venous blood into the right atrium.

DISTRIBUTION OF BLOOD FLOW

The lungs receive blood supply from the pulmonary arteries (which contain systemic venous blood from the right ventricle) and bronchial arteries (which contain oxygenated blood from the left ventricle). The pulmonary artery emerges from the right ventricle and divides into right and left main pulmonary arteries anterior to the carina of the trachea (Fig. 8.8). The pulmonary arteries divide into branches corresponding to the divisions of the bronchial tree and supply the pulmonary arterioles. The pulmonary circulation is a low pressure system with

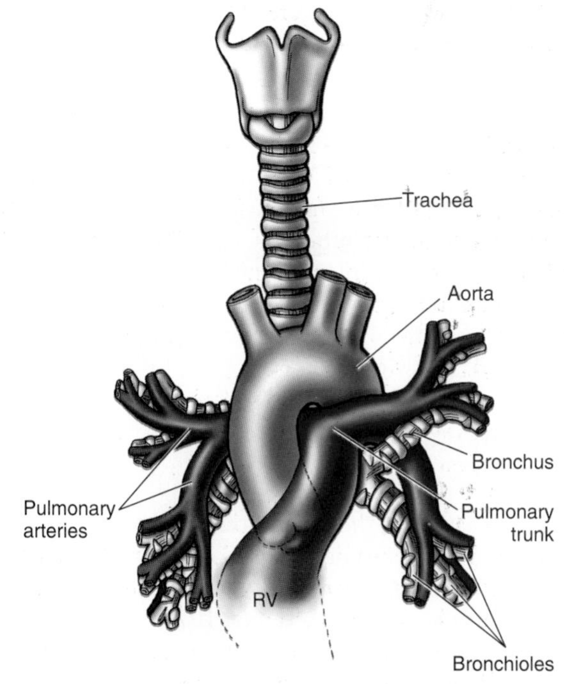

Figure 8.8. Diagram of the major pulmonary arteries which originate from the right ventricle (RV). Branches of the pulmonary artery are located adjacent to bronchi/bronchioles.

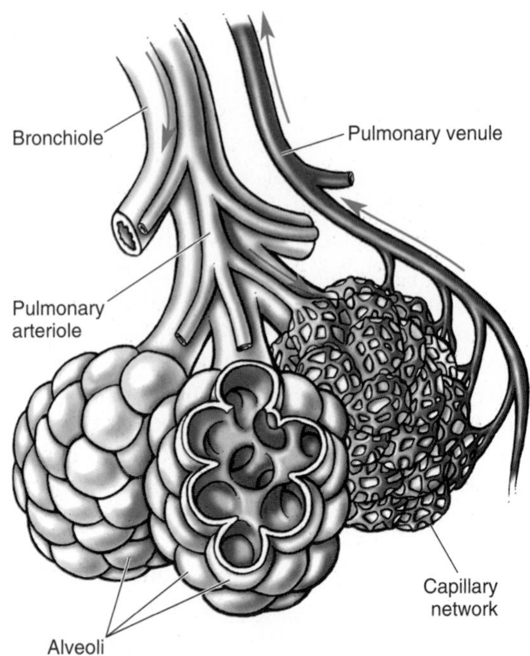

Figure 8.9. Diagram of the functional respiratory unit. It consists of a bronchiole and corresponding blood supply (pulmonary arteriole carries deoxygenated blood, while pulmonary venule carries oxygenated blood). The rich capillary network supplies the alveoli for the purpose of gas exchange.

a normal mean pressure of approximately 15 mm Hg at rest. The majority of blood flow to the alveoli is derived from the pulmonary circulation whereas the bronchial arteries supply the walls of the bronchi and bronchioles to the level of the alveoli. Pulmonary arterioles divide into pulmonary capillaries which form networks in the walls of the alveoli where gas exchange occurs.

Oxygenated blood is carried from the pulmonary capillaries by pulmonary veins which form the main pulmonary veins that empty into the left atrium. The pulmonary veins also receive blood from the bronchial circulation (which does contribute to gas exchange) and accounts for a right-to-left shunt that normally occurs in the lungs and includes up to 5% of cardiac output.

GAS EXCHANGE

Functional Respiratory Unit

Gas exchange in the lungs occurs at the alveolar-capillary membrane located within the anatomical area called the functional respiratory unit (Fig. 8.9). As illustrated in Figure 8.9, the terminal bronchiole enters the center of the functional respiratory unit accompanied by a pulmonary arteriole carrying deoxygenated blood from the body tissues and muscles. The arteriole divides into a rich network of pulmonary capillaries that enter the alveolar walls and drain into pulmonary veins/venules.

Table 8.2. Major Cells of the Alveolus

- Alveolar epithelial cells
- Type I - covers most of the alveolar surface
- Type II - produces surfactant
- Interstitial cells
- Endothelial cells - line the pulmonary capillary
- Alveolar macrophages - resides within the alveolus; can phagocytose bacteria and particulates

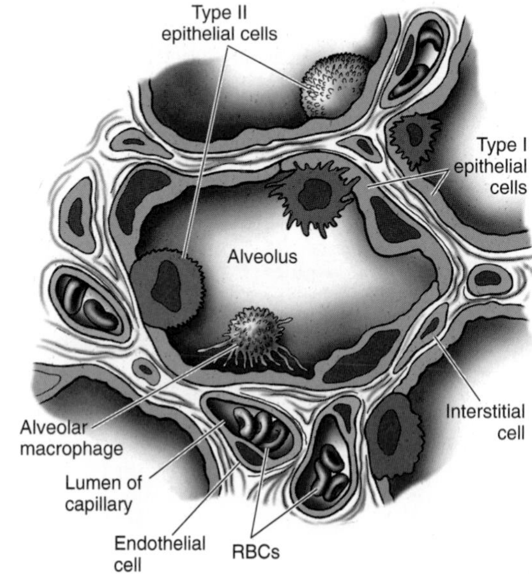

Figure 8.10. The major cells of the alveolus include epithelial cells (Types I and II), endothelial cells of the pulmonary capillary, and alveolar macrophages. Also shown are lumen of capillary with red blood cells (RBCs).

Alveolus

The alveolus consists of five major cells (Table 8.2). Most of the alveolar surface is covered by a thin layer of type I epithelial cells. The alveolar capillary membrane consists of the alveolar epithelium, the interstitium containing the basement membrane, and the pulmonary capillary endothelial cells (Fig. 8.10). Type II epithelial cells are located primarily at the junctions of alveolar walls and produce surfactant that consists of a mixture of phospholipids and lipid binding apoproteins. A thin layer of surfactant lines the alveolus and functions to lower the surface tension in the alveolus. This helps to keep the alveolus open and to prevent collapse.

LUNG CLEARANCE AND DEFENSES

Because the respiratory tract is in direct contact with ambient air and the atmosphere, the lung is at risk for potential injury from inhalation of particles, gases, and fumes.

Particle Deposition

The deposition of airborne particles into the lungs depends on size, density, travel distance, relative humidity, and breathing pattern. In general, particles greater than 10 mm in diameter impact in the upper respiratory tract. Particles between 2 and 10 mm in diameter are carried in the airstream into the lower respiratory tract where they impact in the bronchial tree. Particles between 0.5 and 3 mm are deposited in the gas exchange areas (functional respiratory unit).

Mucociliary Escalator

In the main bronchi the mucociliary apparatus is formed by ciliated epithelial cells, mucus-producing goblet cells, and mucus glands. Inhaled particles may impact on the mucus layer which is the transport medium for the rhythmic movement of the cilia to move the mucus up the bronchial tree toward the larynx (Fig. 8.5). Material may then be coughed up or swallowed. The transport rate of the mucociliary escalator is about 3 mm/minute so that approximately 90% of particles directly deposited on the mucus layer are cleared within 2 hours. The velocity of transport of the mucociliary escalator increases from the peripheral to the central airways. Inhalation of toxic fumes, severe air pollution, and exposure to cigarette smoke may disrupt the normal wave patterns or may cause cilia to stop beating (impaired transport).

Alveolar Macrophages

The mucociliary escalator does not extend into the alveolus. Therefore, the principal alveolar defense is the alveolar macrophage. This resident cell can phagocytose (ingest) bacteria and non-living particulates. Following phagocytosis, bacteria may be killed, and particles may be digested by enzymes within the cellular lysosomes. Alveolar macrophages can also release mediators (cytokines) which recruit and activate other inflammatory cells.

Lymphatic Drainage

A third method of clearance and defense is the lymphatic transport system. Lymphatic vessels in the functional respiratory unit converge in the interlobular septa. Lymphatics also line pulmonary arteries and veins as well as bronchi and converge at the pulmonary hila where hila lymph nodes are located. Lymphatic fluid from the left and right lungs drains into the thoracic duct and the right lymphatic duct, respectively. These lymphatic vessels enter the systemic venous circulation at the junction of the subclavian and internal jugular veins.

References

1. Nilsestuen J. Pulmonary physiology. In: Berghuis P, Cohen N, Decker M, Gettinger A, Myrabo K, Nilsestuen J, Strohl K, Yount J, eds. *Respiration.* Redmond, WA: SpaceLabs, Inc, 1992:1–11.
2. Carrin B. Development and structure of the normal human lung. In: Turner-Warwick M, Hodson ME, Corrinm B, Kerr IH, eds. *Clinical Atlas: Respiratory Diseases.* Philadelphia: J.B. Lippincott, 1989:1–14.
3. Staub NC, Albertine KH. Anatomy of the lungs. In: Murray JF, Nadel JA, eds. *Textbook of Respiratory Medicine,* Vol 1, 2nd ed. Philadelphia: W.B. Saunders Co, 1994:3–25.
4. Berger AJ. Control of breathing. In: Murray JF, Nadel JA, eds. *Textbook of Respiratory Medicine,* Vol 1, 2nd ed. Philadelphia: W.B. Saunders Co, 1994:199–218.
5. Light RW. *Pleural Diseases* 2nd ed. Philadelphia: Lea & Febiger, 1990:1–7.

1, 3–5

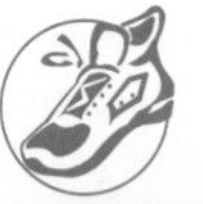

12, 13, 43,
44, 45, 46, 55

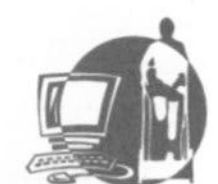

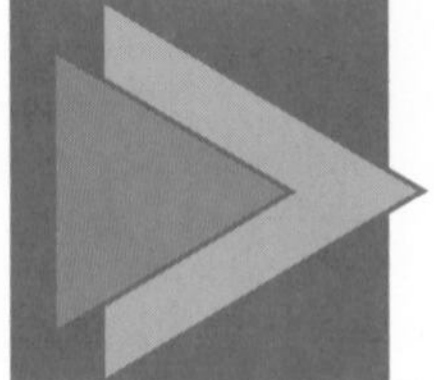

CHAPTER 9
MUSCULOSKELETAL ANATOMY

Reed Humphrey

A major objective of exercise training is to improve musculoskeletal fitness. The physiological adaptation of muscle to exercise training is manifested through improvements in muscle force production, cardiovascular endurance, and resistance to injury. Inherent in designing effective training programs is a thorough understanding of muscle structure and function. This chapter provides a brief overview of the fundamentals of musculoskeletal anatomy. For further study, the reader is referred to a variety of excellent sources (1–5)

BASIC STRUCTURE OF BONE, SKELETAL MUSCLE, AND CONNECTIVE TISSUE

Beyond supporting soft tissue, protecting internal organs, and acting as an important source of nutrients and blood constituents, bone serves as the rigid levers for locomotion. The skull, vertebral column, sternum and ribs are considered the **axial skeleton,** and the remaining bones, particularly those of the upper and lower limbs, are considered the **appendicular skeleton.** The major bones of the body are illustrated in Figure 9.1. An outer, fibrous layer of connective tissue attaches the bone to muscles, deep fascia, and joint capsules. Just beneath the outer layer is a highly vascular inner layer that contains cells for the creation of new bone. Both the inner and outer layers, which line the outside of bones, are referred to as the **periosteum.**

The periosteum is continuous with tendons and adjacent articulated structures, serving to anchor muscle to bone. Tendons are likewise continuous with the outer layer of connective tissue covering muscle, the **epimysium**. The macroscopic anatomy of muscle is illustrated in Figure 9.2. Individual skeletal muscles comprise a varying number of muscle bundles referred to as fasciculi (an individual bundle is called a fasciculus). Fasciculi are likewise covered and separated by **perimysium**. Individual muscle fibers are enveloped by the **endomysium.** Just beneath the endomysium is the thin, membranous **sarcolemma,** the cell membrane which serves to enclose the cellular contents of the muscle fiber including nuclei, local stores of fat and glucose (in the form of glycogen), enzymes, contractile proteins, and other specialized structures, such as the mitochondria. The major muscles of the body are illustrated in Figures 9.3 and 9.4.

Approximately 5% of skeletal muscle is composed of high-energy phosphates, key minerals and energy sources needed for force production. Another 20% of muscle is made up of protein, principally the contractile elements, **myosin, actin** and **tropomyosin.** The largest component of skeletal muscle is water, comprising 75% of total muscle composition (6). Physical training results in significant alteration of these constituents, depending on the specific training stimulus.

Given the wide shift in blood supply shunted to active skeletal muscle during vigorous exercise, a highly competent vascular bed must exist throughout. Likewise, the body has the ability to enhance blood supply through formation of new capillary networks, secondary to endurance or aerobic training.

STRUCTURE AND FUNCTION OF JOINTS IN MOVEMENT

Table 9.1 summarizes commonly used terms of motion, while Figure 9.5 illustrates major movements. Consistent use of these terms is essential to avoid confusion. The effective interaction of bone and muscle to produce movement is somewhat dependent upon joint function. Joints are the articulations between bones, and along with bones and ligaments, comprise the articular system. **Ligaments** are tough, fibrous connective tissue anchoring bone to bone. Joints are typically classified as **fibrous,** wherein bones are united by fibrous tissue, **cartilaginous** (cartilage or a fibrocartliaginous anchor), or **synovial,** in which the joint cavity is enclosed by a fibrous articular capsule and an inner synovial membrane lining. The cavity is filled with synovial fluid, which pro-

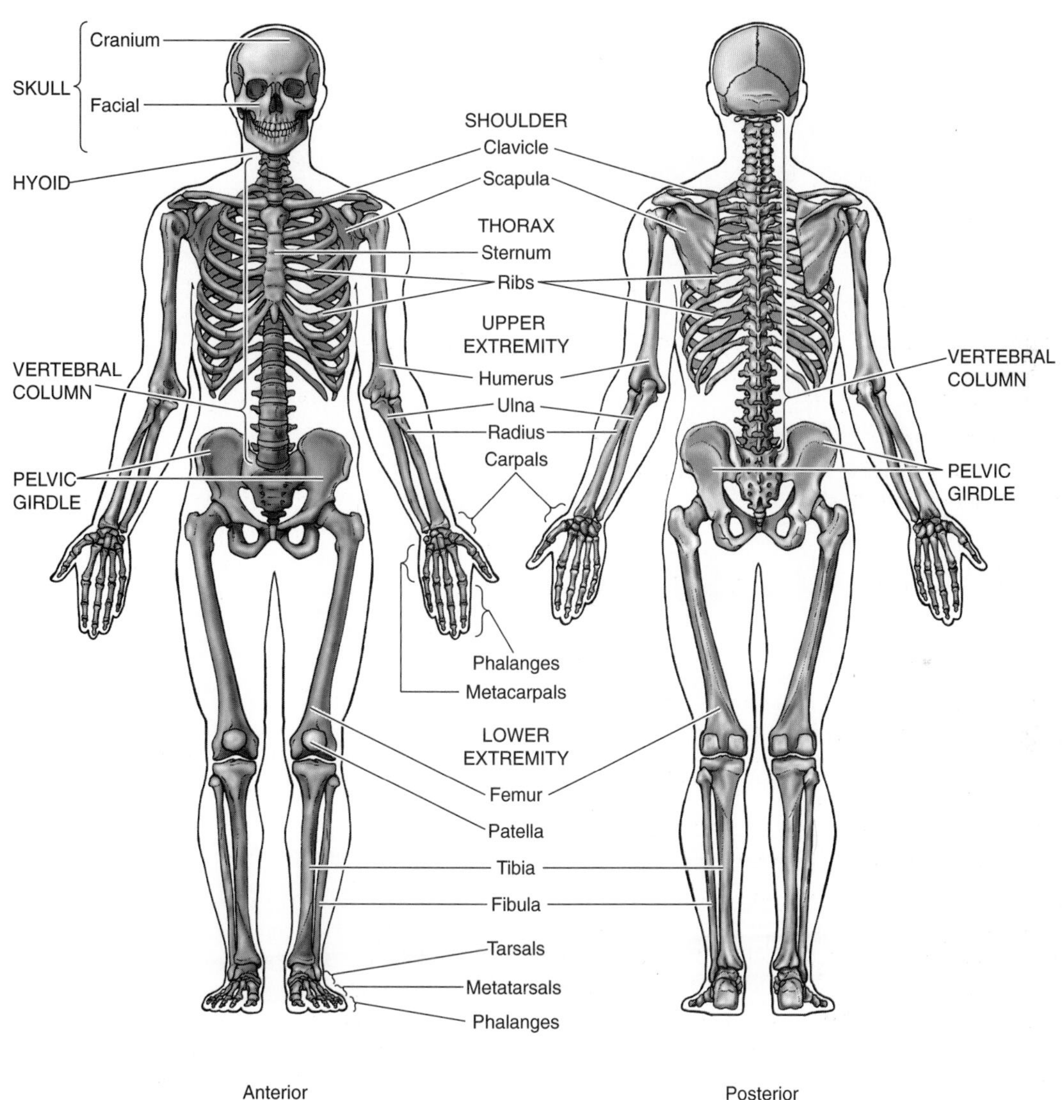

Figure 9.1. Divisions of the skeletal system. (With permission from Tortora G, Anagnostakos N. *Principles of Anatomy and Physiology.* 6th ed. New York: Harper & Row, 1992:163.)

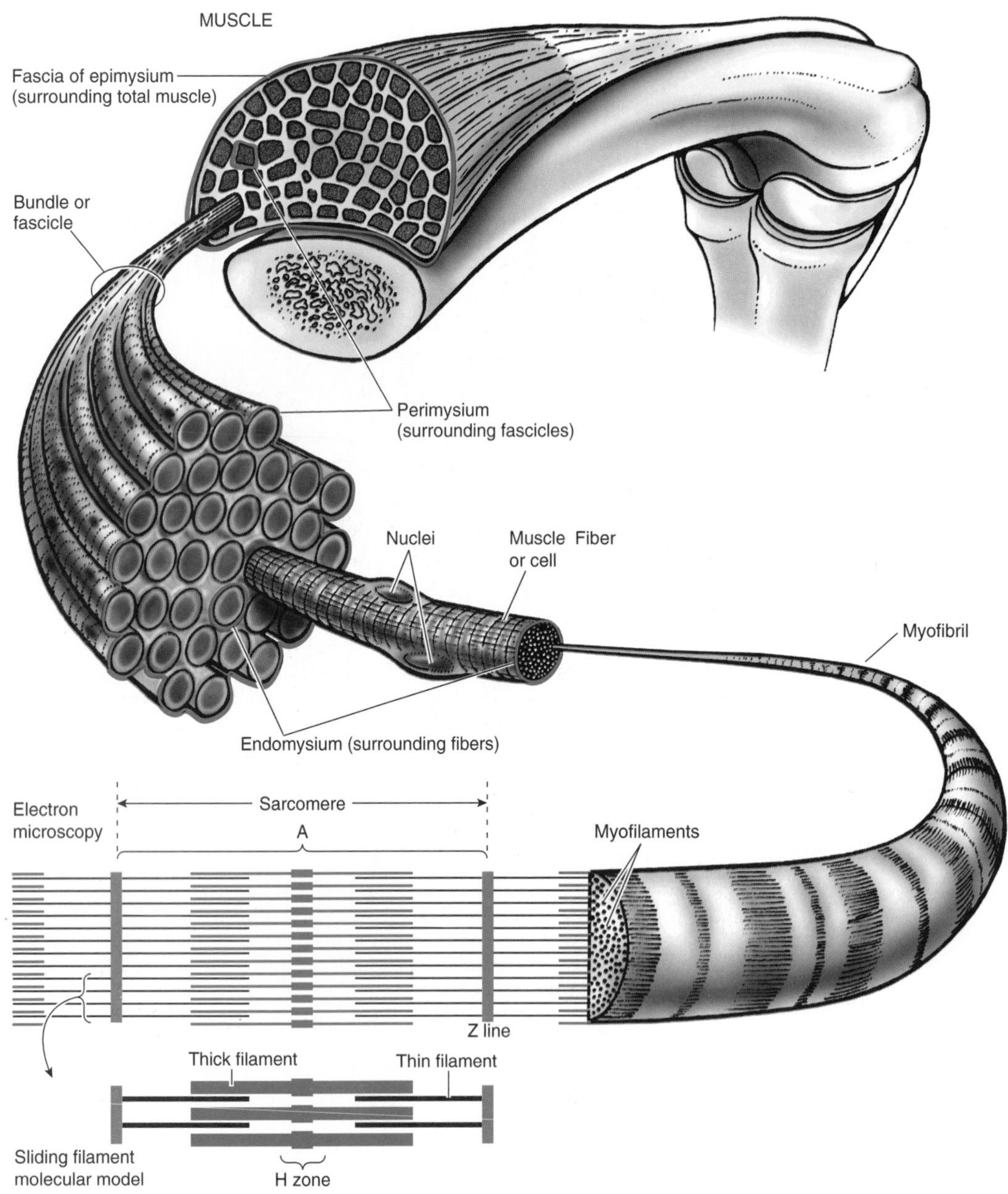

Figure 9.2. Cross section of skeletal muscle and the arrangement of its connective tissue wrappings.

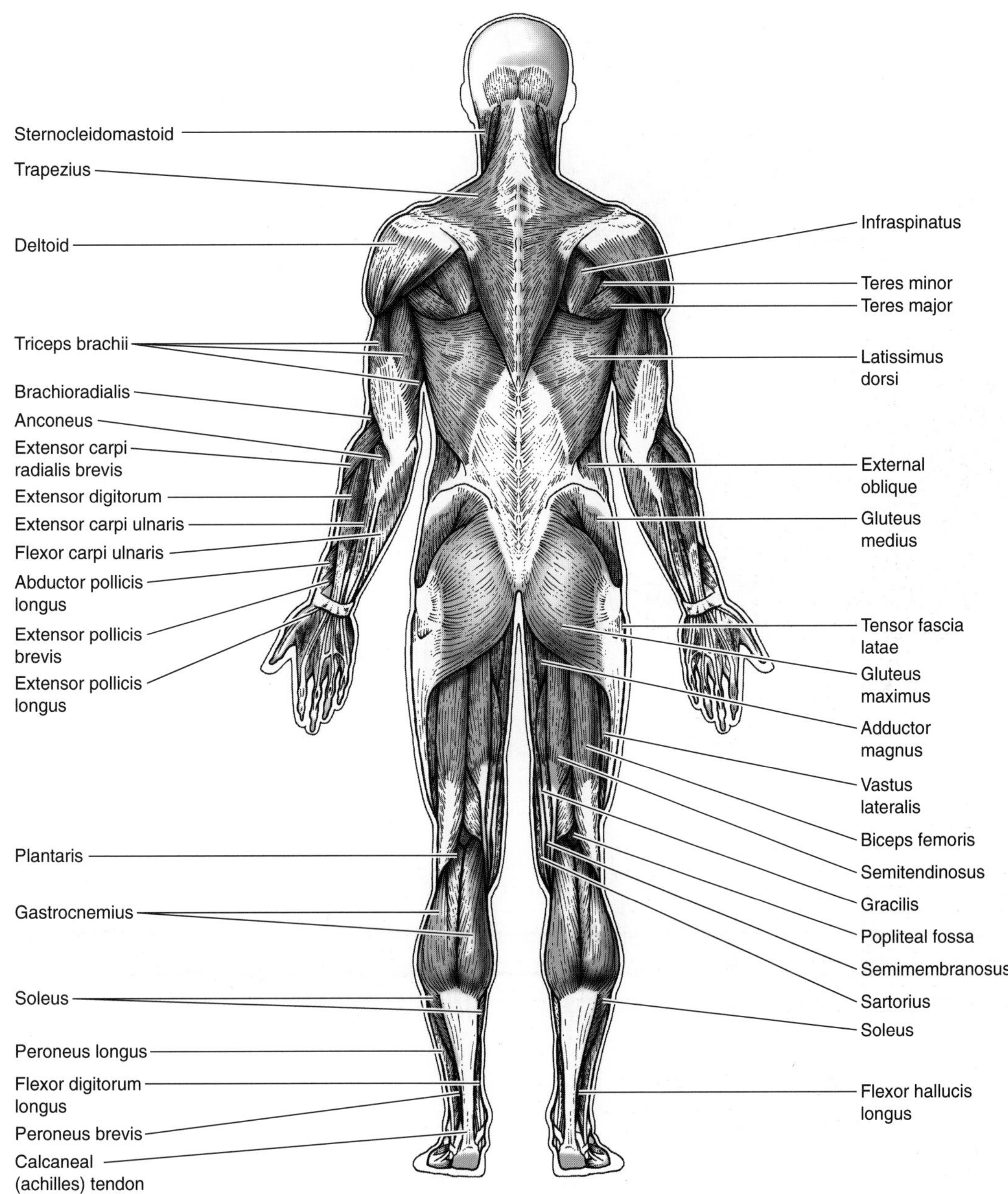

Figure 9.3. Diagrammatic posterior view of superficial muscles. (With permission from Tortora G, Anagnostakos N. *Principles of Anatomy and Physiology*. 6th ed. New York: Harper & Row, 1992:265.)

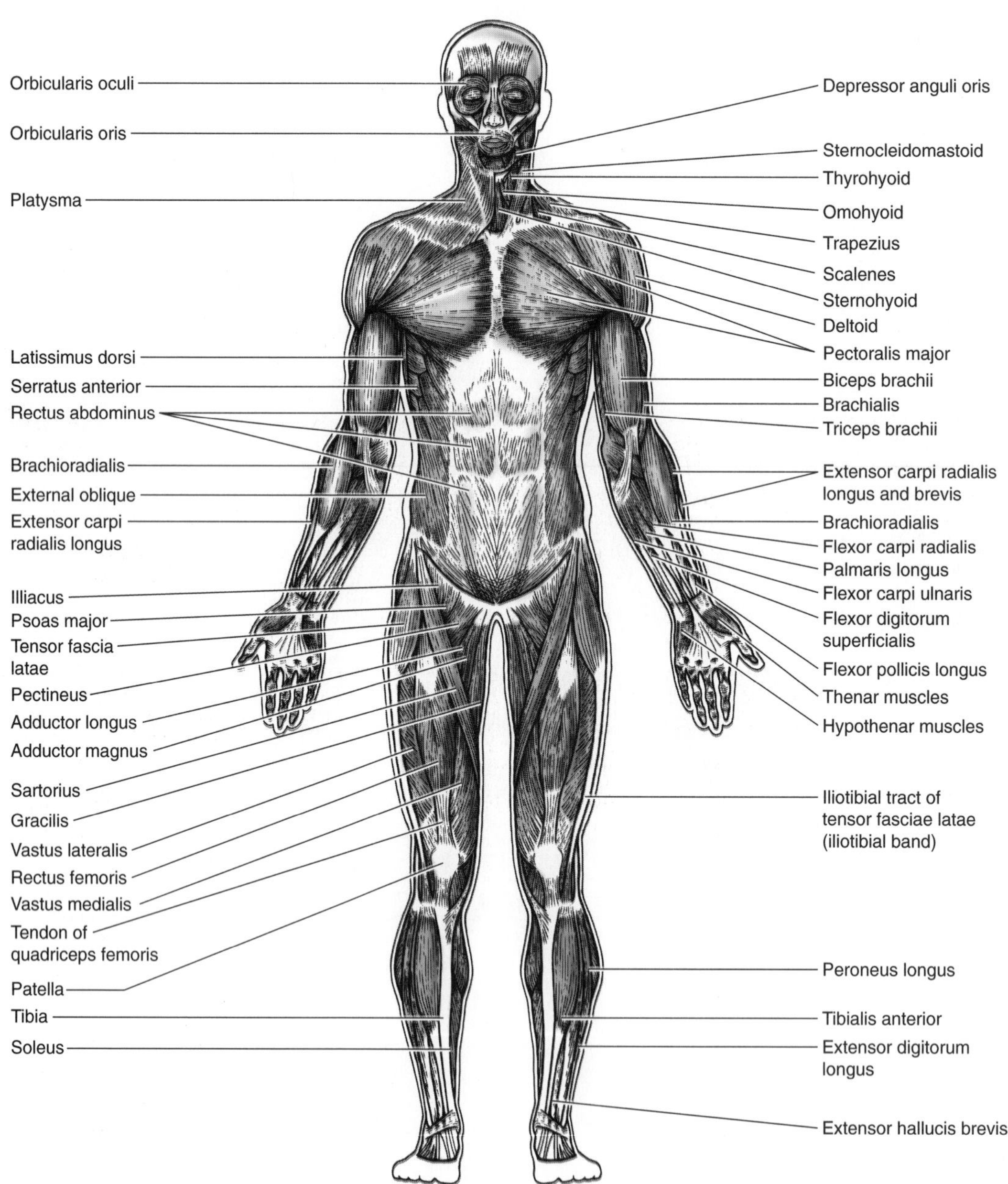

Figure 9.4. Diagrammatic anterior view of superficial muscles. (With permission from Tortora G, Anagnostakos N. *Principles of Anatomy and Physiology*. 6th ed. New York: Harper & Row, 1992:266.)

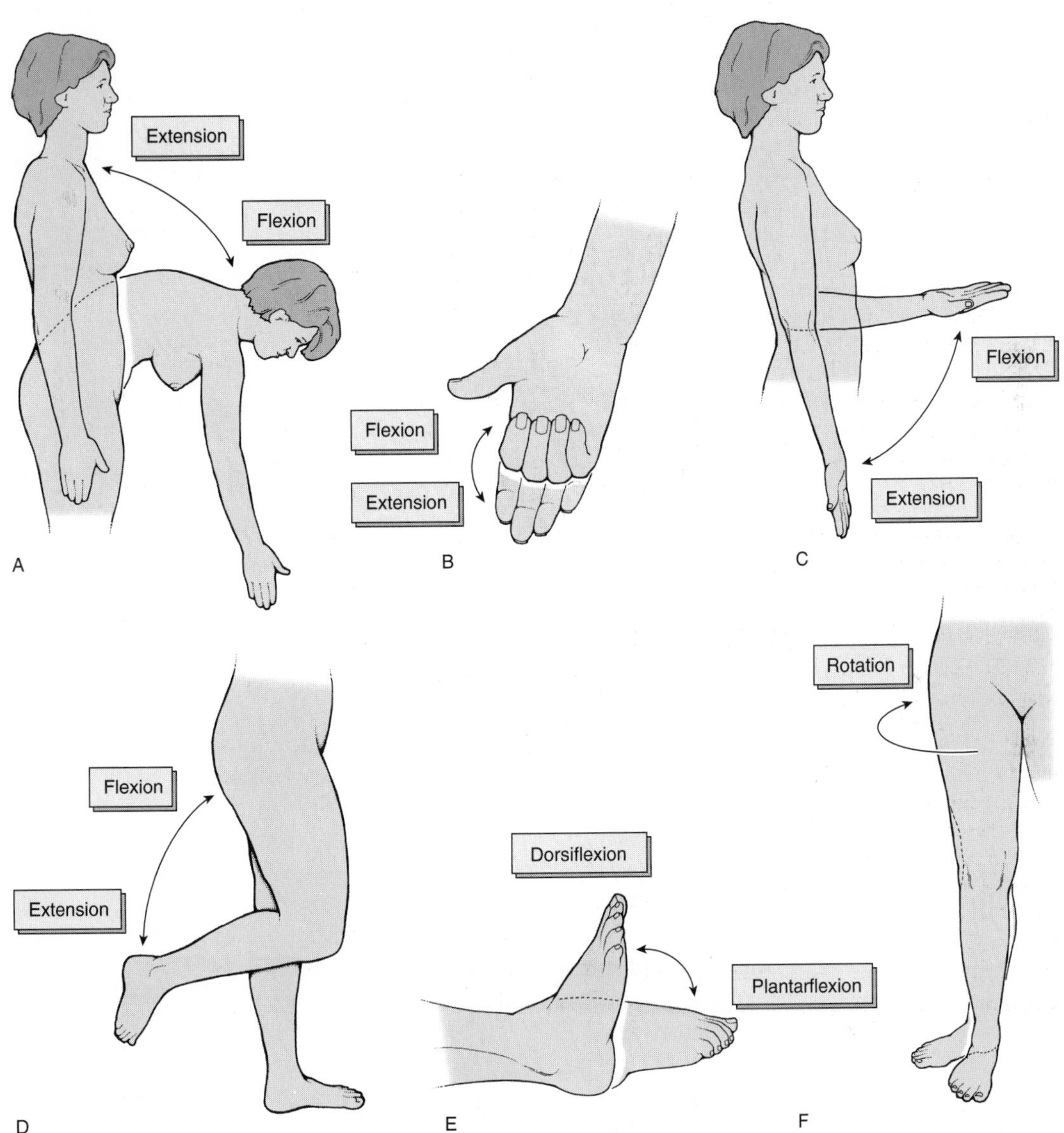

Figure 9.5. **A** to **E**, Flexion and extension of various parts of the body. **F**, Rotation of the lower limb at the hip joint. (With permission from Moore KL. *Clinically Oriented Anatomy*. 3rd ed. Baltimore: Williams & Wilkins, 1992.

Table 9.1. Commonly Used Terms of Movement[a]

TERM	EXPLANATION OF TERM AND EXAMPLE OF ITS USE
Flexion	*Bending* or decreasing the angle between body parts (e.g., flexing the elbow joint)
Extension	*Straightening* or increasing the angle between body parts (e.g., extending the knee joint)
Abduction	*Moving away from the median plane* (e.g., abducting the upper limb)
Adduction	*Moving toward the median plane* (e.g., adducting the lower limb)
Rotation	*Moving around the long axis* (e.g., medial and lateral rotation of the lower limb)
Circumduction	*Circular movement* combining flexion, extension, abduction, and adduction (e.g., circumducting the upper limb)
Eversion	*Moving the sole of the foot away from the median plane* (e.g., when the lateral surface of the foot is raised)
Inversion	*Moving the sole of the foot toward the median plane* (e.g., when you examine the sole of your foot to remove a splinter)
Supination	*Rotating the forearm and hand laterally* so that the palm faces anteriorly (e.g., when a person extends a hand to beg)
Pronation	*Rotating the forearm and hand medially* so that the palm faces posteriorly (e.g., when a person pats a child on the head)
Protrusion	*Moving anteriorly* (e.g., sticking the chin out)
Retrusion	*Moving posteriorly* (e.g., tucking the chin in)

[a] With permission from Moore KL. *Clinically Oriented Anatomy*. 3rd Ed. Baltimore: Williams & Wilkins, 1992.

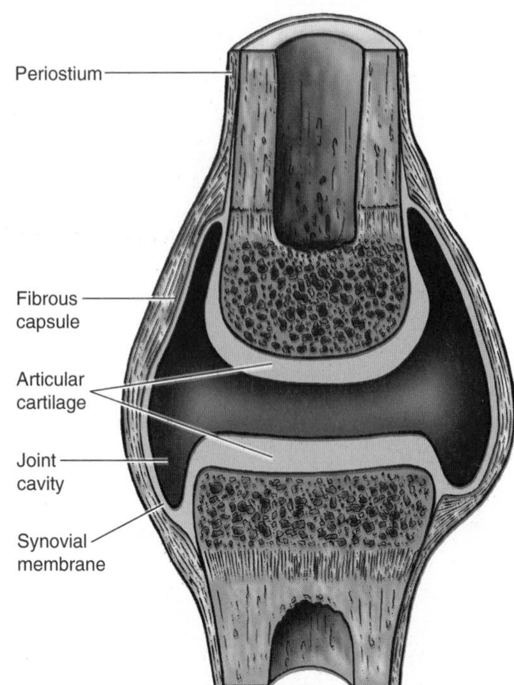

Figure 9.6. A synovial joint. (With permission from Moore KL. *Clinically Oriented Anatomy*. 3rd ed. Baltimore: Williams & Wilkins, 1992.)

vides constant lubrication during human movement to minimize the wearing effects of friction on the cartilaginous covering of the articulating bones. Figure 9.6 illustrates this unique capsular arrangement that is important to the exercise professional. Table 9.2 summarizes the joint classifications and examples in the human body.

Joints are typically well-perfused by numerous arterial branches and are innervated by branches of those nerves supplying the adjacent muscle and overlying skin. Proprioceptive feedback is an important joint sensation, as is pain, because of the high density of sensory fibers located in the joint capsule. This feedback is of obvious importance in regulating human movement and in injury prevention.

The degree of movement within a joint is typically referred to as the range of motion (ROM). ROM can be active (AROM), the range that can be reached by voluntary movement, or passive (PROM), that range that can be achieved by external means (an examiner or device, for example). Joints are typically limited in range by the articulations of bones (as in the limitation of elbow extension by the olecranon process of the ulna), ligamentous arrangement, and soft tissue limitations, as occurs in elbow or knee flexion.

Movement at one joint may influence the extent of movement at adjacent joints, as a number of muscles and other soft tissue structures cross multiple joints. For example, finger flexion decreases in the presence of wrist flexion due to the crossing of multiple joints by muscles that function to flex both the wrist and fingers. Tables 9.3 and 9.4 summarize major joint movements and the associated muscles producing those movements.

MUSCLE FIBER CONTRACTION AND FIBER TYPES

Skeletal muscles are controlled by the central nervous system (CNS) at higher centers and the individual spinal segments, and by proprioceptive structures (e.g., muscle spindles, Golgi tendon organs) inherent to the muscle and tendon complex. The integration is both complex and remarkably efficient. While never conclusively proven, the preponderance of scientific evidence indicates that, when stimulated to contract, muscle shortens or lengthens because the myosin and actin myofilaments slide past each other up to the point of minimum contact without changing their individual length. The contact between filaments is known as "cross-bridging" and controls the shortening or lengthening of muscles during contractile movements. Table 9.5 summarizes the sliding filament theory (7). This continual process of forwarding

Table 9.2. **Classification of Joints in the Human Body**

JOINT CLASSIFICATION	FEATURES, EXAMPLES
FIBROUS	
Sutures	Tight union unique to the skull
Syndesmosis	Interosseous membrane between bones (e.g., the union along the shafts of the radius and ulna, tibia and fibula)
Gomphosis	Unique joint at the tooth socket
CARTILAGINOUS	
Primary (synchondroses; hyaline cartilaginous)	Usually temporary to permit bone growth and typically fuse; some do not (e.g., at the sternum and rib [costal cartilage])
Secondary (symphyses; fibrocartiliaginous)	Strong, slightly moveable joints (e.g., intervertebral discs, pubic symphysis)
SYNOVIAL	
Plane	Gliding and sliding movements (e.g., acromioclavicular joint)
Hinge (ginglymus)	Uniaxial movements (e.g., elbow, knee extension and flexion)
Ellipsoidal (condyloid)	Biaxial joint (e.g., radiocarpal extension/flexion at the wrist)
Saddle	Unique joint that permits movements in all planes, including opposition (e.g., the carpometacarpal joint of the thumb)
Ball and Socket	Multiaxial joints that permit movements in all directions (e.g., hip and shoulder joints)
Pivot	Uniaxial joints that permit rotation (e.g., humeroradial joint)

Table 9.3. **Major Movement of the Upper Extremity[a]**

REGION	ACTION(S)	PRINCIPAL MUSCLE(S)
Scapula	Fixation	Serratus anterior, pectoralis minor, trapezius, levator scapulae, rhomboids
Upper arm	Flexion	Anterior deltoid, pec major (clavicular head)
	Extension	Latissimus dorsi, pec major (sternocostal head)
	Abduction	Middle deltoid, supraspinatus
	Adduction	Latissimus dorsi, teres major, pec major
	Medial (internal) rotation	Latissimus dorsi, teres major, subscapularis
	Lateral (external) rotation	Infraspinatus, teres minor
Lower arm	Flexion	Biceps brachii, brachialis, brachioradialis
	Extension	Triceps brachii, anconeus
	Supination	Supinator, biceps brachii
	Pronation	Pronator teres, pronator quadratus
Wrist	Flexion	Flexor carpi radialis, palmaris longus, flexor carpi ulnaris, flexor digitorum superficialis
	Extension	Extensor carpi radialis longus and brevis, extensor digitorum, extensor carpi ulnaris
	Adduction	Flexor and extensor carpi ulnaris
	Abduction	Extensor carpi radialis longus and brevis, flexor carpi radialis

[a] Adapted from Moore K, Agur A. *Essential Clinical Anatomy*. Baltimore: Williams & Wilkins, 1996.

and releasing cross-bridges generates tension, resulting in concentric (shortening), eccentric (lengthening) or isometric (static) force development. Force production continues as long as the muscle is stimulated, but the ability of the muscle to perform may be limited by intrinsic factors, such as diminished adenosine triphosphate (ATP) production, decreased pH, and accumulation of metabolic by-products.

Three common terms describing muscle contraction are **twitch**, summation and **tetanus. Twitch** refers to a single, brief muscle contraction caused by a single stimulus. **Summation** refers to successive stimuli arriving to a pre-synaptic terminal at a high rate that when summed, result in muscle contraction. This is known as **temporal summation. Spatial** summation occurs when different pre-synaptic terminals on the same nerve are stimulated at the same time, resulting in contraction. **Tetanus** may be defined as muscle fiber stimulation of such high frequency that it is unable to return to its resting length between contractions (6).

The human body has the ability to perform a wide range of physical tasks combining varying composites of speed, power and endurance. No singular type of muscle fiber possesses the characteristics that would allow optimal performance across this continuum of physical challenges. Rather, muscle fibers possess certain characteristics that result in relative specialization. For example, muscle fasciculi of a specific fiber type are selectively recruited by the body for speed and power tasks of short duration, while others are recruited for endurance tasks of long duration and relatively lower intensity. When the challenge requires elements of speed or power, but also has an endurance component, yet another type of muscle fiber is recruited.

These different fiber types, which are described more specifically later, should not be thought of as mutually exclusive. In fact, intricate recruitment and switching occurs in muscle over the performance of many tasks, and fibers designed to be optimal for one type of task can still contribute to the performance of another. The net

Table 9.4. Major Movement of the Lower Extremity[a]

REGION	ACTION(S)	PRINCIPAL MUSCLE(S)
Abdomen	Flexion and rotation of trunk	External and internal oblique
	Flexion	Rectus abdominus
Back	Laterally bend and rotate head	Splenius (capitus and cervicis) - acting unilaterally
	Extension of head and neck	Splenius - acting bilaterally
	Extension of vertebral column	Erector spinae - acting bilaterally (flexion when contracting eccentrically)
	Lateral bending of vertebral column	Erector spinae - acting unilaterally
Thigh	Flexion at hip joint	Iliopsoas
	Extension	Gluteus maximus, hamstrings (semitendinosus, semimembranosus, long head of biceps femoris)
	Abduction and flexion	Tensor fasciae latae, sartorius
	Adduction and medial rotation	Gluteus medius and minimus
	Adduction	Adductor longus, brevis, magnus; gracilis
	Lateral rotation	Piriformis, obturator internis
Lower	Flexion	Hamstrings
Leg	Extension	Quadriceps femoris (rectus femoris, vastus lateralis, medialis and intermedius)
Foot	Dorsiflexion	Tibialis anterior, extensor digitorum longus; extensor hallucis longus, peroneus tertius
	Plantarflexion	Gastrocnemius, soleus, tibialis posterior, flexor digitorum longus, flexor hallucis longus
	Eversion	Peroneus longus and brevis
	Inversion	Tibialis anterior and posterior

[a] Adapted from Moore K, Agur A. *Essential Clinical Anatomy*. Baltimore: Williams & Wilkins, 1996.

Table 9.5. Sliding Filament Summary of Muscle Contraction and Relaxation

RESTING MUSCLE
Calcium ions are bound to the sarcoplasmic recticulum (SR)
Tropomyosin-troponin complex blocks attachment sites for myosin
ATP is bound to myosin heads
MUSCLE CONTRACTION
Nerve impulse exceeding resting potential spreads across sarcolemma and down transverse tubules, causing release of calcium from the SR
Calcium binds with troponin, which permits actin and myosin to form cross bridges
Myosin ATPase is activated, splitting ATP; this transfer of energy causes movement of the myosin cross bridges, generating tension
Cross bridges uncouple when ATP binds to the myosin bridge
RELAXATION
Coupling and uncoupling continue until calcium concentration becomes insufficient
When the nerve impulse ceases, calcium is taken up by the SR; actin and myosin return to a resting state

Table 9.6. Muscle Fiber Composition in Selected Populations[a]

SPORT	% TYPE I (SLOW TWITCH)	% TYPE II (FAST TWITCH)
Distance runners	60–90	10–40
Track sprinters	25–45	55–75
Weight lifters	45–55	45–55
Shot putters	25–40	60–75
Non-athletes	47–53	47–53

[a] With permission from Powers SK, Howley ET. *Exercise Physiology*. Dubuque: WC Brown, 1990:160.

result is a functioning muscle that can respond to a wide variety of tasks, and, while the composition of the muscle might lend itself to performing best in endurance activities, it still can accomplish speed and power tasks to a lesser degree.

Fortunately, for the great majority of physical tasks encountered in everyday living, the human body can respond adequately. In the presence of muscle impairment, specific training regimens may restore muscle performance to normal function. Likewise, normal function can be enhanced through exercise training to accomplish physical tasks that are in excess of the demands of daily living, such as athletics (8, 9).

Over the years, there has been a fair amount of controversy about the classification of muscle fiber types (10). In addition, there are questions about whether these types can change in response to an intervention such as endurance training (11–14). In either case, there is general agreement that, relative to exercise performance, two distinct fiber types–Type I (slow twitch) and Type II (fast twitch) and their proposed subdivisions–have been identified and classified by contractile and metabolic characteristics (15, 16). To illustrate the variation in fiber types within the population, Table 9.6 lists fiber type distribution in elite athletes relative to the normal population.

Type I Muscle Fibers

The characteristics for type I muscle fibers, listed in Table 9.7, are consistent with muscle fibers that are fa-

Table 9.7. Structural and Functional Characteristics of Slow-Twitch (ST) and Fast Twitch (FT_A and FT_B) Muscle Fibers

	Fiber Type		
Characteristics	ST	FT_A	FT_B
Neural Aspects			
Motoneuron size	Small	Large	Large
Motoneuron recruitment threshold	Low	High	High
Motor nerve conduction velocity	Slow	Fast	Fast
Structural Aspects			
Muscle fiber diameter	Small	Large	Large
Sarcoplasmic reticulum development	Less	More	More
Mitochondrial density	High	High	Low
Capillary density	High	Medium	Low
Myoglobin content	High	Medium	Low
Energy Substrates			
Phosphocreatine stores	Low	High	High
Glycogen stores	Low	High	High
Triglyceride stores	High	Medium	Low
Enzymatic Aspects			
Myosin-ATPase activity	Low	High	High
Glycolytic enzyme activity	Low	High	High
Oxidative enzyme activity	High	High	Low
Functional Aspects			
Twitch (contraction) time	Slow	Fast	Fast
Relaxation time	Slow	Fast	Fast
Force production	Low	High	High
Energy efficiency, "economy"	High	Low	Low
Fatigue resistance	High	Low	Low
Elasticity	Low	High	High

Courtesy of Fox EL, Bowers RW, Foss ML: *The Physiological Basis of Physical Education and Athletics*. 4th Ed. p 110. Dubuque: WC Brown, 1989.

tigue-resistant. Thus, type I fibers are selected for activities of lower intensity and longer duration. Within whole muscle, type I motor units asynchronously contract; that is, in addition to their inherent fatigue-resistance, endurance is prolonged by the constant switching that occurs to assure freshly-charged muscle as the exercise stimulus continues. Sedentary males and females have approximately 50% type I fibers and this distribution is generally equal throughout the major muscle groups of the body (17). In endurance athletes, the percentage of type I fibers is greater, but this is thought to be largely genetic predisposition, despite some evidence suggesting that prolonged exercise training can alter fiber type (18, 19).

Essentially, those most successful at endurance activities generally have a higher proportion of type I fibers and this is most likely due to genetic factors, supplemented through appropriate exercise training. From a metabolic perspective, type I fibers are those frequently referred to as "aerobic," since the generation of energy for continued muscle contraction is met through the ongoing oxidation of available foodstuffs. Thus, with minimal accumulation of anaerobically produced metabolites, continued muscle contraction is favored in type I fibers.

Type II Muscle Fibers

At the opposite end of the continuum, individuals who achieve the greatest success in power and higher-intensity speed tasks usually have a greater proportion of type II muscle fibers distributed through the major muscle groups. Since force generation is so important, type II fibers shorten and develop tension considerably faster than type I fibers (20). These fibers are typically thought of as type IIB fibers, the "classic" fast twitch fiber. Metabolically, these fibers are the classic anaerobic fibers, in that they rely on energy sources intrinsic to the muscle, not the fuels used by type I fibers, as previously described. When an endurance component is introduced, such as in events lasting upwards of several minutes (e.g., 800 to 1500 meter races), a second type of fast twitch fiber, type IIA, is recruited. As noted in Table 9.7, the type IIA fibers represent a transition of sorts between the needs met by the type I and type IIB fibers. Metabolically, while type IIA fibers have the ability to generate a good deal of force, they likewise have some aerobic capacity, although not to the degree of type I fibers. This

Table 9.8. Adaptation in Skeletal Muscle Relative to Specific Training Regimens[a]

Muscle Fiber Type	Type I (Slow Twitch)		Type II (Fast Twitch)	
Variables	Resistance	Endurance	Resistance	Endurance
% Composition	nc or ?	nc or ?	nc or ?	nc or ?
Fiber size	+	nc or +	++	nc
Contractile property	nc	nc	nc	nc
Oxidative capacity	nc	++	nc	+
Anaerobic capacity	? or +	nc	? or +	nc
Glycogen content	nc	++	nc	++
Capillary density	?	+	?	? or +
Blood flow during work	?	? or +	?	?
Fat oxidation	nc	++	nc	+

nc = no change; ? = unknown; + = moderate increase; ++ = large increase

[a] Adapted from Gollnick PD, Sembrowich WI. Adaptations in human skeletal muscle as a result of training. In: Amsterdam E, ed. *Exercise and Cardiovascular Health and Disease*. New York: Yorke Medical Books, 1977:90; and from McArdle W, Katch F, Katch V. *Exercise Physiology*. 4th ed. Baltimore: Williams & Wilkins, 1996:334.

is a logical and necessary bridge between the types of muscle fibers and the body's ability to meet the variety of physical tasks imposed. Reference to the existence of a the type IIC fiber is necessary in a complete description of human muscle fiber types. The IIC fiber has been described as a rare and undifferentiated muscle fiber type that is likely involved in re-innervation of impaired skeletal muscle (21).

▶ SUMMARY

In summary, a profile of skeletal muscle is comprised of varying amounts of type I, IIA and IIB muscle fibers, the quantity and distribution of which is largely genetic. While some controversy exists regarding the conversion of fiber types through disuse or training and in the splitting and/or generation of muscle fibers, what is certain about exercise training and fiber type is that metabolic adaptations are significantly enhanced by specific training. These, along with secondary adaptations, are described in Table 9.8.

References

1. Moore KL. *Clinically Oriented Anatomy.* 3rd ed. Baltimore: Williams & Wilkins, 1992.
2. Olson TR. *A.D.A.M. Student Atlas of Anatomy.* Baltimore: Williams & Wilkins, 1996.
3. Agur AMR. *Grant's Atlas of Anatomy.* 9th ed. Baltimore: Williams & Wilkins, 1991.
4. Moore KL, Agur MR. *Essentials of Clinical Anatomy.* Baltimore: Williams & Wilkins, 1996.
5. Hall-Craggs ELB. *Anatomy as a Basis for Clinical Medicine.* 3rd ed. London: Williams & Wilkins, 1995.
6. McArdle WD, Katch F, Katch V. *Exercise Physiology: Energy, Nutrition And Human Performance.* 4th Ed. Baltimore: Williams & Wilkins, 1996.
7. Huxley HE: The structural basis of muscular contraction. *Proc Royal Soc Med* 178:131–149, 1971.
8. Coggan AR, Spina RJ, King DS, Rodgers MA, Brown M, Nemeth PM, Holloszy JO. Skeletal muscle adaptations to endurance training in 60- to 70-yr-old men and women. *J Appl Physiol* 72:1780–1786, 1992.
9. Jansson E, Kaijser L. Muscle adaptation to extreme endurance training in man. *Acta Physiol Scand* 100:315, 1977.
10. Armstrong RB. Muscle fiber recruitment patterns and their metabolic correlates. In: Horton ES, Terjung RL, eds. *Exercise, Nutrition and Energy Metabolism.* New York: Macmillan, 1988.
11. Gollnick P, Armstrong R, Sembrowich W, Shepard R, Saltin B. Glycogen depletion pattern in human skeletal muscle fiber after heavy exercise. *J Appl Physiol* 34:615–618, 1973.
12. Chi MM-Y, Hintz CS, Coyle EF, Martin WH III, Ivy JL, Nemeth PM, Holloszy JO, Lowry OH. Effects of detraining on enzymes of energy metabolism in individual human muscle fibers. *Am J Physiol* 244:C276–C287, 1983.
13. Jacobs I, Esbjornsson M, Slyvan C, Holm I, Jansson E. Sprint training effects on muscle myoglobin, enzymes, fiber types, and blood lactate. *Med Sci Sports Exerc* 19:368–374, 1987.
14. Jansson E, Sjodin B, Tesch P. Changes in muscle fiber type distribution in man after physical training. *Acta Physiol Scand* 104:235–237, 1978.
15. Brooke MH, Kaiser KK. Muscle fiber types: how many and what kind? *Arch Neurol* 23:369–379, 1970.
16. Edstrom L, Nystrom B. Histochemical types and sizes of fibers of normal human muscles. *Acta Neurol Scand* 45: 257–269, 1969.
17. Fox EL, Bowers RW, Foss ML. *The Physiological Basis of Physical Education and Athletics.* 4th ed. Dubuque, IA: WC Brown, 1989.
18. Burke F, Cerny F, Costill D, Fink W. Characteristics of skeletal muscle in competitive cyclists. *Med Sci Sports Exerc* 9: 109–112, 1977.
19. Costill D, Daniels J, Evans W, Fink W, Krahenbuhl G, Saltin B. Skeletal muscle enzymes and fiber composition in male and female track athletes. *J Appl Physiol* 40:149–154, 1976.
20. Vrbova G. Influence of activity on some characteristic properties of slow and fast mammalian muscles. *Exerc Sport Sci Rev* 7:181–213, 1979.
21. Komi PV, Karlsson J. Skeletal muscle fiber types, enzyme activities and physical performance in young males and females. *Acta Physiol Scand* 103:210, 1978.

4, 28 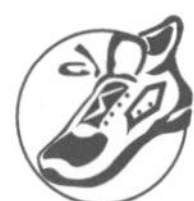 15 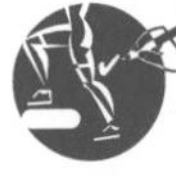 143 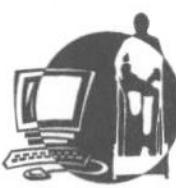 286, 287, 288, 289, 290, 374, 375, 379, 415, 417 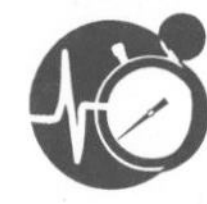 295, 407 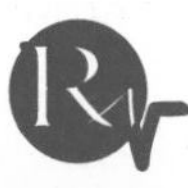

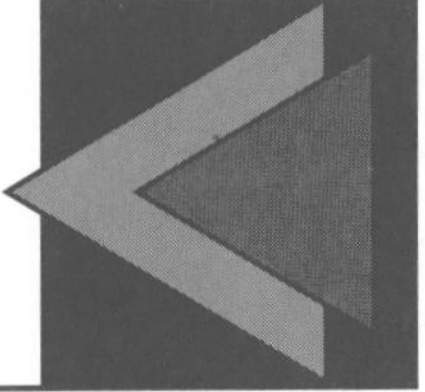

CHAPTER 10
SURFACE ANATOMY

Richard W. Latin

Exercise professionals are routinely required to make measurements and assessments based on external body locations or dimensions. Knowledge of basic surface anatomy is essential to determining pulses, electrocardiogram (ECG) lead placements, blood pressures, anthropometric dimensions, performing cardiopulmonary resuscitation (CPR), and emergency defibrillation. The surface anatomy related to these procedures is presented in this chapter.

DEFINITIONS OF ANATOMICAL LOCATIONS

The following are terms and their definitions related to anatomical locations (1):

1. Anterior (ventral): the front of the body (Fig. 10.1).
2. Anatomical position: the body is erect with feet together, with the upper limbs hanging at the side, palms of the hands facing forward, thumbs facing away from the body, and fingers extended. Typically, all anatomical references to the body relate to this position (Fig. 10.2).
3. Distal: farther from any reference point (Fig. 10.1).
4. Inferior: away from the head (Fig. 10.2).
5. Lateral: away from the superior-inferior axis or mainline of the body (Fig. 10.2).
6. Medial: toward the superior-inferior axis of the body (Fig. 10.2).
7. Posterior (dorsal): refers to the back of the body (Fig. 10.1).
8. Proximal: closer to any point of reference (Fig. 10.1).
9. Superior: toward the head (Fig. 10.2).

DEFINITIONS OF COMMON MOVEMENT TERMINOLOGY

The following are terms and their definitions related to human movement (2):

1. Abduction: movement away from the superior-inferior axis or mainline of the body when in the anatomical position (Fig. 10.3—Hip abduction).
2. Adduction: movement toward the superior-inferior axis or mainline of the body when in the anatomical position (Fig. 10.3—Hip adduction).
3. Circumduction: movement in which the distal end of a bone inscribes a circle with no shaft rotation (Fig. 10.4—Shoulder circumduction).
4. Extension: movement that increases the joint angle between two articulating bones (Fig. 10.5—Elbow extension).
5. Flexion: movement that decreases the joint angle between two articulating bones (Fig. 10.5—Elbow flexion).
6. Hyperextension: movement in the direction of extension that positions a joint angle beyond normal extension (Fig. 10.6—Shoulder hyperextension).
7. Pronation: movement that produces rotation on the axis of a bone. When applied specifically to the forearm, the palm of the hand would face downward (Fig. 10.7—Forearm pronation).
8. Supination: movement that produces rotation on the axis of a bone. When applied specifically to the forearm, the palm of the hand would face upward (Fig. 10.7—Forearm supination).
9. Rotation: movement of a segment that produces rotatory action around its own long axis (Fig. 10.8—Neck rotation).

ANATOMICAL SITES FOR ECG LEAD PLACEMENT

Two of the more useful and popular ECG lead systems, the Mason-Likar 12-Lead and the Bipolar Lead, are described below.

Mason-Likar 12-Lead System

The Mason-Likar 10 electrode placement system allows for conventional 12-lead exercise ECG. The stan-

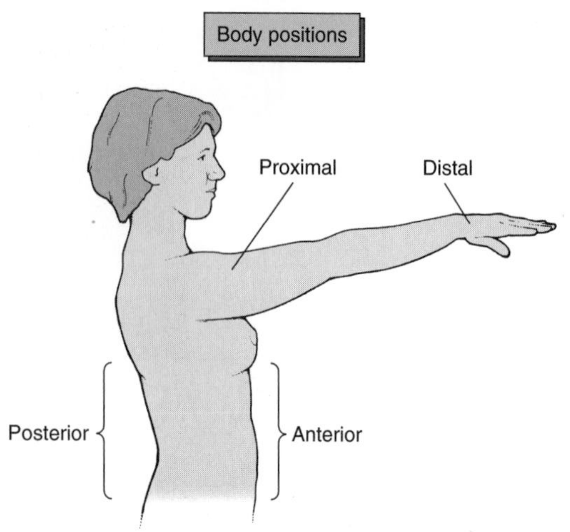

Figure 10.1. Anterior (ventral): the front of the body.

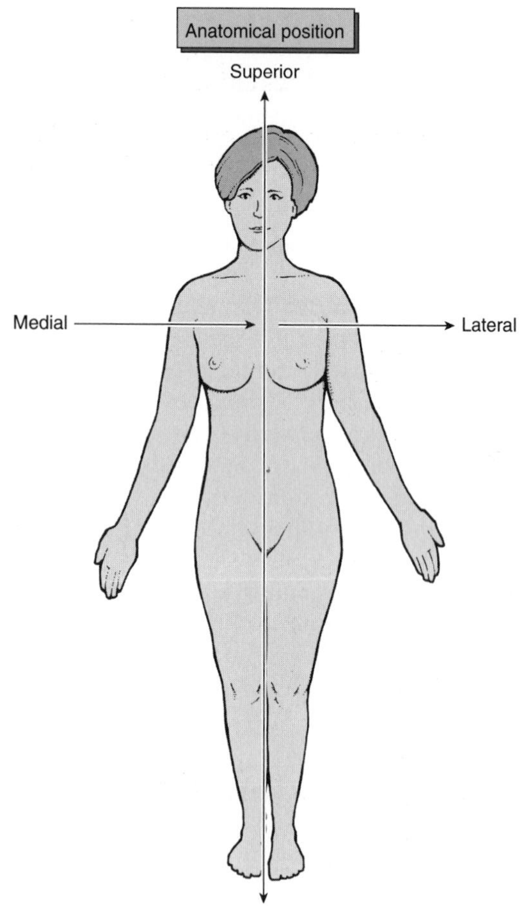

Figure 10.2. Anatomical position: the body is erect with feet together, with the upper limbs hanging at the side, palms or the hands facing forward, thumbs facing away from the body, and fingers extended. Typically, all anatomical references to the body relate to this position.

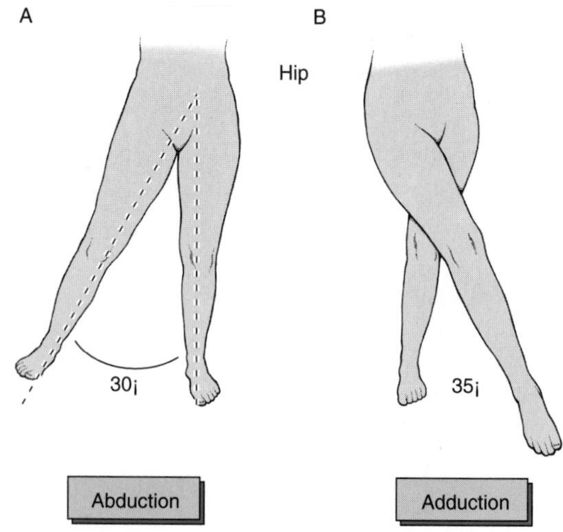

Figure 10.3. **A**, Abduction: movement away from the superior-inferior axis or mainline of the body when in the anatomical position (hip abduction). **B**, Adduction: movement toward the superior-inferior axis or mainline of the body when in the anatomical position (hip adduction).

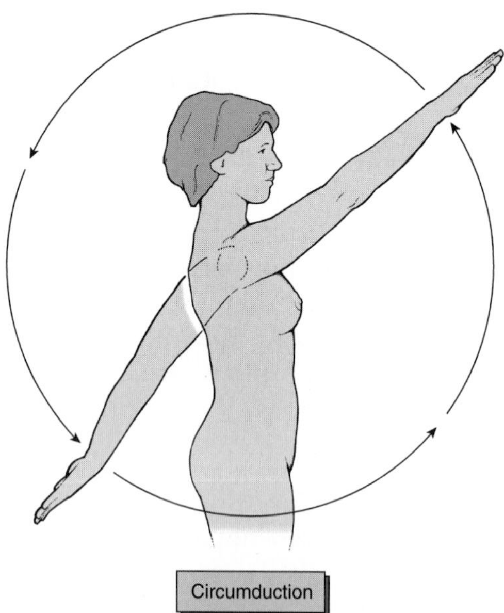

Figure 10.4. Circumduction: movement in which the distal end of a bone inscribes a circle with no shaft rotation (shoulder circumduction).

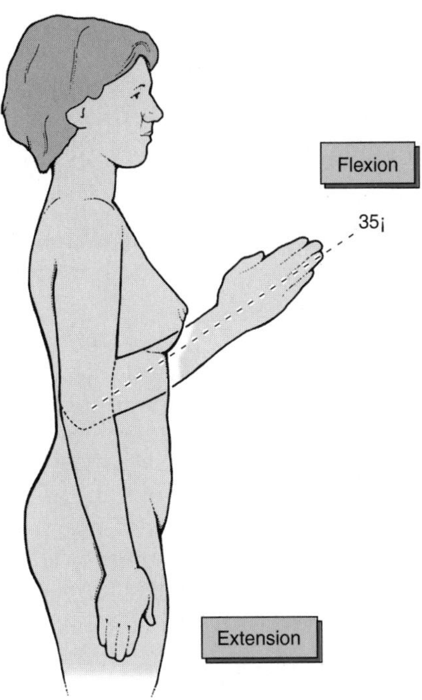

Figure 10.5. Extension: movement that increases the joint angle between two articulating bones (elbow extension).

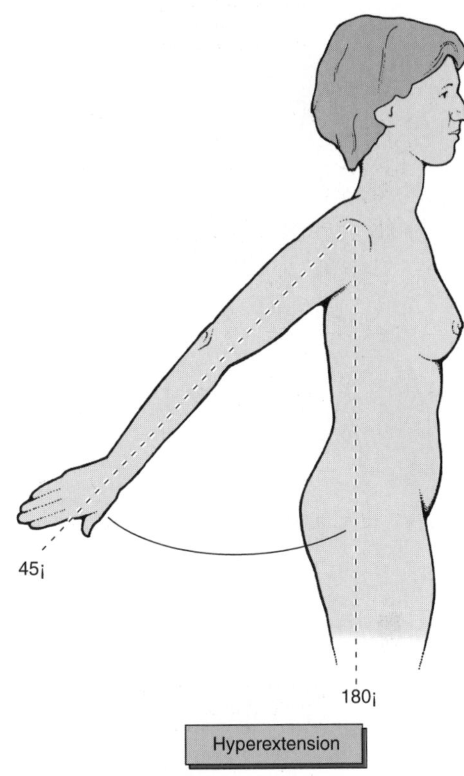

Figure 10.6. Hyperextension: movement in the direction of extension that positions a joint angle beyond normal extension (shoulder hyperextension).

A

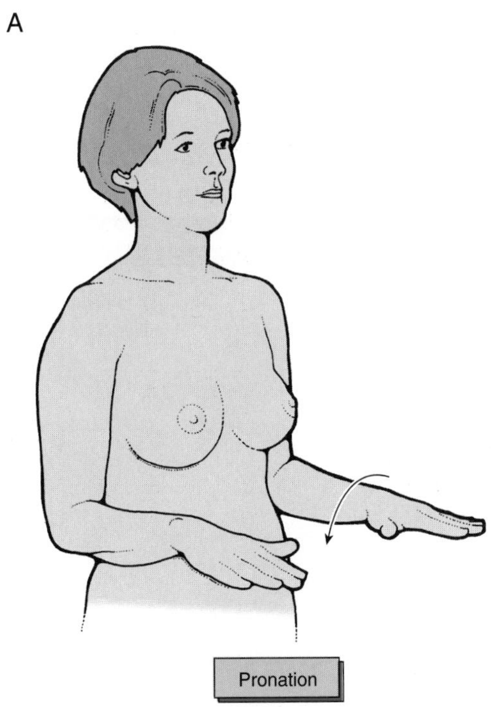

B

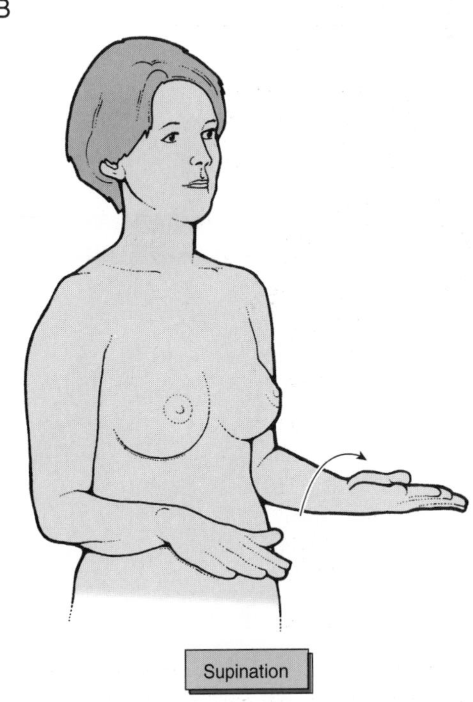

Figure 10.7. **A**, Pronation: movement that produces rotation on the axis of a bone. When applied specifically to the forearm, the palm of the hand would face downward (forearm pronation). **B**, Supination: movement that produces rotation on the axis of a bone. When applied specifically to the forearm, the palm of the hand would face upward (forearm supination).

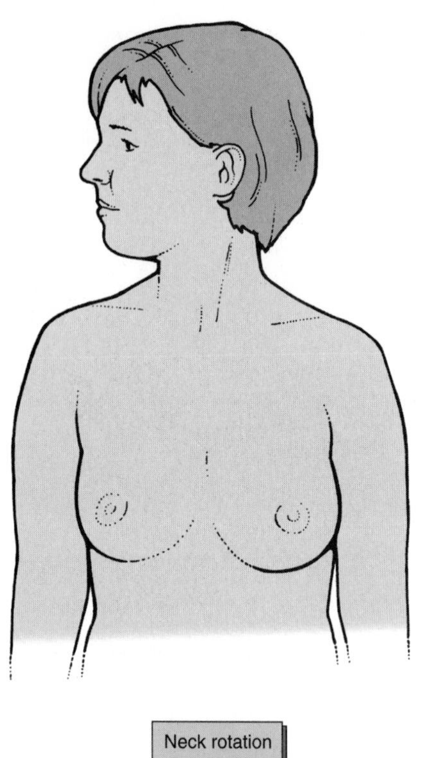

Figure 10.8. Rotation: movement of a segment that produces rotatory action around its own long axis (neck rotation).

dard limb electrodes, which are placed on the medial side of the ankles and palm side of the wrists for a standard 12-lead ECG, are replaced by electrodes on the torso. The location of these electrodes can be seen in Figure 10.9 and are described below (3, 4):

1. Right Arm (RA): upper right arm/chest region immediately below the distal end of the clavicle.
2. Left Arm (LA): upper left arm/chest region immediately below the distal end of the clavicle.
3. Right Leg (RL): lower right abdominal region, immediately above the iliac crest, midclavicular line.
4. Left Leg (LL): lower left abdominal region, immediately above the iliac crest, midclavicular line.

If leg electrodes need to be moved due to excessive subcutaneous fat or electrical interference from electrode belt box friction, avoid placing them on the rib cage or regions of the torso with less body fat. Any alteration in recommended positions should be noted.

The location of the precordial ("V") electrodes can also be seen in Figure 10.9 and are described below (5):

1. V_1: on the right sternal border in the 4th intercostal space. The 4th intercostal space is found by locating the right sternoclavicular joint and placing the index finger in the space immediately below the first rib. This is the 1st intercostal space. Proceed down the sternum until the 4th space is found.
2. V_2: on the left sternal border in the 4th intercostal space.
3. V_3: at the midpoint on a straight line between V_2 and V_4.

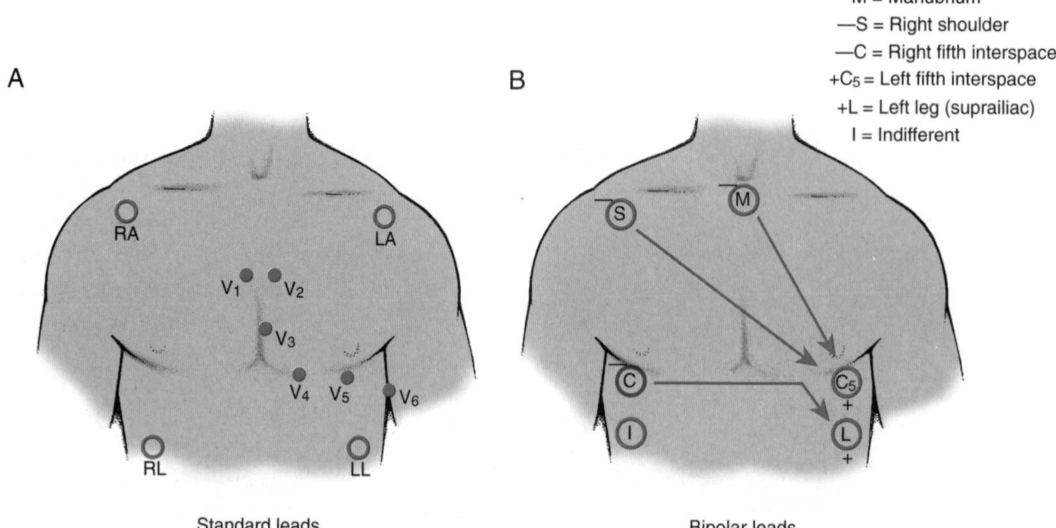

Figure 10.9. Lead Placement. **A**, Standard placement. **B**, Bipolar placement.

4. V_4: on the 5th intercostal space, midclavicular line.
5. V_5: on the anterior axillary line, immediately horizontal to V_4.
6. V_6: on the midaxillary line, immediately horizontal to V_4 and V_5.

Bipolar Lead Systems

Bipolar lead systems are commonly used for exercise tests where extensive ECG data are of less importance, such as physical fitness exercise testing or determination of exercise heart rate. There are numerous bipolar lead configurations. One conventional electrode placement, the CM-5 configuration, places the negative electrode at the manubrium and the positive electrode at precordial lead V_5. The manubrium is located at the proximal articulations of the clavicles with the sternum. The locations of these and other bipolar leads may be seen in Figure 10.9.

ANATOMICAL SITES FOR BLOOD PRESSURE DETERMINATION

Measuring arterial blood pressure is a routine procedure prior to, during, and following an exercise test. The most common method used is brachial artery auscultation. This technique requires the use of a stethoscope, a manometer (which may be either an aneroid or mercury design), and an inflatable cuff of the appropriate width and length. Recommended cuff and bladder dimensions are the following (6):

1. Child (arm girth 13 to 20 cm): 8 cm wide × 13 cm long.
2. Adult (arm girth 24 to 32 cm): 13 cm wide × 24 cm long.
3. Large adult: (arm girth 32 to 42 cm): 17 cm wide × 32 cm long.

Most cuffs have an arterial reference indicator near the center of the cuff that is placed securely over the brachial artery. The lower edge of the cuff should be about 1 inch above the antecubital space, which is located on the frontal aspect of the elbow. The brachial artery courses through a groove formed by the bifurcation of the triceps and biceps brachii muscles on the medial aspect of the arm. It should be palpated with the first two fingers at the medial antecubital space, since this is the location for the diaphragm of the head of the stethoscope. The stethoscope head should be held firmly in this position with moderate pressure. There are usually only nominal differences in blood pressures taken on right or left arms. Additionally, novices at taking exercise blood pressures may find it helpful to mark the location of the stethoscope head for quick repositioning during testing. The position of the stethoscope head and pressure cuff is seen in Figure 10.10.

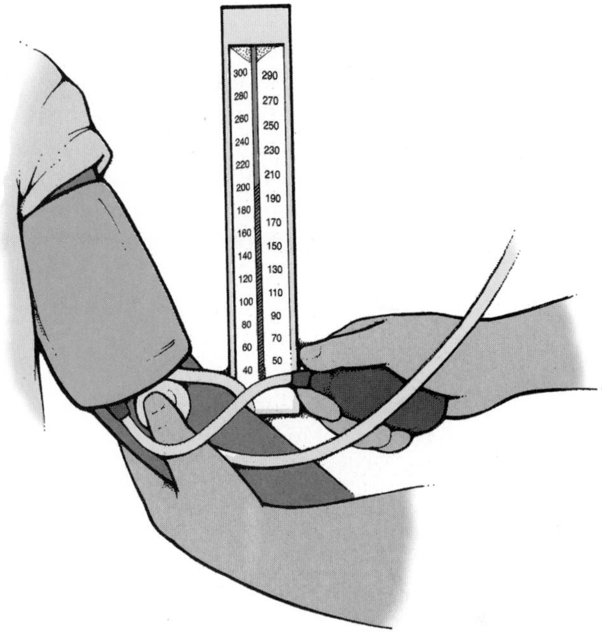

Figure 10.10. Positions of the stethoscope head and pressure cuff.

ANATOMICAL SITES AND METHODS FOR OBTAINING PERIPHERAL PULSES

Exercise professionals may measure peripheral pulses to obtain an index of resting heart rate, training bradycardia, or aerobic exercise intensity. Large, superficial arteries are preferred for pulse determination since they are easily palpable. Two conventional palpation sites are the common carotid and radial arteries.

Carotid Pulse

The common carotid artery sites are similarly located on both sides of the frontal aspect of the neck. Each are in the groove formed by the larynx (Adam's apple) and the sternocleidomastoid muscles (large muscles on the side of the neck) just below the mandible (lower jawbone) (1). The carotid pulse is taken by placing the first two fingers in the groove and pressing gently inward. An illustration of this site and technique is seen in Figure 10.11. Care should be taken when using this site because baroreceptors in the carotid sinus may be sensitive to pressure which can result in a reduction in heart rate in some individuals (7, 8). In extreme cases, blood flow may be occluded to the point that causes lightheadedness or fainting. The possibility of fainting or feeling lightheaded is of greater concern when taking the pulse immediately after exercise rather than at rest or during activity (9).

Radial Pulse

The radial artery courses deeply on the lateral (thumb side) aspect of the forearm and becomes superficial near the distal head of the radius (1). By placing the first two fingers over this region and gently pressing, the radial pulse can be palpated. Figure 10.12 illustrates this location. Radial pulses can be difficult to obtain with individuals who have large amounts of subcutaneous fat over the palpation site.

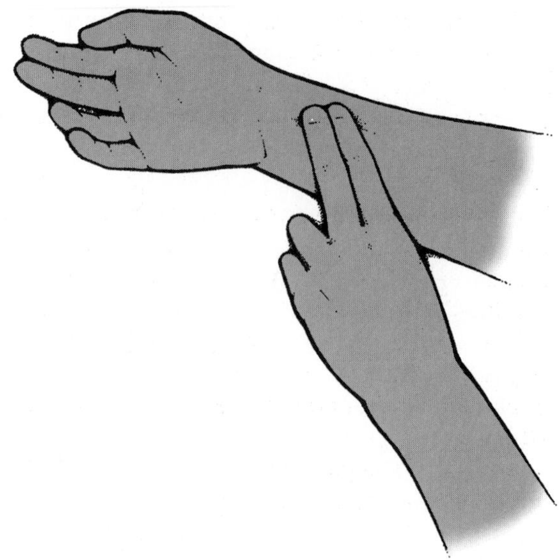

Figure 10.12. By placing the first two fingers over this region and gently pressing, the radial pulse may be palpated.

Other Pulse Sites

Pulses can also be taken at any arterial site. The location and palpation site for the brachial artery was presented in the section on blood pressure. Other arterial palpation sites include temporal (temple region of skull), popliteal (behind the knee), femoral (inguinal fold of groin), and dorsal pedis (top of foot). Lower extremity pulses can provide information about the adequacy of peripheral blood flow.

Taking Pulses

The number of seconds a pulse is counted depends on the purpose of the pulse count and the degree of accuracy required. For example, a 6-second pulse count results in an error of 10 beats per minute if a one beat error is made in counting. The error can be decreased by taking longer pulse counts. For rest and during exercise, 15-second pulse counts are recommended although it may be difficult to obtain an accurate pulse count during some forms of exercise. In those cases, it is acceptable to stop exercising and obtain a pulse immediately. Because post-exercise heart rate decreases quickly, a 6 or 10-second pulse is recommended.

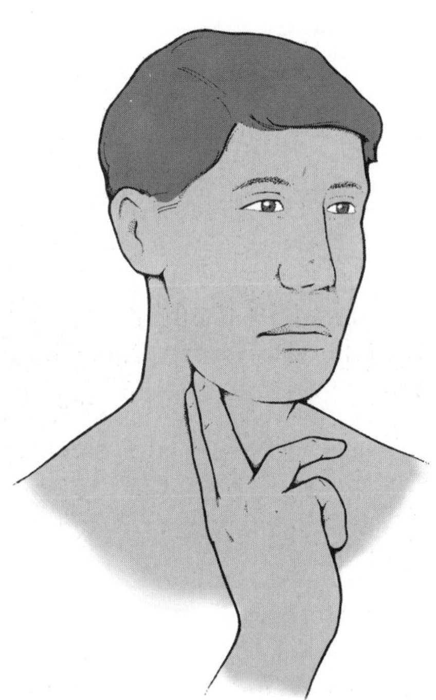

Figure 10.11. The carotid pulse is taken by placing the first two fingers in the groove and pressing gently inward.

ANATOMICAL SITES FOR ANTHROPOMETRIC MEASUREMENTS

Anthropometric measurements are those made on external body dimensions. These measures include weight, height, skinfold thickness, and body diameters including lengths and girths. A relationship exists between what can be measured externally and the distribution of internal fat and fat-free tissue. Therefore, relatively accurate estimations of body composition can be obtained by making as few as two or three simple measurements. Body composition prediction equations based on anthropometric measurements are only estimates of values that might otherwise be attained with a laboratory technique (10). Because most equations are based on skinfolds or body girths, only selected locations for these measurements will be presented.

Skinfold Thickness

Approximately half of the body fat is subcutaneous. Therefore, differences in skinfold thickness may be used to estimate the total amount of body fat. All skinfolds should be taken on the right-hand side. Two to three measurements should be taken at each site, averaging those within 1 mm of one another. The following are anatomical locations for selected skinfold sites (5):

1. Abdominal: Vertical fold; 2 cm to the right of the umbilicus (Fig. 10.13).
2. Biceps: Vertical fold; on the anterior aspect of the arm over the belly of the biceps muscle, 1 cm above the level used to mark the triceps site (Fig. 10.14).
3. Chest/Pectoral: Diagonal fold; one-half the distance between the anterior axillary line and the nipple (men) or one-third the distance between the anterior axillary line and the nipple (women) (Fig. 10.15).
4. Medial Calf: Vertical fold; at the maximum girth of the calf on the midline of the medial border (Fig. 10.16).
5. Midaxillary: Vertical fold; on the midaxillary line at the level of the xiphoid process of the sternum (Fig. 10.17).
6. Subscapular: Diagonal fold (45°), 1 to 2 cm below the inferior angle of the scapula (Fig. 10.18).
7. Suprailiac: Diagonal fold; in line with the natural angle of the iliac crest taken in the anterior axillary line immediately superior to the iliac crest (Fig. 10.19).
8. Thigh: Vertical fold; on the anterior midline of the thigh, midway between the proximal border of the patella and the inguinal fold (Fig. 10.20).
9. Triceps: Vertical fold; on the posterior midline of the upper arm, halfway between the acromion and olecranon processes, with the arm held freely at the side (Fig. 10.21).

Body Circumferences

All girths should be taken on the right-hand side with a tension regulated fiberglass or metal tape. Two to three

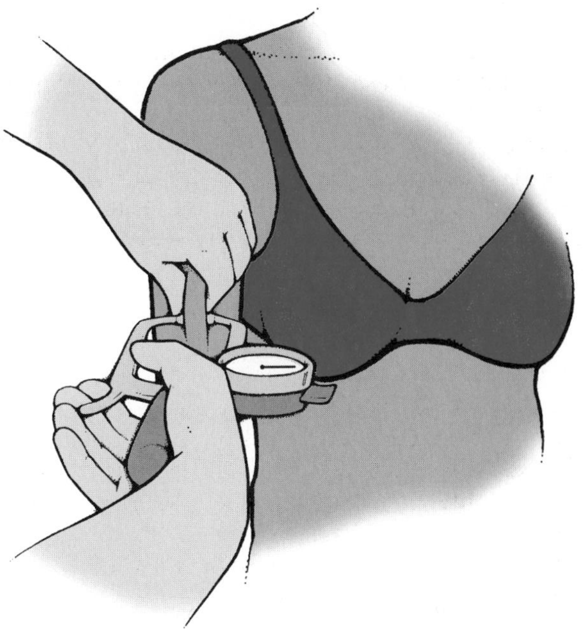

Figure 10.14. Biceps: Vertical fold; on the anterior aspect of the arm over the belly of the biceps muscle, 1 cm above the level used to mark the triceps site.

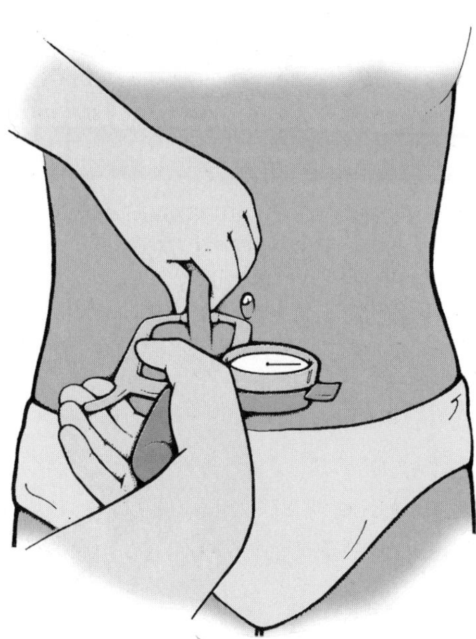

Figure 10.13. Abdominal: Vertical fold; 2 cm to the right of the umbilicus.

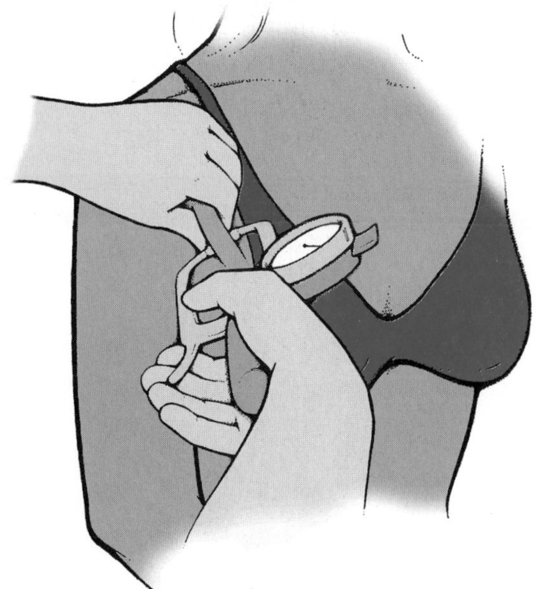

Figure 10.15. Chest/Pectoral: Diagonal fold; one-half the distance between the anterior axillary line and the nipple (men) or one-third the distance between the anterior axillary line and the nipple (women).

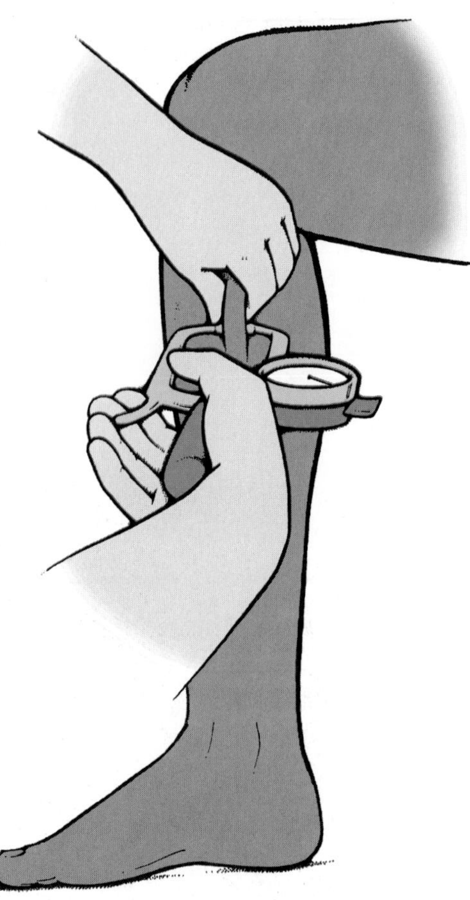

Figure 10.16. Medial Calf: Vertical fold; at the maximum girth of the calf on the midline of the medial border.

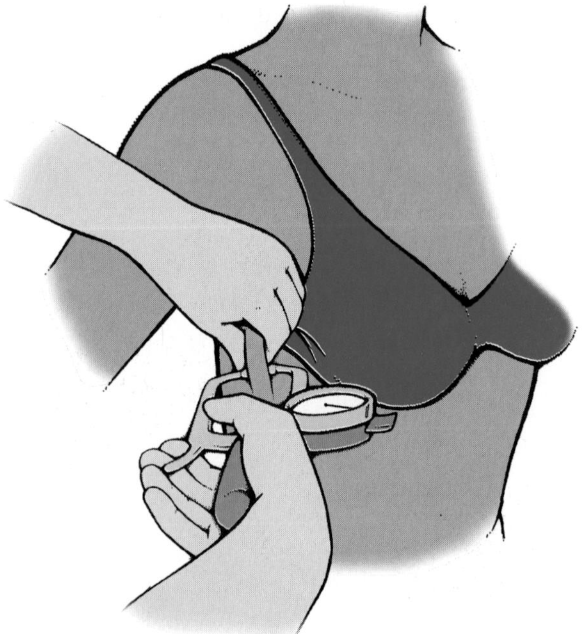

Figure 10.17. Midaxillary: Vertical fold; on the midaxillary line at the level of the xiphoid process of the sternum.

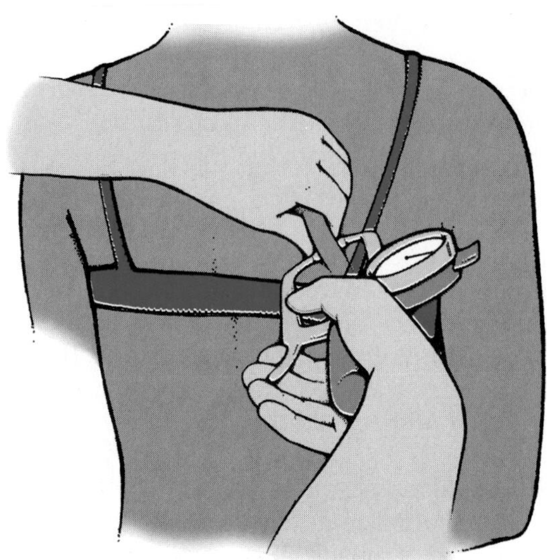

Figure 10.18. Subscapular: Diagonal fold (45°), 1 to 2 cm below the inferior angle of the scapula.

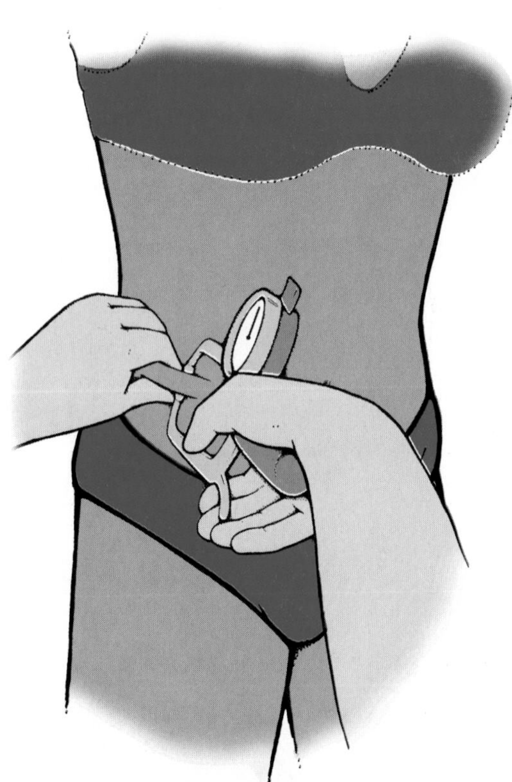

Figure 10.19. Suprailiac: Diagonal fold; in line with the natural angle of the iliac crest taken in the anterior axillary line immediately superior to the iliac crest.

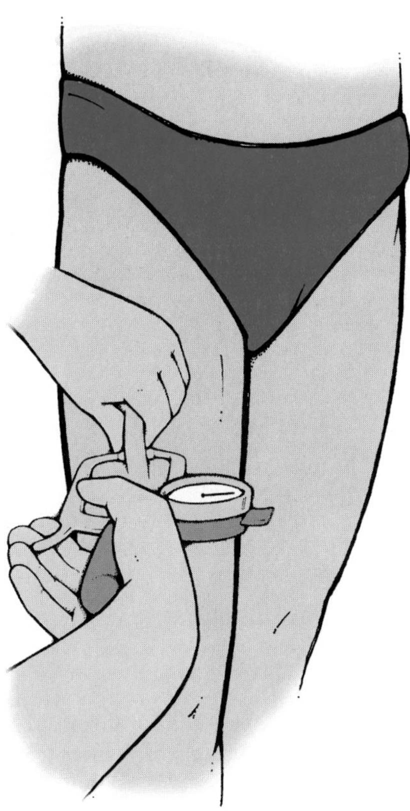

Figure 10.20. Thigh: Vertical fold; on the anterior midline of the thigh, midway between the proximal border of the patella and the inguinal fold.

measurements should be taken at each site, averaging those within 1 cm of one another. The following are anatomical locations for selected girth sites (5):

1. Abdomen: At the level of the umbilicus (Figure 10.22).
2. Arm: Midway between the acromion and olecranon processes with the arm in anatomical position (Fig. 10.23).
3. Calf: At the maximum girth between the knee and ankle joint (Fig. 10.24).

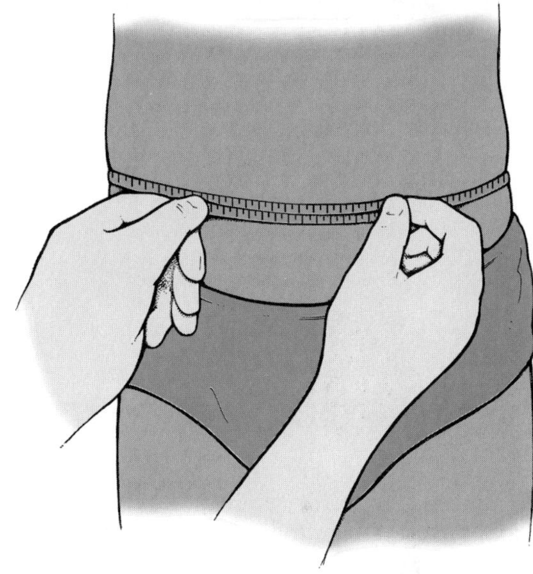

Figure 10.22. Abdomen: At the level of the umbilicus.

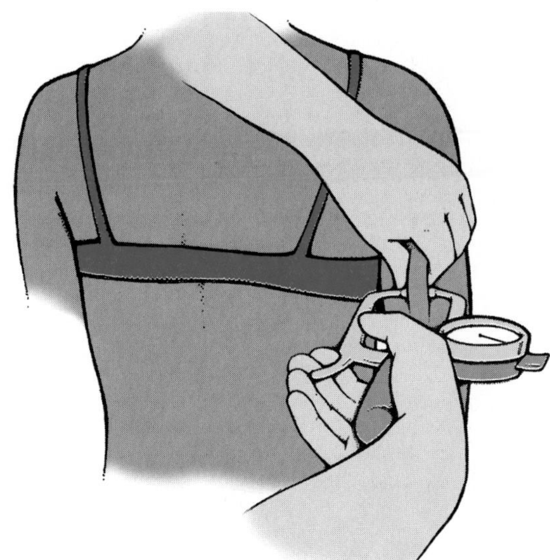

Figure 10.21. Triceps: Vertical fold; on the posterior midline of the upper arm, halfway between the acromion and olecranon processes, with the arm held freely at the side.

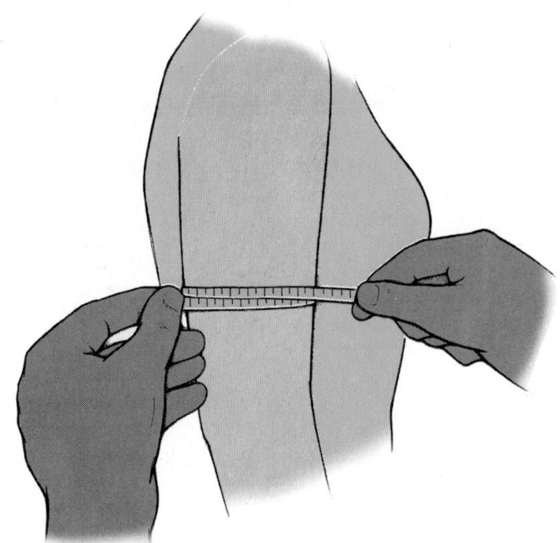

Figure 10.23. Arm: Midway between the acromion and olecranon processes with the arm in anatomical position.

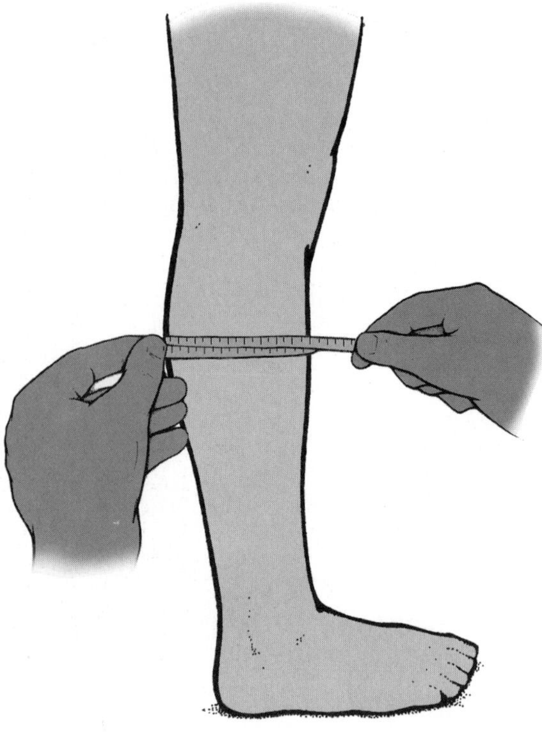

Figure 10.24. Calf: At the maximum girth between the knee and ankle joint.

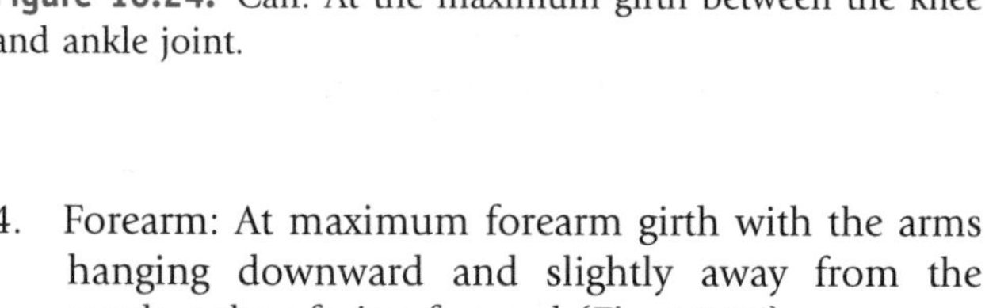

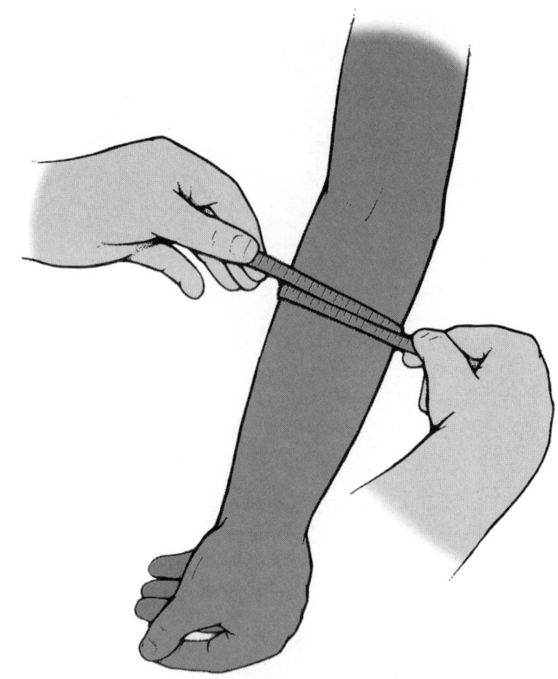

Figure 10.25. Forearm: At maximum forearm girth with the arms hanging downward and slightly away from the trunk, palms facing forward.

4. Forearm: At maximum forearm girth with the arms hanging downward and slightly away from the trunk, palms facing forward (Fig. 10.25).
5. Hips: At the maximal girth of the hips or buttocks region, above the gluteal fold (Fig. 10.26).
6. Thigh: At the maximal girth of the thigh (below the gluteal fold) with the legs slightly apart (Fig. 10.27).
7. Waist: At the narrowest part of the torso (above the umbilicus and below the xiphoid process) (Fig. 10.28).

ANATOMICAL LANDMARKS FOR CARDIOPULMONARY RESUSCITATION AND ELECTRICAL DEFIBRILLATION

All exercise professionals should be trained in CPR as well as institutional procedures for handling emergencies. These skills should be routinely practiced. Below are descriptions of landmarks used for CPR and electrical defibrillation.

CPR

The American Heart Association recommends the following procedures to locate the correct hand position for cardiac compressions (11). Trace along the lower border of the ribs with the middle and index fingers up to the xiphoid notch. The middle finger should be placed in the notch with the index finger next to it. This is to avoid

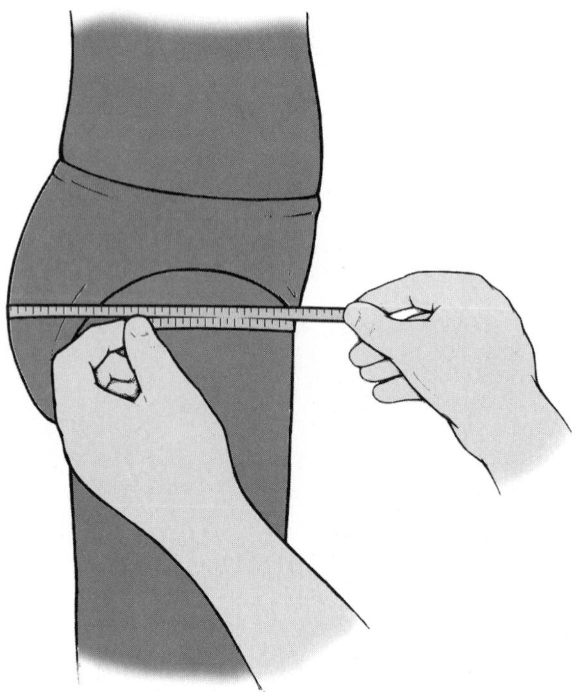

Figure 10.26. Hips: At the maximal girth of the hips or buttocks region, above the gluteal fold.

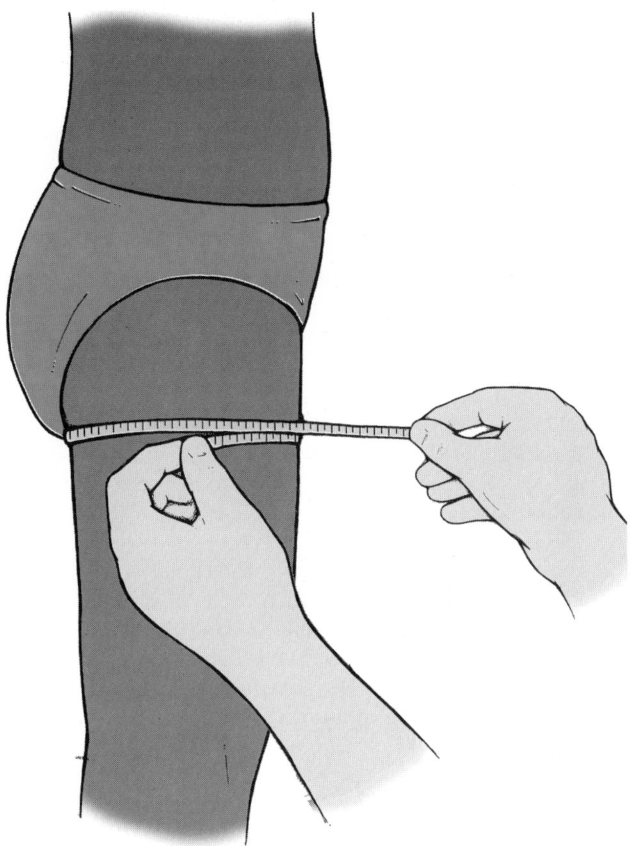

Figure 10.27. Thigh: At the maximal girth of the thigh (below the gluteal fold) with the legs slightly apart.

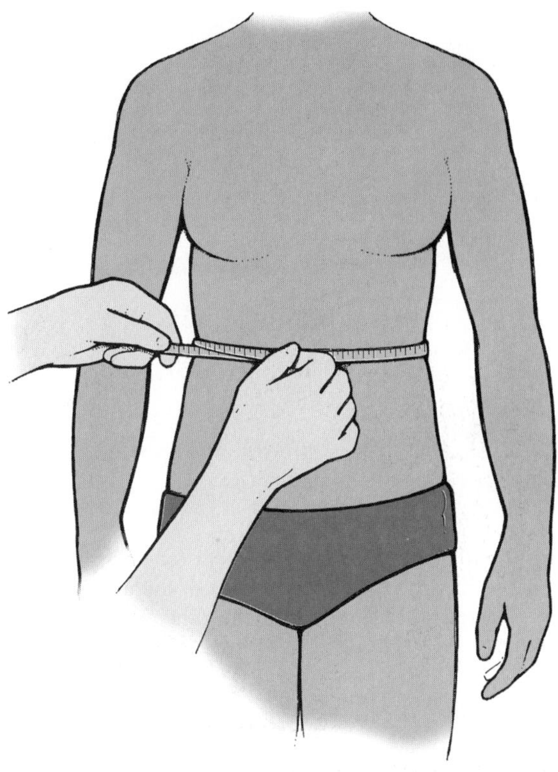

Figure 10.28. Waist: At the narrowest part of the torso (above the umbilicus and below the xiphoid process).

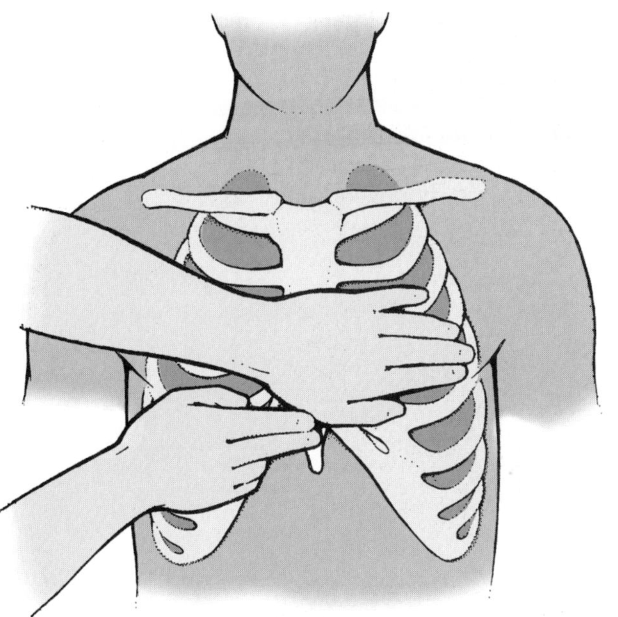

Figure 10.29. The correct hand position for cardiac compressions.

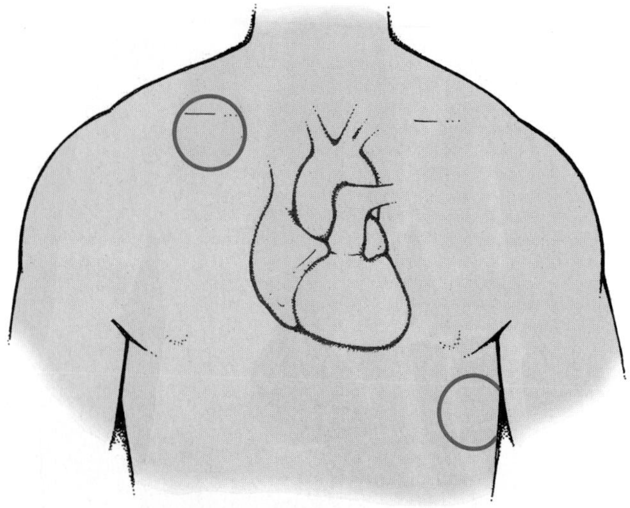

Figure 10.30. The standard placement for defibrillation electrodes is one immediately to the right of the upper part of the sternum below the clavicle and the other to the left of the nipple with the electrode center in the midaxillary line.

placing any direct compressive force on the xiphoid process. The heel of the opposite hand should be positioned next to the index finger on the body of the sternum. Once the hand is positioned, the heel of the other hand is then placed on top of it. The rescuer should compress the chest vertically with the fingers interlaced. The correct hand position can be seen in Figure 10.29.

Electrical Defibrillation

The standard placement for defibrillation electrodes is one immediately to the right of the upper part of the sternum below the clavicle and the other to the left of the nipple with the electrode center in the midaxillary line. These sites may be seen in Figure 10.30. Another acceptable configuration is formed with the anterior electrode over the left apex and the posterior electrode in the right infrascapular region. Placing defibrillating electrodes near a pacemaker generator should be carefully avoided so as to circumvent damage or malfunction (11).

References

1. Spence AP. *Basic Human Anatomy*. Reading, MA: Benjamin Cummings Publishing Co, 1982.
2. Cooper JM, Adrain M, Glassow RB. *Kinesiology*. St. Louis: C.V. Mosby Co, 1982.
3. Hanson P: Clinical exercise testing. In: Strauss RH, ed. *Sports Medicine*. Philadelphia: W.B. Saunders, 1984.
4. Froelicher VF. *Exercise and the Heart: Clinical Concepts*. St Louis: Yearbook Medical Publishers: 1987:17–27.
5. American College of Sports Medicine. *Guidelines for Exercise Testing and Prescription*. Baltimore: Williams & Wilkins, 1995.
6. Perloff D, Grim C, Flack J, Frohlich ED, Hill M, MacDonald M, Morgenstern BZ. Human blood pressure determination by sphygmomanometry. *Circulation* 88:2460–70, 1993.
7. White JR. EKG changes using carotid artery for heart rate monitoring. *Med Sci Sports Exerc* 9:88–94, 1977.
8. Boone T, Frentz KL, Boyd NR. Carotid palpitation at two exercise intensities. *Med Sci Sports Exerc* 17:705–709, 1985.
9. Gardner GW, Danks DI, Scharfsienin L. Use of carotid pulse for heart rate monitoring (abstract). *Med Sci Sports Exerc 11*:111, 1979.
10. Lohman TG, Roche AF, Martorell R, eds. *Anthropometric Standardization Reference Manual*. Champaign, IL: Human Kinetics Publishers, 1991.
11. American Heart Association. Guidelines for cardiopulmonary resuscitation and emergency cardiac care. *JAMA 268*: 2199–2241, 1992.

Sugested Readings

Ellestad MH. *Stress Testing: Principles and Practice*. Philadelphia: F.A. Davis, 1986.

Golding LA, Meyers CR, Sinning WE, eds. *Y's Way to Physical Fitness*. Champaign, IL: Human Kinetics Publishers, 1989.

Marieb EN. *Human Anatomy and Physiology*. Redwood, CA: Benjamin/Cummings Publishing Co., Inc., 1992.

Maud PJ, Foster C, eds. *Physiological Assessment of Human Fitness*. Champaign, IL: Human Kinetics Publishers, 1995.

Reid JG, Thomson JM. *Exercise Prescription for Fitness*. Englewood Cliffs, NJ: Prentice-Hall, 1985.

Wilmore J, Costill D. *Physiology of Sport and Exercise*. Champaign, IL: Human Kinetics Publishers, 1995.

SECTION THREE

BIOMECHANICS

SECTION EDITOR: *Mark Williams, PhD, FACSM*

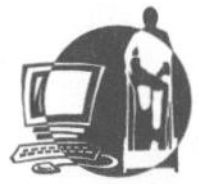

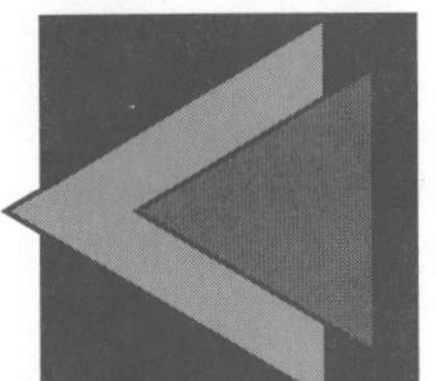

CHAPTER 11
Mechanical Load on the Body

Joseph Hamill

Biomechanics is the application of the principles of physics to the study of biological systems. A common focus of the discipline is the application of mechanics to human movement. While the human body is comprised of a number of different types of tissue, each one of these tissues is subjected to forces during motion. The forces to which these tissues are exposed are generally referred to as "loading." This is a collective term describing all external forces acting on the system.

BIOMECHANICAL PRINCIPLES

Forces and Torques

In order for movement of a segment or body to occur, a force must be applied. A force is an interaction of two objects that produces a change in the state of motion of an object. A force may cause an object to move, to accelerate or decelerate, to change direction of movement, or to stop. In most situations, multiple forces act concurrently on either a segment or the total body. In these cases, the concept of net force is important. A net force is the sum of all concurrent forces. For example, at a given joint, there are a number of muscles that cross the joint resulting in either flexion or extension actions. Each individual muscle that crosses the joint can exert a force with the result of possible simultaneous flexor and extensor forces. If the total force of the flexor muscles is greater than the total force of the extensor muscles, the net force is flexor.

A force has four characteristics, two of which are defined because a force is a vector. These characteristics are magnitude and direction. The remaining two characteristics are the line of action and the point of application of the force. The point of application of a force is the location at which the force acts on the body. The line of action is the line passing through the point of application in the direction of the action. The unit of force is called a Newton.

Depending upon how forces are applied, they may cause specific types of motion referred to as: 1) pure translation or straight line motion; 2) pure rotation or angular motion; or 3) general motion or a combination of both translation and rotation motion. When a force is applied such that its line of action is directly through the center of mass of an object, the resulting motion is pure translation. When pure translation occurs, all points of the body move through the same distance in the same time interval.

In order for a pure rotation to take place, two equal and opposite forces must act at a distance from an axis of rotation and not through the center of mass of the body. The product of a force and the perpendicular distance from the line of action of the force to the axis of rotation is called a moment of force or a torque. The most common unit of torque is the Newton-meter (N·m). Each of the two forces results in a torque about the same axis of rotation with each causing translation and rotation. Since the forces act in opposite directions, the translation from each force cancels the other. Pure rotation, however, results because each torque produces a rotation in the same direction. The pairs of forces arranged to produce pure rotation are referred to as a force couple.

In causing both translation and rotation to occur, a force must be applied such that the line of action passes through any point other than the center of mass of a free body. Such a force is called an eccentric force and results in a torque. A single force causing a torque results in both a rotation and a translation in the direction of the force application or general motion of the body. In most instances, the forces that act on the human body and result in movement are of this type.

Newton's Laws of Motion

The three Laws of Motion promulgated by Sir Isaac Newton (1642–1727) describe the interaction of forces on a body that result in movement. These laws are known as:

1. The law of inertia.
2. The law of acceleration.
3. The law of action-reaction.

The law of inertia states that "a body continues in its state of rest, or of uniform motion in a straight line, unless a force acts upon it." Mathematically, this law can be expressed as: If $\Sigma F = 0$, then $v =$ constant; that is, if the sum of the forces acting on a body is zero, the velocity will not change. To produce motion of an object that is at rest, a force must be applied. Likewise, to stop or alter a motion, a force must be applied to the object. The inertia of an object describes the resistance to motion and is directly related to the amount of matter (mass) of the object.

The second law, the law of acceleration, states that "a body acted on by an external force moves such that the force is equal to the time rate of change of linear momentum." This gives us the expression:

$$\mathbf{F} = \frac{\Delta(\mathrm{mv})}{\Delta \mathbf{t}}$$

where **F** is the net force, $\Delta(\mathrm{mv})$ is the change in linear momentum (mass × velocity) and $\Delta \mathbf{t}$ is the change in time. However, this law is probably more commonly expressed as: "a force applied to an object causes an acceleration of the object that is proportional to the force and inversely proportional to the mass of the object." This statement results in the well-known expression: **F** = **ma;** where **F** is the net force acting on the object, **m** is the mass of the object, and **a** is the resulting acceleration of the object. This statement provides a cause-effect relationship. The force, "**F**," can be thought of as the cause while the result can be thought of as the acceleration of the mass the force acts upon, "**ma.**"

The third of Newton's laws states that "for every action there is an equal and opposite reaction." This law can be expressed mathematically as: $F_{AB} = -F_{BA}$. When objects A and B interact, object A produces an effect on B. In turn, the second object, B, produces an equal and opposite effect on A. This law illustrates that forces never act in isolation and, in fact, act in pairs. For example, during locomotion, the foot exerts a force each time it contacts the ground. The ground, however, exerts an equal and opposite force on the foot. The force that the ground exerts on the individual is referred to as the **ground reaction force.**

FORCES ACTING DURING HUMAN MOVEMENT

Forces result from the interaction of biological systems and their environment. These forces have many classifications; those that are most often considered in the analysis of human movement are:

- Body weight
- Ground reaction force
- Joint reaction force and bone-on-bone force
- Friction
- Muscle force
- Elastic force

Body Weight

Gravity is the attractive force of the earth on an object and the magnitude of this attraction is the **body weight** of the object. Since body weight is a force, it is measured in Newtons. Body weight is proportional to mass because it is the product of the mass of the object and the acceleration due to gravity (9.81 m/sec^2).

Ground Reaction Force

As described previously, the **ground reaction force** is provided by the surface upon which the movement occurs and is a direct application of Newton's third law of motion–action–reaction. The ground reaction force changes in magnitude, direction, and point of application during the contact period with the surface and can be measured with a force platform. The ground reaction force can be resolved into orthogonal components referred to as the vertical, anteroposterior, and mediolateral components. These components have a greater magnitude during running than during walking; the magnitude is also affected by the running speed (1). It should be noted that the ground reaction force is the net force acting at the center of an individual's mass and reflects the force necessary to accelerate the total body center of mass.

Joint Reaction Force

In biomechanical analyses, a single segment is often examined isolated from other segments. In this case, the **joint reaction force** acting across a joint must be considered. According to Newton's third law, equal and opposite forces must act on each segment that constitute the joint. In most situations, the magnitude of the joint reaction force is unknown, but can be calculated given the appropriate kinematic, kinetic, and anthropometric data (2). The joint reaction force does not, however, reflect the actual force between the proximal bony surface of one segment and the distal bony surface of the other segment. This force, known as the **bone-on-bone force** is the sum of the joint reaction force and the muscle, tendon, and ligament forces pulling the joint together. To estimate the bone-on-bone force, very sophisticated calculations must be done since estimates of the joint reaction force and the individual muscle and ligamentous forces are required (3).

Friction

Friction is a force acting parallel to two surfaces in contact and acts in the opposite direction of the motion or impending motion (Fig. 11.1). **Translational friction** determines how much horizontal force is required to cause one surface to slide over the other surface. The friction force (F_f) is proportional to the normal force between the surfaces and is expressed as $F_f = \mu N$; where μ is the **coefficient of friction** and N is the **normal force** (force perpendicular to the surface). The coefficient of friction is a dimensionless number with larger numbers indicating a greater interaction between the surfaces. The maximum coefficient of friction of the impending motion is the static coefficient of friction; it is greater than the dynamic coefficient of friction measured when the two surfaces are actually moving. **Rotational friction** determines how much force must be applied as a torque to cause one surface to pivot on another. Rotational friction does not have a coefficient of friction but relies on the relative value of the **free moment of rotation** between the two surfaces. The moment of rotation is derived from Coulomb's Law and expressed as:

$$M = \mu_d \int_A p(\gamma, \theta) \cdot \gamma^2 \, \Delta\gamma \, \Delta\theta$$

where **M** is the moment of rotation, μ_d is the translational coefficient of friction, **p** is the vertical pressure, γ and θ are polar coordinates, and **A** is the contact area (4). This expression also illustrates that the translational and rotational components of friction are not independent parameters.

Muscle Force

The role of muscle in the human body is to exert a force on the bone resulting in segment movement. While a force is often defined as a push or a pull, a muscle can only generate a pulling or tensile force. Muscle forces thus act unidirectionally. To accomplish movements at joints, opposing pairs of muscles must act. In most biomechanical analyses, it is assumed that the muscle force acting across a joint is the net force of a number of individual muscles. It is also assumed that the point of application of the muscle force is a single point. Both of these assumptions are not quite correct, but are made to ease the computation of the muscle force. The net muscle force can be calculated using an inverse dynamics approach (5). To compute the force of individual muscles requires a sophisticated mathematical model although some researchers have placed force transducers directly onto the tendon of a muscle to measure muscle forces directly (6–8).

The force that a muscle can exert is dependent on a number of mechanical factors along with the internal contractile state of the muscle. The first of these factors is the force-length relationship. This relationship indicates the force that a muscle can exert at different muscle lengths. The functional significance of this relationship is seen when determining the torque (the product of force and moment arm) generated by the muscle at each joint angle. Researchers have generated angle-torque curves for many muscles and have found that the torque varies as a function of joint angle (9, 10). There appears, however, to be an optimal joint angle at which the muscle can generate a maximal active contraction.

The second factor is the force-velocity relationship. The torque that a muscle can exert depends on the rate of change of muscle length; that is, on the velocity of the muscle contraction. When a muscle performs a concentric contraction, the torque generated is less than that of an isometric contraction (velocity = 0) and the velocity is greater. As the velocity of shortening increases, the amount of torque that can be generated decreases. During eccentric contractions, the torque generated is greater than that of an isometric contraction.

Elastic Force

Elastic forces are generated by the return of a deformed material to its original state. The amount that a material can be stretched depends on the nature of the material and the magnitude of the force that stretches the material. This relationship is described in the following equation: $F = k\,x$; where **F** is the force that stretches the material, **k** is the stiffness of the material, and **x** is the amount that the material was stretched. The stiffness of the material, **k**, ranges from very stiff to very compliant. Compliant materials can be deformed more than stiff materials and therefore can generate a greater elastic force.

The elasticity of bio-materials such as muscle, tendon, and ligament can be tested with the results plotted on a **stress-strain curve. Stress** (θ) is defined as the force per unit area or the load placed on the bone and has units of Newtons/cm^2. **Strain** (ϵ) is defined as the change in length divided by the initial length and is presented as a percent. Figure 11.2 illustrates an idealized stress-strain curve. When a bio-material is stressed and remains below its yield point, that is, within its **elastic region,** it undergoes no permanent change. However, when the material is stressed such that it is stretched into its **plastic region,** there are permanent changes to the structure of

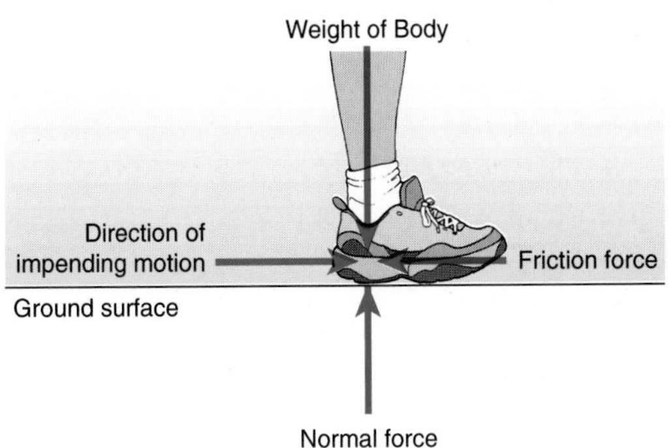

Figure 11.1. Illustration of translational friction force during foot contact of a running stride.

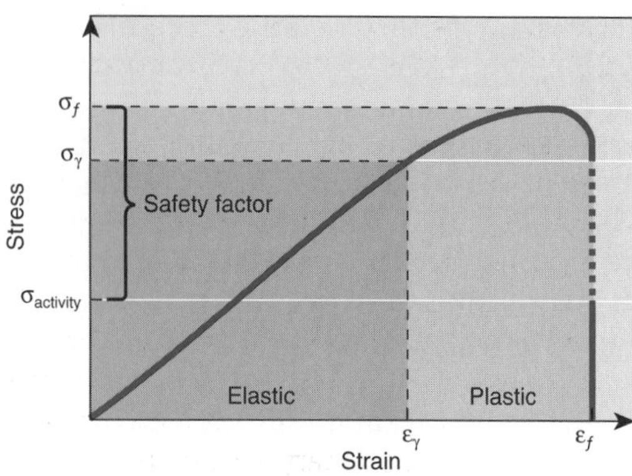

Figure 11.2. An idealized stress-strain curve. The elastic region is bounded by the yield point (designated by ϵ_y, θ_y). The plastic region is bounded by the yield point and the failure point (designated by ϵ_f, θ_f). Note that the stress of normal activity is much less than either the yield or failure points. The difference between the yield and failure points is the safety factor. (With permission from Biewener AA, ed. *Biomechanics: Structures and Systems.* Oxford: Oxford University Press, 1992.)

the material. If the deformation continues, the material will ultimately fail. The stress point in normal activity is generally much less than the yield point and thus, the difference between the stress point of normal activity and the failure point is regarded as the safety factor (11). Biomaterials that can be stretched are like a spring and can impart a force when they return to their original length. This force is due to the potential energy stored in the spring and is referred to as an elastic force (12, 13).

APPLICATIONS TO HUMAN MOVEMENT

It has been suggested that there is an optimal window of loading that healthy individuals should maintain and that loading above this window presents the risk of injury (14). However, this window has not been defined and it is difficult to estimate the load on the body for various activities (15). Nevertheless, the result of the loading on the body depends on three factors: the magnitude of the force, the rate at which the force is applied, and the repetition of load application. During normal activity, the **magnitude of the force** on tissue is within a range that will not cause tissue (e.g.,bone) to fail as in a traumatic situation and in fact, can be associated with positive effects, particularly when **rate at which the force is applied** is also considered (16). The greater the rate of loading, the more load can be withstood before failure. Loading rate is clinically relevant because it determines both the fracture pattern and the surrounding soft tissue damage at fracture.

The third factor is **load repetition.** Again, load repetition generally does not result in injury during normal activity although it has been suggested that repeated impacts such as the collision of the foot and ground during locomotion can result in microtrauma. To this point, it has been reported that repeated impacts can cause trabecular microfractures and cartilage and knee joint degeneration that is consistent with osteoarthritis (17–19).

The human body has a number of mechanisms by which load is attenuated. These include structures such as the fat pads on the plantar surface of the foot, articular cartilage in the joints, bone, and soft tissue surrounding the bone. There are also particular motions of the segments that attenuate shock. In the lower extremity, these include knee flexion, sub-talar pronation, and ankle dorsiflexion. Under normal conditions, these motions are effective. However, it has been suggested that structural abnormalities in conjunction with repeated activity patterns result in injury. An individual with a structural abnormality such as a forefoot varus, for example, has a greater likelihood of excessive motion at the sub-talar joint (20). Excessive motion of the sub-talar joint has been linked to soft tissue injuries of the knee (21). This research suggests that structural abnormalities cause a mis-timing of the lower extremity joint actions resulting in soft tissue injury. These injuries are not specifically related to the load imposed, but in response to the load imposed on mis-aligned structures.

One particular source of loading on the body is the ground reaction force. Figure 11.3 illustrates the vertical ground reaction force component during heel-toe running. The first peak on this curve, occurring within 50 msec of contact, is a high frequency peak (> 5 Hz), and is referred to as the **passive peak** or the **impact peak** (22). This peak is relatively high in magnitude but the loading rate is very high. The second peak is a low frequency peak (< 5 Hz), and is referred to as the **active peak.** The active peak is a high magnitude peak but with a relatively low loading rate. The impact peak has been related to both the etiology of lower extremity injuries and to further orthopedic problems.

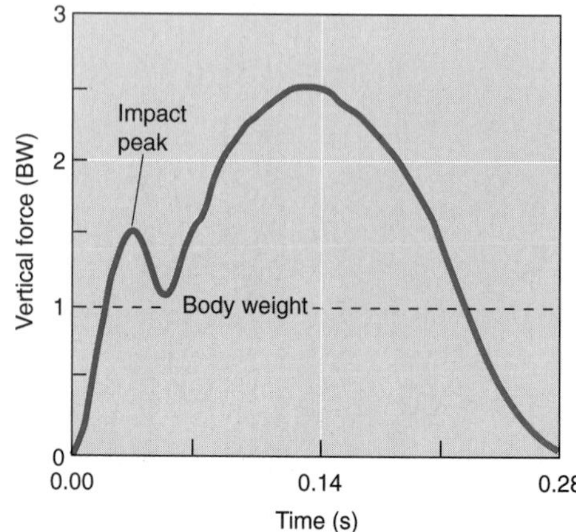

Figure 11.3. Vertical ground reaction force component during heel-toe running.

The vertical ground reaction force component has been reconstructed from positional data to gain a better understanding of the impact peak (4). Using this method, researchers partitioned the vertical ground reaction force component and related the contributions of various body segments to the total force. It was illustrated that the passive peak of the vertical component was mainly borne by the lower extremity of the support leg. Therefore, the lower extremity of the support leg was the major shock bearing and shock absorbing structure during running.

The impact force resulting from the collision of the foot and the ground produces an acceleration in the body that is transmitted throughout the skeletal system in the form of a **shock wave.** This shock wave travels through the skeletal system much like a sound wave travels through a solid object, taking about 10 msec to reach the head. As the wave travels through the body it is attenuated by the body structures and by the kinematics of the body. Figure 11.4 illustrates profiles of the impact shock on the distal medial tibia and the head during the support phase of a running stride. In these profiles, the input shock, measured in g's (where 1 g = 9.81 m/sec^2), has a peak of 4.0 g while the peak shock at the head is approximately 1.0 g.

The importance of attenuating the shock wave before it reaches the head may also have implications for the motor control of gait. If the level of the shock wave is not attenuated adequately, then the shock wave may affect motion of the head. The head houses both the visual and the vestibular systems that contribute to the environmental information that is essential for the organization of efficient gait. It has been postulated that an unattenuated shock wave would disrupt these systems and possibly impair the control of the locomotor pattern (23).

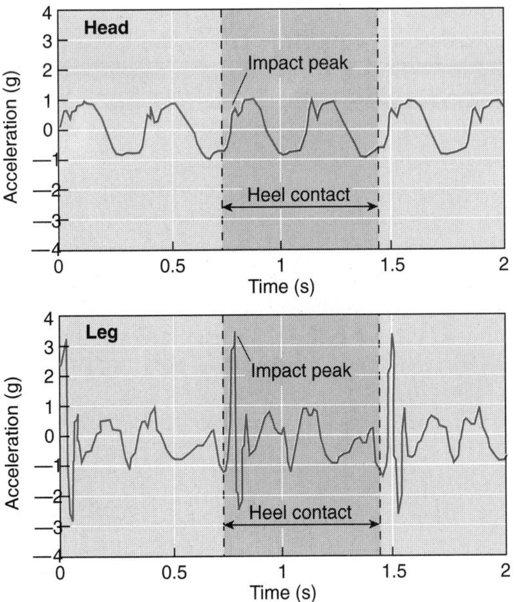

Figure 11.4. Impact shock on the leg and the corresponding shock on the head during heel-toe running.

There are a number of factors that influence the load on the body during locomotion. Increases in load can be seen in situations of increased locomotor speed or increased stride length at a constant speed, and in activities which produce higher peak impact forces, such as running downhill. In downhill running, the center of mass of the runner falls a greater distance resulting in a greater impact. Thus, the lower extremity must absorb this added shock. The primary mechanism for attenuating this added impact is increased flexion of the knee during the initial portion of the support phase (24). Controlling this increased flexion are the quadriceps muscles of the anterior thigh. Although the quadriceps are knee extensors, they act eccentrically during this portion of support. Repeated eccentric activity over a prolonged period of time such as that experienced in downhill running has been related to myofibril and connective tissue damage. This damage has been linked to delayed-onset muscle soreness (25).

It would appear that altering kinematics may reduce the impact force to the system. As was suggested previously, increasing the degree of knee flexion is one alternative. However, there are trade-offs to this strategy. As an example, increasing the knee flexion angle at midstance ("Groucho running") indeed reduces the impact shock on the body (the shock transmission from the ankle to the head was decreased to less than 20% of its original value) (26). However, the cost of such a strategy is an increased rate of energy utilization such that this style of running is responsible for a 50% increase in steady-state oxygen consumption.

The load on the human body may appear to be deleterious to the various tissues, but loading can also beneficial. Bone has the ability to remodel by altering its size, shape, and structure to meet the demands of loads. Thus, bone can gain or lose cancellous and cortical bone in response to the level of the stress placed on it. For example, a positive correlation between body weight and bone mass exists (27). Increasing body weight increases bone mass because the added weight constitutes an added mechanical stress on the bone. On the other hand, prolonged weightlessness such as that experienced in space travel has been found to decrease bone mass (28). Similarly, when there is a partial or total immobilization of the lower extremity, the limb is not subjected to the normal mechanical stresses and bone is absorbed.

▶ SUMMARY

Force is the interaction of an object with its surroundings. Newton's three Laws of Motion form the basis for classical mechanics and explain the interactions between objects. The mechanical load on the human system is defined as the sum of the external forces on the system. The forces that constitute the load on the system depend on how the system is defined. For the most part, these are:

1. body weight
2. ground reaction force
3. joint reaction force
4. muscle force
5. elastic force.

External forces applied to the body (loading) depend on three factors: the magnitude of the force, the rate at which the force is applied, and the repetition of load application. The load on the system can have both a deleterious effect in causing injury or degeneration of the musculoskeletal system as well as a beneficial effect such as in the remodeling of bone. Fortunately, in the case of the former, the human body has a number of mechanisms by which load can be attenuated.

References

1. Munro CF, Miller DI, Fuglevand AJ. Ground reaction forces in running: a reexamination. *J Biomech* 20:147–155, 1987.
2. Winter DA. Moments of force and mechanical power in jogging. *J Biomech* 16:91–97, 1983.
3. An KN, Kwak BM, Chao EY, Morrey BF. Determination of muscle and joint forces: a new technique to solve the indeterminate problem. *J Biomech Eng* 106:364–367, 1984.
4. Schaepfer FE, Unold E, Nigg BM. The frictional charcateristics of tennis shoes. In: Nigg BM, Ker BA, eds. *Biomechanical Aspects of Sport Shoes and Playing Surfaces.* Calgary, Alberta: University of Calgary, 1983:153–160.
5. Paul JP. Bioengineering Studies of the Forces Transmitted by Joints—II. In: Kenedi RM, ed. *Biomechanics and Related Bioengineering Topics.* Oxford: Pergamon Press, 1965.
6. Crowninshield RD, Brand RA. A physiologically based criterion of muscle force prediction in locomotion. *J Biomech* 14:793–801, 1981.
7. Caldwell GE, Chapman AE. The general distribution problem: a physiological solution which includes antagonism. *Hum Move Sci* 10:355–392.
8. Gregor RJ, Komi PV, Jarvinen M. Achilles tendon forces during cycling. *Int J Sport Med* 8:9–14, 1987.
9. Marsh E, Sale DG, McComas AJ, Quinlan, J. The influence of joint position on ankle dorsiflexion in humans. *J Appl Physiol* 51:160–167, 1981.
10. Sale DG, Quinlan J, Marsh E, McComas AJ, Belanger AY. Influence of joint position on ankle plantar flexion in humans. *J Appl Physiol* 52:1636–1642, 1982.
11. Biewener AA, ed. *Biomechanics: Structures and Systems.* Oxford: Oxford University Press, 1992
12. Asmussen E, Bonde-Peterson F. Apparent efficiency and storage of elastic energy in human muscles during exercise. *Acta Physiol Scand* 92:537–545, 1974.
13. Komi PV, Bosco C. Utilization of stored elastic energy in leg extensor muscles by men and women. *Med Sci Sports Exerc* 10:261–265, 1978.
14. Nigg BM, Cole GK, Bruggeman GP. Impact forces during heel-toe running. *J Appl Biomech* 11:407–432, 1995.
15. Forwood MR, Burr DB. Physical activity and bone mass: exercise in futility? *Bone Min* 21:89–112, 1993.
16. Nordin M, Frankel VH. *Basic Biomechanics of the Musculoskeletal System.* 2nd ed. Philadelphia: Lea & Febiger, 1989.
17. Simon SR, Radin EL, Paul IL, Rose RM. The response of joints to impact loading-II invivo behavior of subchondral bone. *J Biomech* 5:267–272, 1972.
18. Radin E L, Parker HG, Pugh JW, Steinberg RS, Paul IL, Rose RM. Response of joints to impact loading-III. *J Biomech* 6: 51–57, 1973.
19. Voloshin A, Wosk J. An in vivo study of low back pain and shock absorption in the human locomotor system. *J Biomech* 15:21–27, 1982.
20. Holt KG, Hamill J. Running injuries and treatment: a dynamic approach. In: Sammarco GJ, ed. *Rehabilitation of the Foot and Ankle.* St. Louis: Mosby, 1995:241–258.
21. Hamill J, Bates BT, Holt KG. Timing of lower extremity joint actions during treadmill running. *Med Sci Sports Exerc* 24(7):807–813, 1992.
22. Nigg BM. Biomechanical aspects of running. In: BM Nigg BM ed. *Biomechanics of Running Shoes.* Champaign, IL: Human Kinetics Publishers, 1986:1–25.
23. Hamill J, Derrick TR, Holt KG. Shock attenuation and stride frequency during running. *Hum Move Sci* 14:45–60, 1995.
24. Buczek FL, Cavanagh PR. Stance phase knee and ankle kinematics and kinetics during level and downhill running. *Med Sci Sports Exerc* 22:669–677, 1990.
25. Schwane JA, Johnson SR, Vandenakker CB, Armstrong RB. Delayed-onset muscular soreness and plasma CPK and LDH activities after downhill running. *Med Sci Sports Exerc* 15:51–56, 1983.
26. McMahon TA, Valiant G, Frederick EC. Groucho running. *J Appl Physiol* 62:2326–2337, 1987.
27. Exner GU, Prader A, Elasser U, Ruegsegger P, Anliker M. Bone densitometry using computed tomography. Part I: selected determination of trabecular bone density and other bone mineral parameters. Normal values in children and adults. *Br J Radiol* 52:14–23, 1979.
28. Rambaut PC, Johnston RS. Prolonged weightlessness and calcium loss in man. *Acta Astronautica* 6:1113–1122, 1979.

6 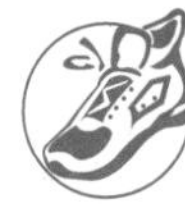 14  16, 17 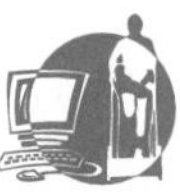 291, 292, 293 

CHAPTER 12
BIOMECHANICS AND PHYSIOLOGY OF POSTURE AND GAIT

Mark D. Grabiner and Philip E. Martin

Maintenance of posture and locomotion are, to varying degrees, critical components of all land-based exercise and athletic activities. The biomechanics and physiology of posture and locomotion have been among the most extensively studied of human activities. The purposes of this chapter are to 1) introduce the exercise professional to biomechanical and physiological issues associated with postural control and gait, and 2) provide a basis for understanding the experimental methods used to make quantitative biomechanical and physiological measurements associated with postural control and gait, the outcome variables, the interpretation of the variables, and the limitations of the interpretations. The reference list provides sources through which detailed treatment of many of the concepts may be explored. The first part of this chapter presents a framework of biomechanical fundamentals as they relate to the biomechanics of postural control and postural stability. The second part of this chapter presents some of the basic relationships between the biomechanics and physiology of gait, specifically as they relate to the topic of economy.

POSTURAL CONTROL AND STABILITY

The continuum of human performance that includes standing, walking, and running share many common neuromuscular and biomechanical mechanisms to which other motor tasks are subservient. Two of these mechanisms are postural control and stability.

Postural Control

Postural control is defined as the ability to predict, detect, and encode any change in posture; select and adapt a response; and execute the response within the biomechanical constraints of the body and the physical constraints of the environment (1). There are at least three conditions during which the postural control system must function. The first is simply maintaining postural stability against the force of gravity. The second is maintaining postural stability in the presence of self-initiated motions, such as lifting a weight. The third is maintaining postural stability in response to externally applied loads or forces, such as being tackled.

Postural control is dependent upon a number of systems that provide feedback to the central nervous system (CNS). The feedback arises from the vestibular, visual, and somatosensory systems. This feedback is processed by the central nervous system which subsequently generates muscle activation signals necessary for postural corrections. The vestibular system feedback, housed in the inner ear, provides information related to head position and motion with respect to gravity. The visual system provides information related to head position and motion relative to an external coordinate system. The somatosensory system comprises a number of elements including muscles, joints, and skin. Receptors in muscles and joints provide information related to the position and motion of joints. Mechanoreceptors in the skin, for example, those in the plantar surface of the foot, provide information regarding pressure allowing the body to accommodate to swaying that occurs while standing.

The systems that provide postural feedback are redundant and one of the tasks faced by the CNS is to decode all the incoming signals to determine the status of the system. For example, while in a car, the movement of another vehicle detected by virtue of peripheral vision indicates only general motion. Often, one cannot immediately determine whether the perceived motion is that of the vehicle in which one is seated or that of the second vehicle. However, without shifting one's gaze, feedback from the vestibular system can signal whether the head has experienced an acceleration. If so, the perceived motion can be attributed, in part, to motion of the vehicle in which the person is riding.

Postural Stability

In a broad sense, stability refers to whether a system (body) returns to its original stable position or motion or another stable position or motion after it has been subjected to a perturbation (disturbance). Postural stability generally refers to body stability during upright standing conditions. It has traditionally been characterized as a function of the center of gravity or the center of pressure relative to the base of support. The center of gravity is a point about which all the mass of a body can be considered to reside. The base of support is defined by the size and shape of the contact area between the body segments that are in contact with the supporting surface (floor or ground). For a person standing barefoot on a flat supporting surface, the base of support is the outline of the area encompassed by the feet. If the horizontal position of the center of gravity is located within the dimensions of the base of support, then the basic requirement for static postural stability is satisfied.

The location of the center of gravity is a function not only of the mass of the body, but also the manner in which the mass is distributed or oriented. For example, the location of the center of gravity shifts anteriorly and superiorly as a person simply flexes the shoulder joints to 90°. From a practical standpoint, estimation of the location of the center of gravity can be time consuming and associated with error. Fortunately, the use of force plates makes the quantification of static postural stability somewhat straight-forward. Quantifying postural stability using force plate data relies to a great extent on determining the center of pressure rather than the center of gravity. The center of pressure is a single point on the surface of a force plate through which the resultant vertical force acts. Motion of the center of pressure reflects, but does not mirror, motion of the center of gravity. However, during conditions in which the center of pressure lies within the boundaries of the base of support, the basic requirements for static postural stability are satisfied.

Although descriptions of common laboratory and clinical tests are available, measuring postural control and postural stability poses numerous challenges (2). Laboratory tests have been criticized as having little clinical relevance and in some cases little biomechanical relevance. On the other hand, clinical tests have been criticized as having less than satisfactory sensitivity. An example of such difficulties is the general acceptance that physiological changes associated with the normal aging process result in an increase in the amplitude of static postural sway and that this increased postural sway is associated with the increased incidence of falling in the elderly. Recent scientific investigation does not necessarily support these contentions (3). Postural stability has been demonstrated to be substantially greater in younger than older subjects (3). However, measures of static postural sway and stability are not correlated in either age group. In elderly subjects, the correlation between static postural sway and static stability was 0.23, indicating little relationship between these attributes (3).

Thus, force plate measurement of static postural sway may lack the sensitivity to provide consistently meaningful information regarding the status of the postural control system. However, stability limits appear to discriminate between age groups to a much greater extent and may better reflect the characteristics of a postural perturbation, the reaction to which, is a stepping response.

Dynamic Posturography

Clinically, it is important to assess the status of the vestibular, visual, and somatosensory components of the postural control system, both individually and as an integrated whole. One of the measurement standards that has emerged for this purpose is called dynamic posturography (4). Dynamic posturography uses a computer-controlled platform on which the subject stands. The platform is enclosed by a "visual surround" that serves both to provide a consistent visual stimulus and to visually isolate the subject from the environment. Both the platform which the subject stands on and the visual surround may be moved, under control of the computer, which alters the fidelity of a particular feedback source. By systematically manipulating the type of feedback used to determine the extent of postural stability (the Sensory Organization Test [SOT]), the relative contribution of each feedback system to postural stability can be derived. An equilibrium quotient (EQ) for each system manipulation representing an index of postural stability is computed.

Research findings using such methods are consistent with the previously discussed results regarding the failure of static postural sway measured on a force plate to differentiate between young and old subjects. The data illustrate that systematic reduction of sensory feedback has a substantial effect on the EQ. Further, the effects of aging tend to amplify the effects of the SOT conditions. Compared to eliminating visual feedback, diminishing somatosensory feedback (sway referencing) results in a larger reduction of the EQ. The largest EQ reduction appears to be elicited during conditions in which the vestibular system is taxed to the greatest extent.

A second variable, called the Balance Strategy Score (BSS) is also computed for the various types of feedback of the SOT. The BSS relates to the motor pattern used by a subject to maintain postural stability. There are three basic motor strategies for correction of anterior-posterior postural perturbations; the ankle strategy, the hip strategy, and the stepping strategy. The specific strategy selected by normal adults depends on the surface upon which the subject is standing and the magnitude of the perturbation. The ankle strategy, which is the most commonly implemented, controls body sway by generating moments about the ankle joint. The ankle strategy is effective when the support surface is large and firm enough to resist the ankle joint movements. Normally the ankle strategy is used to counteract perturbations that are applied slowly and are of low magnitude. An ankle strategy is most useful when the amplitude of body sway does not approach the limit, where a loss of balance is likely. A hip strategy is used in response to larger, more rapidly applied perturbations occurring when the support surface is compliant or smaller than the surfaces of the feet. A hip strategy is employed quite often when a loss of balance is imminent. During conditions in which neither an ankle or hip strategy is effective in restoring postural stability, a stepping response is selected to establish a new and stable posture.

Lastly, dynamic posturography includes a motor coordination test (MCT). During the MCT, large anterior and posterior translations, and toes-up and toes-down rotations are applied to the subject through movement/rotation of the platform. The purpose of the MCT is to assess the activation of the lower extremity and trunk muscles that are stretched by the platform motion and which muscles contribute to the restoration of postural stability. For example, an ankle strategy in response to a perturbation that rotates the subject forward (a backward surface translation), is associated with a distal-to-proximal activation pattern of the posterior ankle, thigh, and trunk muscles. A hip strategy, associated with a perturbation in the same direction, however, elicits activation of anterior trunk and thigh muscles. The sequence of muscle activation in response to specific perturbations, as well as the latencies of the activations (from perturbation to onset of muscle activation) can be substantially affected by normal aging as well as neuromuscular disorders.

While dynamic posturography measures postural stability during static upright posture and is considered a "gold standard," true dynamic postural stability is a somewhat elusive quantity because the easily quantified criterion for static stability (i.e., center of pressure within the boundaries of the base of support) is not easily applied. For example, during walking, specifically during the swing phase of gait, the center of pressure falls outside of the boundaries of the support foot for up to 80% of the time. A body is considered dynamically stable if active and passive disturbances can be predicted and detected, if responses to the disturbances can be selected, and if the selected responses can be executed. However, unlike static postural stability, a mathematical description of the previous statement describing dynamic stability has not been formulated. Given that most falls and injuries occur during gait, ascending or descending stairs, or rising from chairs, it seems reasonable, if not expedient, to include dynamic motor tasks in the description of postural stability (1).

The range of measurement techniques, instruments and variables, and the potential for uncertainty relative to interpreting the measurements in a functional context confront the exercise practitioner with something of a conundrum that is related to both the availability of many expedient measurement methods and the inability to generalize from testing conditions to conditions of daily living. Guidelines have been developed that are useful in the decision making process that relate to the selection of the task(s), the selection of the perturbation(s), and the selection of outcome variables (5). It is suggested that the tasks selected should represent the normal spectrum of movement and, in particular, challenge the postural control system. Similarly, the selection of the perturbation should be based upon the extent to which the system is challenged and to which type feedback is provided regarding the performance of the postural control system. Outcome variables should be selected based upon the ability to identify performance deficits and provide diagnostic information. However, these recommendations represent the "ideal" and serve as a goal for research efforts. For the exercise professional, they serve as a reminder that effective measurement, interpretation, and application of postural control data can prove difficult.

RELATIONSHIPS BETWEEN ECONOMY AND LOCOMOTION BIOMECHANICS

Inter-individual Variation in Movement Economy

Economy is measured by the steady-state oxygen consumption for a given submaximal task. This measure of the aerobic demand is typically normalized to the body weight of the individual, particularly for tasks in which upright posture must be maintained and body weight supported by the musculature. This measure is expressed as milliliters of oxygen consumed per minute of exercise per unit of body weight (ml/kg/min). Occasionally economy is expressed per unit of distance traveled (e.g., ml/km/kg) when comparing the economy for different speeds of movement (e.g., different walking or running speeds). Numerous research reports have demonstrated that the economy of motion for a given task tends to vary widely among individuals. It should be stressed that this between-individual variation in economy exists independently of neurological and musculoskeletal deficiencies and diseases that may have large deleterious effects on movement economy.

In describing normal variation in economy among a group of young, healthy adults by correlating the aerobic demands observed for one task against those for another task, it has been noted that individuals clearly were neither economical nor uneconomical for all types of physical activity (6). Economy tends to be task specific and thus may be governed in part by biomechanical factors which define the movement technique used by an individual to perform a certain task.

Despite the commonly held belief that biomechanical factors help to explain economy differences between individuals, the extent to which these differences can be attributed to biomechanics is not well defined. Assuming that selected biomechanical factors are related to movement economy, the subsequent question becomes one of whether or not lasting changes in movement patterns can be produced so that movement economy is improved. The following sections attempt to highlight the relationships that have been observed between movement economy and a few selected kinematic, kinetic, and structural factors, and the practical implications of these relationships when measuring economy and prescribing exercise. The reader is referred to several published reviews for further information on the topic (7–10).

Speed of Movement

The speed at which an individual moves is one of the simplest and most fundamental biomechanical descriptors of movement. As an example, preferred walking speed is a good indicator of the debilitating effects caused by knee injury and of the general decline in physical performance capabilities of elderly adults (11, 12). Thus, preferred walking speed should not be overlooked as one simple marker that offers insight into the movement capabilities of an individual, especially when evaluating individuals whose exercise capacity has been limited by disease, injury, and/or normal aging. The average preferred walking speed of healthy, young adults is approximately 1.45 m/sec while that for healthy, elderly adults (approximately 70 years of age) is approximately 1.30 m/sec. The preferred walking speeds of young and old adults has also been shown to be subtly associated with physical activity status. Individuals pursuing a physically active lifestyle tend to possess self-selected walking speeds that are slightly higher (approximately 0.1 to 0.2 m/sec higher) than sedentary individuals (13).

When evaluating gait economy, it is obvious that increasing the speed of movement results in increased rates of oxygen consumption for both walking and running. Altering the speed of walking or running is one of the most common ways of modifying the intensity of the task in exercise evaluations. Many economy comparisons between individuals or groups presented in the research literature have been made at fixed speeds of walking or running with aerobic demand expressed in ml/in/kg. Any confounding effect that speed may have on economy comparisons is thereby eliminated through use of a common test speed. On the other hand, having a subject walk or run at a preferred speed during an economy or biomechanical evaluation of gait has the appeal of assessing an individual under exercise conditions that are typical of those used by the individual on a daily basis and that are within the exercise capabilities of the individual.

One problem of using preferred speeds of locomotion during gait evaluations is that there is a speed-related confound that cannot be ignored. From an economy perspective, a U-shaped speed-economy relationship (Fig. 12.1) exists for walking when aerobic demands for a wide range of walking speeds are expressed relative to distance traveled (ml/km/kg). In other words, there is a speed of walking (approximately 1.3 to 1.4 m/sec) for adults that minimizes the aerobic demand required to walk a given distance (14, 15). At walking speeds both higher and lower than this intermediate speed, the cost to traverse a given distance is increased. This effect of speed is most apparent at particularly low and high speeds of walking. For example, it has been demonstrated that energy expenditure (cal/kg/m) was minimized at approximately 1.25 m/sec but that the speed-energy expenditure curve was nearly flat at approximately 1.1 to 1.4 m/sec (13).

In contrast to walking, the energy cost to run a given distance is reasonably similar for a given individual across a range of running speeds. While Figure 12.1 sug-

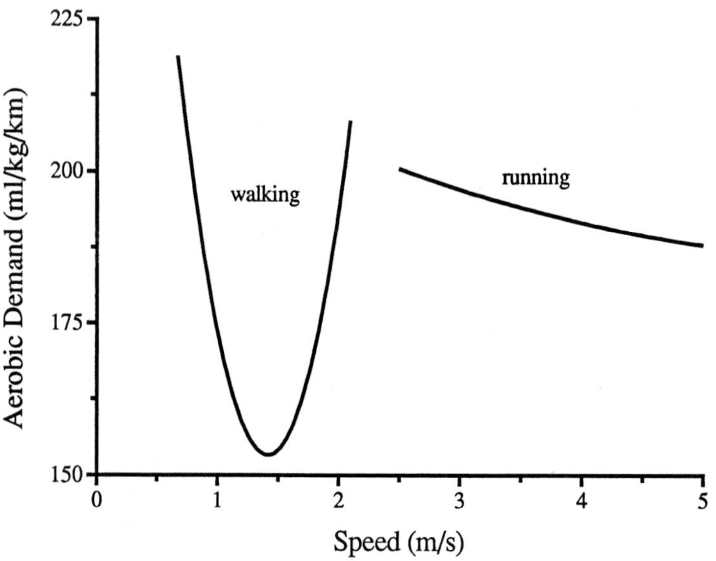

Figure 12.1. The aerobic demand to walk a given distance (ml/kg/km) is affected substantially by walking speed. The most economical walking speed is approximately 1.3 to 1.4 m/sec. In contrast, the aerobic demand to run a given distance is affected minimally by speed.

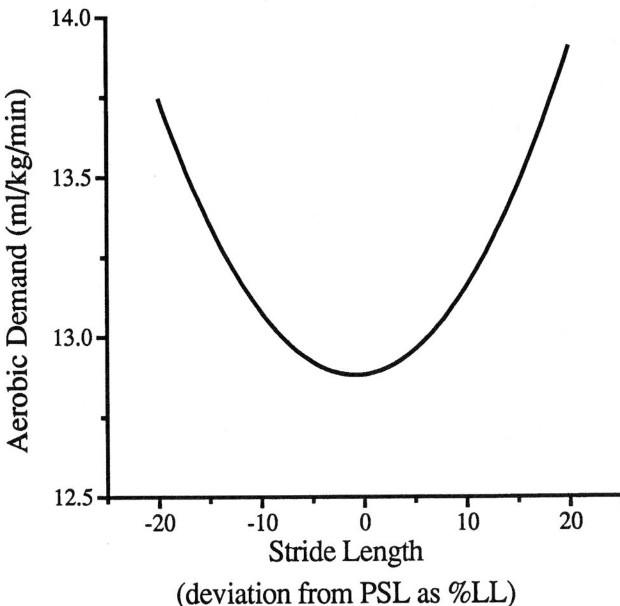

Figure 12.2. The aerobic demand for walking (shown here) and running is affected significantly by stride length and rate. For most individuals, as stride length is either increased or decreased (ergo, stride rate is decreased or increased, respectively) from the preferred stride length (PSL), expressed as a percentage of leg length (%LL), aerobic demand increases.

gests that there is a subtle decline in the aerobic demand per kilometer traveled as running speed increases, the slope of the speed-economy curve for running can vary somewhat from slightly negative as shown to slightly positive depending on the individual subject, specific subject group, and range of speeds examined. The important point is that the speed confound is of far less concern when assessing running economy if the energy demand is met aerobically.

From a biomechanics perspective, comparing gait patterns becomes particularly challenging when comparisons are not being made at a common walking or running speed. The reason for this is that nearly all kinematic and kinetic descriptors of gait are speed-dependent. For example, it is well established that as walking speed increases, factors such as stride length, joint angular velocities, peak values for ground reaction forces and new moments about joints of the lower extremity, and activation levels of numerous leg muscles all tend to increase, while other factors such as stride time and related temporal descriptors of the gait pattern tend to decrease. Thus, while existing technology and methods offer the potential to describe a wide range of biomechanical characteristics of walking or running patterns, assessing specific deficiencies in gait is compromised, or at least substantially complicated, by the absence of speed control.

Stride Length/Rate

Stride length is defined as the distance traveled by the body during one full cycle of motion (e.g., from the instant of left foot contact until the subsequent left foot contact). Stride rate or cadence, which is the reciprocal of stride time, represents the number of strides completed per unit of time. The average speed or velocity of walking or running is then reflected simply as the product of stride length and rate.

The effect that stride length and rate have on gait economy during steady-state submaximal exercise lends itself to simple experimental assessment because of this relationship and our ability to control velocity by using a treadmill. The protocol used most frequently involves first determining the preferred stride length and rate for a particular velocity, followed by steady-state aerobic demand assessments at a series of stride length and rate combinations that deviate from the preferred condition. This is accomplished by having an individual match the stepping rate to an audible signal so that desired stride rate and stride length conditions are produced. When this experimental manipulation is conducted, a curvilinear stride length/rate-economy curve results (Fig. 12.2). The aerobic demand of walking or running at a controlled speed tends to increase nonlinearly as optimal (preferred) stride length or rate is changed (16).

The preferred and most economical stride length/rate combinations are usually in close agreement with one another, suggesting that most individuals naturally achieve their optimal stride length and rate combination through some unknown mechanism. One practical implication of this outcome is that a coach is generally ill-advised to manipulate stride length and rate for the purpose of improving economy and running performance unless aerobic demand data specifically confirm an uneconomical running pattern. In addition, research suggests that there is no meaningful relationship between the most economical stride length and leg length, indicating that it is not possible to predict the most economical stride length from physical dimensions.

The reason for the U-shaped stride length/rate-economy response is probably associated with fundamental muscle force and power generating capabilities. Based on fundamental mechanical properties of muscle, it is well known that the force generating capacity of muscle falls non-linearly as the velocity of shortening increases (17). When plotting power (the product of muscle force and the velocity of shortening) as a function of the velocity of shortening, the capacity of muscle to generate power is greatest when muscle fiber velocity is approximately one-third of maximum shortening velocity. Changes in stride length and rate require concomitant changes in the rates of muscle lengthening and shortening, the rate of force development, and the demand for muscular power output, all of which should affect aerobic demand.

MOVEMENT KINETICS: GROUND REACTION FORCES AND MECHANICAL POWER

Ground Reaction Forces

The ground reaction force, which reflects the net effect of muscular action and segment accelerations while the body is in contact with the ground, has been studied extensively by gait specialists. There is surprisingly little research, however, that provides insight into the relationships between gait economy and ground reaction force features. Existing research suggests that only moderate to weak relationships exist between ground reaction force characteristics and economy (9). More economical runners exhibit significantly lower first peaks in the vertical component of the ground reaction force and also tend to have smaller antero-posterior and vertical peak forces and more of a rearfoot striking pattern. It is speculated that the need to provide cushioning during early contact may have an important effect on the demands placed on the muscles, which in turn may affect economy. When landing on the forefoot, an individual may need to rely more heavily on musculature to assist with cushioning the impact. In contrast, the footwear and skeletal structures of a rearfoot striker may play greater roles in cushioning and supporting the body during early contact.

Mechanical Power

Aerobic demand represents a global measure of the physiological demand of walking or running. One example of a global estimate of muscular effort from a biomechanics perspective is mechanical power output. Assuming that a substantial portion of the aerobic demand of gait is associated with muscles performing mechanical work (i.e., actively shortening or lengthening), then mechanical power should be an effective predictor of gait economy. This is certainly true when the aerobic demand and mechanical power are studied for a wide range of walking or running speeds. As walking or running speed increases, both aerobic demand (ml/min/kg) and mechanical power increase in direct proportion to speed. This is not surprising since both aerobic demand and power output are viewed as markers of exercise intensity. Research has shown, however, that measures of mechanical power explain only a small amount of the inter-individual variation in gait economy when examining a single speed of walking or running (13). This may be due to the fact that there are a multitude of factors, biomechanical and otherwise, that affect gait economy, and that the relative importance of these factors is likely to vary from individual to individual. In addition, methods of estimating mechanical power output of the body have their own limitations that negatively affect their accuracy as an estimate of muscular effort.

FLEXIBILITY AND GAIT ECONOMY

One fundamental component of physical fitness is musculoskeletal flexibility. Intuitively, one would speculate that better flexibility, particularly within the trunk and lower extremities, would have a positive effect on gait economy. This notion is consistent with a widely held view that increasing flexibility is desirable for optimal running performance and may also contribute to reduced incidence of certain types of musculoskeletal injury. Poorer flexibility, on the other hand, could result in a modified gait pattern (e.g., shorter stride length and higher stride rate) that is less economical or in increased muscular effort to produce the same gait pattern because of increased resistance to motion near the extremes of the range of motion. This interpretation is compatible with the observations that: (1) gait economy is known to be adversely affected by advancing age in adults and by lower extremity orthopedic pathologies, and (2) musculoskeletal flexibility tends to decline with old age and joint pathologies.

Interestingly, however, is the observation that higher "non-pathologic musculoskeletal tightness" was modestly related to lower aerobic demands (i.e., better economy) during walking and jogging (19). The average aerobic demand for a third of the study sample that was determined to be the most flexible was approximately 10% higher than that for the least flexible third of the sample. It was speculated that less flexible individuals may benefit economically from greater elastic energy contributions and a reduced need to use active musculature to neutralize unproductive or undesired movements. These rather limited and counterintuitive observations suggest a need for additional research on the specific effects of musculoskeletal flexibility on gait economy in various subject populations.

MODIFICATION OF ECONOMY VIA TRAINING AND MOVEMENT EDUCATION

Based on the preceding discussions, the reader should be left with the impression that the association between gait kinematics and kinetics and economy is complex and far less definitive than intuition or common beliefs may suggest. Nevertheless, it is possible through careful testing to identify individuals who display uneconomical gait patterns, such as runners who overstride excessively. From an economy perspective, such individuals may clearly benefit from changes in their pattern of motion. However, there are conflicting findings from studies attempting to describe the effect of training and education on moment economy (20–22). From these limited analyses, it is apparent that the question regarding the ability to significantly improve economy through biomechanical training remains unanswered.

▶ SUMMARY

For the exercise professional, biomechanics and physiology represent two of the foundational bricks in the science of exercise. These two disciplines have considerable overlap relative to postural control and gait. This overlap has been briefly presented in this chapter by first linking the physiology of the postural control system to the mechanics of static and dynamic postural stability, and then linking the economy of the biomechanics of walking and running. Some of the uncertainties associated with each area that impacts the utility of the measures for the exercise professional were identified. These uncertainties are related to the technology and models used to collect and analyze research data, the complexity and disparity of human motor performance, and the trade-off between cost and accessibility for various methods of assessment. These uncertainties provide an impetus for continued research and development that ultimately will yield practical applications.

References

1. Horak FB, Shupert CL, Mirka A. Components of postural dyscontrol in the elderly: a review. *Neurobiol Aging* 10:727–738, 1989.
2. Berg K. Balance and its measure in the elderly: a review. *Physiother Can* 41:240–246, 1989.
3. Martin PE, Grabiner MD, Collins JJ, Messier SP, Ashto-Miller JA. Postural control and gait deficiencies in older adults. *Med Sci Sports and Exerc* 28(5 Suppl):S150, 1996.
4. Wolfson L, Whipple R, Derby CA, Amerman P, Murphy T, Tobin JN, Nashner L. A dynamic posturography study of balance in healthy elderly. *Neurology* 42:2069–2075, 1992.
5. Patla AE, Frank JS, Winter DA. Balance control in the elderly: implications for clinical assessment and rehabilitation. *Can J Public Health* 83:S29-S33, 1992.
6. Daniels JT, Scardina NJ, Foley P. $V0_2$ submax during five modes of exercise. In: Bachl N, Prokop L, Sucket R, eds. *Proceedings of the World Congress on Sports Medicine.* Vienna: Urban & Schwartzenberg, 1984:604–615.
7. Cavanagh PR, Kram R. Mechanical and muscular factors affecting the efficiency of human movement. *Med Sci Sports Exerc* 17:326–331, 1985.
8. Martin PE, Morgan DW. Biomechanical considerations for economical walking and running. *Med Sci Sports Exerc* 24:467–474, 1992.
9. Morgan DW, Martin PE, Krahenbuhl GS. Factors affecting running economy. *Sport Med* 7:310–330, 1989.
10. Williams KR, CavanaghPR. Relationship between distance running mechanics, running economy, and performance. *J Appl Physiol* 63:1236–1245, 1987.
11. Andriacchi TP, Ogle JA, Galante JO. Walking as a basis for normal and abnormal gait measurements. *J Biomech* 10: 261–268, 1977.
12. Himann JE, Cunningham DA, Rechnitzer PA, Patterson DH. Age-related changes in speed of walking. *Med Sci Sports Exerc* 20:161–166, 1988.
13. Martin PE, Heise GD, Morgan DW. Interrelationships between mechanical power, energy transfers, and walking and running economy. *Med Sci Sports Exerc* 25:508–515, 1993.
14. Ralston HJ. Energy-speed relation and optimal speed during level walking. *Arbeitsphysiologica* 17:277–283, 1958.
15. Martin PE, Rothstein DE, Larish DD. Effects of age and physical activity status on the speed-aerobic demand relationship of walking. *J Appl Physiol* 73:200–206, 1992.
16. Cavanagh PR, Williams KR. The effect of stride length variation on oxygen uptake during distance running. *Med Sci Sport Exerc* 14:30–35, 1982.
17. Hill AV. The maximum work and mechanical efficiency of human muscles, and their most economical speed. *J Physiol* 56:19–41, 1922.
18. Gleim GW, Stachenfeld NS, Nicholas JA. The influence of flexibility on the economy of walking and jogging. *J Orthop Res* 8:814–823, 1990.
19. Petray CK, Krahenbuhl GS. Running training, instruction on running technique, and running economy in 10-year old males. *Res Quarterly Exerc Sport* 56:251–255, 1985.
20. Messier SP, Cirillo KJ. Effects of a verbal and visual feedback system on running technique, perceived exertion and running economy in female novice runners. *J Sport Sci* 7:113–126, 1989.
21. Morgan DW, Martin PE, Craig M, Caruso C, Clifton R, Hopewell R. Effect of stride length optimization on the aerobic demand of running. *J Appl Physiol* 77:245–251, 1994.

7, 8, 75, 159, 161, 167 185 293

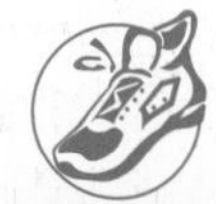
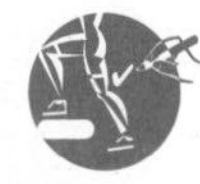

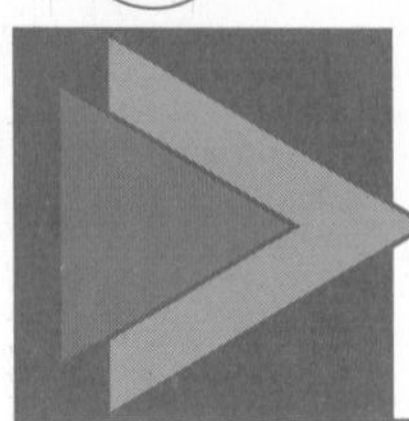

CHAPTER **13**

Low Back Exercises: Prescription for the Healthy Back and When Recovering from Injury

Stuart M. McGill

Low back and abdominal exercises are prescribed for a variety of reasons, but primarily for rehabilitation of the injured low back, prevention of injury, and/or as a component of fitness training programs. The objective of exercise prescription is to stress both damaged tissue and other healthy supporting tissues to promote tissue repair, while avoiding further excessive loading that can exacerbate existing structural weakness. While knowledge of tissue forces during exercise is important to avoid further injury, choosing the optimal load requires a blend of "art" and "science." In general, the better exercise programs are designed to train the motor control system to activate the spine stabilizers, then to progress with endurance training and, finally, to enhance strength and flexibility. The professional challenge is to make wise decisions from the balance of laboratory and clinical experience. This chapter describes the causes of low back injuries, the scientific support for certain types of exercises to train the low back, the specific exercises documented to challenge muscle, enhance performance, and minimize spine loading, and discusses several caveats for exercise prescription to enhance the chance of positive outcome.

The focus of this chapter is on developing the safest exercises for daily maintenance of low back health and has been compiled with several scientific manuscripts and book chapters by the author along with the most recent developments in back health.

EXERCISE AND LOW BACK PAIN

The reported effectiveness of various training and rehabilitation programs for the low back is quite variable, with some claiming great success while others report no success, or even negative results (1, 2). In fact, some training programs appear to harm the lower back of some individuals. The cause of this tissue damage has been attributed to excessive torso flexion, disadvantageous muscle lengths in some postures, inappropriate orientation of internal structures of the torso with respect to the legs, and other reasons (3–7). The discrepancy regarding the effectiveness and safety of exercise programs in various reports may be due to the prescription of inappropriate exercises caused by a lack of understanding of the tissue loading that results during various tasks (8). Exercise professionals sometimes unknowingly formulate programs that create excessive loads and exacerbate the damage. While specific exercises have been recommended for their capacity to maximize muscle activity in the past, virtually none have examined the safety by quantifying individual spine tissue forces (9, 10). The exercises reviewed in this chapter were evaluated on a tissue loading, injury criterion.

Many studies report loss of strength, flexibility, and endurance associated with low back injury. However, whether these deficits are the cause or the result of low back disease is not distinguishable from these data, which makes the findings open to misinterpretation. Very few longitudinal studies are available, although one such study clearly demonstrated "more fit" firefighters had fewer injuries than their "less fit" colleagues (11).

Several hypotheses can be considered to explain the general role of exercise on maintaining low back tissue health and optimizing the repair process. There is powerful evidence which demonstrates that exercise:

- Stimulates tissue hypertrophy
- Slows (possibly reverses) several degenerative conditions
- Enhances the nutritional benefit to the disc
- Is efficacious in treating the injured back compared to surgical intervention, bedrest, or simple flexibility programs (12–15)

In addition, the success of a carefully formulated exercise program that includes progressive "stabilization exercise routines," emphasizing muscle cocontraction with the spine in a neutral posture, has been documented (16).

While hip flexibility has been shown to be important, spine flexibility has never been shown to enhance the outcome of low back exercise programs for those with low back injury, nor reduce the risk of future injury in healthy populations.

ANATOMY

The lumbar spine is comprised of five vertebrae, each separated by intervertebral discs and two facet joints posteriorly. While the vertebrae are often considered rigid and most of the motion takes place in the discs, both the discs and vertebrae act as shock absorbers (Fig. 13.1) (17). While the ligaments are not shown in Figure 13.1, they connect adjacent vertebrae and become strained at the end range of spine motion. Some specific functional aspects of the anatomy are discussed later.

In upright standing, there is a natural curve in the low back called lordosis. Despite the common belief that hyperlordosis (an extended lumbar spine) is linked to low back pain, this is not true. Rather, standing hypolordosis and hyperlordosis are indications of biological variability and are only problematic in the most extreme cases. Nonetheless, certain individuals may develop inappropriate muscle balance and flexibility about the hips, low back, and knees which can result in increased loading of these areas during the performance of both athletic and daily activities if the level of lordosis is not controlled. Avoiding the end range of motion (in the spine) during activity can reduce the risk of several types of injury.

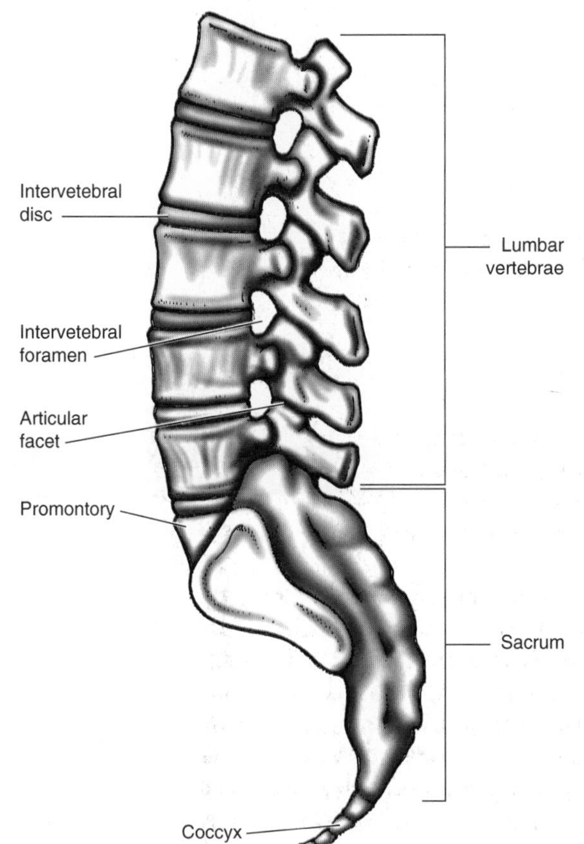

Figure 13.1. The lumbar spine consists of 5 vertebrae with intervening discs. It has a normal lordotic curve, which is a position of elastic equilibrium and lowest stress. (Adapted with permission from White AM, Anderson R, eds. *Conservative Care of Low Back Pain.* Baltimore: Williams & Wilkins, 1991.)

HOW SPECIFIC INJURIES OCCUR

Understanding the cause of injury is important for appropriate prescription of exercise and the development of injury avoidance strategies. There is a tendency among those reporting or describing the back injury to identify a single specific event as the cause of the damage, such as lifting and twisting with a box. This description of low back injury is common, particularly among the occupational/medical community who are often required to identify a single event when filling out injury reporting forms. However, relatively few low back injuries occur from a single event; rather, the culminating injury event was preceded by a history of excessive loading which gradually, but progressively, reduced the level of tolerance to tissue failure (18). Thus other scenarios where sub-failure loads can result in injury are probably more important. For example, the ultimate failure of a tissue (i.e., injury) can result from accumulated trauma produced by either repeated application of load (and failure from fatigue) or of a sustained load that is applied for long duration or repetitively applied (and failure from deformation and strain). Thus, the injury process may not always be associated with loads of high magnitude. Injury to specific low back structures are described below.

Vertebrae

A number of studies over the years demonstrate that a neutral spine under compressive load results in bony failure, specifically end plate fracture occurring together with damage to underlying trabeculae (Fig 13.2) (19, 20). Furthermore, repeated loading reduces the ultimate strength so that bony failure occurs at lower levels (21). Disc herniation is an extremely rare occurrence when the spine motion unit is compressed in a neutral posture (i.e., neutral lordosis—not flexed, laterally bent, or twisted). High velocity compression results in often catastrophic vertebral burst fractures, although this is not associated with non-impact exercise (22).

Disc Herniation

Disc herniation from a one-time application of load is extremely difficult to produce in the laboratory although it has been described with the application of compression to a spine deviated into hyperflexion and

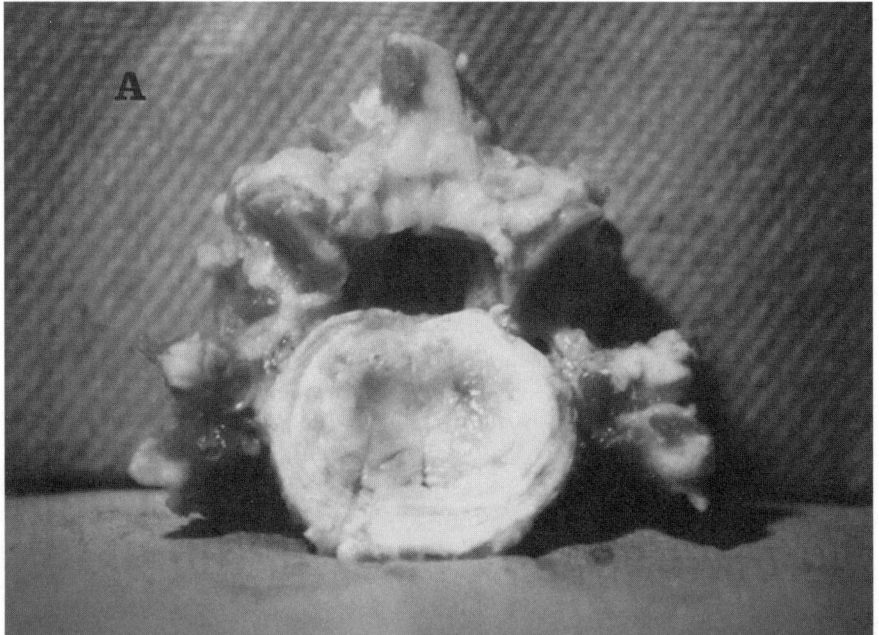

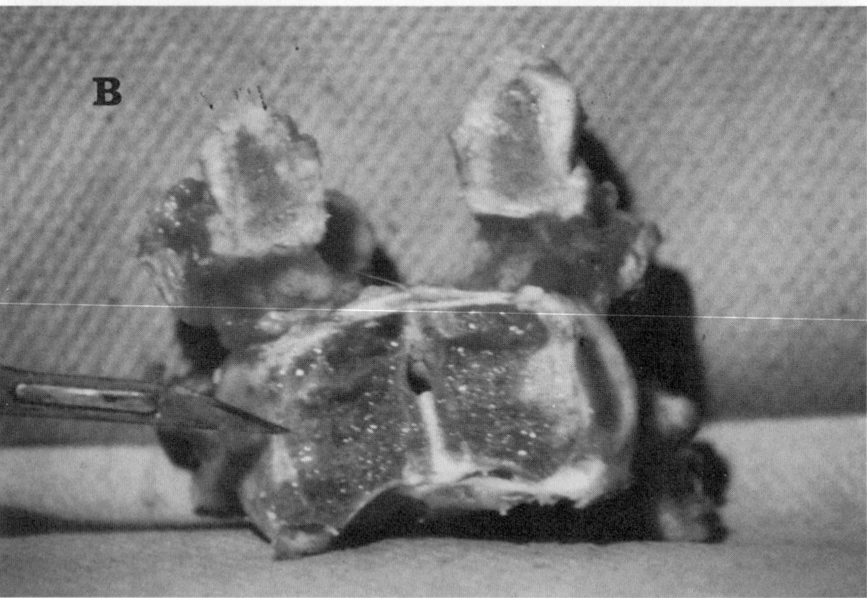

Figure 13.2. End plate fracture (A) and intrusion of nuclear material (shown at the tip of the scalpel) into the vertebral body (B) from compressive loading of a spine in a neutral posture. These are porcine specimens from the University of Waterloo laboratory.

lateral bending (23). Herniation is more consistently produced under many cycles of combined compression, flexion, and torsional loading and tends to occur in younger specimens with no visible gross signs of degeneration (24–26). Epidemiological data also links herniation with sedentary occupations and the sitting posture (27). Older disks appear not to have enough fluid to "flow," leading to herniation, and older spines appear not to exhibit "classic extrusion" of nuclear material, but rather are characterized by delamination of the anulus layers and radial cracks, which appear to progress with repeated loading (28, 29). In summary, it appears that disc herniation is the result of cyclic loading, or prolonged and sustained loading, in deviated spine postures. The notion that disc herniation in an occupational or athletic setting is the result of a single event appears unlikely.

Ligaments

A similar story unfolds with bony failure and ligamentous injury. It has been noted that soft tissue injuries are much more common during high energy traumatic events such as automobile collision (30). Other research in both human and animal specimens loaded at slow load rates in bending and shear suggest that, most frequently, excessive tension in the longitudinal ligaments results in avulsion (tearing away) or bony failure as the ligament pulls some bone away near its attachment (31, 32). Slower strain rates produce more ligament avulsion injuries while faster strain rates result in more ligamentous failure to the fiber bundles (in the middle region of the ligament).

Another clinical report found that approximately 20% of cadaveric spines possessed visibly ruptured interspinous ligaments (in their middle, not at their bony attachment) and that dorsal and ventral positions, together with supraspinous, remained intact (33). Given the oblique fiber direction of the interspinous complex (Fig. 13.3), a very likely scenario to damage this ligament would be slipping, falling, and landing on the buttocks (causing a high ligament loading rate), driving the pelvis forward on impact, and creating a posterior shearing of the lumbar joints when the spine is fully flexed. The interspinous ligament is a major load bearing tissue in this example of high energy loading where anterior shear displacement is combined with full flexion (34).

Given the available data, it would appear that torn ligaments of the spine during lifting or other non-impact activities, particularly to the interspinous complex, is more uncommon than common. Rather, it appears much more likely that ligament damage occurs during a more traumatic event, such as during a fall with direct impact on the spine, which leads to joint laxity and acceleration of subsequent arthritic changes. The possibility of crushing the interspinous ligament complex, in forced hyperextension (hyperlordosis), has also been noted (22).

Facets and Neural Arch

The facets and neural arch appear to withstand moderate shearing load and fail under shear loading and torsional loading and hyperextension (35, 36). Epidemiologically, failure of the neural arch and pars interarticularis is common among athletes who rapidly

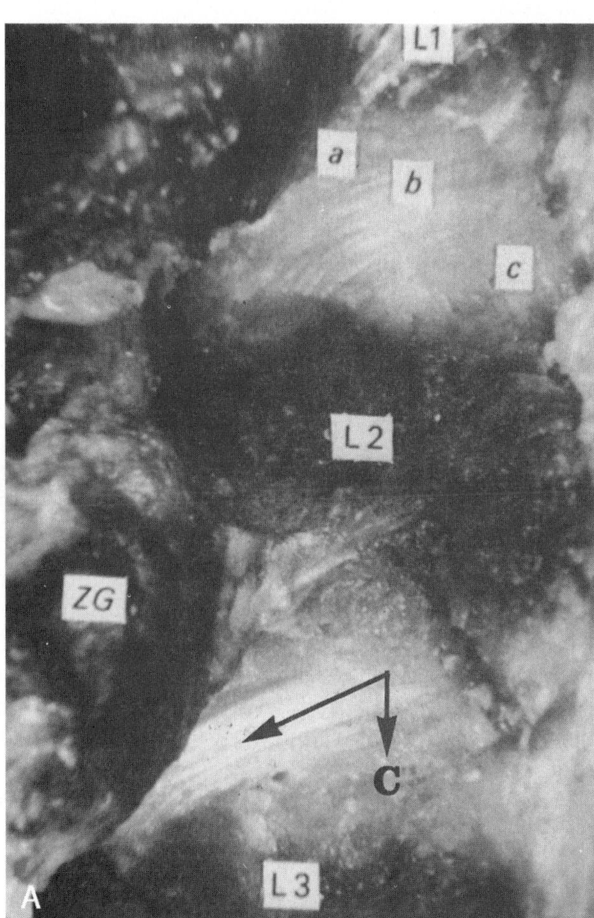

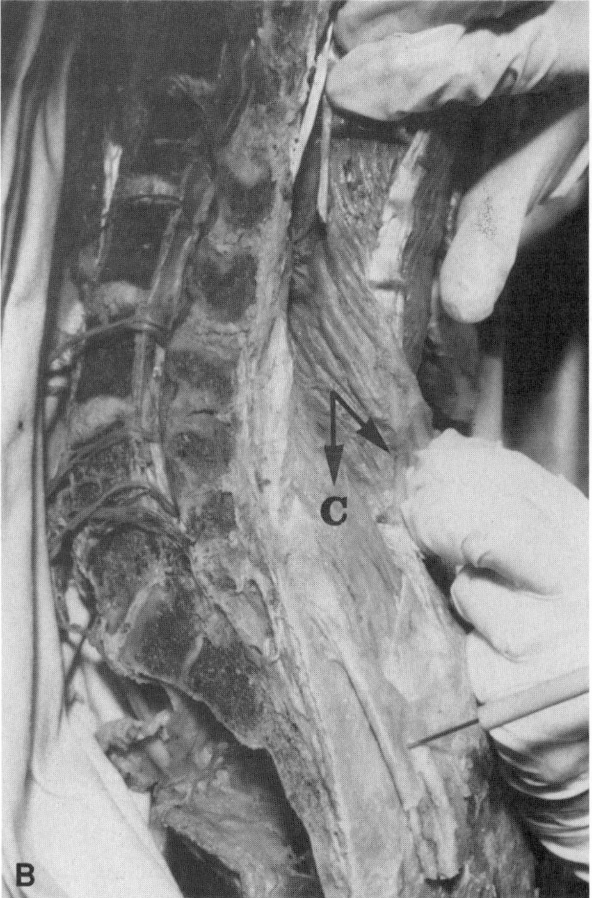

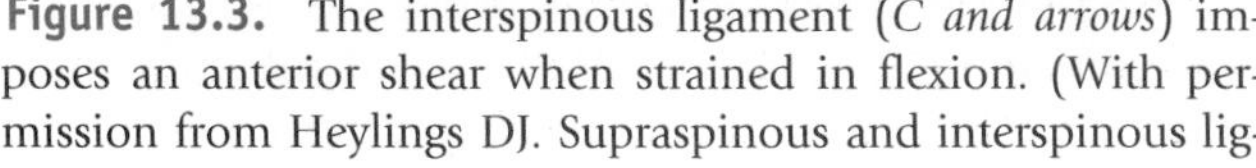

Figure 13.3. The interspinous ligament (*C and arrows*) imposes an anterior shear when strained in flexion. (With permission from Heylings DJ. Supraspinous and interspinous ligaments of the human lumbar spine. *J Anat* 123:127–131, 1978.)

cycle between flexion and extension suggesting strain reversals of the flexible arch promotes fatigue and eventually failure (37, 38).

LUMBAR POSTURE AND INJURY AVOIDANCE

Many injuries are associated with the end of range of motion of the spine. Thus, based on knowledge of how injury occurs, it appears that a neutral spine (neutral lordosis) may reduce the risk of many injuries. Shifts in tissue loading, as predicted from a modelling approach, have dramatic effects on shear loading of the intervertebral column and injury risk. First, the dominant direction of some of the small muscles acting on the spine can produce a posterior shear force on the superior vertebra. In contrast, the interspinous ligament complex generates forces in the opposite direction which imposes an anterior shear force on the superior vertebra. During this type of activity, spine posture determines the interplay between passive tissues (ligaments) and muscles, which ultimately modulates the risk of several types of injury. For example, if a load is held in the hands with the spine fully flexed (thus achieving little activity, and tension, in the extensors) and with all spinal joints motionless so that the low back moment remains the same, the ligaments seem to add to the anterior shear which is of concern relative to risk of injury. However, if a more neutral lordotic posture is adopted and the extensor musculature is activated at the same time, there is support for the anterior shearing action of gravity on the upper body and hand-held load, thus reducing shear load. In this example, the spine is at much greater risk of sustaining shear injury than compressive injury, simply because the spine is fully flexed or at the end range of motion.

In summary, evidence from tissue-specific injury generally supports the notion of a neutral spine (neutral lordosis) when performing loading tasks to minimize the risk of low back injury. There is no evidence to support conscious effort to perform "pelvic tilts" (i.e., hyperlordosis or lumbar flexion) during lifting or exertion.

METHODS TO EVALUATE SPECIFIC EXERCISES

It is important to understand the applications, and conversely the limitations, of scientific laboratory approaches for investigating tissue loading in vivo that are used to quantify better exercises. Basically, two types of methodologies are used: the method of obtaining individual tissue forces, and specific data collection procedures with human subjects. Because the low back system is an extremely complex mechanical structure and direct measurement of tissue forces in vivo is not feasible, the only tenable option for tissue load prediction is to use sophisticated modelling approaches. However, there are several issues that must be addressed including the need for anatomic detail, a method to reconcile the inherent variability of the many unknown forces among the significant load bearing structures, and development of methods that enable the prediction of loads in deep (and inaccessible) muscles and supporting ligaments (39–41).

SCIENCE AND LOW BACK EXERCISE

The following example illustrates the need for quantitative analysis in evaluating the safety of certain exercises (41–43). There has been considerable emphasis on the need to perform sit-ups and other flexion exercises with the knees flexed. Several hypotheses have suggested that this disables the psoas and/or changes the line of action of psoas. Recent magnetic resonance imaging (MRI)-based data demonstrated that psoas line of action does not change due to lumbar or hip posture (except at the lumbosacral joint) as the psoas laminae attach to each vertebrae and "follow" the changing orientation of spine (44). There is no doubt that psoas is shortened with the flexed hip, modulating force production.

But the question remains, is there a reduction in spine load with the legs bent? Recent data suggested no major difference in lumbar load as the result of bending the knees (45). However, excessive compressive loads certainly raises a question of safety. This type of quantitative analysis is necessary to demonstrate that the issue of performing sit-ups using bent knees or straight legs is probably not as important as the issue of whether to prescribe sit-ups at all.

EXERCISE RECOMMENDATIONS

The following examples of exercises have been formally evaluated and selected based on tissue loading evidence and knowledge of how injury occurs to specific tissues. It is not possible to universally recommend only those low back exercises with the highest muscle challenge and the lowest compressive cost indices. Several exercises are required to train all the muscles of the lumbar torso and the exercises which best suit the individual depend on a number of variables, such as fitness level, training goals, history of previous spinal injury, and other factors specific to the individual. However, depending on the purpose of the exercise program, several principles apply. For example, an individual beginning a post-injury program is better advised to avoid loading the spine throughout the range of motion while a trained athlete may indeed achieve higher performance levels by doing so.

Selection of the following exercises was biased toward safety, that is, minimizing spine loading during muscle challenge. Therefore a "neutral" spine (neutral lordosis, neither hyperlordotic or hypolordotic) is emphasized while the spine is under load. A general rule is to preserve the normal low back curve (similar to that of upright standing). A caveat for this generalization is that the curve may be modified by patients to enter or maintain a "pain-free" zone while performing these exercises. Performing a "pelvic tilt" during some of these exercises has previously been recommended, but (as stated above) is not justified since pelvic tilt increases spine tissue loading and takes the spine out of static-elastic equilibrium. Therefore, it is unwise to recommend the pelvic tilt when challenging the spine. Exercises in the following sections have been evaluated and chosen based on tissue loading evidence and the knowledge of how injury occurs to specific tissues.

Aerobic Exercise

The mounting evidence supporting the role of aerobic exercise in both reducing the incidence of low back injury and also in the treatment of low back patients is quite convincing (11, 41). Recent investigation into loads sustained by the low back tissues during walking confirm very low levels of supporting tissue load coupled with mild, but prolonged, activation of the supporting musculature (46). Epidemiological evidence also clarifies the effects of aerobic exercise. A large study examined age related changes to the lumbar spines of elderly people as a function of life long activity level (12). Those who were runners had no differences in spine changes measured from MRI images while weight lifters and soccer players were characterized with more disc degeneration and bulges.

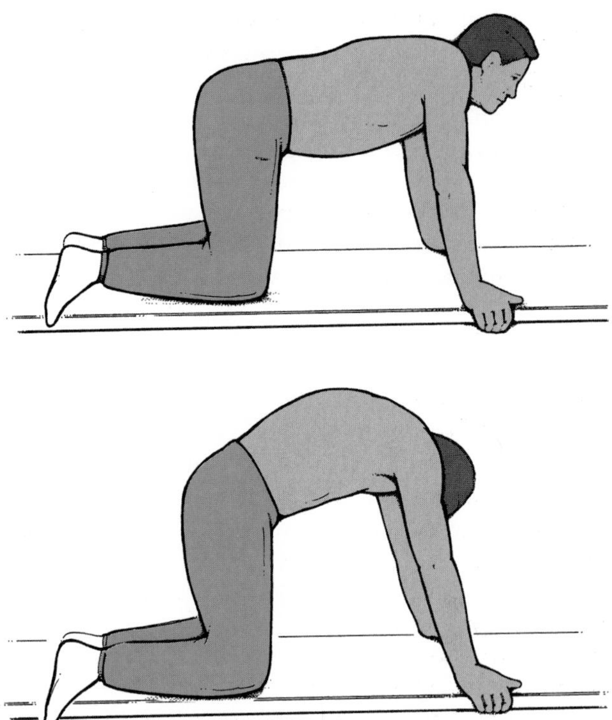

Figure 13.4. The "cat stretch" is performed by slowly cycling from full spine flexion to full extension. Spine mobility is emphasized rather than pressing at the end range of motion. This exercise provides motion for the spine with very low loading of the intervertebral joints.

Flexibility Exercise

Emphasis on spine flexibility depends on the injury history and exercise or fitness goals. Generally, for the injured back, spine flexibility should not be emphasized until the spine has stabilized and has undergone strength and endurance conditioning. Despite the notion held by some, there is little quantitative data to support a major emphasis on trunk flexibility to improve back health and lessen the risk of injury. In fact, some exercise programs that have included loading of the torso throughout the range of motion (in flexion-extension, lateral bend, or axial twist) have had negative results and greater spine mobility has been, in some cases, associated with low back problems (8, 47–50). Further, spine flexibility has been shown to have little predictive value for future low back problems (49, 51). The most successful programs emphasize trunk stabilization throughout exercise with a neutral spine, and emphasize mobility at the hips and knees (16, 52, 53).

For these reasons, specific torso flexibility exercises should be limited to unloaded flexion extension (the cat stretch) for those concerned with safety or for non-athletes (spine flexibility may be of greater desirability in athletes who have never suffered back injury). The spine may be cycled through full flexion and extension in a slow, smooth motion (Fig. 13.4). Emphasizing a neutral spine throughout, hip and knee flexibility may be achieved with the following maneuvers: hip mobility, standing hip extension, standing hip flexion, and slow lunges (for hip mobility) (Figs. 13.5 and 13.6).

Strength and Endurance Exercise

While it is well documented that those with previous back injuries have lower muscle strength and endurance performance, very few studies have linked reduced strength and endurance with the risk of a subsequent first time low back injury. The few results available suggest that endurance has a much greater prophylactic value than strength (54). Furthermore, emphasis placed on endurance should precede specific strengthening exercise in a gradual progressive exercise program (i.e., longer duration, lower effort exercises).

Abdominal Exercise (anterior and lateral)

There is no single abdominal exercise that challenges all of the abdominal musculature. Thus, the prescription of more than one single exercise is required. Calibrated intramuscular and surface electromyogram evidence suggests that the various types of curl-ups challenge mainly rectus abdominis and that psoas and obliques (internal and external oblique, transverse abdominis) activity is low (41, 45). Sit-ups (both straight-leg and bent-knee) are characterized by higher psoas activation and higher low back compression while leg raises cause even higher activation and also spine compression (Table 13.1).

The challenge to the psoas is lowest during curl-ups, followed by higher levels during the horizontal isometric side support. While bent knee sit-ups were characterized by larger psoas activation than straight leg sit-ups, the highest psoas activity is observed during leg raises and hand-on-knee flexor isometric exertions. It is interesting to note that the "press-heels" sit-up, which has been hypothesized to activate hamstrings and neurally inhibit psoas, actually increased psoas activation (55). Biomechanically, active hamstrings create a hip extensor moment requiring more hip flexor activity from the psoas, resulting in a higher compressive penalty on the spine.

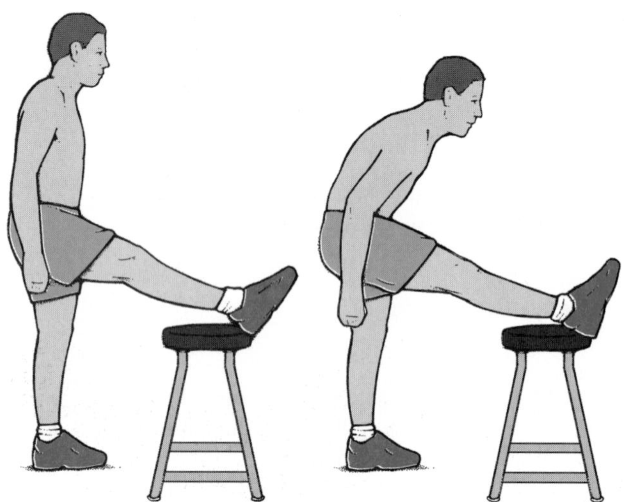

Figure 13.5. Hip mobility is enhanced with standing flexion and extension. The left panel illustrates the correct "neutral" spine while the right panel shows an **incorrect flexed spine**.

One exercise not often performed, but one that has merit, is the horizontal side support which challenges the lateral obliques without high lumbar compressive loading. In addition, this exercise produces high activation levels in the quadratus lumborum which is a significant stabilizer of the spine (56). Graded activity in the rectus abdominis and in each of the components of the abdominal wall changes with each of these exercises demonstrating that there is no single best task for the abdominals.

Clearly, curl-ups activate the rectus abdominis, but produce relatively lower oblique activity. Several other clinically relevant findings are as follows:

1. Psoas activation is dominated by hip flexion demands and psoas activity is not consistent with either lumbar sagittal moment (flexor-extensor torque) or spine compression demands, although there is some question regarding the often cited idea that the psoas is a lumber spine stabilizer.
2. Quadratus lumborum activity is consistent with lumbar sagittal moment and compression demands, suggesting a larger role in stabilization.

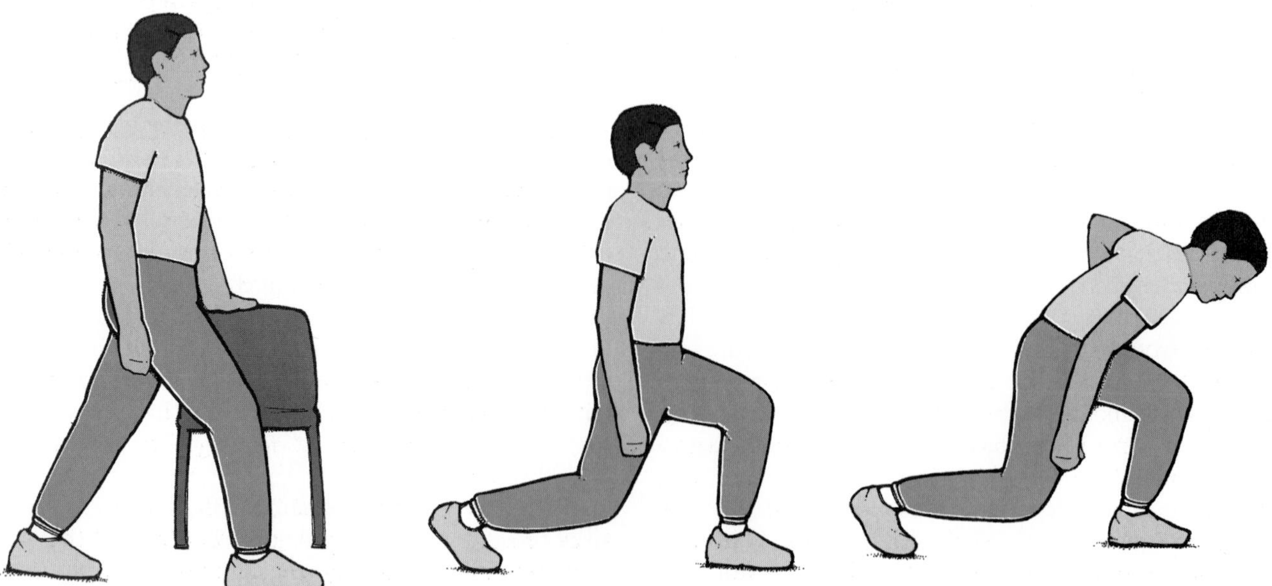

Figure 13.6. Hip mobility, strength, and endurance are challenged with slow lunges. The torso remains upright throughout the lunge effort, while emphasis is placed on a "neutral" spine during hip exercises to focus the stretch over the hip and knee joints (middle panel). The **incorrect flexed spine** is shown in the right panel.

Table 13.1. Low Back Moment, Muscle Activity, and Lumbar Compressive Load During Several Types of Abdominal Exercises

		Muscle Activation		
	Moment (Nm)	Rectus Abdominis (% MVC)	External Oblique	Compression (N)
Straight Leg Situp	148	121	~70	3506
Bent Leg—Situp	154	103	70	3350
Curlup Feet Anchored	92	87	45	2009
Curlup Feet Free	81	67	38	1991
Quarter Situp	114	78	42	2392
Straight Leg Raise	102	57	35	2525
Bent Leg Raise	82	35	24	1767
Cross-knee Curlup	112	89	67	2964
Hanging Straight Leg	107	112	90	2805
Hanging Bent Leg	84	78	64	3313
Isometric Side Support	72	48	50	2585

Note: MVC contractions were isometric. Activation values higher than 100% are often seen during dynamic exercise.

3. Psoas activation is relatively high (greater than 25% maximal voluntary contraction) during push-ups, suggesting cautious concern for the low back injured.

A good choice for abdominal exercises in the early stages of training or rehabilitation consists of several variations of curl-ups for rectus abdominis and isometric, horizontal side support (with the body supported by the knees and upper body supported by one elbow on the floor) to challenge the abdominal wall in a way that imposes minimal compressive penalty to the spine. The level of challenge with the isometric, horizontal side support can be increased by supporting the body with the feet rather than the knees.

Specific recommended low back exercises are shown (Figs. 13.7 and 13.8): the curl-up with the hands under the low back stabilizes the pelvis and assists in preserving a neutral lordosis (lumbar curvature); and the horizontal isometric side support (again with the spine in a neutral posture) uses either the knees or feet for support.

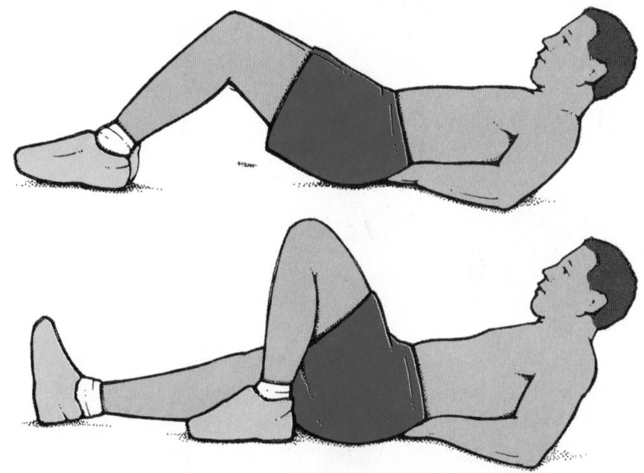

Figure 13.7. The curlup, where the head and shoulders are raised off the ground with the hands under the lumbar region to help stabilize the pelvis and support the neutral spine (top panel). A variation is to only bend one leg while the other straight leg assists in pelvic stabilization and preservation of a "neutral" lumbar curve (bottom panel).

Back Extensors Exercise

Most traditional extensor exercises are characterized by high spine loads which result from externally applied compressive and shear forces (either from free weights or resistance machines). The single leg extension hold while on the hands and knees minimizes external loads on the spine, but produces spine extensor moment (and small isometric twisting moments) which activates the extensors (Fig. 13.9). Activation is sufficiently high on one side of the extensors to facilitate training but the total spine load is reduced since the contralateral extensors are producing lower forces. Switching legs trains both sides of the extensors. Simultaneous leg extension with contralateral arm raise increases the unilateral extensor muscle challenge but also significantly increases lumbar compression.

The often-performed exercise of laying prone on the floor and raising the upper body and legs off the floor is contraindicated for anyone at risk of low back injury or reinjury. In this task the lumbar region pays a high compression penalty to a hyperextended spine which transfers load to the facets and crushes the interspinous ligament (noted earlier as an injury mechanism). This

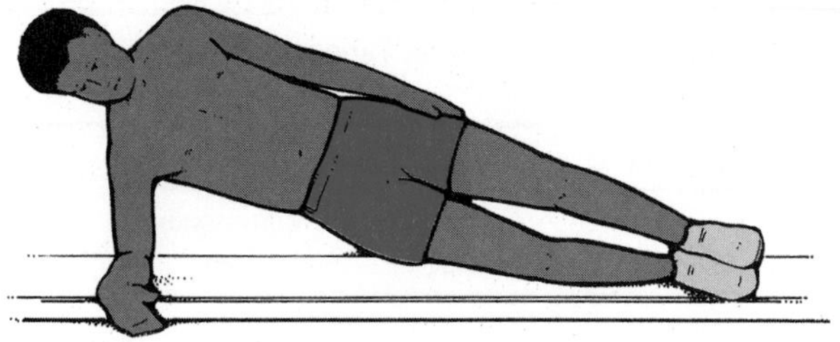

Figure 13.8 The horizontal isometric side support. Supporting the lower body with the knees on the floor reduces the demand further for those who are more concerned with safety while supporting the body with the feet increases the muscle challenge and spine load.

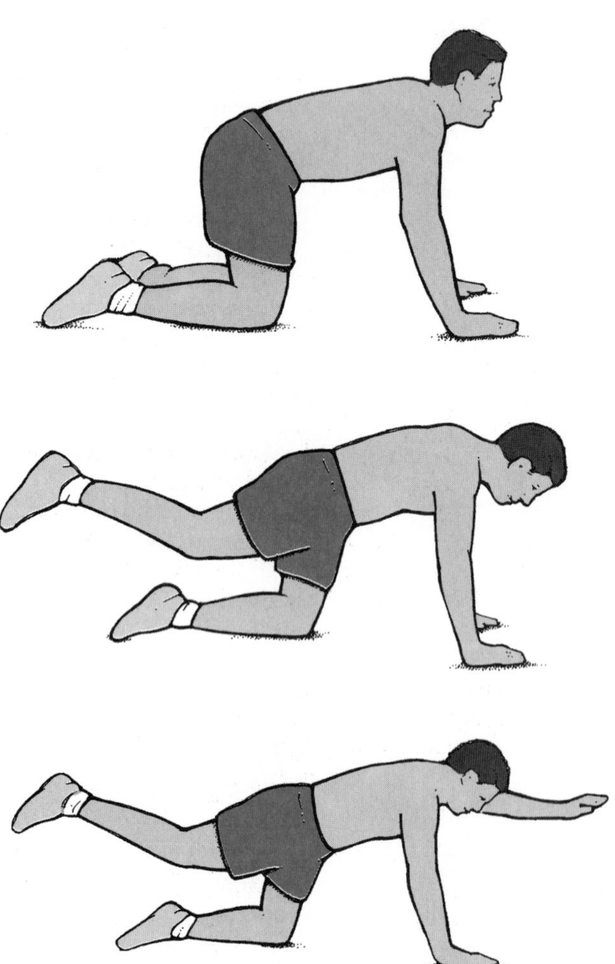

Figure 13.9. Single leg extension holds, while on the hands and knees, produces mild extensor activity and lower spine compression (< 2500N). Raising the contralateral arm increases extensor muscle activity but also spine compression to levels over 3000N.

type of data illustrates that exercise professionals must design programs with a wide range of objectives and with detailed attention to the effects of such exercises on back health.

The Use of Abdominal Belts

A review of the effects of wearing an abdominal belt is summarized in the following:

1. Those who have never had a previous back injury appear to have no additional protective benefit from wearing a belt.
2. It appears that those who have had an injury while wearing a belt, risk a more severe injury.
3. Belts give people the perception that they can lift more and may, in fact, enable them to lift more.
4. Belts appear to increase intra-abdominal pressure and blood pressure.
5. Belts appear to change the lifting styles of some people to either increase or decrease the loads on the spine (57).

In summary, given the assets and liabilities to belt wearing, they are not recommended for routine exercise participation.

Exercise Prescription Guidelines for the Low Back

The following is a list of general caveats for prescribing low back exercises:

1. While there is a common belief that exercise sessions should be performed at least 3 times per week, it appears low back exercises have the most beneficial effect when performed daily (58).
2. The "no pain-no gain" axiom does not apply when exercising the low back, particularly when applied to weight training (though scientific and clinical wisdom suggests that the opposite is true).
3. While specific low back exercises have been described in this chapter, general exercise programs that also combine cardiovascular components (like walking) have been shown to be more effective in both rehabilitation and injury prevention (46).
4. Diurnal variation in the fluid level of the intervertebral discs changes the stresses on the disc throughout the day (discs are more hydrated early in the morning after rising from bed). It would be very unwise to perform full range spine motion while under load, shortly after rising from bed (22).
5. Low back exercises performed for maintenance of health need not emphasize strength, with high-load, low repetition tasks. Rather, more repetitions of less demanding exercises assist in the enhancement of endurance and strength. There is no doubt that back injury can occur during seemingly low

level demands (such as picking up a pencil) and that the risk of injury from motor control error can occur. While the chance of motor control errors resulting in inappropriate muscle forces can increase with fatigue, there is also evidence documenting the changes in passive tissue loading with fatiguing lifting (59). Given that endurance has more protective value than strength, strength gains should not be overemphasized at the expense of endurance (54).

6. There is no such thing as an ideal set of exercises for all individuals. Training objectives must be identified (they may include reducing the risk of injury, optimizing general health and fitness, or maximizing athletic performance) and the most appropriate exercises chosen. While science cannot evaluate the optimal exercises for each situation, the combination of science and clinical experiential wisdom must be utilized to enhance low back health.
7. Patience and compliance are important aspects of all low back exercise programs. Increased function and reducing pain may not occur for up to 3 months (60).

ACKNOWLEDGMENT

The author wishes to acknowledge the help of several colleagues who have contributed to the collection of works reported here: Daniel Juker, MD, Craig Axler, MSc, Jacek Cholewicki, PhD, Michael Sharratt, PhD, John Seguin, MD, Vaughan Kippers, PhD, and in particular, Robert Norman, PhD. Also, the continual financial support from the Natural Science and Engineering Research Council, Canada has made this series of work possible.

References

1. Koes BW, Bouter LM, Beckerman H, et al. Physiotherapy exercises and back pain: a blinded review. *Br Med J* 302: 1572–1576, 1991.
2. Battie MC, Bigos SJ, Fisher LD, et al. The role of spinal flexibility in back pain complaints within industry: a prospective study. *Spine* 15:768–773, 1990.
3. Nachemson A, Morris JM. Invivo measurements of intradiscal pressure. *J Bone Joint Surg* 46A:1077–1080, 1964.
4. Nachemson A. The load on lumbar disks indifferent positions of the body. *Clin Orthop* 45:107–112, 1966.
5. Halpern AA, Bleck EE. Sit-up exercises: an electromyographic study, *Clin Orthop* 145:172–178, 1979.
6. Vincent WJ, Britten SD. Evaluation of the curl-up–a substitute for the bent knee sit-up. *J Phys Ed Rec* Feb:74–75, 1980.
7. Jette M, Sidney K, Cicutti N. A critical analysis of sit-ups: a case for the partial curl-up as a test of abdominal muscular endurance. *Can J Phys Ed Rec* Sept-Oct:4–9, 1984.
8. Malmivaara A, Hakkinen U, Aro T, et al. The treatment of acute low back pain–bed rest, exercises, or ordinary activity? *N Engl J Med* 332:351–355, 1995.
9. Walters CE, Partridge MJ. Electromyographic study of the differential action of the abdominal muscles during exercise, *Am J Phys Med* 36:259–268, 1957.
10. Flint MM. Abdominal muscle involvement during performance of various forms of sit-up exercises: electromyographic study. *Am J Phys Med* 44:224–234, 1965.
11. Cady LD, Bischoff DP, O'Connell ER, et al. Strength and fitness and subsequent back injuries in firefighters. *J Occup Med* 21(4):269–272, 1979.
12. Videman T, Sarna S, Crites-Battie M, et al. The long term effects of physical loading and exercise lifestyles on back-related symptoms, disability, and spinal pathology among men, *Spine* 20(b):669–709, 1995.
13. Videman T. Experimental models of osteoarthritis: the role of immobilization. *Clin Biomech* 2:223–229, 1987.
14. Holm S, Nachemson A. Variations in the nutrition of the canine intervertebral disc induced by motion. *Spine* 8:866–874, 1983.
15. Nachemson A. Newest knowledge of low back pain: a critical look. *Clin Orthop* 279:8–20, 1992.
16. Saal JA, Saal JS. Nonoperative treatment of herniated lumbar intervertebral disc with radiculopathy: an outcome study. *Spine* 14:431–437, 1989.
17. Roaf R. A study of the mechanics of spinal injuries. *J Bone Joint Surg* 42B:810, 1960.
18. McGill SM. ISB Keynote Lecture–The biomechanics of low back injury: Implications on current practice in industry and the clinic. *J Biomech* 30:465–475, 1997.
19. Brinkmann P, Biggemann M, Hilweg D. Prediction of the compressive strength of human lumbar vertebrae. *Clin Biomech* 4(Suppl 2), 1989.
20. Fyhrie DP, Schaffler MB. Failure mechanisms in human vertebral cancellous bone. *Bone* 15:105–109, 1994.
21. Hansson TH, Keller T, Spengler D. Mechanical behaviour of the human lumbar spine II: Fatigue strength during dynamic compressive loading. *J Orthop Res* 5:479–487, 1987.
22. Adams MA, Dolan P. Recent advances in lumbar spine mechanics and their clinical significance. *Clin Biomech* 10:3–19, 1995.
23. Adams MA, Hutton WC. Prolapsed Intervertebral disc: A hyperflexion injury. *Spine* 7:184–191,1982.
24. Gordon SJ, Yang KH, Mayer PJ, et al. Mechanismof disc rupture–a preliminary report. *Spine* 16:450–456, 1991.
25. Yang KH, Byrd AJ, Kish VL, et al. Annulus fibrosus tears–an experimental model. *Orthop Trans* 12:86–87, 1988.
26. Adams MA, Hutton WC. Gradual disc prolapse. *Spine* 10: 524–531, 1985.
27. Videman T, Nurminen M, Troup JD. Lumbar spinal pathology in cadaveric material in relation to history of back pain. Occupation and physical loading. *Spine* 15:728–740, 1990.
28. Wilder DG, Pope MH, Frymoyer JW. The biomechanics of lumbar disc herniation and the effect of overload and instability. *J Spine Dis* 1:16–32, 1988.
29. Goel VK, Monroe BT, Gilbertson LG, et al. Interlaminar shear stresses and laminae-separation in a disc: finite element analysis of the L3-L4 motion segment subjected to axial compressive loads. *Spine* 20:689–698, 1995.
30. King AI. Injury to the thoraco-lumbar spine and pelvis. In: Nahum AM, Melvin JW, eds. *Accidental Injury, Biomechanics and Presentation.* New York: Springer-Verlag, 1993.
31. Noyes FR, De Lucas JL, Torvik PJ. Biomechanics of ligament failure: an analysis of strain-rate sensitivity and

mechanisms of failure in primates. *J Bone Joint Surg* 56A: 236–253, 1974.

32. Yoganandan H, Pintar R, Butler J, et al. Dynamic response of human cervical spine ligaments. *Spine* 14:1002–1110, 1989.
33. Rissanen PM. The surgical anatomy and pathology of the supraspinous and interspinous ligaments of the lumbar spine with special reference to ligament ruptures. *Acta Orthop Scand* (46 Suppl), 1960.
34. Heylings DJ. Supraspinous and interspinous ligaments of the human lumbar spine. *J Anat* 123:127–131, 1978.
35. Cripton P, Berlemen U, Visarino H, et al. Response of the lumbar spine due to shear loading. In: *Injury Prevention Through Biomechanics*. Symposium proceedings, May 4–5, Wayne State University, 1985.
36. Adams MA, Hutton WC. The relevance of torsion to the mechanical derangement of the lumbar spine. *Spine* 6: 241–248, 1981.
37. Wiltse LL, Widell EM, Jackson DW. Fatigue fracture: the basic lesion in isthmic spondylolisthesis. *J Bone Joint Surg* 57A:17–22, 1975.
38. Hardcastle P, Annear P, Foster D. Spinal abnormalities in young fast bowlers. *J Bone Joint Surg* 74B(3):421–425, 1992.
39. McGill SM. A myoelectrically based dynamic three-dimensional model to predict loads on lumbar spine tissues during lateral bending. *J Biomech* 25:395–414, 1992.
40. Cholewicki J, McGill SM. Mechanical stability of the invivo lumbar spine: Implications for injury and chronic low back pain. *Clin Biomech* 11:1–15, 1996.
41. Juker D, McGill SM, Kropf P, et al. Quantitative intramuscular myoelectric activity of lumbar portions of psoas and the abdominal wall during a wide variety of tasks. *Med Sci Sports Exerc* (in press).
42. Callaghan J, Gunning J, McGill SM. Choosing the best low back extensor exercise for the back injured. *Phys Ther* (in press).
43. Axler CT, McGill SM. Choosing the best abdominal exercises based on knowledge of tissue loads. *Med Sci Sports Exerc* 29:804–811, 1997.
44. Santaguida L, McGill SM. The psoas major muscle: A three-dimensional mechanical modelling study with respect to the spine based on MRI measurement. *J Biomech* 28(3): 339–345, 1995.
45. McGill SM. The mechanics of torso flexion: situps and standing dynamic flexion manoeuvres. *Clin Biomech* 10(4): 184–192, 1995.
46. Nutter P. Aerobic exercise in the treatment and prevention of low back pain. *Occup Med* 3:137–145, 1988.
47. Callaghan JP, Patla A, McGill SM. 3D analysis of spine loading during gait. Proceedings from American Society for Biomechanics meeting, Atlanta, GA. Oct. 17–19, 1996.
48. Nachemson A. Newest knowledge of low back pain: a critical look. *Clin Orthop* 279:8-20, 1992.
49. Biering-Sorensen F. Physical measurements as risk indicators for low back trouble over a one year period. *Spine* 9: 106–109, 1984.
50. Burton AK, Tillotson KM, Troup JD. Variation in lumbar sagittal mobility with low back trouble. *Spine* 14:584–590, 1989.
51. Battie MC, Bigos SJ, Fischer LD, et al. The role of spinal flexibility in back pain complaints within industry: A prospective study. *Spine* 15:768–773, 1990.
52. Bridger RS, Orkin D, Henneberg M. A quantitative investigation of lumbar and pelvic postures in standing and sitting: Interrelationships with body position and hip muscle length. *Int J Ind Ergonom* 9:235–244, 1992.
53. McGill SM, Norman RW. Low Back Biomechanics in industry–the prevention of injury. In: Grabiner MD, ed. *Current Issues of Biomechanics*. Champaign, IL: Human Kinetics Publishers, 1992.
54. Luoto S, Heliovaara M, Hurri H, et al. Static back endurance and the risk of low back pain. *Clin Biomech* 10:323–324, 1995.
55. Spring H. Kraft-Theorie und praxis. New York: Thieme Stuttgardt, 1990.
56. McGill SM, Juker D, Kropf P. Quantitative intramuscular myoelectric activity of quadratus lumborum during a wide variety of tasks. *Clin Biomech* 11(3):170–172, 1996.
57. McGill SM. Abdominal belts in industry: A position paper on their assetts, liabilities and use. *Am Ind Hyg Assoc J* 54: 752–754, 1993.
58. Mayer TG, Gatchel RJ, Kishino N, et al. Objective assessment of spine function following industrial injury: A prospective study with comparison group and one-year follow up. *Spine* 10:482–493, 1985.
59. Potvin JR, Norman RW. Can fatigue compromise lifting safety: Proc. NACOB II. The Second North American Congress on Biomechanics, August 24–28, 1992:513–514.
60. Manniche C, Hesselsoe G, Bentzen L, et al. Clinical trial of intensive muscle training for chronic low back pain. *Lancet* 24:1473–1476, 1988.

SECTION FOUR

EXERCISE PHYSIOLOGY

SECTION EDITOR: *Tom LaFontaine, PhD, FACSM*

18, 19, 21 33, 44, 55 313

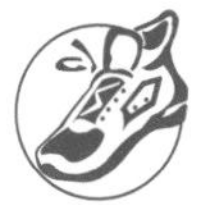
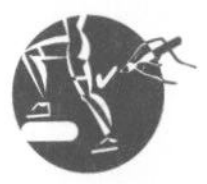

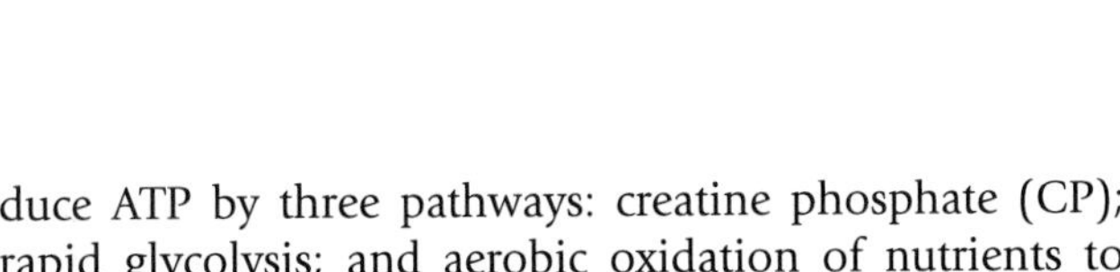

CHAPTER 14
FUNDAMENTALS OF EXERCISE METABOLISM

Scott R. Powers and John M. Lawler

At rest, a 70 kg human has an energy expenditure of about 1.2 kilocalories per minute (kcal/min); less than 20% of this resting energy expenditure is attributed to skeletal muscle. However, almost all changes occurring in the body during exercise are related to the increase in energy metabolism largely within the contracting skeletal muscle. For example, cardiac output and heart rate increase as a direct linear function of whole body metabolism. To meet the demands on the heart there is a fourfold increase in myocardial blood flow and oxygen consumption.

During intense exercise, total energy expenditure may increase 15 to 25 times above resting values, resulting in a caloric expenditure of approximately 18 to 30 kcal/min. Most of this increase is used to provide energy for exercising muscles which may increase energy requirement by a factor of 200 (1). Therefore, daily caloric expenditure can be changed dramatically by simply altering the amount of physical activity performed during a day. The focus of this chapter is on muscle bioenergetics and exercise metabolism. A detailed review of bioenergetics and exercise metabolism is provided in the suggested readings section of this chapter.

ENERGY FOR MUSCULAR CONTRACTION

Adenosine Triphosphate (ATP)

Skeletal muscle contractions are powered by the energy released through hydrolysis of high-energy compound adenosine triphosphate (ATP) to form adenosine diphosphate (ADP) and inorganic phosphate (Pi). This reaction is catalyzed by the enzyme myosin ATPase:

$$ATP \xrightarrow{\text{(myosin ATPase)}} ADP + Pi + energy$$

The amount of ATP directly available in muscle at any time is small and, thus, it must be re-synthesized continuously if exercise continues for more than a few seconds. Muscle fibers contain the metabolic machinery to produce ATP by three pathways: creatine phosphate (CP); rapid glycolysis; and aerobic oxidation of nutrients to carbon dioxide (CO_2) and H_2O.

Creatine Phosphate (CP)

The CP system involves the transfer of high-energy phosphate from CP to rephosphorylate ATP from ADP as follows:

$$ADP + CP \xrightarrow{\text{(creatine kinase)}} ATP + C$$

This system is very rapid because it involves only one enzymatic step (i.e., one chemical reaction); however, CP exists in finite quantities in cells, thus the total amount of ATP that can be produced is limited. Oxygen (O_2) is not involved in the rephosphorylation of ADP to ATP in this reaction, and thus the CP system is considered anaerobic (without O_2).

Rapid Glycolysis

When glycolysis is rapid, it is capable of producing ATP without involvement of O_2. Glycolysis is the degradation of carbohydrate (glycogen or glucose) to pyruvate or lactate and involves a series of enzymatically catalyzed steps (Fig. 14.1). The net energy yield of glycolysis, without further oxidation through aerobic metabolism, is 2 or 3 ATP through substrate level phosphorylation. The net ATP production is 2 ATP when glucose is the substrate and 3 ATP when glycogen is the substrate. Although the process of glycolysis does not involve the use of O_2 and is considered anaerobic, pyruvate can readily participate in aerobic production of ATP when O_2 is available in the cell. Therefore, in addition to being an anaerobic pathway capable of producing ATP without O_2, glycolysis can also be considered the first step in the aerobic degradation of carbohydrate.

Lactic Acid

Historically, rising blood lactate levels during exercise have been considered an indication of increased anaer-

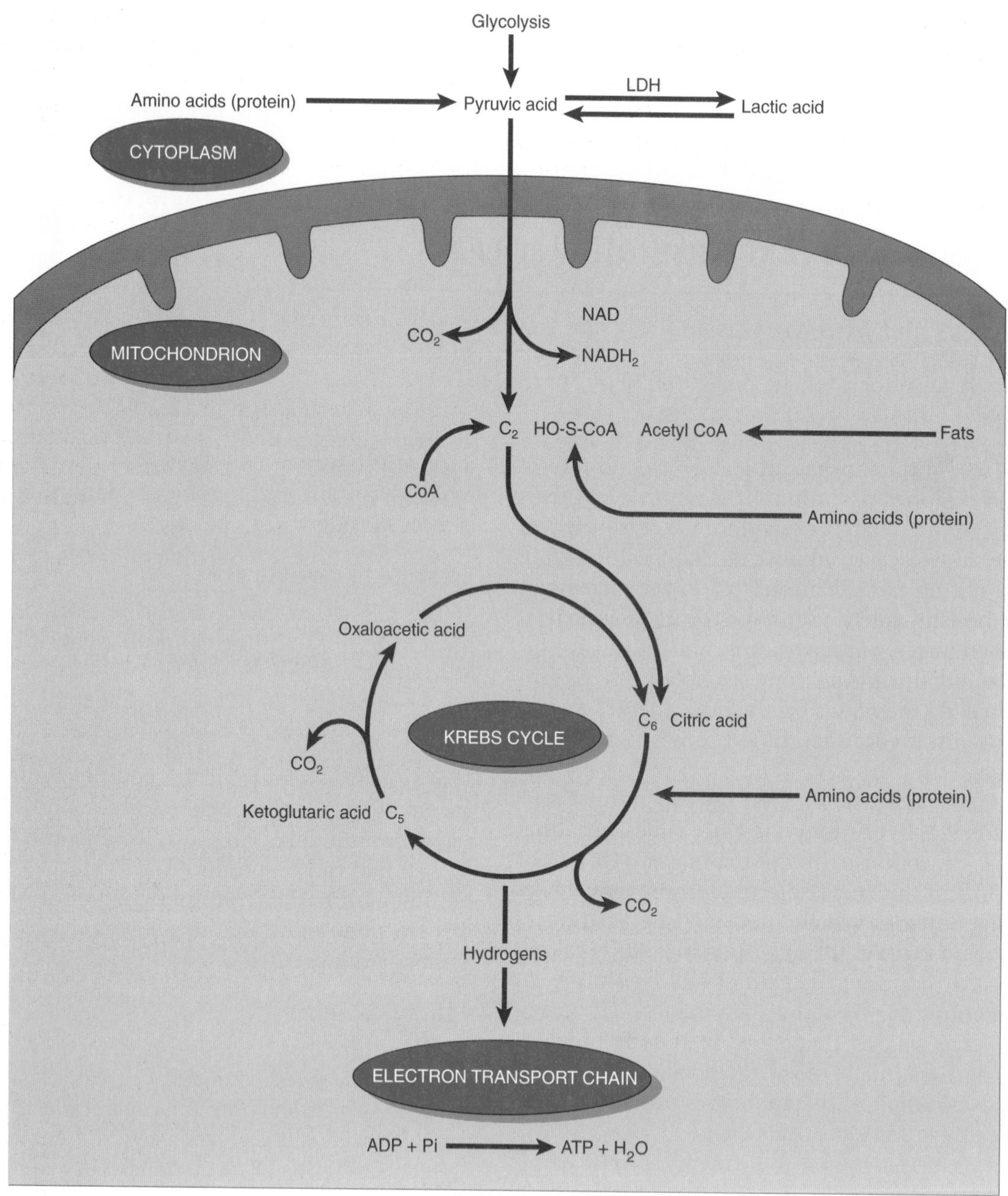

Figure 14.1. Relationship between glycolysis, the Krebs cycle, and the electron transport chain.

obic metabolism within the contracting muscle due to a lack of oxygen. However, the hypoxia theory is controversial. Whether the end product of glycolysis is pyruvate or lactate depends on several factors. If O_2 is not available in the mitochondria to accept hydrogen released during glycolysis, pyruvate must accept hydrogen to form lactate as an end product so that glycolysis can proceed. In addition, if glycolytic flux is extremely rapid, hydrogen production may exceed the transport capability of those shuttle mechanisms which move hydrogens from the cytoplasm (called sarcoplasm in muscle) into the mitochondria where oxidative phosphorylation occurs.

When glycolytic hydrogen production exceeds the mitochondria transport capability, pyruvate must again accept the hydrogens to form lactate so glycolysis can continue. During exercise, epinephrine (adrenaline) levels in the blood are elevated which stimulates muscle glycogenolysis (breakdown of glycogen for fuel) and, thus, increases the rate of glycolysis.

When at rest and during low exercise intensities ($<$ 40% of maximal aerobic capacity), slow-twitch muscle fibers are recruited predominantly. As the exercise intensity increases, more fast-twitch fibers are recruited. This recruitment pattern has an important influence on lactic acid production. Conversion of pyruvate to lactate (and vice versa) is catalyzed by the enzyme lactate dehydrogenase (LDH), which exists in several forms (isozymes). Fast-twitch muscle fibers contain an LDH isozyme that favors the formation of lactate, whereas slow-twitch fibers contain an LDH form that promotes less conversion of pyruvate to lactate or even conversion of lactate to pyruvate. Therefore, more lactate formation occurs in fast-twitch fibers during exercise simply because of the type of LDH isozyme present, independent of O_2 availability in the muscle. Finally, fast twitch fibers have higher activities of glycolytic enzymes than do slow twitch fibers, indicating a greater potential of substrate flux through glycolysis.

In summary, debate continues over the mechanism(s) responsible for muscle lactate production during exercise. It seems possible that any one or a combination of these possibilities (as well as lack of oxygen) might provide an explanation for muscle lactate production during exercise. The most important consequence of elevated lactic acid levels is the contribution to muscle fatigue. However, it is important to note that blood lactate can also be used as a fuel by muscles during and following exercise which can influence blood concentrations of lactate. A detailed discussion of this topic is available from other sources (2–4).

Aerobic Oxidation

The final metabolic pathway for ATP production combines two complex metabolic processes (i.e., Krebs cycle and electron transport chain) and is located inside the mitochondria. Oxidative phosphorylation uses O_2 as the final hydrogen acceptor to form H_2O and ATP. Unlike glycolysis, aerobic metabolism can use fat, protein, and carbohydrate as substrate to produce ATP. The interaction of these nutrients is illustrated in Figure 14.1.

Conceptually, the Krebs cycle can be considered a "primer" for oxidative phosphorylation. Entry into the Krebs cycle begins with the combination of acetyl-CoA and oxaloacetic acid to form citric acid. The primary purpose of the Krebs cycle is to remove hydrogens from four of the reactants involved in the cycle. The electrons from these hydrogens follow a chain of cytochromes (electron transport chain) in the mitochondria and the energy released from this process is used to rephosphorylate ADP to form ATP. Oxygen is the final acceptor of hydrogen to form H_2O and this reaction is catalyzed by cytochrome oxidase (Fig. 14.1). Oxidation of carbohydrates via the Krebs cycle and the electron transport chain results in a total of 36 ATP per unit of glucose substrate or 38 ATP per unit of glycogen substrate. A more detailed review of oxidative phosphorylation can be found in other sources (5).

Fat Metabolism

Oxidation of fat provides acetyl CoA as substrate for the Krebs cycle and is possible through aerobic metabolism. Note that glycolysis can also interact with the Krebs cycle in the presence of O_2 by the conversion of pyruvate to form acetyl-CoA. Fat or triglycerides are lipids broken down to fatty acids and glycerol by hormone-sensitive lipase, which is inhibited by insulin and activated by catecholamines and growth hormone. Glycerol can be metabolized through glycolysis or used to make glucose. Free fatty acids enter the blood to be used as fuel in a process known as β-oxidation or they may be used as a precursor in the production of many substances such as cholesterol. Fat metabolism and transport in the blood have important influences on many health related problems such as obesity and heart disease. Fatty acids must be activated using ATP and coenzyme A (CoA) in order to enter the mitochondria for oxidation. In the mitochondrial matrix, β-oxidation proceeds sequentially by cleaving off two carbon atoms at a time forming acetyl CoA, the substrate for the Krebs cycle. A 16 carbon fatty acid such as palmitate yields 129 ATPs.

REGULATION OF BIOENERGETIC PATHWAYS

The bioenergetic pathways that result in production of cellular ATP are under very precise control. This control is achieved by regulation of one or more regulatory (allosteric) enzymes which catalyze one-way reactions. Rate-limiting enzymes exist in each of the aforementioned bioenergetic pathways and can be "up-regulated" or "down-regulated" depending upon demand for ATP. In other words, the catalytic activity of allosteric enzymes is regulated by cellular modulators. Two of the most important modulators of bioenergetic regulatory enzymes are cellular concentrations of ATP and ADP. For example, creatine phosphate breakdown is regulated by creatine kinase activity. Creatine kinase activity is elevated when cytoplasmic concentrations of ADP increase and ATP levels decrease. Conversely, creatine kinase activity is inhibited by high cellular ATP levels. This type of negative feedback control is common among bioenergetic pathways in the muscle fiber.

The rate-limiting enzyme in glycolysis is phosphofructokinase (PFK). PFK is located early in the glycolytic pathway and, similar to the regulation of creatine kinase, PFK activity is increased by a rise in cellular ADP concentration and a decrease in ATP levels. PFK activity is inhibited by a variety of factors including high cellular concentrations of hydrogen ions, citrate, and ATP.

Although oxidative phosphorylation is under complex control, it is clear that key enzymes in the Krebs cycle (i.e., isocitrate dehydrogenase) and electron transport chain (i.e., cytochrome oxidase) are regulated, in part, by cellular levels of ATP, ADP, and Ca^{2+}. An increase in cellular levels of ADP promotes oxidative phosphorylation while high concentrations of ATP inhibit this process, which is similar to the control schemes presented for the creatine phosphate system and glycolysis. A more detailed discussion of oxidative phosphorylation is available (5).

METABOLIC RESPONSES TO EXERCISE

The importance of the interaction of the aforementioned metabolic pathways in the production of ATP during exercise should be emphasized. In reality the energy to perform most types of exercise comes from a combination of anaerobic/aerobic sources, not one exclusively (Fig. 14.2). The contribution of anaerobic sources (PC system and glycolysis) to exercise energy metabolism is inversely related to the duration and intensity of the activity. The shorter and more intense the activity, the greater the contribution of anaerobic energy production; whereas, the longer the activity and the lower the intensity, the greater the contribution of aerobic energy production. Although proteins can be used as a fuel for aerobic exercise, carbohydrates and fats are the primary energy substrates during exercise in a healthy, well-fed individual. In general, carbohydrates are used as the primary fuel at the onset of exercise and during high intensity work (6–8). However, during prolonged exercise of low to moderate intensity (longer than 30 minutes), a gradual shift occurs from carbohydrate toward an increasing reliance on fat as a substrate (Fig. 14.3) (8, 9). The greatest amount of fat use occurs at about 60% of maximal aerobic capacity ($\dot{V}O_2max$). A detailed discussion outlining the interplay of substrates during exercise is available from several sources (6–13). A brief discussion of the metabolic response to various types of exercise follows.

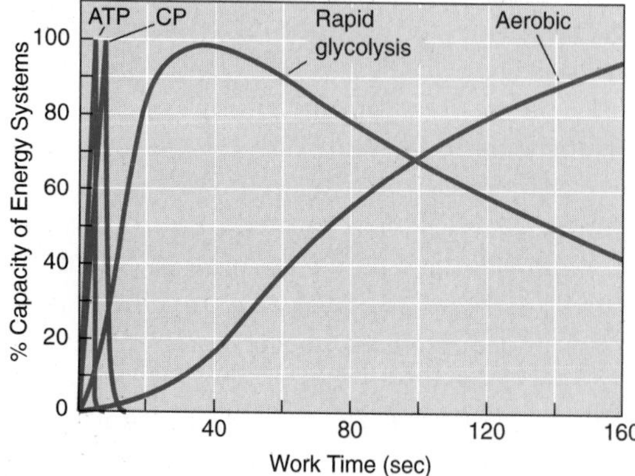

Figure 14.2. Interaction between anaerobic and aerobic energy sources during exercise including ATP, creatine phosphate, rapid glycolysis, and aerobic (oxidative phosphorylation). Note that energy to perform short-term high intensity exercise comes primarily from anaerobic sources whereas energy for muscular contraction during prolonged exercise comes from aerobic metabolism.

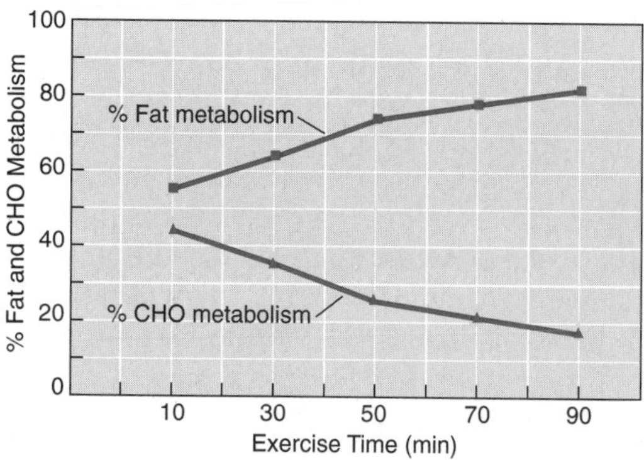

Figure 14.3. Alterations in substrate utilization during prolonged submaximal (~60% $\dot{V}O_2max$) exercise. CHO = carbohydrate. (With permission from Powers S, Byrd R, Tulley R, et al. Effects of caffeine ingestion on metabolism and performance during graded exercise. *Eur J Appl Physiol* 50:301, 1983.)

Short-term High Intensity Exercise

The energy to perform short-term high intensity exercise (i.e., 5 to 60 seconds duration) such as weight lifting or sprinting 400 meters comes primarily from anaerobic pathways. Whether the ATP production is dominated by the PC-ATP system or glycolysis depends upon the duration of the muscular effort. In general, energy for all activities lasting less than 5 seconds comes from the ATP + CP system. In contrast, energy to perform a 200 meter sprint (i.e., 30 seconds) would come from a combination of the ATP + CP system and anaerobic glycolysis, with glycolysis predominating. The transition from the CP system to glycolysis is not an abrupt change but rather a gradual shift from one pathway to another as the duration of the exercise increases.

As illustrated in Figure 14.2, exercise bouts lasting longer than 45 seconds use a combination of the CP system, glycolysis, and oxidative phosphorylation. For example, the energy required to sprint 400 meters (i.e., 60 seconds) would come primarily from anaerobic pathways (~70%) while the remaining ATP production would be provided by aerobic metabolism (~30%). The principal fuel used during this type of exercise are carbohydrates (glycogen) stored in muscle (14).

Transition from Rest to Light Exercise

In the transition from rest to light exercise, oxygen uptake kinetics follow a mono-exponential pattern, reaching a steady state generally within 1 to 4 minutes (Fig. 14.4) (15). The time required to reach a steady state increases at higher work rates and is longer in untrained individuals compared to aerobically trained individuals. Because oxygen uptake does not increase instantaneously to steady state at the onset of exercise, it is implied that

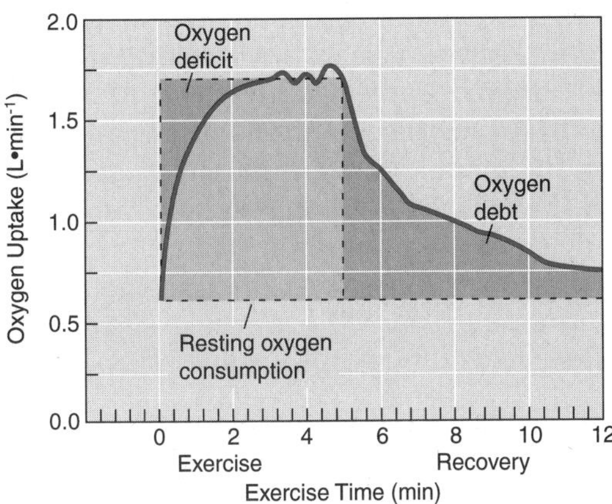

Figure 14.4. Oxygen uptake dynamics at onset and offset of exercise. See text for details.

anaerobic energy sources contribute to the required $\dot{V}O_2$ at the beginning of exercise. Indeed, evidence exists that both the CP system and glycolysis contribute to the overall production of ATP at the onset of muscular work (16). Once a steady state is obtained, however, the ATP requirements are met by aerobic metabolism. The term "O_2 deficit" has been used to describe inadequate O_2 consumption at the onset of exercise (Fig. 14.4). Similar to short-term heavy exercise, the principal fuel used during the transition from rest to light exercise is muscle glycogen (12).

Prolonged Submaximal Exercise

A steady-state $\dot{V}O_2$ can usually be maintained during 10 to 60 minutes of submaximal continuous exercise. Two exceptions to this rule exist. First, prolonged exercise in a hot and humid environment results in a steady "drift upward" of $\dot{V}O_2$ during the course of exercise (17). Second, continuous exercise at a high relative work load results in a slow rise in $\dot{V}O_2$ across time similar to that in observed during exercise in a hot environment. In both cases, this drift probably occurs because of a variety of factors (i.e., rising body temperature and increasing blood catecholamines) (18, 19).

As depicted in Figure 14.3, both carbohydrate and fat are used as substrates during prolonged exercise. As mentioned previously, during prolonged low and moderate intensity exercise, there is a gradual shift from carbohydrate metabolism toward the use of fat as a substrate. The percentage contribution of fat versus carbohydrate as energy substrate during prolonged exercise is determined by a complex interaction between the exercise intensity, nutritional status of the individual, state of training, and the duration of the activity.

Progressive Incremental Exercise

Figure 14.5 illustrates the oxygen uptake during a progressive-incremental exercise test. Note that oxygen uptake increases as a linear function to work rate until $\dot{V}O_2$max is reached. After reaching a steady state, ATP used for muscular contraction during the early stages of an incremental exercise test comes primarily from aerobic metabolism. However, as the exercise intensity increases, blood levels of lactate rise (Fig. 14.6). Although much controversy surrounds this issue, many investigators believe that this lactate "inflection" point represents a point of increasing reliance upon anaerobic metabolism.

Although the precise terminology is controversial, this sudden increase in blood lactate levels—termed the "anaerobic threshold" or "lactate threshold"—has important implications for the prediction of performance and perhaps exercise prescription. For example, it has been shown that the anaerobic threshold used in combination with other physiological variables (i.e., $\dot{V}O_2$max) is a

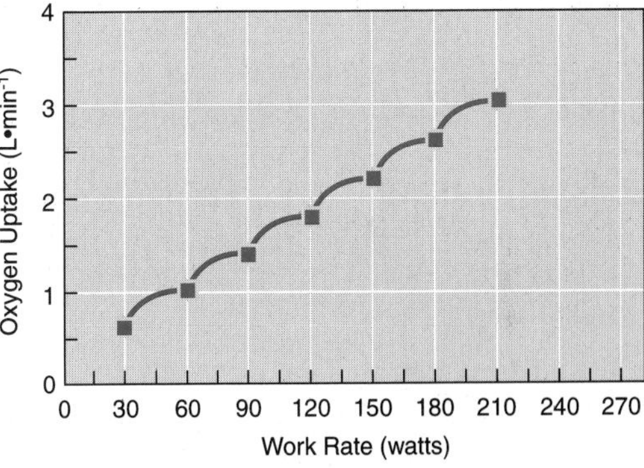

Figure 14.5. Changes in oxygen uptake as a function of work rate during incremental exercise.

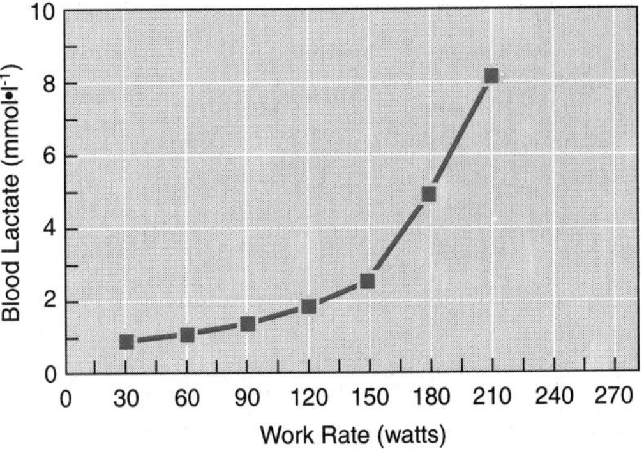

Figure 14.6. Changes in blood lactate concentrations as a function of work rate during incremental exercise.

useful predictor of success in distance running (20, 21). The lactate threshold might also prove to be a useful marker of the transition from moderate to heavy exercise for subjects and, thus, could be useful in exercise prescription.

Recovery from Exercise

Oxygen uptake remains elevated above resting levels for several minutes during recovery from exercise (Fig. 14.4). This elevated post-exercise O_2 consumption has traditionally been termed the "oxygen debt," but more recently the term, "elevated post exercise oxygen consumption (EPOC)" has been applied (18). In general, post-exercise metabolism is higher following high-intensity exercise than after light or moderate work. Furthermore, post-exercise $\dot{V}O_2$ remains elevated longer after prolonged exercise compared to shorter-term exertion. The mechanisms to explain these observations are probably linked to the fact that both high intensity and prolonged exercise results in higher body temperatures, greater ionic disturbance and higher plasma catecholamines than in light or moderate, short-term exercise (18).

MEASUREMENT OF METABOLISM AND OXYGEN CONSUMPTION

Traditionally, whole body metabolism is measured using one of two different strategies: direct calorimetry and indirect calorimetry (22). The principles behind these two strategies can be explained by the following relationship:

$$\underset{\text{(Indirect calorimetry)}}{Foodstuffs + O_2} \rightarrow \underset{\text{(Direct calorimetry)}}{Heat + CO_2 + H_2O}$$

Heat is liberated as a consequence of cellular respiration and cell (e.g., muscular) work. Thus, heat production by the body allows a direct assessment of metabolism. Direct calorimetry requires a subject be placed in an airtight chamber. As heat is released, the temperature inside the chamber rises. Typically, a circulating jacket of water is used to transfer heat to the environment and allows a means of determining the metabolic rate (in joules or kilocalories).

Although direct calorimetry is a very precise technique, construction of large chambers for measurement of metabolic rate in humans is often prohibitively expensive. Additionally, heat produced by exercise equipment can complicate measurements using direct calorimetry. The principle of indirect calorimetry uses the measurement of O_2 consumption ($\dot{V}O_2$) to determine metabolic rate. Using this method metabolic rate (in kcal) can be estimated using the following formula:

$$metabolic\ rate\ (kcal/min) = \dot{V}O_2(l/min) \times [4.0 + RQ]$$

where: RQ = $\dot{V}CO_2/\dot{V}O_2$ (respiratory quotient).

The most common method of measuring oxygen consumption uses open-circuit spirometry (Fig. 14.7). Volume of inspired oxygen is measured using a dry gas meter, turbine, or pneumatic. A one-way valve directs air through the mouth. Gas fractions are then sampled and measured by O_2 and CO_2 analyzers on the expired side. Typically, analog voltages from the gas meter and analyzers are converted to digital information and fed into a microcomputer with $\dot{V}O_2$ calculated using the Haldane transformation of the Fick equation:

$$\dot{V}O_2 = V_I \times F_IO_2 - V_I \times ([1 - F_EO_2 - F_ECO_2]/[1 - F_IO_2 - F_ICO_2]) \times F_EO_2$$

where: V_I = inspired ventilation
F_IO_2 = inspired oxygen fraction = 0.2093
F_ICO_2 = inspired carbon dioxide fraction = 0.0003
F_EO_2 = expired oxygen fraction
F_ECO_2 = inspired carbon dioxide fraction

ENERGY COST OF ACTIVITIES

The energy cost of many types of physical activity has been established. Appendix A lists some physical activities and their associated energy expenditures expressed in kilocalories per minute. Activities that are vigorous and involve large muscle groups usually result in more energy expended than those activities that use small muscle mass or require limited exertion. The estimates of energy expenditure listed in Table 6.1 were obtained by measuring oxygen cost of these activities in an adult population.

Clinicians often use the term "metabolic equivalent" (MET) to describe exercise intensity. A single MET is equivalent to the amount of energy expended during 1 minute of rest. Therefore, exercise at a metabolic rate that is five times the resting $\dot{V}O_2$ rate is equivalent to 5 METs. In a strict sense, the absolute energy expenditure during exercise at a 5 MET intensity would depend on the body size of the individual (i.e., a large individual would likely have a larger resting $\dot{V}O_2$ when compared to a smaller individual). For simplicity, individual differences in resting energy expenditures are often overlooked and 1 MET is considered equivalent to a $\dot{V}O_2$ of 3.5 ml/kg/min. Hence, 1 MET represents an energy expenditure of approximately 1.2 kcal/min for a 70 kg person.

▶ SUMMARY

Exercise metabolism is a reflection of each metabolic pathway as it contributes to the increased energy demands of activity and work. Substrates for energy production include carbohydrate, fat and, perhaps, protein. The mix of these substrates during exercise metabolism is dependent upon the intensity and du-

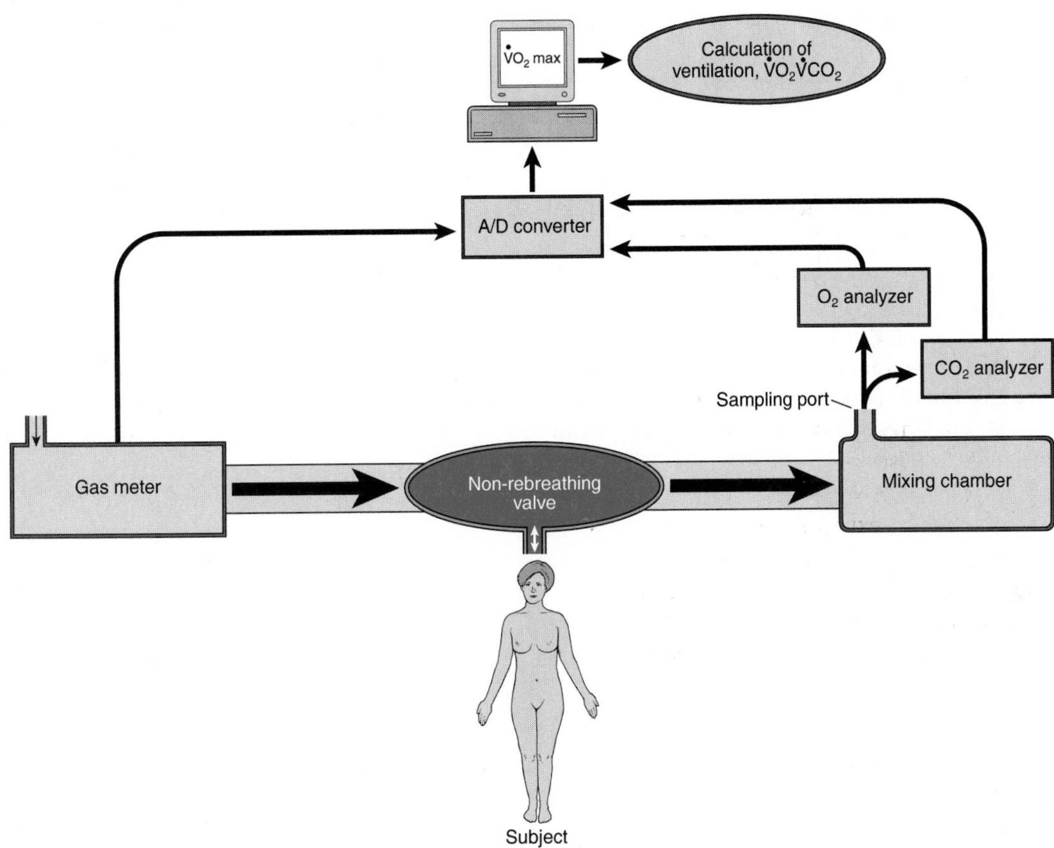

Figure 14.7. Open-circuit spirometry system interfaced with computer technology.

ration of exercise as well as the conditioning of the individual.

References

1. Armstrong R. Biochemistry: Energy liberation and use. In: Strauss RS, ed. *Sports Medicine and Physiology.* Philadelphia: W.B. Saunders, 1979.
2. Graham T. Mechanisms of blood lactate increase during exercise. *Physiologist* 27:299, 1984.
3. Katz A, Sahlin K. Oxygen in regulation of glycolysis and lactate production in human skeletal muscle. *Exerc Sport Sci Rev* 18:1, 1990.
4. Stainsby W, Brooks G. Control of lactic acid metabolism in contracting skeletal muscles during exercise. *Exerc Sport Sci Rev* 18:29, 1990.
5. Senior A. ATP synthesis by oxidative phosphorylation. *Physiol Rev* 68:177, 1988.
6. Gollnick P, Riedy M, Quintinskie J, Bertocci L. Differences in metabolic potential of skeletal muscle fibres and their significance for metabolic control. *J Exp Biol* 115:191, 1985.
7. Gollnick P. Metabolism of substrates: Energy substrate metabolism during exercise and as modified by training. *Fed Proc* 44:353, 1985.
8. Newsholme E. The control of fuel utilization by muscle during exercise and starvation. *Diabetes* 28(Suppl 1):1, 1979.
9. Powers S, Riley W, Howley E. Comparison of fat metabolism between trained men and women during prolonged aerobic work. *Res Q Exerc Sport* 51:427, 1980.
10. Holloszy J, Coyle E. Adaptations of skeletal muscle to endurance exercise and their metabolic consequences. *J Appl Physiol* 56:831, 1984.
11. Holloszy J. Utilization of fatty acids during exercise. In: Taylor AW, Gollnick PD, Green HJ, et al, eds. *Biochemistry of Exercise VII.* Champaign, IL: Human Kinetics Publishers, 1990.
12. Stanley W, Connett R. Regulation of muscle carbohydrate metabolism during exercise. *FASEB J* 5:2155, 1991.
13. Bonen A, McDermott J, Tan M. Glucose transport in muscle. In: Taylor AW, Gollnick PD, Green HJ, et al, eds. *Biochemistry of Exercise VII.* Champaign, IL: Human Kinetics, 1990.
14. Powers S, Byrd R, Tulley R, et al. Effects of caffeine ingestion on metabolism and performance during graded exercise. *Eur J Appl Physiol* 50:301, 1983.
15. Powers S, Dodd S, Beadle R. Oxygen uptake kinetics in trained athletes differing in VO_2max. *Eur J Appl Physiol* 54: 306, 1985.

16. diPrampero P, Boutellier U, Pietsch P. Oxygen deficit and stores at onset of muscular exercise in humans. *J Appl Physiol* 55:146, 1983.
17. Powers S, Howley E, Cox R. Ventilatory and metabolic reactions to heat stress during prolonged exercise. *J Sports Med* 22:32, 1982.
18. Gaesser G, Brooks G. Metabolic bases of excess post-exercise oxygen consumption: A review. *Med Sci Sports Exerc* 16:29, 1984.
19. Powers S, Howley E, Cox R. A differential catecholamine response during prolonged exercise and passive heating. *Med Sci Sports Exerc* 14:435, 1982.
20. Farrell PA, Wilmore JH, Coyle EF, et al. Plasma lactate accumulation and distance running performance. *Med Sci Sports Exerc* 11:338, 1979.
21. Powers S, Dodd S, Deason R, et al. Ventilatory threshold, running economy and distance running performance of trained athletes. *Res Q Exerc Sport* 51:179, 1983.
22. Powers SK, Howley ET. *Exercise Physiology.* Madison, WI: Brown & Benchmark Publishers, 1994.

Suggested Readings

Brooks G, Fahey T. *Exercise Physiology: Human Bioenergetics and its Applications.* New York: John Wiley & Sons, 1984.

Holloszy J. Muscle metabolism during exercise. *Arch Phys Med Rehab* 63: 231, 1982.

Mathews C, van Holde K. *Biochemistry.* Redwood City: Benjamin Cummings, 1990.

McArdle W, Katch F, Katch V. *Exercise Physiology.* Philadelphia: Lea & Febiger, 1991.

Powers S, Howley E. *Exercise Physiology: Theory and Application to Fitness and Performance.* Dubuque: William C. Brown, 1990.

18, 19, 24, 25, 29, 176 · 33, 37, 40, 50, 51, 52, 53 · 57, 58 · 296, 297, 298, 300, 301 · 307, 310, 311, 313, 339, 430, 431

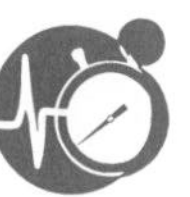

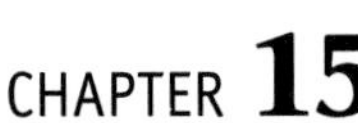

CHAPTER **15**

Normal Cardiorespiratory Responses to Acute Aerobic Exercise

Barry A. Franklin

The energy requirements of exercising human muscle may increase substantially in the transition from rest to maximal physical exertion. Because the available stores of adenosine triphosphate (ATP) are limited and capable of providing energy to maintain vigorous activity for only several seconds, ATP must be constantly resynthesized to provide continuous energy production (Fig. 15.1). Therefore, exercising muscle must possess a large capacity for increasing metabolic rate in order to produce sufficient ATP so that increased activity can continue. Energy production relies heavily on the respiratory and cardiovascular systems for the delivery of oxygen and nutrients and for the removal of waste products to maintain the internal equilibrium of cells.

The purpose of this chapter is to review the normal cardiorespiratory responses to acute aerobic exercise with specific reference to energy systems, hemodynamics, posture, maximal oxygen consumption ($\dot{V}O_2max$), the anaerobic threshold, dynamic versus isometric exertion, arm versus leg exercise, myocardial oxygen consumption, and the effects of physical conditioning. This information is vital to the understanding of the role of exercise physiology in the interpretation of diagnostic and functional exercise testing and the prescription of exercise in health and disease.

ENERGY SYSTEMS FOR EXERCISE

Adenosine triphosphate is broken down enzymatically inside cells into adenosine diphosphate (ADP) and phosphate (P) to provide energy for muscle contraction and the generation of force, as summarized by the reaction:

$$ATP + H_2O \rightarrow ADP + P + energy$$

Although not all ATP is formed aerobically, it should be emphasized that the amount of ATP yielded by anaerobic glycolysis is extremely small (Table 15.1) (1). Nevertheless, anaerobic mechanisms provide a rapid source of ATP, which is particularly important at the beginning of any exercise bout and during high intensity activity that can only be sustained for a brief period of time. As duration of exercise increases, the relative contribution of anaerobic energy sources decreases (Fig. 15.2) (2).

The aerobic system requires adequate delivery and use of O_2 and uses glycogen, fats, and proteins as energy substrates. It can sustain high rates of ATP production for muscular energy. The relative contribution of anaerobic and aerobic metabolism is dependent upon O_2 consumption (respiration), delivery (cardiovascular) and use (muscular extraction) at rates commensurate with the energy demands of activity.

ACUTE CARDIORESPIRATORY RESPONSES TO EXERCISE

Many cardiorespiratory and hemodynamic mechanisms function collectively to support increased aerobic requirements of physical activity. The overall effect of changes in heart rate (HR), stroke volume, cardiac output, blood flow, blood pressure, arteriovenous oxygen difference, and pulmonary ventilation is to oxygenate blood that is delivered to the active tissues.

Heart Rate

Heart rate increases in a linear fashion with the workrate and oxygen uptake during dynamic exercise. The increase in HR during exercise occurs primarily at the expense of diastole (filling time), rather than systole (Fig. 15.3) (3). Thus, at high exercise intensities, diastolic time may be so short as to preclude adequate ventricular filling. The magnitude of the HR response is related to age, body position, fitness, type of activity, the presence of heart disease, medications, blood volume, and environmental factors such as temperature and humidity. In contrast to systolic blood pressure, which usually increases with age, maximum attainable HR decreases with age. The equation, 220 − age, provides an approxima-

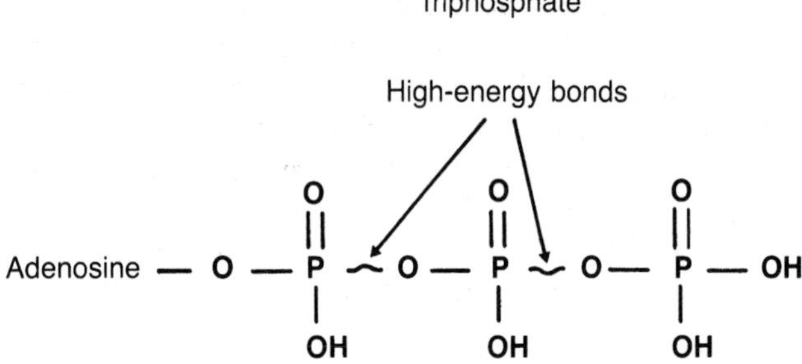

Figure 15.1. Simplified structure of an ATP molecule. The ~ symbol represents the high-energy bonds.

Table 15.1. Characteristics of the Two Mechanisms by Which ATP is Formed[a]

Mechanism	Food or Chemical Fuel	Oxygen Required?	Relative ATP Yield
Anaerobic			
Phosphocreatine	Phosphocreatine	No	Extremely limited
Glycolysis	Glycogen (glucose)	No	Extremely limited
Aerobic			
Krebs cycle and electron transport system	Glycogen, fats, proteins	Yes	Large

[a] Adapted from Mathews DK, Fox EL. *The Physiological Basis of Physical Education and Athletics,* 3rd ed. Philadelphia: WB Saunders 1981.

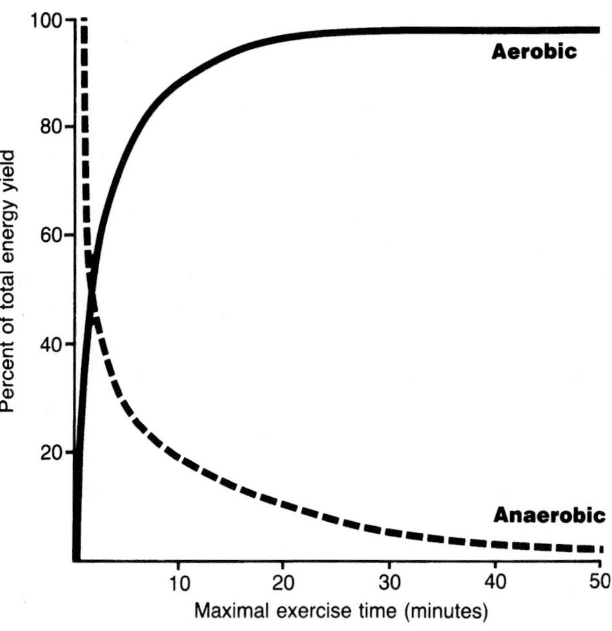

Figure 15.2. Relative contribution of aerobic and anaerobic metabolism during physical activity of increasing duration. In intense activities lasting 1½ to 2 minutes, the ATP-CP and lactic acid energy systems generate approximately 50% of the energy, while aerobic metabolism supplies the remainder. A distance runner, on the other hand, derives essentially 98% of his energy from aerobic metabolism during a 50-minute training run.

tion of the maximum HR in healthy men and women, but the variance for any fixed age is considerable (standard deviation ~ ± 10 beats/minute).

Stroke Volume

The stroke volume (SV) (volume of blood ejected per heart beat) is equal to the difference between end-diastolic volume (EDV) and end systolic volume (ESV). The former is determined by HR, filling pressure, and ventricular compliance, whereas the latter is dependent on two variables: contractility and afterload. Thus, a greater diastolic filling (preload) will increase SV. In contrast, factors that resist ventricular outflow (afterload) will result in a reduced SV.

SV at rest in the upright position generally varies between 60 and 100 ml/beat among healthy adults, while maximum SV approximates 100 to 120 ml/beat. During exercise, SV increases curvilinearly with the workrate until it reaches near maximum at a level equivalent to approximately 50% of aerobic capacity, increasing only slightly thereafter (4). Within physiological limits, enhanced venous return increases EDV, stretching cardiac muscle fibers and increasing force of contraction (Frank-

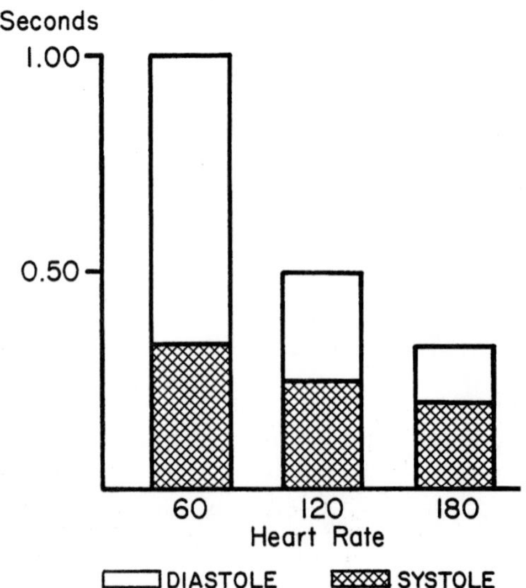

Figure 15.3. Relationship of systolic and diastolic time to heart rate (HR). Since coronary blood flow predominates during diastole, with increased HR, as during exercise, diastolic (perfusion) time is disproportionately shortened. (Adapted from Dehn MM, Mullins CB. Physiologic effects and importance of exercise in patients with coronary artery disease. *J Cardiovasc Med* 2:365–387, 1977.)

Starling mechanism). There is an increase in ejection fraction:

$$\textit{ejection fraction} = [SV/EDV] \times 100$$

Ejection fraction is normally 65% ± 8%, resulting from both the Frank-Starling mechanism and decreased ESV (Fig. 15.4) (5). The latter is due to increased ventricular contractility, secondary to catecholamine mediated sympathetic stimulation. The magnitude of these changes depends on several variables, including ventricular function, body position, and the intensity of exercise. Moreover, at a higher HR, stroke volume may actually decrease due to the disproportionate shortening in diastolic filling time (Fig. 15.3) (3, 6).

Cardiac Output

The product of SV and HR determines cardiac output. Cardiac output in healthy adults increases linearly with increased workrate, from a resting value of approximately 5 l/min to a maximum of about 20 l/min during upright exercise. However, maximum values of cardiac output are dependent upon many factors including age, posture, body size, presence of cardiovascular disease, and the level of physical conditioning. At exercise intensities up to 50% $\dot{V}O_2max$, the increase in cardiac output is facilitated by increases in HR and SV (4). Thereafter, the increase results almost solely from the continued rise in HR.

Arteriovenous Oxygen Difference

Oxygen extraction by tissues reflects the difference between oxygen content of arterial blood (~20 ml O_2/100 ml/dl at rest) and the oxygen content of venous blood (~ 15 ml O_2/dl), yielding a typical arteriovenous oxygen difference (CaO_2-CvO_2) at rest of 5 ml O_2/dl. This approximates a utilization coefficient of 25%. During exercise to exhaustion, the mixed venous oxygen content typically decreases to 5 ml/dl blood or lower, thus widening the arteriovenous oxygen difference from 5 to 15 ml/dl blood, corresponding to a utilization coefficient of 75% (4).

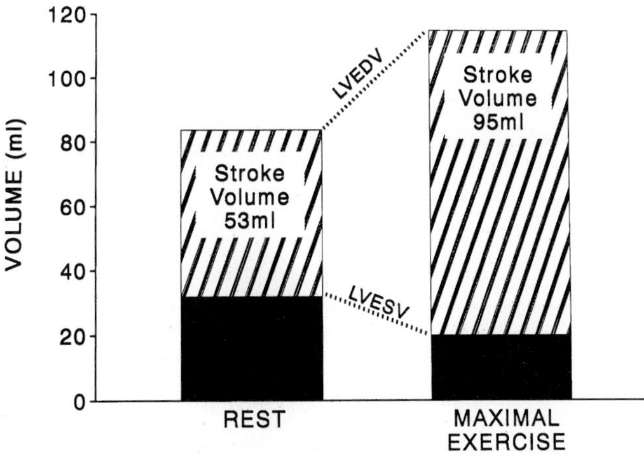

Figure 15.4. Changes in stroke volume from rest to maximal upright exercise is shown in young, healthy men. LVEDV = left ventricular end-diastolic volume; LVESV = left ventricular end-systolic volume. (Adapted from Poliner LR, Dehmer GJ, Lewis SE, et al. Left ventricular performance in normal subjects: A comparison of the responses to exercise in the upright and supine position. *Circulation* 62:528–534, 1980.)

Blood Flow

At rest, 15% to 20% of the cardiac output is distributed to the skeletal muscles, the remainder goes to visceral organs, the heart, and the brain (7). However, during exercise as much as 85% to 90% of the cardiac output is selectively delivered to working muscle and shunted away from the skin and the splanchnic, hepatic, and renal vascular beds. Myocardial blood flow may increase four to five times with exercise, whereas blood supply to the brain is maintained at resting levels (8).

Blood Pressure

There is a linear increase in systolic blood pressure (SBP) with increasing levels of exercise, approximating 8 to 12 mm Hg per metabolic equivalent (MET) where 1 MET = 3.5 ml O_2/kg/min. Maximal values typically reach 190 to 220 mm Hg (9). Nevertheless, maximal SBP should not be greater than 260 mm Hg (10). Diastolic blood pressure (DBP) may decrease slightly or remain unchanged; thus, pulse pressure (SBP minus DBP) generally increases in direct proportion to the intensity of exercise.

Because blood pressure is directly related to cardiac output and peripheral vascular resistance, it provides a noninvasive way to monitor the **inotropic** performance or pumping capacity of the heart. Until automated devices are adequately validated, the blood pressure response to exercise should be taken manually with a cuff and a stethoscope (10). A SBP that fails to rise or falls with increasing work loads may signal a plateauing or decreasing cardiac output, respectively (11). Exercise testing should be terminated in persons demonstrating exertional hypotension (SBP toward the end of a test decreasing below baseline standing level and/or SBP decreasing 20 mm Hg or more during exercise after an initial rise). This response has been shown to correlate with myocardial ischemia, left ventricular dysfunction, and an increased risk of cardiac events during follow-up (12). In one study, men with a maximal SBP $<$ 140 mm Hg had a 15-fold increase in the annual rate of sudden death compared with those whose pressures exceeded 200 mm Hg (13).

Pulmonary Ventilation

Pulmonary ventilation ($\dot{V}_E$), the volume of air exchanged per minute, generally approximates 6 l/min at rest in the average sedentary adult male. At maximal exercise, however, $\dot{V}_E$ often increases 15 to 25-fold over resting values. During mild-to-moderate exercise intensities, $\dot{V}_E$ is increased primarily by increasing tidal volume, whereas increases in the respiratory rate are more important to augment $\dot{V}_E$ during vigorous exercise. For the most part, the increase in pulmonary ventilation is directly proportional to the increase in somatic oxygen consumed ($\dot{V}O_2$) and carbon dioxide produced ($\dot{V}CO_2$). However, at a critical exercise intensity (usually 47% to 64% of the $\dot{V}O_2$max in healthy untrained individuals and 70% to 90% of the $\dot{V}O_2$max in highly trained subjects), $\dot{V}_E$ increases disproportionately relative to $\dot{V}O_2$, paralleling the abrupt nonlinear increases in serum lactate and $\dot{V}CO_2$ (14, 15). This suggests that pulmonary ventilation is, perhaps, regulated more by the requirement for carbon dioxide removal than by oxygen consumption and that ventilation is not normally a limiting factor to aerobic capacity.

POSTURAL CONSIDERATIONS

Posture has an effect on venous return and preload, particularly during brief bouts of physical exertion. At rest, EDV is highest when the body is recumbent. It decreases progressively as one shifts into sitting and standing postures, respectively. During exercise in the supine position, EDV remains largely unchanged. Thus, alterations in preload have little influence in increasing SV in this type of exercise. During exercise in the upright posture, EDV increases at intensities less than 50% $\dot{V}O_2$max. However, at higher exercise intensities, end-diastolic and SVs may decrease in some subjects (16, 17).

Prolonged upright exercise at a constant workrate places an increasing load on the heart (cardiovascular drift). Although the aerobic requirement of the exercise does not change, there is a progressive decrease in venous return, leading to a reduction in SV and a progressive rise in HR. The resulting tachycardia may be attributed, at least in part, to alterations in sympathetic blood flow control mechanisms, increased shunting of blood to the periphery (skin) for cooling, and decreased central blood volume (particularly in warm environments).

MAXIMAL OXYGEN CONSUMPTION

The most widely recognized measure of cardiopulmonary fitness is the aerobic capacity or $\dot{V}O_2$max. This variable is defined physiologically as the highest rate of oxygen transport and use that can be achieved at maximal physical exertion. Somatic oxygen consumption ($\dot{V}O_2$) may be expressed mathematically by a rearrangement of the Fick equation:

$$\dot{V}O_2 = HR \times SV \times (a\text{-}vDO_2)$$

where:
$\dot{V}O_2$ = Oxygen consumption$_2$ (ml/kg/min)
Heart rate = Heart rate (bpm)
Stroke volume = Stroke volume (ml/beat)
($a\text{-}vDO_2$) = arteriovenous oxygen difference

Thus, it is apparent that both central (i.e., cardiac output) and peripheral (i.e., arteriovenous oxygen difference) regulatory mechanisms affect the magnitude of body oxygen consumption.

Typical circulatory data at rest and during maximal exercise in a healthy, sedentary 30-year-old man and a similarly aged world-class endurance athlete are shown in Table 15.2. The absolute resting oxygen consumption (250 ml/min) divided by body weight (70 kg) gives the resting energy requirement, 1 MET (~3.5 ml/kg/minute). This expression of resting $\dot{V}O_2$, believed to originate from the work of Balke, is extremely important in exercise physiology, being independent of body weight and aerobic fitness (18). Furthermore, multiples of this value are often used to quantify respective levels of energy expenditure. For example, running at a 6-mph pace requires 10 times the resting energy expenditure, thus the aerobic cost is 10 METs or 35.0 ml/kg/min.

The 10-fold increase in oxygen transport and use in the sedentary individual is contrasted by a 23-fold increase in the endurance athlete, corresponding to a

Table 15.2. Hypothetical Circulatory Data at Rest and during Maximal Exercise for a Sedentary Man and a World-Class Endurance Athlete: 30-Year-Old Subjects

Condition	Oxygen Consumption (l/min)	Oxygen Consumption (ml/kg/min)	Cardiac Output (l/min)	Heart Rate (beats/min)	Stroke Volume (ml/beat)	Arteriovenous Oxygen Difference (ml/dl blood)
Sedentary Man (70 kg)						
Rest	0.25	3.5	6.1	70	87	4.0
Maximal Exercise	2.50	35.0	17.7	190	93	14.0
World-Class Endurance Athlete (70 kg)						
Rest	0.25	3.5	6.1	45	136	4.0
Maximal Exercise	5.60	80.0	35.0	190	184	16.0

$\dot{V}O_2$max of 35 ml/kg/min and 80 ml/kg/min, respectively. Increased aerobic capacity in trained athletes appears primarily as the result of increased maximal cardiac output, due to a greater increment in HR and SV, rather than an increased peripheral extraction of oxygen. Because there is little variation in maximal HR and maximal systemic arteriovenous oxygen difference with training, $\dot{V}O_2$max virtually defines the pumping capacity of the heart. Therefore, it is of major importance in the cardiovascular evaluation of the individual.

$\dot{V}O_2$max may be expressed on an absolute or relative basis, that is, in liters per minute, reflecting total body energy output and caloric expenditure (i.e., 1 liter ~ 5 kilocalories [kcal]), or by dividing this value by body weight in kilograms. Because large persons usually have a large absolute oxygen consumption by virtue of larger muscle mass, the latter allows a more equitable comparison between individuals of different body mass. This variable, when expressed as milliliters of oxygen per kilogram of body weight per minute (ml/kg/min) or as METs, is widely considered the single best index of physical work capacity or cardiorespiratory fitness (19).

Determination of the $\dot{V}O_2$max

Maximal oxygen consumption is usually determined by measuring the volume and oxygen content of expired air, corrected to standard temperature and pressure dry (STPD), using the following equation:

$$\dot{V}O_2 = \dot{V}_E\ (F_IO_2 — F_EO_2)$$

where: $\dot{V}_E$ = expired air (l/min)
F_EO_2 = directly measured fraction O_2 in expired air
F_IO_2 = directly measured fraction O_2 in inspired air (normally 0.2093)

Traditionally, $\dot{V}O_2$ has been measured using an open circuit or Douglas bag technique. However, several automated systems are available to measure $\dot{V}O_2$ and related respiratory variables during exercise testing.

Because it is often inconvenient to measure the $\dot{V}O_2$max directly, physiologists have sought to estimate aerobic capacity from the peak treadmill speed and grade, or cycle ergometer workrate, expressed as kilogram meters per minute. The conventional "Bruce" test is perhaps the most familiar and widely employed treadmill protocol with normative data on oxygen consumption so that aerobic capacity may be estimated from the workload attained (Fig. 15.5) (20). However, when a multistage protocol, like Bruce, is used to predict the $\dot{V}O_2$max, aerobic capacity may be markedly overestimated (21). One recent advance in test methodology that can overcome many of the limitations of incremental exercise is ramping (22, 23). Ramp protocols involve a nearly continuous and uniform increase in aerobic requirements that replaces the "staging" used in conventional exercise tests. With ramping, the gradual increase in demand allows a steady rise in cardiopulmonary responses.

ANAEROBIC (VENTILATORY) THRESHOLD

The onset of metabolic acidosis during exercise, traditionally determined by serial measurements of blood lactate, can be noninvasively determined by assessment of expired gases during exercise testing, specifically pulmonary ventilation ($\dot{V}_E$) and carbon dioxide production ($\dot{V}CO_2$) (24). Theoretically, gas exchange anaerobic threshold (AT) signifies the peak workrate or oxygen consumption at which the energy demands exceed circulatory ability to sustain aerobic metabolism. The phys-

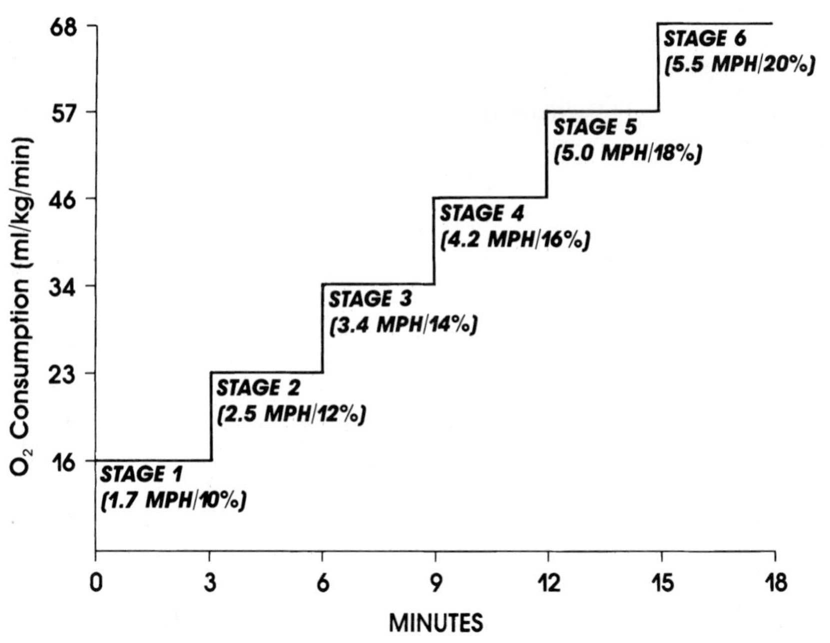

Figure 15.5. The standard Bruce treadmill protocol showing progressive stages (speed, percentage grade) and the corresponding aerobic requirement, expressed as ml/kg/min.

iology underlying the AT may be attributed, at least in part, to buffering of lactic acid by sodium bicarbonate in the blood, so that CO_2 is released in excess of that produced by muscle metabolism, providing an additional stimulus for ventilation. These biochemical alterations are summarized by the following reaction:

$$\underset{\text{(Lactic acid)}}{HLa} + \underset{\text{(sodium bicarbonaate)}}{NaHCO_3} \rightarrow \underset{\text{(sodium lactate)}}{NaLa} + \underset{\text{(carbonic acid)}}{H_2CO_3} + H_2O + CO_2$$

Accordingly, values for $\dot{V}_E$ and CO_2 production increase out of proportion to the intensity of exercise performed (Fig. 15.6) suggesting an abrupt increase in serum lactate (14). This method correlates well with the lactate method and obviates the need to measure lactate in repeated blood samples. An increase in the ventilatory equivalent for oxygen ($\dot{V}_E/\dot{V}O_2$) during exercise without a corresponding change in the ventilatory equivalent for CO_2 ($\dot{V}_E/\dot{V}CO_2$) has also been reported to be sensitive and reliable for determining the AT (25). There is, however, controversy surrounding the mechanisms responsible for the AT (26). Increased lactate production may result from mechanisms not related to inadequate oxygen delivery. Another theory is that inflections in $\dot{V}_E$ and $\dot{V}CO_2$ are due to inadequate buffering at a fixed metabolic intensity, even when lactate production and oxygen uptake continue to rise linearly.

The AT from respiratory gas measurements is often expressed as a percentage of the $\dot{V}O_2$max. For example, a highly trained athlete with a $\dot{V}O_2$max of 4.25 l/min whose break point in $\dot{V}_E$ occurs at 3.20 l/min, has an AT corresponding to 75% of aerobic capacity (Fig. 15.7). This athlete should be able to maintain exercise intensities below 75% of $\dot{V}O_2$max using a predominance of aerobic processes. Moreover, such exertion should be accomplished without inducing a significant increase in blood lactic acid and muscle fatigue. Although the AT typically corresponds to 55% ± 8% of the $\dot{V}O_2$max in healthy untrained individuals, it normally occurs at a higher percentage of the $\dot{V}O_2$max (i.e., 70% to 90%) in physically trained subjects (14, 15).

The $\dot{V}O_2$max is recognized as an important predictor of performance in endurance events. However, several studies now suggest that the highest percentage of the $\dot{V}O_2$max that can be used over an extended duration, without incurring significant increase in arterial lactate, may represent an even more important determinant of cardiorespiratory performance (15, 27). This suggests that the AT may be critical in determining optimal pace during endurance events.

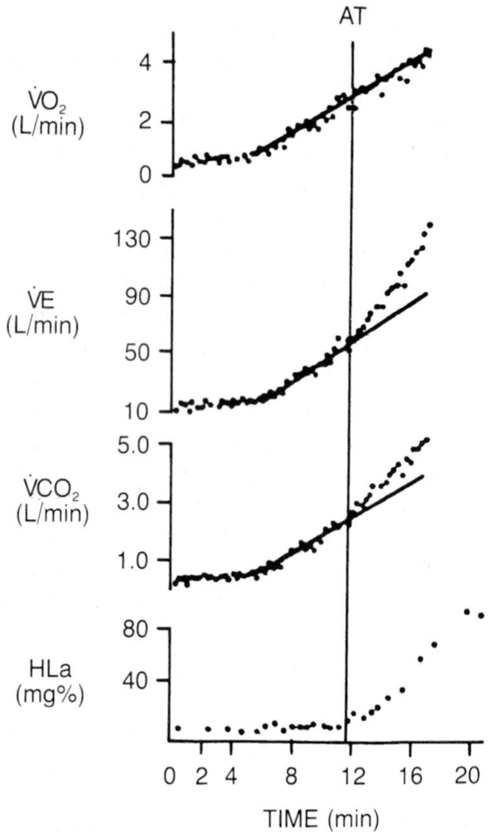

Figure 15.6. Relationship between intensity of exercise (oxygen consumption, $\dot{V}O_2$) and simultaneous, abrupt nonlinear increases in serum lactate (HLa), CO_2 production ($\dot{V}CO_2$), and pulmonary ventilation ($\dot{V}_E$) occurring at the anaerobic threshold (AT). Exercise was initiated at minute 4. (Adapted from Davis JA, Vodak P, Wilmore JH, et al. Anaerobic threshold and maximal aerobic power for three modes of exercise. *J Appl Physiol* 41:544-550, 1976.)

DYNAMIC (ISOTONIC) VERSUS ISOMETRIC (STATIC) EXERTION

Dynamic or isotonic activity (physical exertion characterized by rhythmic, repetitive movements of large

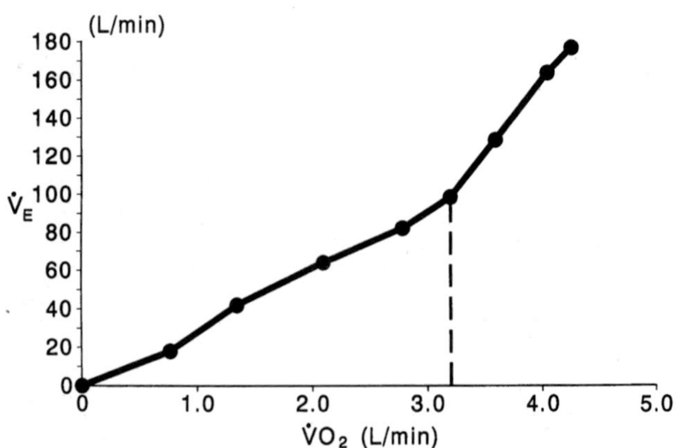

Figure 15.7. Relationship between intensity of exercise ($\dot{V}O_2$) and simultaneous, abrupt nonlinear increase in minute ventilation, signifying the anaerobic threshold. In this subject, the breakpoint occurred at 3.20 l/min, corresponding to 75% of measured $\dot{V}O_2$max (4.25 l/min).

muscle groups) results in increased oxygen consumption and HR that parallels the intensity of activity as well as an increase in SV. There is a concomitant, progressive increase in SBP with maintenance of or a slight decrease in the DBP, increasing pulse pressure.

Blood is shunted from the viscera to working skeletal muscle, where increased oxygen extraction increases systemic a-vO_2 diff. Thus, dynamic exercise imposes a volume load on the myocardium, which is the basis for a "cardiac training effect." In contrast, isometric exertion involves sustained muscle contraction against a fixed load or resistance with no change in length of the involved muscle group or joint motion.

The cardiovascular response to isometric exertion is apparently mediated by a neurogenic mechanism (28). Activities involving less than 20% of the maximum voluntary contraction (MVC) of the involved muscle group evoke a modest increase in SBP, DBP, and HR. During contractions greater than 20% of the MVC, HR increases in relation to the tension exerted, and there is an abrupt and precipitous increase in SBP. The SV remains essentially unchanged except at high levels of tension (> 50% MVC), where it may decrease. The result is a moderate increase in cardiac output, which is nevertheless high for the accompanying magnitude of increased metabolism. Despite the increased cardiac output, blood flow to the noncontracting muscle does not significantly increase, probably because of reflex vasoconstriction. The combination of vasoconstriction and increased cardiac output causes a disproportionate rise in systolic, diastolic, and mean blood pressure. Thus, a significant pressure load is imposed on the heart, presumably to increase perfusion to the active (contracting) skeletal muscle. A comparison of the relative hemodynamic responses to dynamic and isometric exercise is shown in Table 15.3.

The magnitude of the pressor response to isometric exertion depends on tension exerted relative to the greatest possible tension in the muscle group (% MVC), as well as muscle mass involved (29, 30). Thus, a relatively mild isometric contraction by weakened upper extremities may evoke an excessive pressor response. The increased myocardial demands are camouflaged by the relatively low aerobic requirements, so the usual warning signs of overexertion (tachycardia, sweating, dyspnea) may be absent. In persons who have an ischemic left ventricle, a marked pressure increase may lead to threatening ventricular arrhythmias, significant ST-segment depression, angina pectoris, ventricular decompensation and, in rare instances, sudden cardiac death (31).

Table 15.3. Comparison of the Relative Hemodynamic Responses to Dynamic and Static Exertion

	Dynamic (isotonic)	Static (isometric)
Cardiac output	+ + + +	+
Heart rate	+ +	+
Stroke volume	+ +	0
Peripheral resistance	−	+ + +
Systolic blood pressure	+ + +	+ + + +
Diastolic blood pressure	0 −	+ + + +
Mean arterial pressure	0 +	+ + + +
Left ventricular work	Volume Load	Pressure Load

Legend: + increase, − decrease, 0 unchanged

ARM VERSUS LEG EXERCISE

At a fixed power output (kgm/min or watts [W]), HR, SBP and DBP, the product of the HR times SBP (rate-pressure product), $\dot{V}_E$, $\dot{V}O_2$, respiratory exchange ratio, and blood lactate concentration are higher, while SV and AT (the latter expressed as a percentage of aerobic capacity) are lower during arm exercise compared with leg exercise (32). Since cardiac output is nearly the same in arm and leg exercise at a fixed oxygen uptake, elevated blood pressure during arm exercise is believed to reflect increased peripheral vascular resistance. During maximal effort, physiological responses are usually greater during leg exercise than arm exercise, except when subjects are limited in ability to perform leg work by neurologic, vascular, or orthopedic impairment of the lower extremities (33).

The disparity in cardiorespiratory and hemodynamic response to arm exercise versus leg exercise at identical workrates appears to be due to several factors. Mechanical efficiency (i.e., the ratio between the output of external work and caloric expenditure, or $\dot{V}O_2$) is lower during arm exercise than leg exercise (33). This may reflect the involvement of smaller muscle groups and the static effort required with arm work, which increases $\dot{V}O_2$ but does not affect the external work output. The higher rate-pressure product and estimated myocardial oxygen consumption at a fixed external workrate for arm work compared with leg work (Fig. 15.8) is believed to reflect increased sympathetic tone during arm exercise, perhaps mediated by reduced SV with compensatory tachycardia, concomitant isometric contraction, vasoconstriction in the non-exercising leg muscles, or all of these factors (34).

Maximal oxygen consumption ($\dot{V}O_2$max) during arm exercise in men and women generally varies between 64% and 80% of leg $\dot{V}O_2$max (32). Similarly, maximal cardiac output is lower during arm exercise compared with leg exercise, whereas the maximal HR, SBP, and rate-pressure product are comparable or slightly lower during arm exercise. The latter, however, has relevance to arm exercise training recommendations, particularly training intensity. Accordingly, an arm exercise prescription that **assumes** a maximal heart rate equivalent to leg exercise testing may result in an overestimation of the training HR. As a general guideline, the prescribed HR for leg training should be reduced by approximately 10 beats/min for arm training (35).

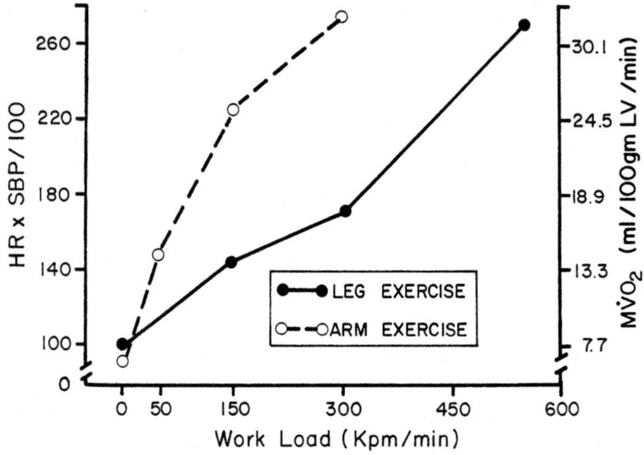

Figure 15.8. Mean rate-pressure product and estimated myocardial oxygen consumption ($M\dot{V}O_2$) during arm (*dashed line*) and leg (*solid line*) exercise. $M\dot{V}O_2$ is estimated from its hemodynamic correlates, heart rate (HR) multiplied by systolic blood pressure (SBP). (Adapted from Schwade J, Blomqvist CG, Shapiro W. A comparison of the response to arm and leg work in patients with ischemic heart disease. *Am Heart J* 94:203–208, 1977.)

MYOCARDIAL OXYGEN CONSUMPTION

Determinants of myocardial oxygen consumption ($M\dot{V}O_2$) include HR, myocardial contractility, and the tension or stress developed in the ventricular wall. Wall tension reflects a combination of SBP and ventricular volume and is inversely related to myocardial wall thickness (Fig. 15.9). During exercise, increased HR is the major contributor to increased myocardial oxygen demand. In contrast, oxygen supply is primarily facilitated by increased coronary blood flow, enabled by decreased coronary vascular resistance with only a modest increase in an already substantial myocardial oxygen difference.

Several investigators have reported excellent correlations between measured $M\dot{V}O_2$, (expressed as milliliters of oxygen per 100 gram of left ventricle per minute), HR and rate-pressure product; where $M\dot{V}O_2 = 0.28$ HR—14 ($r = 0.88$) or $M\dot{V}O_2 = ([0.14 \times HR \times SBP)/100]—6.3)$ ($r = 0.92$) (36, 37). HR alone is limited in ability to assess $M\dot{V}O_2$, especially when SBP is markedly elevated; this may occur during upper-extremity work involving isometric or isodynamic efforts.

Exercise-induced angina and significant ST-segment depression ($\geq$1 mm) usually occur at the same rate-pressure product in an individual with ischemic heart disease. This suggests the existence of an "ischemic threshold," at which myocardial oxygen demand exceeds myocardial oxygen supply. The rate-pressure product also provides an estimate of maximal workload that the left ventricle can perform. It has been suggested that an

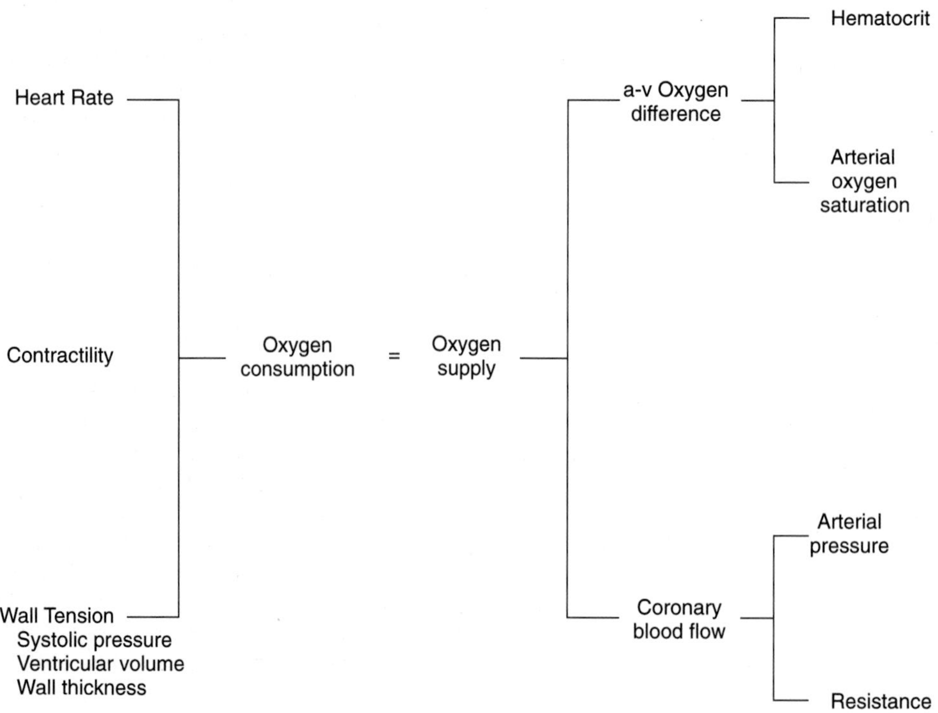

Figure 15.9. Determinants of myocardial oxygen demand and supply.

adequate rate-pressure product during maximal exercise is greater than 25,000; however, this may be influenced by age, clinical status, and medications, especially beta-blockers (10).

References

1. Mathews DK, Fox EL. *The Physiological Basis of Physical Education and Athletics,* 3rd ed. Philadelphia: W.B. Saunders, 1981.
2. Åstrand PO, Rodahl K. *Textbook of Work Physiology.* New York: McGraw-Hill Book Co, 1970:304.
3. Dehn MM, Mullins CB. Physiologic effects and importance of exercise in patients with coronary artery disease. *J Cardiovasc Med* 2:365–387, 1977.
4. Mitchell JH, Blomqvist G. Maximal oxygen uptake. *N Engl J Med* 284:1018–1022, 1971.
5. Poliner LR, Dehmer GJ, Lewis SE, et al. Left ventricular performance in normal subjects: A comparison of the responses to exercise in the upright and supine position. *Circulation* 62:528–534, 1980.
6. Ferguson RJ, Faulkner JA, Julius S, et al. Comparison of cardiac output determined by CO_2 rebreathing and dye-dilution methods. *J Appl Physiol* 25:450–454, 1968.
7. Rowell LB. Circulation. *Med Sci Sports* 1:15–22, 1969.
8. Zobl EG, Talmers FN, Christensen RC, et al. Effect of exercise on the cerebral circulation and metabolism. *J Appl Physiol* 20:1289–1293, 1965.
9. Naughton J, Haider R. Methods of exercise testing. In: Naughton JP, Hellerstein HK, Mohler IC, eds. *Exercise Testing and Exercise Training in Coronary Heart Disease.* New York: Academic Press, 1973, p 79.
10. ACSM. *Guidelines for Exercise Testing and Prescription,* ACSM's 5th ed. Baltimore; Williams & Wilkins, 1995: 97.
11. Comess KA, Fenster PE. Clinical implications of the blood pressure response to exercise. *Cardiology* 68:233–244, 1981.
12. Franklin BA. Diagnostic and functional exercise testing: Test selection and interpretation. *J Cardiovasc Nurs* 10:8–29, 1995.
13. Irving JB, Bruce RA, DeRouen TA. Variations in and significance of systolic pressure during maximal exercise (treadmill) testing: Relation to severity of coronary artery disease and cardiac mortality. *Am J Cardiol* 39:841–848, 1977.
14. Davis JA, Vodak P, Wilmore JH, et al. Anaerobic threshold and maximal aerobic power for three modes of exercise. *J Appl Physiol* 41:544–550, 1976.
15. Costill DL. Physiology of marathon running. *JAMA* 221: 1024–1029, 1972.
16. Ginzton LE, Conant R, Brizendine M, et al.Effect of long-term high intensity aerobic training on left ventricular volume during maximal upright exercise. *J Am Coll Cardiol* 14: 364–371, 1989.
17. Concu A, Marcello C. Stroke volume response to progressive exercise in athletes engaged in different types of training. *Eur J Appl Physiol* 66:11–17, 1993.
18. Balke B. Experimental studies on the functional capacities of middle-aged and aging persons. *J Okla Med Assoc* 54: 120–123, 1961.
19. Buskirk E, Taylor HL. Maximal oxygen intake and its relation to body composition, with special reference to chronic physical activity and obesity. *J Appl Physiol* 2:72–78, 1957.
20. Bruce RA, Kusumi F, Hosmer D. Maximal oxygen intake and nomographic assessment of functional aerobic impairment in cardiovascular disease. *Am Heart J* 85:546–562, 1973.
21. Franklin BA. Pitfalls in estimating aerobic capacity from exercise time or workload. *Appl Cardiol* 14:25–26, 1986.
22. Myers J, Buchanan N, Walsh D, et al. Comparison of the ramp versus standard exercise protocols. *J Am Coll Cardiol* 17:1334–1342, 1991.
23. Myers J, Buchanan N, Smith D, et al. Individual ramp treadmill: Observations on a new protocol. Chest 101: 236S-241S, 1992.
24. Wasserman K, Whipp BJ, Koyal SN, et al. Anaerobic threshold and respiratory gas exchange during exercise. *J Appl Physiol* 35:236–243, 1973.
25. Davis JA, Frank MH, Whipp BJ, et al. Anaerobic threshold alterations caused by endurance training in middle-aged men. *J Appl Physiol* 46:1039–1046, 1979.
26. Brooks GA. Anaerobic threshold : review of the concept and directions for future research. *Med Sci Sports Exerc* 17: 22–31, 1985.
27. Costill DL, Thomason H, Roberts E. Fractional utilization of the aerobic capacity during distance running. *Med Sci Sports Exerc* 5:248–252, 1973.
28. Lind AR, Taylor SH, Humphreys PW, et al. The circulatory effects of sustained voluntary muscle contraction. *Clin Sci* 27:229–244, 1964.
29. Lind AR, McNichol GW. Muscular factors which determine the cardiovascular responses to sustained and rhythmic exercise. *Can Med Assoc J* 96:706–715, 1967.
30. Mitchell JH, Payne FC, Saltin B, et al. The role of muscle mass in the cardiovascular response to static contractions. *J Physiol* 309:45–54, 1980.
31. Atkins JM, Matthews OA, Blomqvist CG, et al. Incidence of arrhythmias induced by isometric and dynamic exercise. *Br Heart J* 38:465–471, 1976.
32. Franklin BA. Exercise testing, training and arm ergometry. *Sports Med* 2:100–119, 1985.
33. Fardy PS, Webb D, Hellerstein HK. Benefits of arm exercise in cardiac rehabilitation. *Phys Sportmed* 5:30–41, 1977.
34. Schwade J, Blomqvist CG, Shapiro W. A comparison of the response to arm and leg work in patients with ischemic heart disease. *Am Heart J* 94:203–208, 1977.
35. Franklin BA, Vander L, Wrisley D, et al. Aerobic requirements of arm ergometry: Implications for exercise testing and training. *Phys Sportsmed* 11:81–90, 1983.
36. Kitamura K, Jorgenson CR, Gobel FL, et al. Hemodynamic correlates of myocardial oxygen consumption during upright exercise. *J Appl Physiol* 32:516–522, 1972.
37. Nelson RR, Gobel FL, Jorgensen CR, et al.Hemodynamic predictors of myocardial oxygen consumption during static and dynamic exercise. *Circulation* 50:1179–1189, 1974.

38, 50, 51, 53  86 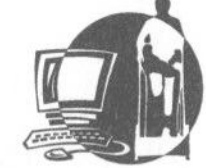 296, 298, 301, 331, 334 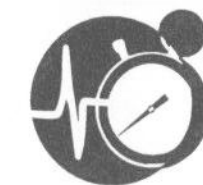 303, 310, 339, 340 

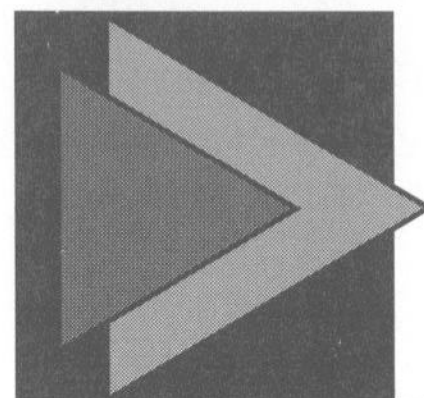

CHAPTER 16

ABNORMAL CARDIORESPIRATORY RESPONSES TO ACUTE AEROBIC EXERCISE

Barry A. Franklin

Three types of exercise can be used to stress the circulatory and ventilatory systems: dynamic, isometric, and a combination of the two (isodynamic). Dynamic exercise is associated with a volume load on the heart and appropriate increases in cardiac output and oxygen uptake. Isometric exercise, on the other hand, imposes a disproportionate pressure load on the left ventricle relative to the somatic aerobic requirements. Surprisingly, superimposing static on dynamic effort appears to attenuate the magnitude of cardiovascular stress, because the relationship between myocardial oxygen supply and demand is favorably altered.

The acute cardiorespiratory responses to these forms of exercise have both immediate value, for evaluating the suitability of physical activity, and prognostic implications in regard to morbidity and mortality. These data extend the clinical information obtained from other sources (history and physical examination, resting electrocardiogram [ECG], blood chemistry profile), and can be used to identify the primary mechanism underlying exercise intolerance and are useful in assessing a change in clinical status or the effectiveness of various interventions (1). The latter may include exercise training, pharmacotherapy, or revascularization procedures such as angioplasty or coronary artery bypass surgery. In this chapter normal and abnormal cardiorespiratory responses to acute aerobic exercise will be reviewed, with specific reference to clinical exercise testing, the value of gas exchange data, associated ECG and hemodynamic responses, symptoms, isometric and isodynamic exertion, and patients with chronic disease.

CLINICAL EXERCISE TESTING

Dynamic exercise testing is one of the most common evaluations performed in the assessment of persons with known or suspected coronary artery disease (CAD). The test is based primarily on the ECG response to exercise. One millimeter or more of ST-segment depression at 80 msec beyond the J point is considered an indicator of myocardial ischemia (2). However, other variables, including angina pectoris, threatening ventricular arrhythmias, exertional hypotension, and aerobic fitness, expressed as exercise duration, metabolic equivalents (METs), or peak power output (kilogram meters per minute) are also related to subsequent cardiovascular morbidity and mortality. In addition, recent studies suggest that blood lactate concentration at peak exercise appears to be a strong independent predictor of CAD in men (3, 4).

Unfortunately, the conventional exercise ECG has significant limitations in the diagnosis of occult CAD (5), with an approximate sensitivity and specificity of 75% and 85%, respectively. In some persons, exercise-induced ST segment depression suggests myocardial ischemia and underlying heart disease when, in fact, no disease is present. This scenario, termed a false-positive response, occurs predominantly in populations with a low pretest likelihood of CAD (e.g., young adults, asymptomatic women). Conversely, when a patient is found to have significant CAD and fails to demonstrate exercise-induced ST segment depression, the test is classified as a false-negative test.

Pre- and Post-test Probability of Coronary Disease

Probability tables based on age, gender, the presence of major coronary risk factors (cigarette smoking, hypertension, abnormal lipid/lipoprotein profile, sedentary lifestyle) and related clinical information (ECG, family history) can be used to estimate likelihood ("Bayesian" analysis) of having significant CAD even before an exercise test (6). However, the most meaningful and profound alterations in pre-test probability of CAD are caused by symptomatology. Atypical angina pectoris raises the pre-test probability for significant angiographic coronary disease to 50% in a middle-aged man or postmenopausal woman, whereas typical angina raises it to 90% (7).

These estimates are helpful in deciding whether a diagnostic exercise test is clinically warranted and in clarifying the post-test likelihood of CAD. When the pretest risk of CAD is high, as is the case with a history of typical angina, or very low, as in asymptomatic patients or those with nonanginal pain, a normal or abnormal exercise ECG response has little influence on the post-test likelihood of disease. Accordingly, exercise testing has the greatest impact in persons with an intermediate likelihood of CAD, that is, in those with atypical angina. For example, probability tables suggest that a 55-year-old man with exertional jaw and back pain (atypical angina) has a 59% likelihood of significant CAD before exercise testing. After an exercise ECG, post-test likelihood of CAD is either 90% or 30% according to the presence or absence, respectively, of significant ST segment depression (8). Thus, by applying Bayesian analyses, the need for additional diagnostic studies (e.g., exercise testing with myocardial perfusion imaging, exercise echocardiography) can be defined more intelligently.

Value of Gas Exchange Data: Differential Diagnosis

The value of clinical exercise testing is not limited to assessing potential indices of myocardial ischemia, suggesting significant CAD. By permitting simultaneous assessment of respiratory gas exchange data, which has been simplified by the availability of computerized systems, cardiopulmonary exercise testing can be especially helpful in the differential diagnosis of exertional dyspnea and fatigue (1). Moreover, in patients with coexistent cardiovascular and pulmonary disease, it can be used to identify the dominant factor limiting exercise tolerance. Differences in body size, muscle mass, age, gender, habitual level of activity and physical conditioning account for much of the physiological variation in maximal oxygen consumption ($\dot{V}O_2$max). It is adversely affected by disease and disuse (10). Decreases in aerobic capacity are often subtle; thus, it is possible for a large percentage of the $\dot{V}O_2$max to be lost before the ability to perform daily activities becomes noticeably compromised (Fig. 16.1) (11).

With cardiopulmonary exercise testing, it is now possible to objectively evaluate and classify chronic heart failure on the basis of oxygen consumption at the anaerobic (ventilatory) threshold (AT) and at maximal exercise ($\dot{V}O_2$max). Weber and Janicki demonstrated that treadmill $\dot{V}O_2$max correlates with cardiac reserve, expressed as the maximum cardiac index (Table 16.1) (12). Others, however, suggest that the accuracy and generalizability of this classification scheme is limited, because it is necessary to relate aerobic performance to expected values for matched, healthy individuals. Bruce et al. developed the concept of functional aerobic impairment (FAI) for this purpose (13). The FAI is the percentage difference between observed $\dot{V}O_2$max, (measured directly or estimated) and the $\dot{V}O_2$max predicted for a healthy person of the same age, gender, and habitual activity status. Average predicted values of $\dot{V}O_2$max according to age for active and sedentary men and women are shown in Table 16.2.

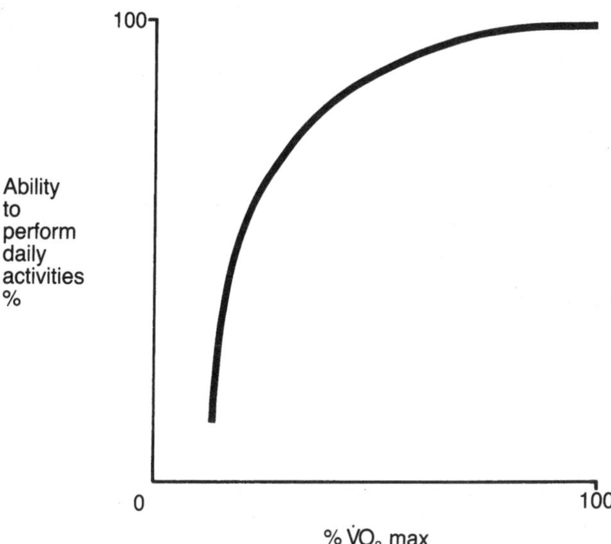

Figure 16.1. The reserve physiological capacity of the oxygen transport system is such that it is possible for much of the aerobic capacity ($\dot{V}O_2$max) to be lost before the demands of daily living become compromised. This appears to be particularly true among sedentary individuals. (Adapted from Jones NL, Campbell EJM. *Clinical Exercise Testing.* Philadelphia: WB Saunders, 1981:2.)

Table 16.1. Weber's Classification of Functional Impairment in Aerobic Capacity and Anaerobic Threshold[a]

Class	Severity	$\dot{V}O_2$max (mL/kg/min)	AT ($\dot{V}O_2$max, mL/kg/min)
A	mild to none	> 20	> 14
B	mild to moderate	16–20	11–14
C	moderate to severe	10–16	8–11
D	severe	6–10	5–8
E	very severe	< 6	< 4

[a] Adapted from Weber KT, Janicki JS. Cardiopulmonary exercise testing for evaluation of chronic cardiac failure. *Am J Cardiol* 55(Suppl A):22A–31A, 1985.

FAI can be calculated from the following formula:

$$\%FAI = \frac{\text{Predicted } \dot{V}O_2max - \text{Observed } \dot{V}O_2max}{\text{Predicted } \dot{V}O_2max} \times 100$$

The normal value for the FAI is 0%; this indicates that the $\dot{V}O_2$max is 100% of the age- and gender-predicted value and that there is no functional impairment. Negative values for FAI signify above-average fitness. The degree of FAI can be categorized as mild (27% to 40%),

Table 16.2. Average $\dot{V}O_2$max Values (ml/kg/min) for Healthy Active and Sedentary Men and Women According to Age[a]

	Men		Women	
Age (years)	Active 69.7– (0.612 × years)	Sedentary[b] 57.8– (0.445 × years)	Active 42.9– (0.312 × years)	Sedentary[b] 42.3– (0.356 × years)
20	57.5	48.9	36.7	35.2
22	56.2	48.0	36.0	34.5
24	55.0	47.1	35.4	33.8
26	53.8	46.2	34.8	33.0
28	52.6	45.3	34.2	32.3
30	51.3	44.5	33.5	31.6
32	50.1	43.6	32.9	30.9
34	48.9	42.7	32.3	30.2
36	47.7	41.8	31.7	29.5
38	46.4	40.9	31.0	28.8
40	45.2	40.0	30.4	28.1
42	44.0	39.1	29.8	27.3
44	42.8	38.2	29.2	26.6
46	41.5	37.3	28.5	25.9
48	40.3	36.4	27.9	25.2
50	39.1	35.6	27.3	24.5
52	37.9	34.7	26.7	23.8
54	36.7	33.8	26.1	23.1
56	35.4	32.9	25.4	22.4
58	34.2	32.0	24.8	21.7
60	33.0	31.1	24.2	20.9
62	31.8	30.2	23.6	20.2
64	30.5	29.3	22.9	19.5
66	29.3	28.4	22.3	18.8
68	28.1	27.5	21.7	18.1
70	26.9	26.7	21.1	17.4

[a] $\dot{V}O_2$max for any age can be predicted using the above-referenced regression equations from reference #13.

[b] Defined as subjects who do not exert themselves sufficiently to develop sweating at least once a week.

moderate (41% to 54%), marked (55% to 68%), and extreme (>68%). The concept of FAI is particularly useful in making serial evaluations of individuals as well as comparisons with peers.

Several approaches have been suggested for the differential diagnosis of exercise intolerance (exertional dyspnea), using gas exchange data to identify the predominant circulatory or ventilatory limitation (1). One widely-recognized method examines $\dot{V}O_2$peak and AT as a function of the predicted $\dot{V}O_2$max and considers these variables in sequential fashion, as shown in Fig. 16.2 (14, 15). If $\dot{V}O_2$peak is ≥ 85% of the predicted value, exertional symptoms are likely to be attributed to anxiety, obesity, mild cardiopulmonary disease, or combinations thereof. If $\dot{V}O_2$peak is low and AT and "breathing reserve" are normal, exertional intolerance is likely to be due to poor effort, deconditioning, or coronary disease. In contrast, this scenario coupled with a low breathing reserve suggests a ventilatory limitation. As expected, low $\dot{V}O_2$peak and low AT are attributed to circulatory impairment or mixed lesions, depending on the normality of the breathing reserve. This algorithm is attractive in scope, but clearly depends on the validity of the formulas used to classify these variables.

ECG RESPONSES TO EXERCISE TESTING

ECG responses to graded exercise tests should be interpreted according to the magnitude and configuration of ST segment displacement and the presence of supraventricular and ventricular dysrhythmias. Such information is useful in evaluating clinical status as well as the efficacy of selected interventions, including coronary revascularization and medications.

ST Segment Depression

Traditionally, exercise-induced ST segment depression (especially > 1 mm horizontal or downsloping) has been considered diagnostic of myocardial ischemia and suggestive of CAD. McHenry et al. found the ST segment index, that is, the algebraic sum of the ST J segment depression in millimeters and the ST slope in millivolts per second, to be a valid and reliable method to assess exercise-induced myocardial ischemia, as confirmed by angiographically-documented CAD (16). A negative index (i.e., < 0) is considered abnormal, provided that the magnitude of ST segment depression (from the baseline to the J point) is at least 1.0 mm (Fig. 16.3). Recently, exercise-induced QRS prolongation has also been shown to be a marker of myocardial ischemia in patients with CAD (17).

ST Segment Elevation

Although ST segment elevation is an infrequent (0.1% prevalence) and often disregarded ECG response, it is widely regarded as an ominous finding, especially in the absence of a previous Q wave infarction. The finding usually reflects wall motion abnormalities and associated left ventricular dysfunction in patients with a history of myocardial infarction and/or Q waves in the lead corresponding to the ST segment elevation (18, 19). However, exercise-induced ST segment elevation in the absence of a previous myocardial infarction (not over diagnostic Q waves) suggests severe transmural ischemia, is arrhythmogenic, and localizes the artery where there is spasm or a critical lesion (20, 21).

Dysrhythmias

Infrequent atrial or ventricular ectopic beats and short runs of supraventricular tachycardia commonly occur during exercise testing and do not appear to have diag-

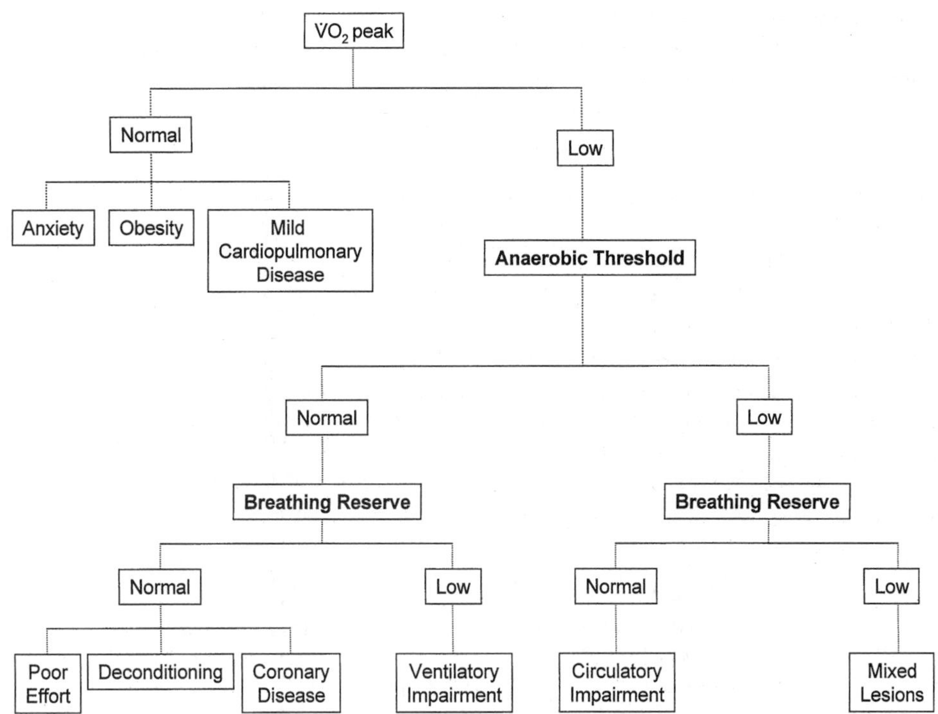

Figure 16.2. Flow chart for differential diagnosis of exertional dyspnea. (Adapted from Wasserman K, Hansen JE, Sue DY, et al. *Principles of Exercise Testing and Interpretation.* Philadelphia: Lea & Febiger, 1987; Zavala DC. *Manual on Exercise Testing: A Training Handbook.* Iowa City: University of Iowa Press, 1985.)

nostic or prognostic significance for CAD. Similarly, the provocation or suppression of ventricular dysrhythmias during exercise testing does not necessarily signal the presence or absence of CAD, respectively (22). Threatening forms of ventricular ectopy are even more likely to be associated with significant CAD and a poor prognosis in the presence of ischemic ST-segment depression (23).

HEMODYNAMIC RESPONSES

The evaluation of hemodynamic responses, specifically heart rate (HR) and blood pressure, has been shown to enhance the predictive value of exercise studies.

Heart Rate

A patient with a reduced HR response during exercise, in the absence of ß-blocker or calcium channel blocker therapy, is said to have chronotropic incompetence which may be expressed as the peak heart rate attained, chronotropic index (ratio of heart rate reserve to metabolic reserve), or the percent of age-predicted maximal heart rate achieved (24, 25). Traditionally this is identified by the failure of the exercise heart rate to rise to within two standard deviations (~ 20 beats/minute) of the age-predicted response to exercise, assuming the subject was highly motivated. This finding during exercise, even as an isolated anomaly, has been shown to predict the presence and angiographic severity of CAD and is associated with a higher subsequent morbidity and mortality rate (25–27).

Systolic Blood Pressure

The normal systolic blood pressure response to incremental exercise is a progressive rise, typically 10 ± 2 mm Hg/MET, with a possible plateau at peak exercise. Exertional hypotension is defined as failure of the systolic blood pressure to rise, a drop below the pre-test value (at standing rest), or a decrease of ≥ 20 mmHg during exercise, after an initial rise. This abnormal response may be attributed to chronic ventricular dysfunction, exercise-induced myocardial ischemia causing left ventricular dysfunction, or papillary muscle dysfunction and mitral regurgitation, and is associated with an increased risk of cardiac events during follow-up (28, 29).

Diastolic Blood Pressure

Diastolic blood pressure generally remains unchanged or decreases slightly during progressive exercise. Although an increase of more than 15 mmHg during treadmill testing may be an indicator of severe CAD, it is more likely a marker for labile hypertension (30).

SYMPTOMS

It is important to note all symptoms that occur during and after the exercise test, especially substernal pressure that radiates across the chest to the left arm, jaw, back, or lower neck areas. Anginal symptoms can be rated by

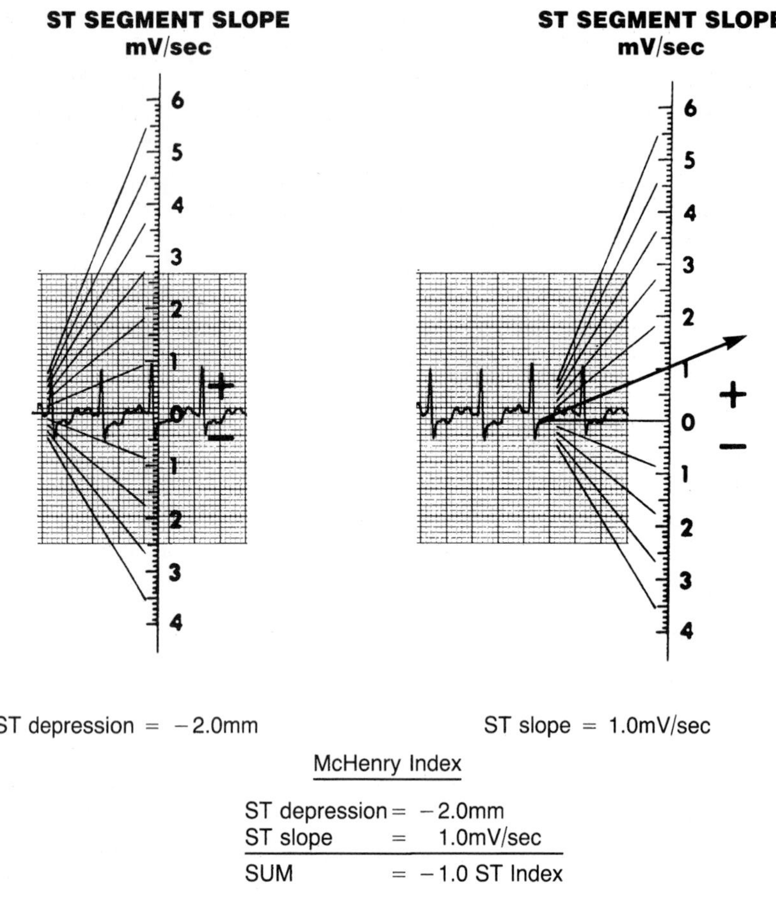

Figure 16.3. Example showing calculation of the ST segment index by using a transparent overlay to determine the ST segment slope and depression. An abnormal ECG response with upsloping ST segment depression is shown.

the patient on a scale of 1–4 ("perceptible, but mild" to "severe"); however, ratings of > 2 (moderate) are generally used as end points for testing. Patients with angina during exercise, with or without concomitant ST segment depression, are at increased risk of subsequent coronary events (31).

STATIC AND ISODYNAMIC EXERTION

The myocardial demands imposed by static (isometric) or high-resistance effort may exceed those for low-resistance, dynamic exercise. Because the pressor response to static exertion is proportionate to the relative intensity (percent of maximal voluntary contraction [MVC]), duration of effort, and muscle mass involved, a relatively mild static contraction in an isolated, weak muscle group may evoke an excessive pressor response, despite relatively small increases in heart rate, somatic oxygen consumption, and cardiac output (32, 33).

Although static or combined static/dynamic (isodynamic) exercise has been traditionally discouraged in patients with CAD, it appears that these types of exertion may be less hazardous than once presumed, particularly in patients with normal or near-normal aerobic fitness and left ventricular function (34). Despite earlier reports that static exercise may precipitate arrhythmias, the appearance of new wall motion abnormalities and sudden cardiac death (rare), several studies now indicate that nonsustained isometric exercise, regardless of the percentage MVC used, generally fails to elicit angina pectoris, ischemic ST-segment displacement, or threatening ventricular arrhythmias among clinically stable coronary patients (35–37). The rate-pressure product and estimated myocardial oxygen demands are lower during static than during maximal dynamic exercise, primarily due to a lower peak heart rate response (37). Increased subendocardial perfusion, secondary to elevated diastolic blood pressure, may also contribute to the lower incidence of ischemic ST-segment depression and/or angina pectoris during static or isodynamic efforts. Furthermore, the myocardial oxygen supply/demand relationship appears to be favorably altered by superimposing static on dynamic effort, so that the magnitude of ST-segment depression is reduced at a given rate-pressure product (Fig. 16.4) (36, 38). These findings are changing the cautious attitude toward static and isodynamic exertion (and resistance training) for coronary patients, particularly in regard to vocational counseling and exercise prescription.

Since it is virtually impossible to participate in normal daily activities without engaging in some static efforts, realistic testing should include an evaluation of the physiological response to static forms of exercise, especially for patients at moderate-to-high risk. This applies to individuals involved in occupations with static requirements (carrying loads, operating a jackhammer, carpentry) as well as those involved in resistance training and selected recreational activities. Rather than arbitrarily proscribing such activities, the response to such predominantly static activities should be assessed and recommendations given regarding minimizing adverse responses. For example, a shoulder strap for carrying weights or luggage with wheels and an extendable handlebar can be recommended to minimize static efforts in selected patients.

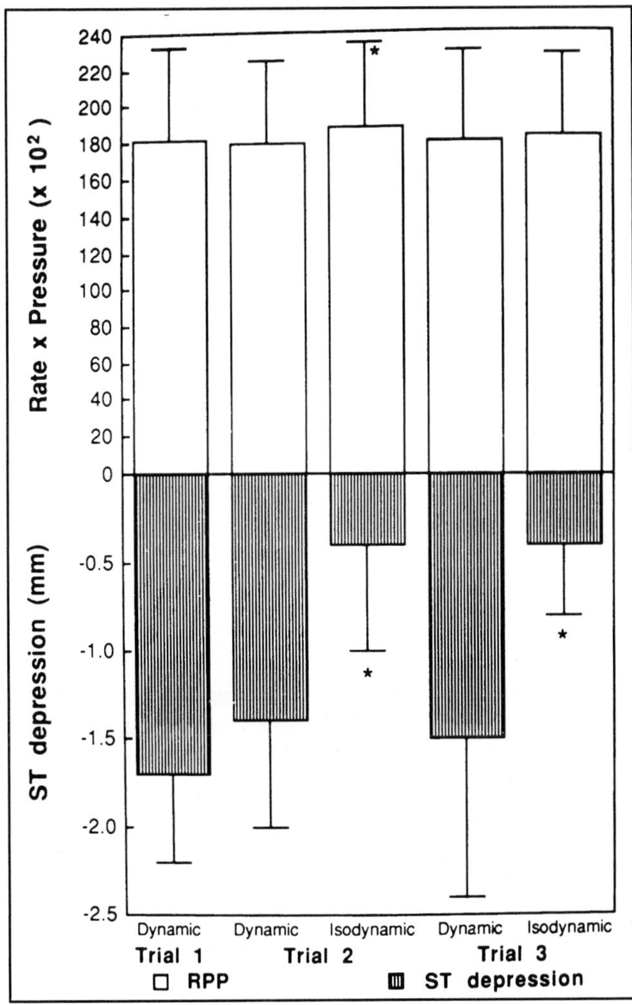

Figure 16.4. (Top) Rate-pressure product (RPP). (Bottom) Corresponding ST segment depression. Trial 1 is baseline dynamic exercise. Trials 2 and 3 are dynamic and isodynamic exercise. Values are mean ± SD. *P < 0.001 for differences between dynamic and isodynamic exercise trials. (With permission from Bertagnoli K, Hanson P, Ward A. Attenuation of exercise-induced ST depression during combined isometric and dynamic exercise in coronary artery disease. *Am J Cardiol* 65:314–317, 1990.)

PATIENTS WITH CHRONIC DISEASE

The electrocardiographic, cardiorespiratory, and hemodynamic responses to acute aerobic exercise may be markedly altered in patients with chronic disease. This section briefly reviews these anomalies, with specific reference to patients with cardiopulmonary disease, hypertension, diabetes, obesity, and peripheral vascular disease.

Coronary Artery Disease

Typical circulatory data at rest and during maximal exercise in a healthy sedentary man and a patient with CAD are shown in Table 16.3. The 10-fold increase in oxygen consumption at maximal exercise ($\dot{V}O_2max$) in the sedentary man is contrasted to a 6-fold increase in the cardiac patient. The reduced oxygen transport capacity in the cardiac patient is primarily due to diminished cardiac output (stroke volume and/or heart rate) rather than a reduction in peripheral extraction of oxygen.

In some patients, a primary limitation appears to be decreased contractile force of the left ventricle due to residual myocardial ischemia or necrosis, causing a progressive decrease in ejection fraction and stroke volume with exercise. This may be manifested as exertional hypotension during progressive exercise (28). In others, cardiac output may be limited by the restriction in the rise of heart rate due to intrinsic disease of the SA or AV node, resulting in chronotropic impairment, or to the appearance of adverse signs and/or symptoms that preclude exercising at a higher work rate or intensity.

Pathophysiologic evidence suggests that increased aerobic requirements imposed by progressive isotonic exercise may induce myocardial ischemia or electrical instability in patients with CAD. By increasing myocardial oxygen consumption and simultaneously shortening diastole and coronary perfusion time, exercise may evoke a transient oxygen deficiency in subendocardial tissue which may be exacerbated by a decrease in venous return secondary to an abrupt cessation of exercise. Intracellular sodium/potassium imbalance, catecholamine excess, and increased circulating free fatty acids may also be arrhythmogenic (Fig. 16.5). This scenario, in the presence of documented or occult CAD, may precipitate angina pectoris, ischemic ST-segment depression, threatening ventricular arrhythmias, or combinations thereof.

Table 16.3. Hypothetical Circulatory Data at Rest and during Maximal Exercise for a Sedentary Man and a Patient with Heart Disease

Condition	Oxygen Consumption (l/min)	Oxygen Consumption (ml/kg/min)	Cardiac Output (l/min)	Heart Rate (beats/min)	Stroke Volume (ml/beat)	Arteriovenous Oxygen Difference (ml/dl blood)
Sedentary Man (70 kg)						
Rest	0.25	3.5[a]	6.1	70	87	4.0
Maximal Exercise	2.50	35.0	17.7	190	93	14.0
Cardiac Patient (70 kg)						
Rest	0.25	3.5[a]	6.1	82	74	4.0
Maximal Exercise	1.50	21.5	10.4	165	66	13.6

[a] 3.5 ml/kg/min = 1 metabolic equivalent (MET); average resting metabolic rate expressed per unit body weight.

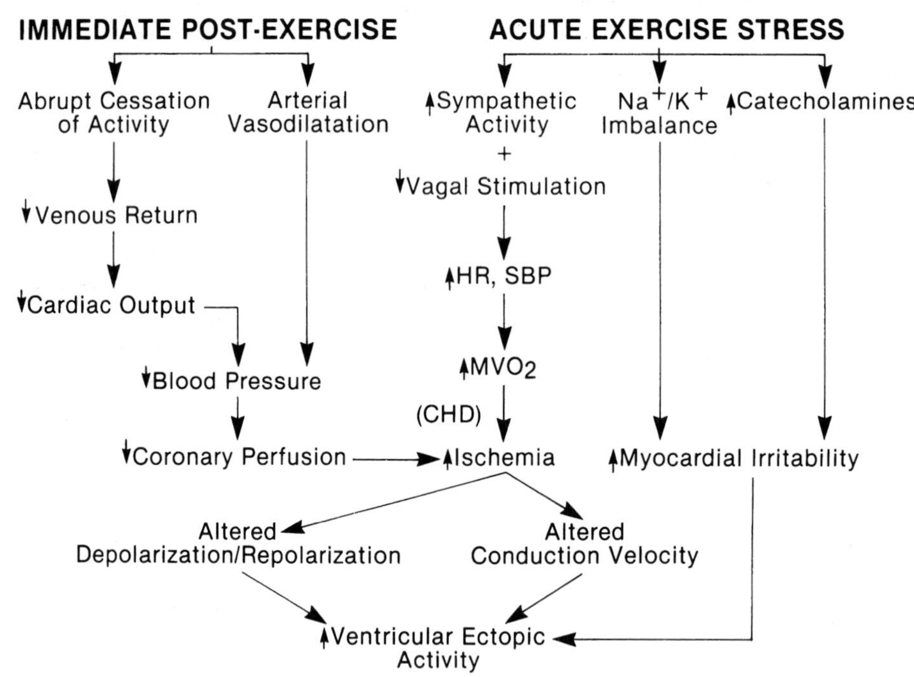

Figure 16.5. Physiologic alterations accompanying acute exercise and recovery, and their possible sequelae. CHD = coronary heart disease; HR = heart rate; MVO_2 = myocardial oxygen uptake; Na^+/K^+ = sodium/potassium ion; SBP = systolic blood pressure.

Pulmonary Disease

Patients with a ventilatory limitation to exercise become fatigued when limits of "breathing reserve" are reached, yet the cardiovascular system may remain largely unchallenged (1). Two reasons have been suggested for the premature exhaustion of breathing reserve (12, 14, 15). First, maximum ventilatory volume (MVV) is reduced by obstruction of air flow, restriction of lung volumes, or both. Second, ventilation-perfusion abnormalities increase physiological dead space, so that a higher minute ventilation ($\dot{V}_E$) at peak exercise is required to maintain gas exchange. In addition, arterial oxygen desaturation is often observed at peak exercise in patients with pulmonary disease, but not in healthy subjects or patients with CAD.

Hypertension

Preliminary exercise testing is strongly recommended prior to vigorous exercise training in persons with a history of hypertension (above 140/90 mm Hg). It should be emphasized, however, that hypertensive patients frequently take diuretics which, by virtue of the potential association with hypokalemia, may cause spurious ST-segment depression (39). Hypertensive patients may also demonstrate ECG evidence of left ventricular hypertrophy, with or without "strain," which confounds the interpretation of the exercise ECG with respect to myocardial ischemia (40). Thus, exercise induced ST-segment depression should be interpreted with caution and additional studies obtained to differentiate true and false positive responses. Follow-up exercise testing with concomitant rest and post-stress myocardial perfusion imaging may be particularly helpful in this regard.

Although those with hypertension generally exhibit above normal systolic and diastolic blood pressure during exercise, most studies report no difference in the relative blood pressure increase between mildly hypertensive subjects and normotensive controls. In other words, it appears that blood pressure is simply "reset" and maintained at higher levels, regardless of whether the subject is at rest, performing static handgrip, or treadmill exercise at varying percentages of maximum functional capacity (Fig. 16.6) (41). Other patients with mild hypertension may normalize blood pressure during exercise relative to resting values. This phenomenon is presumably attributed to metabolic vasodilation, which transiently lowers an elevated resting peripheral resistance.

Several studies now suggest that an excessive blood pressure response to dynamic exercise in normotensive subjects may be predictive of future hypertension (42, 43). This applies to both an exaggerated systolic blood pressure rise (> 220 mm Hg) and/or abnormal diastolic pressure (increase of more than 10 mm Hg or > 90 mm Hg).

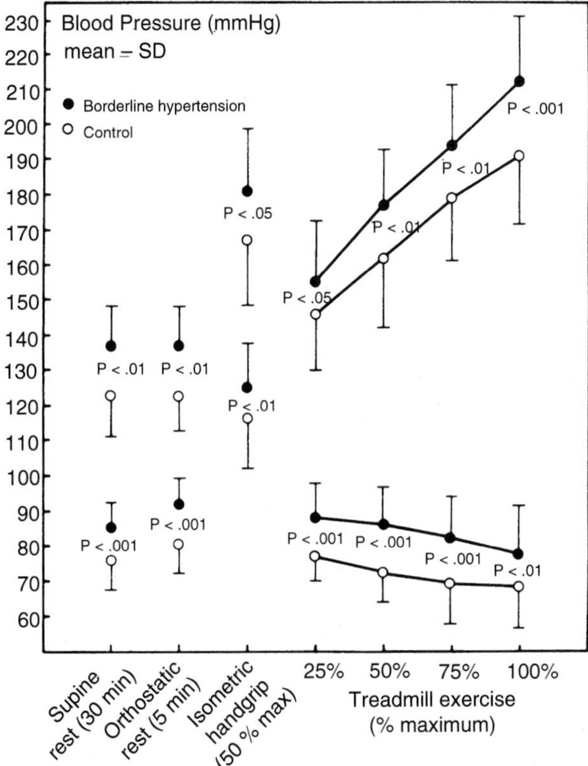

Figure 16.6. Systolic and diastolic blood pressure responses in normal and borderline hypertensive young men during supine rest, orthostatic stress, isometric exertion, and increasing percentages of maximum treadmill exercise capacity. (With permission from Hanson P, Ward A, Painter P. Exercise training for special patient populations. *J Cardiopulm Rehab* 6:104–112, 1986.)

Diabetes

Before providing physical conditioning guidelines to diabetic patients, appropriate baseline studies should be performed to evaluate blood glucose and the potential for underlying CAD. Although treadmill or cycle ergometer testing may be used to assess the exercise ECG and acute cardiorespiratory response to progressive physical exertion, arm ergometry may be preferred in patients with peripheral neuropathy and/or peripheral vascular disease impairment of the lower extremities (44). The presence of autonomic neuropathy may result in chronotropic insufficiency, which may reduce functional capacity, as well as sensitivity of the exercise test.

Obesity

During treadmill testing, obese subjects often demonstrate a higher cardiac output, absolute oxygen consumption (L/min) and minute ventilation at any given work rate (45). Systemic and pulmonary blood pressures and heart rate are also frequently higher in obese than in lean subjects during submaximal exercise (46). Because there is little or no difference in maximal heart rate between overweight and lean subjects, the obese tend to perform a given work task at a higher percentage of maximal heart rate. Although obese persons may have a large, absolute $\dot{V}O_2max$ by virtue of a large muscle mass, aerobic capacity is reduced when expressed relative to body weight (47). Other conditions that may limit exercise performance of obese patients may include heat intolerance, hyperpnea/dyspnea, movement restriction, orthopedic pain, local muscular weakness, balance problems and anxiety (45).

Peripheral Vascular Disease

Patients with peripheral vascular disease (PVD) experience discomfort, ischemic pain (claudication), or fatigue in the legs with walking. Like angina, claudication pain is attributed to a discrepancy between oxygen supply and demand in working muscle. This pain typically occurs in the calf, can be graded in severity from I-IV ("established, but minimal" to "excruciating and unbearable"), and disappears quickly with the cessation of walking. Accordingly, it is generally the "limiting factor" to performance in this patient population, since both circulatory and ventilatory systems may remain relatively unstressed at peak exercise or volitional fatigue.

Treadmill testing is the exercise modality of choice when patients with suspected PVD are being evaluated for diagnostic purposes (i.e., with Doppler studies) (48). On the other hand, when the assessment of CAD is the primary focus, arm ergometry may be preferred because many of these patients achieve suboptimal levels of cardiac stress during conventional treadmill or cycle ergometer testing (44).

▶ SUMMARY

Abnormal responses to exercise can be used to diagnose and classify persons undergoing exercise evaluation. Physiological changes that deviate from normal or that contrast markedly with normal response can be diagnostic of disease states leading to exercise intolerance. Categorizing functional status, the reason for the abnormal response and the response itself may explain the intolerance and lead to identification of those disease states.

References

1. Neuberg GW, Friedman SH, Weiss MB, et al. Cardiopulmonary exercise testing: The clinical value of gas exchange data. *Arch Intern Med* 148:2221–2226, 1988.
2. Franklin BA. Diagnostic and functional exercise testing: Test selection and interpretation. *J Cardiovasc Nurs* 10:8–29, 1995.
3. Barthélémy JC, Roche F, Gaspoz JM, et al. Maximal blood lactate level acts as a major discriminant variable in exercise testing for coronary artery disease detection in men. *Circulation* 93:246–252, 1996.
4. Cannon RO III, Lesch M. The search for a better exercise test: A self-fulfilling prophecy? *Circulation* 93:205–207, 1996.
5. Laslett LJ, Amsterdam EA. Management of the asymptomatic patient with an abnormal ECG. *JAMA* 252:1744–1746, 1984.
6. Diamond GA, Forrester JS. Analysis of probability as an aid in the clinical diagnosis of coronary artery disease. *N Engl J Med* 300:1350–1358, 1979.
7. Froelicher VF, Quaglietti S. *Handbook of Exercise Testing.* Boston: Little, Brown and Co, 1996:127–128.
8. Epstein SE. Implications of probability analysis on the strategy used for non-invasive detection of coronary artery disease. *Am J Cardiol* 46:491–499, 1980.
9. Buskirk E, Taylor HL. Maximal oxygen intake and its relation to body composition, with special reference to chronic physical activity and obesity. *J Appl Physiol* 2:72–78, 1957.
10. Mitchell JH, Blomqvist G. Maximal oxygen uptake. *N Engl J Med* 284:1018–1022, 1971.
11. Jones NL, Campbell EJM. *Clinical Exercise Testing.* Philadelphia: WB Saunders, 1981:2.
12. Weber KT, Janicki JS. Cardiopulmonary exercise testing for evaluation of chronic cardiac failure. *Am J Cardiol* 55(Suppl A):22A–31A, 1985.
13. Bruce RA, Kusumi F, Hosmer D. Maximal oxygen intake and nomographic assessment of functional aerobic impairment in cardiovascular disease. *Am Heart J* 85:546–562, 1973.
14. Wasserman K, Hansen JE, Sue DY, et al. *Principles of Exercise Testing and Interpretation.* Philadelphia: Lea & Febiger, 1987.
15. Zavala DC. *Manual on Exercise Testing: A Training Handbook.* Iowa City: University of Iowa Press, 1985.
16. McHenry PL, Phillips JF, Knoebel SB. Correlation of computer-quantitated treadmill exercise electrocardiogram with arteriographic location of coronary artery disease. *Am J Cardiol* 30:747–752, 1972.
17. Michaelides A, Ryan JM, VanFossen D, et al. Exercise-induced QRS prolongation in patients with coronary artery disease: a marker of myocardial ischemia. *Am Heart J* 126: 1320–1325, 1993.
18. Chaitman BR, Waters DD, Théroux P, et al. ST-segment elevation and coronary spasm in response to exercise. *Am J Cardiol* 47:1350–1358, 1981.
19. Bruce RA, Fisher LD, Pettinger M, et al. ST segment elevation with exercise: a marker for poor ventricular function and poor prognosis. *Circulation* 77:897–905, 1988.
20. Chahine RA, Lowery MH, Bauerlein EJ. Interpretation of the exercise-induced ST-segment elevation. *Am J Cardiol* 72: 100–101, 1993.
21. Yasue H, Omote S, Takizawa A, et al. Comparison of coronary arteriographic findings during angina pectoris associated with S-T elevation or depression. *Am J Cardiol* 47: 539–546, 1981.
22. Califf RM, McKinnis RA, McNeer JF, et al. Prognostic value of ventricular arrhythmias associated with treadmill exercise testing in patients studied with cardiac catheterization for suspected ischemic heart disease. *J Am Coll Cardiol* 2: 1060–1067, 1983.
23. Fuller T, Movahed A. Current review of exercise testing: application and interpretation. *Clin Cardiol* 10:189–200, 1987.
24. Ellestad MH, Wan MK. Predictive implications of stress testing: follow-up of 2700 subjects after maximum treadmill stress testing. *Circulation* 51:363–369, 1975.
25. Brener SJ, Pashkow FJ, Harvey SA, et al. Chronotropic response to exercise predicts angiographic severity in patients with suspected or stable coronary artery disease. *Am J Cardiol* 76:1228–1232, 1995.
26. Lauer MS, Okin PM, Larson MG, et al. Impaired heart rate response to graded exercise: prognostic implications of chronotropic incompetence in the Framingham Heart Study. *Circulation* 93:1520–1526, 1996.
27. Ellestad MH. Chronotropic incompetence: The implications of heart rate response to exercise (compensatory parasympathetic hyperactivity?). *Circulation* 93:1485–1487, 1996.
28. Comess KA, Fenster PE. Clinical implications of the blood pressure response to exercise. *Cardiology* 68:233–244, 1981.
29. Irving JB, Bruce RA, De Rouen TA. Variations in and significance of systolic pressure during maximal exercise (treadmill) testing: relation to severity of coronary artery disease and cardiac mortality. *Am J Cardiol* 39:841–848, 1977.
30. Sheps DS, Ernst JC, Briese FW, et al. Exercise-induced increase in diastolic pressure: indicator of severe coronary artery disease. *Am J Cardiol* 43:708–712, 1979.
31. Cole JP, Ellestad MH. Significance of chest pain during treadmill exercise: correlation with coronary events. *Am J Cardiol* 41:227–232, 1978.

32. Lind AR, McNichol GW. Muscular factors which determine the cardiovascular responses to sustained and rhythmic exercise. *Can Med Assoc J* 96:706–715, 1967.
33. Mitchell JH, Payne FC, Saltin B, et al. The role of muscle mass in the cardiovascular response to static contractions. *J Physiol* 309:45–54, 1980.
34. Fardy PS. Isometric exercise and the cardiovascular system. *Physician Sportsmed* 9:43–56, 1981.
35. DeBusk RF, Valdez R, Houston N, et al. Cardiovascular responses to dynamic and static effort soon after myocardial infarction: Application to occupational work assessment. *Circulation* 58:368–375, 1978.
36. DeBusk RF, Pitts W, Haskell W, et al. Comparison of cardiovascular responses to static-dynamic and dynamic effort alone in patients with ischemic heart disease. *Circulation* 59:977–984, 1979.
37. Ferguson RJ, Cote P, Bourassa MG, et al. Coronary blood flow during isometric and dynamic exercise in angina pectoris patients. *J Cardiac Rehab* 1:21–27, 1981.
38. Bertagnoli K, Hanson P, Ward A. Attenuation of exercise-induced ST depression during combined isometric and dynamic exercise in coronary artery disease. *Am J Cardiol* 65: 314–317, 1990.
39. Georgopoulos AJ, Proudfit WL, Page IH. Effect of exercise on electrocardiogram of patients with low serum potassium. *Circulation* 23:567–572, 1961.
40. Schlant RC, Blomqvist CG, Brandenburg RO, et al. Guidelines for exercise testing. *Circulation* 74:653A–667A, 1986.
41. Hanson P, Ward A, Painter P. Exercise training for special patient populations. *J Cardiopulm Rehab* 6:104–112, 1986.
42. Wilson N, Meyer E. Early prediction of hypertension using exercise blood pressure. *Prev Med* 10:62–68, 1981.
43. Dlin R, Hanne N, Silverberg DS, et al. Follow-up of normotensive men with exaggerated blood pressure response to exercise. *Am Heart J* 106:316–320, 1983.
44. Franklin BA. Exercise testing, training and arm ergometry. *Sports Med* 2:100–119, 1985.
45. Foss ML, Lampman RM, Watt E, et al. Initial work tolerance of extremely obese patients. *Arch Phys Med Rehab* 56: 63–67, 1975.
46. Alexander JK. Obesity and cardiac performance. *Am J Cardiol* 14:860–865, 1964.
47. Goodman C, Kenrick M. Physical fitness in relation to obesity. *Obesity/Bariatric Med* 4:12–15, 1975.
48. Berglund B, Eklund B. Reproducibility of treadmill exercise in patients with intermittent claudication. *Clin Physiol* 1: 253–256, 1981.

22, 24, 25 39, 52, 53 57, 58 301 312 313

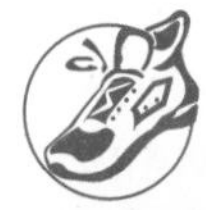

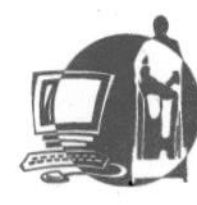
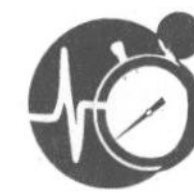

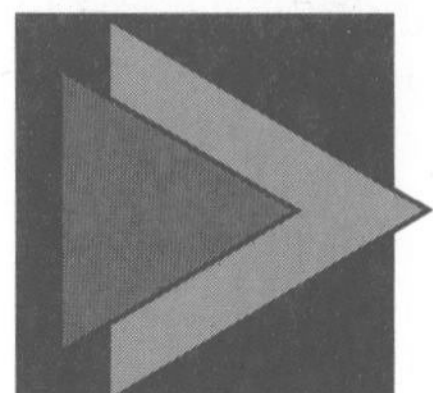

CHAPTER 17
CARDIORESPIRATORY ADAPTATIONS TO EXERCISE

Barry A. Franklin and Jeffrey L. Roitman

Physical inactivity is now classified as a major contributing risk factor for heart disease, with an overall weight for preventive value similar to elevated blood cholesterol, cigarette smoking, and hypertension (1). Moreover, longitudinal studies have shown that higher levels of aerobic fitness are associated with a lower mortality from heart disease even after statistical adjustments for age, coronary risk factors, and family history of heart disease (Fig. 17.1) (2). These findings, and other recent reports in persons with and without heart disease, have confirmed an inverse association between aerobic capacity and cardiovascular mortality (3–8).

Endurance exercise training increases functional capacity and provides relief of symptoms in a majority of patients with coronary artery disease (CAD). This is particularly important since most patients with clinically manifest CAD have a subnormal functional capacity (50% to 70% age, gender-predicted) and some may be limited by symptoms at relatively low levels of exertion. Improvement in function appears to be mediated by increased central and/or peripheral oxygen transport and supply, while relief of angina pectoris may result from increased myocardial oxygen supply, decreased oxygen demand, or both.

This chapter reviews the cardiorespiratory adaptations to regular aerobic exercise in health and disease, with specific reference to alterations at submaximal and maximal exercise, gender differences (and similarities), variables influencing exercise trainability, the role of training specificity, and responses in conditioned and unconditioned subjects.

SUBMAXIMAL AND MAXIMAL EXERCISE

Cardiovascular Changes

Cardiovascular changes induced by physical training during submaximal and maximal exercise are summarized in Table 17.1. Most exercise studies on healthy subjects demonstrate 20% ± 10% increases in aerobic capacity ($\dot{V}O_2max$), with the greatest relative improvements among the most unfit (9). Because a fixed submaximal workrate has a relatively constant aerobic requirement, the physically trained individual works at a lower percentage of $\dot{V}O_2max$, with greater reserve after exercise training. Enhanced oxygen transport, particularly increased maximal stroke volume and cardiac output, has traditionally been regarded as the primary mechanism underlying the increase in $\dot{V}O_2max$ with training.

The effects of chronic exercise training on the autonomic nervous system act to reduce myocardial demands at rest and during exercise. Exercise bradycardia may be attributed to an intracardiac mechanism (an effect directly on the myocardium, e.g., increased stroke volume during submaximal work) or an extracardiac mechanism (e.g., alterations in trained skeletal muscle) or both. The result is reduced heart rate and systolic blood pressure at rest and at any fixed oxygen uptake or submaximal workrate.

The increased oxidative capacity of trained skeletal muscle appears to offer a distinct hemodynamic advantage. Lactic acid production and muscle blood flow are decreased at a fixed external work load, whereas submaximal cardiac output and oxygen uptake are unchanged or slightly reduced. As a result, there are compensatory increases in arteriovenous oxygen difference ($a\text{–}vDO_2$) at submaximal and maximal exercise (Table 17.1).

Respiratory Changes

Several respiratory adaptations result from physical conditioning regimens. Although ventilation generally does not limit exercise in apparently healthy individuals, in elite athletes the limits of ventilation may be reached at $\dot{V}O_2max$ (10). Maximal minute ventilation is augmented by increased tidal volume and breathing frequency and is controlled by neural and chemical factors and by sensory mechanisms within the lungs and breathing muscles. There is also increased ventilatory ef-

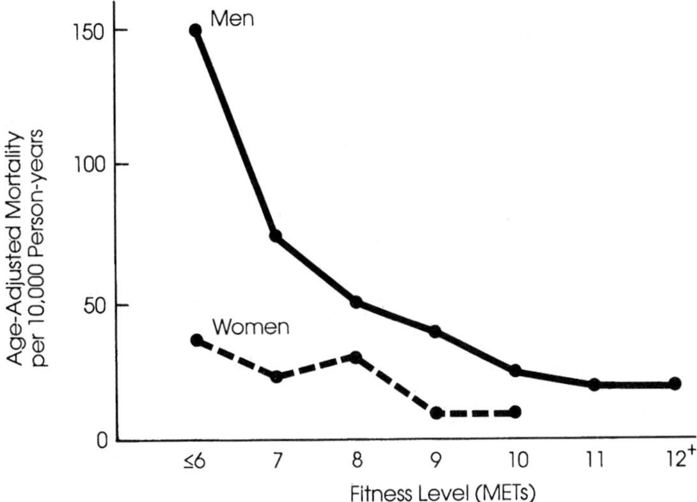

Figure 17.1. Age-adjusted, all-cause mortality rates per 10,000 person-years of follow-up by physical fitness (METs) achieved during maximal treadmill exercise testing. (Adapted from Blair SN, Kohl HW III, Paffenbarger RS, et al. Physical fitness and all-cause mortality: a prospective study of healthy men and women. *JAMA* 262:2395–2401, 1989.)

Table 17.1. Physiological Responses to Aerobic Conditioning in Untrained Individuals

VARIABLE[1]	UNIT OF MEASURE	RESPONSE
$\dot{V}O_2max$	ml/kg/min	↑
Resting Heart Rate	beats/min	↓
Exercise Heart Rate (submax)	beats/minute	↓
Maximum Heart Rate	beats/min	↔ (or slight ↓)
$A\text{-}V_{O_2diff}$	ml O_2/100 ml blood	↑
Maximum Minute Ventilation	liters/minute	↑
Stroke Volume	ml/beat	↑
Cardiac Output	liters/min	↑
Blood Volume (resting)	liters	↑
Systolic Blood Pressure	mm Hg	↔ (or slight ↑)
Blood Lactate	ml/100 ml blood	↑
Oxidative Capacity Skeletal Muscle	multiple variables[2]	↑

[1] at maximum exercise unless otherwise specified.
[2] represents increases in skeletal muscle mitochondrial number and size, capillary density, and/or oxidative enzymes.
↑ = increase
↓ = decrease
↔ = no change

ficiency as substantiated by a reduced ventilatory equivalent for oxygen ($\dot{V}_E/\dot{V}O_2$) in trained as compared with untrained individuals. Ventilation increases linearly with $\dot{V}O_2$ up to about 50% $\dot{V}O_2max$, after which the increase is proportionately greater than the increase in work rate or $\dot{V}O_2$ (10, 11). Physically trained persons demonstrate larger lung volumes and diffusion capacity at rest and during exercise than their sedentary counterparts.

Ventilation is either unaffected or only modestly affected by cardiorespiratory training. Maximal ventilatory capacity may be increased by exercise training, but it is unclear that this provides any advantage other than increased buffering capacity for lactate. Submaximal ventilation is probably not affected, but may be decreased in some circumstances due to decreased production of lactate coinciding with decreased need to buffer lactate and, therefore, decreased ventilation (11). Moreover, studies in subjects with and without heart disease have demonstrated increases in the ventilatory threshold after an exercise intervention with associated decreases in blood lactate during submaximal work loads (12, 13).

GENDER-SPECIFIC IMPROVEMENT AND TRAINABILITY

The salutary effects of chronic endurance training in men are well documented. However, numerous studies now provide ample data on $\dot{V}O_2max$, cardiovascular hemodynamics, body composition, and serum lipids of middle-aged and older women, as well as changes with physical conditioning. The results demonstrate that women with and without CAD respond to aerobic training in much the same way as men when subjected to comparable programs in terms of frequency, intensity, and duration of exercise (Fig. 17.2) (14, 15). Improvement is negatively correlated with age, habitual physical activity, and initial $\dot{V}O_2max$ (which is generally lower in women than men) and positively correlated with conditioning frequency, intensity, and duration (16).

There are, however, large inter-individual differences in the effects of physical conditioning independent of age, initial capacity, or conditioning program. These individual variations in response to aerobic exercise training may be due to childhood patterns of activity, state of conditioning at the initiation of the program, or degree of physiological aging. Body compositional differences in trainability may also play an important role with respect to the results of physical conditioning.

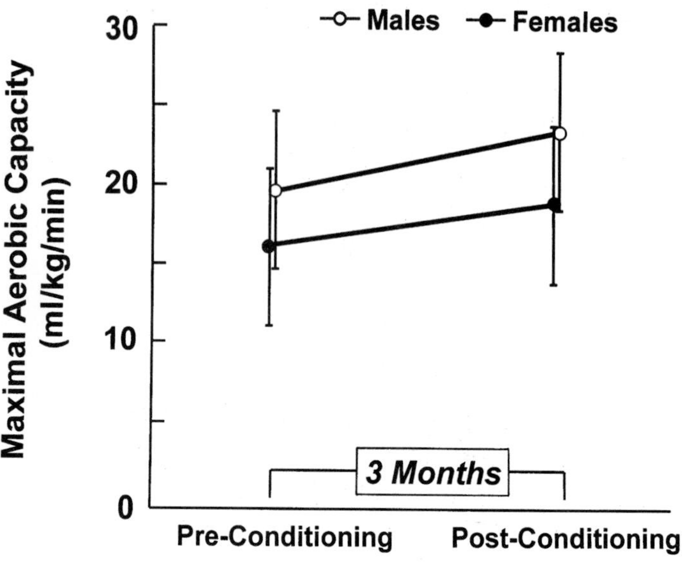

Figure 17.2. Aerobic capacity before and after physical conditioning in older (≥ 62 years) men and women with coronary heart disease. Maximal oxygen consumption (ml/kg/min) increased by 19% and 17% in the men and women, respectively (both $p < 0.001$). (Adapted from Ades PA, Waldmann ML, Polk DM, et al. Referral patterns and exercise response in the rehabilitation of female coronary patients aged ≥62 years. *Am J Cardiol* 69:1422–1425, 1992.)

Obese women demonstrate lower aerobic capacity (per-kilogram body weight), altered cardiovascular hemodynamics, and elevated serum lipids compared to leaner women (17). This initial varied profile may serve to modify the outcome of an aerobic conditioning program with respect to the magnitude of quantitative change.

SPECIFICITY OF TRAINING

Decreased heart rate at rest and during fixed submaximal work rates, with an inherent reduction in myocardial aerobic requirements, is a well-documented adaptation to endurance exercise training. This response is believed to reflect intracardiac and/or extracardiac mechanisms. The former is attributed to enhanced stroke volume with a compensatory decrease in sympathetic stimulation and heart rate, the latter to alterations in the central nervous system, adaptations in trained muscles, or both (18, 19). Evidence supporting an extracardiac or peripheral mechanism includes an unchanged heart rate response or a considerably less marked bradycardia during exercise involving non-trained muscles.

Numerous studies of normal subjects and cardiac patients have investigated the cardiorespiratory and metabolic adaptations of trained versus untrained muscle to physical conditioning. Results generally demonstrate little or no crossover of arm and leg training. After endurance training of one limb or set of limbs, several investigators report increased $\dot{V}O_2max$ and anaerobic (ventilatory) threshold or decreased heart rate (Fig. 17.3), blood lactate, pulmonary ventilation, ventilatory equivalent, blood pressure, and perceived exertion during submaximal exercise in trained, but not untrained limbs (19, 20). These "limb-specific" training effects imply that a substantial portion of the conditioning response is attributed to extracardiac or peripheral factors such as alterations in blood flow and cellular and enzymatic adaptations in the trained limbs alone (21–23).

On the other hand, studies in both normal subjects and cardiac patients indicate some "transfer effects" (i.e., increased $\dot{V}O_2max$ or reduced submaximal exercise heart rate in untrained limbs), providing evidence for central circulatory adaptations to endurance training (24, 25). Although the conditions under which the crossover of arm and leg training may vary, there is evidence suggesting that the initial fitness, as well as the intensity, frequency, and duration of training may be important variables in determining the extent of cross-training benefits from arms to legs and vice versa (26).

The limited degree of cardiovascular and metabolic crossover from one set of limbs to another appears to discount the general practice of restricting aerobic conditioning to the lower extremities alone. Many recreational and occupational activities require sustained arm work to a greater extent than leg work. Consequently, individuals who rely on upper extremities for vocational or leisure-time pursuits should train arms as well as legs, with the expectation of improved cardiorespiratory, hemodynamic, and perceived exertion responses to both forms of effort. Specially designed arm ergometers or combined arm-leg ergometers are particularly beneficial for upper extremity training. Other equipment suitable for upper body training includes rowing machines, wall pulleys, vertical climbing devices, and cross-country skiing simulators.

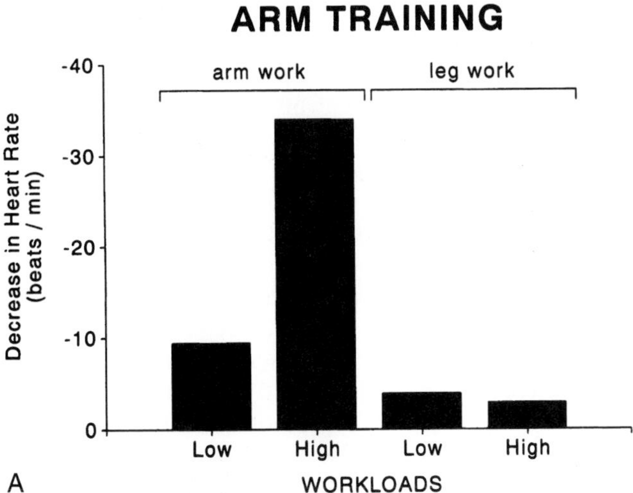

Figure 17.3. A, Arm training using a cycle ergometer markedly decreased the heart rate response during arm exercise at low and high work loads, whereas the heart rate reduction during leg work was small. B, Similarly, leg training markedly decreased the heart rate during leg work, whereas the heart rate reduction during arm work was minimal. (Adapted from Clausen JP, Trap-Jensen J, Lassen NA. The effects of training on the heart rate during arm and leg exercise. *Scand J Clin Lab Invest* 26:295–301, 1970.)

Trainability of Arms Versus Legs

Arm training for persons with and without heart disease is now widely accepted as an integral component of a comprehensive physical conditioning program. Until recently, however, few data were available regarding the relative trainability of the upper extremities. Franklin et al. reported the effects of a 6-week aerobic circuit training program on 13 post-myocardial infarction patients that involved alternating upper and lower extremity exercise devices for 15 minutes each at an intensity of 70% to 85% of peak heart rate (27). Post-conditioning rate-pressure products during submaximal arm and leg ergometry were similarly decreased, while arm and leg $\dot{V}O_2max$ increased 13% and 11%, respectively (Fig. 17.4). These findings suggest that the upper extremities respond to aerobic exercise conditioning in the same qualitative and quantitative manner as the lower extremities.

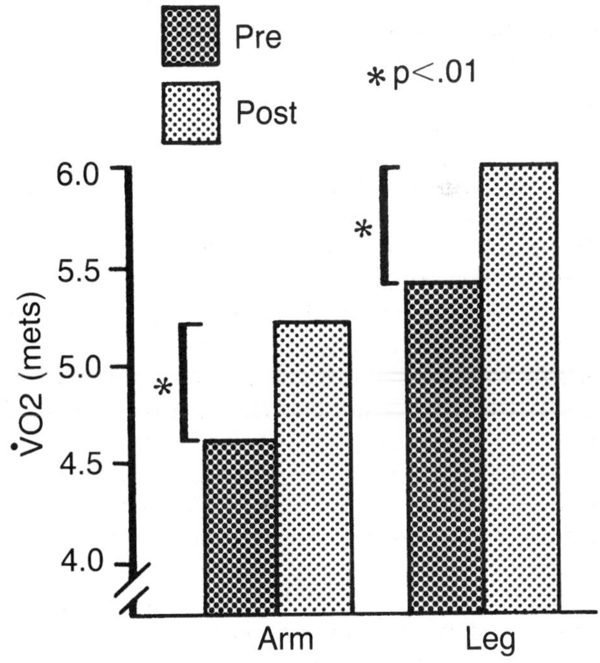

Figure 17.4. Mean $\dot{V}O_2max$ values, expressed as metabolic equivalents (METs; 1 MET = 3.5 ml/kg/min), during arm and leg exercise testing before and after training in men with previous myocardial infarction. (Adapted from Franklin BA, Vander L, Wrisley D, et al. Trainability of arms versus legs in men with previous myocardial infarction. *Chest* 105:262–264, 1994.)

CONDITIONED AND UNCONDITIONED RESPONSE

Adaptation to cardiorespiratory endurance exercise may be shown by contrasting responses to exercise in conditioned and unconditioned persons. The central effects (cardiorespiratory) of regular exercise (training) are manifested in several ways. The net outcome of increased ability to deliver oxygen to working muscle and to use nutrients at the cellular level is to increase $\dot{V}O_2max$. Changes in heart rate, stroke volume, CaO_2-$C\bar{v}O_2$, cardiac output, blood lactate and ventilation each contribute to increased $\dot{V}O_2max$ and to increased metabolic efficiency of the trained person. Table 17.1 summarize the cardiorespiratory adaptations to exercise in conditioned and unconditioned persons.

Heart Rate

The heart rate response plays a critical role in the delivery of oxygen to working skeletal muscle. Heart rate increases during exercise to assist in augmenting cardiac output. The increase is initially caused primarily by neural influences, but as maximum exercise is approached, the increase is also influenced by neurohormonal and chemical factors. Resting heart rate is restrained by the vagus nerve ("vagal tone") and vagal tone appears to be increased at rest, decreasing resting heart rate by approximately 10 to 15 beats/minute, whereas sympathoadrenergic drive (circulating catecholamines, particularly norepinephrine) is attenuated during exercise (18). Increased heart rate during exercise is influenced by mechanical receptors, sympathetic stimulation and the release of vagal tone (11, 28, 29). Exercise in unconditioned persons causes a proportionately greater increase in heart rate at any fixed submaximal work rate than in conditioned persons.

Heart rate and stroke volume both contribute to cardiac output. In untrained persons, heart rate plays a more significant role because of the ability to induce relatively large changes in rate, as opposed to limited changes in stroke volume, which may be restricted by deconditioning. Heart rate, therefore, increases proportionately more during graded exercise and is higher at any given level of submaximal exercise in unconditioned persons (11, 30). Maximal heart rate is unchanged or slightly decreased (3 to 10 beats/min) after aerobic conditioning (31). The latter is probably attributed to two training adaptations: cardiac hypertrophy via an increase in the size of the ventricular cavity and decreased sympathetic drive.

Stroke Volume

Stroke volume, the second factor used in determining cardiac output, increases during exercise secondary to increased venous return (Frank-Starling mechanism) and to increased contractile state (perhaps by neurohormonal influences) (11, 28, 32–35). The left ventricle is able to contract with greater force during exercise, in part due to increased end-diastolic volume and enhanced mechanical ability of myocardial fibers to produce force (36, 37). It is also likely that chronic cardiovascular exercise training strengthens myocardial tissue and enables more forceful contraction (11, 28, 38, 39). The result is augmented ejection of end diastolic volume or increased ejection fraction.

Comparatively, cardiorespiratory training allows conditioned individuals to increase ejection fraction to a greater degree than their sedentary counterparts, hence stroke volume is higher in conditioned individuals at any fixed or relative, submaximal work load (39). The increased stroke volume from training allows conditioned individuals to exercise at similar absolute and relative work loads at a lower heart rate, thus decreasing the myocardial oxygen demand of submaximal exercise (33, 35). The increase in ejection fraction is approximately 5% to 10% during maximal exercise.

Normal ventricular wall thickness and enlarged end-diastolic volume are consistently reported after endurance exercise training, with attendant increases in rest and exercise stroke volume (40). Cardiovascular morphologic characteristics, including central blood volume and total hemoglobin, also increase with physical conditioning (41). Both of these variables are closely correlated with the $\dot{V}O_2max$.

Cardiac Output

Maximum cardiac output is significantly higher in trained than in untrained individuals, primarily because of the ability to increase stroke volume (28, 38, 39). Increased cardiac output during exercise is initially influenced by both heart rate and stroke volume, but stroke volume plateaus at approximately 40% to 60% $\dot{V}O_2max$ and increased heart rate is the sole contributor to increasing cardiac output thereafter. This is particularly evident in trained individuals with the ability to increase stroke volume significantly (39). It is generally accepted that cardiac output is essentially unchanged at any fixed submaximal workload before and after training and between conditioned and unconditioned individuals (38).

Arteriovenous Oxygen Difference

The final contributor to increased oxygen consumption during exercise is $a\text{–}vDO_2$. The difference between arterial and venous content of oxygen in blood reflects the ability of skeletal muscle tissue to extract oxygen (38, 42). Chronic training enhances the metabolic machinery within muscle, thereby enhancing the ability to use (i.e., extract) oxygen that is transported in circulating blood. Increased ability to deliver oxygen to working skeletal muscle and to remove and use it for generating energy is a hallmark of aerobic training.

Conditioned individuals have greater ability to use oxygen at the cellular level than unconditioned persons, but $a\text{–}vDO_2$ is similar in trained and untrained persons at submaximal levels of exercise until near $\dot{V}O_2max$ is reached. $a\text{–}vDO_2$ is greater at maximum exercise in trained than untrained persons.

Systolic Blood Pressure

Resting blood pressure is modulated by a number of factors including cardiac output, general vasomotor tone (peripheral resistance) and arterial elasticity (28). Systolic blood pressure increases in a relatively linear fashion with cardiac output (and $\dot{V}O_2$) during exercise Blood pressure can be expressed as follows:

$$BP \sim CO \times TPR$$

where: BP = blood pressure
CO = cardiac output
TPR = total peripheral resistance

Primary control of blood pressure is exerted centrally by neural mechanisms affecting peripheral arterioles, which control peripheral resistance, and the arteriolar bed metabolites produced during exercise (38, 43). There is vasoconstriction in some areas during exercise (sphlancnic areas, for example) and vasodilatation in others (skeletal muscle and myocardium); the net effect is decreased vasomotor tone and peripheral resistance (28, 36). Systolic blood pressure increases during progressive exercise in healthy individuals due to increased cardiac output. Increased cardiac output maintains systolic blood pressure despite decreased peripheral resistance from arterial dilatation (11). Diastolic blood pressure remains constant or may decrease slightly in both conditioned and unconditioned individuals.

At any fixed submaximal workload, conditioned individuals demonstrate comparable or lower systolic blood pressure than untrained individuals. Relative to $\dot{V}O_2$max, systolic blood pressure is lower in trained than untrained people.

Blood Lactate

Lactic acid (lactate) is a by-product of anaerobic glycolysis. Though "anaerobic threshold" can be defined by many different criteria, lactate threshold is commonly associated with the onset of significant anaerobic contribution to exercise metabolism. Blood lactate is buffered during exercise to maintain a tolerable acid-base balance. However, it begins to increase significantly when production exceeds buffering capacity of the blood. It is at this point that ventilation increases disproportionately and exercise begins to be perceived as more uncomfortable (10, 38).

Endurance exercise training improves oxidative capacity of skeletal muscle by stimulating increases in the size and number of skeletal muscle mitochondria, as well as increases in muscle myoglobin content, oxidative enzymes, and capillary density (44). Conditioned individuals have lower lactate at any fixed submaximal workrate since they produce less and buffer more of the lactic acid produced (11, 38). However, at $\dot{V}O_2$max, lactic acid levels are significantly higher in conditioned individuals after training since there is increased capacity to buffer and to tolerate lactate. At fixed submaximal work rate, lactic acid is lower after training in trained than untrained individuals, thus training increases lactate threshold (Fig.

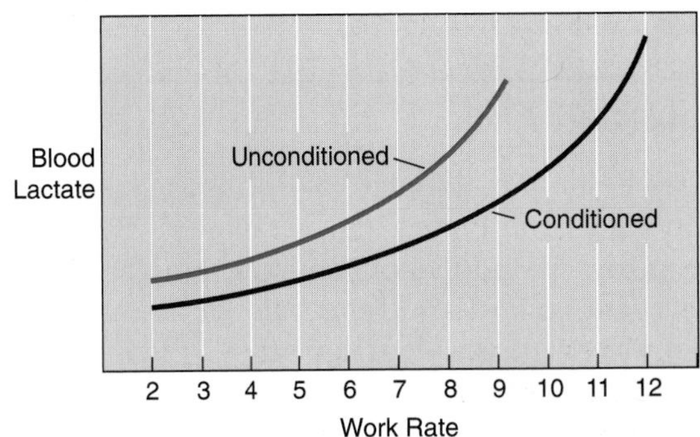

Figure 17.5. Blood lactate concentration during progressive exercise in conditioned vs. unconditioned persons. Note that the conditioned response typically exhibits lower lactate concentrations at any given work rate than unconditioned, but has higher maximum lactate at $\dot{V}O_2$max.

Table 17.2. Factors Influencing the Training Response

VARIABLE(S)	COMMENT
Prolonged bed rest	Results in physiological deconditioning, including a significant reduction in $\dot{V}O_2$max
Intensity, frequency, and duration of training	Improvement in aerobic capacity generally demonstrates a positive correlation to these variables
Age, habitual physical activity, and initial $\dot{V}O_2$max	Improvement generally demonstrates an inverse relationship with these variables; however, recent studies suggest that older and younger adults demonstrate comparable exercise trainability
Adherence to the exercise prescription	Parallels the magnitude of improvement in cardiorespiratory function
Detraining	When physical conditioning is stopped or reduced, training-induced cardiorespiratory and metabolic adaptations are reversed to varying degrees over time
Coronary artery disease	Severity or progression of disease may present an obstacle to improvement
Left ventricular dysfunction[a]	Exercise training appears to be generally safe and effective in this patient population
Beta-blockade	Patients may derive considerable physiological benefit from exercise training in the presence of both cardioselective and nonselective beta blockers, despite a reduced training heart rate
Calcium antagonists	No adverse effect on exercise trainability

[a] Ejection fraction $\leq$ 35%

17.5). Other variables affecting the training response are summarized in Table 17.2).

▶ SUMMARY

Exercise training induces many physiological changes that make a conditioned individual more efficient, more able to deliver and use oxygen and nutrients and resist fatigue. The conditioning effect also offers some protection against cardiovascular mortality and enhances ability to perform activities of daily living.

References

1. Fletcher GF, Balady G, Blair SN, et al. Statement on exercise: benefits and recommendations for physical activity programs for all Americans. *Circulation* 94:857–862, 1996.
2. Blair SN, Kohl HW III, Paffenbarger RS, et al. Physical fitness and all-cause mortality: a prospective study of healthy men and women. *JAMA* 262:2395–2401, 1989.
3. Vanhees L, Fagard R, Thijs L, et al. Prognostic significance of peak exercise capacity in patients with coronary artery disease. *J Am Coll Cardiol* 23:358–363, 1994.
4. Blair SN, Kohl HW III, Barlow CE, et al. Changes in physical fitness and all-cause mortality: a prospective study of healthy and unhealthy men. *JAMA* 273:1093–1098, 1995.
5. Blair SN, Kampert JB, Kohl HW III, et al. Influences of cardiorespiratory fitness and other precursors on cardiovascular disease and all-cause mortality in men and women. *JAMA* 276:205–210, 1996.
6. Barlow CE, Kohl HW III, Gibbons LW, et al. Physical fitness, mortality and obesity. *Int J Obesity* 19:S41–S44, 1995.
7. Paffenbarger RS, Hyde RT, Wing AL, et al. The association of changes in physical-activity level and other lifestyle characteristics with mortality among men. *N Engl J Med* 328:538–545, 1993.
8. Sandvik L, Erikssen J, Thaulow E, et al. Physical fitness as a predictor of mortality among healthy, middle-aged Norwegian men. *N Engl J Med* 328:533–537, 1993.
9. Pate RR, Pratt M, Blair SN, et al. Physical activity and public health. A recommendation from the Centers for Disease Control and Prevention and the American College of Sports Medicine. *JAMA* 273:402–407, 1995.
10. Beck KC, Johnson BD. Pulmonary adaptations to dynamic exercise. In: Durstine JL, ed. *Resource Manual for Guidelines for Exercise Testing and Prescription.* 2nd ed. Baltimore: Williams & Wilkins, 1993.
11. Durstine JL, Pate RR, Branch JD. Cardiorespiratory responses to acute exercise. In: Durstine JL, ed. *Resource Manual for Guidelines for Exercise Testing and Prescription.* 2nd ed. Baltimore: Williams & Wilkins, 1993.
12. Davis JA. Anaerobic threshold: review of the concept and directions for future research. *Med Sci Sports Exerc* 17:6–21, 1985.
13. Sullivan MJ, Higginbotham MB, Cobb FR. Exercise training in patients with chronic heart failure delays ventilatory anaerobic threshold and improves submaximal exercise performance. *Circulation* 79:324–329, 1989.
14. Ades PA, Waldmann ML, Polk DM, et al. Referral patterns and exercise response in the rehabilitation of female coronary patients aged ≥62 years. *Am J Cardiol* 69:1422–1425, 1992.
15. Getchell LH, Moore JC. Physical training: comparative responses of middle-aged adults. *Arch Phys Med Rehab* 56: 250–254, 1975.
16. Franklin BA, Bonzheim K, Berg T. Gender differences in rehabilitation. In: Julian DG, Wenger NK, eds. *Women and Heart Disease.* London: Martin Dunitz Ltd, 1997:151–171.
17. Franklin B, Buskirk E, Hodgson J, et al. Effects of physical conditioning on cardiorespiratory function, body composition and serum lipids in relatively normal-weight and obese middle-aged women. *Int J Obesity* 3:97–109, 1979.
18. Frick M, Elovainio R, Somer T. The mechanism of bradycardia evoked by physical training. *Cariologia* 51:46–54, 1967.
19. Clausen JP, Trap-Jensen J, Lassen NA. The effects of training on the heart rate during arm and leg exercise. *Scand J Clin Lab Invest* 26:295–301, 1970.
20. Rasmussen B, Klausen K, Clausen JP, et al. Pulmonary ventilation, blood gases, and blood pH after training of the arms or the legs. *J Appl Physiol* 38:250–256, 1975.
21. Davies CTM, Sargeant AJ. Effects of training on the physiological responses to one- and two-leg work. *J Appl Physiol* 38:377–381, 1975.
22. Henriksson J, Roitman JS. Time course of changes in human skeletal muscle succinate dehydrogenase and cytochrome oxidase activities and maximal oxygen uptake with physical activity and inactivity. *Acta Physiol Scand* 99:91–97, 1977.
23. Saltin B, Nazar K, Costill DL, et al. The nature of the training response: Peripheral and central adaptations to one-legged exercise. *Acta Physiol Scand* 96:289–305, 1976.
24. Clausen JP, Klausen K, Rasmussen B, et al. Central and peripheral circulatory changes after training of the arms or legs. *Am J Physiol* 225:675–682, 1973.
25. Thompson PD, Cullinane E, Lazarus B, et al. Effect of exercise training on the untrained limb exercise performance of men with angina pectoris. *Am J Cardiol* 48:844–850, 1981.
26. Lewis S, Thompson P, Areskog NH, et al. Transfer effects of endurance training to exercise with untrained limbs. *Eur J Appl Physiol* 44:25–34, 1980.
27. Franklin BA, Vander L, Wrisley D, et al. Trainability of arms versus legs in men with previous myocardial infarction. *Chest* 105:262–264, 1994.
28. Astrand PO, Rodahl K. *Textbook of Work Physiology: Physiological Bases of Exercise.* 4th ed. New York: McGraw-Hill, 1986.
29. Kenney WL. Parasympathetic control of resting heart rate: relationship to aerobic power. *Med Sci Sports Exerc* 17:451–455, 1985.
30. Rowell LB. Human cardiovascular adjustments to exercise and thermal stress. *Physiol Rev* 54:75–159, 1974.
31. Fox E, Bartels R, Billings C, et al. Intensity and distance of interval training programs and changes in aerobic power. *Med Sci Sports* 5(1):18–22, 1973.
32. Bevegard BS, Shepherd JT. Regulation of the circulation during exercise in man. *Physiol Rev* 47:178–213, 1967.
33. Longhurst JC, Kelly AR, Gonyea WJ, et al. Chronic training with static and dynamic exercise: Cardiovascular adapta-

tion and response to exercise. *Circ Res* 48(6Pt2):I171–I178, 1981.

35. Levine BD, Lane LD, Buckey JC, et al. Left ventricular pressure-volume and Frank-Starling relations in endurance athletes: Implications for orthostatic tolerance and exercise performance. *Circulation* 84:1016, 1991.
36. Blomqvist CG, Saltin B. Cardiovascular adaptations to physical training. *Ann Rev Physiol* 45:169–189, 1983.
37. Perski A, Tzankoff SP, Engel BT. Central control of cardiovascular adjustments to exercise. *J Appl Physiol* 58:431–435, 1985.
38. Rerych, SK, Sholz PM, Sabiston DC, et al. Effects of exercise training on left ventricular function in normal subjects: A longitudinal study by radionuclide angiography. *Am J Cardiol* 45:244–252, 1980.
39. McArdle WD, Katch FI, Katch VL. *Exercise Physiology: Energy, Nutrition and Human Performance.* 3rd ed. Philadelphia: Lea & Febiger, 1991.
40. Smith ML, Mitchell JH. Cardiorespiratory adaptations to exercise training. In: Durstine JL, ed. *Resource Manual for Guidelines for Exercise Testing and Prescription.* 2nd ed. Baltimore: Williams & Wilkins, 1993.
41. Morganroth J, Maron B, Henry W, et al. Comparative left ventricular dimensions in trained athletes. *Ann Intern Med* 82:521–524, 1975.
42. Oscai L, Williams B, Hertig B. Effect of exercise on blood volume. *J Appl Physiol* 24(5):622–624, 1968.
43. Holoszy JO. Adaptations of skeletal muscle to endurance exercise. *Med Sci Sports Exerc* 7:155–164, 1975.
44. Rowell LB. General principles of vascular control. In: *Human Circulation: Regulation During Physical Stress.* New York: Oxford University Press, 1986.
45. Hermansen L, Wachtlova M. Capillary density of skeletal muscle in well-trained and untrained men. *J Appl Physiol* 30(6):860–863, 1971.

22, 26, 32

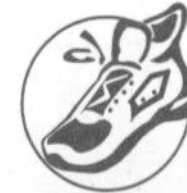

33, 37, 38, 44, 47, 50, 179

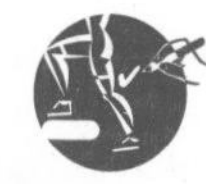

55

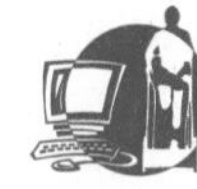

313

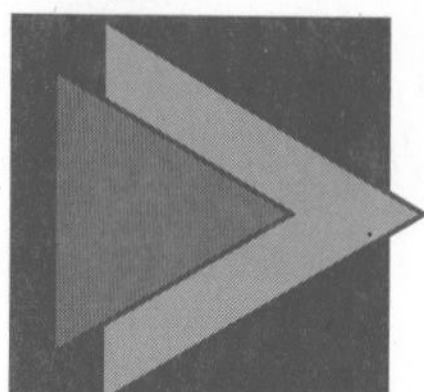

CHAPTER **18**

Factors Affecting the Acute Neuromuscular Responses to Resistance Exercise

William J. Kraemer and Jill A. Bush

Resistance training is repeated exposure to an acute exercise stimulus that is specific and characterized by various factors which define the physiological and biomechanical demands. Understanding the factors that affect acute resistance exercise stimuli is important in gaining insight into different resistance training protocols. Acute physiological changes are directly related to the configuration of external demands of resistance exercise and resistance exercise protocols must be specific to the physiological systems targeted.

PHYSIOLOGY OF RESISTANCE EXERCISE

Neuromuscular Activation

The stimulus for muscle activation comes from a high level, central control command signal originating from the premotor cortex and the motor cortex. The signal is relayed through a lower level controller (brainstem and spinal cord) and transformed into a specific motor unit activation pattern. To perform a specific task, the required motor units meet specific demands for force production by activating associated muscle fibers (1, 2). Various feedback loops exist which modify force production, as well as provide communication to other physiological systems (e.g., the endocrine system). The high and low level commands can be modified by feedback from peripheral sensory or higher central command.

Motor Unit Activation

The functional unit of the neuromuscular system is called the "motor unit" (3). It consists of the motoneurone and the muscle fibers it innervates. Motor units range in size from a few to several hundred muscle fibers. Muscle fibers from different motor units can be anatomically situated adjacent to each other, and therefore a muscle fiber may be actively generating force while the adjacent fiber moves passively with no direct neural stimulation. When maximal force is required, all available motor units are activated. Another adaptive mechanism affected by heavy resistance training is the muscle force affected by different motor unit firing rates and/or frequencies.

Motor unit activation is also influenced by the "size principle." This principle is based on the observed relationship between motor unit twitch force and recruitment threshold. Specifically, motor units are recruited in order, according to recruitment thresholds and firing rates, resulting in a continuum of voluntary force. Thus, most muscles contain a range of motor units (Type I and Type II fibers) and force production can span wide levels. Maximal force production requires not only the recruitment of all motor units including "high threshold" motor units, but also recruitment at sufficiently high firing rate to produce maximal force. It has been theorized that untrained individuals may not be able to voluntarily recruit the highest threshold motor units or maximally activate muscles. Further, electrical stimulation has been shown to be more effective in eliciting gains in untrained or injury rehabilitation scenarios suggesting further inability to activate all available motor units. Thus, training adaptation develops the ability to recruit a greater percentage of motor units when required.

Few exceptions to the size principle have been identified, however, some advanced weight lifters or athletes may not require the order of recruitment stipulated by the size principle. It may be possible to inhibit lower threshold, yet activate higher threshold motor units, to enhance rate of force development and power production. This theory emanates from observations during rapid, stereotyped movements and voluntary eccentric muscle action in humans. The central nervous system can also limit force by engaging inhibitory mechanisms which are protective. Thus, training may result in changes in fiber recruitment order or reduced inhibition which assists in the performance of certain types of muscle actions.

Muscle Fiber Types

Several different nomenclatures have been used to classify skeletal muscle fibers, including color (red or white), contraction speed (fast or slow twitch), oxidative or glycolytic enzyme content (fast glycolytic, fast-oxidative glycolytic, or oxidative), combination schemes (fast glycolytic), and myosin ATPase content (Type I, IIa, IIb).

It is evident that a great deal of plasticity exists with regard to exercise-induced changes in muscle (4–6). This is due in part to a complex yet readily adaptable group of contractile and regulatory proteins. Studies have focused on the myosin molecule and examination of fiber types. Fiber typing by myosin ATPase has been the most popular classification system (4–6). Figure 18.1 illustrates the continuum of human muscle fiber types from the most oxidative (Type I) to the least oxidative (Type IIB) fibers.

Three major types of polypeptide chains constitute the myosin molecule including a heavy chain and two different types of light chains. The complexity of the system allows for different expression of isomyosin forms with different heavy and light chain compositions. The differential myosin expression is of interest since it is related to muscle function and adaptation. A link between the mATPase fiber type distribution and myosin heavy chain content in skeletal muscle has been investigated by examining relationships for entire biopsy samples or single fibers. The relative percentage of myosin heavy chain (MHC I, MHC IIa, MHC IIb) is highly correlated with the corresponding percentage of muscle fiber types (I, IIA, IIB) in both men and women (7).

Muscle Soreness

Muscle soreness may occur after an acute resistance training session. The exact mechanisms of muscle soreness remain speculative. It is typically observed after excessively intense resistance training. It is most dramatic in less experienced or novice weight lifters. However, experienced weight lifters experience soreness with novel exercise or excess intensity progression.

Several investigations demonstrate that eccentric exercise precipitates delayed onset muscle soreness (DOMS). Ecentric contractions may damage the basic ultrastructure of the muscle cell. The focal point of the damage is the Z-disk, a structural component that anchors the contractile protein actin.

The loss of structural integrity of the Z-disks may be the stimulus leading to the associated symptoms. The appearance of DOMS ranges from 24–48 hours after exercise and may last up to 10 days. Symptoms of DOMS include localized muscular stiffness, tenderness, local edema, limited range of motion due to edema, and pain (which varies from low-grade ache to severe pain). Severity and location of discomfort specifically relates to the muscles used. The reason for increased soreness associated with eccentric training is unclear. However, one bout of eccentric exercise appears to result in protection from excessive soreness from another for up to 5–6 weeks in untrained or novice individuals. Thus, a slow progression in intensity is critical to limit soreness. It appears that excessive soreness develops from using resistance greater than the concentric 1 repetition maximum (RM).

PRINCIPLES OF RESISTANCE TRAINING PROGRAMS

The primary principles related to adaptation within the neuromuscular system during resistance training are specificity, progressive overload, and program variation.

Specificity

The principle of specificity states that resistance training should match the specific demands of the performance task. The concept of overload to enhance strength performance is a basic principle of progressive resistance training. A number of concepts of specificity exist (8).

Speed of contraction relates to the speed of movement. Speed is important as an acute program variable since it affects the safety of performing a specific movement (9). An intermediate training velocity is best if the aim is to increase strength at all velocities. Thus, for general strength, an intermediate training velocity is recommended through lifting and lowering the weight in a controlled manner. However, training at a fast velocity results in slightly greater gains in strength and power at the fast velocity than training at a slow velocity. Thus, velocity specific training is appropriate for athletes during selected periods.

Greater speed of movement requires proper equipment for safety. It has been shown that "speed reps" (i.e., loads of 30–45% of 1 RM) should not be performed when the weight is at the end of a limb (e.g., bench press, arm curls, etc.) since protective mechanisms will decelerate the joint through activation of antagonist and inhibition of agonist muscles. If the goal is to develop ability to accelerate through the range of motion, then the mass must be released. Plyometric exercises, such as medicine ball throws, free weight exercises in which the bar moves vertically, or sophisticated machines which catch the weight as it is released are safest and most effective. In addition, different modes of resistance such as isokinetic, pneumatic, or hydraulic machines which do not accelerate through the range of motion can be used to enhance speed. Appropriate exercises are required to train appropriate patterns of muscle activation (10).

Muscle group specificity requires that strength be developed through training of that muscle group. Increased elbow flexor and extensor strength requires exercises for both groups in a resistance program.

Metabolic specificity is also important in training. If the task requires high levels of muscular endurance, then

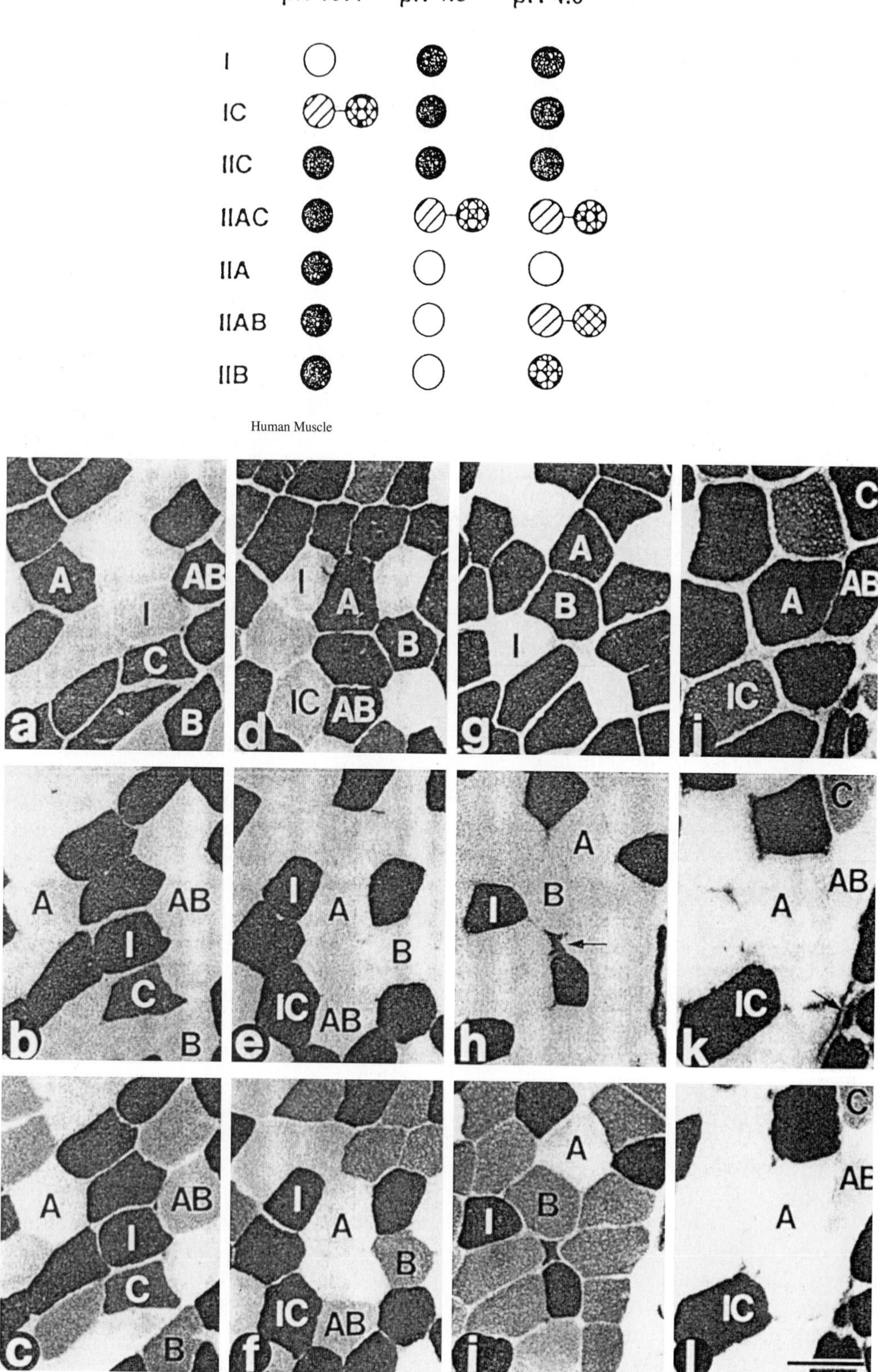

Figure 18.1. Myosin ATPase Classification System. Staining profile and example fiber micrograph at 4.6 pH+ . (Courtesy of Dr. Robert Staron, Ohio University, Athens, OH.)

metabolic demands must be matched in training. Increased ability to perform anaerobic exercise requires reduced length of rest periods to stimulate anaerobic glycolysis and associated increased blood lactate. Likewise, increased aerobic capacity requires longer duration, lower intensity training.

Progressive Resistance

Adaptations from resistance training depend on the increased demands placed on the neuromuscular system (4, 8, 11). Progressive resistance exercise refers to continual increases in stress placed on the muscle as training induces greater ability to produce and sustain force.

Ploutz et al. demonstrated the importance of increasing resistance by using 1 RM for training. Strength increased by 14%, and cross-sectional area increased by 5% in trained left quadriceps, while strength increased by 7% and cross-sectional area did not change in right, untrained quadriceps (12). This illustrates that neural factors mediate much of the improvement in 1 RM strength-induced adaptation. Additionally, in trained quadriceps, reduced muscle activation required to lift a given resistance seen in the post-training state demonstrated that less muscle is activated as strength increases with training, unless resistance is also progressively increased.

Periodization

Variation in the volume and intensity of training, or periodization, is important for optimal strength gain (8, 10). Much of the early research focused on the concept that there is an optimal combination of sets and repetitions that induces increased strength. Such an optimal combination probably does not exist, rather varying resistance, the number of sets, and the number of repetitions is associated with greater strength increase. The most popular term for changing acute program variables is "periodization." Periodization is planned variation in acute program variables.

Selye's general adaptation syndrome underlies the concept of periodization. This theory proposes three phases of adaptation during acute stress (i.e., resistance exercise): shock, adaptation, and staleness. The first stage, shock, occurs after the initiation of a novel stimulus (resistance exercise or new resistance), resulting in development of syndromes of maladaptation (soreness for example) and a resultant performance decrement. The second phase, the adaptation phase, occurs during repeated training exposure to the stimulus and results in increased performance. In the third phase adaptation has occurred and the same stimulus does not produce further adaptation. Performance may plateau in this phase and for further adaptation to occur, a change in stimulus or rest must be imposed.

Programs that do not provide sufficient variation and rest, result in a classic plateau of training or, perhaps, decreased performance (i.e., overtraining). Periodization can help avoid staleness and/or overtraining by allowing for adequate rest so that the exercise stimulus-response is maintained. Thus, variation in exercise stimulus becomes an important factor for consistent improvements in performance capacity.

The classic form of periodization breaks the training program into specific time periods. The longest period is the macrocycle (about one year). The macrocycle can be divided into periods called mesocycles (generally 3–4 months each). A mesocycle may be further divided into a microcycle of approximately 2–6 weeks. Each training phase has a specific goal and is a planned part of the total program. This type of training was originally designed for track and field and weight lifting to assist competitors in "peaking." Further, only large muscle groups were normally periodized. Others have learned the benefits of such training and have adapted periodization for use in other sports and fitness activities. There are two different models for periodization of training.

Classic Periodization Model

The goals of a program determine the number of training cycle phases and it is thought that several cycles are better than one long cycle, thus the length of each phase typically ranges from 2–4 weeks. Training frequency is typically 3 times per week.

General Pre-Preparation Phase. At least 6–8 weeks are required for general conditioning to allow tolerance of strength training. Proper techniques should be emphasized with little or no resistance. Intensity allowing 12–15 repetitions, low volume (1 or 2 sets), and limited numbers of exercises are ideal for this phase. Exercises may be added as proper technique is demonstrated. Large muscle group exercises are generally periodized and small muscle group exercises are performed at a slightly higher intensity (8–10 RM), but can also be periodized. A length of 2–4 weeks is used for all of the following cycles.

Preparation Phase. This is the first phase of a formal training cycle. The number of exercises and initial tolerance should be established in the previous cycle. An intensity allowing 12–15 repetitions in 3–4 sets with a 1–2 minute rest (between sets and exercises) is used. This is a high volume, low intensity stimulus.

Strength Phase. A resistance allowing 3–5 repetitions in 2–3 sets with 2–2.5 minute rest periods between sets and exercises is used. Technique is emphasized along with progression of resistance.

Power Phase. This phase uses resistance allowing 8–10 repetitions in 2–3 sets with 1–2 minute rest periods between sets and exercises. Again, technique is emphasized along with progression. Plyometric exercise or modalities such as isokinetics, pneumatics, and hydraulics can be added to the program for speed specificity at this point.

TRANSITION PHASE. This period is used for active rest (i.e., performing endurance rather than resistance exercise).

This phase can range from a few days to a couple of weeks depending upon the program and the amount of prior training.

Non-Linear Periodization Model

Non-linear or undulating models for periodization are becoming more common. This model is non-linear because larger resistance changes than those commonly used in linear models are used. The non-linear model varies exercise within 1–2 week periods between light, moderate, and heavy, and even very heavy resistance, for appropriate exercises (e.g., core exercises). It begins with a general pre-preparation phase identical to that previously discussed. Then, for example, an 8–10 RM (moderate resistance) on the first training day of the week, 3–5 RM (heavy) on the next day, and 12–15 RM (light) on the third day for a 12-week period. The 12 week cycle is followed by a short, active rest or transition phase and repeated. This model may be most appropriate for team and individual sports where peaking is not of primary importance because many competitions may take place in a season. A higher volume of training can be performed when light and moderate resistances are used and both training intensity and volume vary dramatically on a daily basis.

ACUTE PROGRAM VARIABLES

Several factors, termed acute program variables, affect configuration of resistance exercise stimuli. In 1983, Kraemer developed an approach for evaluating a single workout using five global variables as follows (8, 10):

- Choice of exercise
- Order of exercises
- Number of sets
- Rest periods
- Intensity of resistance

The acute program variables describe all possible single training sessions and determine acute physiological response to resistance exercise. A training session is designed by manipulating each variable and the training session is specific to the combination effect of the acute program variables (8, 10, 13).

Choice of Exercise

The basis for choice of exercise relates to movement pattern and equipment (e.g., multi-joint versus single joint; machine vs. free weights; isokinetic vs. constant external resistance; slow vs. faster velocity etc.). Further, each time joint angle changes, the pattern of muscle tissue activation changes. Based on the needs analysis, exercises should be selected that stress both designated muscles and joint angles. Exercises can also be arbitrarily designated as **primary exercises** and **assistance exercises. Primary exercises** train prime movers in a particular movement and are typically major muscle group exercises (e.g., squat, bench press). **Assistance exercises** train smaller muscle groups and aid in the movement produced by the prime movers (e.g., triceps press, lat pull down, biceps curls, etc.). Often assistance exercises are classified as single joint or isolated exercise movements.

Exercises can also be classified as **structural** or **isolation. Structural exercises** include whole body lifts requiring coordinated action of multiple muscle groups. Power cleans, power snatches, deadlifts, and squats are examples of structural, whole body, closed kinetic chain exercises. Exercises can also be classified as multiple joint exercises, which use more than one joint in the movement. For example, the bench press which involves movement of both the elbow and shoulder joints is a multi-joint exercise. Other examples of multiple-joint exercises are lat pull downs, military press, and leg press. **Isolation exercises** isolate a muscle group and are considered to be single-joint exercises. Bicep curls, sit-ups, knee extensions, and knee curls are good examples of isolated or single joint exercises.

Order of Exercise

The order of exercises in resistance training programs typically consists of performing large muscle prior to small muscle exercises. It has been demonstrated that by exercising the larger muscle groups first, a higher intensity of exercise can be achieved. Multi-joint exercises (e.g., squats) are performed first followed by smaller muscle group exercises (e.g., hamstring curls). Thus, order profiles focus on gaining a greater training effect for the large muscle groups by enhancing the amount of resistance that can be lifted.

Ordering of exercises also involves the sequence used in circuit weight training protocols. For example, it is important to consider whether to perform a leg exercise followed by another leg exercise or to proceed to another muscle group. Inherent in this decision is the concept of pre-exhaustion. Pre-exhaustion is characterized by performing smaller muscle group exercise prior to larger muscle group. This method produces fatigue within the muscle group using isolation exercises prior to structural exercises. Arm-to-leg ordering allows for some recovery of arm muscles while legs are exercised and this is the most common order used in circuit weight training. Novice lifters are more likely to be less tolerant of pre-exhaustion and arm-to-arm or leg-to-leg exercise in circuit weight training due to high blood lactate concentrations (10–14 mmol/L), especially with short rest periods (10 seconds) (14).

One final consideration for order of exercises is fitness level. The order of exercise can have a significant impact on the intensity level of a training session and care should be taken to avoid excessive intensity for beginning lifters who may be less conditioned.

Number of Sets

The number of sets is directly related to training results. For general fitness, one set is used at the initiation of a training program, progressing to three or four sets. It has been suggested that multiple-set, periodized systems (planned variation in sets, repetitions and volume over a training period) are most effective for continued development of strength and local muscular endurance (8). Change in strength appears to be similar between one, two, or three sets of 10–12 RM during the first several weeks or months of training in untrained individuals when programs are not periodized. Thus, in a long-term training program, periodized multiple set programs should be used.

Multiple sets of an exercise present a training stimulus during each set. Once initial fitness levels have been improved, multiple presentation of the stimulus is required to gain additional physiological benefit. Exercise volume (sets × repetitions × intensity) is vital to progression in each specific exercise, especially in individuals who have participated in several months of training (4, 5, 8). The interaction of sets and variation in training or "**periodized training**" may also help augment training adaptations.

Rest Periods

The length of the rest period between sets and exercises is often overlooked in exercise prescription. The rest period is a primary determinant of the overall intensity and influences the amount of resistance that can be used. It also significantly affects neuromuscular and metabolic demands. Rest periods determine how much of the ATP-PC (immediate) energy source is recovered and how high lactate concentrations increase in muscle and blood (14–17). Figures 18.2 and 18.3 show the effects of rest period length on blood lactate and growth hormone responses, respectively, in men and women.

The data indicates that, for the same load (10 RM resistance) and total work, length of rest period dictates changes in the blood. In addition, heavier resistance does not always result in higher blood lactate concentrations, but rather the total amount of work performed and the duration of the force demands placed on the muscle actually determines blood lactate concentrations. For example, 10 RM allows more repetitions and longer sets, yet exercise remains at a relatively high percentage of the 1 RM (75–85% of 1 RM), therefore higher lactate concentrations may result than from 1 or 2 RM exercises. Practically, it has been demonstrated that short rests are associated with greater psychological anxiety and fatigue. The psychological ramifications of using short rest periods should be carefully weighed when designing a training session. The anxiety appears to be due to dramatic

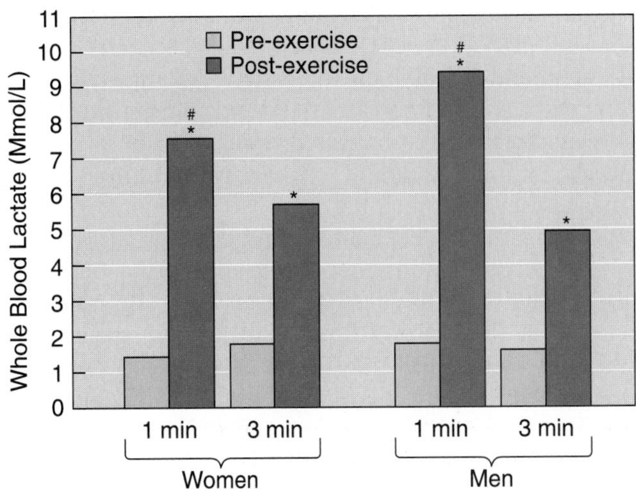

Figure 18.2. Pre- to post-exercise (peak value) response of blood lactate to short (1 min) and long (3 min) rest period in men and women. * = $P < 0.05$ from corresponding pre-exercise value and # from corresponding 3 min rest period length. (Adapted from Kraemer WJ, Fleck SJ, Dziados JE, et al. Changes in hormonal concentrations following different heavy resistance exercise protocols in women. *J Appl Physiol* 75(2): 594–604, 1993; Kraemer WJ, Marchitelli L, McCurry D, et al. Hormonal and growth factor responses to heavy resistance exercise. *J Appl Physiol* 69(4):1442–1450, 1990.)

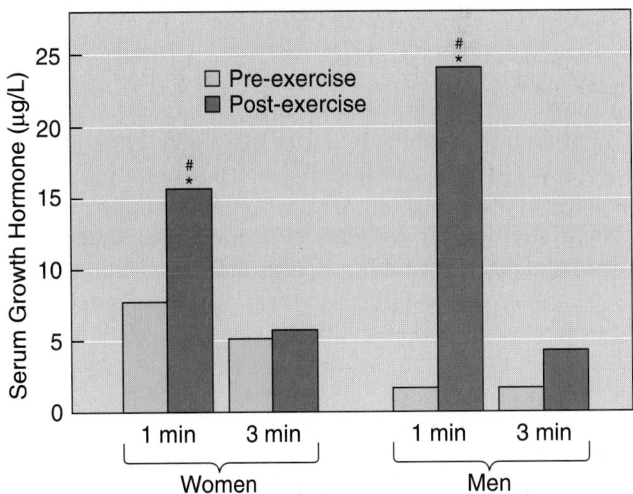

Figure 18.3. Pre- to post-exercise (peak value) response of growth hormone to short (1 min) and long (3 min) rest period in men and women. * = $P < 0.05$ from corresponding pre-exercise value and # from corresponding 3 min rest period length. (Adapted from Kraemer WJ, Fleck SJ, Dziados JE, et al. Changes in hormonal concentrations following different heavy resistance exercise protocols in women. *J Appl Physiol* 75(2): 594–604, 1993; Kraemer WJ, Marchitelli L, McCurry D, et al. Hormonal and growth factor responses to heavy resistance exercise. *J Appl Physiol* 69(4):1442–1450, 1990.)

metabolic demands of short rest workouts (i.e., 1 minute or less) (18).

Frequent use of high intensity workouts with short rest periods and heavy resistance should be introduced slowly. Tolerance of increased muscle and blood lactate levels and development of effective acid-base buffer mechanisms are required to offset associated adverse symptomatology (e.g., nausea and dizziness) (8, 14).

Short rest periods are also characteristic of circuit weight training, but resistances are typically moderate (i.e., 40% to 60% of 1 RM) (8, 10). When rest periods are decreased to less than 1 minute, intensity is significantly reduced, except in highly trained bodybuilders (7). It should be noted that symptoms such as nausea and emesis do not indicate a quality workout, but rather represent adverse symptoms of exceeding the ability to tolerate acid-base changes.

Intensity of Resistance

The amount of resistance used for a specific exercise is, perhaps, the most important variable in resistance training. It is probably the major stimulus related to changes in strength and local muscular endurance. The use of RM (the specific resistance which allows a specific number of repetitions) may be the easiest method to determine resistance. The RM continuum (Fig. 18.4) relates resistances to the broad training effects derived. It appears that RM resistances of six or less have the greatest effect on strength or maximal power output. RM resistances of 20 and above show the greatest effect on muscular endurance measures.

As resistances decrease from the strength stimulus zone, gains in strength diminish. The strength gains achieved above 25 RM resistances are small or non-existent and, when they occur, may be related to enhanced motor performance or learning effects. Pre-training status must be considered in evaluating strength improvement. The higher the pre-training level, the lower the percentage increase in the strength with training (8).

Another method for determining resistances uses a percentage of 1 RM (e.g., 70% of the 1 RM). This method requires that maximal strength, in various lifts be evaluated regularly. If 1 RM is not assessed regularly, the percentage used in training decreases, therefore training intensity is reduced.

Percentages of 1 RM are often used in training for competitive Olympic lifts, such as the clean and jerk, snatch, and pulls. Such lifts require coordinated movements and optimal power development to result in correct lifting technique. They cannot be performed at a "true" RM or to failure. Therefore, % 1 RM allows correctly calculated resistances for such lifts. In addition, for those in which a Valsalva maneuver is contraindicated (e.g., cardiac patients) typically use a specific number of reps at a % of 1 RM.

Interestingly, studies indicate that the relationship between % of 1 RM and number of repetitions that can be performed with the resistance do not agree with the RM zones for optimal training (Fig. 18.4). This relationship varies with the amount of muscle mass required to perform the exercise (i.e., leg press requires more muscle recruitment than a leg extension). For example, using 80% of 1 RM typically results in the performance of greater than 10 repetitions, especially for large muscle group exercises such as the leg press. Thus, number of repetitions must be carefully monitored to maintain resistance in the optimal training zone. Large muscle group exercises appear to require a higher percentage of 1 RM to maintain the strength RM zone (e.g., 10 and under) (8).

Theoretical Repetition Continuum

Loading Effects	Local Muscular Endurance	Power	Strength
Repetition Maximum	25 ⟷ 12 ⟷	10 ⟷ 5	⟷ 1

Figure 18.4. Theoretical Repetition continuum for loading effects.

Summary

A single resistance training session can be described by acute program variables. The configuration of these variables allows for a specific amount of exercise stimulus. Exercise sessions should be designed to meet training goals and to provide training variation. Because so many different combinations are possible, a variety of sessions can be developed. Cognizance of the importance of each acute program variable is vital to understanding factors which affect acute physiological stress and, ultimately, the chronic adaptations to resistance training. There is a need for program variation to avoid overtraining. A reasonable guideline is to avoid increases in repetitions or volume of training of more than 2.5–5% at one time (8).

MUSCULAR STRENGTH AND ENDURANCE

The fitness characteristics of muscular performance typically targeted by a resistance training program include:

Local muscular endurance—the ability of a muscle or muscle group to perform repeated muscle actions against a submaximal resistance, and

Muscle strength—the ability of a muscle or muscle group to produce maximal force at a given velocity of movement.

Within the concept of muscle strength, power should also be considered. Power is defined as:

$$\frac{\text{Force} \times \text{Distance}}{\text{Time}}$$

The ability to engage and produce force early in the activation pattern (rate of force production) is becoming recognized as an important feature of the acute functional ability of muscle (9, 10). This concept is shown in a typical force time curve in Figure 18.5. Although maximum strength may be the same, the rate of force development to maximum is faster in some individuals. The ability to engage the muscle in a shorter period of time seems to be important not only for sports performance, but also for daily challenges such as reacting to loss of balance, climbing stairs, or picking up a bag of groceries and putting it on a shelf (8).

ISOMETRICS

Isometrics, or static resistance training, occurs when contractions result in no apparent change in the length of the muscle, and thus no movement. This type of resistance training is usually performed against an immovable object such as a wall or a weight machine loaded beyond maximal concentric strength. Isometrics is also performed when a weak muscle group contracts against a strong muscle group.

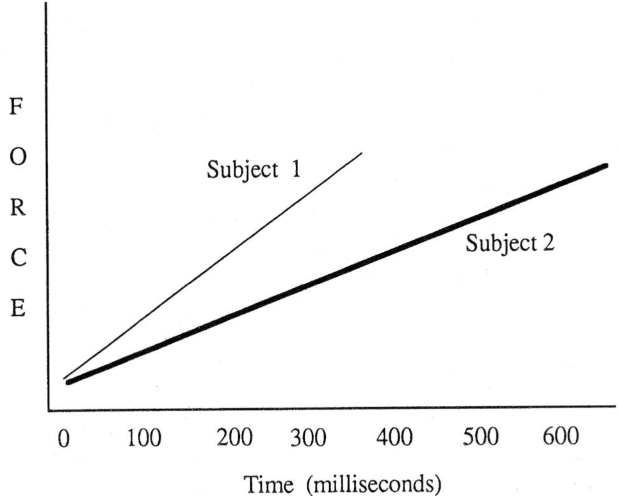

Figure 18.5. Typical force time curve. Two individuals are shown with equal maximal force capabilities but with different rates of force production (Subject 1 high rate of force production).

Isometric specificity is the result of isometric training. If isometric training is assessed isometrically, large strength gains are apparent; however, if progress is assessed using concentric or eccentric methods, little or no increase in strength may be demonstrated. Specificity, in this case, is related to recruitment of muscles and motor units specific to the activity. Increases in isometric strength are related to the frequency, duration, intensity, and number of exercises performed. Most studies using isometric training manipulate several variables simultaneously making it difficult to evaluate any single factor. Some recommendations concerning isometric training are possible, however.

Increases in strength can be achieved with submaximal isometric muscle exercises. However, research supports the use of maximal voluntary muscle actions (MVMA) as more effective for increasing strength (8). The majority of research has utilized MVMAs of 3–10 seconds duration and a relatively small number of exercises per day. The length of time a muscle is activated is directly related to strength increase. Optimal gains in strength also result from either fewer, long duration muscle actions or more short duration exercises. The strength gain from isometric training occurs predominantly at the joint angle at which the isometric training is performed (joint angle specificity). There is, however, carry over of strength increase up to at least ±20° of the training angle. Isometric training is enhanced by visual feedback.

The safety of isometric training is well established. However, the Valsalva maneuver can occur (as in all resistance training), but should be discouraged, especially in individuals with cardiovascular disease because of the resulting exaggerated blood pressure response (systolic and diastolic).

HEMODYNAMIC RESPONSES TO ACUTE RESISTANCE EXERCISE

Heart Rate and Blood Pressure

Heart rate and blood pressure increase during dynamic resistance exercise using machines, free weights, or isokinetics, although peak blood pressure response is higher during weight training in which a concentric and an eccentric phase occur compared to isokinetic exercise (19). Blood pressure and heart rate may increase quite dramatically, with peak blood pressures of 320/250 mm Hg and heart rates of 170 beats per minute for a two-legged leg press at 95% of 1 RM during a set to voluntary concentric failure with a Valsalva maneuver. Heart rate and blood pressure response is also significant when the Valsalva maneuver is limited.

Peak blood pressure and heart rate normally occur during the last several repetitions of a set to voluntary concentric failure and are higher during sets at submaximal resistance to voluntary failure than at 1 RM. In dynamic resistance exercise, increased blood pressure, but not heart rate occurs during the concentric as compared to the eccentric portion of a repetition. In addition blood pressure increases with active muscle mass, but the increase is not linear (19).

Stroke Volume and Cardiac Output

Stroke volume (determined by electrical impedance) is not significantly elevated above resting during the **concentric** phase of resistance training exercise with or without a Valsalva maneuver. However, during the **eccentric** phase, stroke volume is significantly increased above rest (with or without a Valsalva maneuver) and is significantly greater than during the concentric phase of a repetition (19).

During both the concentric and eccentric phases of a repetition, cardiac output may be increased. Cardiac output during squat exercise may increase to approximately 20 L during the eccentric phase, but only 15 L during the concentric phase. However, during exercise involving smaller muscle mass (e.g., knee extension), cardiac output may elevated above resting only during the eccentric phase. The differing response between eccentric and concentric phases may result in no overall change from rest in mean cardiac output and stroke volume during exercise involving a small muscle mass. Heart rate is not significantly different between the concentric and eccentric phases. Stroke volume is significantly greater during the eccentric compared to the concentric phase of a repetition. Therefore, increased cardiac output during the eccentric compared to the concentric phase is due to increased stroke volume.

CALORIC COST OF RESISTANCE EXERCISE

The caloric cost of resistance exercise can be increased both during and after exercise. The caloric costs of an acute exercise session have been studied in a variety of protocols from single exercises to multiple exercise circuits. The caloric cost ranges from 14–75 kcal/kg/day. It appears that the caloric cost of resistance exercise is related to the amount of muscle mass activated (choice of exercises), the length of the rest period, the intensity of the exercise, and the ability to tolerate higher volumes of total work (20).

▶ SUMMARY

The acute physiological stress of the neuromuscular system during resistance exercise is related to external demands. These demands are created by acute program variables which dictate the acute resistance exercise protocol. Careful consideration of the variables affecting the demands allows optimization of the exercise prescription in resistance exercise.

References

1. Edgerton VR, Roy RR, Gregor RJ, et al. Muscle fiber activation and recruitment. In: Knuttgen HG, Vogel JA, Poortmans S, eds. *Biochemistry of Exercise.* Champaign, IL: Human Kinetics, 1983:31–49.
2. Faulkner J, Claflin D, McCully K. Power output of fast and slow fibers from human skeletal muscles. In: Jones N, McCartney N, McComas A, eds. *Human Muscle Power.* Champaign, IL: Human Kinetics, 1986:81–90.
3. Noth J. Motor units. In: Komi PV, ed. *Strength and Power in Sport.* Oxford, England: Blackwell Scientific Publications, 1992:21–28.
4. Staron RS, Hikida RS. Histochemical, biochemical, and ultrastructural analyses of single human muscle fibers with special reference to the C fiber population. *J Histochem Cytochem* 40:563–568, 1992.
5. Staron RS, Karapondo DL, Kraemer WJ, et al. Skeletal muscle adaptations during the early phase of heavy-resistance training in men and women. *J Appl Physiol* 76:1247–1255, 1994.
6. Staron RS, Leonardi MJ, Karapondo DL, et al. Strength and skeletal muscle adaptations in heavy-resistance trained women after detraining and retraining. *J Appl Physiol* 70: 631–640, 1991.
7. Fry AC, Allemeier CA, Staron RS. Correlation between percentage fiber type area and myosin heavy chain content in human skeletal muscle. *Eur J Appl Physiol* 68:246–251, 1994.
8. Fleck SJ, Kraemer WJ. *Designing Resistance Training Programs.* 2nd ed. Champaign, IL: Human Kinetic Publishers, 1997.
9. Newton RU, Kraemer WJ. Developing explosive muscular power: Implications for a mixed methods training strategy. *J Strength Cond* 16:20, 1994.
10. Kraemer WJ, Koziris LP. Muscle strength training: Techniques and considerations. Phys Ther Pract, 2:54–68, 1992.
11. Sale DG. Neural adaptation to strength training. *In:* Komi P, ed. *Strength and Power in Sports. The Encyclopaedia of Sports Medicine.* Oxford, England: Blackwell Scientific Publications, 1992:249–265.
12. Ploutz LL, Tesch PA, Biro RL, et al. Effect of resistance training on muscle use during exercise. *J Appl Physiol* 76:1675–1681, 1994.
13. Kraemer WJ, Baechle TR. Development of a strength training program. In: Allman FL, Ryan AJ, eds. *Sports Medicine,* 2nd ed. Orlando: Academic Press 1989:113–127.
14. Kraemer WJ, Noble BJ, Culver BW, et al. Physiologic responses to heavy-resistance exercise with very short rest periods. *Int J Sports Med* 8:247–252, 1987.
15. Kraemer WJ, Fleck SJ, Dziados JE, et al. Changes in hormonal concentrations following different heavy resistance exercise protocols in women. *J Appl Physiol* 75:594–604, 1993.
16. Kraemer WJ, Marchitelli L, McCurry D, et al. Hormonal and growth factor responses to heavy resistance exercise. *J Appl Physiol* 69:1442–1450, 1990.
17. Kraemer WJ, Gordon SE, Fleck SJ, et al. Endogenous anabolic hormonal and growth factor responses to heavy re-

sistance exercise in males and females. *Intl J Sports Med* 12: 228–235, 1991.

18. Tharion WJ, Rausch TM, Harman EA, et al. Effects of different resistance exercise protocols on mood states. *J Appl Sci Res* 5:60–65, 1991.
19. Fleck SJ. Cardiovascular response to strength training. In: Komi P, ed. Strength and Power in Sports. *The Encyclopaedia of Sports Medicine.* Oxford, England: Blackwell Scientific Publications, 1992:305–315.
20. Stone MH. Weight gain and weight loss. In: Bacchle TR, ed. *Essentials of Strength Training and Conditioning.* Champaign, IL: Human Kinetics, 1994:231–237.

22, 25, 26, 27, 61, 163, 164, 176

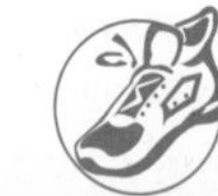

37, 38, 39, 47, 48, 52, 182

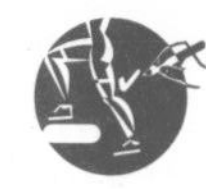

55

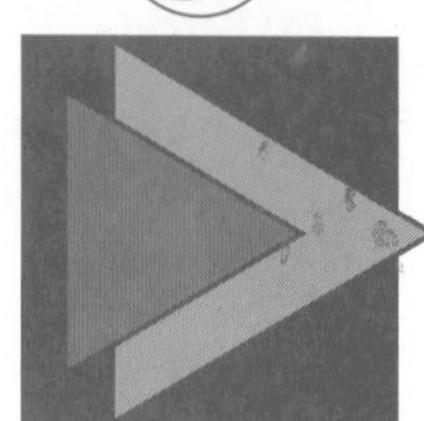

CHAPTER 19

Chronic Musculoskeletal Adaptations to Resistance Training

William J. Kraemer, Jeff S. Volek, and Steven J. Fleck

Both acute and chronic physiological changes occur with resistance exercise. An acute response usually results in an immediate change, whereas a chronic change is a function of the response to a repeated exercise stimulus. The term "adaptation" refers to the physiological process by which adaptation to physical training occurs. Ultimately, the adaptation to training determines whether resistance training is effective and whether a higher level of physiological function and/or performance is possible. Since resistance exercise protocols can be differentially configured to present a variety of demands, training adaptations appear to be specific to the type of protocol used. The specificity is related to the particular pattern of neuromuscular activation required to perform a resistance exercise. In turn, this neuromuscular stimulation activates a variety of other systems (e.g., endocrine, cardiovascular) which act to support the adaptive changes in the neuromuscular system. The sequence of adaptational events is initiated with the first exercise session and follows a time course specific to the individual and the type of protocol used.

Studies of chronic adaptations to resistance training have come primarily from training programs of less than 4 months duration. Table 19.1 summarizes adaptations from heavy resistance training (i.e., resistances greater than 80% of 1 repetition maximum [RM]). The purpose of this chapter is to discuss these adaptations which are important to understanding program design for resistance training.

MUSCLE ENLARGEMENT

Hypertrophy

One of the most prominent adaptations to a properly designed and implemented strength training program is muscle growth. Increased muscle size has been primarily attributed to muscle fiber hypertrophy (increased size of individual fibers) (1). Only fibers activated during training are subject to this adaptational response. The mechanisms of muscle enlargement are unclear, but it is a multivariate phenomenon that impacts the genetic machinery. Initial increases in water content, changes in the type of muscle proteins and eventual increases in contractile proteins are supported and signaled by a host of systematic trophic influences from hormones to nutrition. Clearly, resistance exercise disrupts or damages certain muscle fibers which later undergo repair and remodeling. This process may well involve many regulatory mechanisms (e.g., hormonal and metabolic) interacting with the training status as well as the availability of protein.

Increased muscle size is generally attributed to hypertrophy of existing muscle fibers. Muscle fiber hypertrophy is thought to occur through remodeling of protein within the cell and increased size and number of myofibrils. Furthermore, increases in the number of contractile filaments (actin and myosin) and sarcomeres contribute to increased muscle fiber size and, ultimately, intact muscle. It has been suggested that the packing density of actin, but not myosin, increases as the contractile proteins are added to the outside of the myofibril without altering cross-bridge configuration. The contractile proteins and fluid (sarcoplasma) in muscle fibers turn over every 7–15 days (2). Resistance training influences this process by affecting the quality (i.e., the type of protein) and quantity (i.e., the absolute amount) of contractile proteins produced.

Changes in types of muscle protein, such as myosin heavy chains, begin with the initiation of heavy resistance training (3). As training continues, the quantity of contractile protein increases as muscle fibers develop increased cross-sectional area. It appears that longer training (>8 sessions) is required to increase contractile protein content in all muscle fibers to demonstrate significant muscle fiber hypertrophy. Ultimately, the amount of muscle fiber hypertrophy that occurs is dependent upon the upper genetic limits for cell size. All fibers appear to hypertrophy, but not to the same extent.

Table 19.1. Physiological Adaptations Associated with Chronic Resistance Training in Humans

Variable	Directional Change in Adaptation
Performance	
Muscle strength & endurance	Increases
Aerobic power	No change
Maximal rate of force development	Increases
Vertical jump	Increases
Anaerobic power	Increases
Sprint speed	Improves
Muscle fibers	
Fiber size	Increases
Capillary volume density	No change or decreases
Mitochondrial volume density	Decreases
Myosin Heavy Chains	
Fast	Increases
Slow	No change or decreases
Enzyme activity	
Creatine phosphokinase	Increases
Myokinase	Increases
Phosphofructokinase	Increases
Metabolic energy stores	
Stored ATP	Increases
Stored creatine phosphate	Increases
Stored glycogen	Increases
Intramuscular triglycerides	May increase
Connective tissue	
Ligament strength	? (theoretically increases)
Tendon strength	? (theoretically increases)
Collagen content	? (theoretically increases)
Bone density	? (theoretically increases)
Body composition	
% body fat	Decreases
Fat-free mass	Increases
Neuroendocrine	
Growth hormone (acute exercise)	Increases
Growth hormone (chronic)	No change or decrease
Testosterone (acute & chronic)	Increases
Cortisol (acute)	Increases
Cortisol (chronic)	No change
Cardiovascular	
Heart rate	No change or decrease
Heart size	Increase
Blood pressure	Decreases
Max VO_2	No change
Serum lipids	
Total Cholesterol	Decreases
HDL	Increases
LDL	Decreases or no change
Triglycerides	Decreases
Neuromuscular	
Activation of synergistic muscles	Increases
Inhibition of antagonistic muscles	Increases
Neural protective mechanisms	Decreases
Motor neuron excitability	Increases

The amount of enlargement is dependent upon the type of muscle fiber and the pattern of recruitment (4). It is believed that in Type II muscle fibers, the hypertrophy involves increased rate of protein synthesis and in Type I muscle fibers, decreased rate of degradation is responsible (2).

Hyperplasia

Although controversial, it has been suggested that increased muscle size may also be due to muscle fiber hyperplasia (increased number of muscle fibers). Hyperplasia, following resistance training has not been demonstrated in humans due to methodological difficulties (e.g., unavailability of whole muscle for examination), but it has been shown in response to various exercise protocols in both birds and mammals (1, 5). Hyperplasia was first implicated in adaptation to resistance training in laboratory animals. Critics of the hyperplasia hypothesis claim that methods of evaluation, damage to muscle samples, and degenerating muscle fibers account for the observed hyperplasia. Later studies, even while attempting to correct for such problems, continue to demonstrate increases in muscle fiber number. Though no clear evidence supports hyperplasia in humans, there are indications that it may occur.

One theory advanced to explain hyperplasia is activation of satellite cells (i.e., reserve cells located outside the muscle fiber plasma membrane). Although activation of satellite cells (and subsequent regeneration of new fibers) is generally thought to occur in response to fiber injury or death, the possibility exists that new muscle fibers may be formed as an adaptation to "mild damage" caused by intensive resistance training. While hyperplasia in humans may not be the primary adaptational response of muscle fibers, it may represent an adaptation to resistance training that occurs when some fibers reach a theoretical "upper limit" in cell size. Very intense, long-term training may make some Type II muscle fibers primary candidates for such an adaptational response. If hyperplasia does occur, it probably accounts for only a small portion (5–10%) of the increase in muscle size.

MUSCLE FIBER TRANSFORMATION

Much plasticity exists with regard to changes in muscle with exercise due, in part, to the complex, yet readily adaptable group of myosin contractile and regulatory proteins. The majority of resistance exercise research has focused on the myosin molecule and examination of fiber types. Changes in muscle mATPase also indicates associated changes in the myosin heavy chain (MHC) content (6). A continuum of muscle fiber types exist and transformation (e.g., Type IIB to Type IIA) within a particular subtype is a common adaptation to resistance training (7). Figure 19.1 illustrates the transformation process occurring in heavy resistance training in the mus-

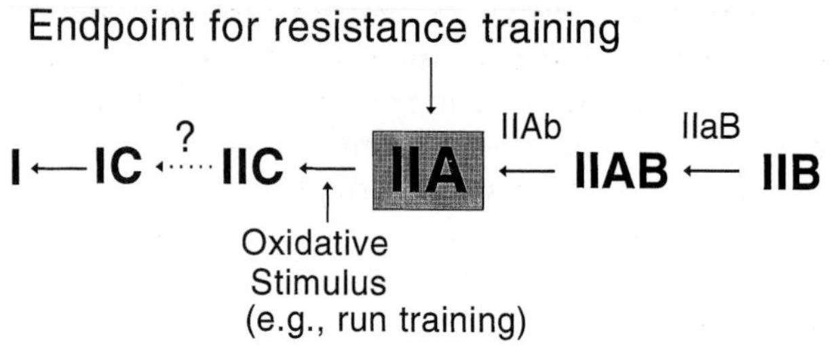

Endpoint for resistance training

I ← IC ←?… IIC ← **IIA** ← IIAB ← IIB

(IIAb, IIaB; Oxidative Stimulus (e.g., run training) → IIC)

Figure 19.1. The process of muscle fiber type transformation is presented. Changes in myosin ATPase and myosin heavy chain proteins underlie this process.

cle fiber subtypes. Using this classification scheme for evaluating changes in sub-type, it is doubtful that, under normal training conditions, muscle fibers transform from Type II to Type I. However, movement along the continuum within a fiber type clearly occurs (for reviews, see the Suggested Readings).

It appears that as soon as a Type IIB muscle fiber is stimulated, it begins a process of transformation toward the Type IIA profile by changing the quality of proteins and expressing different types and amounts of mATPase. Thus, following resistance training, very few Type IIB fibers remain. These alterations in the muscle fiber types are supported by MHC analyses with the replacement of MHC IIB with MHC IIA chains. Muscle fiber type conversions may occur very early during training (as early as 4 sessions). **Conversions of fast fiber types do not appear to be related to the rate of change of the cross-sectional area (over the short or long-term).** In addition, some evidence indicates women may experience these conversions more quickly than men.

The shift from Type IIB to Type IIA is reversed during detraining. Further, it appears that when resistance training is restarted, the conversion from Type IIB to Type IIA is quicker relative to starting in an untrained state. Thus, Type IIB fibers appear to be a non-recruited pool of fibers which improve in oxidative ability when recruited for high threshold types of activities (i.e., heavy resistance exercise). In general, the proportion of Type I muscle fibers and MHC I composition remain unchanged with resistance training. The extent that this muscle fiber remodeling contributes to muscle strength is unknown; however, gradual increases in number and size of myofibrils and perhaps the fast fiber type conversions of Type IIB to IIA may contribute to force production. Thus, while nervous system alterations may be the most dramatic effects mediating strength and power changes early in training, many other changes occur in the remodeling of muscle fibers in the early phase of training which may influence when hypertrophy reaches a critical threshold. Therefore, the "quality" of the protein type being generated due to the influence of resistance training is an important aspect of muscular development.

Information gained from studies examining the compatibility of performing strength and aerobic training simultaneously demonstrate that muscle fiber adaptations occur differentially compared to the adaptive response when performing single-mode training (4). Thus, the mechanisms of adaptation to resistance exercise are dependent upon the global exercise stimuli presented to the activated musculature. Such changes may begin to have an impact on performance within 3 months of initiating training.

CONNECTIVE TISSUE

Physical activity also increases the size and strength of ligaments, tendons, and bone. Ligaments, tendons, and bones must adapt in order to support the greater forces generated by skeletal muscles in order to prevent injury. Bone tends to adapt more slowly (6–12 months for changes in bone density) than muscle (8). Both the attachment site of a ligament or tendon and the muscle-tendinous junction are frequent sites of injury. Research involving laboratory animals demonstrates that, with endurance-type training, the amount of force necessary to cause separation at these areas increases (9). It is probable that resistance training produces similar results.

The connective tissue sheath that surrounds the entire muscle (epimysium), groups of muscle fibers (perimysium), and individual muscle fibers (endomysium) may also adapt to resistance training. These sheaths form the framework that supports an overload. Compensatory hypertrophy induced in the muscle of laboratory animals also causes an increase in the collagen content of the sheaths. Surprisingly, body builders do not differ from age-matched control subjects in the relative amount of connective tissue in the biceps brachii. Thus, connective tissue sheaths appear to increase at the same rate as muscle tissue. Furthermore, resistance training has been demonstrated to increase the thickness of hyaline cartilage on the articular surfaces of bone. One major function of hyaline cartilage is to act as a shock absorber between the bony surfaces of a joint. Increasing the thickness of this cartilage may facilitate the improved shock absorption.

ENZYMATIC ADAPTATIONS

The human body derives energy from three sources; the phosphagen or ATP-PC system, the glycolytic or lactic acid system, and the oxidative or aerobic system. Enzyme activity of the phosphagen energy source (creatine phosphokinase and myokinase) has been demonstrated to increase in humans due to isokinetic training and in rats due to isometric training. Enzymatic changes associated with the phosphagen energy source appear to be linked to the duration of exercise bouts (i.e., no change with bouts $\leq$ 6 seconds). However, little or no change in creatine phosphokinase and myokinase has been observed due to resistance training (10). Thus, the type of training program affects enzymatic adaptation. Neither of the glycolytic enzymes (phosphofructokinase or lactic dehydrogenase) appear to be affected by heavy resistance training (11, 12).

Increases in aerobic enzyme activity are reported with isokinetic and isometric training in humans and with isometric training in rats. These changes may also be dependent upon the duration of individual exercise bouts. However, aerobic enzymes obtained from pooled samples of weight-trained muscle fibers do not demonstrate increased activity (10). Nevertheless, increases in oxidative enzymes have been demonstrated to be higher in Type IIA fibers than in Type IIB fibers. This may be due to the fact that Type IIB fibers represent a non-recruited population of Type II muscle fibers and, when activated, increase oxidative enzymes and begin to converge toward a Type IIA fiber. Body builders using training with high volume, short rest periods, and moderate resistance have higher citrate synthase activity in Type II fibers than other types of lifters who train with heavier loads and longer rest periods (10). Again, the type of program may influence the magnitude of enzyme change. An enzyme associated with all three energy sources, myosin ATPase, undergoes minor changes in pooled muscle fibers (10). The fact that various types of myosin ATPase exist may suggest that interconversion of the type of myosin ATPase is more important than change in the absolute concentration.

ENERGY SUBSTRATES

The final source of energy for muscular activity is ATP that is ultimately derived from intramuscular phosphagens (phosphocreatine and ATP), carbohydrate (muscle glycogen and blood glucose), and lipids (plasma fatty acids and intramuscular triglycerides). In humans it has been demonstrated that strength training increases resting intramuscular concentrations of phosphocreatine and ATP. However, this finding is not supported by other studies, even when significant amounts of muscle fiber hypertrophy occur (13). Recent evidence that creatine supplementation expands the total creatine content of muscle (~20–30%), even in trained individuals, appears to support the concept that training induces only small changes even though stores can be improved by supplementation.

Resistance training for 5 months may increase intramuscular glycogen stores. However, muscle glycogen content does not change during resistance training (13). The aerobic energy system uses glycogen (from hepatic and intramuscular sources), triglycerides (from intramuscular and adipose tissue sources), and some protein to produce ATP; endurance training also enhances intramuscular storage and mobilization of triglycerides. Whether resistance training induces similar adaptations is equivocal, since increased triglyceride use has been observed in the triceps, but not in the quadriceps after training. Thus, there may be differences in the response of different muscle groups with respect to triglyceride storage and mobilization.

Although dietary practices and type of program may affect triglyceride concentrations, it may be speculated that, because most resistance training programs are anaerobic, intramuscular concentrations of triglycerides are minimally affected by resistance training. Storage and mobilization of energy within the body is highly dependent on nutritional status and recent food consumption. Thus, both acute and chronic dietary intake influence potential adaptations associated with energy substrate availability and use.

Myoglobin content of muscle may decrease with resistance training (13). Thus, it has been postulated that long-term strength training may depress myoglobin content and, therefore, the ability of muscle fibers to extract oxygen. Again, the initial state of training and the specific type of program may influence the effect of resistance training on myoglobin content.

CAPILLARY SUPPLY AND MITOCHONDRIAL DENSITY

Oxidative metabolism is supported by capillary supply and the concentration of cellular mitochondria. Capillarization may be enhanced with resistance training of untrained subjects. Capillaries per unit area and per fiber are significantly increased in response to different types of heavy resistance training (i.e., combinations of concentric and eccentric muscle actions). Olympic weight lifters and power lifters exhibit lower, and body builders higher, capillary density compared to untrained men. This may, in part, be due to the larger fibers exhibited by weight lifters and power lifters contributing to an area dilution. Thus, high-intensity/low-volume strength training (i.e., Olympic weight lifting or power lifting) actually decreases capillary density, whereas low-intensity/high-volume strength training (i.e., body building) increases capillary density. As with the selective hypertrophy of Type II fibers, increased capillaries appears to be linked to the intensity and volume of resistance training. However, the time course of changes in capillary density appears to be slow since studies have demonstrated that 6–12 weeks may not stimulate capillary growth beyond normal untrained levels (14).

Increased capillary density may facilitate performance of low intensity weight training by increasing blood supply to active muscle. The short rest periods used by body builders during sessions result in large increases in blood lactate concentrations (1–2 mmol/L to > 20 mmol/L). Increased capillary density may increase the ability to remove lactate, and thereby improve the ability to tolerate training under highly acidic conditions. This theory is supported by the ability of body builders to use heavier resistance under the same lactate conditions compared to power lifters whose blood lactate concentrations (in heavy resistance training) are rarely above 4 mmol/L; therefore the physiological stimulus to increase capillarization may not be as great in heavy resistance training (15).

Few studies have examined the effect of resistance training on mitochondrial density. Similar to capillaries per muscle fiber, mitochondrial density decreases with resistance training due to dilution effects of muscle fiber hypertrophy. The observation of decreased mitochondrial density is consistent with the minimal demands for oxidative metabolism during most resistance training programs. The functional significance of this morphological alteration remains unclear.

NEURAL ADAPTATIONS

Following a resistance training, the correlation between increases in strength and changes in whole muscle cross-sectional area, limb circumference, and muscle fiber cross-sectional area is low, indicating that other factors are responsible for gains in strength (3). This is especially true during the initial weeks of training. On the basis of this type of evidence, it has been concluded that neural factors profoundly influence muscular force production. Such neural factors are related to the following processes:

- Increased neural drive to muscle,
- Increased synchronization of motor units,
- Increased activation of the contractile apparatus, and
- Inhibition of protective mechanisms of the muscle (i.e., golgi tendon organs).

Scientists have investigated the neural drive to muscle using integrated electromyogram (EMG) techniques (16–18). This technique measures electrical activity within muscles and nerves and indicates the amount of neural drive to a muscle (i.e., the number and amplitude of impulses). Evidence suggests that the amount of muscle required to be activated following resistance training is less than that required to perform the same exercise protocol prior to training. This reduction in the amount of muscle needed to move a given resistance (post-training) demonstrates that, unless resistance is progressively increased, less muscle will be activated as muscular strength increases.

Since less neural drive is required to produce a given submaximal force after training, there is either improved activation of muscle or a more efficient recruitment pattern of muscle fibers. Since no improvement in activation of muscle after training has been demonstrated, some suggest that more efficient recruitment order may play an important role in increased force production in trained muscle. Furthermore, there is evidence suggesting that these neural adaptations are specific to certain muscle fibers and therefore may contribute to increased force output in some, but not all, muscles.

After the initial neural adaptations, muscle hypertrophy becomes the predominant factor in increased strength, especially for younger men. Sale described this dynamic interplay of neural and hypertrophic factors (19). A significant increase in neural factor adaptation is observed over the time course used for most resistance training studies (e.g., 6–10 weeks). As duration of training increases (>10 weeks), muscle hypertrophy eventually occurs and contributes more than neural adaptations to strength and power gain. Eventually muscle hypertrophy also reaches a maximum and plateaus. The development of whole muscle image systems (e.g., MRI and CAT scans) has confirmed that fiber changes do not necessarily reflect the magnitude of change in whole muscle. Whole muscle must be frequently stimulated at several different angles of movement to activate all available tissue over the cross-sectional area. Nevertheless, strength and power gains derived from the "progressively and properly" loaded and activated musculature appear to be bounded by a genetic upper limit of neuromuscular adaptation. Although neural adaptations account for much of the strength increase early in a resistance training program, strength and power improvement in advanced resistance trained athletes (i.e., Olympic weight lifters) may be due to neural factors (18).

Morphological changes in the human nervous system with heavy resistance training are unclear. Evidence suggests that exercise increases the area of the neuromuscular junction (NMJ) and that this adaptation is differentially influenced by the intensity of exercise (19, 20). High-intensity, endurance exercise appears to result in more dispersed, irregularly shaped synapses, while low intensity training results in more compact, symmetrical synapses. High intensity training also induces a greater total length of NMJ branching compared to low intensity exercise. Thus, it may be hypothesized that heavy resistance training produces morphological changes in the NMJ. These changes may be of greater magnitude than adaptations to endurance training due to the differences in required quanta of neurotransmitter involved with the recruitment of high threshold motor units.

NEUROENDOCRINE ADAPTATIONS

The close association of hormones to the nervous system make the neuroendocrine system potentially one of the most important physiological systems related to resistance training adaptations. Chronic adaptations in the neuroendocrine system are important in mediating many of the anabolic (tissue building) and catabolic (tissue breakdown) effects on muscle protein. The endocrine system also plays an important support function for adaptational mechanisms ultimately leading to enhanced muscular force production (21–24).

Hormones mediate changes primarily through metabolic or trophic effects on nerve and muscle cells. The alteration of metabolism (usually protein) and the molecular mechanisms associated with cell transport phenomena must then be translated to enhanced synthesis, reduced degradation, or augmentation of the functional structure or secretory products leading to enhanced muscle mass and/or improved force production. Endocrine function is highly integrated with nutritional status, training status, and other external factors (e.g., stress, sleep, disease) which affect the remodeling and repair processes. Much of the work in the area of hormonal changes with resistance exercise has focused on the alteration of concentrations of hormones in circulating blood. Differential alterations in hormones have been observed to be a function of type of exercise protocol and associated physiological demands. The challenge is to link physiological response to chronic adaptation (e.g., muscle hypertrophy and strength).

The primary anabolic hormones are testosterone, growth hormone, and insulin-like growth factor I (IGF-I), while the primary catabolic hormones are cortisol and catecholamines. Resistance training increases resting and exercise-induced testosterone concentrations. The response of testosterone appears to be determined by the mode, intensity, and duration of the training program. In contrast, resistance training does not appear to alter resting concentrations of growth hormone, however, exercise-induced increases in growth hormone may be enhanced in trained individuals. There is less information available concerning the responses of IGF-I, cortisol, and the catecholamines to resistance training. There is some evidence to indicate that a well conditioned athlete will experience a less pronounced increase in cortisol during exercise than an unconditioned athlete (25).

Acute increases in circulating concentrations of hormones are differentially sensitive to manipulations of the acute program variables in a resistance training session. For example, the highest growth hormone concentrations (Beta-endorphin and cortisol) are observed when short-rest (1 min), 10 RM multiple sets (3 sets) of exercises are performed. Testosterone appears responsive to both high intensity (5 RM), long rest (3 min) resistance exercise protocol, as well as a 10 RM, short rest protocol (25). The following factors are important determinants of the hormonal response to resistance exercise:

- Amount of muscle mass recruited,
- Intensity of the workout,
- Amount of rest between sets and exercises,
- Total volume of work, and
- Training level of the individual.

The view of the endocrine system response to resistance exercise has been somewhat limited to molecular forms that can be detected with an antibody mediated assay (immunoreactive molecular forms), thus eliminating various molecular forms which are not immunoreactive (e.g., various forms of growth hormone). Finally, the understanding of receptors on the target tissue for various hormones is developing. It is now understood that the receptors can be differentially regulated in different fiber types in response to different types of exercise (20). These responses at the target level determine whether a hormonal message is realized at the level of individual cells.

CARDIOVASCULAR ADAPTATIONS

Cardiovascular adaptations, as with other adaptations to resistance training, are affected by training volume and intensity. Cardiovascular adaptations are due to the training stimulus on the cardiovascular system, and thus, are different from muscular adaptations to resistance training. In general, the differences are due to the requirement to pump a large volume of blood at a relatively low pressure during endurance type exercise and a relatively small volume of blood at a high pressure during resistance training.

Heart Rate and Blood Pressure

Strength-trained athletes have average or lower than average resting heart rates (26). Short-term resistance training studies result in either significant (5–12%) or no significant decrease in resting heart rate (27). Decreased resting heart rate due to physical training is attributed to a combination of decreased sympathetic and increased parasympathetic stimulation to the heart. Short-term training studies on men also demonstrate no change or slightly decreased resting systolic and diastolic blood pressures (26, 27). Decreased resting blood pressure is probably due to decreased body fat, decreased body salt and alterations in the sympathetic drive to the heart. Rate-pressure product, an estimate of myocardial work and oxygen consumption, has been shown to decrease significantly as a result of resistance training. This indicates a decreased myocardial oxygen consumption and is normally viewed as a positive adaptation to training. Despite evidence to the contrary, there is a common misconception that resistance training results in hypertension. Hypertension, when it occurs in resistance trained athletes, is most likely related to essential hypertension, chronic overtraining, use of steroids, large increases in muscle mass or increases in total body weight (27).

Stroke Volume

Highly resistance-trained men have normal or above normal absolute resting stroke volumes. However, relative to body surface area or lean body mass, resting stroke volume of highly resistance-trained men is not significantly different from normal. Greater than normal absolute stroke volume is due to a significantly greater left ventricular diastolic diameter, indicating increased ventricular filling and a normal ejection fraction. A long training period and/or a high training volume are probably required to increase absolute resting stroke volume (26).

Peak Oxygen Consumption ($\dot{V}O_2$peak)

Heavy resistance training may induce small increases (5–10%) in peak oxygen consumption ($\dot{V}O_2$peak) in contrast to 15–20% increases in $\dot{V}O_2$peak which occur with traditional endurance training. Again, the volume of work appears to be critical for stimulating an adaptational response in aerobic power. For example, circuit weight training (e.g., 12–15 repetition sets at 40–60% of 1 RM) with short rest periods (15–30 seconds) have been shown to increase $\dot{V}O_2$peak marginally (i.e., 5–10%). The $\dot{V}O_2$peak of competitive Olympic weight lifters, power lifters and bodybuilders range from 41 to 55 ml/kg/min (22). The mechanism by which resistance training induces small increases in $\dot{V}O_2$peak may be related to a true aerobic training effect. It is possible that certain training programs (e.g., circuit training and Olympic weight training) may reach a minimum threshold for improving $\dot{V}O_2$peak. Alternatively, increased cardiac output at peak aerobic workloads may explain the small improvements in $\dot{V}O_2$peak. Collectively this information indicates that a resistance training program designed to increase $\dot{V}O_2$peak should consist of a high volume with relatively short rest periods between sets and exercises.

Left Ventricular Mass

An increase in left ventricular mass can be associated with either increased wall thickness or chamber size. Increased ventricular wall thickness is an adaptation to intermittent elevated blood pressure during resistance training. Increased left ventricular chamber size or volume is an indication of volume overload on the heart and is a common adaptation observed in endurance athletes. Most studies on highly resistance-trained athletes, as well as short term training studies show absolute left ventricular mass, left ventricular and intraventricular septal wall thickness to be increased in both bodybuilders and weight lifters (26). However, only bodybuilders have a significantly greater-than-normal left ventricular end-diastolic dimension (i.e., both systolic or diastolic chamber dimensions). Thus, in body builders, increased left ventricular mass is due to both greater left ventricular wall thickness and chamber size, whereas in weight lifters, it is predominantly due to a greater than normal wall thickness. It is important to note that these differences are greatly reduced or non-existent relative to body surface area or lean body mass. Factors related to increased left ventricular wall thickness include caliber of athlete, whether or not sets are carried to concentric failure, and size of muscle mass involved in the exercises.

Lipid Profile

The effect of resistance training on the lipid profile is controversial. Resistance trained men demonstrate normal, higher, and lower than normal high-density lipoprotein cholesterol (HDL-C), low-density lipoprotein cholesterol (LDL-C), total cholesterol and total cholesterol-to-HDL-C ratio (22). Data on the lipid profile in strength trained women are also mixed. The lipid profile of body builders is similar to that of runners, while power lifters have lower HDL-C and higher LDL-C values than runners, when body fat, age and steroid use (steroid use lowers HDL-C concentrations) are considered. Other factors, such as nutrition and genetics, probably account for much of the variability in serum lipids. However, resistance training can positively affect this profile. High volume programs with short rest periods between sets and exercises are probably most effective for positive effects on lipid profile.

Body Composition

Body composition changes occur in short-term resistance training programs (6–24 weeks) (28). In general, strength training induces decreased body fat and increased body mass and fat-free mass in both men and women using dynamic, constant external resistance, variable resistance, and isokinetic training with programs involving a variety of combinations of exercises, sets, and repetitions. Because of the variation in the numbers of sets, repetitions, exercises, and relatively small body composition changes, it is impossible to reach definitive conclusions regarding the optimal program for decreasing percent fat and increasing fat-free mass. The largest increases in fat-free mass are slightly greater than 3 kg (6.6 lb) in 10 weeks of training. This is equivalent to a fat-free mass increase of ~0.66 lb per week. Though some coaches desire huge gains in body mass for athletes during the off-season, this may not be possible, if the added body mass is to be muscle mass.

▶ SUMMARY

Adaptations in resistance training focus on the development and maintenance of the neuromuscular units required for force production. Training neuromuscular units affects many other physiological systems (e.g., connective tissue, cardiovascular system, and the endocrine system). Training programs are specific to the types of adaptation which occur. Activation of specific patterns of motor units in training dictate which tissue and how other physiological systems are affected by exercise training. The time course of the development of the neuromuscular system appears to be predominated in the early phase by neural factors with associated changes in types of contractile protein. In the later phase, increased muscle protein and the contractile unit begins to contribute to the changes in performance capacity. A host of other factors can affect adaptations such as functional capabilities of the individual, age, nutritional status, and behavioral factors (e.g., sleep, health habits). Optimal adaptation appears to be related to the use of specific resistance training programs to meet individual training objectives.

References

1. MacDougal JD. Hypertrophy or Hyperplasia. In: Komi P, ed. *Strength and Power in Sports. The Encyclopaedia of Sports Medicine.* Oxford England: Blackwell Scientific Publishers, 1992:230–238.
2. Goldspink C. Cellular and molecular aspects of adaptation in skeletal muscle. In: Komi P, ed. *Strength and Power in Sports. The Encyclopaedia of Sports Medicine.* Oxford England: Blackwell Scientific Publishers, 1992:211–229.
3. Staron RS, Karapondo DL, Kraemer WJ, et al. Skeletal muscle adaptations during the early phase of heavy-resistance training in men and women. *J Appl Physiol* 76:1247–1255, 1994.
4. Kraemer WJ, Patton J, Gordon SE, et al. Compatibility of high intensity strength and endurance training on hormonal and skeletal muscle adaptations. *J Appl Physiol* 78: 976–989, 1995.
5. Antonio J, Gonyea WJ. Muscle fiber splitting in stretch-enlarged avian muscle. *Med Sci Sports Exerc* 26:973–977, 1994.
6. Fry AC, Allemeier CA, Staron RS. Correlation between percentage fiber type area and myosin heavy chain content in human skeletal muscle. *Eur J Appl Physiol* 68:246–251, 1994.
7. Staron RS. Correlation between myofibrillar ATPase activity and myosin heavy chain composition in single human muscle fibers. *Histochem* 96:21–24, 1991.
8. Conroy BP, Kraemer WJ, Maresh CM. Bone mineral density in elite junior weight lifters. *Med Sci Sports Exerc* 25:1103–1109, 1993.
9. Tipton CM, Matthes RD, Maynard JA, et al. The influence of physical activity on ligaments and tendons. *Med Sci Sports* 7:165–175, 1975.
10. Tesch PA. Short- and long-term histochemical and biochemical adaptations in muscle. In: Komi P, ed. *Strength and Power in Sports. The Encyclopaedia of Sports Medicine.* Oxford: Blackwell Scientific Publishers, 1992:239–248.
11. Komi PV, Karlsson J, Tesch P, et al. Effects of heavy resistance and explosive-type strength training methods and mechanical, functional and metabolic aspects of performance. In: Komi PV, ed. *Exercise and Sports Biology. International Series on Sports Sciences.* Champaign, IL: Human Kinetics, 1982:99–102.
12. Tesch PA, Komi PV, Häkkinen K. Enzymatic adaptations consequent to long-term strength training. *Intl J Sports Med* 8(Suppl):66–69, 1987.
13. Tesch PA, Thorsson A, Colliander EB. Effects of eccentric and concentric resistance training on skeletal muscle substrates, enzyme activities and capillary supply. *Acta Physiol Scand* 140:575–580, 1990.
14. Tesch PA, Thorsson A, Kaiser P. Muscle capillary supply and fiber type characteristics in weight and power lifters. *J Appl Physiol* 56:35–38, 1984.
15. Kraemer WJ, Noble BJ, Clark MJ, et al. Physiological responses to heavy-resistance exercise with very short rest periods. *Intl J Sports Med* 8:247–252, 1987.
16. Häkkinen K. Neuromuscular adaptation during strength training, again, detraining and immobilization. *Crit Rev Phys Rehab Med* 6:161–198, 1994.
17. Häkkinen K. Neuromuscular and hormonal adaptations during strength and power training. A review. *J Sports Med* 29:9–26, 1989.
18. Häkkinen K, Parkarinen A, Alen M, et al. Neuromuscular and hormonal adaptations in athletes to strength training in two years. *J Appl Physiol* 65:2406–2412, 1988.
19. Sale DG. Neural adaptation to strength training. In: Komi P, ed. *Strength and Power in Sports. The Encyclopaedia of Sports Medicine.* Oxford, England: Blackwell Scientific Publishers, 1992:249–265.
20. Deschenes MR, Maresh CM, Armstrong LE, et al. Endurance and resistance exercise induce muscle fiber type specific responses in androgen binding capacity. *J Steroid Biochem Molec Biol* 50(3/4):175–179, 1994.
21. Deschenes MR, Maresh CM, Crivello JF, et al. The effects of exercise training of different intensities on neuromuscular junction morphology. *J Neurocytol* 22:603–615, 1993.
22. Kraemer WJ. Endocrine responses to resistance exercise. *Med Sci Sports Exerc* 20(Suppl):S152–S157, 1988.
23. Kraemer WJ. Endocrine responses and adaptations to strength training. In: Komi PV, ed. *The Encyclopaedia of Sports Medicine: Strength and Power.* Oxford, England: Blackwell Scientific Publishers, 1992:291–304.
24. Kraemer WJ. Hormonal mechanisms related to the expression of muscular strength and power. In: Komi PV, ed. *The Encyclopaedia of Sports Medicine: Strength and Power.* Oxford, England: Blackwell Scientific Publishers, 1992:64–76.
25. Deshenes MR, Kraemer WJ, Maresh CM, et al. Exercise-induced hormonal changes and their effects upon skeletal muscle tissue. *Sports Med* 12:80–93, 1991.
26. Fleck SJ. Cardiovascular adaptations to resistance training. *Med Sci Sports Exerc* 20:S146–S151, 1988.
27. Fleck SJ. Cardiovascular response to strength training. In: Komi PV, ed. *The Encyclopaedia of Sports Medicine: Strength and Power in Sport.* Oxford, England: Blackwell Scientific Publications, 1992:305–315.
28. Kraemer WJ, Fleck SJ. *Designing Resistance Training Programs.* 2nd ed. Champaign, IL: Human Kinetic Publishers, 1987:153–157.

Suggested Readings

Stone MH, Fleck SJ, Triplett NT, et al. Health- and performance-related potential of resistance training. *Sports Med* 11:210–231, 1991.

Strength and Power in Sport: The Encyclopedia of Sports Medicine. Komi PV, ed. Oxford, England: Blackwell Scientific Publications, 1992.

32 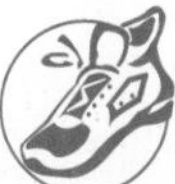 56 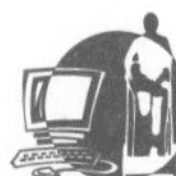

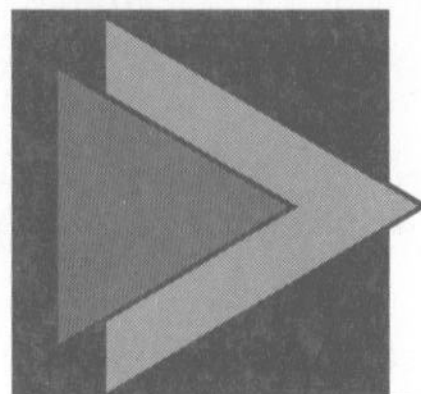

CHAPTER 20
MECHANISMS OF MUSCULAR FATIGUE

Mark Davis and Robert Fitts

The etiology of muscle fatigue has interested exercise scientists for more than a century, yet definitive fatigue agent(s) have yet to be identified. The problem is complex because muscle fatigue may result from deleterious alterations in the muscle (peripheral fatigue) and/or from changes in the neural input to the muscle (central fatigue). The latter may be mediated by central and/or peripheral changes. Furthermore, the nature and extent of muscle fatigue clearly depends on the type, duration, and intensity of exercise, the fiber type composition of the muscle, individual fitness level, and environmental factors. For example, fatigue experienced in high intensity, short duration exercise is dependent on factors differing from those precipitating fatigue in endurance activity. Similarly, fatigue during tasks involving heavily loaded contractions (e.g., weight lifting) probably differs from that produced during relatively unloaded movement (running and swimming). Finally, the often debilitating fatigue that accompanies viral or bacterial infections, recovery from injury or surgery, chronic fatigue syndrome, depression, sleep deprivation, and jet lag probably has little to do with the muscles themselves and likely involve factors within the central nervous system (CNS).

For the purpose of this review, muscle fatigue is defined as the loss of force or power output in response to voluntary effort leading to reduced performance. This definition illustrates the likelihood that both central and peripheral factors may be involved. Central fatigue is the progressive reduction in voluntary drive to motor neurons during exercise, whereas peripheral fatigue is the loss of force and power that is independent of neural drive. This chapter focuses primarily on muscle fatigue resulting from two general types of activity: short-duration, high-intensity and endurance exercise. However, it should be noted and remembered that muscle fatigue is a common phenomenon that confronts daily activities in ways that may be unrelated to athletic participation. This chapter includes a brief review of current theories and important supportive experimental results. Detailed discussions can be found in earlier reviews (1–5).

SHORT-DURATION, HIGH INTENSITY EXERCISE

Fatigue during short duration, high intensity exercise may result from impairment anywhere along the chain of command from upper brain areas to contractile proteins (Fig. 20.1). Although the preponderance of evidence suggests that a dysfunction within the muscle itself is the most likely cause of fatigue under these circumstances, central deficits in motor drive may also occur.

Peripheral Mechanisms

It is clear that the primary sites of fatigue are located within the muscle and do not generally involve peripheral nerves or the neuromuscular junction (NMJ). The observation that fatigued muscles generate the same tension whether stimulated directly or by the motor nerve argues against NMJ fatigue.

There are several possible sites within the excitation-contraction (E-C) coupling components of a muscle cell where alteration during heavy exercise may induce fatigue. With fatigue, the resting membrane potential is frequently altered and the action potential (AP) amplitude and duration are depressed and prolonged, respectively (6, 7). The membrane mechanism of muscle fatigue hypothesizes that K^+ efflux, Na^+ influx and inhibition of the Na^+-K^+ pump cause cell depolarization, a reduced AP amplitude and, in some cells, complete inactivation (8). These may inhibit subsequent steps in E-C coupling, reduce propagation of the impulse into the T-tubules, and inhibit Ca^{++} release, thus affecting the strength of contraction (4, 5).

Fatigued muscle frequently shows prolonged twitch duration and reduced peak rate of tension development (9). A prolonged twitch duration reflects a similar prolongation in the time course of the increase in intracellular levels of Ca^{++} (Ca^{++} transient) which is suggestive

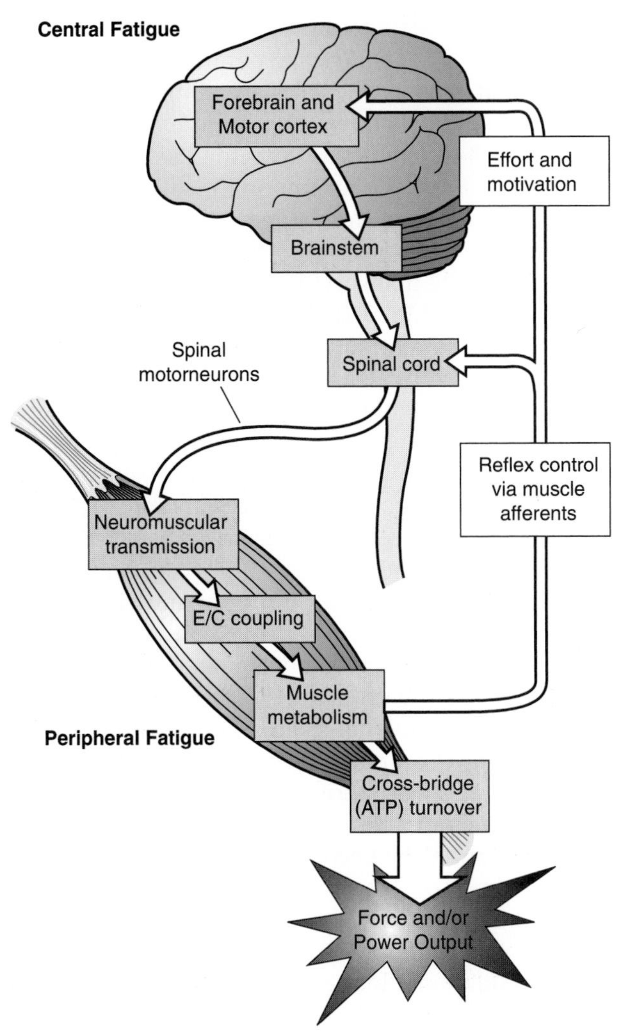

Figure 20.1. The chain of command for muscular contraction. Impairment along this pathway may be associated with fatigue.

of a reduced rate of release and/or re-uptake of Ca^{++} by the sarcoplasmic reticulum (SR). Such changes could take place for any number of reasons. Several investigators have demonstrated that the amplitude of the Ca^{++} transient decreases as fatigue develops (10, 11). Additionally, fatigue could result from a direct effect on the contractile proteins.

High intensity exercise involves an energy demand that exceeds maximal aerobic power and, thus requires a high level of anaerobic metabolism. Consequently, the levels of high-energy phosphates, ATP, and phosphocreatine (PC) decrease, and levels of inorganic phosphate (Pi), ADP, lactate, and the H^+ ion increase as fatigue develops. All of these changes are possible fatigue-inducing agents and each has been studied extensively (4, 5, 12).

Adequate tissue ATP levels must be maintained to avoid fatigue because this substrate supplies the immediate source of energy for force generation. ATP is required for the sodium-potassium pump to function. Additionally, ATP stabilizes the SR Ca^{++} release channel and is a substrate of the SR ATPase, thus is required in the process of Ca^{++} release and re-uptake by the SR. A disturbance in any of these processes could lead to muscle fatigue; however, a cause and effect relationship between low cell ATP and muscle fatigue has not been demonstrated (13, 14).

PC levels decrease with contractile activity and some suggest that low muscle PC levels may induce fatigue (15). The decline in PC concentration and tension during contractile activity, however, follow different time courses, making a casual relationship unlikely (13). The possibility exists that a critically low PC level may disrupt the PC-ATP shuttle system and slow the rate of ADP rephosphorylation to ATP which could lead to a critically low ATP at various sub-cellular sites including:

The sarcolemma Na^+-K^+ pump;
The SR Ca^{++} release channel;
The SR pump; and
The crossbridges.

However, this is not likely because:

1. Single cell analysis shows that the lowest post-fatigue cell ATP concentrations are 100-fold higher than that required for full crossbridge activation (16).
2. Various levels of fatigue are generally associated with equal ATP and PC values.
3. The highest ATP utilization rate (and thus ATP synthesis) is observed in the exercise model producing the lowest force (17).
4. Cell ATP concentration rarely drops below 60–70% of the pre-exercise level even in cases of extensive fatigue (4).

Therefore, the evidence suggests that fatigue produced by other factors reduces the ATP utilization rate before ATP becomes limiting.

ADP, Pi, and H^+ ions increase during intense contractile activity and may cause fatigue by direct inhibition of hydrolysis of ATP (18–20). The hydrogen ion is a particularly interesting potential fatigue agent because it could produce fatigue at numerous sites. In addition to a direct inhibition of the crossbridge actomyosin ATPase and ATP hydrolysis, a build-up in the intracellular H^+ ion (decreased intracellular pH, abbreviated pHi) could induce fatigue by any of the following:

1. Inhibiting phosphofructokinase and thus the glycolytic rate.
2. Competitive inhibition of Ca^{++} binding to troponin C reducing crossbridge activation.

3. Inhibiting the SR ATPase reducing Ca^{++} re-uptake and subsequently Ca^{++} release (21).

A major source of H^+ ion production during intense muscular activity is anaerobic production of lactic acid. Although lactic acid has long been implicated as a source of fatigue (22), the general consensus is that fatigue results from the elevated number of H^+ ions.

Early work gave credence to the concept that elevated H^+ concentration inhibits glycolysis (22, 23). However, it was not until recently that a definitive relationship was found in both skeletal and cardiac muscle (24, 25). Decreasing pH (7.4 to 6.2) not only reduces maximal tension, but also increases the threshold of free Ca^{++} required for contraction (24, 25). Fast-twitch fibers are more sensitive to the acidotic depression of maximal tension than slow muscle fibers (25).

This is supported by the fact that elevated H^+ ion concentration, which inhibits the ATPase, can decrease the maximum speed of shortening (Vmax) as well as Po during recovery (26, 27). Force recovers in two phases—a short, rapid phase (about 30 sec) followed by a slower, relatively prolonged phase of recovery (about 50 min) (14, 26). The rapid phase of force recovery is probably explained by reversal of a non-H^+ ion-mediated alteration in E-C coupling. The second, slower phase of recovery probably results, in part, from the removal of the excess intracellular H^+ ion.

Changes in pH may also affect Ca^{++} regulation by disturbing SR Ca^{++} release and/or re-uptake (27, 28). Changes in free H^+ ion may also affect the Ca^{++} binding properties which, by itself, would alter the Ca^{++} transient and force output.

It has been suggested that an increased $H_2PO_4^-$ concentration can induce fatigue by inhibiting the cross-bridge transition from the low to the high force state (20, 29). The primary support for this hypothesis comes from the observation that high Pi reduces peak force during the development of, and recovery from, fatigue as well as a close inverse relationship between Pi and force in this state (16, 20).

Central Nervous System Mechanisms

The potential role of the CNS in fatigue is usually addressed in studies involving the twitch interpolation technique (30). In these experiments, the maximum muscular force that a subject can elicit voluntarily is compared to that elicited by supramaximal electrical stimulation of the nerve or muscle itself. Many of these studies demonstrate that superimposing a supramaximal electrical stimulus does not usually increase maximal voluntary contractions of isolated muscle during fatiguing exercise in well practiced and highly motivated subjects (2). These data are often used to conclude that reduced CNS drive is not a factor in muscular fatigue. However, many of these studies may have lacked the sensitivity to detect small reductions in central drive (30). There are also several examples in which this clearly was not the case (31–33). The preponderance of evidence suggests that sensory feedback can inhibit motor unit discharge rates at the level of the motor neuron in the spinal cord (34). This is known as the "Sensory Feedback Hypothesis." However, an important contribution from reduced central drive from upper brain regions cannot be excluded.

The possibility that specific brain mechanisms can reduce the magnitude of descending motor drive has received the least attention as a possible mediator of muscular fatigue even though willingness to maintain central motor drive (e.g., willingness to maintain a maximal effort) probably contributes to fatigue in most people during activities of daily life. It has been postulated that, because failure to produce the necessary force during fatigue is usually preceded by increased perceived effort, the CNS processes are at least as likely to contribute to fatigue as are those that lie within the muscle (3).

Most evidence of central fatigue comes from studies often dismissed because of inadequate practice of the task or because the effect may represent alterations in "psychological factors" like attention, motivation, and perceptions of effort and pain. For example, it has been shown that force generation and electromyogram (EMG) activity during repeated maximal voluntary contractions may be enhanced by encouragement (35). Fatigue may also be more pronounced in subjects who are concentrating on performance compared to being distracted (36). The motivation issue has also been addressed in a series of studies in which rats were motivated to run on a treadmill by electrical stimulation of a reward system in the brain (37–39). Run time to fatigue is significantly longer in well acclimated, but untrained, rats during pleasurable stimulation of brain versus electric shocks (38). The specific mechanisms of this effect have not been elucidated, but they are not likely to be due to cardiovascular or metabolic alterations.

Decreased motivation in conjunction with increased perceived exertion may also explain chronic debilitating fatigue affecting individuals with "effort syndromes," such as chronic fatigue syndrome (CFS) (40–42). It has been demonstrated that isolated muscle function is normal in CFS patients, but that the level of perceived exertion is much higher than expected (41). CFS patients appear to have normal muscle metabolism, muscle membrane function, and E-C coupling, but have an inability to fully activate skeletal muscle prior to exercise, which increases abnormally after 25 minutes of submaximal isometric exercise (40). It is likely, therefore, that the primary defect in CFS patients is an abnormality in the perception of effort translating into inability/unwillingness to reach and/or maintain the level of effort (central drive) necessary to achieve maximal performance during heavy work involving whole body or large muscle groups. Therefore, it appears that there is a significant central component to muscle fatigue in CFS, although it is too early to determine the level of the defect within the CNS.

It is only recently that direct evidence of reduced motor drive within the brain during fatiguing contractions has become evident. The most convincing evidence comes from studies in humans using a new technique called transcranial magnetic stimulation (TMS) (43). Recent reports provide good evidence of inhibition of central motor drive following fatiguing exercise (44–47). The electrical stimulus reaching the muscle following magnetic stimulation of the motor cortex (motor-evoked potential) is suppressed following fatiguing exercise. Recently, a prolonged silent period following TMS has been demonstrated (46). These changes are not influenced by muscle afferent feedback and can result from altered voluntary drive to the motor cortex as well as intrinsic cortical processes (45, 46). The genesis of central fatigue may involve inadequate neural drive by the motor cortex at the highest levels of the brain.

ENDURANCE EXERCISE

Numerous factors have been linked to fatigue resulting from prolonged endurance activity, including depletion of muscle and liver glycogen, decreases in blood glucose, dehydration, and increases in body temperature. Undoubtedly, each of these factors contributes to fatigue to a varying degree, the relative importance depending on environmental conditions and the nature of the activity. Mechanisms involving various neurotransmitters and neuromodulators have also recently been proposed to explain possible CNS involvement in fatigue during prolonged exercise. This section reviews some of these potential fatigue factors. In particular, carbohydrate depletion, alterations in SR function, and increased brain serotonin will be discussed.

Glycogen Depletion

It has long been suggested that the rate of carbohydrate utilization is dependent on the intensity of work. This belief was based on the observation that the respiratory exchange ratio (RER) increases from rest to exercise. The early theories have been confirmed by direct measurements of glycogen use at different work intensities (12, 48). The rate of body carbohydrate usage is dependent not only on intensity, but also on the state of fitness. At a fixed work load, trained individuals have a lower RER, deplete glycogen more slowly, and can work longer than untrained individuals (48). High carbohydrate diets and ingestion of carbohydrate drinks during exercise can delay fatigue by increasing the availability and oxidation of carbohydrates (49). These observations support the hypothesis that depletion of carbohydrate stores is causative of muscular fatigue during endurance activity. However, the exact mechanism is not known. Low muscle glycogen concentration may reduce NADH production and electron transport, drain intermediates of the Krebs cycle, and/or reduce fat oxidation. The effects of which would be to inhibit ATP production and cause fatigue (5, 50).

It is also possible that central fatigue may occur in conjunction with carbohydrate depletion during prolonged exercise. Carbohydrate ingestion throughout exercise may attenuate the onset of negative CNS changes involving serotonin (discussed in more detail later in this chapter) (51). However, the effects of carbohydrate feedings on central fatigue mechanisms and the well-established beneficial effects on the contracting muscle are difficult to distinguish (49). It seems apparent that future efforts should focus on the mechanisms by which glycogen depletion causes fatigue.

Other Factors

Glycogen depletion is probably not an exclusive fatigue factor during endurance exercise. Other potential candidates include disruption of important intracellular organelles, such as the mitochondria, the SR, or the myofilaments (5). The role of mitochondrial damage in fatigue is controversial (5, 52).

The contractile proteins and, in particular, myofibril ATPase activity appear relatively resistant to change with endurance exercise (5, 9). Ca^{++} uptake by the SR vesicles, however, is depressed in the slow and fast-twitch red region of the vastus lateralis which is suggestive of uncoupling of the transport or a "leaky" membrane allowing Ca^{++} flux back into the intracellular fluid. In addition to these functional changes, it has been demonstrated that exhaustive endurance exercise structurally damages the SR (5, 28). The exact nature of this change and its effect on muscle function has not been elucidated.

In one study, a prolonged swim produced a significant decrease in glycogen concentration in slow type I, fast type IIa, and fast type IIb fibers of muscles, but the type IIb fibers exhibited no fatigue and no change in any of the contractile or biochemical properties measured (9). The apparent explanation is that the type IIb (fast white glycolytic) fiber is recruited less frequently during endurance activity, but glycogen use is similar to other fiber types despite fewer total contractions. It is apparent that muscle fatigue during endurance activity is somehow related to the degree of muscle use and is not entirely dependent on glycogen depletion.

In some cases, fatigue is characterized by a period of prolonged recovery where force may be depressed for days. This type of fatigue is frequently referred to as low frequency fatigue (LFF) (53). Recent evidence suggests that it is caused by disruption of the E-C coupling process, perhaps due to excessive production of reactive oxygen species and/or prolonged exposure to high levels of intracellular Ca^{++} (54, 55).

The long recovery period following LFF may be related to the time required for refolding of damaged proteins or the replacement of degraded proteins (54). Protein degradation could produce swelling and, thus, lead to muscle soreness. This possibility is supported by results of structural studies in which muscle soreness is related to changes in various intracellular organelles. The time course of recovery from muscle soreness (days) exceeds that observed for most forms of fatigue, but correlates well with recovery from LFF and reflects the time required to synthesize new muscle proteins.

Of the many proposed causes of central fatigue during prolonged exercise, the role of brain serotonin has generated the most interest. Interesting new theories have been proposed that implicate various neurotransmitters such as norepinephrine, dopamine, acetylcholine, and serotonin (2). However, a review of the mechanisms involved in the control of brain serotonin synthesis and turnover at rest and during exercise (Fig. 20.2), along with its well known influence on depression, sleepiness, mood, and pain make it a particularly attractive candidate (2).

Evidence to support a role for brain serotonin in central fatigue during prolonged exercise is beginning to emerge. Concentrations of serotonin and 5-HIAA (a major metabolite) increase in several brain regions during prolonged exercise and peak at fatigue (56, 57). The administration of serotonin agonist and antagonist drugs decreases and increases, respectively, run times to fatigue in the absence of any apparent peripheral markers of muscle fatigue (56, 58, 59).

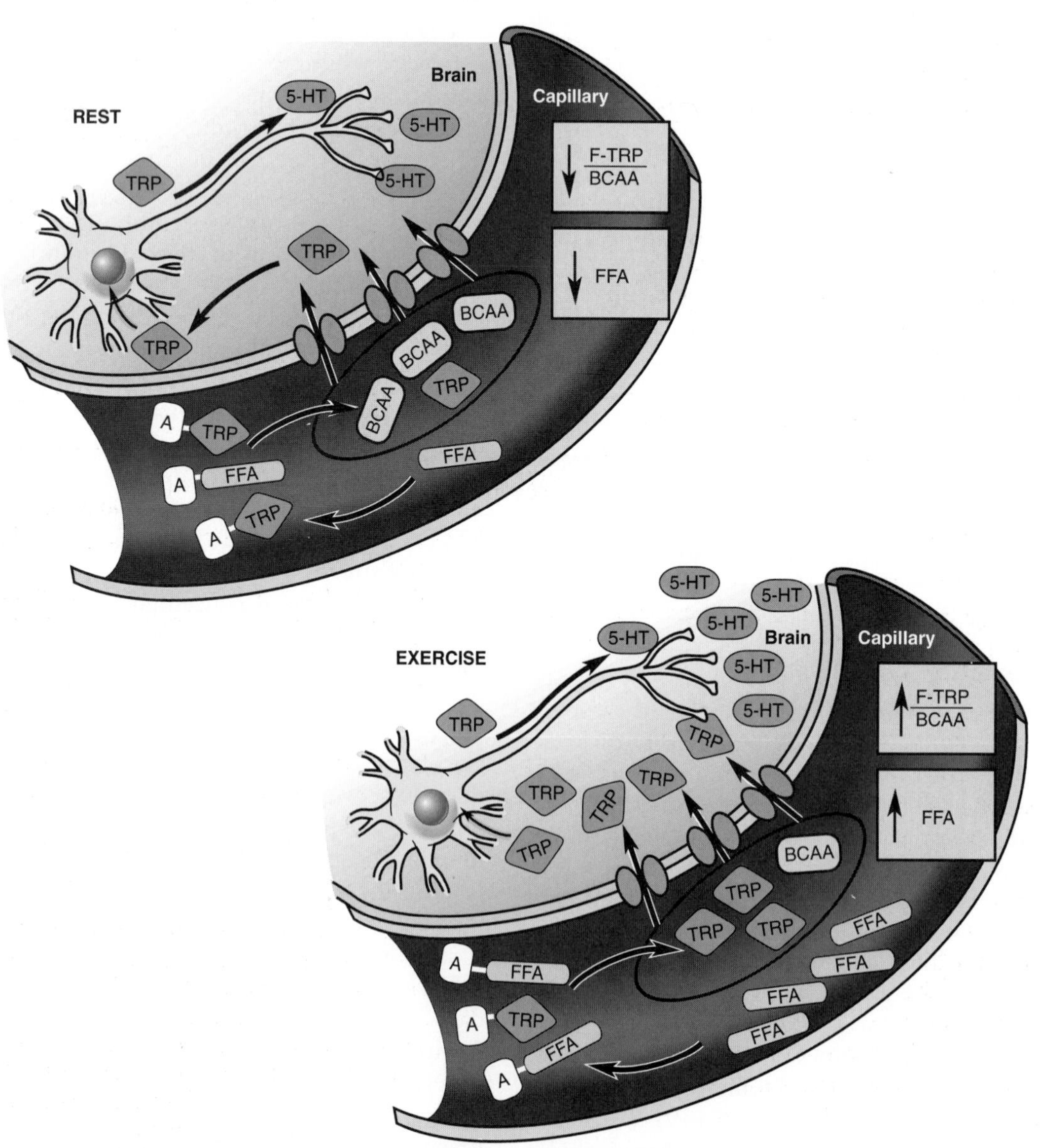

Figure 20.2. An illustration of the mechanisms involved in the control of brain serotonin synthesis and turnover at rest and during exercise. The well known influence of thesemechanisms on depression, sleepiness, mood, and pain make this a likely candidate for a center of fatigue.

▶ SUMMARY

The studies and findings described in this chapter illustrate the complex nature of fatigue. Both central nervous system and muscle mechanisms are likely to contribute to fatigue. After short duration, high-intensity exercise, recovery in force production usually occurs in two components that are probably caused by separate mechanisms: 1) A rapidly reversible non-H^+ ion-mediated perturbation, perhaps related to changes in E-C coupling, and 2) A slower change that is probably mediated by H^+ and Pi ions. The potential mechanisms of the deleterious effects of the H^+ and Pi ions are described. Reduction in central motor drive occurring at the highest levels of the brain can also accompany fatigue, but this aspect is much less well studied and the mechanisms have not been elucidated.

In prolonged endurance exercise, the depletion of skeletal muscle carbohydrate stores frequently occurs and it appears as though muscle glycogen depletion is an important factor in fatigue. Additionally, minimal levels of muscle glycogen metabolism may be important in maintaining essential Krebs cycle intermediates. Undoubtedly, other factors are involved, however, because muscle glycogen depletion can exist without fatigue and visa versa. Disruption of muscle protein, particularly the E-C coupling complex, has been shown to be associated with LFF. This process may be mediated by elevated levels of reactive oxygen species (free radicals) and/or intracellular Ca^{++}. Increased brain serotonin metabolism has also been implicated in central fatigue under these circumstances.

Practical Application

It is clear that exercise training reduces fatigue. The principles of specificity suggest that fatigue suppression applies to the specific intensities, durations, and modes of exercise regularly used in the training program, although some crossover effects may be possible. Training may somehow affect the basis of these components of fatigue. While the exact mechanisms may not be entirely clear, regular, specific exercise training reduces the onset and the effects of fatigue on the activities. In endurance exercise a number of factors are involved, including glycogen depletion which can be delayed by ingesting carbohydrates both before and during exercise. In this case, training may contribute by enhancing intracellular metabolic machinery, thus increasing cellular ability to use nutrients and produce energy. While other mechanisms also contribute to fatigue in endurance activity, the practical application of those mechanisms is, at this point, unclear.

References

1. Bigland-Ritchie B, Rice CL, Garland SJ, et al. Task-dependent factors in fatigue of human voluntary contractions. In: Gandevia SC, Enoka RM, McComas AJ, et al, eds. *Fatigue: Neural and Muscular Mechanisms.* New York: Plenum Press, 1995:361–380.
2. Davis JM, Bailey SP. Possible mechanisms of central nervous system fatigue during exercise. *Med Sci Sports Exerc* 29: 45–57, 1997.
3. Enoka RM, Stuart DG. Neurobiology of muscle fatigue. *J Appl Physiol* 72:1631–1648, 1992.
4. Fitts RH. Cellular mechanisms of muscle fatigue. *Physiol Rev* 74:49, 1994.
5. Fitts RH. Cellular, molecular, and metabolic basis of muscle fatigue. In: Rowell LB, Shephard JT, eds. *Handbook of Physiology: Section 12: Regulation and Integration of Multiple Systems.* New York: Oxford University Press, 1996,
6. Lannergren J, Westerblad H. Force and membrane potential during and after fatiguing, continuous high-frequency stimulation of single Xenopus muscle fibers. *Acta Physiol Scand* 128:35 , 1986.
7. Metzger JM, Fitts RH. Fatigue from high and low frequency muscle stimulation: Role of sarcolemma action potentials. *Exp Neurol* 93:320, 1986.
8. Sjogaard G. Role of exercise-induced potassium fluxes underlying muscle fatigue: a brief review. *Can J Physiol Pharmacol* 69:238, 1990.
9. Fitts RH, Courtright JB, Kim DM, et al. Muscle fatigue with prolonged exercise: Contractile and biochemical alterations. *Am J Phy[illegible]iol* 242:C65, 1982.
10. Allen DG, Lee [illegible] Westerblad H. Intracellular calcium and tension in is[illegible]d single muscle fibers from Xenopus. *J Physiol* 415:4[illegible]989.
11. Westerblad H[illegible]en DG. Changes of myoplasmic calcium concentration [illegible]ing fatigue in single mouse muscle fibers. *J Gen Physiol* 9[illegible]15, 1991.
12. Bergstrom J. Muscle electrolytes in man. *Scand J Clin Lab Invest* 14(Suppl 68), 1962.
13. Fitts RH, Holloszy JO. Lactate and contractile force in frog muscle during development of fatigue and recovery. *Am J Physiol* 231:430, 1976.
14. Fitts RH, Holloszy JO. Effects of fatigue and recovery on contractile properties of frog muscle. *J Appl Physiol* 45:899, 1978.
15. Sahlin K, Edstrom L, Sjoholm H. Force, relaxation and energy metabolism of rat soleus muscle during anaerobic contraction. *Acta Physiol Scand* 129:1, 1987.
16. Thompson LV, Fitts RH. Muscle fatigue in the frog semitendinosus: role of high energy phosphates and P(I). *Am J Physiol* 263:C803, 1992.
17. Berstrom M, Hultman E. Energy cost and fatigue during intermittent electrical stimulation of human skeletal muscle. *J Appl Physiol* 65:1500, 1988.
18. Cooke R, Franko K, Luciana GB, et al. The inhibition of rabbit skeletal muscle contraction by hydrogen ions and phosphate. *J Physiol* 395:77, 1988.
19. Godt RE, Nosek TM. Changes of intracellular milieu with fatigue or hypoxia depress contraction of skinned rabbit skeletal and cardiac muscle. *J Physiol* 412:155, 1989.
20. Nosek TM, Fender KY, Godt RE. It is deprotonated inorganic phosphate that depresses force in skinned skeletal muscle fibers. *Science* 236:191, 1987.
21. Nakamura Y, Schwartz A. The influence of hydrogen ion concentration on calcium binding and release by skeletal muscle sarcoplasmic reticulum. *J Gen Physiol* 59:22, 1972.

22. Hill AV. The absolute value of the isometric heat coefficient T1/H in a muscle twitch, and the effect of stimulation and fatigue. *Proc R Soc Lond B Biol Sci* 103:163, 1928.
23. Sahlin K, Harris RC, Nylind B, et al. Lactate content and pH in muscle samples obtained after dynamic exercise. *Pflugers Arch* 367:143, 1976.
24. Fabiato A, Fabiato F. Effects of pH on the myofilaments and the sarcoplasmic reticulum of skinned cells from cardiac and skeletal muscles. *J Physiol* 276:233, 1978.
25. Metzger JM, Moss RL. Greater hydrogen ion-induced depression of tension and velocity in skinned single fibres of rat fast rather than slow muscles. *J Physiol* 393:727, 1987.
26. Metzger JM, Fitts RH. Role of intracellular pH in muscle fatigue. *J Appl Physiol* 62:1392, 1987.
27. Thompson LV, Balog EM, Fitts RH. Muscle fatigue in frog semitendinosus: role of intracellular pH. *Am J Physiol* 263: C1507, 1992.
28. Byrd SK, McCutcheon LJ, Hodgson DR, et al. Altered sarcoplasmic reticulum function after high-intensity exercise. *J Appl Physiol* 67:2072,1989.
29. Wilkie DR. Muscular fatigue: effects of hydrogen ions and inorganic phosphate. *Fed Proc* 45:2921, 1986.
30. Allen GM, Gandevia SC, McKenzie DK. Reliability of measurements of muscle strength and voluntary activation using twitch interpolation. *Muscle and Nerve* 18:593–600, 1995.
31. Bigland-Ritchie B, Furbush B, Woods JJ. Fatigue of intermittent submaximal voluntary contractions: central and peripheral factors. *J Appl Physiol* 61:421–429, 1986.
32. Garner SH, Sutton JR, Burse RL, et al. Operation Everest II: Neuromuscular performance under conditions of extreme simulated altitude. *J Appl Physiol* 68:1167–1172, 1990.
33. Westing SH, Cresswell AG, Thorstensson A. Muscle activation during maximal voluntary eccentric and concentric knee extension. *Eur J Appl Physiol* 62:104–108, 1991.
34. Bigland-Ritchie B. EMG/Force relations and fatigue of human voluntary contractions. *Exer Sports Sci Rev* 9:75–117, 1981.
35. Rube N, Secher NH. Paradoxical influence of encouragement on muscle fatigue. *Eur J Appl Physiol* 46:1–7, 1981.
36. Asmussen E. Muscle fatigue. *Med Sci Sports Exerc* 11:313–321, 1979.
37. Burgess JM, Davis JM, Wilson SP, et al. Effects of intracranial self-stimulation on selected physiological parameters in rats. *Am J Physiol* 264:R149–R155, 1993.
38. Burgess ML, Davis JM, Borg TK, et al. Intracranial self-stimulation motivates treadmill running in rats. *J Appl Physiol* 71:1593–1597, 1991.
39. Burgess ML, Davis JM, Borg TK, et al. Exercise training alters cardiovascular and hormonal responses to intracranial self-stimulation. *J Appl Physiol* 75:863–869, 1993.
40. Kent-Braun SK, Weiner MW, Massie B, et al. Central basis of muscle fatigue in chronic fatigue syndrome. *Neurology* 43:125–131, 1993.
41. Lloyd AR, Gandevia SC, Hales JP. Muscle performance, voluntary activation, twitch properties and perceived effort in normal subjects and patients with the chronic fatigue syndrome. *Brain* 114:85–98, 1991.
42. Lloyd AR, Hales JP, Gandevia SC. Muscle strength, endurance and recovery in the post-infection fatigue syndrome. *J Neurol Neurosurg Psych* 51:1316–1322, 1988.
43. Gandevia SC. Insights into motor performance and muscle fatigue based on transcranial stimulation of the human motor cortex. *Clin Exp Pharm Physiol* 23:957–960, 1996.
44. Brasil-Neto JP, Pascual-Leone A, Valls-Sole J, et al. Postexercise depression of motor evoked potentials: a measure of central nervous system fatigue. *Exp Brain Res* 93:181–184, 1993.
45. Gandevia S, Gabrielle MA, Butler JE, et al. Supraspinal factors in human muscle fatigue: evidence for suboptimal output from the motor cortex. *J Appl Physiol* 490:520–536, 1996.
46. Taylor JL, Butler JE, Allen GM, et al. Changes in motor cortical excitability during human muscle fatigue. *J Appl Physiol* 490:519–528, 1996.
47. Zanette G, Bonato C, Polo A, et al. Long-lasting depression of motor-evoked potentials to transcranial magnetic stimulation following exercise. *Exp Brain Res* 107:80–86, 1995.
48. Saltin B, Karlsson J. Muscle glycogen utilization during work of different intensities. In: Pernow P, Saltin B, eds. *Muscle Metabolism During Exercise.* New York-London: Plenum, 1971.
49. Wagenmakers AJ, Bechers EJ, Brouns F, et al. Carbohydrate supplementation, glycogen depletion, and amino acid metabolism during exercise. *Am J Physiol* 260:E883–890, 1991.
50. Davis JM, Bailey SP, Woods JA, et al. Effects of carbohydrate feedings on plasma free-tryptophan and branched-chain amino acids during prolonged cycling. *Eur J Appl Physiol* 65:513–519, 1992.
51. Coggan AR, Coyle EF. Carbohydrate ingestion during prolonged exercise: effects on metabolism and performance. In: *Exercise and Sports Sciences Reviews.* Baltimore: Williams & Wilkins, 1991:1–40.
52. Nimmo MA, Snow DH. Time course of ultrastructural changes in skeletal muscle after two types of exercise. *J Appl Physiol* 52:910, 1982.
53. Edwards RH, Hill DK, Jones DA, et al. Fatigue of long duration in human skeletal muscle after exercise. *J Physiol* 272:769, 1977.
54. Brotto MA, Nosek TM. Hydrogen peroxide disrupts calcium release from the sarcoplasmic reticulum of rat skeletal muscle fibers. *J Appl Physiol* 81:731,1996.
55. Chin ER, Allen DG. The role of elevations in intracellular [calcium] in the development of low frequency fatigue in mouse single muscle fibers. *J Physiol* 491:813,1996.
56. Bailey SP, Davis JM, Ahlborn EN. Neuroendocrine and substrate responses to altered brain 5-HT activity during prolonged exercise to fatigue. *J Appl Physiol* 74:3006–3012, 1993.
57. Meeusen R, Thorre K, Chaouloff F, et al. Effects of tryptophan and/or acute running on extracellular 5-HT and 5-HIAA levels in the hippocampus of food-deprived rats. *Brain Res* 740:245–252,1996.
58. Bailey SP, Davis JM, Ahlborn EN. Brain serotonergic activity affects endurance performance in the rat. *Intl J Sports Med* 6:330–333, 1993.
59. Wilson WM, Maughan RJ. Evidence for a possible role of 5-hydroxytryptamine in the genesis of fatigue in man: administration of paroxetine, a 5-HT re-uptake inhibitor, reduces the capacity to perform prolonged exercise. *Exp Physiol* 77:921–924, 1992.

55 41, 52

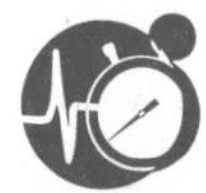

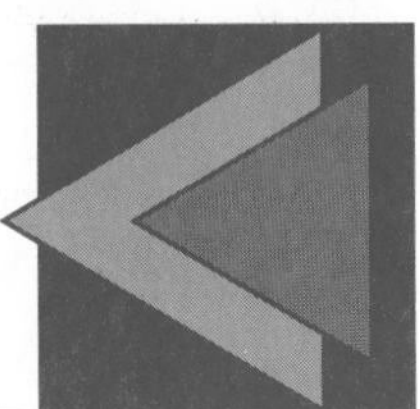

CHAPTER **21**

Deconditioning and Retention of Adaptations Induced by Endurance Training

Edward F. Coyle

The human organism possesses an amazing ability to respond to the stimulus of regular exercise. After several weeks of training, specific systems (e.g.; cardiovascular, muscular, nervous) that are stressed display physiological adaptations which improve tolerance for the specific type of exercise encountered in training. The level of adaptation and the magnitude of improvement in exercise tolerance is proportional to the potency of the training stimuli.

Although training promotes a variety of physiological adaptations, long periods of inactivity (i.e., detraining) are associated with reversal of many of these adaptations. The "reversibility concept" holds that, when physical training is stopped or reduced, systems readjust in accordance with diminished physiologic stimuli. The focus of this chapter is on the time course of loss of adaptations to endurance training as well as on the possibility that certain adaptations persist, to some extent, when training is stopped. Because endurance exercise training generally improves cardiovascular function and promotes metabolic adaptations within exercising skeletal musculature, the reversibility of these specific adaptations is considered.

CARDIOVASCULAR DETRAINING

Maximal Oxygen Uptake

Endurance training induces increased in maximal oxygen uptake ($\dot{V}O_2max$), cardiac output, and stroke volume (1, 2). When sedentary people participate in a 6–10 week, low-intensity training program, $\dot{V}O_2max$ increases by 6–10% and may remain at this level for 2–3 weeks after cessation of low intensity training (3, 4). However, prolonged detraining (8–10 weeks) results in a return of $\dot{V}O_2max$ to pretraining level (5). Moderate endurance training increases $\dot{V}O_2max$ by 10–20%, yet $\dot{V}O_2max$ may decline to pre-training levels when training is stopped (6–9). $\dot{V}O_2max$ declines rapidly during the first month of inactivity, whereas a slower decline to untrained levels occurs during the second and third months of detraining (6–9). Therefore, the available evidence suggests that increases in $\dot{V}O_2max$ produced by endurance training resulting from exercise of low to moderate intensity and duration are totally reversed after several months of detraining and a sedentary lifestyle.

Studies involving already-trained endurance athletes who cease training have allowed study of the reversibility of physiological adaptation and whether long-term, intense endurance training results in a persistent maintenance of $\dot{V}O_2max$ (10). Figure 21.1 illustrates the time course of decline in $\dot{V}O_2max$, maximal stroke volume, heart rate and arteriovenous oxygen (a-vO_2) difference induced from detraining after intense training for approximately 10 years.

$\dot{V}O_2max$ value was relatively high initially in these trained subjects (62 ml/kg/min) and it declined 16% after 84 days of detraining. A rapid decline of (7%) occurred in the first 12–21 days with a subsequent decline (9%) during days 21–84. The rapid, early decline in $\dot{V}O_2max$ was associated with a reduction in maximal stroke volume and cardiac output, despite increased heart rate (Fig. 21.1). Most of the decline in stroke volume occurred during the first 12 days of inactivity. Adaptive increases in maximal heart rate partially compensated for loss of stroke volume. The decline in $\dot{V}O_2max$ during the 21–84 days was associated with a decline in maximal a-vO_2 difference.

The 84-day period of detraining resulted in stabilization of $\dot{V}O_2max$ and maximal stroke volume. Thus, subjects appeared to have detrained for a sufficient length of time to display a complete readjustment of cardiovascular response in accordance with a sedentary lifestyle. Maximal stroke volume during upright exercise in detrained subjects is the same as that observed in those who had never engaged in endurance training (Table 21.1). This finding does not necessarily imply decreased cardiovascular function. Although maximal cardiac output and stroke volume declined to untrained levels,

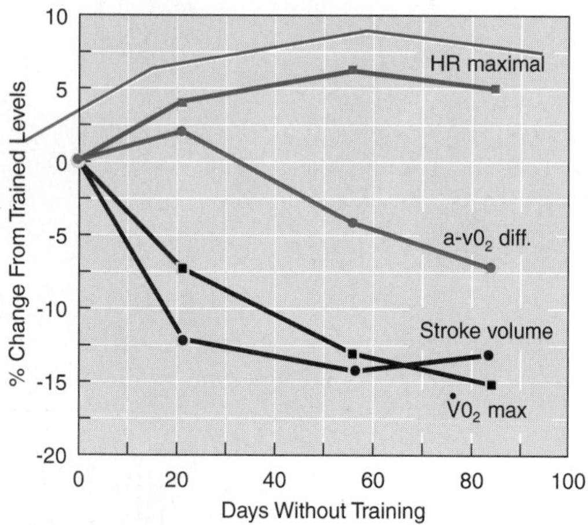

Figure 21.1. Effects of detraining upon percent change in stroke volume during exercise, maximal O_2 uptake ($\dot{V}O_2$max), maximal heart rate (HR), and maximal arteriovenous O_2 difference (a-vO_2 diff.). (Modified from Coyle EF, et al. Time course of loss adaptations after stopping prolonged intense endurance training. *J Appl Physiol* 57:1857–1864, 1984.)

Table 21.1. Responses of Highly Trained Individuals After 3 Months of Detraining Compared to Sedentary Controls

	Sedentary Control	% of Sedentary Control: Trained	% of Sedentary Control: Detrained 3 Months
$\dot{V}O_2$max (ml/kg/min)	43.3	143%*	117%†
Stroke Volume (ml)	128	120%*	101%†
a-vO_2 diff at max (ml/100 ml)	12.6	122%	116%†
Citrate Synthase Activity (mol/kg/hr)			
Whole Muscle of Both Fiber Types	4.1	243%*	149%*†
Type I Fibers	4.8	140%*	108%†
Type II Fibers	2.6	246%*	180%†
Capillary Density (cap/mm^2)	318	146%*	150%*

Trained responses are expressed as a percentage of sedentary control values. * Higher ($p < 0.05$) than sedentary control. † Detrained lower than trained: $p < 0.05$. (Modified from Coyle EF, et al. Time course of loss adaptations after stopping prolonged intense endurance training. *J Appl Physiol* 57:1857–1864, 1984; Coyle EF, Martin WH, Bloomfield SA, et al. Effects of detraining on responses to submaximal exercise. *J Appl Physiol* 59:853–859, 1985; Costill DL, et al. Metabolic characteristics of skeletal muscle during detraining from competitive swimming. *Med Sci Sports Exerc* 17:339–343, 1985.)

$\dot{V}O_2$max in detrained subjects remained 17% higher than untrained individuals, primarily because of an elevation of maximal a-vO_2 difference. The persistent elevation of $\dot{V}O_2$max in detrained subjects as a result of augmented ability of exercising musculature to extract oxygen may be related to maintenance of increased capillary density and only partial loss of increased muscle mitochondria derived from training.

Stroke Volume and Heart Size

Prolonged and intense endurance training promotes increased heart mass, whereas detraining results in decreased heart mass (1, 11, 12). Whether training-induced increases in ventricular volume and myocardial wall thickness regress totally with inactivity is not known. Athletes who become sedentary have enlarged hearts and elevated $\dot{V}O_2$max in contrast to people who have never trained (13).

The rapid decline in stroke volume is a striking effect of detraining in endurance-trained individuals. Martin et al. measured stroke volume during exercise with echocardiography in trained subjects, in both upright and supine position, and after 21 and 56 days of inactivity (Fig. 21.2) (14). The decline in stroke volume during upright cycling was associated with parallel reductions in diameter of the left ventricle at end-diastole (LVEDD). When subjects were evaluated during exercise in the supine position, a condition that usually augments ventricular filling because of the drainage of blood from the elevated legs, reduction in LVEDD was minimal. As a result, stroke volume during exercise in the supine position was maintained within a few percent of trained levels during the 56-day detraining period (Fig. 21.2). These observations indicate that ventricular filling is an important factor for stroke volume during exercise and, when it declines, perhaps due to reductions in blood volume, stroke volume also declines. Furthermore, it is also possible that training-induced increases in stroke volume may be partially due to increases in cardiac filling as a result of increases in blood volume.

Endurance-training in rats promoted significant increases in heart mass that were, essentially, completely reversed after 3–7 weeks of detraining (12, 15). Endurance-trained athletes also experience decreased heart mass after 3–8 weeks of detraining associated with a reduced posterior and septal wall thickness of the left ventricle (11, 14). However, it appears that these reductions do not lower stroke volume during submaximal exercise when ventricular filling is high (supine exercise) (14).

Cullinane et al. found that 10 days of detraining did not alter $\dot{V}O_2$max or echocardiographically determined left ventricular mass (16). Furthermore, Pavlik et al. reported that 60 days of detraining resulted in no reduction in left ventricular end-diastolic diameter at rest (17).

Blood Volume

It appears that rapid, detraining-induced reduction of stroke volume during exercise in the upright position is related to decreased blood volume (Fig. 21.3) (18). Intense exercise training usually results in increased blood volume (approximately 500 ml) through expansion of plasma volume (19, 20). This adaptation is gained after

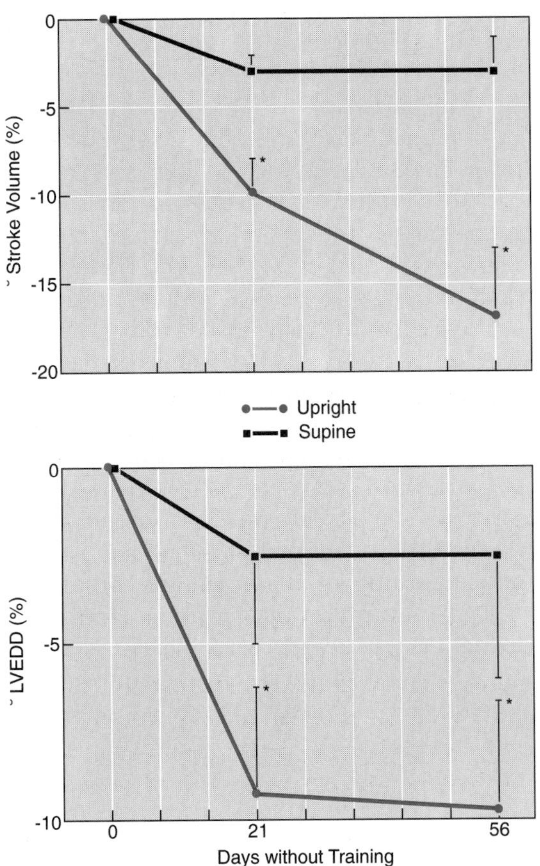

Figure 21.2. Percentage decline in exercise stroke volume (A) and left ventricular end diastolic diameter (LVEDD) (B) during exercise in upright and supine postures when trained and after 21 and 56 days of inactivity. * = responses in upright position are significantly (p < 0.05) lower than in supine position and lower than when trained. (With permission from Martin WH, Coyle EF, Bloomfield SA, et al. Effects of physical deconditioning after intense training on left ventricular dimensions and stroke volume. *J Am Coll Cardiol* 7:982–989, 1986.)

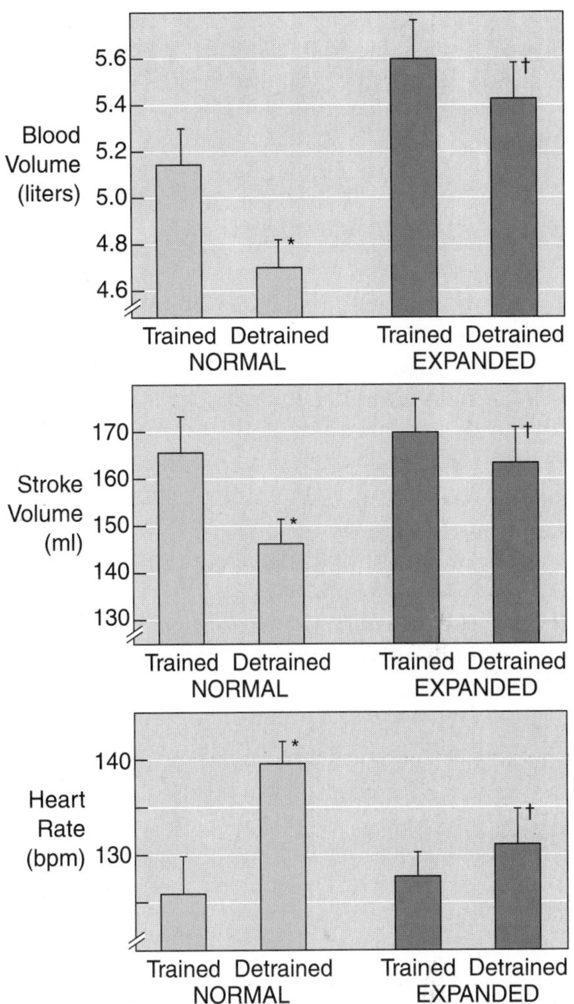

Figure 21.3. Responses to upright exercise with normal and expanded blood volume when trained and detrained. Significantly different from trained normal (* = p < 0.05). Detrained with expanded blood volume significantly different from detrained with normal blood volume († = p < 0.05). (With permission from Coyle EF, Hemmert MK, Coggan AR. Effects of detraining on cardiovascular responses to exercise. Role of blood volume. *J Appl Physiol* 60:95–99, 1986.)

only a few bouts of exercise and is quickly reversed when training ceases (18–20). The decline in stroke volume and increased heart rate during submaximal exercise, normally accompanied by several weeks of detraining, can be reversed and returns to near trained levels when blood volume expands to levels similar to trained subjects (Fig. 21.3) (18).

Since stroke volume during exercise is maintained at near trained levels when blood volume is adequate, the filling capacity left ventricle may not be significantly altered by detraining. If ventricular mass declines, myocardial thinning rather than reduction in LVEDD may be responsible (14). Thus, reduction in intrinsic cardiovascular function, at least during submaximal exercise is apparently minimal after several weeks of inactivity in previously intensely trained men (18). The large reduction in stroke volume during exercise in the upright position is largely a result of reduced blood volume and not deterioration of heart function (18).

Heart Rate During Maximal and Submaximal Exercise

Maximal heart rate increases markedly with detraining, indicating some cardiovascular compensation which may offset a large reduction in blood volume and stroke volume. Coyle et al. observed increased maximal heart rate after 3 and 12 weeks of inactivity (Fig. 21.1) (10). These results generally agree with the findings of others (16, 21). Heart rate also increases markedly during exercise at any given submaximal intensity during detraining. For example, 12 days of inactivity have been shown to increase heart rate from 158 to 170 beats per minute, and eventually to 184 beats per minute after 84 days of detraining (22).

DETRAINING AND MUSCLE METABOLISM

Enzymes of Energy Metabolism

Endurance exercise training induces enzymatic adaptations in exercising musculature resulting in slower rates of glycogen use and lactate production and improved endurance during submaximal exercise (23). Increased activity of mitochondrial enzymes, resulting in increased ability to metabolize fuels in the presence of oxygen is another important adaptation of endurance training. Moderate endurance training (2–4 months) increases mitochondrial enzyme activity by 20–40% (8, 24). When moderate training ceases and the stimuli for adaptation are removed, increases in mitochondrial activity are quickly and totally reversed. Mitochondrial activity returns to pretraining levels within 28–56 days after cessation of training (8, 10, 25).

Figure 21.4 illustrates a pattern of change in enzyme activity in individuals who trained intensely for 10 years and ceased for 84 days (26). Mitochondrial enzyme activity in trained subjects (citrate synthase, succinate dehydrogenase, malate dehydrogenase, and §-hydroxyacyl-CoA dehydrogenase), which is initially twofold higher than in untrained persons, declines progressively during the first 56 days of detraining and then stabilizes at levels that are 50% higher than sedentary control subjects. Others have also reported similar declines in mitochondrial activity with detraining (25, 27). Figure 21.4 indicates that the half-life of decline is approximately 12 days (50% decline in 12 days). Therefore, prolonged and intense training, in contrast to training lasting only a few months, appears to result in a partial loss of mitochondrial enzyme activity, thus a persistent elevation of activity above untrained persons (detrained citrate synthase activity in trained individuals is 149% of sedentary controls, see Table 21.1). This elevation occurs almost entirely because of a persistent 80% elevation in the mitochondrial enzyme activity in fast twitch muscle fibers (26). The mechanism for this persistent elevation in mitochondrial activity of fast twitch fibers from detrained endurance athletes is unclear. One possibility is that fast twitch fibers were more readily recruited to contract during daily activities of a sedentary lifestyle in detrained

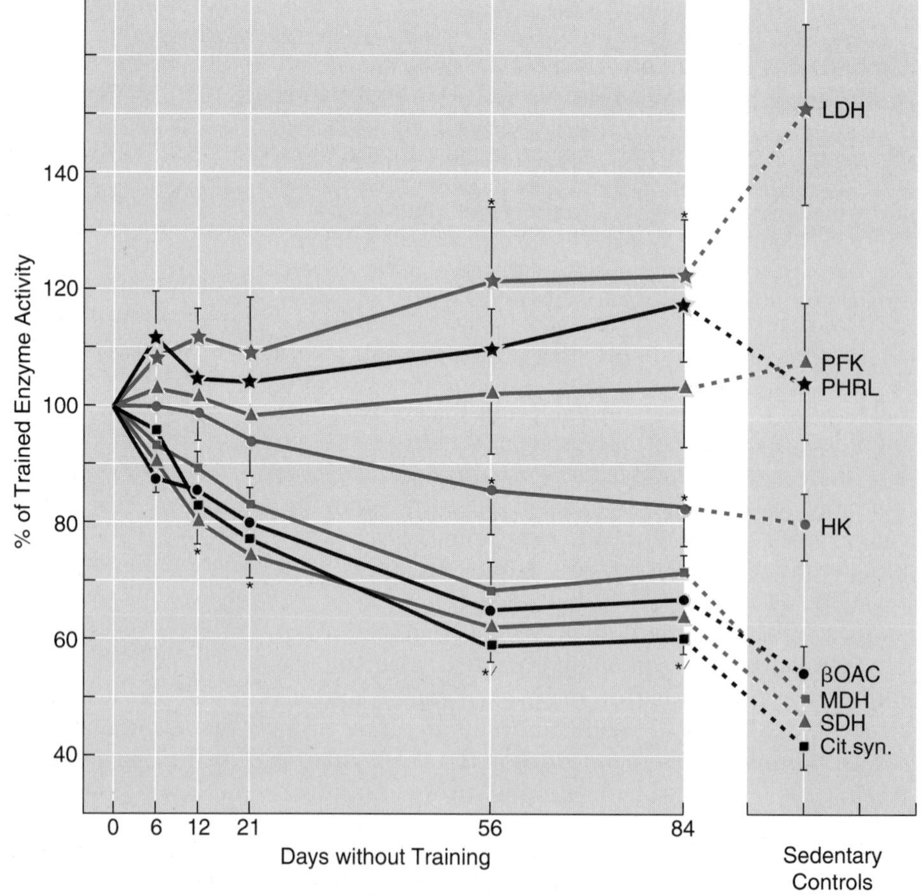

Figure 21.4. Enzyme activity during detraining compared to sedentary controls. Values expressed as percentage of trained values. Cit. syn., citrate synthase; SDH, succinate dehydrogenase; MDH, malate dehydrogenase; βOAC, β-hydroxyacyl-CoA dehydrogenase; HK, hexokinase; LDH, total lactate dehydrogenase; PHRL, phosphorylase; PFK, phosphofructokinase. * = significantly different from trained ($p < 0.05$); † = significantly different from 21 days ($p < 0.01$); à = control significantly different from 84 days ($p < 0.05$);† ‡ = control significantly different from 84 days ($p < 0.001$). (With permission from Coyle EF, Martin WH, Bloomfield SA, et al. Effects of detraining on responses to submaximal exercise. *J Appl Physiol* 59:853–859, 1985.)

persons. Other explanations including neuromuscular factors or even that these individuals are atypical and predisposed to higher fast twitch mitochondrial activity are also possibilities, although less likely (10, 26).

Muscle Capillarization

Endurance training promotes increased capillarization of exercising musculature, which theoretically both prolongs transit time of blood flow through muscle and reduces diffusion distance, thus improving availability of oxygen and nutrients to muscle as well as improving removal of metabolic waste. Moderate endurance training lasting several months increases muscle capillarization by 20–30% (8, 28). However, it appears that 8 weeks of detraining can fully or partially reverse increases in capillarization (8, 29). More prolonged and intense training increases muscle capillary density by 40–50% from untrained levels and this high degree of capillarization may be maintained for up to 3 months of detraining (Table 21.1) (10, 28).

MUSCULAR ADAPTATIONS PERSISTING WITH DETRAINING

Detrained responses in skeletal muscle of highly trained athletes regularly engaged in intense exercise over several years seems to differ from those who have trained a short duration. With cessation of prolonged, intense training, no loss of increased muscle capillarization occurs for at least 3 months although such a loss does occur when moderate training is stopped. Cessation of moderate training results in complete reversal of training-induced increases in mitochondrial enzyme activity, whereas only a partial decline (therefore, a persistent elevation above untrained levels) occurs with cessation of exercise after prolonged, intense endurance training (10, 22, 26).

It is likely that the relatively high $\dot{V}O_2$max observed in detrained athletes is partially due to genetics, hence untrained values are higher than normal, predisposing endurance activities. However, it also seems likely that some persistent muscular adaptation contributes to a relatively high a-vO_2 difference and maximal oxygen uptake (Table 21.1). It has also been observed that detrained subjects display an ability to exercise at a relatively high percentage of $\dot{V}O_2$max before becoming fatigued or experiencing increased blood lactate (22). The ability to exercise at a higher percentage of $\dot{V}O_2$max, in the detrained state, reflects maintenance of muscular adaptations (high capillary density and mitochondria in fast twitch muscle fibers).

REDUCED TRAINING RATHER THAN DETRAINING

Detraining implies total cessation of exercise, therefore removal of stimuli for adaptation. Detraining produces more marked effects than reduced training, which may maintain cardiovascular and metabolic adaptations more effectively. Indeed, Hickson has demonstrated that $\dot{V}O_2$max and heart size are maintained at trained levels when training frequency is reduced from 6 to 2 days/week, provided that intensity is sufficiently high (85–100% $\dot{V}O_2$max) (30).

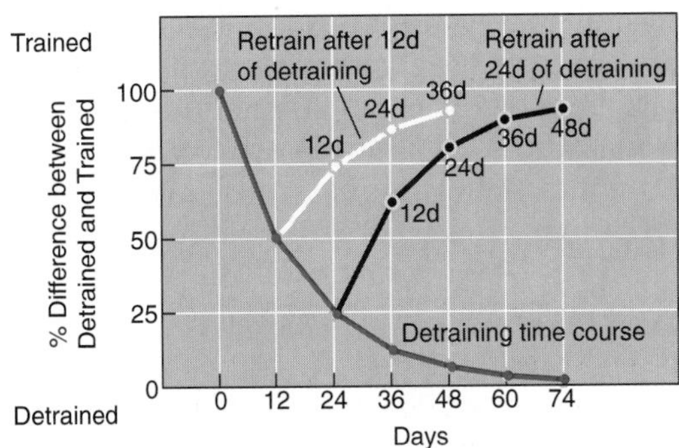

Figure 21.5. Theoretical time course of decline in mitochondrial enzyme activity and endurance performance ability with detraining, as well as rate of increase when training is resumed after 12 days or 24 days of detraining.

DETRAINING AND RETRAINING OF MUSCLE MITOCHONDRIA

While it seems logical that detrained subjects, who display only partial loss of adaptations, should be able to retrain to former levels more rapidly, this has never been directly studied in a controlled setting. Detrained former athletes seem to maintain morphological adaptations (heart size and muscle capillarization), which require years to develop, for at least 3 months. Detraining primarily causes reductions in blood volume and mitochondrial enzyme activity and it appears that blood volume is restored with several weeks of retraining (19, 20). Therefore, the limiting factor determining the time course of retraining seems likely to be the rate of increase in mitochondrial enzyme activity. As previously stated, the half-life of decline in mitochondrial enzyme activity is approximately 12 days (Fig. 21.5); therefore, 12 days of detraining requires at least 36 days of re-training to restore previous levels of mitochondrial activity. It appears that a longer period of retraining is required to restore the mitochondrial adaptations lost from a given period of detraining (3:1). Reduced training will attenuate this loss, therefore off season training should be encouraged.

▶ SUMMARY

When physical training ceases (detraining), systems readjust in accordance with diminished physiological stimuli and many training-induced adaptations are reversed. Available evidence suggests that increases in $\dot{V}O_2max$ produced by endurance training of low to moderate intensities and durations are totally reversed after several months of detraining. After several years of intense training, detraining is associated with significant reductions (5–15%) in stroke volume and $\dot{V}O_2max$ during the first 12–21 days. These changes do not indicate deterioration of myocardial function, but instead largely result from reduced blood volume and venous return. $\dot{V}O_2max$ of endurance athletes continues to decrease during 21–56 days of detraining because of reductions in maximal a-vO_2 difference. These reductions are associated with a loss of mitochondrial enzyme activity within trained skeletal muscle, which decreases with a half-life of approximately 12 days. Endurance athletes, however, do not regress to levels displayed by individuals who have never trained. Prolonged, intense endurance training is associated with persistent elevation of mitochondrial enzyme activity, skeletal muscle capillarization, maximal a-vO_2 difference, and $\dot{V}O_2max$.

References

1. Blomqvist CG, Saltin B. Cardiovascular adaptations to physical training. *Ann Rev Physiol* 45:169–189, 1983.
2. Rowell LB. Human cardiovascular adjustments to exercise and thermal stress. *Physiol Rev* 54:75–159, 1974.
3. Henriksson J, Reitman JS. Time course of changes in human skeletal muscle succinate dehydrogenase and cytochrome oxidase activities and maximal oxygen uptake with physical activity and inactivity. *Acta Physiol Scand* 99:91–97, 1977.
4. Moore RL, Thacker EM, Kelley GA, et al. Effect of training/detraining on submaximal exercise responses in humans. *J Appl Physiol* 63:1719–1724, 1987.
5. Orlander J, Kiessling KH, Karlsson J, Ekblom B. Low intensity training, inactivity and resumed training in sedentary men. *Acta Physiol Scand* 101:351–362, 1977.
6. Fringer MN, Stull GA. Changes in cardiorespiratory parameters during periods of training and detraining in young adult females. *Med Sci Sports* 6:20–25, 1974.
7. Fox EL, et al. Frequency and duration of interval training programs and changes in aerobic power. *J Appl Physiol* 38: 481–484, 1975.
8. Klausen K, Andersen LB, Pelle I. Adaptive changes in work capacity, skeletal muscle capillarization and enzyme levels during training and detraining. *Acta Physiol Scand* 113:9–16, 1981.
9. Drinkwater BL, Horvath SM. Detraining effects on young women. *Med Sci Sports Exerc* 4:91–95, 1972.
10. Coyle EF, et al. Time course of loss adaptations after stopping prolonged intense endurance training. *J Appl Physiol* 57:1857–1864, 1984.
11. Ehsani AA, Hagberg JM, Hickson RC. Rapid changes in left ventricular dimensions and mass in response to physical conditioning and deconditioning. *Am J Cardiol* 42:52–56 1978.
12. Hickson RC, Hammons GT, Holloszy JO. Development and regression of exercise-induced cardiac hypertrophy in rats. *Am J Physiol* 236:H268–H272, 1979.
13. Saltin B, Grimby GG. Physiological analysis of middle-aged and old former athletes: Comparison with still active athletes of the same ages. *Circulation* 38:1104–1115, 1968.
14. Martin WH, Coyle EF, Bloomfield SA, et al. Effects of physical deconditioning after intense training on left ventricular dimensions and stroke volume. *J Am Coll Cardiol* 7:982–989, 1986.
15. Craig BW, Martin G, Betts J, et al. The influence of training-detraining upon the heart, muscle and adipose tissue of female rats. *Mech Aging Dev* 57:49–61, 1991.
16. Culliname EM, Sady SP, Vadeboncoeur L, et al. Cardiac size and $\dot{V}O_2max$ do not increase after short-term exercise cessation. *Med Sci Sports Exerc* 18:420–424, 1986.
17. Pavlik G, Bachl N, Wollein W, et al. Resting echocardiographic parameters after cessation of regular endurance training. *Int J Sports Med* 7:226–231, 1986.
18. Coyle EF, Hemmert MK, Coggan AR. Effects of detraining on cardiovascular responses to exercise. Role of blood volume. *J Appl Physiol* 60:95–99, 1986.
19. Convertino VA, et al. Exercise training-induced hypervolemia: Role of plasma albumin, renin, and vasopressin. *J Appl Physiol* 48:665–669, 1980.
20. Green HJ, et al. Alterations in blood volume following short-term supramaximal exercise. *J Appl Physiol* 56:145–149, 1984.
21. Houston ME, Bentzen H, Larsen H. Interrelationships between skeletal muscle adaptations and performance as studied by detraining and retraining. *Acta Physiol Scand* 105:163–170, 1979.
22. Coyle EF, Martin WH, Bloomfield SA, et al. Effects of detraining on responses to submaximal exercise. *J Appl Physiol* 59:853–859, 1985.
23. Holloszy JO, Coyle EF. Adaptations of skeletal muscle to endurance exercise and their metabolic consequences. *J Appl Physiol* 56:831–838, 1984.
24. Henriksson J, Reitman JS. Time course of changes in human skeletal muscle succinate dehydrogenase and cytochrome oxidase activities and maximal oxygen uptake with physical activity and inactivity. *Acta Physiol Scand* 99:91–97, 1977.
25. Costill DL, et al. Metabolic characteristics of skeletal muscle during detraining from competitive swimming. *Med Sci Sports Exerc* 17:339–343, 1985.
26. Chi MM-Y, Hintz CS, Coyle EF, et al. Effects of detraining on enzymes of energy metabolism in individual human muscle fibers. *Am J Physiol* 244:C276–C287, 1983.
27. Wibom RE, et al. Adaptation of mitochondrial ATP production in human skeletal muscle to endurance training and detraining. *J Appl Physiol* 73:2004–2010, 1992.
28. Ingjer F. Capillary supply and mitochondrial content of different skeletal muscle fiber types in untrained and endurance-trained men: A histochemical and ultrastructural study. *Eur J Appl Physiol* 40:197–209, 1979.
29. Schantz PG. Plasticity of human skeletal muscle with specific reference to effects of physical training on enzyme levels of the NADH shuttles and phenotypic expression of slow and fast myofibrillar proteins. *Acta Physiol Scand* 558(Suppl):1–62, 1986.
30. Hickson RC, et al. Reduced training intensities and loss of aerobic power, endurance and cardiac growth. *J Appl Physiol* 58:492-499, 1985.

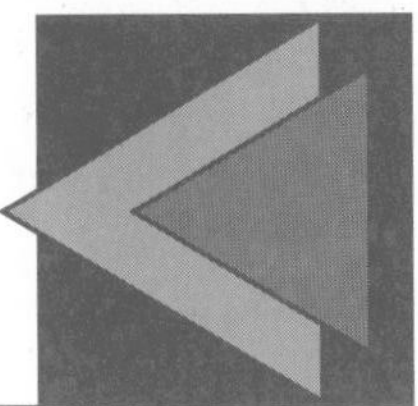

CHAPTER **22**

Deconditioning and Bed Rest: Induced Effects on Bone Health

Susan A. Bloomfield

Just as physical training induces an integrated adaptive response (physiological adaptation), so too does cessation of active training (detraining) or the more restricted activity of bed rest. The magnitude of decrement observed in both muscle and bone depends on the training status prior to detraining or bed rest, as well as the severity and duration of reduced activity relative to habitual activity. The atrophy of skeletal muscle by the end of a 6-week period of casting (e.g., after orthopedic injury) is obvious; unseen, but no less insidious, is the effect of immobilization on bone mass and calcium metabolism. Similar effects on bone, including measurable changes in bone mineral density (BMD), are observed at multiple anatomic sites during strict bed rest.

Most people experience detraining or some enforced inactivity many times over a lifespan and, more rarely, prolonged bed rest due to illness or injury. Clinicians and exercise professionals should be aware of the multiple deleterious effects of enforced inactivity. Decrements in bone mass and bone strength may predispose individuals to injury and, in extreme cases, premature onset of osteoporosis if activity is resumed too quickly.

Studies of healthy male volunteers subjected to prolonged bed rest or casting of limbs allows determination of the effects of restricted activity separated from effects of illness or injury commonly associated with bed rest or immobilization. Many changes observed in these studies also apply to adaptations observed during prolonged exposure to the microgravity of spaceflight and diminished use of lower limb musculature. Extreme musculoskeletal changes are observed in clinical populations, such as individuals with spinal cord injury or paralytic polio, but co-existing pathologic sequelae may complicate comparisons with healthy individuals subjected to even strict immobilization.

This discussion focuses on data from studies and effects of detraining, bed rest, or immobilization on bone mass and calcium metabolism in adult humans (recent review articles provide more detailed information) (1, 2). Bone mass is particularly important because it predicts bone strength relatively well. In addition to the metabolic function as a calcium reservoir, the key function of bone is the ability to resist fracture. Bone mass is most often assessed by non-invasive measurement of BMD, which is the most frequently used surrogate measure of bone strength in humans. Calcium metabolism can be assessed by following changes in urinary excretion of calcium, absorption of calcium by the gut, and, more rarely, deposition of calcium in bone; assays of endocrine regulators of serum calcium provide valuable information, as well.

CHANGES WITH DETRAINING

There are relatively few longitudinal studies yielding information on whether gains in bone mass achieved with training are lost with subsequent detraining. Dalsky et al. demonstrated complete reversal of training-induced increases in lumbar spine BMD in post-menopausal women who trained vigorously for 22 months (3). After an additional 8 months of sedentary living, spine BMD returned to baseline levels (Fig. 22.1). Simply reducing the weekly hours of weight bearing exercise may produce significant decrements in mineral content of lumbar spine trabecular bone in active men and women over the age of 50 (4). In young women, gains in lower limb BMD acquired after 1 year of unilateral resistance training are essentially lost within 3 months of detraining (5). It is doubtful, however, that brief periods of reduced training in healthy young adults (< 40 years) result in functionally meaningful decrements of BMD, given that increases in BMD with moderate to vigorous intensity exercise in healthy adults are minimal (1–3, 6).

ADAPTIVE CHANGES WITH BED REST

Reduction in weight-bearing muscle activity during bed rest invariably produces significant changes in cal-

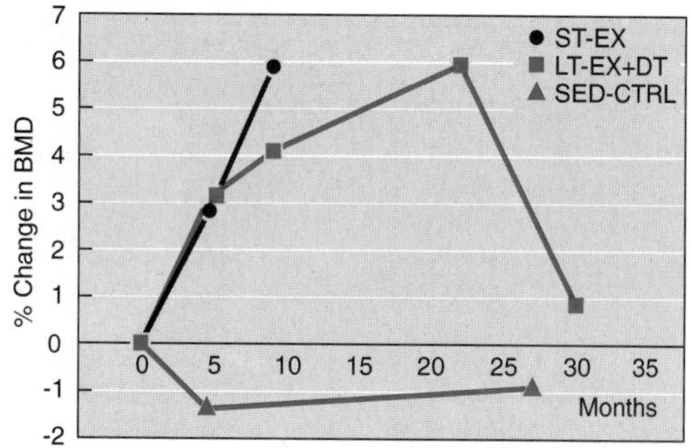

Figure 22.1. Gains in lumbar spine bone mineral density (BMD) with training for 9 months (ST-EX) and 22 months (LT-EX) and subsequent loss of BMD in those exercisers re-measured after 8 months of sedentary living. ST-EX = short-term exercise, LT-EX = long-term exercise & detraining, SED-CTRL = sedentary control. (Adapted from Dalsky G, Stocke KS, Ehsani AA, et al. Weight-bearing exercise training and lumbar bone mineral content in postmenopausal women. *Ann Intern Med* 108:824, 1988.)

cium balance and, some weeks later, changes in bone mass. The external dimensions of bone in bed-rested adults do not change, but gradual loss of bone mineral content and organic matrix and some thinning of cancellous bone plates and cortical walls is eventually noted.

Calcium Balance

Maintaining normal bone mass requires a balance between resorption of existing bone and formation of new bone. Prolonged bed rest appears to disrupt this balance with either an absolute increase in resorption or a proportionately greater increase in resorption than in formation (when both activities are stimulated). Bone calcium released into general circulation by increased resorptive activity transiently increases serum calcium allowing increased urinary excretion of calcium which is mediated by the endocrine system, including parathyroid hormone (PTH) and other substances. This resorption-driven hypercalciuria is uniformly observed in bed rested individuals, peaking at 60% above ambulatory values after 5–7 weeks of bed rest (7). A concomitant increase in fecal calcium also contributes to negative calcium balance suggesting a reduction in intestinal calcium absorption. This has been verified with calcium balance studies in humans, in whom true calcium absorption by the gut decreases from 31% (while ambulating) to 24% after bed rest (8).

It is important to note that endocrine changes are not the primary events causing loss of bone mineral. That is, reduced mechanical usage produces a net increase in bone resorption by osteoclasts; the mobilization of bone calcium itself seems to drive certain endocrine responses to mediate the increased calcium load. Intestinal calcium absorption is regulated by 1,25 dihydroxyvitamin D (1,25-D), and indirectly by PTH. In healthy men subjected to bed rest, no change or a decrease in serum PTH concurrent with a negative calcium balance has been observed; serum 1,25-D decreased or did not change (8–11). On the other hand, patients with acute spinal cord injury and functionally complete immobilization of affected limbs have consistently low PTH and low 1,25-D serum levels and presumably reduced intestinal calcium absorption (12, 13).

Bone Mass

Negative calcium balance secondary to disuse eventually results in decreased bone mass. Krolner first observed the deleterious effects of therapeutic bed rest (combined with traction) in lumbar disc disease patients, who experienced mean BMD loss of 0.9% per week in the lumbar spine (14). Healthy individuals, however, appear to experience slower rates of bone loss (4% after 17 weeks) even with strict bed rest (15). Figure 22.2 summarizes changes in bone mass with increasing durations of disuse.

Bony sites in weight bearing lower limbs appear to be the most susceptible to bone loss secondary to disuse. Loss of BMD at the calcaneus (10%) is double that observed at the femoral neck (4%) and spine (4%) after 17 weeks of strict bed rest (Fig. 22.3) (15). By contrast, over the same time period, no significant changes are noted in the radius of the forearm. The relative composition of bone is also likely to affect the rate of loss of bone at a particular anatomic site. Cancellous (trabecular) bone, with its greater surface area per volume, is particularly susceptible to increased activity of bone-resorbing osteoclasts during periods of reduced mechanical loading. For example, the proximal tibia (higher content of cancellous bone) is susceptible to more rapid bone loss with disuse than the cortical shaft (16–18). Loss of cortical bone occurs if disuse is of sufficient duration (16). Cortical bone accounts for the major component of increased fragility of osteopenic bone (19).

Analyses of bone biopsy and changes in biochemical markers of bone formation and resorption from bed rest subjects provide insight into tissue-level mechanisms for disuse bone loss. Biopsy data from healthy males subjected to 120 days of bed rest revealed no significant change in indices of cancellous bone mass and surprisingly subtle changes in bone cell activities (20, 21). Changes in thickness and density of trabecular plates, with some indication of increased bone resorption, suggest that chronic unloading in healthy adults may exert effects primarily on bone architecture, which may reduce bone strength independent of change in bone mass. These changes, after bed rest, might be quite different in lower limb bone (e.g., proximal tibia) as opposed to the non-weight bearing iliac crest, where bone biopsies are typically taken.

Changes in biochemical markers of bone resorption or formation might better indicate more global changes

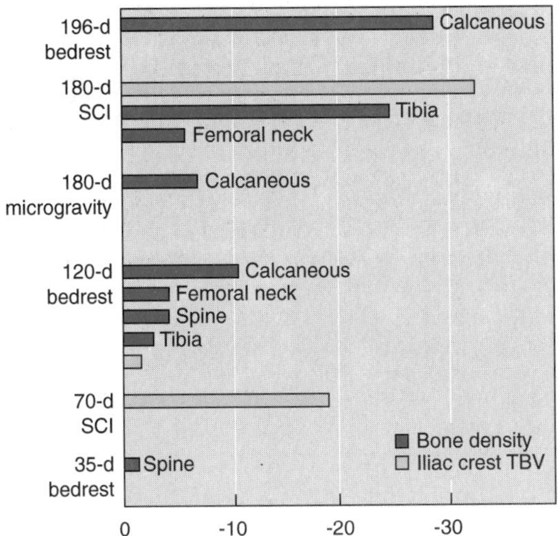

Figure 22.2. Decrements in trabecular bone volume (TBV), determined from iliac crest biopsies, and bone mineral density at various sites observed after bed rest, exposure to microgravity, or spinal cord injury (SCI). (Adapted from LeBlanc AD, Schneider VS, Evans HJ, et al. Bone mineral loss and recovery after 17 weeks of bed rest. *J Bone Miner Res* 5:843, 1990; Biering-Sørensen F, Bohr HH, Schaadt OP. Longitudinal study of bone mineral content in the lumbar spine,the forearm and the lower extremities after spinal cord injury. *Eur J Clin Invest* 20:330, 1990; Minaire P, Meunier P, Edouard C, et al. Quantitative histological data on disuse osteoporosis: comparison with biological data. *Calcif Tissue Res* 17:57, 1974; Vico L, Chappard D, Alexandre C, et al. Effects of a 120-day period of bed-rest on bone mass and bone cell activities in man: attempts at countermeasure. *Bone Miner* 2:383, 1987; LeBlanc A, Schneider V, Krebs J, et al. Spinal bone mineral after 5 weeks of bed rest. *Calcif Tissue Int* 41:259, 1987; Schneider VS, McDonald J. Skeletal calcium homeostasis and countermeasures to prevent disuse osteoporosis. *Calcif Tissue Int* 36:S151, 1984.)

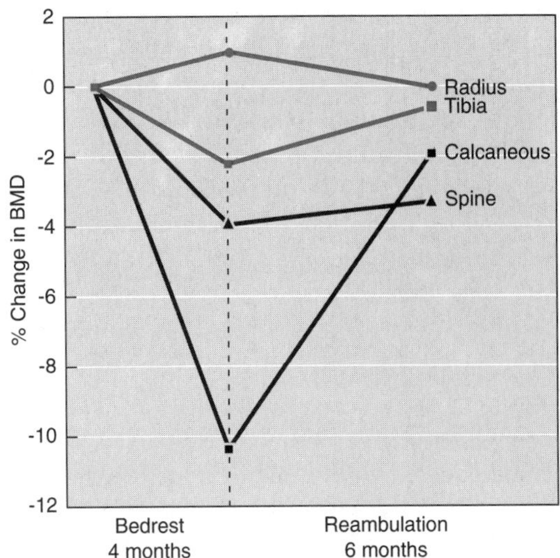

Figure 22.3. Alterations in bone mineral density (BMD), expressed as % change from baseline, during 4 months of bed rest and 6 months of reambulation in able-bodied young men. (Adapted from LeBlanc AD, Schneider VS, Evans HJ, et al. Bone mineral loss and recovery after 17 weeks of bed rest. *J Bone Miner Res* 5:843, 1990.)

in the skeleton with bed rest. Biochemical components of collagen fibril cross-links, released when bone matrix is resorbed, increase within 4 days of bed rest in healthy adult males. However, one biochemical marker for bone formation does not increase during the same period of bed rest, indicating unchanged formation concurrent with elevated resorptive activity (22). Interestingly, some markers of bone resorption remain elevated for up to 6 weeks during re-ambulation after a period of bed rest. This suggests that elevated resorption rates continue after activity resumes (11, 22).

These changes in healthy men contrast with findings in patients with spinal cord injury (SCI), in whom iliac crest cancellous bone volume decreases by 33% in the first 6 months after the injury (19). Maximal hypercalciuria observed in patients with acute SCI is 2–4 times greater than in healthy men at bed rest; disrupted calcium metabolism can persist for up to 12 months postinjury (12). Factors unique to SCI (changes in bone blood flow or bone fluid pH) probably accentuate changes in bone cell activities noted in healthy men on bed rest. Bone mineral densities of the femoral neck, distal femur, and proximal tibia in individuals with longstanding SCI average 65%, 48%, and 45%, respectively, of healthy values (18, 23). Interestingly, BMD of the lumbar spine in persons with SCI remains within normal range (18, 23). Continued load bearing on the spine, or even impact force incurred during chair transfer, appears to provide sufficient mechanical stimulus to maintain bone mass in the spine.

REMOBILIZATION: CAN LOST BONE BE REGAINED?

Recovery of lost bone mass, and reversal of presumed decreases in resistance to fracture, require at least twice as long as the duration of disuse. Cancellous bone mass lost in dogs whose hindlimbs were immobilized for 32 weeks, was not fully regained after 28 weeks of remobilization (24). In young, healthy rats treadmill running during remobilization after 3 weeks of hindlimb immobilization appeared to restore normal cancellous bone architecture (25). This effect needs confirmation in skeletally mature animals.

There is little data on recovery of bone mass after disuse in humans. Recovery is limited and very slow, although it varies among anatomical sites. A residual deficit in BMD of the calcaneus has been observed in astronauts 5 years after repeated exposures to microgravity (26). Loss of density at lumbar spine and femoral neck following 17 weeks of bed rest seems to be unaffected by 6 months of normal weight-bearing activity (Fig. 22.3) (15). BMD of the calcaneus and proximal tibia, however, appears to rebound adequately in this population. The residual deficit in BMD (−6 to −11%) noted in the lower limb of men 9 years after tibial shaft fracture, as well as a 12% lower spine BMD, implies that some BMD loss sustained after serious orthopedic injuries may be permanent unless rehabilitation efforts are especially vigorous (27).

PRACTICAL IMPLICATIONS

It is doubtful that changes in bone mass of bed rest subjects have any immediate impact on functional work capacity, as do decrements in muscle strength and endurance upon return to normal weight-bearing activity. Of greater concern is increased risk for bone fracture, particularly after muscle strength is regained and resumed activity imposes higher forces on relatively weak osteopenic bone. There also is a potential increase in risk for clinically relevant osteoporosis later in life.

For each bony site there is a critical bone density that constitutes a **fracture** threshold; that is, bone at densities below this threshold is susceptible to fracture with minimal trauma. It is also probable that, during a period of bed rest, the age-related bone loss all adults over 40 years experience may be temporarily accelerated. The result would be an increased decline in bone mass over time and earlier arrival at fracture threshold at the bony site. Elderly individuals are more likely to experience prolonged bed rest with illness or injury and are more likely to be closer to a fracture threshold before a period of bed rest begins. The severe osteopenia in hip fracture, for example, almost certainly is worsened in prolonged immobilization during recovery (28).

Reduced BMD after bed rest significantly increases risk of bone fracture with even minor falls in older individuals. Concurrent decrements in muscle strength and balance after bed rest exacerbate the likelihood of falling once ambulating begins (29, 30). Hip fractures in elderly individuals can be life-threatening and mortality in the first year after hip fracture, usually from complications of prolonged immobility, is not unusual (31). For survivors, decreased mobility detracts significantly from functional capacity and general quality of life.

There are many practical implications of musculoskeletal changes with bed rest for exercise professionals to consider (Table 22.1). Clearly, the highest priority should be avoidance of prolonged immobility. Periods of bed rest mandated by medical conditions should be limited to as short a duration as possible. Even short periods of weight bearing each day during a period of bed rest may help minimize disuse changes.

During remobilization, emphasis of training in muscle groups most significantly affected by relative disuse, should be implemented using a conservative progressive overload program. Training to improve dynamic balance and postural stability should be incorporated early in the remobilization period to reduce risk of falling, especially in the elderly. Given the slower time course of recovery of bone mass relative to muscle mass, awareness of the increased risk of fracture in remobilizing individuals after prolonged bed rest is important. The imbalance between muscle strength and bone strength is greatest when muscle strength has returned to normal and before bone mass is fully restored. These concerns are magnified in the frail elderly who may enter a period of bed rest with little reserve of bone or muscle mass.

Table 22.1. Guidelines for Exercise Professionals Working with Severely Detrained or Bed-Rested Individuals

Emphasize strength training of back and lower limb postural muscle groups
Back extensors
Quadriceps and associated hip extensors
Ankle extensors (soleus and gastrocnemius)
Use gradual, progressive, overload starting at appropriately low intensities
Incorporate training for postural stability and dynamic balance during walking, particularly if the client is elderly
Be aware of increased risk of bone fracture even after muscle strength is normalized, especially in osteopenic-prone individuals (estrogen-deficient women, elderly)

▶ SUMMARY

There are effective training regimens for improving muscle strength and both static and dynamic balance. Aggressive use of these regimens, adapted in intensity and rate of progression, may make a major contribution to bone health by minimizing risk of fracture after a period of prolonged disuse or bed rest. Regular exercise training should be incorporated into the lifestyle thereafter to attempt to regain as much bone mass as possible, although it is unclear, at present, whether all bone lost can be replaced.

References

1. Bloomfield SA. Changes in musculoskeletal structure and function with prolonged bed rest. *Med Sci Sports Exer* 29: 197, 1997.
2. Uebelhart D, Demiaux-Domenech B, Roth M, et al. Bone metabolism in spinal cord injured individuals and in others who have prolonged immobilization. A review. *Paraplegia* 33:669, 1995.
3. Dalsky G, Stocke KS, Ehsani AA, et al. Weight-bearing exercise training and lumbar bone mineral content in postmenopausal women. *Ann Intern Med* 108:824, 1988.

4. Michel, BA, Lane NE, Bloch DA, et al. Effect of changes in weight-bearing exercise on lumbar bone mass after age fifty. *Ann Med* 23:397, 1991.
5. Vuori I, Heinonen A, Seivänen H, et al. Effects of unilateral strength training and detraining on bone mineral density and content in young women: a study of mechanical loading and deloading on human bones. *Calcif Tissue Int* 55: 59, 1994.
6. Forwood MR, Burr DB. Physical activity and bone mass: exercises in futility? *Bone Miner* 21:89, 1993.
7. Arnaud, SB. Effects of inactivity on bone. In: Sandler H, Vernikos J, eds. *Inactivity: Physiological Effects*. Orlando, FL: Academic Press, Inc, 1986:56.
8. LeBlanc A, Schneider V, Spector E, et al. Calcium absorption, endogenous excretion, and endocrine changes during and after long-term bed rest. *Bone* 16:301S, 1995.
9. Ruml LA, Dubois SK, Roberts ML, et al. Prevention of hypercalciuria and stone-forming propensity during prolonged bedrest by alendronate. *J Bone Miner Res* 10:655, 1995.
10. Arnaud SB, Sherrard DJ, Maloney N, et al. Effects of 1-week head-down tilt bed rest on bone formation and the calcium endocrine system. *Aviat Space Environ Med* 63:14, 1992.
11. Van der Wiel HE, Lips P, Nauta J, et al. Biochemical parameters of bone turnover during ten days of bed rest and subsequent mobilization. *Bone Miner* 13:123, 1991.
12. Bergmann P, Heilporn A, Schoutens A, et al. Longitudinal study of calcium and bone metabolism in paraplegic patients. *Paraplegia* 15:147, 1977–1978.
13. Stewart AF, Adler M, Byers CM, et al. Calcium homeostasis in immobilization: an example of resorptive hypercalciuria. *N Engl J Med* 306:1136, 1982.
14. Krolner B, Toft B. Vertebral bone loss: an unheeded side effect of therapeutic bed rest. *Clin Sci* 64:537, 1983.
15. LeBlanc AD, Schneider VS, Evans HJ, et al. Bone mineral loss and recovery after 17 weeks of bed rest. *J Bone Miner Res* 5:843, 1990.
16. LeBlanc A, Marsh C, Evans H, et al. Bone and muscle atrophy with suspension of the rat. *J Appl Physiol* 58:1669, 1985.
17. Young DR, Niklowitz WJ, Brown RJ, et al. Immobilization-associated osteoporosis in primates. *Bone* 7:109, 1986.
18. Biering-Sørensen F, Bohr HH, Schaadt OP. Longitudinal study of bone mineral content in the lumbar spine, the forearm and the lower extremities after spinal cord injury. *Eur J Clin Invest* 20:330, 1990.
19. Minaire P, Meunier P, Edouard C, et al. Quantitative histological data on disuse osteoporosis: comparison with biological data. *Calcif Tissue Res* 17:57, 1974.
20. Vico L, Chappard D, Alexandre C, et al. Effects of a 120-day period of bed-rest on bone mass and bone cell activities in man: attempts at countermeasure. *Bone Miner* 2: 383, 1987.
21. Palle S, Vico L, Bourrin S, et al. Bone tissue response to four month antiorthostatic bedrest: a bone histomorphometric study. *Calcif Tissue Int* 51:189, 1992.
22. Lueken SA, Arnaud SB, Taylor AK, et al. Changes in markers of bone formation and resorption in a bed rest model of weightlessness. *J Bone Miner Res* 8:1433, 1993.
23. Bloomfield SA, Mysiw WJ, Jackson RD. Bone mass and endocrine adaptations to training in spinal cord injured individuals. *Bone* 19:61, 1996.
24. Jaworski ZF, Uhthoff HK. Reversibility of nontraumatic disuse osteoporosis during its active phase. *Bone* 7:431, 1986.
25. Bourrin S, Palle S, Genty C, et al. Physical exercise during remobilization restores a normal bone trabecular network after tail suspension-induced osteopenia in young rats. *J Bone Miner Res* 10:820, 1995.
26. Tilton FE, DeGioanni JJ, Schneider VS. Long-term follow-up of Skylab bone demineralization. *Aviat Space Environ Med* 51:1209, 1980.
27. Kannus P, Järvinen M, Seivänen H, et al. Osteoporosis in men with a history of tibial fracture. *J Bone Miner Res* 9: 423, 1994.
28. Heaney RP. The natural history of vertebral osteoporosis. Is low bone mass an epiphenomenon? *Bone* 13:S23, 1992.
29. Dudley GA, Duvoisin MR, Convertino VA, Buchanan P. Alterations of the *in vivo* torque-velocity relationship of human skeletal muscle following 30 days exposure to simulated microgravity. *Aviat Space Environ Med* 60:659, 1989.
30. Dupui P, Montoya R, Costes-Salon MC, et al. Balance and gait analysis after 30 days – 6 degrees bed rest: influence of lower-body negative-pressure sessions. *Aviat Space Environ Med* 63:1004, 1992.
31. Cummings SR, Rubin SM, Black D. The future of hip fractures in the United States. Numbers, costs and potential effects of postmenopausal estrogen. *Clin Orthop* 252:163, 1990.

76 41 87 309

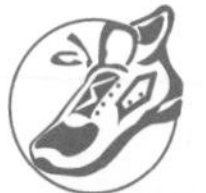  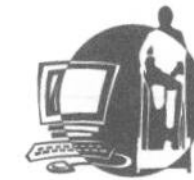 

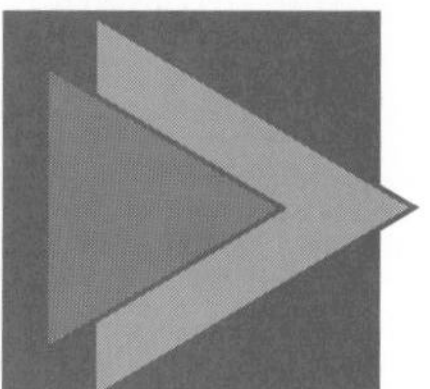

CHAPTER 23

Deconditioning and Bed Rest: Musculoskeletal Response

Gary A. Dudley and Lori L. Ploutz Snyder

Reductions in physical activity are common occurrences that affect almost everyone and are associated with physiological consequences. It is important to understand musculoskeletal adaptations to reduced physical activity so that functional ability can be predicted and appropriate exercise can be prescribed during disuse or rehabilitation. Decreased muscle activity can result from detraining, bed rest, casting, use of crutches, paralysis, aging, or even the microgravity of space flight. The effects of reduced muscular activity are not confined to diseased or disabled populations, but can also affect elite athletic performance or weekend athletes.

The term **decreased muscle activity** refers to reductions in intensity and/or amount of total daily activity performed by a muscle or muscle group. Note that detraining (returning to a sedentary life style after training) does not evoke the same adaptive response as 1 month of bed rest in a sedentary person. The magnitude of the adaptive response to decreased activity depends on relative change in muscle use. For example, bed rest of previously sedentary individuals for 1 month causes greater skeletal muscle atrophy than does cessation of resistance training for the same period (1, 2). Muscle atrophy (reduction in muscle size) from disuse, in this case, is a normal response, not a maladaptation.

TYPES AND DEFINITIONS OF REDUCED USE (UNLOADING)

Detraining

Detraining is that time following the cessation of training in which previously observed adaptations are gradually reduced or lost (3–5). Detraining in athletes often occurs during the off-season when normal training routines are interrupted. Detraining is most often observed in previously sedentary individuals who participate in exercise for several weeks or months, then discontinue participation.

Bed Rest

Periods of bed rest are commonly associated with disease processes, thus it is difficult to determine the exact cause of muscular adaptation. However, bed rest has been used as an experimental model of muscle unloading in healthy individuals to rule out underlying disease and yields similar results as casting or use of crutches (1, 6–10).

Casting

Skeletal muscle adaptations occur as a result of immobilizing a joint with casting. A unique feature to casting is that a joint is typically in a fixed position with the intent of immobilizing injured tissue which also immobilizes muscle at a constant length. Muscles immobilized in a shortened position undergo more severe atrophy than muscles casted in a neutral or lengthened position (11, 12). Furthermore, after several weeks of casting, joint stiffness may be observed and must be considered when prescribing exercise for injured patients.

Crutches

The use of crutches may or may not also be associated with casting. While a casted lower limb often necessitates crutches, minor injuries (sprains and strains) may not require casting, but may require nonweight-bearing. Human lower limb suspension is also used as an experimental technique to study adaptations to unloading (13–19).

Paralysis

Many diseases lead to partial or total paralysis. Spinal cord injuries are responsible for varying degrees of muscle paralysis, often in previously young and active individuals. While it is often difficult to discern how a disease process interacts with muscle disuse to produce functional changes, spinal cord injury is unique in that affected muscles may still be innervated, yet receive no input from higher nervous centers. Thus, muscles are innervated by intact motor neurons but are seldom activated except for spasm (20–25).

Space Flight

Though few individuals participate in space flight, studies of reduced muscle use have been inspired by lack of understanding of the effect of gravity on skeletal muscle. Astronauts adapt muscle function following space flight (26, 27). The mechanism(s) responsible for compromised function and countermeasures or rehabilitation procedures are unknown.

Aging

Decreases in skeletal muscle size and strength occur with increasing age (28, 29). The largest decrements in muscular strength occur after age 50. Decrements average 15% during the 6th and the 7th decades of life and reach 30% per decade thereafter. Much of the reduction in strength is due to a reduction in muscle mass. There is controversy regarding whether these changes are inherent to the aging process, due to reductions in muscle use associated with increasingly sedentary lifestyle, and/or other disease processes.

CONSEQUENCES OF REDUCED USE (UNLOADING) ON SKELETAL MUSCLE

Morphological

Regardless of the method of unloading, the predominant adaptive response to decreased use is skeletal muscle atrophy. Atrophy is the process whereby muscle size is reduced, almost exclusively due to reductions in the contractile proteins actin and myosin (30). Reduction in muscle size may occur through reduced cross-sectional area of individual fibers, a decrease in fiber number, or a combination of these two processes. In unloading of a few weeks to a month, a decrease in fiber cross-sectional area is responsible. This is based on the finding that, after 6 weeks of lower limb suspension, the decrease in average fiber cross-sectional area in vastus lateralis muscle (-14%) was comparable to the decrease in average cross-sectional area of the muscle (-15%) (18). In contrast, reduced fiber numbers due to functional denervation and fiber atrophy appears to contribute to the decreased muscle mass associated with aging (29).

For the first several weeks of disuse, atrophy is almost linearly related to duration and extent of unloading and differs among muscles depending on function (Fig. 23.1). Generally, atrophy is most severe in muscles that are involved in weight bearing and postural control; extensor muscles are typically more severely affected than flexor muscles (8, 18). Likewise, it has recently been shown that the atrophic response of thigh adductor muscles to unloading is intermediate to that of extensor and flexor muscles (Table 23.1) (31). Of particular concern are muscles of the thigh and calf. These are critical in normal ambulation and show marked atrophy in nonweightbearing conditions. Generally, unloading the quadriceps femoris (knee extensor) muscle group causes reduced cross sectional area of about 0.4% per day of unloading (Fig. 23.1).

The atrophic response to detraining appears to occur at least as slowly as the hypertrophic response to training (about 1% per week) (2–5). Thus, the atrophic response to resistance training cessation appears to be slower than to unloading in previously sedentary individuals. There-

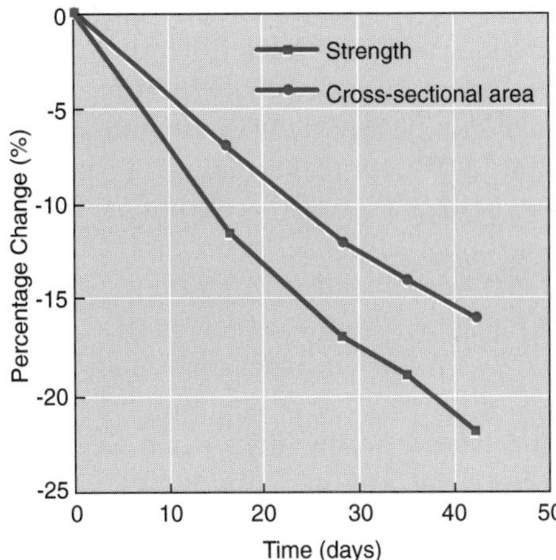

Figure 23.1. Time course of change in knee extensor strength and muscle cross sectional area following unweighting using limb suspension. (Data adapted from Berg HE, Dudley GA, Haggmark T, et al. Effects of lowerlimb unloading on skeletal muscle mass and function in humans. *J Appl Physiol* 70:1882, 1991; Adams GR, Hather BM, Dudley GA. Effect of short-term unweighting on human skeletal muscle strength and size. *Aviat Space Environ Med* 65:1116, 1994; Hather BM, Adams GR, Tesch PA, et al. Skeletal muscle responses to lower limb suspension in humans. *J Appl Physiol* 72:1493, 1992; Ploutz-Snyder LL, Tesch PA, Crittenden DJ, et al. Effect of unweighting on skeletal muscle use during exercise. *J Appl Physiol* 79:168, 1995.)

Table 23.1. Muscle Cross Sectional Area Following 6 Weeks of Unloading

Muscle Group	% Change in Size
Knee extensor	16%
Knee flexor	7%
Knee adductors	9%

Data adapted from Hather BM, Adams GR, Tesch PA, et al. Skeletal muscle responses to lower limb suspension in humans. *J Appl Physiol* 72:1493, 1992; Berg H. Effects of unloading on skeletal muscle mass and function in man. Dissertation, Karolinska Institute, Stockholm 1996.

fore, with respect to muscle atrophy, detraining in exercising individuals is less deleterious than in bedridden, previously sedentary individuals. A short period of detraining may not be especially detrimental, but a bed rest patient should attempt reambulation as early as possible.

In lower mammals, fiber type composition may influence the atrophic response to unloading, however, this has not been demonstrated in humans. Human skeletal muscle, in general, does not present clear segmentation of fiber type as found in lower mammals (32). Fast and slow fibers of human vastus lateralis and soleus muscles show comparable atrophy after 4 to 6 weeks of bed rest (1). Likewise soleus muscle, predominantly slow in humans, does not appear to exhibit greater atrophy after 6 weeks of unloading than the gastrocnemius muscle (18).

Fiber type composition of muscle, especially the relative area of muscle occupied by any given fiber type, has a marked effect on energy demands of contraction. Fast fibers evoke substantially greater energy demand per unit of contractile material compared to slow fibers, and therefore require greater energy supply to sustain contraction. If a muscle becomes relatively faster due to preferential slow fiber atrophy with unloading, the result is increased energy demand per unit of force development and, all other factors being unchanged, increased relative fatigue. Muscle also becomes faster if slow fibers are transformed to fast fibers during unloading. Neither process appears to occur in humans during 4–6 weeks of unloading (1, 9, 14, 16, 18). Thus the energy demand of contraction is apparently not altered during several weeks of unloading in humans. If relative fatigue is increased with short-term unloading in humans, less efficient recruitment and/or compromised energy supply may be responsible.

In contrast to unloading of otherwise healthy individuals, detraining appears to alter fast-twitch fiber in subtype populations (2, 5). Studies show that resistance training evokes a decrease in percent of type IIb fibers and a concomitant increase type IIa fibers in human skeletal muscle. When training is stopped, fiber type composition reverts to that evident prior to training (5). Considered in light of the aforementioned results, it appears that type IIb fibers in human muscle serves as a reserve for type IIa fibers during increased loading, but that at least short term unloading does not provide sufficient stimulus to increase the proportion of these fibers (which are subject to easy fatigue).

The extent to which atrophy occurs depends in large part on the duration and extent of reduced use. Most studies use several weeks unloading. Patients with permanent paralysis, such as in spinal cord injury, exhibit about 50% reduction in muscle size and a shift to almost completely fast muscle after a year of complete muscle disuse (21–24). Although this has not been experimentally documented, it suggests a nadir of atrophic response to disuse. In addition, it appears that with extreme, prolonged unloading, the energy demand of contraction increases and resulting in reduced resistance to fatigue.

Following 6 weeks of unloading of the vastus lateralis muscle, the number of capillaries surrounding each fiber is unchanged, thus capillaries per unit area of muscle (capillary density) actually increases (18). However, in moderate to severe denervation of human gastrocnemius muscle, capillaries per fiber is reduced in proportion to the degree of fiber atrophy, thus capillary density is unchanged (33). This suggests that fiber atrophy exceeds capillary loss during initial weeks of unloading and, thereafter, loss of capillaries normalizes capillary density. In either case, it seems that the diffusional characteristics of capillary/muscle milieu is not compromised by unloading.

Metabolic

The influence of unloading on metabolic characteristics of human skeletal muscle has received less attention than atrophy and reduced strength. Homogenates of muscle biopsies show decreased concentrations of enzyme markers of aerobic oxidative capacity after unloading, while anaerobic enzymes of energy supply do not seem to change (1, 14). Reduced enzymes associated with aerobic capacity may reflect preferential loss of contractile protein with unloading (i.e., aerobic oxidative enzyme content per fiber volume may not change and the anaerobic enzyme content may actually increase) (26, 30). Nonetheless, fiber atrophy results in lower total mitochondrial content, so absolute muscular endurance is compromised by unloading (10, 14). This also suggests that relative muscular endurance is not significantly effected by unloading (14). However, preferential loss of contractile protein requires the remaining muscle to work against greater absolute load. This work is accomplished with reduced total capacity for aerobic-oxidative energy supply because mitochondrial content is lower.

Unlike short-term unloading, spinal cord injury appears to reduce mitochondrial content, not only because of the atrophy these patients present, but also because there are fewer mitochondria per unit volume of contractile machinery (21). This limited ability for aerobic-oxidative energy supply may, in part, account for poor fatigue resistance evident after spinal cord injury (20, 21).

Strength and Local Muscular Endurance

Unloading results in reduced muscular strength, regardless of the type of action or movement performed or the method of strength expression (6–10, 13–19, 34). Strength reduction is nearly linearly related to the duration of unloading and extent of muscle atrophy for the first few weeks (Fig. 23.1). Atrophy accounts for a large part, but not all, of decreased force production, suggesting that the ability to activate muscle is also compromised by unloading (see below). This is interesting because marked force during eccentric, isometric and slow-speed, concentric muscle contraction is believed to be controlled by some neural inhibitory mechanisms (35, 36). However, the relative decline in strength is comparable across speeds and types of muscle actions, thus increased inhibition is not responsible for reduced voluntary activation, or if so, the reduction is uniform across speeds and types of muscle actions (6, 9, 13, 17).

The lack of shape change in the speed-torque relationship with short-term unloading may suggest that muscle fiber type composition is not altered. However, as transformation to a "faster" muscle occurs with long-term, extreme unloading, an increased ability to maintain force, as speed increases during concentric actions, should be evident (35). This finding has been reported after long-term space flight (26). However, 120 days of unloading (of otherwise healthy individuals) did not alter relative rise time during surface electrical stimulation of the triceps surae muscle group, suggesting that myofibrillar actomyosin ATPase activity is not altered by 3 months of disuse (34). Likewise, time to peak tension for a twitch of tibialis anterior muscle has been reported comparable between spinal cord injured patients and healthy controls, suggesting that calcium kinetics are not markedly altered by long term unloading (20). Comparable twitch mechanics in spinal cord injured patients and healthy controls may be interpreted to infer that fiber type composition of muscle and, thereby, myofibrillar actomyosin ATPase activity are not altered by spinal cord injury. Martin et al. reports this finding in patients with spinal cord injuries (21). Thus, a muscle appears "faster" in spinal cord injured patients than controls, yet is comparable to healthy individuals for myofibrillar actomyosin ATPase activity and mechanical function.

The magnitude of strength reduction is also specific to muscle group, with weight bearing muscles most affected (Table 23.2). For knee extensors, decline in strength averages about 0.6% per day. In contrast, the first dorsal interosseus hand muscle is relatively resistant to adaptation after 3–5 weeks of immobilization (37).

Table 23.2. Muscle Strength Following 5 Weeks of Unweighting

Muscle Group	% Change in Strength
Knee extensor	20%
Knee flexor	8%
Ankle extensor	26%
Ankle flexor	10%

Data adapted from Gogia PP, Schneider VS, LeBlanc AD, et al. Bed rest effect on extremity muscle torque in healthy men. *Arch Phys Med Rehabil* 69:1030, 1988; LeBlanc A, Gogia P, Schneider V, et al. Calf muscle area and strength changes after five weeks of horizontal bed rest. *Am J Sports Med* 16:624, 1988.

Neuromuscular

Decreased strength with reduced use has consistently been shown to be greater than that explained by muscle atrophy (19). An exception to this concept has been reported after short-term space flight. Muscle strength decreases in proportionately similar amounts, or perhaps less than fiber size after 5 or 11 days of unloading (about 15% vs 20%) (26). This implies increased ability to recruit muscle and/or greater specific tension (force per unit muscle size). Neither has been reported in studies of unloading at normal gravity (9, 10, 30). Thus, neuromuscular impairment may occur after unloading.

Electromyographic (EMG) studies demonstrate that maximal firing rate and maximal integrated EMG activity are decreased and periods of silent EMG activity appear during maximal voluntary contractions after unloading (38). The ability to recruit high threshold motor units also seems to be compromised (10). The greater relative decline in strength than size suggests more muscle might be used to perform a given submaximal task. This has recently been reported using magnetic resonance imaging (MRI) and supports EMG analyses where greater numbers of motor units are required to develop submaximal force (9, 15, 19, 39).

The exercise professional should account for these neuromuscular adaptations to unloading in exercise prescription for subjects recovering from reduced muscular activity. Submaximal loads that were once easily accomplished require more absolute muscle involvement. Additionally, individuals may not have visible muscle atrophy, but may be particularly weak due to irregularities in motor control.

VULNERABILITY TO MUSCLE DAMAGE

Recently it has been shown that unloading lower limb skeletal muscle for 5 weeks increases vulnerability to eccentric, exercise-induced dysfunction and muscle injury (39). Following 5 weeks of unloading one lower limb, strength is reduced by 20%. Submaximal eccentric exercise performed by the already weakened limb results in further reductions in strength. There are no changes in strength in contralateral, weight bearing muscle. MRI, obtained 3 days after eccentric exercise, demonstrated muscle damage over the unloaded cross-sectional area while none was evident in the contralateral weight bearing limb.

These results are of practical importance to the exercise professional. Dysfunction and injury during reloading may be sufficient to prolong recovery. In the previous study, 10 days after the eccentric exercise, strength remained reduced by 20% (pre-unloading). Low-intensity exercise should be used with care initially during reambulation to minimize muscle dysfunction and injury.

Increased vulnerability to exercise-induced muscle injury has also been reported in elderly (28). Whether this is due to aging and/or low physical activity is not known, but when starting an exercise program, caution is recommended.

POSSIBLE COUNTERMEASURES

There is little data regarding efficacy of various countermeasures designed to prevent muscle atrophy and dysfunction or to enhance recovery during disuse. Endurance activity enhances fatigue resistance of skeletal muscle during unloading. Electrical stimulation of tibialis anterior muscle for 45 minutes to 2 hours per day in complete spinal cord injured patients evoked a marked increase in ability to maintain force during contraction. This response is attributed in part to increased muscle fiber aerobic-oxidative enzyme content (20, 21). Endurance activation does not increase fiber size. Resistance-like exercise (high-force intermittent stimulation) in spinal cord injured patients or ladder climbing in hindlimb suspended rats, however, has been shown to increase muscle size, yet not improve endurance (23, 25, 40). Designing a program combining some aspects of endurance and high force conditioning, whether evoked by electrical stimulation or voluntary means may be helpful in these cases (41). Data supporting this have been reported in cardiomyoplasty (42).

Although it is not clear to what extent disuse is responsible for neuromuscular dysfunction in the elderly, it is clear that resistance exercise training can be used by individuals to increase strength and muscle mass (29). This may enhance performance of activities of daily living, decrease severity and occurrence of fall related injury, and delay onset of disease.

Retraining

Short-term retraining after detraining appears to return muscle strength and size to that of the previously trained state (5). However, it appears that there is less deconditioning than expected during detraining and more rapid adaptation after resuming training than expected.

References

1. Hikida RS, Gollnick PD, Dudley GA, et al. Structural and metabolic characteristics of human skeletal muscle following 30 days of simulated microgravity. *Aviat Space Environ Med* 60:664, 1989.
2. Hather BM, Bruce M, Tesh PA, et al. Influence of eccentric actions on skeletal muscle adaptations to resistance training. *Acta Physiol Scand* 143:177, 1991.
3. Narici MV, Roi GS, Landoni L, et al. Changes in force, cross-sectional area and neural activation during strength training and detraining of the human quadriceps. *Eur J Appl Physiol* 59:310, 1989.
4. Houston ME, Froese EA, Valeriote P, et al. Muscle performance, morphology and metabolic capacity during strength training and detraining: a one leg model. *Eur J Appl Physiol* 51:25, 1983.
5. Staron RS, Leonardi MJ, Karapondo DL, et al. Strength and skeletal muscle adaptations in heavy-resistance-trained women after detraining and retraining. *J Appl Physiol* 70: 631, 1991.
6. Dudley GA, Duvoisin MR, Convertino VA, et al. Alterations of the in vivo torque-velocity relationship of human skeletal muscle following 30 days exposure to simulated microgravity. *Aviat Space Environ Med* 60:659, 1989.
7. Gogia PP, Schneider VS, LeBlanc AD, et al. Bed rest effect on extremity muscle torque in healthy men. *Arch Phys Med Rehabil* 69:1030, 1988.
8. LeBlanc A, Gogia P, Schneider V, et al. Calf muscle area and strength changes after five weeks of horizontal bed rest. *Am J Sports Med* 16:624, 1988.
9. Berg HE, Larsson L, Tesch PA. Lower limb skeletal muscle function after 6 weeks of bedrest. *J Appl Physiol* 82:182–188, 1996.
10. Duchateau J. Bed rest induces neural and contractile adaptations in triceps surae. *Med Sci Sports Exerc* 27:1581, 1995.
11. Goldspink DF, Morton AJ, Loughna P, et al. The effect of hypokinesia and hypodynamia on protein turnover and the growth of four skeletal muscles of the rat. *Pflugers Arch* 407:333, 1986.
12. Pattullo MC, Cotter MA, Cameron NE, et al. Effects of lengthened immobilization on functional and histochemical properties of rabbit tibialis anterior muscle. *Exptl Physiol* 77:433, 1992.
13. Berg HE, Dudley GA, Haggmark T, et al. Effects of lower-limb unloading on skeletal muscle mass and function in humans. *J Appl Physiol* 70:1882, 1991.
14. Berg HE, Dudley GA, Hather BM, et al. Work capacity and metabolic and morphologic characteristics of the human quadriceps muscle in response to unloading. *Clin Physiol* 13:337, 1993.
15. Berg HE, Tesch PA. Changes in muscle function in response to 10 days of lower limb unloading in humans. *Acta Physiol Scand* 157:63–70, 1996.
16. Adams GR, Hather BM, Dudley GA. Effect of short-term unweighting on human skeletal muscle strength and size. *Aviat Space Environ Med* 65:1116, 1994.
17. Dudley GA, Duvoisin MR, Adams GR, et al. Adaptations to unilateral lower limb suspension in humans. *Aviat Space Environ Med* 63:678, 1992.
18. Hather BM, Adams GR, Tesch PA, et al. Skeletal muscle responses to lower limb suspension in humans. *J Appl Physiol* 72:1493, 1992.
19. Ploutz-Snyder LL, Tesch PA, Crittenden DJ, et al. Effect of unweighting on skeletal muscle use during exercise. *J Appl Physiol* 79:168, 1995.
20. Stein RB, T Gordon T, Jefferson J, et al. Optimal stimulation of paralyzed muscle after human spinal cord injury. *J Appl Physiol* 72:1393, 1992.
21. Martin TP, Stein RB, Hoeppner PH, et al. Influence of electrical stimulation on the morphological and metabolic

properties of paralyzed muscle. *J Appl Physiol* 72:1401, 1992.

22. Taylor PN, Edwins BJ, Fox B, et al. Limb blood flow, cardiac output and quadriceps muscle bulk following spinal cord injury and the effect of training for the Odstock functional electrical stimulation standing system. *Paraplegia* 31: 303, 1993.
23. Pacy PJ, Evans RH, Halliday D. Effect of anaerobic and aerobic exercise promoted by computer regulated functional electrical stimulation (FES) on muscle size, strength and histology in paraplegic males. *Pros Ortho Intl* 11:75, 1987.
24. Round JM, Barr FM, Moffat B, et al. Fibre areas and histochemical fibre types in the quadriceps muscle of paraplegic subjects. *J Neurol Sci* 116:207, 1993.
25. Rabischong F, Ohanna F. Effects of functional electrical stimulation (FES) on evoked muscular output in paraplegic quadriceps muscle. *Paraplegia* 30:467, 1992.
26. Edgerton VR, Zhou MY, Ohira Y, et al. Human fiber size and enzymatic properties after 5 and 11 days of spaceflight. *J Appl Physiol* 78:1733, 1995.
27. LeBlanc A, Rowe R, Schneider V, et al. Regional muscle loss after short duration spaceflight. *Aviat Space Environ Med* 66: 1151, 1995.
28. Manfredi TG, Fielding RA, O'Reilly KP, et al. Plasma creatine kinase activity and exercise-induced muscle damage in older men. *Med Sci Sports Exerc* 23:1028, 1991.
29. Tseng BS, Marsh DR, Hamilton MT, et al. Strength and aerobic training attenuate muscle wasting and improve resistance to the development of disability with aging. *J Gerontol Series A* 50A(Spec issue):113, 1995.
30. Kandarin, SC, Boushel RC, Schulte LM. Elevated interstitial fluid volume in rat soleus muscles by hindlimb unweighting. *J Appl Physiol* 71:910, 1991.
31. Berg H. Effects of unloading on skeletal muscle mass and function in man. Dissertation, Karolinska Institute, Stockholm 1996.
32. Roy RR, Baldwin KM, Edgerton VR. The plasticity of skeletal muscle effects of neuromuscular activity. *Exerc Sports Sci Rev* 19:269, 1991.
33. Carpenter S, Karpati G. Necrosis of capillaries in denervation atrophy of human skeletal muscle. *Muscle Nerve* 5: 250, 1982.
34. Koryak Y. Contractile properties of the human triceps surae muscle during simulated weightlessness. *Eur J Appl Physiol* 70:344, 1995.
35. Harris RT, Dudley GA. Factors limiting force during slow, shortening actions of the quadriceps femoris muscle group in vivo. *Acta Physiol Scand* 152:63, 1994.
36. Westing SH, Seger H, Thorstensson A. Effects of electrical stimulation on eccentric and concentric torque-velocity relationships during knee extension in man. *Acta Physiol Scand* 140:17, 1990.
37. Fuglevand AJ, Bilodeau M, Enoka RM. Short-term immobilization has a minimal effect on the strength and fatigability of a human hand muscle. *J Appl Physiol* 78:847, 1995.
38. Duchateau J, Hainaut K. Effects of immobilization on contractile properties, recruitment and firing rates of human motor units. *J Physiol* 422:55, 1990.
39. Ploutz-Snyder LL, Tesch PA, Hather BM, et al. Vulnerability to dysfunction and muscle injury after unloading. *Arch Phys Med Rehabil* 77:773–777, 1996.
40. Herbert ME, Roy RR, Edgerton VR. Influence of one-week hindlimb suspension and intermittent high load exercise on rat muscles. *Exptl Neurol* 102:190, 1988.
41. Cavanagh, PR, Davis BL, Miller TA. A biomechanical perspective on exercise countermeasures for long term spaceflight. *Aviat Space Environ Med* 63:482, 1992.
42. Badylak SF, Hinds M, Geddes LA. Comparison of three methods of electrical stimulation for converting skeletal muscle to a fatigue resistant power source suitable for cardiac assistance. *Ann Biomed Engr* 18:239, 1990.

201 30,189 345

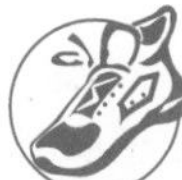

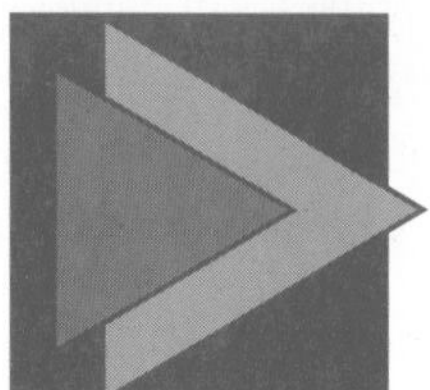

CHAPTER **24**

ENVIRONMENTAL CONSIDERATIONS: HEAT AND COLD

Thomas E. Bernard

The prevailing thermal environment can profoundly change the physiological response to exercise and increase the risk of an environmentally-related disorder. An understanding of the inter-relationships between thermal environment and exercise allows better management of risk for heat or cold disorders during exercise by exercise professionals.

The physiological response to heat and cold are different and the disorders associated with each stressor differ fundamentally. This chapter presents the interaction between the environment and exercise, disorders that may occur, and a management plan for managing adverse environmental stress.

HEAT STRESS

Heat stress is the combination of environmental conditions, metabolic rate, and clothing that increases core temperature. The traditional approach to study and assess heat stress is to describe the balance that must be achieved between all sources of heat gain and heat loss (1–3). If a balance cannot be achieved, then risk for excessive core temperature increases. A basic understanding of heat exchange is necessary to appreciate the interactions of environment, exercise, and clothing. The risk of a serious heat-related disorder is associated with the level of heat stress and control of risk is based on maintaining health and managing exposure to heat stress.

Heat Balance

The major source of heat gain is internal heat generated by energy metabolism. Approximately 25% of metabolic energy expenditure is actually translated to mechanical work during locomotion (i.e., walking, biking), the remaining 75% is released as heat in contracting muscle (1). As metabolic rate increases to meet increasing demands of exercise, the rate of internal heat generation also increases. Rate of energy expenditure can be estimated using tables or equations (1, 4). An average man (73 kg) walking on a level surface at 1.6 m/s (3.5 mph) has a metabolic rate of about 350 Watts (1).

Sweat Evaporative Cooling

The major avenue of heat loss is evaporative cooling through evaporation of sweat from the skin surface. Evaporative cooling by secreting water onto the skin surface through eccrine sweat glands is one response to heat stress. As water absorbs heat from the skin, it changes from liquid to vapor. The vapor is carried away by surrounding air. Because the heat of vaporization is quite high, small amounts of sweat remove relatively large amounts of heat. Specifically, the evaporation of 0.5 liters of sweat per hour is sufficient to remove the 350 Watts of excess heat in the preceding walking example (2).

If sufficient volumes of sweat are produced quickly enough and evaporation is not impeded, then thermal balance is maintained and core temperature does not rise. This scenario does not occur for several reasons. First, there are physiological limits to sweat evaporation. In the short-term, it is not reasonable to expect a sustained sweat rate >1 L/hr. In the long-term (several hours), rate of evaporation may be further reduced by dehydration (5).

The physiological limit to volume of sweat produced varies by state of acclimation, aerobic fitness, and genetically among individuals (2). Acclimation (also known as acclimatization) is a physiological adjustment that occurs naturally with repeated exposures to heat stress during exercise. Acclimation increases rate of sweating, shortens onset time, and conserves sodium. Resulting benefits include reduced cardiovascular strain and lower core temperature for the same level of heat stress. Most improvement occurs over the initial 3–5 days, with smaller additional improvements over the subsequent 2–7 days (1, 2). As a rule, 1 day of acclimation is lost for every 3 days away from exercise in heat stress, or in the case of illness, 1 day is lost per day of illness. Aerobic fitness is the single best indicator of ability to tolerate heat stress. On the other hand, about 1 in 20 people are heat "intolerant" for unknown reasons (6).

Secondly, the physical limits to rate of evaporative cooling are due to environmental conditions and clothing (1, 3, 7). The primary drive for evaporative cooling is the difference in water vapor pressures on skin and in air. If the difference is small, rate of evaporative cooling is decreased; if the difference is large, the evaporation rate can be sufficient to balance even high rates of metabolic heat. Water vapor pressure on the skin is relatively constant. The vapor pressure of water in air is the primary source of difference in environmental contribution to heat stress. It is for this reason that humidity is an important factor in heat stress. Air movement, as well as humidity, modifies rate of evaporative cooling. If air movement is 2–3 m/sec (4–6 mph), maximum rate of evaporative cooling is achieved; higher speeds do not increase evaporative cooling appreciably (8).

Clothing

Clothing further restricts maximum rate of evaporative cooling. If clothing is placed between skin and environment, the result is decreased cooling ability through evaporation of sweat (2, 7). Under some circumstances, clothing effects are negligible. For example, if air is very dry (low humidity) or if metabolic rate is low, rate of sweat evaporation through clothing is sufficient to allow adequate cooling. The resistance clothing offers to sweat evaporation depends on surface area covered, intrinsic nature of the fabric, number of layers, and construction of the ensemble. To minimize the effect of clothing, the following are important:

- The covered surface area should be as small as is reasonable
- The fabric should be light-weight, open weave (or other material freely allowing water vapor to pass through)
- Trapped air spaces from multiple layers should be minimized
- The construction should be loose with openings to allow air easy movement around and through the clothing.

At the other extreme is clothing that covers most of the body, is impermeable to water vapor (e.g., plastic or rubber rain clothing), and is tightly fitting around openings for arms, legs, and head. Under these conditions, little evaporative cooling can occur.

Convection and Radiation

Other factors that modify overall heat stress are convection and radiation. When the air temperature is greater than skin temperature (nominally 35°C or 95°F), additional heat is added by convection. Conversely, when air temperature is approximately 35°C or lower, some heat is lost by convection. Rate of convection is enhanced by air movement and reduced by clothing insulation. Infrared radiation from the sun and warm/hot surfaces increases heat stress, while cool surfaces reduce heat stress. Clothing insulation reduces rate of heat flow (in either direction) by radiation. Convection and radiation combined usually account for less than 20% of either heat gain or heat loss during exercise.

Physiological Response

The physiological response to heat stress is reflected in body temperature, heart rate, and sweating. Metabolic heat raises temperature of working muscle and circulating blood transports heat to the central organs, causing a rise in core temperature. Additional blood flow carries excess heat to the skin. To move heat from working muscle to the skin, cardiac output increases and blood flow is shunted from splanchnic and renal circulation (9).

HEAT-RELATED DISORDERS

The normal and acceptable response to heat stress includes elevated core temperature, increased heart rate, and water loss due to sweating. Left unchecked, however, these responses may lead to heat-related disorders, as well as psychomotor and cognitive performance decrements. The disorders of particular importance during exercise are the following:

- heat cramps,
- heat syncope,
- dehydration,
- heat exhaustion, and
- heat stroke (1–3).

Table 24.1 lists these disorders and describes signs, symptoms, and first aid. These features of heat disorders should be understood by exercise professionals. Preventive measures are described below.

Heat Cramps and Syncope

Heat cramps are most likely to occur during or after sustained exercise with profuse sweating. Cramps usually appear in fatigued calf or abdominal muscles. Heat syncope may result from dehydration or excessive pooling of blood in peripheral vascular beds. The subsequent hypotension may cause familiar "black-out" symptoms. Recovery is relatively quick and most are generally aware of the occurrence. In addition to adequate hydration, risk for syncope can be reduced by avoiding prolonged standing or rapid transition to an upright posture.

Dehydration and Heat Exhaustion

Dehydration and heat exhaustion are more likely to occur in the unacclimated and in those who ignore hy-

Table 24.1. Heat-related Disorders Including the Symptoms, Signs, and First Aid

Heat Cramps
- Symptom
  - Painful muscle cramps, especially in abdominal or fatigued muscles
- Sign
  - Incapacitating pain in voluntary muscles
- First Aid
  - Rest in cool environment
  - Drink salted water (0.5% salt solution)
  - Massage muscles

Heat Syncope
- Symptoms
  - Blurred vision (gray-out)
  - Fainting (brief) (black-out)
- Sign
  - Brief fainting or near-fainting behavior
  - Normal temperature
- First Aid
  - Lay on back in cool environment
  - Drink water

Dehydration
- Symptoms
  - No early symptoms
  - Fatigue/weakness
  - Dry mouth
- Signs
  - Loss of work capacity
  - Increased response time
- First Aid
  - Fluid and salt replacement

Heat Exhaustion
- Symptoms
  - Fatigue
  - Weakness
  - Blurred vision
  - Dizziness, headache
- Signs
  - High pulse rate
  - Profuse sweating
  - Low blood pressure
  - Insecure gait
  - Pale face
  - Collapse
  - Body temperature: Normal to slightly increased
- First Aid
  - Lay down flat on back in cool environment
  - Drink water
  - Loosen clothing

Heat Stroke
- Symptoms
  - Chills
  - Restless
  - Irritable
- Signs
  - Red face
  - Euphoria
  - Shivering
  - Disorientation
  - Erratic behavior
  - Collapse
  - Unconsciousness
  - Convulsions
  - Body temperature ≥ 40°C (104°F)

First Aid
- Immediate, aggressive, effective cooling
- Transport to hospital

dration practices or early warning signs. In competitive sports, a 5% loss of body weight is not unusual (1, 2). Losses greater than 1.5% should be followed by a period of recovery and rehydration.

Heat Stroke

Heat stroke is a medical emergency and the least suspicion that it may be present justifies an immediate and aggressive response. The risk for heat stroke is greatest among those who abuse alcohol or drugs, who are highly motivated and ignore symptoms of heat exhaustion, or who are heat intolerant (i.e., do not acclimate).

MANAGEMENT OF HEAT STRESS DURING EXERCISE

Exercise in warm or hot environments always carries risk of heat disorder. Risk is increased if exercise is vigorous or clothing is improper or excessive. Managing risk depends on recognition of external factors and adjusting exercise intensity and/or duration appropriately. In addition, there are personal protective practices to follow that can minimize effects of heat stress. This section describes the ways to minimize risk of heat-related disorders during exercise.

External Factors

The wet bulb globe temperature (WBGT) is an environmental index, originally developed for the military and widely accepted for use in occupational health and athletics (1–3). This index accounts for limits of humidity on evaporative cooling by incorporating a wet bulb temperature (T_{wb}, WBT, or WB) and radiation and convection by including a globe temperature (T_g or GT). The dry bulb (air) temperature (T_{air}, T_{db}, DB, or DBT) is also used for exercise in direct sunlight. Instrumentation for directly measuring the WBGT is commercially available. For exposures to direct sunlight:

$$WBGT_{out} = 0.7\ T_{wb} + 0.2\ T_g + 0.1\ T_{db}.$$

When the day is overcast or when the exercise is in the shade or indoors:

$$WBGT_{in} = 0.7\ T_{wb} + 0.3\ T_g.$$

If the instrumentation is not available, WBGT can be estimated (Table 24.2) from air temperature and any one of several measures of humidity, adjusting for direct sunlight. Dew point temperature (T_{dp}) is the best indicator of humidity for outside applications. It is often reported by local news outlets and remains relatively constant during the day (if weather is stable), therefore, it is not required to be "current."

For indoor or outdoor environments, wet bulb temperature can be easily measured by adapting a typical liquid-in-glass or electronic thermometer with a temperature sensitive "bulb." Alternatively, for indoor

Table 24.2. Tables for Estimation of WBGT from Air Temperature and Either (1) Dew Point Temperature, (2) Wet Bulb Temperature, or (3) Relative Humidity. Note that estimated values must be increased by 4°F if exercise is in direct sunlight

Estimate of WBGT (°F) from Air Temperature (T_{air}) and Dew Point Temperature (T_{dp})

T_{DP} °F	T_{air} (°F) 60	65	70	75	80	85	90	95	100	105	110	T_{dp} °C
95	86	88	90	91	93	95	97	99	101	103	105	35
90	80	83	85	87	89	91	93	95	97	99	101	32
85	76	78	80	83	85	87	89	91	93	96	98	28
80	72	74	77	79	81	83	86	88	90	93	95	27
75	69	71	73	76	78	81	83	85	88	90	92	24
70	66	65	71	73	76	78	80	83	85	88	90	21
65	63	66	68	71	73	76	78	81	83	86	88	18
60	61	64	66	69	71	74	76	79	82	84	87	16
55	60	62	64	67	70	72	75	77	80	83	85	10
50	58	60	62	66	68	71	74	76	79	81	84	13
45	58	59	62	64	67	70	72	75	78	80	83	7
40	56	58	61	63	66	69	71	74	77	80	82	4
35	54	57	60	62	66	68	71	73	76	79	82	2
30	53	56	59	62	64	67	70	73	75	78	81	−1
T_{air} (°C)	**16**	**18**	**21**	**24**	**27**	**29**	**32**	**35**	**38**	**41**	**43**	

For outdoor exercise, WBGT can be estimated from the current air temperature an the dew point temperature that has been recorded in the last few hours.

If the exercise occurs in direct sunlight, add 4°F to the estimated WBGT.

Estimate of WBGT (°F) from Air Temperature (T_{air}) and Wet Bulb Temperature (T_{wb})

T_{WB} °F	T_{air} (°F) 60	65	70	75	80	85	90	95	100	105	110	T_{wb} °C
94	84	86	87	88	90	91	93	94	96	97	99	34
92	82	84	85	87	88	90	91	93	94	96	97	33
90	81	83	84	86	87	89	90	92	93	95	96	32
88	80	81	83	84	86	87	89	90	92	93	95	31
86	78	80	81	83	84	86	87	89	90	92	93	30
84	77	78	80	81	83	84	86	87	89	90	92	29
82	75	77	78	80	81	83	84	86	87	89	90	28
80	74	76	77	79	80	82	83	85	86	88	89	27
78	73	74	76	77	79	80	82	83	85	86	88	26
76	71	73	74	76	77	79	80	82	83	85	86	24
74	70	71	73	74	76	77	79	80	82	83	85	23
72	68	70	71	73	74	76	77	79	80	82	83	22
70	67	69	70	72	73	75	76	78	79	81	82	21
64	66	67	69	70	72	73	75	76	78	79	81	20
T_{air} (°C)	**16**	**18**	**21**	**24**	**27**	**29**	**32**	**35**	**38**	**41**	**43**	

For inside or outside, WBGT can be estimated from the current air temperature and the current wet bulb temperature.

If the exercise occurs in direct sunlight, add 4°F to the estimated WBGT.

(continued)

Table 24.2. *(Continued)*

Estimate of WBGT (°F) from Air Temperature (T_{air}) and Relative Humidity (%)

RH °F	T_{air} (°F) 60	65	70	75	80	85	90	95	100	105	110	RH °C
95	60	65	70	75	80	85	90	95	100	105	110	94
90	60	64	69	74	79	85	90	95	100	105	110	90
85	59	64	68	73	78	83	89	95	100	105	110	85
80	59	63	68	72	77	82	88	93	99	105	110	80
75	58	62	67	71	76	81	86	92	98	103	110	75
70	58	62	66	71	76	80	85	90	96	102	108	70
65	57	61	68	70	74	79	84	88	94	100	105	65
60	57	60	66	69	73	78	83	87	93	98	103	60
55	56	60	64	68	72	77	81	86	91	96	101	55
50	55	59	63	67	71	75	80	84	89	94	99	50
45	55	58	62	66	70	74	79	83	88	92	97	45
40	54	58	62	65	69	73	77	82	88	90	95	40
35	54	57	61	64	68	72	76	80	84	89	93	35
30	53	57	60	64	67	71	76	79	83	87	91	30
25	53	56	59	63	66	70	73	77	81	85	89	25
20	52	55	58	62	65	69	72	76	79	83	87	20
15	51	54	58	61	64	67	71	74	76	81	85	15
10	51	54	57	60	63	68	69	73	76	79	82	10
T_{air} (°C)	**16**	**18**	**21**	**24**	**27**	**29**	**32**	**36**	**38**	**41**	**43**	

For inside or outside, WBGT can be estimated from the current air temperature and current relative humidity. Note: Relative humidity is very sensitive to air temperature

If the exercise occurs in direct sunlight, add 4°F to the estimated WBGT.

environments or if dew point is unknown, percent relative humidity (%rh) can be used. The value for %rh **must** be current with air temperature. Knowing air temperature and either dew point temperature, wet bulb temperature, or relative humidity, Table 24.2 can be used to estimate WBGT. If exercise occurs in direct sunlight or on a partly cloudy day, then 4°F is added to the value of WBGT to account for the effects of the sun. Adjustments for state of acclimation, metabolic demands and clothing are required (Table 24.3) (1, 3).

Methods to reduce the level of heat stress include the following:

- Reducing exercise intensity (reduces metabolic rate),
- Rescheduling exercise to cooler times of day or to cooler places, and
- Reducing the amount of clothing.

Personal Protective Practices

Personal protective practices are steps an individual can take to minimize risk of heat disorder (3). Table 24.4

Table 24.3. **Guidance Based on Estimated or Measured Values of Enviromental WBGT Adjusted for Acclimation State, Metabolic Rate, and Clothing**

Adjustments for External Factors

Step 1. Determine environmental WBGT.
Step 2. If not acclimated (no recent heat stress exposure)-add 3°F.
Step 3. If the metabolic rate is light (eg, walking)-subtract 2°F.
If the metabolic rate is heavy (eg, sustained running)-add 2°F.
Step 4. If clothing is multiple layers-add 6°F.
If clothing is impermeable to water-add 15°F.

Level of Heat Stress

- WBGT Description
- < 80°F No Appreciable Heat Stress
- 80–85°F Low Heat Stress: Implement Personal Protective Practices
- 86–88°F Moderate Heat Stress: Increased risk; assure adequate breaks; avoid strenuous exercise
- > 88°F High Heat Stress: Significant risk; consider cancellation of exercise

Table 24.4. Personal Protective Practices to Reduce Risk for Heat Disorder

- Seek relief from heat stress exposure with sensation of extreme discomfort, lightheadedness, nausea, headache, loss of coordination, or weakness.
- Maintain adequate hydration by drinking small amounts of water, sports drinks, diluted citrus-flavored drinks, diluted iced tea, etc. at frequent intervals. (A weight loss of 2% of body weight in 1 day is evidence of dehydration.)
- Maintain a healthy lifestyle through sound diet, adequate sleep, and avoiding drug abuse.
- Avoid heat stress exposure and exercise during acute illness (eg, fever, nausea, vomiting, diarrhea).
- Seek medical advice if diagnosed with a chronic disease (disease or treatment may reduce heat tolerance).
- Reduce expectations if no recent exercise in warm or hot environments.

lists some common personal protective practices. Physiological monitoring is a useful method to assess heat. Oral temperature is a reasonably good measure under certain conditions. Oral temperature can be taken 10–15 minutes after fluid intake or strenuous exercise. Temperatures < 38°C are considered safe, temperatures > 38.5°C indicate the need for immediate relief from exposure. Temperatures between 38°C and 38.5°C suggests that relief is indicated. (Some clinical thermometers employ an infrared detector to estimate tympanic temperature; because hot environments and placement affect the outcome, use these units with caution.)

Heart rate is an easily assessed index of heat strain. Recovery heart rate, assessed approximately 1 minute after discontinuing exercise is a simple and useful method. If recovery heart rate is < 110 beats per minute (bpm), heat stress is not excessive; if the recovery heart rate is > 110 bpm, relief is recommended (11). The use of heart rate monitors with an alarm for heart rate based on an acceptable limit in non-heat stress conditions (e.g., 75% of maximum heart rate) is another protective method (12).

If exercise involves cycles of exercise and recovery, use of either oral temperature or recovery heart rate (or both) may be used to assess length of the exercise and/or recovery period. Elevation of either temperature or heart rate indicates that exercise should be shortened or the recovery period extended.

COLD STRESS

Cold stress is the combination of environment, metabolic rate and clothing that results in heat loss from the core as a whole or from localized areas (2, 3, 13). Cold-related disorders include hypothermia and varying degrees of local tissue damage (1–3, 13). Again, control of cold stress is accomplished through managing risk factors.

Heat Balance

Like heat stress, cold stress is described as a thermal balance between heat gained from metabolism and heat lost to the environment by convection, radiation, and evaporation, as well as conduction (3). The problem, rather than heat accumulation however, is net loss.

The sole source of heat gain during cold stress is metabolic heat released during muscular work along with basal biological processes. As exercise demands increase, rate of heat gain from metabolism increases. If the rate of metabolic heat decreases due to fatigue or changes in demand, a disorder is more likely (13).

Heat Loss

Heat is lost primarily by convection due to the difference between skin and ambient temperature (2, 13, 14). The rate of convection increases with air movement from wind or motion through the air (e.g., cycling or running). Sitting or laying on a cold, solid surface, may cause heat loss by conduction. Cyclic exercise and rest in which there is accumulation of heat and sweating under clothing may be associated with heat loss through evaporation. Additional loss by radiant heat flow to colder surfaces is also possible.

Clothing

Proper clothing is the primary mechanism for achieving thermal balance during cold stress (13, 14). The amount of insulation that clothing affords is described in units called "clo." A wool business suit has an insulating value of approximately 1 clo. Generally, each 1/4 inch of clothing adds one clo of insulation. Figure 24.1 illustrates the relationship among air temperature, metabolic rate, and clothing in maintaining thermal balance (14). The insulating quality of clothing decreases precipitously when it becomes wet.

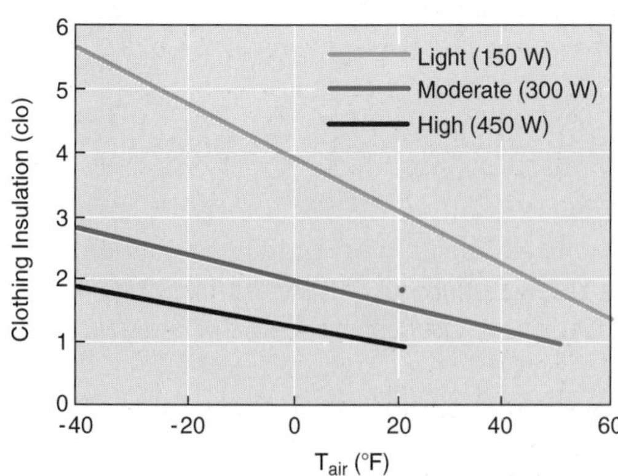

Figure 24.1. Relationship between air temperature and adequate clothing insulation for three levels of exercise.

Sometimes, clothing is sufficient to protect from hypothermia, but exposed skin is still at risk for excessive local cooling. The major method of heat loss is convection, but conduction via contact with cold objects can also occur. Adequate heating from circulating blood may not be available because of reductions in peripheral blood flow (vasoconstriction) that naturally occur as a mechanism for heat conservation.

COLD-RELATED DISORDERS

Normal physiological response to cold stress is directed toward heat conservation, decreasing peripheral circulation and increasing metabolic rate. These mechanisms, however, are not adequate for most cold stress exposure and behavioral thermal regulation is crucial for preventing cold-related disorders. Cold-related disorders can be systemic or local. Table 24.5 list of some common cold-related disorders along with symptoms, signs, and steps for first aid (1–3, 13).

Systemic

The systemic cold disorder is hypothermia. Mild cases are marked by shivering and cold sensation in extremities. Progression is associated with unstable cardiac function followed by central nervous system depression. Mild cases can be addressed by simple first aid, but moderate to severe hypothermia requires medical attention.

Local Disorders

Acute, local disorders are associated with localized tissue freezing (frostbite) or cooling (frostnip and trench foot). Frostbite can occur only when ambient temperature is < −1°C (30°F): it is marked by actual crystallization of water in tissue and subsequent destruction of cells. Because of the risk of further complication, significant cases of frostbite should be referred to medical personnel. Frostnip and trench foot are skin disorders resulting from extreme cooling of the skin and underlying tissue, but without actual freezing of water in the tissue. The distinguishing characteristic between frostnip and trench foot is the presence of damp clothing accelerating heat loss.

Table 24.5. Cold-related Disorders Including Symptoms, Signs and First Aid

Hypothermia
- Symptoms
  - Chills
  - Fatigue or drowsiness
  - Pain in the extremities
- Signs
  - Euphoria
  - Slurred speech
  - Slow, weak pulse
  - Shivering
  - Collapse and/or unconsciousness
  - Body core temperature < 35°C (95°F)
- First Aid
  - Move to warm area and remove wet clothing
  - Modest external warming
  - Drink warm, carbohydrate-containing fluids
  - Transport to hospital

Frostbite
- Symptoms
  - Burning sensation at first
  - Coldness, numbness, tingling
- Signs
  - Skin color white or grayish yellow to reddish violet to black
  - Blisters
  - Response to touch depends on depth of freezing
- First Aid
  - Move to warm area and remove wet clothing
  - External warming (e.g., warm water)
  - Drink warm, carbohydrate-containing fluids if conscious
  - Treat as a burn, do not rub affected area
  - Transport to hospital

Frostnip
- Symptoms
  - Possible itching or pain
- Signs
  - Skin turns white
- First Aid
  - Similar to frostbite

Trench Foot
- Symptoms
  - Severe pain
  - Tingling, itching
- Signs
  - Edema
  - Blisters
  - Response to touch depends on depth of freezing
- First Aid
  - Similar to frostbite

MANAGEMENT OF COLD STRESS DURING EXERCISE

Environmental conditions, especially air temperature and air speed, along with exercise demands are considered in management of cold stress. Ultimately, cold stress is managed through personal protective practices (3).

Evaluation of Cold Stress

Air temperature alone has utility for predicting degree of cold stress, but the role of air motion in facilitating loss of heat is also of importance. The Equivalent Chill Temperature (ECT) accounts for both air temperature and motion. ECT translates a combination of air temperature and motion into an equivalent air temperature with no air motion. Table 24.6 is used to determine ECT. The table provides guidance with regard to overall risk of experiencing a cold-related disorder with an emphasis on exposed skin (1, 3). Table 24.7 provides guidelines for cold stress as a function of air temperature (T_{air}) and ECT. Generally, some risk may be present with exercise at air temperatures < 50°F.

Table 24.6. Table for Determining Equivalent Chill Temperature (ECT) in °F from Air Temperature and Air Motion

Air Speed		Air Temperature (°F)											
		50	40	30	20	10	0	−10	−20	−30	−40	−50	−60
mph	m/s	Equivalent Chill Temperature (ECT) (°F)											
0	0.0	50	40	30	20	10	0	−10	−20	−30	−40	−50	−60
5	2.2	48	37	27	16	6	−5	−15	−26	−36	−47	−57	−68
10	4.5	40	28	16	4	−9	−24	−33	−46	−58	−70	−83	−95
15	6.7	36	22	9	−5	−18	−32	−45	−58	−72	−85	−99	−112
20	8.9	32	18	4	−10	−25	−39	−53	−67	−82	−96	−110	−121
25	11	30	16	0	−15	−29	−44	−59	−74	−88	−104	−118	−133
30	13	28	13	−2	−18	−33	−48	−63	−79	−94	−109	−125	−140
35	16	27	11	−4	−20	−35	−51	−67	−82	−98	−113	−129	−145
> 35	>16	26	10	−6	−21	−37	−53	−69	−85	−100	−116	−132	−148
		Little Danger If exposures with dry skin are less than 60 min. Caution: Avoid false sense of security.				**Increasing Danger** Exposed flesh may freeze within 1 min.			**Great Danger** Flesh may freeze within 30 sec.				

Caution: Trench foot may occur anywhere on this chart.

Developed by the US Army Research Institute of Environmental Medicine, Natick MA

Table 24.7. Cold Stress Guidance Based on Air Temperature (T_{air}) and Equivalent Chill Temperature (ECT)

Risk	T_{air}(°F)<	ECT (°F)<
Decreases in manual dexterity	60	
Hypothermia (no special clothing)	50	50
Hypothermia (with special clothing)	see Figure 24.1	
Frostnip		−22
Frostbite	30	
Prolonged contact with objects	30	
Incidental contact with objects	19	

Table 24.8. Personal Protective Practices to Reduce the Risk for Cold Disorders

- Seek relief from cold stress exposure with sensation of extreme discomfort especially in extremities, fatigue or weakness, or loss of coordination.
- Frequently drink warm, non-caffeinated fluids containing carbohydrates.
- Anticipate, wear, and adjust (as necessary) proper clothing.
- Change wet clothing immediately, especially if the air temperature is < 36°F.
- Plan exercise to avoid fatigue at a location removed from a warm recovery station.
- Maintain a healthy lifestyle through sound diet, adequate sleep, and avoiding drug abuse.
- Seek medical advice for repeated or unusual intolerance to cold, such as repeated episodes of frostnip, appearances of welts, or severe shivering. Medical approval for exercise at ECT < −11°F is recommended.

(Appropriate practices are recommended for exercise at air temperatures below 50°F.)

Personal Protective Practices

Personal responsibility is key for successful management of cold stress. Table 24.8 provides minimal protective practices for risk management of cold-related disorders (3).

▶ SUMMARY

Environmental stressors such as heat and cold can significantly affect exercise and can also be dangerous if uncontrolled. Adequate preventive precautions for both heat and cold are possible and should be known by exercise professionals. Situations requiring medical attention are not infrequent and immediate referral of problems can be important.

References

1. McArdle D, Katch FI, Katch VL, eds. *Exercise Physiology*, 4th ed. Philadelphia: Lea & Febiger, 1996.
2. Pandolf B, Sawka MN, Gonzalez RG, eds. *Human Performance Physiology and Environmental Medicine at Terrestrial Extremes.* Carmel, IN: Cooper Publishing Group, 1986.
3. Bernard E. Thermal Stress. In: Plog BA, ed. *Fundamentals in Industrial Hygiene.* Itasca, IL: National Safety Council, 1996.
4. Eastman Kodak Company. *Ergonomic Design for People at Work, Volume 2.* New York: Van Nostrand Reinhold, 1986.

5. International Organization for Standardization (ISO). Hot environments-Analytical determination and interpretation of thermal stress using calculation of required sweat rate. Geneva: ISO 7933, 1989.
6. Wyndham CH, Strydom NB, Benade JS, et al. Heat stroke risk in unacclimatized and acclimatized men of different maximum oxygen intakes working under hot humid conditions. Chamber of Mines Research Report No 12/72, Johannesburg, South Africa: Chamber of Mines of South Africa, 1972.
7. Parsons KC. *Human Thermal Environments.* Bristol, PA: Taylor & Francis Inc, 1993.
8. Kamon E, Avellini BD. Wind speed limits to work under hot environments for clothed men. *J Appl Physiol* 46:340–349, 1979.
9. Rowell LB. *Human Cardiovascular Control.* Cary, NC: Oxford University Press, 1994.
10. Kenney WL, Humphrey RH, Bryant CX, et al, eds. ACSM's Guidelines for Exercise Testing and Prescription, 5th ed. Baltimore: Williams & Wilkins, 1995.
11. Bernard TE, Kenney WL. Heart rate recovery. American Industrial Hygiene Conference, 1988.
12. Humen DP, Boughner DR. Evaluation of commercially available heart rate monitors. *Can Med Assoc J* 131:585–589, 1984.
13. Holmér I. Cold Stress. Part I—Guidelines for the practitioner, and Part II—The scientific basis (knowledge base) for the guide. *Intl J Indust Ergonomics* 14:139–159, 1994.
14. Holmér I. Assessment of cold stress in terms of required clothing insulation—IREQ. *Intl J Indust Ergonomics* 3:159–166, 1988.

30, 189 345

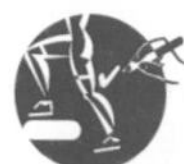

CHAPTER 25

Exercise and the Environment: Altitude and Air Pollution

George Havenith and Michael Holewijn

The condition of ambient air, which is inhaled into the lungs for respiratory gas exchange, is of great importance for exercise capacity, physiological performance and general health. Two main characteristics of ambient air are discussed in this chapter: density, which changes with altitude, and contaminants, generally referred to as air pollution. It is necessary to be aware of possible hazards since exposure to altitude and polluted air can have profound effects on physical performance and can cause serious illness even in well-trained individuals.

HIGH TERRESTRIAL ALTITUDE

Considerable evidence exists that altitude training is beneficial in preparation for competition at altitude, therefore many athletes spend considerable resources training at altitude. However, the value of this training for increasing performance at sea level is controversial. The lack of consensus may be attributed to differences in duration of exposure to altitude, elevations of training, and initial fitness levels (1). Recent studies indicate that, under specific conditions, intermittent altitude exposure might have some beneficial effects for sea-level performance (2, 3). In this section, physiological responses that occur at altitudes up to 3,000 m are discussed. Above 3,000 m, the negative effects of prolonged exposure to hypoxia outweigh the potential positive training effects of exposure to hypoxia (4).

Physiological Responses

The amount of oxygen bound to hemoglobin in red blood cells depends on the partial pressure of oxygen in the inspired air (P_IO_2). P_IO_2 decreases as a result of declines in barometric pressure with increasing altitude at constant oxygen percentage (Table 25.1). There is a fall in the arterial oxygen saturation (PaO_2) with the decline in P_IO_2 and thus in the amount of oxygen available. Acute exposure to reduced oxygen saturation triggers several compensatory mechanisms to increase oxygen transfer to tissue. Following these acute reactions acclimatization occurs with more fundamental adaptations.

Acute Physiological Responses

One of the most significant physiological compensatory reactions during acute exposure above 1,200 m, is increased pulmonary ventilation (hypoxic ventilatory response [HVR]) at rest and during exercise. Chemoreceptors in arterial blood vessels are stimulated and signals are sent to the brain to increase ventilation. The increase in pulmonary ventilation is primarily associated with an increase in tidal volume, but with prolonged exposure or higher altitude, breathing frequency also increases. Hyperventilation substantially increases the arterial oxygen saturation. Increased ventilation also leads to "wash out" of carbon dioxide in the blood. Therefore, uncompensated respiratory alkalosis (higher pH) may develop. This respiratory alkalosis can cause a "left shift" of the oxygen-hemoglobin dissociation curve resulting in a higher arterial oxygen saturation, a second compensatory mechanism (5). Finally, during early altitude exposure, reduced oxygen pressure is compensated for by small increases in cardiac output. This is primarily due to an increased heart rate, since stroke volume is constant or even slightly reduced at rest and during submaximal and maximal exercise.

Despite acute responses that compensate for lower oxygen tension at altitude, arterial oxygen saturation is decreased (Fig. 25.1). The magnitude of desaturation is directly related to altitude and exercise intensity. The primary pulmonary factor leading to increasing desaturation with increasing exercise intensity is limited alveolar-end-capillary diffusion. The result is an almost linear decrease of maximal oxygen uptake at a ratio of 10% per 1,000 m altitude above 1,500 m (6). Since the oxygen uptake required by a fixed submaximal workload is not affected by altitude, the result is higher relative exercise intensity for any given workload.

Muscular strength or muscular endurance seem unaffected during acute exposure to altitude. However, subtle

Table 25.1. Barometric Pressure (for a standard atmosphere) and Inspired Partial Oxygen Pressure for Five Altitudes, Accounting for the Pressure of Water Vapor in the Lungs (47 mm Hg)

Altitude (m)	Barometric Pressure (mm Hg)	Inspired Oxygen Pressure (P_IO_2)
0	760	149
1500	627	123
2000	596	115
2500	627	107
3000	522	100

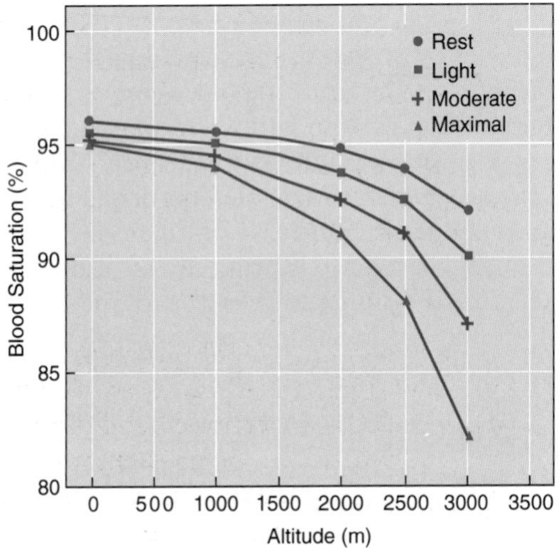

Figure 25.1. The effect of altitude and exercise levels on arterial oxygen saturation.

neuropsychological effects associated with acute mountain sickness can occur at altitudes of 3,000 m within 6 hours of exposure. Above 4,500 m, the deterioration for most mental functions may be considerable, although large inter-individual variation exists (7). These neuropsychological effects may, in turn, affect muscular strength and endurance.

Long-term Physiological Responses (Acclimatization)

With prolonged stay at altitude (days to weeks), acclimatization occurs. This includes adjustments at the pulmonary, circulatory, and muscle tissue (cellular) level. Within 3–4 days, the increase in resting ventilatory rate at moderate altitude (± 3,000 m) is stabilized at 40% above sea-level values. The increase in exercise ventilation rate also stabilizes, but in a longer time frame depending on exercise intensity and altitude. After acclimatization, pulmonary ventilation during exercise can increase 100% over sea level controls. This increase is more pronounced at heavier workloads (8).

Red cell production increases (polycythemia) within 2 weeks, leading to a 4–12% increase in hemoglobin (9). Increased red blood cell production is the result of a substantial increase in erythropoietin (EPO) hormone concentration (9). Maximum levels of EPO (produced in the kidney) occur within the first few days, followed by a gradual fall to sea level concentration within a month. Hematocrit (ratio of red blood cells to total blood volume) and blood viscosity increase due to the polycythemia, but a substantial reduction of plasma volume during the first weeks at altitude (up to 15% at 3,500 m) has the greatest early impact on hematocrit (5, 8).

With increasing acclimatization to altitude, cardiac output at rest and during sub-maximal and maximal exercise is reduced, due to decreased stroke volume. This process is complete within 2 weeks. The decrease in maximal stroke volume, which may be considered a negative side effect, is probably due to increased blood viscosity and lower filling pressure leading to a decreased venous return. Acclimatization to altitude does not change heart rate during submaximal exercise (it remains elevated) (8). However, chronic hypoxia seems to lower maximal heart rate depending on altitude and duration of exposure (10).

It is unclear whether systemic oxygen transport is altered with acclimatization by changes in the shape and position of the oxygen dissociation curve. The concentration of 2,3-diphosophoglycerate (2,3-DPG) in red blood cells increases, shifting the dissociation curve to the right and facilitating unloading of oxygen from hemoglobin to tissue (8). This positive effect can be "overruled" by the opposite effect of systemic alkalosis. The net effect of both mechanisms is unknown.

In skeletal muscle, capillary density, mitochondrial number, and tissue myoglobin concentration increase so that in exercising muscle, chronic hypoxic exposure results in an improved peripheral oxygen uptake. There is increased mobilization and use of free fatty acids, sparing muscle glycogen and increasing endurance time (11).

As a result of these physiological adaptations with acclimatization, physical work capacity ($\dot{V}O_2$max and endurance) at altitude improves and, at moderate altitude, may nearly reach sea level values with adequate acclimatization time. Generally, about 2–3 weeks are needed to adapt to moderate altitude. For each 600 m increase, an additional week is required. It should be noted that all of the above adaptive changes are reversible on return to sea level and within a month after ending exposure, adaptation is lost (5).

TRAINING AT ALTITUDE

There are coaches and athletes who can provide "evidence from the practice" supporting the use of altitude training to enhance performance at sea-level. Until recently, few well-controlled studies were available showing consistent improvement in sea-level performance due to altitude training. Differences in type of athlete, altitude level, training, and testing method do not allow some of the improvements to be attributed solely to altitude residence (3). Recently some beneficial effect of altitude training has been suggested for elite athletes, who have reached a "plateau" (3).

"Altitude" training can be performed by training at altitude, by using gas mixtures (with lower partial oxygen pressure [pO_2]) or training in a hypobaric chamber. Each of these methods has advantages and disadvantages. Hypobaric chambers are sparsely available and hypoxic gas mixtures interfere with high training intensities due to flow and other equipment limitations; therefore, "simulated" altitude training has rarely been conducted except for research purposes.

Care should be taken to choose adequate altitude level since the relationship between altitude and magnitude of physiological adaptation depends on the physiological variable in question. Adaptations aimed at changing the oxygen transport are related to level of oxygen saturation. The most significant adaptations are seen when training is done at 2,000–2,500 m altitude (3). It should be emphasized that the concept of "higher is better" may be compromised by severe side-effects of exposure to high altitude. Altitudes above 4,000 m are known to result in loss of body mass, due to initial loss of water and subsequent loss of fat and muscle mass (4).

One of the major disadvantages that mitigates potential beneficial effects of altitude training is the necessary reduction in training workload. Due to reduction in aerobic power, elite athletes may not reach and sustain normal training workloads during altitude residence (3, 12). In the initial days after arrival at altitude, training sessions of short duration (e.g., moderate to high intensity with prolonged rest intervals) can be performed at sea level intensities. Aerobic exercise in the first week of acclimatization should be restricted to short durations, but within 2 weeks, training workload can be increased and maximal training performance can be achieved within 3–4 weeks of residence (13). Prolonged, high intensity exercise during initial exposure should be avoided to minimize exercise-induced decrease of EPO production, which would delay increased red blood cell formation (9). Performance in activities with a large anaerobic component, which involve rapid body displacement, may actually be slightly improved because of decreased air resistance and lower gravitational forces. Special attention should be given to control of caloric and fluid intake. In order to meet increased iron demand due to increased red blood cell formation, supplemental oral iron intake in combination with vitamin C and vitamin E should be initiated 2–3 weeks before ascent and continued 2–4 weeks afterwards (9).

Recently, alternatives for altitude training have been suggested. A primary reason for the absence of performance improvement in altitude training is reduced training intensity and volume. In order to avoid this, intermittent exposure or training in hypobaric chambers has been recommended. The time outside the chamber can be used to obtain a normal daily training volume. In this way positive adaptations to hypoxia (increases in hemoglobin, hematocrit, capillary density, and altered substrate use) without negative effects of prolonged altitude exposure (loss of muscle and body mass, reduction of plasma volume, reduction of maximal heart rate) may be obtained (1). In five of six studies of subjects living at sea-level and exercising at (simulated) altitude, enhanced performance at both sea-level and altitude has been reported. (2).

HIGH ALTITUDE ILLNESS

Exposure to high altitude can lead to a number of illnesses, varying in seriousness. The speed of ascent and the absolute altitude are primary determinants of the incidence of altitude illness. Those exercising in, or exposed to altitude (athletes and coaches) should anticipate the hazards and prepare through prevention and recognition of symptoms.

Acute Mountain Sickness

Acute mountain sickness (AMS) is characterized by severe headache and often accompanied by nausea, vomiting, decreased appetite, weariness, and sleep disturbances (14). AMS begins 6–12 hours after arrival, usually peaks on the second or third day, and disappears on the fourth or fifth day (15). AMS normally appears above 2,500 m and the frequency of AMS increases with altitude and rate of ascent. Generally, above 3,000 m, 24 hours of acclimatization should be acquired for every 300 m altitude gain (15). Although AMS is self limiting, persistence of symptoms may require medical treatment. If AMS is not at least partially resolved within 2–3 days, descent is the only effective treatment. Supplemental oxygen and pharmacological treatment (acetazolamide, furosemide, analgesics) may be necessary for severe cases.

High Altitude Pulmonary Edema

High altitude pulmonary edema (HAPE) is considered a progression in the severity of AMS, associated with pulmonary edema (15). The onset may be subtle and symptoms include dyspnea, fatigue, chest pain, tachycardia, coughing, and cyanosis of lips and extremities. As HAPE progresses, affected individuals may cough frothy or blood-tinged sputum (14). This complication can be fatal if not treated promptly. Children and young adults are at higher risk of developing HAPE than adults and immediate medical attention is necessary. Evacuation to lower altitude is essential. Individuals with a history of HAPE appear to be more susceptible to subsequent bouts upon return to altitude.

High Altitude Cerebral Edema

High-Altitude Cerebral Edema (HACE) may develop when the rate of ascent is too fast. The symptoms of HACE include severe headache, fatigue, vomiting, nausea, ataxia, and changes of mental status (14). The incidence of HACE is low (1%), but HACE is potentially fatal if untreated. In cases of symptoms of cerebral edema, direct medical care with immediate evacuation to low altitude and supplemental oxygen is recommended (16).

Preventing Altitude Sickness

Preventing AMS is achieved by adjusting the amount and rate of ascent. Options include an interrupted ascent with time (days) to acclimatize at successive altitudes before reaching final elevation or limiting daily gain in altitude to 300 m or less. Initially, unacclimatized subjects should avoid vigorous exercise. Further, adequate hydration and a high carbohydrate diet may aid prevention. Acetazolamide is currently the only FDA approved drug for altitude sickness. Since acetazolamide may affect exercise performance, it is contraindicated when training at altitude. Prophylactic administration of acetazolamide may be effective (14).

AIR POLLUTION

Air pollution can also affect exercise performance and health. Though nature contributes through ozone (O_3) from lightning, dust and sulfuric oxides (SO_x) from volcano activity and other "natural pollutants," the problem with polluted air is widespread since the start of the industrial revolution. Specific pollutants that affect human welfare reflect industrial development. Organizers of sporting events or exercisers are more frequently confronted with problems related to exercising in polluted air. Both large sporting events and daily activity are performed in major cities which are usually sites with the highest pollution levels. Additionally, with indoor training and sports events, the infiltration of outdoor air pollution may be significant. Furthermore, the indoor environment may actually add to the problem with specific indoor air pollutants emitted by the occupants, the activities and building materials.

There are two major groups of pollutants—primary and secondary. Primary pollutants are directly attributable to a source of pollution, such as carbon monoxide (CO), sulfur oxides (SO_x), nitrogen oxides (NO_x), hydrocarbons and particulates (dust, smoke, and soot). Secondary pollutants result from an interaction of the environment (sunlight, moisture, other pollutants) with primary pollutants. These include O_3, aldehydes, sulfuric acid (H_2SO_4), and peroxy-acetyl-nitrate (PAN). Polluted city air commonly contains both primary and secondary pollutants.

General Effector Mechanisms

The effect of pollutants is, in part, related to level of penetration. This "dosage" is determined by exposure time, concentration of pollutant in inspired air, ventilation rate, temperature and humidity of inspired air, and route of inspiration (the nose versus the mouth). Pollution primarily affects the respiratory tract. This tract provides a large surface area for contact by the pollutant. The mucous membranes of the nose remove large particles and highly soluble gases effectively (e.g., 99.9% of inhaled SO_2) preventing them from affecting deeper airways and lung tissue. However, smaller particles and agents with low solubility pass through this barrier easily. During exercise, where mouth breathing plays an important role, this air filtration process is less efficient and more pollutants reach the lungs, traverse the diffusion surface, and enter the blood and body tissues. Tissues pollutants can have several effects during their course through the body, including:

- Irritation of the airways, which may lead to bronchoconstriction and, therefore, increased airway resistance
- Reduction of alveolar diffusion capacity
- Reduction of oxygen transport capacity.

Other effects of pollutants that can indirectly affect exercise performance are irritation of eyes (PAN and formaldehyde) and skin. Short term effects of exposure to pollutants, rather than long term exposure is discussed below.

Outdoor Pollution

Geographical distribution of outdoor pollution is strongly related to the presence of industry and population density. Automobiles, trucks, busses, aircraft, industrial sources, and combustion of fossil fuels are major sources for carbon monoxide, sulfur and nitrogen oxides, hydrocarbons and particles. Areas with equal production of pollutants do not necessarily have equally polluted air or smog because climate and topography play major roles. River and mountain valleys generally have greater smog levels than hill tops and plains. High temperature and humidity typically promote photochemical smog with associated high O_3 levels. For example, in the Los Angeles area, such smog, enhanced by summer winds towards the surrounding mountains, is a common phenomenon (17). Low temperature with a concomitant increase in fuel consumption for heating, and high humidity (fog, rain) promotes a different type of fog, in which high sulfur oxide concentrations combined with particulate matter are converted into sulfuric acid (acid rain) and sulfates. The most famous fog of this type is the "London fog," which produced a large number of deaths in 1952 (4,000 in a 4 day period) (18). Such fog can be persistent when temperature inversion occurs—a condition brought about by little wind and a layer of cool (polluted) air trapped beneath a layer of warmer air.

Specific Pollutants

Carbon Monoxide (CO)

In urban areas, carbon monoxide (CO) is the most common pollutant. It plays a role in indoor events due to emissions from equipment (usually gas-powered), but is more commonly associated with motor vehicle exhaust outdoors. The ambient concentration of CO tends to be highest during peak traffic flow and at low temperatures (Fig. 25.2) (18). The primary effect of CO is the formation of carboxyhemoglobin (COHb) due to its high affinity (> 200 times that of oxygen) for hemoglobin (Hb). Exposure to 100 parts per million (ppm) CO for 8 hours leads to over 12% COHb. COHb is difficult to dissociate and it impedes oxygen transport from lungs to cells (19). CO also reduces release of oxygen from Hb in tissues due to a leftward shift in the lower end of the oxygen dissociation curve (20). COHb concentrations above 20% are required to produce these effects. However, during submaximal exercise, little effect has been observed. Such values are generally higher than those found in typically polluted air. At COHb concentrations below 20%, compensation occurs by augmenting heart rate, cardiac contractility, and cardiac output.

During maximal exercise, both exercise time and $\dot{V}O_2max$ are inversely related to CO concentration. The critical concentration for reduced $\dot{V}O_2max$ is near 4.3% COHb (approximately 100 ppm CO in inhaled air for 2 hours) which, when considering that COHb concentration during prolonged exposure to heavy traffic can reach 5%, is of practical importance (21). Individuals with coronary artery disease may be at risk during submaximal exercise. During exercise at COHb concentrations above 6% , arrhythmias have been observed and concentrations of 2% COHb have been shown to decrease exercise time to the onset of angina. Smokers have higher baseline levels of COHb (> 4%). However, since the CO gradient between lungs and blood during ambient exposure is lower than for nonsmokers, the additional negative effect of CO from air pollution is less than for nonsmokers (17).

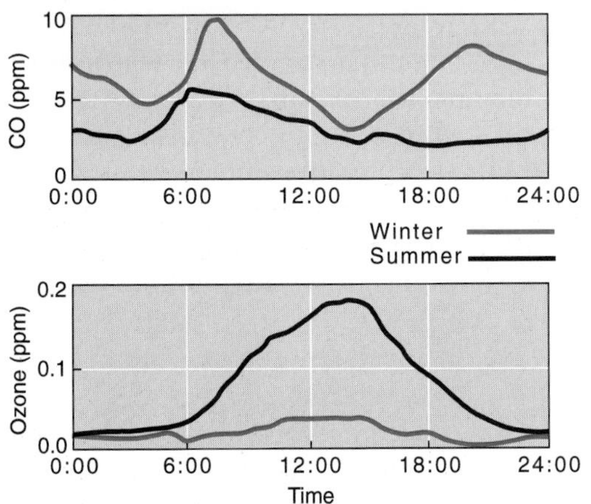

Figure 25.2. Daily and seasonal fluctuations in carbon monoxide and ozone concentrations in the Los Angeles area. (With permission from McCafferty W. *Air Pollution and Athletic Performance.* Springfield IL: Charles Thomas Publishers, 1981.)

Sulfur Oxides (SO_x)

Sulfur oxides, mainly in the form of SO_2 or acid sulfides, have their main influence through irritation of the upper respiratory tract, which can cause reflex bronchoconstriction and increased airway resistance. Nose breathing strongly reduces this effect compared to mouth breathing, since nasal mucosa removes up to 99.9% of SO_2 before it reaches sensitive bronchial areas (22). Ambient air values of SO_2 do not normally reach concentrations that have important effects on lung function in normal, healthy subjects (23). In submaximal exercise, pulmonary function starts to be affected between 1 and 3 ppm; threshold values for maximal exercise are unknown. However, athletes in competition may be at risk due to extreme pulmonary ventilation and concomitant mouth breathing. Scrubbing in the upper respiratory tract may be less effective, thus more pollutant is able to reach sensitive areas. People with reactive airway disease (asthma) are nearly five times more sensitive to SO_2 than those without. Sensitivity is exacerbated by cold and/or dry air (22).

Nitrogen Oxides (NO_x)

Of the nitrogen oxides, only nitrogen dioxide (NO_2) and nitric acid vapor (HNO_3) have been studied in humans. Acute exposure to extreme concentrations of NO_2 (200–4000 ppm) can be dangerous and result in death. During submaximal exercise (below 50% $\dot{V}O_2max$) no effect has been observed for concentrations up to 1-2 ppm, which is rarely exceeded in the atmosphere. Effects of higher concentrations are unknown. HNO_3 inspiration up to a concentration of 500 micrograms/m^3 (0.18 ppm) has not been shown to cause any proximal airway or distal lung injury, nor has it been shown to increase airway resistance (24).

Particulate Matter (Aerosols, Soot, Dust, and Smoke)

Particulate matter is solid or liquid particles found in air. The physiological effect of minute particles in exercising humans has not been evaluated. Normally bronchoconstriction is associated with particulate inhalation. The penetration of particulates into the respiratory system is related to particle size (17). Particles < 3 μm may reach alveoli, while those between 3 and 5 μm usually settle in areas of the upper respiratory tract. Particles > 5 μm are normally removed by coughing, sneezing, and ciliary action, and do not reach the respiratory tract at all. Thus, particles < 5 μm can be associated with bronchial inflammation, congestion or ulceration. The shift from nose to mouth breathing during exercise increases the amount of particulates reaching the alveoli.

There are a large number of aerosols and their effect on exercise performance is usually related to airway irritation. The most common aerosols are sulfate aerosols, which seem to have minimal adverse effects. Sulfuric acids have minimal adverse effects, except when prolonged exposure occurs, or there are large particles and/or high ambient relative humidity. Nitrate aerosols have minimal to no effect and saturated and unsaturated aldehydes have minimal effects other than irritation (formaldehyde, acrolein, and crotonaldehyde are examples).

Ozone (O_3)

The production of the secondary pollutant O_3 involves sunlight (UV) or electrical arcs and, therefore, concentration is highest during daytime (Fig. 25.2). In contrast to the O_3 in the upper atmosphere, O_3 at ground level can create a health risk. Most inhaled O_3 is absorbed by mucous membranes in the respiratory tract. The dose is dependent on inspiratory concentration, lung ventilation level and duration of exposure. Symptoms related to O_3 exposure include throat irritation, cough, nausea, inability to take a deep breath, headaches and sub-sternal pain. Such symptoms predominate in asthmatics. O_3 poisoning has been reported in welders (secondary to electrical arcs) exposed to 9.2 ppm. Inhalation of 50 ppm O_3 for 30 minutes may be fatal.

During light to moderate submaximal exercise, lasting several hours, exposures to 0.3–0.45 ppm O_3 have resulted in decrements in pulmonary function (reduced force vital capacity [FVC] and forced expiratory volume [FEV_1]) and increased subjective discomfort. However, no limitation of cardiorespiratory function has been observed. Adverse reactions have been observed at O_3 concentrations as low as 0.08 to 0.12 ppm after prolonged exposure (7 hours) (25). These concentrations are not unusual in ambient air. During heavy submaximal and, perhaps maximal exercise, inspiration of 0.2–0.3 ppm O_3 may be limiting due to respiratory discomfort and associated changes in pulmonary function (shallow, rapid breathing) (20). Repeated exposure to O_3 (3–5 days) leads to desensitization with a reduction in O_3 related symptoms. Whether suppression of natural defense mechanism is compatible with long term health is questionable (18).

Peroxy-Acetyl-Nitrate (PAN)

The effects of the secondary pollutant, PAN, formed from NO_x and organic compounds have been studied for concentrations up to 0.27 ppm. Concentrations up to this level did not result in significant effects during either submaximal or maximal exercise. The threshold value is apparently higher, yet unknown. PAN concentration in the atmosphere rarely exceeds 0.1 ppm however (23). Eye irritation can occur at lower concentrations than 0.27 ppm.

Indoor Pollution

Since many buildings where exercise and sports events are performed are ventilated with unfiltered outside air, the indoor air is also polluted. The choice of site for air intake can have a substantial effect on indoor air quality. Indoor air is also characterized by a wide spectrum of compounds, occurring at low levels, emanating from building materials, furniture, carpeting, office equipment, human metabolism and tobacco smoke. The major indoor substances of concern for human health are:

- Soil gases (radon, gas from landfills, such as methane, CO_2, hydrogen sulfide, and volatile organic compounds (VOC) from building materials),
- Combustion products (leakage from garage spaces, cooking areas, heating appliances–CO, NO_2),
- Tobacco smoke,
- Formaldehyde (from particle boards containing urea-formaldehyde resin-based adhesives or urea-formaldehyde foam insulation), and
- Metabolic gases (humans, animals)

Most of these substances have long term effects on health. Others, rather than being toxic hazards, present more of a nuisance odor.

Of the substances not previously described, short term effects at realistic pollution levels are found from exposure only to formaldehyde, VOC, and tobacco smoke. Formaldehyde is a colorless, reactive gas with a pungent smell. Its effect on humans is irritation of eyes and respiratory system and it may affect exercise performance (26). Human response to VOC in indoor air involves acute or sub-acute inflammatory-like reactions of skin or mucous membranes, or sub-acute and weak stress-like reactions. The most commonly occurring and rapidly experienced effects of tobacco smoke are irritation of mucous membranes of eyes, nose and throat. Circulating smoke in the environment is also an important source of CO for non-smokers, resulting in a COHb concentration of up to 3%, resulting in irritation and discomfort in up to 20% of those exposed to 2 ppm (19, 26).

Interactions

Air commonly contains several pollutants and the presence of more than one can result in interactions which can make it additive, synergistic or nullifying. Several combinations (CO and PAN, O_3 and SO_2, SO_2 and NO_2) have been shown to produce additive effects, but additional research is needed. Further, interaction can occur between a pollutant and other environmental stressors such as heat, cold and high altitude. Heat stress has generally been shown to be a more significant stressor than air pollution and additive effects have been observed for heat stress and CO, PAN and O_3 (21). Low relative humidity may facilitate adverse effects of O_3, whereas high relative humidity may facilitate adverse effects of SO_2 and NO_2 (18).

Humidity also plays an important role in the determination of indoor air quality. High humidity stimulates growth of bacteria, dust mites, molds and other fungi, which may cause allergy and malodorous smells. Occasionally these organisms breed in, and are distributed by, poorly maintained humidifiers and air conditioning systems. High humidity also enhances the emission of chemicals from building materials. Conversely, low humidity causes dryness and facilitates irritation of skin and mucous membranes in some individuals. Indoor humidity levels between 30–70%, without condensation in cold spots, usually does not cause these types of problems. (26). Breathing cold air (< 0°C) can result in reflex bronchoconstriction, especially in individuals with reactive airways. In addition the combination of cold air and a pollutant, such as SO_2 may to have a synergistic effect.

Interaction of pollutants with exercise at high altitudes has been studied only for CO. This combination is relatively common due to incomplete combustion of fuels at altitude. The combination of low pO_2 and competition between O_2 and CO for Hb binding sites seems additive rather than synergistic and may have negative effects on performance (17). Smokers appear to be less affected by the combination of moderate altitude and low COHb levels (4%) (17).

Table 25.2. National Ambient Air Quality Standards (NAAQS) as Provided by the Environmental Protection Agency. For those Pollutants with High Hourly or Daily Fluctuations Longer Duration Averages and Short Term Peak Level Limits are Provided. The Numbers Correspond to a Pollution Standards Index (PSI) of 100

Pollutants	Time Period For Averaging	Standard Limit Level
Carbon Monoxide	8 hour	9 ppm
	1 hour	35 ppm
Ozone	1 hour	0.12 ppm
	8 hour	0.08 ppm
Nitrogen Dioxide (NO_2)	AAM	0.053 ppm
Sulfur Dioxide (SO_2)	AAM	80 micrograms/m^3
	24 hours	365 micrograms/m^3
Particulates (PM-2.5) (< 2.5 micron diameter)	AAM	15 micrograms/m^3
	24 hours	65 micrograms/m^3
Particulates (PM-10) (< 10 micron diameter)	AAM	50 micrograms/m^3
	24 hours	150 micrograms/m^3

AAM = annual arithmetic mean

Prevention

Avoidance of exposure is the primary method for preventing acute and long term adverse effects of outdoor pollutants. Timing and selection of optimal location for exercise and moderating intensity and duration are key factors (21). Knowledge of daily and seasonal patterns and fluctuations (Fig. 25.2) is important when planning an event involving high intensity exercise. Avoiding periods and areas with heavy traffic can minimize CO exposure. Summer and early autumn afternoons are unfavorable for O_3 exposure.

Information on air pollution can be acquired from local meteorological authorities which often provide a Pollutant Standards Index (PSI), developed by the En-

Table 25.3. The Pollution Standards Index (PSI) and Implications for Short Term Health Effects

Index Value	PSI Descriptor	General Health Effects	Cautionary Statements
Up to 50	Good	None for the general population.	None required.
50 to 100	Moderate	Few or none for the general population.	None required.
100 to 200	Unhealthful	Mild aggravation of symptoms among susceptible people, with irritation symptoms in the healthy population.	Persons with existing heart or respiratory ailments should reduce physical exertion and outdoor activity. General population should reduce vigorous outdoor activity.
200 to 300	Very Unhealthful	Significant aggravation of symptoms and decreased exercise tolerance in persons with heart or lung disease; widespread symptoms in the healthy population.	Elderly and persons with existing heart or lung disease should stay indoors and reduce physical activity. General population should avoid vigorous outdoor activity.
over 300	Hazardous	Early onset of certain diseases in addition to significant aggravation of symptoms and decreased exercise tolerance in healthy persons. At PSI levels above 400, premature death of ill and elderly persons may result. Healthy people experience adverse symptoms that affect normal activity.	Elderly and persons with existing diseases should stay indoors and avoid physical exertion. At PSI levels above 400, general population should avoid outdoor activity. All people should remain indoors, keeping windows and doors closed, and minimize physical exertion.

vironmental Protection Agency (EPA). The PSI converts measured pollutant concentration to a number on a scale from 0–500. The critical number is 100, since this corresponds to the threshold established under the Clean Air Act (Table 25.2) (23). A PSI above 100 indicates pollution in an unhealthful range. PSI places maximum emphasis on acute health effects (24 hours or less), rather than chronic effects, making it useful for exercise planning. It does not incorporate interactions between pollutants. See Table 25.3 for information on the PSI (23).

The important factors for controlling exposure to indoor pollution include: selecting an optimal location for air intake, using low-emission building materials, regularly cleaning and use of "low dust" floor coverings, clean ventilation and air conditioning systems, and sufficiently high, fresh air ventilation rate. More specifically, exercise centers (or fitness facilities) require higher ventilation rates than offices and living quarters. A CO_2 concentration limit of 1000 ppm at an outdoor concentration of 350 ppm is often used as an indicator for adequate ventilation. At that level, 80% of the users are satisfied with air quality. A level of 650 ppm CO_2 is needed to increase satisfaction to 90% (26). Indoor exercise areas should maintain the lowest CO_2 concentration practically possible.

▶ SUMMARY

The environmental effects of altitude and air pollution can affect exercise and athletic performance. Physiological adaptation or maladaptation (in the case of altitude sickness or exposure to air pollution) is often a factor in fitness, exercise, and training programs. While some effects of altitude can be overcome with chronic adaptations to training at altitude, prevention of harmful effects of pollution is often a function of avoiding and/or minimizing exposure.

References

1. Favier R, Spielvogel H, Desplanches D, et al. Training in hypoxia vs. training in normoxia in high-altitude natives. *J Appl Physiol* 78: 2286–2293, 1995.
2. Levine BD, Roach RC, Houston CS. Work and training at altitude. In: Sutton JR, Coates G, Houston CS, eds. *Hypoxia and Mountain Medicine.* Burlington, VT: Queen City Printers, 1992:192–201.
3. Levine BD, Stray-Gundersen J. A practical approach to altitude training. *Intl J Sports Med* 13:S209–S212, 1992.
4. Kayser B. Nutrition and energetics of exercise at altitude. Theory and possible practical implications. *Sports Med* 17: 309–323, 1994.
5. Åstrand PO, Rodahl K. Textbook of Work Physiology. *Physiological Bases of Exercise.* Chicago: McGraw-Hill, 1986.
6. Buskirk ER. Decrease in physical working capacity at high altitude. In: Hegnauer AH, Natick MA, eds. *Biomedicine of High Altitude.* US Army Research Institute of Environmental Medicine, 1969:204–222.
7. Cudaback DD. Four-KM altitude effects on performance and health. *Pub Astronom Soc Pac* 96:463–477, 1984.
8. Young A, Young PA, Young AJ, et al. Human acclimatization to high terrestrial altitude. In: Pandolf KB, Swaka MN, Gonzalez RR, eds. *Human performance Physiology and Environmental Medicine at Terrestrial Extremes.* Indianapolis: Benchmark Press Inc, 1988:497–545.
9. Berglund B, High-altitude training. Aspects of hematological adaptation. *Sport Med* 14:289–303, 1992.
10. Savard GK, Areskog NH, Saltin B. Cardiovascular response to exercise in human following acclimatization to extreme altitude. *Acta Physiol Scand* 154:499–509, 1995.
11. Bigard AX, Brunet A, Guezennec CY, Monod H. Skeletal muscle changes after endurance training at high. *J Appl Physiol* 71:2114–2121, 1991.
12. Levine BD, Stray-Gundersen J. Altitude training does not improve running performance more than equivalent training near sea level in trained runners. *Med Sci Sports Exerc* 24:1992.
13. Martin DE, The challenge of using altitude to improve performance. In: Nebiole P, et al, eds. *New Studies in Athletics.* 9(2): 1994.
14. Malconian MK, Rock PB. Medical problems related to altitude. In: Pandolf KB, Swaka MN, Gonzalez RR, eds. *Human Performance Physiology and Environmental Medicine at Terrestrial Extremes.* Indianapolis: Benchmark Press Inc, 1988.
15. Ward MP, Milledge JS, West JB. *High Altitude Medicine and Physiology.* New York: Chapman & Hall Ltd, 1989.
16. Hamilton AJ, Cymerman A, Black P. High altitude cerebral edema. *Neurosurgery* 19:841–849, 1986.
17. Haymes EM, Welss CL. *Environment and Human Performance,* Champaign, IL: Human Kinetics Publishers, 1986.
18. McCafferty W. *Air pollution and athletic performance.* Springfield IL: Charles Thomas Publishers, 1981.
19. Peterson JE, Stewart RD. Absorption and elimination of carbon monoxide by inactive young men. *Arch Environ Health* 21:165–171, 1970.
20. Folinsbee LJ. Air pollution and exercise. In: Welsh, et al, eds. *Current Therapy in Sports Medicine 1985-1986.* Toronto: CV Mosby, 1985.
21. Cedaro R. Environmental factors and exercise performance: a review. II Air pollution. *Excel* 8:161–166, 1992.
22. Anderson O. Dodging the deadly cocktail. *Running Magazine* 1989 Oct;68:42–43.
23. Environmental Protection Agency, Public information provided on the World Wide Web server: http://www.epa.gov/ 1992.
24. Aris R, Christian D, Hearne PQ, et al. Effects of Nitric Acid Vapor Alone, and in Combination with Ozone, in Exercising, Healthy Subjects as Assessed by Bronchoalveolar and Proximal Lavage; Report No: ARB/R-94/552 San Francisco General Hospital, CA. Center for Occupational and Environmental Health, 1994.
25. Horstman DH, Folinsbee LJ, Ives PJ, et al. Ozone concentration and pulmonary response relationships for 6.6-hour exposures with five hours of moderate exercise to 0.08, 0.10, and 0.12 ppm. *Am Rev Resp Dis* 142:1158–1163, 1990.
26. Bienfait D, Fanger PO, Fitzner K, et al. European Concerted Action Report No. 11: Guidelines for ventilation requirements in buildings, Office for publications of the European communities, Brussels, 1992.

SECTION FIVE

Coronary Artery Disease

SECTION EDITOR: *Tom LaFontaine, PhD, FACSM*

78	82, 84	330, 331	346, 349	358
	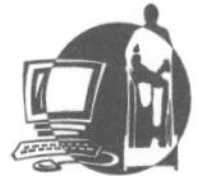	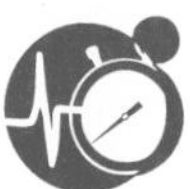		

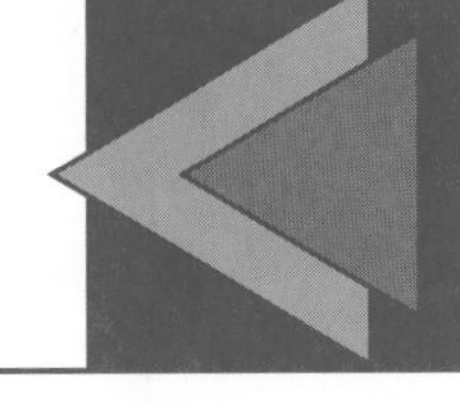

CHAPTER 26
CORONARY ATHEROSCLEROSIS

Ray W. Squires

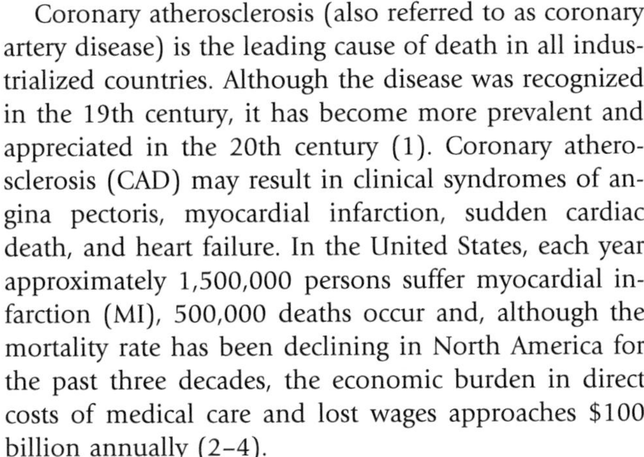

Coronary atherosclerosis (also referred to as coronary artery disease) is the leading cause of death in all industrialized countries. Although the disease was recognized in the 19th century, it has become more prevalent and appreciated in the 20th century (1). Coronary atherosclerosis (CAD) may result in clinical syndromes of angina pectoris, myocardial infarction, sudden cardiac death, and heart failure. In the United States, each year approximately 1,500,000 persons suffer myocardial infarction (MI), 500,000 deaths occur and, although the mortality rate has been declining in North America for the past three decades, the economic burden in direct costs of medical care and lost wages approaches $100 billion annually (2–4).

CAD is not necessarily an inevitable consequence of genetic predisposition and aging. Multiple, powerful risk factors due to lifestyle are operative as evidenced by marked variation in the incidence of coronary heart disease around the world (5). This is powerfully illustrated by the observation that migrants, on leaving a geographic area of low incidence of cardiovascular mortality, assume the higher incidence of the new country (6).

Arteries undergo anatomic changes associated with the aging process, such as thickening of the intima, loss of elastic connective tissue, and increase in diameter (7). These natural changes occur throughout the arterial tree and are referred to as **arteriosclerosis.** In contrast, **atherosclerosis** (atherosis, or soft "gruel-like"; sclerosis, or "hard collagenous") is a pathologic phenomenon resulting in potentially obstructive lesions located primarily in coronary, carotid, iliac, and femoral arteries, as well as the aorta (3). The disease is multifactorial and is incompletely understood, at present. Several risk factors, characteristics which increase probability of developing disease, have been identified and are discussed elsewhere. This chapter summarizes what is currently known about CAD.

THE NORMAL CORONARY ARTERY

Arteries are lined by a single layer of metabolically active cells, the **endothelium,** which serves as a barrier between blood and the arterial wall (Fig. 26.1). Endothelial cells are connected to each other and are attached to a basement membrane (8). They are selectively permeable and control passage of substances from blood into the arterial wall. Various receptors, such as those for low-density lipoprotein and growth factors, are located on endothelial cells. The endothelium is also capable of producing several vasoactive substances, such as prostacyclin (a vasodilator and inhibitor of platelet aggregation), angiotensin converting enzyme (important in vasoconstriction), and connective tissue molecules (8, 9). When intact, the endothelium produces endothelial-derived relaxing factor (nitric oxide) which is released into both the lumen and the arterial wall. This factor inactivates platelets, inhibits adhesion of cells from blood to the arterial wall, and inhibits migration and proliferation of smooth muscle cells (10). These amazing cells are also capable of manufacturing a form of platelet-derived growth factor which stimulates growth of connective tissue and smooth muscle. Endothelial cells can produce substances capable of dissolving blood clots, such as plasminogen, or factors which promote clotting (e.g., von Willebrand factor) (11). Under normal conditions, the endothelium protects against the development of atherosclerosis, but when endothelium is deranged, it plays a critical role in the development of the disease.

Underneath the endothelial basement membrane is the **intima,** consisting of a thin layer of connective tissue with an occasional smooth muscle cell (Fig. 26.1). The intima is the area of the arterial wall where the lesions of atherosclerosis form (8).

The **media** contains most of the smooth muscle cells of the arterial wall, in addition to elastic connective tissue, and is located underneath the intima, between the internal and external elastic laminae (Fig. 26.1). Advanced atherosclerosis is characterized by proliferation of

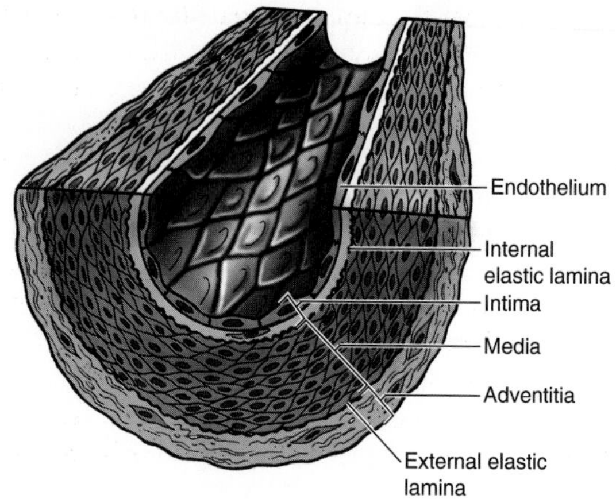

Figure 26.1. The normal coronary artery wall. (With permission from Ross R, Glomset J. The pathogenesis of atherosclerosis. *N Engl J Med* 295:369, 1976.)

smooth muscle cells derived from the media. The vascular smooth muscle responds to various vasoactive stimuli, such as prostacyclin, which cause vasoconstriction and vasodilation. The smooth muscle cells also possess receptors for substances including low-density lipoprotein, insulin, and platelet-derived growth factor (12, 13). Smooth muscle cells located in the arterial wall are capable of functioning as contractile cells or, when properly stimulated, as synthetic cells (capable of the manufacture of substances) (14). When in the synthetic mode of action, these cells are sensitive to various growth-promoting factors, become involved in formation of fibrous connective tissue, and are directly involved in the process of atherosclerosis.

The **adventitia** is the outermost layer of the arterial wall and consists of collagen, elastin, fibroblasts (cells capable of forming connective tissue), and a few smooth muscle cells (Fig. 26.1). This layer is highly vascularized (its blood supply comes from small vessels called the vasa vasorum) and provides the media and intima with oxygen and nutrients (8).

ATHEROGENESIS: RESPONSE TO INJURY

The initial event in the atherosclerotic process is endothelial derangement or injury from substances contained in blood with a subsequent **inflammatory response** resulting in proliferation (growth) of tissue within the arterial wall which may result in obstruction of blood flow (8, 11). The process may begin in childhood and progress over many years before symptoms occur. Progression of the disease is clearly not predictable or linear over time.

Injury to endothelial cells may result from multiple causes, such as (11, 15–20):

- Tobacco smoke and other chemical irritants from tobacco
- Hypertension and the resultant turbulent blood flow and increased shear stress
- Hypercholesterolemia, particularly oxidized low density lipoprotein
- Glycated substances resulting from diabetes mellitus
- Vasoconstrictor substances
- Immune complexes
- Homocysteine
- Viral or bacterial infection

Injury may result in **endothelial dysfunction,** potentially leading to impaired vasodilation and increased propensity for vasospasm, increased permeability to lipoproteins and other blood-borne substances, and increased adhesiveness of endothelial cells which leads to increased platelet deposition and increased **thrombogenesis** as well as increased adhesion of glycoproteins. Low-density lipoproteins (LDLs) may also alter surface characteristics of endothelial cells, thus potentiating adherence of cells and other substances to the arterial wall.

Platelets adhere to injured endothelium (**platelet aggregation**), form small blood clots (**mural thrombi**), and release growth factors and vasoactive substances. Atherosclerosis thrives in a hyperthrombotic state. Platelets, after adhering to endothelium, release thromboxane A2, a potent vasoconstrictor which may cause additional vascular injury (8, 11). A hyperthrombotic state may represent a genetic trait or may result from excessive blood catecholamine concentration (mediators are smoking, psychosocial stress, etc.) (21, 22). In addition, impaired ability to dissolve intra-arterial thrombi (**fibrinolysis**) may be a result of smoking, a sedentary life-style, or from elevated levels of lipoprotein (a) [Lp(a)], an atherogenic lipoprotein related to LDL (23).

Lipids from the blood, primarily carried by LDL, enter the arterial wall and may be taken up by endothelial or other cells which augment the oxidized state of LDL, further increasing cell adherence to endothelium. Monocytes from blood may adhere to the endothelium, accumulate cholesterol, and become transformed into a distinctly different type of cell, the macrophage (8). Macrophages convert mildly oxidized LDL into highly oxidized LDL which enters cells more readily than the less-oxidized form.

Growth factors, such as platelet-derived growth factor, enhance monocyte binding to the endothelium, increase the number of LDL receptors, thus induce increased binding of LDL and increased deposition of cholesterol into the arterial wall and macrophages (8, 12). Growth factors cause increased growth of certain tissues (**mitogenic effect**) as well as the migration of cells into the area of injury (**chemotactic effect**). In response to growth factors, **smooth muscle** cells and **fibroblasts** (a type of relatively undifferentiated connective tissue cell that can synthesize fibrous tissue) migrate from media to intima (8, 24). Some of these cells, in addition to macrophages, accumulate cholesterol, forming **foam cells** which release cholesterol into extracellular space, giving rise to **fatty streaks,** which are the earliest visually detectable lesion of atherosclerosis (Fig. 26.2) (18, 25). The **proliferation** (in both cell number and size) of smooth muscle and fibrous connective tissue appears influenced by several mitogenic factors in addition to platelet derived growth factor (11).

T-lymphocytes (immune system cells) are present in early fatty streaks (26). While their exact role in atherogenesis is uncertain, it appears that the immune system does have a role to play in clinical syndromes resulting from the disease which will be discussed later in the chapter (27).

With continued accumulation of fibrous connective tissue, smooth muscle cells, cholesterol, and other cellular debris, the lesion progresses in size and appearance to a fibromuscular plaque (Fig. 26.2). The plaque may contain a yellow cholesterol core called **atheroma.**

The growth of early atherosclerotic plaque occurs with outward growth of the coronary artery termed "**remodeling**" (27). Thus, **lumen size increases** to compensate for atherosclerotic plaque. The obstructive bulk may rep-

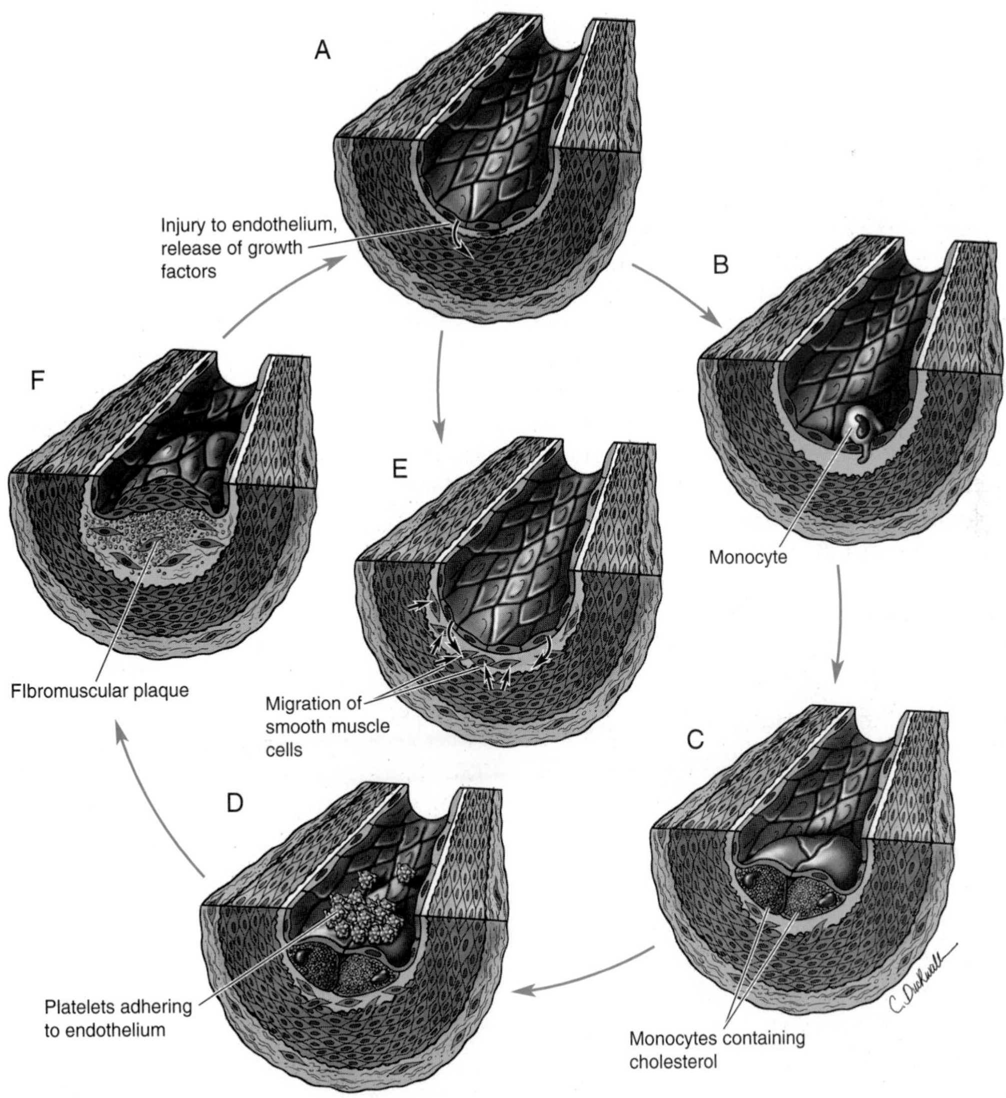

Figure 26.2. The atherosclerotic process-response to injury. **A,** Injury to endothelium with release of growth factors (small arrow). **B,** Monocytes attach to endothelium. **C,** Monocytes migrate to the intima, take up cholesterol, form fatty streaks. **D,** Platelets adhere to the endothelium and release growth factors. **F,** The result is a fibromuscular plaque. An alternative pathway is shown with arrows from **A** to **E** to **F,** with growth factor-mediated migration of smooth muscle cells from the media to the intima (E). (With permission from Ross R. The pathogenesis of atherosclerosis–an update. *N Engl J Med* 314:496, 1986.)

resent up to 40% of the vessel diameter without reduction in inside vessel dimensions. However, if plaque bulk continues to increase, vessel lumen diameter is reduced and obstruction of blood flow occurs (8, 11). **Progression of lesion size does not occur in a stable, linear manner over time (11). Some lesions appear to be relatively stable over many years; while other plaque may progress very quickly within months.**

Plaque rupture with subsequent thrombus formation has been established as a mechanism for rapid progression in plaque size. The **rupture** or **fissuring** of plaque may result from local stress (e.g., turbulent blood flow or vasoconstriction) or chemical factors. Rupture or fissuring exposes the contents of the lesion to blood (11, 28). **Mural thrombi** of varying sizes may form at these sites and thrombi may be incorporated into the plaque during this process. The scenario of plaque rupture, thrombus formation, and incorporation may repeatedly occur giving a layered appearance to the lesion and resulting in considerable progression of the plaque. These highly complicated lesions, which include organized thrombus, are called **advanced atherosclerotic** plaques (Fig. 26.2).

Coronary atherosclerosis affects arteries in an extremely diffuse manner with occasional discrete, localized areas of more pronounced narrowing of the vessel lumen that may produce obstruction of blood flow (29). Selective coronary angiography is considered the best available technique for determining the severity of obstructive coronary atherosclerotic lesions. However, **based upon comparisons of angiographic and autopsy findings, with the exception of complete occlusion of the vessel (100% stenosis), the degree of stenosis is greatly underestimated by angiography due the diffuse nature of the disease process** (30). It should be pointed out that standard coronary angiography provides a **lumenogram** (an image of the size of the lumen) and does not "visualize" the vessel wall where the atherosclerotic process occurs. New imaging techniques, such as intravascular ultrasound, may improve ability to assess extent and severity of coronary atherosclerosis more accurately than standard angiography (31).

Obstructive coronary atherosclerosis (disease severe enough to reduce blood flow) occurs more frequently in the first 4 to 5 cm of the epicardial coronary arteries, although flow-limiting lesions may occur anywhere in the coronary tree (26). Women lag 5–20 years behind men in extent and severity of coronary atherosclerosis (32). The exact reasons for gender differences are not fully understood, but are related to estrogen, since postmenopausal women experience an accelerated course of coronary artery disease unless hormone replacement therapy is instituted.

RISK FACTORS FOR ATHEROSCLEROSIS

Coronary risk factors are associated with increased likelihood that coronary atherosclerosis will develop. Several risk factors have been identified on the basis of epidemiologic studies evaluating common characteristics of persons with the disease (Tables 26.1 and 26.2) (5, 6). Some patients without traditional risk factors develop coronary artery disease, but are less likely to do so. Possible mechanisms of atherogenic effect for some risk factors have been identified, although there is no clear understanding of all possible actions of risk factors. The risk factors for CAD are discussed in detail elsewhere in this book.

NONATHEROSCLEROTIC CORONARY OBSTRUCTION

The vast majority of obstructive coronary artery disease results from atherosclerosis. Non-atherosclerotic coronary obstruction, although uncommon, may result from the following causes (29):

- Coronary vasospasm (primary or cocaine-induced)
- Embolism (thrombi from cardiac valves, calcium, tissue from tumors)
- Primary intracoronary thrombus

Table 26.1. Risk Factors for the Development of Coronary Atherosclerosis

• Cigarette smoking	• High fat diet
• Dyslipidemia	• Menopause
• Hypertension	• Elevated plasma homocysteine
• Sedentary lifestyle	• Psychosocial distress
• Diabetes mellitus/Insulin resistance	• Hemostatic factors
• Family history	• Obesity
• ACE gene abnormalities	• Male gender
	• Increased age

Table 26.2. Dietary Intake of Saturated Fat in Japanese Men Living in Japan, Hawaii, and San Francisco Compared With Death Rates from Coronary Artery Disease

	JAPAN	HAWAII	SAN FRANCISCO
%Kcal from saturated fat	7%	12%	14%
Coronary death rate	1.0	1.7	2.8

Adapted from Tillotson JL, Kato H, Nichaman MZ, et al. Epidemiology of coronary heart disease and stroke in Japanese men living in Japan, Hawaii, and California: methodology for comparison of diet. *Am J Clin Nutr* 26:177, 1973; Kagan A, Harris BR, Winkelstein W Jr, et al. Epidemiologic studies of coronary heart disease and stroke in Japanese men living in Japan, Hawaii, and California: demographic, physical, dietary and biochemical characteristics. *J Chronic Dis* 27:345, 1974.

- Arteritis
- Spontaneous or traumatic coronary vessel dissection
- Congenital abnormalities of the coronary arteries (e.g., anomalous origin of the right or left main coronaries)

CORONARY OBSTRUCTION AFTER CARDIAC INTERVENTIONS

Obstruction of coronary arteries resulting from interventions such as saphenous vein graft bypass surgery, percutaneous transluminal coronary angioplasty (PTCA) or other catheter-based revascularization procedures, and cardiac transplantation is a major problem. Injury to saphenous vein grafts may occur at the time of harvesting, during operative handling, with exposure to high pressure flow of the new location (arterialization), from risk factors such as smoking and/or dyslipidemia, or from other factors (33, 34). Atherosclerotic lesions may develop with intimal thickening, increased smooth muscle cell number and bulk, connective tissue accumulation, and lipid incorporation. At 5 years after surgery, up to 35% of vein grafts are occluded. Internal thoracic artery conduits are not as prone to development of graft atherosclerosis (35).

Angiographic **restenosis** rates of 45% at 6 months have been reported for PTCA (36). Similar or higher restenosis rates are expected for laser angioplasty, atherectomy, and rotablator revascularization. The use of intracoronary stents after PTCA reduces the restenosis rate substantially (37). Restenosis is triggered by arterial injury at the time of catheter treatment. Typically, early thrombosis occurs with release of platelet- and macrophage-derived growth factors which stimulates migration and proliferation of smooth muscle cells resulting in a decrease in vessel lumen size. The lesions of restenosis are not lipid-rich and are not typical atherosclerotic plaques.

After cardiac transplantation, **accelerated graft atherosclerosis** may result in a clinically important reduction of coronary blood flow in less than 1 year. At 3 years after transplantation, approximately 40% of patients are affected (38). The initiating injury to coronary endothelium is probably mediated by the immune system resulting in diffuse, severe, and progressive obstructive lesions. Intimal proliferation occurs with or without lipid deposition. This disease is not classic atherosclerosis.

AGGRESSIVE RISK FACTOR MODIFICATION

Progression of atherosclerosis in native coronary arteries and saphenous vein grafts is related to continued cigarette smoking, elevated blood cholesterol, hypertension, sedentary lifestyle, and an elevated fasting blood glucose concentration (39). It is clear that modification of risk factors through changes in lifestyle can moderate the atherosclerotic process and the stability of the endothelium. This topic is discussed elsewhere in this book in detail.

▶ SUMMARY

Coronary atherosclerosis begins relatively early in life for many persons. It is a multifactorial and complex process. The processes of growth of atherosclerotic lesions, de-stabilization of endothelium, and coagulation are tied together such that single events in the history of lesion development are difficult to pinpoint and explain. However, the resulting disease syndromes of angina pectoris, myocardial infarction, sudden cardiac death, and heart failure affect millions of people and cost billions of dollars.

Prevention of lesion development and its potentially lethal outcomes is of paramount importance (8, 11). Risk factor identification and modification in the children, grandchildren, and siblings of patients with established coronary artery disease is a high priority.

References

1. Report of the Working Group on Arteriosclerosis of the National Heart, Lung, and Blood Institute, Vol 2, DHEW Publication No. (NIH) 82–2035, Washington, D.C., US Government Printing Office, 1981.
2. American Heart Association. 1987 Heart Facts. Dallas: American Heart Association National Center.
3. Gersh BJ, Clements IP. Acute myocardial infarction. A diagnosis and prognosis. In: Giuliani ER, Gersh BJ, McGoon MD, et al, eds. *Mayo Clinic Practice of Cardiology,* 3rd ed. St. Louis: Mosby, 1996.
4. Jones JH, Gotto AM. Prevention of coronary heart disease in 1994: Evidence for intervention. *Heart Dis Stroke* 3:290, 1994.
5. Marmot MG. Epidemiologic basis for the prevention of coronary heart disease. *Bull WHO* 57:331, 1979.
6. Kannel WB. Cardiovascular disease: A multifactorial problem (insights from the Framingham study). In: Pollock ML, Schmidt DH, eds. *Heart Disease and Rehabilitation.* Boston: Houghton Mifflin Professional Publishers, 1979.
7. Li PL. Adaptation of veins to increased intravenous pressure, with special reference to the portal system and inferior vena cava. *J Pathol Bacteriol* 50:121, 1940.
8. Ross R. The pathogenesis of atherosclerosis. In: Braunwald E. *Heart Disease: A Textbook of Cardiovascular Medicine.* 3rd ed. Philadelphia: W.B. Saunders, 1988.
9. Renkin EM. Multiple pathways of capillary permeability. *Circ Res* 41:735, 1977.
10. Schmieder RE, Schobel HP. Is endothelial dysfunction reversible? *Am J Cardiol* 76:117a, 1995.
11. Fuster V, Chesebro JH. Atherosclerosis: Pathogenesis, initiation, progression, acute coronary syndromes, and regression. In: Giuliani ER, Gersh BJ, McGoon MD, et al, eds. *Mayo Clinic Practice of Cardiology.* 3rd ed. St. Louis: Mosby, 1996.

12. Chait A, Ross R, Albers JJ, et al. Platelet-derived growth factor stimulates activity of low density lipoprotein receptors. *Proc Natl Acad Sci USA* 77:4084, 1980.
13. Bowen-Pope DF, Seiffert RA, Ross R. The platelet-derived growth factor receptor. In: Boynton AL, Leffert HL, eds. *Control of Animal Cell Proliferation: Recent Advances. Vol 1.* New York: Academic Press, 1985.
14. Campell GR, Campbell JH. Smooth muscle phenotypic changes in arterial wall homeostasis: Implications for the pathogenesis of atherosclerosis. *Exp Molec Pathol* 42:139, 1985.
15. Ross R, Glomset J. Atherosclerosis and the smooth muscle cell. *Science* 180:1332, 1973.
16. Clowers AW, Reidy MA, Clowers MM. Kinetics of cellular proliferation after arterial injury. I. Smooth muscle growth in the absence of endothelium. *Lab Invest* 49:327, 1983.
17. Faggiotto A, Ross R, Harker L. Studies of hypercholesterolemia in the nonhuman primate. I. Changes that lead to fatty streak formation. *Arteriosclerosis* 4:323, 1984.
18. Fuster V, Pearson TA (Conference Co-chairs). 27th Bethesda conference: Matching the intensity of risk factor management with the hazard for coronary disease events. *J Am Coll Cardiol* 27:957, 1996.
19. Mayer EL, Jacobsen DW, Robinson K. Homocysteine and coronary atherosclerosis. *J Am Coll Cardiol* 27:517, 1996.
20. Muhlestein JB, Hammond EH, Carlquist JF, et al. Increased incidence of chlamydia species within the coronary arteries of patients with symptomatic atherosclerotic versus other forms of cardiovascular disease. *J Am Coll Cardiol* 27:1555, 1996.
21. Rowsell HC, Hegardt B, Downie HB, et al. Adrenaline and experimental thrombosis. *Br J Haematol* 12:465, 1972.
22. Hampton JR, Gorlin R. Platelet studies in patients with coronary artery disease and in their relatives. *Br Heart J* 34: 465, 1972.
23. Scott J. Thrombogenesis linked to atherogenesis at last? *Nature* 341:22, 1989.
24. Ross R, Glomset J, Karija B, et al. A platelet-dependent serum factor stimulates the proliferation of arterial smooth muscle cells in vitro. *Proc Natl Acad Sci USA* 71:1207, 1974.
25. Stary HC. Evaluation of atherosclerotic plaques in the coronary arteries of young adults. *Arteriosclerosis* 3:471a, 1983.
26. Van Furth R. Current view on the mononuclear phagocyte system. *Immunobiology* 161:178, 1982.
27. Libby P. Molecular bases of the acute coronary syndromes. *Circulation* 91:2844, 1995.
28. Chesebro JH, Zoldelyi P, Fuster V. Plaque disruption and thrombosis in unstable angina pectoris. *Am J Cardiol* 68: 9c, 1991.
29. Lie JT. Pathology of coronary artery disease. In: Giuliani ER, Fuster V, Gersh BJ, et al, eds. *Cardiology; Fundamentals and Practice,* 2nd ed. Chicago: Mosby Yearbook, 1991.
30. Arnett EN, Isner JM, Redwood DR, et al. Coronary artery narrowing in coronary heart disease: Comparison of cineangiography and necropsy findings. *Ann Intern Med* 91: 350, 1979.
31. Higano ST, Nishimura RA. Intravascular ultrasound. In: Giuliani ER, Gersh BJ, McGoon MD, eds. *Mayo Clinic Practice of Cardiology.* 3rd ed. St. Louis: Mosby, 1996.
32. Strong JP, McGill HC Jr. The natural history of coronary atherosclerosis. *Am J Pathol* 40:37, 1962.
33. Lie JT, Lawrie GM, Morris CG Jr, et al. Aorto-coronary bypass saphenous vein graft atherosclerosis: Anatomic study of 99 vein grafts from normal and hyperlipoproteinemic patients up to 75 months postoperatively. *Am J Cardiol* 40: 906, 1977.
34. Fuster V, Fay WP, Chesebro JH. Antithrombotic agents in cardiac disease: Platelet inhibitors, anticoagulants, and thrombolytic agents. In: Giuliani ER, Gersh BJ, McGoon MD, eds. *Mayo Clinic Practice of Cardiology.* 3rd ed. St. Louis: Mosby, 1996.
35. Lytle BW, Loop FD, Cosgrove DM, et al. Long-term (5 to 12 years) serial studies of internal mammary artery and saphenous vein coronary bypass grafts. *J Thorac Cardiovasc Surg* 89:248, 1985.
36. Garratt KN, Reeder GS, Holmes DS. Interventional cardiac therapy. In: Giuliani ER, Gersh BJ, McGoon MD, eds. *Mayo Clinic Practice of Cardiology.* 3rd ed. St. Louis: Mosby, 1996.
37. Macaya C, Serruys PW, Ruygrok P, et al. Continued benefit of coronary stenting versus balloon angioplasty: One-year clinical follow-up of benestent trial. *J Am Coll Cardiol* 27: 255, 1996.
38. Rodeheffer RJ, Miller WL, Burnett JC. Pathophysiology of circulatory failure. In: Giuliani ER, Gersh BJ, McGoon MD, eds. *Mayo Clinic Practice of Cardiology.* 3rd ed. St. Louis: Mosby, 1996.
39. Squires RW, Gau GT, Miller TD, et al. Cardiac rehabilitation and cardiovascular health enhancement. In: Giuliani ER, Gersh BJ, McGoon MD, eds. *Mayo Clinic Practice of Cardiology.* 3rd ed. St. Louis: Mosby, 1996.

84 331 47, 349 360

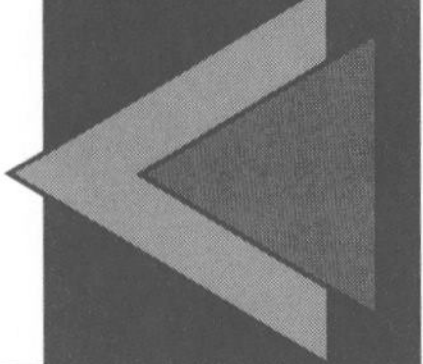

CHAPTER 27
MANIFESTATIONS OF CORONARY ATHEROSCLEROSIS

Ray W. Squires

Coronary atherosclerosis may be present for decades without apparent clinical importance. In some patients, the disease manifests itself through the appearance of stable angina pectoris or by silent (symptomless) ischemia during stress testing. Unfortunately, in other patients the first manifestation is unstable angina, acute myocardial infarction (MI), or sudden cardiac death. This chapter reviews the following topics related to the clinical appearance of coronary atherosclerosis:

- Myocardial blood flow and metabolism
- Myocardial ischemia
- Stable coronary artery disease
- Acute coronary syndromes including MI
- Sudden cardiac death
- Heart failure

MYOCARDIAL BLOOD FLOW AND METABOLISM

Normal cardiac contractile function depends on adequate concentrations of high energy phosphate supplies (primarily adenosine triphosphate [ATP]) in the myocardium. The heart is a highly aerobic organ with an extensive circulatory system and abundant mitochondria (1). The coronary arterial system is well-developed and includes epicardial arteries (Fig. 27.1) which bifurcate into intramyocardial and endocardial branches (Fig. 27.2). At rest, coronary blood flow averages 60–90 ml/min per 100 g of myocardium and may increase five- to sixfold during exercise (2). Under normal conditions, the heart produces ATP using aerobic metabolism and is not adapted to anaerobic energy production. At rest, myocardial oxygen uptake is approximately 8–10 ml O_2/100 g of tissue per minute. During intense exercise, oxygen requirement may increase by 200–300% (3). Because the myocardium extracts nearly all the oxygen from arterial blood which flows through its capillary beds, coronary blood flow is closely regulated to myocardial demand for oxygen (4). Increased myocardial work increases oxygen demand (myocardial oxygen demand is determined by heart rate, contractile state of the left ventricle, end-diastolic pressure, and aortic pressure) and coronary blood flow must increase to provide the necessary oxygen (2).

Blood flow through any regional circulation, including the coronary system, is determined by arterial blood pressure and resistance to flow of blood offered by the vasculature, primarily arterioles, which can change caliber, thus significantly altering resistance to flow (4). Because of the high intramyocardial pressure generated during systole, which partially compresses the coronary arteries, increases vascular resistance, and inhibits forward flow, coronary blood flow to the left ventricle occurs primarily during diastole (Fig. 27.3). Control of coronary blood flow emanates primarily from local myocardial tissue metabolic factors, such as vasodilators (adenosine and prostacyclin) which are released during myocardial contraction (5, 6).

The autonomic nervous system also exerts some effect on myocardial blood flow (7). Sympathetic nervous system stimulation usually results in increased myocardial blood flow due to augmentation of heart rate and contractility (increased myocardial oxygen requirement). However, α receptor-mediated coronary vasoconstriction may occur with sympathetic stimulation if myocardial metabolism is not increased. Parasympathetic nervous system stimulation has been shown to result in coronary vasodilation.

A substantial reduction in internal luminal diameter may occur before decreased blood flow can be measured distal to the narrowed coronary artery segment. When plaque reduces the luminal cross-sectional area by 75% or more, blood flow through the artery is reduced under resting conditions (termed a **hemodynamically significant lesion**) (2). Beyond this level of **critical stenosis,** further small decreases in cross-sectional area of the vessel result in large reductions in flow.

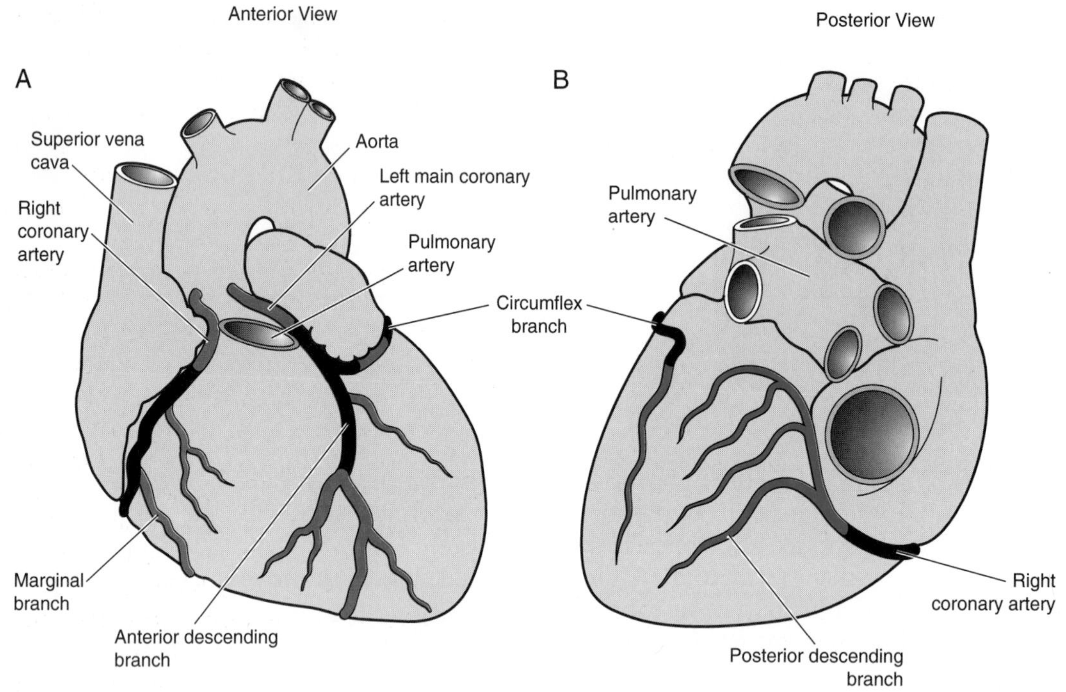

Figure 27.1. The epicardial coronary arteries. Posterior and anterior view. Black segments are prime sites for the development of obstructive atherosclerotic plaques. (With permission from Lie JT. Pathology of coronary artery disease. In: Giuliani ER, Fuster V, Gersh BJ, et al, eds. *Cardiology: Fundamentals and Practice.* St. Louis: Mosby Year Book, 1991.)

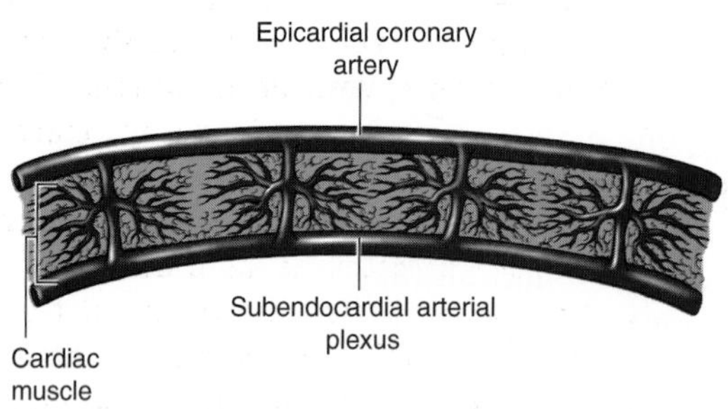

Figure 27.2. Structure of the intramyocardial and subendocardial coronary arteries in relation to the epicardial arteries. (With permission from Guyton AC. *Textbook of Medical Physiology.* 7th ed. Philadelphia: W.B. Saunders, 1986.)

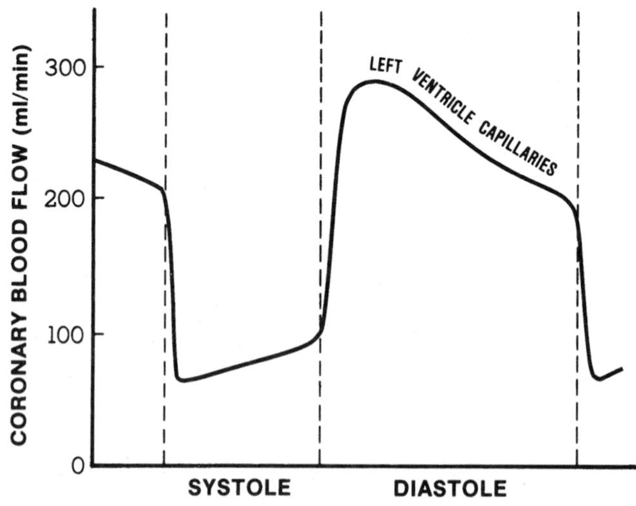

Figure 27.3. Coronary blood flow during systole and diastole. (With permission from Guyton AC. *Textbook of Medical Physiology.* 7th ed. Philadelphia: W. B. Saunders, 1986.)

The reduction in cross-sectional area of a coronary artery may be caused by atherosclerotic plaque exclusively, by vasospasm without obstructive coronary atherosclerosis, by vasospasm superimposed over atherosclerotic plaque, or by platelet aggregation leading to thrombus associated with plaque rupture (discussed in detail later in the chapter) (8, 9).

Coronary vasospasm is defined as a temporary increase in epicardial coronary artery smooth muscle tone (contraction), resulting in reduced luminal cross-sectional area (10). Coronary vasospasm may result from a variety of factors:

Local arterial wall abnormalities, including endothelial cell dysfunction, resulting in exaggerated response to vasoconstrictor agents such as thromboxane A2 and serotonin (released from platelets)
Sympathetic nervous system activity resulting in stimulation of alpha adrenergic receptors in the artery leading to vasoconstriction (e.g., coronary vasoconstriction resulting from exposure to cold)
Blood-borne substances such as epinephrine (which also stimulates the α receptors)

Atherosclerotic arteries are deficient in producing and/or releasing of endothelium-derived relaxing factor (nitric oxide) and may exhibit an exaggerated vasoconstrictor response to blood-borne agents (11). They also have an impaired capacity to vasodilate.

Myocardial ischemia is a pathologic condition in which blood flow to the myocardium is reduced below the demand (oxygen supply < demand) (2, 3). It results in oxygen deprivation accompanied by inadequate removal of metabolites. Three physiologic abnormalities may result from ischemia:

- Hypoxia (insufficient oxygen for the needs of aerobic energy metabolism)
- Accumulation of toxic metabolites
- Development of acidosis

Hypoxia inhibits aerobic metabolism and intracellular stores of ATP may become depleted. Toxic metabolites and acidosis likewise impair myocardial aerobic energy production. This results in a partial shift from the usual aerobic to the uncharacteristic anaerobic production of ATP and a marked increase in the production of lactic acid. Under ischemic conditions, the heart releases lactate into venous blood rather than extracting lactic acid from arterial blood (as it does under nonischemic conditions).

Ischemia may result in progressive abnormalities in cardiac function, referred to as the **ischemic cascade** (12). The first abnormality is stiffening of the left ventricle which decreases diastolic filling (diastolic dysfunction). Second, systolic emptying of the left ventricle becomes impaired. Localized areas of the heart that are ischemic may develop asynergic contraction patterns such as **hypokinesis** (reduced systolic contraction, decreased extent of myocyte shortening), **akinesis** (absent contraction, cessation of myocyte shortening), or **dyskinesis** (paradoxical aneurysmic bulging of an infarcted segment of myocardium during contraction) (13). Under normal conditions, ventricular myocytes shorten during systole and cause chamber walls to thicken and move inward as contraction proceeds. During ischemia, altered systolic function as demonstrated by development of segmental wall motion contraction abnormalities and a reduction in left ventricular ejection fraction and stroke volume may occur. Third, electrocardiographic changes associated with altered repolarization (ST segment depression or elevation, T wave inversion, or pseudonormalization) may occur as a result of nonuniform repolarization through ischemic and surrounding tissue. Ischemia can initiate serious ventricular arrhythmias (ventricular tachycardia and fibrillation). Finally, the patient may develop symptoms of **angina pectoris.**

Angina pectoris is transient, referred cardiac pain resulting from myocardial ischemia (14). Some patients with ischemia, either mild or severe, do not develop pain (**silent ischemia**). However, the majority of patients do develop symptoms if ischemia is moderate to severe. The locations and sensations of angina pectoris are diverse. Pain is usually located in the substernal region, jaw, neck, or arms; although the sensation may occur in the epigastrium and interscapular regions. The characteristic pain is usually described as a feeling of pressure, heaviness, fullness, squeezing, burning, aching, choking, or boring. The pain may vary in intensity and may radiate. If myocardial ischemia leads to increased left ventricular end-diastolic pressure and increased pulmonary vascular pressure, dyspnea (**anginal equivalent**) may result. **Typical angina** is usually provoked by exertion, emotions, cold and heat exposure, meals, and sexual intercourse, and relieved by rest or nitroglycerin. **Atypical angina** refers to similar symptoms, but with some characteristic that is apart from typical angina, such as no relationship with exertion. **Stable angina** is reproducible and predictable in onset, severity, and means of relief. It is believed to result from a fixed stenosis of a coronary artery that limits blood flow in a consistent manner (15). **Unstable angina** is described as new onset of typical angina, increasing frequency or intensity or duration of previously stable angina, or angina that occurs at rest (14). Unstable angina is believed to result from dynamic myocardial ischemia due to development of transient, partially, or completely occlusive platelet thrombi (thrombi that develop and then dissolve) or periodic coronary vasospasm (**variant** or **Prinzmetal's angina**) mediated by local vasoconstrictors such as endothelin, produced by the injured endothelium (16).

With prolonged ischemia, myocyte necrosis (irreversible damage, MI) occurs (12). If the episode of ischemia is relatively brief, contractile abnormalities of the ventricle (discussed above) are reversible. Brief post-ischemic left ventricular dysfunction is called **stunned myocardium** (17). More chronic, but reversible, left ventricular dysfunction is termed **hibernating myocardium** and is the result of ongoing significant, but not lethal (to myocytes) ischemia. In this condition, myocytes remain viable, but exhibit depressed contractile function. This phenomenon appears to be a protective mechanism whereby myocytes reduce oxygen demand when oxygen supply is inadequate for normal function. Elimination of chronic ischemia by revascularization results in a return of normal contractile function, perhaps occurring rapidly or requiring as long as 1 year for resolution (18).

STABLE CORONARY ARTERY DISEASE

Some patients with coronary artery disease have one or more hemodynamically significant lesions which remain anatomically stable over many years. These lesions limit coronary blood flow predictably and reproducibly. Angina pectoris, if present, occurs consistently with various provocative stimuli. These lesions are thought to be advanced, fibrotic, and contain little lipid (19).

ACUTE CORONARY SYNDROMES INCLUDING MI

The syndromes of **unstable angina, non-Q-wave MI, Q-wave MI**, and some instances of **sudden cardiac death** are related to atherosclerotic plaque rupture (vasoconstriction with subsequent occlusive thrombus formation) (15, 20). The duration of thrombotic vessel occlusion is believed to be the critical determinant of the type of coronary event that occurs. Unstable angina is most likely the result of plaque disruption followed by transient (< 10 minutes) vessel occlusion followed by spontaneous thrombolysis (clot dissolution) and vasorelaxation. One postulated mechanism for non-Q-wave MI is a more severe plaque rupture with thrombosis lasting approximately 60 minutes before lysis. Disruption of a large amount of plaque with a fixed thrombus occluding a coronary epicardial artery leads to Q-wave MI. Ischemia resulting from any type of plaque disruption of thrombotic vessel occlusion may result in ventricular tachycardia or fibrillation and sudden cardiac death.

Plaque Rupture Accompanied by Thrombosis

It appears that strength and integrity of the fibrous cap overlying the lipid-rich core of atherosclerotic plaque determines lesion stability (21). Rupture-prone plaques seem to have thin fibrous caps, whereas stable plaques have thicker fibrous caps that protect blood in the lumen from the thrombogenic core. Cytokines, protein mediators of inflammation, are present during various phases of atherogenesis. In particular, interferon gamma from T-cells inhibit collagen synthesis, thus weakening the fibrous cap. Interferon gamma also inhibits smooth muscle cell proliferation and activates the "program of cell death" (apoptosis) and contributes to the relative scarcity of smooth muscle cells in rupture-prone lesions. The forces leading to plaque rupture may be hemodynamic stress, increased blood pressure and/or heart rate, local vasoconstriction, nicotine, or immune complexes. Macrophages located within plaque may release proteases and tumor necrosis factor which may erode plaque from within. After plaque rupture, circulating platelets come in direct contact with the internal environment of plaque which provides a pro-thrombotic state (16, 22).

Angiographic studies demonstrate that rupture-prone plaques are not usually high-grade stenotic lesions. Typically, lesions involved with rupture and thrombus formation are less than 50% occlusive (23). **It must be emphasized that severe obstructive coronary atherosclerosis is not a prerequisite for development of an acute MI.** This explains the finding that many patients who experience acute **MI** do not report a history of angina pectoris before infarction. However, angiographically severe coronary atherosclerosis correlates with the likelihood of an acute coronary event by serving as a marker for angiographically modest, but rupture-prone lesions. Autopsy studies show that many patients have disrupted atherosclerotic plaques but no history of an acute coronary event. Thus, not all plaque ruptures lead to symptomatic events.

Acute MI

Acute MI is necrosis (death) of cardiac myocytes resulting from prolonged myocardial ischemia caused by complete coronary artery occlusion lasting at least 60 minutes (24). The key event in differentiating reversible from irreversible (infarction) cell damage is disruption of the myocyte membrane. This seems to be the lethal event. The myocyte cannot recover if membrane disruption occurs and cytoplasmic contents (e.g., enzymes) spill into the circulation (24).

In a minority of cases, a precipitating event or "trigger" for the infarction may be determined. Events such as the following may trigger MI (25, 26):

- Physical exertion
- Emotional stress, anger
- Surgery associated with substantial loss of blood
- Circadian variation

Slightly more MIs occur in morning hours than at other times, suggesting a potential role for sympathetic nervous system activation at onset of the event (24, 26).

Diagnosis

Acute MI is diagnosed based on symptoms of myocardial ischemia, electrocardiographic (ECG) hallmarks, and evaluation of cardiac enzymes in blood (evidence of myocyte necrosis). ECG-determined regional wall motion abnormalities at rest and myocardial perfusion scanning may also be helpful in making the diagnosis (24, 26).

Signs and Symptoms

Symptoms of acute MI may include chest pain or other anginal pain, gastrointestinal upset, dyspnea, sweating, syncope, or it may be painless (**silent MI**) (26).

Pain is often severe, but all intensities of discomfort may be experienced.

Myocardial infarctions may involve the entire thickness of the ventricle **(transmural infarction)** or only a portion of the wall of the ventricle (**subendocardial infarction**). Transmural infarction can be diagnosed from the ECG in the majority of cases (except in patients with left bundle branch block), but subendocardial infarction cannot be reliably diagnosed from the ECG (26). Transmural myocardial injury produces ST segment elevation on the ECG. During the acute phase of transmural MI, three zones of affected myocardium may be distinguished:

1. Central core of necrosis
2. Surrounding zone of ischemic injury
3. Peripheral area of ischemia

The necrotic core produces a **pathologic Q wave,** the zone of ischemic injury results in **ST segment elevation,** and the peripheral ischemic zone produces an **inverted T wave** (27). Figure 27.4 shows the evolution of ECG changes of acute transmural MI with hyperacute ST segment elevation as the most recognizable abnormality in the early hours, subsequent development of Q waves and T wave inversion, and the return of the ST segment to baseline. Over time, scar tissue of the infarct may shrink and the size of the Q wave may also diminish.

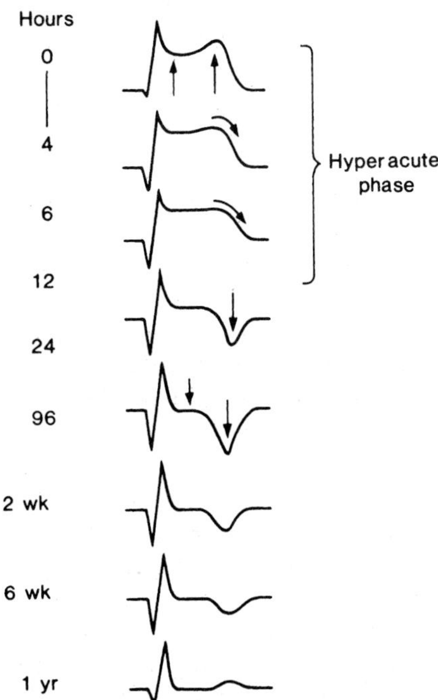

Figure 27.4. The evolution of electrocardiographic changes in Q-wave MI. (With permission from Gau GT. Standard electrocardiography, vectorcardiography and signal-averaged electrocardiography. In: Giuliani ER, Fuster V, Gersh BJ, et al. *Cardiology: Fundamentals and Practice.* St. Louis: Mosby Year Book, 1991.)

Categorizing infarcts as transmural or subendocardial has been replaced by the designation of **Q wave** and **Non-Q wave** based on the ECG. This is because there is no clear relationship between amount of necrosis in the ventricular wall and presence or absence of a Q wave. Also, a pathologic Q wave may be absent when a transmural infarction is present (23). Criteria for anatomic localization of Q wave MIs is provided in Table 27.1.

MI may involve more than one anatomic area simultaneously. Two or more infarctions, some acute and some chronic, may coexist (27). Diagnosis of a Q wave MI from the ECG is difficult or impossible in patients with ECG abnormalities such as left bundle branch block, left ventricular hypertrophy, and Wolff-Parkinson-White syndrome.

Myocardial necrosis results in the disruption of the myocyte membrane and the release of some cytoplasmic contents into blood. Cardiac enzymes released by infarcted areas are useful in diagnosis of acute infarction (26). Lactate dehydrogenase (LDH) catalyzes conversion of pyruvic acid to lactic acid in anaerobic glycolysis. This enzyme is present in most tissues and investigation into the five isoenzymes (different molecular forms of the same enzyme) of LDH is necessary to evaluate myocardial necrosis. More than 50% of LDH is in the form of the isoenzymes LDH-I and LDH-II. Under normal conditions, the blood concentration of LDH-II is greater than that of LDH-I. Within 12–24 hours after onset of MI, level of LDH-I increases dramatically and becomes greater than LDH-II (26, 28).

Creatinine phosphokinase (CK) catalyzes the hydrolysis of creatinine phosphate resulting in release of energy for resynthesis of ATP. This enzyme exists as three isoenzymes: BB, found primarily in the brain and kidney; MM, located in skeletal muscle; and MB, found in the

Table 27.1. Criteria for Q-wave Myocardial Infarction Anatomic Localization

1. Inferior wall MI (usually right coronary artery occlusion): Q-wave (> 40 msec duration, amplitude > 25% of the R wave) in leads II, III, aVf
2. Anterior wall MI (left anterior descending coronary artery occlusion): Q-wave in leads V1-V3 (anteroseptal), QS pattern in leads V1-V3 (anteroseptal), Q-wave in leads V2-V4 (anterior), QS pattern in leads V2-V4 (anterior)
3. Lateral wall MI (usually circumflex coronary artery occlusion): Q-wave in leads V4-V6 or QS pattern in leads V4-V6
4. Posterior wall MI (usually right coronary artery occlusion): prominent R-wave (R>S) in leads V1-V2 with positive T-waves
5. High lateral wall MI (usually circumflex coronary artery occlusion): Q-wave in leads I, aVL, V_5, V_6 or QS pattern in leads I and aVL

heart and, in small amounts, in skeletal muscle. Increased concentration of CK-MB is the most specific enzyme marker for myocardial necrosis (29). CK-MB appears in blood as early as three hours after onset of MI and peaks within 12–24 hours. In the first 24 hours after onset of infarction, only total CK and CK-MB need to be measured for diagnostic purposes. After 24 hours from the onset of suspicious symptoms, peak levels of CK may be past and additional measurement of LDH isoenzymes is usually required (26).

Additional cardiac imaging techniques may be helpful in diagnosis of acute MI (26). Echocardiography may disclose regional wall motion abnormalities of infarction and/or abnormal left ventricular ejection fraction. Radionuclide imaging is helpful in identifying and quantifying area of infarction.

Necrosis of myocytes, as in MI, results in an inflammatory response with infiltration of neutrophils and macrophages (30). Since myocardial cells do not regenerate, infarct healing occurs via scar formation. Depending upon size of the infarction, scar formation may take days to weeks for completion. The scar does not contract, as does normal myocardium. The greater the amount of infarcted myocardium, the larger the scar.

Treatment of MI

Treatment of acute MI includes the following:

- Relief of symptoms
- Reperfusion of the infarct-related artery
- Hemodynamic monitoring and inotropic support with an intra-aortic balloon pump, if required
- Risk factor modification for secondary prevention

Nitroglycerine, oxygen, and morphine may be given to ease pain during infarction. Beta blockers, aspirin, and heparin are commonly given as well. Early reperfusion, ideally within 1–2 hours of symptom onset, with either thrombolytic agents (such as tissue plasminogen activator or streptokinase) or immediate angioplasty may restore normal flow and reduce infarct size (referred to as "myocardial salvage"). Speed of application of reperfusion therapy, after symptom onset, is the critical factor in preventing a large area of necrosis. In some instances, thrombolytic therapy may not result in complete resolution of symptoms and ECG abnormalities, and subsequent angioplasty ("rescue angioplasty") or emergent coronary artery bypass surgery may be performed.

Complications

Serious complications may arise from acute MI and may result in early or late mortality (24, 26). The most common complications are life-threatening ventricular arrhythmias (**ventricular tachycardia, ventricular fibrillation**). Additional potential serious situations include:

- Rupture of the ventricular free wall (occurs most commonly during the first week after infarction in 1–3% of all infarcts)
- Development of a left ventricular aneurysm
- Rupture of the interventricular septum
- Extension or recurrence of infarction
- Severe left ventricular dysfunction leading to heart failure and cardiogenic shock (a downward cascade of cardiac pump failure resulting in further reduction in coronary blood flow due to hypotension and inadequate cardiac output)
- Papillary muscle rupture resulting in severe mitral valve regurgitation
- Pericarditis ("Dressler's syndrome")

Contraction abnormalities of the ventricles are almost universal after MI (24). Diastolic filling abnormalities are commonly seen and represent a stiff, noncompliant ventricle. Systolic contraction abnormalities (asynergic contraction) include hypokinesis, akinesis, and dyskinesis, as previously mentioned may also be present.

MI, particularly in the anterior wall or in other locations with extensive myocardial necrosis, may produce progressive adverse changes over weeks to months (or years) in geometry and contractile function of the ventricle (31). Left ventricular dilation involving both infarcted myocardium (**infarct expansion**) and adjacent noninfarcted tissue (**ventricular remodeling**) may occur. The process may result in progressive thinning of the ventricular wall, enlargement of cardiac chambers, and development of congestive heart failure.

In-hospital mortality for conventionally treated patients after acute MI is approximately 5–10% (26). Annual mortality thereafter averages 5%. However, the following clinical characteristics are associated with a higher risk of reinfarction and death after hospital dismissal (>50%) (32–35):

1. Left ventricular ejection fraction of < 40%; heart failure symptoms during hospitalization.
2. Patients with non-Q-wave infarction experience a hospital mortality than patients with Q-wave infarctions, but are more likely to have recurrent MI within 3 months.
3. Patients exhibiting myocardial ischemia during low-intensity exercise are at increased risk for subsequent cardiac event.
4. Patients with poor exercise capacity, assessed with graded exercise testing (< 4 METs [metabolic equivalents]) are at high risk.
5. Psychosocial stress and social isolation are associated with higher recurrent cardiac event rates.
6. The presence of complex ventricular arrhythmias portends an adverse prognosis.

SUDDEN CARDIAC DEATH

Death due to cardiovascular causes, occuring instantaneously, or within approximately 1 hour of onset of symptoms is termed **sudden cardiac death.** This phenomenon accounts for approximately 50% of all cardiac deaths (36). The majority of sudden cardiac death is due to ventricular arrhythmias, usually ventricular tachycardia degenerating into ventricular fibrillation. The pathophysiology of lethal ventricular arrhythmias may be acute MI, acute myocardial ischemia, chronic MI (scar mediated arrhythmia), left ventricular hypertrophy, or cardiomyopathy. Unfortunately, sudden cardiac death may be the initial manifestation of coronary artery disease in many patients.

Additional causes of sudden cardiac death are less frequent. Such causes include supraventricular tachycardia with a fast ventricular rate, cardiac rupture (usually in the setting of acute MI), pericardial effusion with cardiac tamponade (compression of the heart with subsequent rapid drop in cardiac output), and aortic rupture (36).

HEART FAILURE

MI and/or myocardial ischemia, if extensive in distribution, may lead to left ventricular dysfunction and heart failure (37). **Systolic dysfunction** results in poor contractile performance and is usually diagnosed by below normal left ventricular ejection fraction (normal left ventricular ejection fraction is >50%). **Diastolic dysfunction** is the condition in which the ventricle does not fill at a normal diastolic pressure and results in inadequate left ventricular volume, slow filling, or development of abnormally high ventricular diastolic pressure. Either systolic or diastolic dysfunction (or a combination of both) may result in a below normal cardiac output.

The natural history of heart failure usually includes a variable period of time with an **asymptomatic** stage of depressed left ventricular ejection fraction and cardiomegaly. This progresses to a **minimally symptomatic** stage and finally to a symptomatic stage. The rate of deterioration is variable (38). Common symptoms observed in patients with heart failure include:

- Fatigue, weakness
- Dyspnea, especially with exertion
- Reduced exercise capacity
- Orthopnea and/or paroxysmal nocturnal dyspnea

▶ SUMMARY

Obstructive plaque formation, lesion instability, and thrombosis can lead to a number of coronary syndromes including angina pectoris (stable or unstable), acute MI (Q wave or non-Q wave), heart failure, or sudden cardiac death. The clinical conditions associated with these syndromes indicate that therapeutic modalities which are most appropriate should be administered immediately to increase the possibility of long-term survival.

References

1. Garratt KN, Morgan JP. Pathophysiology of myocardial ischemia and reperfusion. In: Giuliani ER, Fuster V, Gersh BJ, et al, eds. *Cardiology: Fundamentals and Practice.* St. Louis: Mosby Year Book, 1991.
2. Braunwald E, Sobel BE. Coronary blood flow and myocardial ischemia. In: Braunwald E, ed. *Textbook of Cardiovascular Medicine.* 3rd ed. Philadelphia: WB Saunders, 1988.
3. Garratt KN, Morgan JP. Coronary circulation. In: Giuliani ER, Fuster V, Gersh BJ, et al, eds. *Cardiology: Fundamentals and Practice.* St. Louis: Mosby Year Book, 1991.
4. Guyton AC. *Textbook of Medical Physiology.* 7th ed. Philadelphia: WB Saunders, 1986.
5. Rubio R, Wiedimeier VT, Berne RM. Relationship between coronary flow and adenosine production and release. *J Mol Cardiol* 6:561, 1974.
6. Schor K. Possible role of prostaglandins in the regulation of coronary blood flow. *Basic Res Cardiol* 76:239, 1981.
7. Bove AA, Santamore WP. Physiology of the coronary circulation. In: Giuliani ER, Fuster V, Gersh BJ, et al, eds. *Cardiology: Fundamentals and Practice.* St Louis. Mosby Yearbook, 1991.
8. Maseri A. Myocardial ischemia in man: Current concepts, changing views and future investigation. *Can J Cardiol* Suppl A:225A, 1986.
9. Fuster V. Elucidation of the role of plaque instability and rupture in acute coronary events. *Am J Cardiol* 76:24C, 1995.
10. McGoon MD, Fuster V. Coronary artery spasm and vasotonicity. In: Giuliani ER, Fuster V, Gersh BJ, et al, eds. *Cardiology: Fundamentals and Practice.* St. Louis: Mosby Yearbook, 1991.
11. Griffith TM, Lewis MJ, Newby AC, et al. Endothelium-derived relaxing factor. *J Am Coll Cardiol* 12:797, 1988.
12. Hurst JW. Coronary heart disease: the overview of the clinician. In: Wenger NK, Hellerstein HK, eds. *Rehabilitation of the Coronary Patient.* 3rd ed. New York: Churchill Livingstone, 1992.
13. Squires RW, Williams WL. Coronary atherosclerosis and acute myocardial infarction. In: *ACSM's Resource Manual for Guidelines for Exercise Testing and Prescription.* 2nd ed. Philadelphia: Lea & Febiger, 1993.
14. Shub C. Angina pectoris and coronary heart disease. In: Giuliani ER, Fuster V, Gersh BJ, et al, eds. *Cardiology: Fundamentals and Practice.* St. Louis: Mosby Year Book, 1991.
15. Fuster V, Chesebro JH. Atherosclerosis: Pathogenesis, initiation, progression, acute coronary syndromes, and regression. In: Giuliani ER, Gersh BJ, McGoon MD, et al, eds. *Mayo Clinic Practice of Cardiology.* 3rd ed. St. Louis: Mosby, 1996.

16. Assoian RK, Grotendorst GR, Miller DM, et al. Cellular transformation by coordinated action of three peptide growth factors from human platelets. *Nature* 309:804, 1984.
17. Ferrari R. Metabolic disturbances during myocardial ischemia and reperfusion. *Am J Cardiol* 76:17B, 1995.
18. Rahimtoola SH. From coronary artery disease to heart failure: Role of the hibernating myocardium. *Am J Cardiol* 75: 16E, 1995.
19. Maseri A. Introduction to a symposium: From mitochondrial metabolism to coronary artery disease: New trends in the management of myocardial ischemia. *Am J Cardiol* 76: 1B, 1995.
20. Fuster V, Pearson TA. 27th Bethesda conference: Matching the intensity of risk factor management with the hazard for coronary disease events. *J Am Coll Cardiol* 27:957, 1996.
21. Libby P. Molecular bases of the acute coronary syndromes. *Circulation* 91:2844, 1995.
22. Frick RJ, Ostrach LH, Rooney PA, et al. Coronary thrombosis, ulcerated plaques and platelet/fibrin microemboli in patients dying with acute coronary disease. A large autopsy study. *J Invasive Cardiol* 2:199, 1990.
23. Shah PK, Forrester JJ. Pathophysiology of acute coronary syndromes. *Am J Cardiol* 68:16C, 1991.
24. Pasternak RC, Braunwald E, Sobel BE. Acute myocardial infarction. In: Brunwald E, ed. *Textbook of Cardiovascular Medicine.* 3rd ed. Philadelphia: WB Saunders, 1988.
25. Mittleman MA, Maclure M, Sherwood JB, et al. Triggering of acute myocardial infarction by episodes of anger. *Circulation* 92:1720, 1995.
26. Gersh BJ, Clements IP. Acute myocardial infarction: Diagnosis and prognosis. In: Giuliani ER, Gersh BJ, McGoon MD, et al, eds. *Mayo Clinic Practice of Cardiology.* 3rd ed. St. Louis: Mosby, 1996.
27. Gau GT. Standard electrocardiography, vectorcardiography and signal-averaged electrocardiography. In: Giuliani ER, Fuster V, Gersh BJ, et al. *Cardiology: Fundamentals and Practice.* St. Louis: Mosby Year Book, 1991.
28. Agress CM, Kim JH. Evaluation of enzyme tests in the diagnosis of heart disease. *Am J Cardiol* 6:641, 1960.
29. Sobel BE, Shell WE. Serum enzyme determinations in the diagnosis and assessment of myocardial infarction. *Circulation* 45:471, 1972.
30. Edwards WD. Applied anatomy of the heart. In: Giuliani ER, Gersh BJ, McGoon MD, et al, eds. *Mayo Clinic Practice of Cardiology.* 3rd ed. St. Louis: Mosby, 1996.
31. Pfeffer MA, Braunwald E. Ventricular remodeling after myocardial infarction: Experimental observations and clinical implications. *Circulation* 81:1161, 1990.
32. Krone RJ. The role of risk stratification in the early management of a myocardial infarction. *Ann Intern Med* 116: 223, 1992.
33. American College of Sports Medicine. *ACSM's Guidelines for Exercise Testing and Prescription.* 5th ed. Baltimore: Williams & Wilkins, 1995.
34. Frasure-Smith N, Lesperance F, Juneau M. Differentiated long-term impact of in-hospital symptoms of psychological stress after non-q-wave and q-wave acute myocardial infarction. *Am J Cardiol* 69:1128, 1992.
35. Case RB, Moss AJ, Case N, et al. Living alone after myocardial infarction: Impact on prognosis. *JAMA* 267:515, 1992.
36. Osborn MJ. Sudden cardiac death: Mechanisms, incidence, and prevention of sudden cardiac death. In: Giuliani ER, Gersh BJ, McGoon MD, et al, eds. *Mayo Clinic Practice of Cardiology.* 3rd ed. St. Louis: Mosby, 1996.
37. Karon B. Diagnosis and outpatient management of congestive heart failure. *Mayo Clin Proc* 70:1080, 1995.
38. Rodeheffer RJ, Gersh BJ. Dilated cardiomyopathy and the myocarditides. In: Giuliani ER, Gersh BJ, McGoon MD, et al, eds. *Mayo Clinic Practice of Cardiology.* 3rd ed. St. Louis: Mosby, 1996.

361, 362, 365, 366, 409, 413 348, 353, 354, 388 331, 335, 336, 372, 384

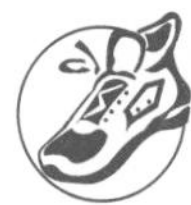

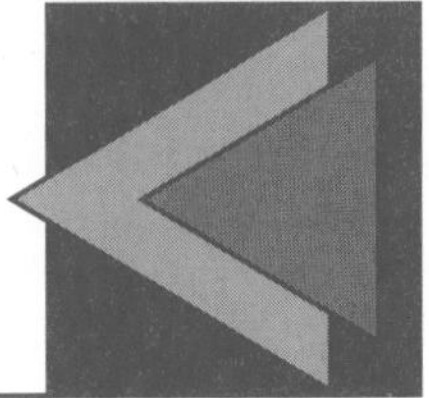

CHAPTER 28

Diagnosis of Coronary Artery Disease

Fredric J. Pashkow and Sharon A. Harvey

The diagnosis of coronary artery disease (CAD) requires using a synergistic mix of traditional medical skills and cutting-edge technology (1). The judicious and appropriate use of tests in evaluating patients for CAD requires clinical judgment and a knowledge of the indications, contraindications, sensitivity, specificity, predictive value and limitations of each test (2). Tests can be used to confirm diagnosis, define coronary anatomy, assess ventricular function and the extent of coronary artery involvement or amount of myocardial damage and, thus, assess prognosis and risk for future event. Typically, using cardiac tests in the diagnosis of CAD begins with the least costly and least invasive test. Abnormal or inconclusive findings then lead the clinician to the next level. Each level of diagnostic testing increases diagnostic accuracy as well as expense. Additionally, as testing becomes more invasive, there is increased risk.

PREDICTIVE ACCURACY OF DIAGNOSTIC TESTS

Calculation of predictive accuracy is based on the incidence of "true" and "false" results. The following are important concepts in understanding the predictive accuracy of diagnostic testing:

1. In a *true-positive* test, the **patient has CAD** and the test is **abnormal.**
2. In a *true-negative* test, the **patient does not have CAD** and the test is **normal.**
3. In contrast, for a *false-positive* test, the **patient does not have CAD,** but the test is **abnormal.**
4. For a *false-negative,* **the patient does have CAD,** but the test is **normal.**

Effective test selection and interpretation of results requires a detailed understanding of the concepts of sensitivity, specificity, predictive accuracy, and relative risk. These values define how effectively a test identifies patents with and without CAD. The predictive ability of a test is significantly influenced by the prevalence of CAD in the population being tested. If the population is skewed toward greater severity of disease, then the test has a higher sensitivity. For example, in the case of exercise testing, there is increased sensitivity in individuals with triple vessel CAD than in those with single vessel CAD. Testing can also have lower specificity if used in individuals more likely to have false-positive results (e.g., exercise testing has lower specificity in women and individuals with mitral valve prolapse because of a higher prevalence of ST-segment changes [false-positive tests] during exercise) (3).

Sensitivity

Sensitivity is the percentage of true-positive tests in patients with CAD. As the rate of false-negative tests increases, sensitivity decreases.

Sensitivity = [(True-Positive Tests)/(True-Positive Tests + False-Negative Tests)] × 100

Specificity

Specificity is the percentage of negative tests in patients who do not have CAD. As the rate of false-positive tests increases, specificity decreases:

Specificity = [(True-Negative Tests)/(True-Negative Tests + False-Positive Tests)] × 100

Predictive Value

The predictive value of an abnormal test is the percentage of patients with an abnormal test who have CAD. It measures the accuracy of the test for identifying patients with disease and is a reflection of demonstrated sensitivity and specificity. Predictive value is dependent on the pre-test likelihood and prevalence of disease in the population being tested. The equation to calculate predictive value for a **positive test** is:

Predictive value = [(True-Positive Tests)/(True-Positive Tests + False-Positive Tests)] × 100

The equation to calculate predictive value for a **negative test** is:

Predictive value = [(True-Negative Tests)/(True-Negative Tests + False-Negative Tests)] × 100

As with sensitivity and specificity, predictive value is improved when additional criteria, other than electrocardiographic (ECG) findings, are used to classify tests as abnormal (i.e., hemodynamic and symptomatic responses).

Relative Risk

Relative risk, or risk ratio, indicates the chance of having disease if the test result is abnormal as opposed to the chance of having disease if the test result is normal.

Risk Ratio = [True-Positive Tests/ All Positive Tests]/[False-Negative Tests/ All Negative Tests]

PATIENT HISTORY

Patient history is a fundamental, yet, critical diagnostic tool. The evocation of a description of classical exertional angina provides diagnostic accuracy that is difficult to exceed with virtually any sophisticated diagnostic technology, particularly as emphasis on cost effectiveness increases (4, 5). Appraisal of ischemic symptoms, such as chest discomfort, is a key factor in differentiating CAD from other cardiovascular and noncardiac diagnoses and is an important guide for selection of appropriate diagnostic testing (6). Bayes' Theorem states that the probability of a hypothesis is variably modified as additional data is considered, that is, if the likelihood of CAD is very low on the basis of coronary risk factors and history, then an abnormal test result is most likely to be a false-positive (7). Clinicians use assessment of pretest probability of having disease to determine whether additional testing will add incremental value for diagnosis.

THE RESTING 12-LEAD ELECTROCARDIOGRAM (ECG)

The resting 12-lead ECG is a surface recording of cardiac electrical potentials. The resting 12-lead ECG provides clinical information regarding the presence or absence of:

- Rhythm abnormalities
- Cardiac conduction disturbances
- Cardiac chamber enlargement
- Pre-excitation syndromes
- Ischemia
- Myocardial infarction (acute, recent, and old)

Any of these findings may be a direct or indirect indication of suspected CAD. Identification of such abnormalities on the resting ECG, particularly if different from previous ECGs, should lead to additional diagnostic tests in order to further define the presence or absence of CAD.

In evaluating CAD, the presence of pathologic Q waves (defined as > 0.04 seconds in duration), the absence of R waves, and the presence of ST-segment elevation are characteristic and, in certain situations, diagnostic of CAD. When determined to be medically stable, such patients require additional functional testing or cardiac angiography to confirm the diagnosis and assess the severity of CAD. The presence of abnormal ST segment depression can be ambiguous, particularly in the presence of hypertrophy, conduction delay, and certain drugs, such as digitalis. Such findings on resting ECG render it uninterpretable for ischemia. Further diagnostic follow-up requires a stress imaging modality (i.e., radionuclide *imaging* or echocardiography) or coronary angiography.

THE EXERCISE ELECTROCARDIOGRAM

Indications for exercise testing are constantly expanding (2, 8, 9). The exercise ECG, used as a screening tool to evaluate asymptomatic patients with at least one major risk factor or as a diagnostic test to evaluate patients with atypical angina assists clinicians in making a preliminary diagnosis of CAD (10, 11). However, use of exercise testing as a screening tool in patients with less than two risk factors can be more misleading than previously thought because of the relatively high rate of false-positive results (12). Therefore, use of the exercise ECG in asymptomatic individuals requires awareness of the limitations of the test and an understanding of Bayesean principles. Low prevalence (approximately 5% in asymptomatic males) of CAD results in a poor predictive value (about 23%) for a positive result, but an excellent predictive value (about 99%) for a negative result (13). For practical purposes, this means that one must regard abnormal screening exercise ECGs in an asymptomatic population with skepticism but negative results may be reassuring (14). Noninvasive diagnostic testing is best used to enhance clinical decision-making in patients with intermediate pre-test probability of having CAD.

The exercise ECG test is an accessible and cost-effective means of assessing cardiac function. Evaluation of hemodynamic and electrocardiographic response to exercise permits prediction of the severity of underlying CAD and prognosis (15–17). Three features, all measurable during either exercise ECG or radionuclide imaging, determine prognosis of CAD:

- The amount of myocardial ischemia
- The amount of left ventricular dysfunction

- The arrhythmic potential of the myocardial substrate

Studies suggest that certain parameters, measurable by exercise testing, provide reliable prediction for outcome after acute coronary events (18, 19). Since survival can be improved only in specific subsets of patients, it is important to carefully select a patient population in whom intervention with catheterization and subsequent revascularization can improve both quality and quantity of life (17, 20). The exercise ECG facilitates identification of patients experiencing an acute ischemic event, thereby improving outcome and providing important prognostic information.

There are significant differences in clinical, ECG, and hemodynamic measurements among patients with increasing coronary disease severity (15). Patients at high risk have more than 0.1 mV of ST-segment depression at < 7 metabolic equivalents (METs), while those at low risk do not have ST-segment depression and are able to exceed 13 METs or achieve a heart rate greater than 160 bpm (16). In patients with known or strongly suspected CAD, an exaggerated exercise blood pressure response, defined as peak systolic pressure ≥ 210 mmHg in men and ≥ 190 mmHg in women, has been shown to be associated with less severe angiographic disease and better prognosis (21). Additionally, impaired chronotropic response has been shown to be predictive of presence and angiographic severity of CAD (22). In a study of healthy men, four exercise test variables were identified to be predictive of subsequent primary coronary events. They were exercise duration < 6 minutes (i.e., < 6 to 7 METs), ≥ 0.1 mV ST-segment depression during recovery, > 10% heart rate impairment, and chest pain during maximal exertion.

Exercise duration provided the greatest risk ratio when applied individually (9). Subjects with one or more primary coronary risk factors and two or more of these variables on an exercise test increased risk ratio to 18 (23). Exercise testing, however, cannot reliably predict location of angiographic CAD. Factors to consider in defining criteria for abnormal studies are summarized in Table 28.1.

Experience has clarified the significance of various findings and methodologies, such as logistic regression, applied in the interpretation of the exercise ECG. For example, it appears that the ST index (a computerized analysis of the ST segment amplitude and ST segment slope) may be better than standard ST segment criteria with respect to diagnosis of CAD, but adds little to multivariate analysis (24). Other principles of performance and interpretation are summarized in Table 28.2.

Table 28.1. Current Criteria for Exercise ECG Interpretation Abnormal Test

- Horizontal or downsloping ST-segment depression ≥ 1 mm, persisting at least 1 minute post-exercise
- ≥ 1.5 mm upsloping ST, both inferior and lateral leads lasting beyond 1 minute into recovery
- Typical pain, ≥ 1.0 mm upsloping ST-depression
- Elevation > 1.0 mm in any lead other than AVR
- Any symptomatic drop in blood pressure, drop in systolic blood pressure below rest blood pressure, drop in heart rate during exercise
- Significant dysrhythmia, exercise induced sustained SVT or VT

Nondiagnostic Test

- ST depression in the face of LVH, LBBB, WPW, nonspecific IVCD, digitalis therapy, or other nonspecific ST-T abnormality
- Ventricular paced rhythm
- Failure to achieve 85% age predicted maximal heart rate (especially if due to submaximal effort)

Normal Test

- Exercise capacity normal for age
- ST segments exhibit less than 1 mm of horizontal or downsloping ST depression (beyond baseline) during exercise or recovery
- Systolic blood pressure increases with each of the first 3 stages of exercise
- Achievement of 85% APMHR or < 85% with normal BP, ST, and symptomatic response in a patient on beta blockers when the test is being performed for evaluation of medical therapy
- Use of "normal except for" to describe potentially important findings that do not meet the abnormal criteria

APMHR = age-predicted maximal heart rate, LVH = left ventricular hypertrophy, LBBB = left bundle branch block, WPW = Wolff-Parkinson-White syndrome, IVCD = intraventricular conduction delay, SVT = supraventricular tachycardia, VT = ventricular tachycardia

Sensitivity and Specificity

The exercise ECG is not sensitive when used alone for diagnosis of CAD. However, the reliability and cost effectiveness for monitoring progression of disease and determining therapeutic efficacy is unequaled by other diagnostic means (8).

The sensitivity and specificity of exercise-induced ST-segment depression can be demonstrated by comparing the results of exercise testing and coronary angiography. The exercise threshold of 0.1 mV horizontal or downsloping ST-segment depression has an approximate 84% specificity for CAD; that is, 84% of those without significant angiographic disease have a normal exercise test. Studies have demonstrated an average 66% sensitivity of exercise testing for significant angiographic CAD (40% for one-vessel disease to 90% for three-vessel disease) (21).

Sensitivity and specificity for each testing laboratory are related to the interpretive criteria used, the disease prevalence in the population, and the definition of "significant" angiographic CAD. The sensitivity of exercise testing is improved when patients are exercised to maximal exertion, multiple lead systems are used, and test data other than ECG response are included as criteria for an abnormal test (i.e., hemodynamic response and

Table 28.2. Principles of Exercise ECG Interpretation

- Ischemic ST-dep normally occurs in the lateral leads (I, V4, V5)
- Changes in both inferior and lateral leads suggests severe CAD
- Isolated inferior or anterior changes or changes in only one lead are often false-positives
- ST changes that resolve within 1 minute of recovery are often false-positives
- ST changes provoked in patients with an abnormal resting ECG are often false-positive
- ST-depression does not localize ischemia to an area of myocardium
- ST-depression without angina suggests milder CAD and lower risk
- ST-depression is not interpretable in LBBB, previous CABG, Q wave myocardial infarction, LVH, digitalis, WPW, or ventricular pacemaker
- ST-elevation over Q wave areas = myocardial damage or aneurysm, over non-Q wave areas means local myocardial ischemia
- Markers of poor prognosis and/or severe CAD:
  - Exertional hypotension: a drop in systolic blood pressure below pre-exercise value
  - Angina that limits exercise
  - Poor exercise capacity (< 6 METS)
  - Downsloping ST depression, especially in recovery
  - ST depression starting at a low double product (< 15,000)
  - ST depression that persists into late recovery

CABG = coronary artery bypass grafting, LVH = left ventricular hypertrophy, WPW = Wolff-Parkinson-White syndrome

symptoms). Sensitivity is also enhanced by reducing criteria for an abnormal ST segment response (i.e., from 0.1 mV to 0.05 mV). However, this also increases the rate of false-positives, thereby sacrificing specificity. Factors that negatively affect sensitivity and specificity are summarized in Tables 28.3 and 28.4 (3). The ability to diagnosis CAD in patients with confounding results is improved with the addition of imaging.

Limitations

A major factor that effects the sensitivity of exercise ECG is the ability to obtain adequate workload and heart rate response. Patients who tolerate testing without complication should be encouraged to exercise to exhaustion. While some patients may not be physiologically able to achieve 100% of age-predicted maximal heart rate (APMHR), others may easily exceed this target. The practice of setting a mandatory termination point at 85% APMHR may prevent the observation of abnormalities occurring at higher workloads. Although the onset of ST changes at high workloads are less diagnostically significant than those occurring during early stages, the data improve sensitivity and merits documentation for future serial test evaluation.

RADIONUCLIDE IMAGING

Radionuclide imaging in combination with exercise or pharmacologic stress is commonly used for diagnosis of CAD (25). Use of radionuclide imaging is indicated in follow-up for patients with abnormal ECG exercise tests, in women with positive tests, in the screening of patients on digitalis and with abnormal resting ECG (i.e., left bundle branch block, left ventricular hypertrophy, Wolffe-Parkinson-White syndrome, intraventricular conduction delay), the assessment of perfusion in angiographically documented CAD, and to study myocardial viability.

Table 28.3. Factors that Lower Sensitivity (False-Negatives)

- Failure to reach 85% age-predicted maximal heart rate
- Medicines that decrease $M\dot{V}O_2$ (e.g., beta & calcium channel blockers)
- Medicines that increase myocardial oxygen supply (e.g., nitrates)
- Equivocal tests called normal
- Failure to use other test data in test interpretation (e.g., chronotropic and inotropic responses, symptoms, and dysrhythmias)
- Single vessel disease
- Good collateral circulation
- Insufficient number of monitoring leads to detect ST changes
- Increased criteria for abnormal ST depression (e.g., 0.2 mV rather than 0.1 mV)
- Technical or observer error

$M\dot{V}O_2$ = myocardial oxygen uptake

Table 28.4. Factors that Lower Specificity (False-Positives)

- Categorization of upsloping ST depression as abnormal
- An abnormal resting ECG (e.g., LBBB, non specific ST-T abnormality)
- Medications that produce ST-T changes (e.g., digitalis)
- Cardiac hypertrophy or cardiomyopathy
- Hypertension
- Female gender
- Mitral valve prolapse
- Low prevalence of CAD in test population
- Wolff-Parkinson-White syndrome
- Pectus excavatum
- Pre-exercise hyperventilation
- Patients with vasospasm
- Hyokalemia and anemia
- Technical or observer error

LBBB = left bundle branch block

Perfusion Imaging

Thallium-201 (Th-201) injected at peak exercise, is proportionally distributed within the myocardium in relation to regional myocardial blood flow and muscle viability. In normal myocardium, imaging following stress shows initial accumulation of the isotope reflecting integrity of regional blood supply. In areas of decreased initial perfusion, peak isotopic concentrations are delayed and associated with slower washout. The presence of transient perfusion defects following exercise that "fill in" with delayed images (obtained within a 4–24 hours after exercise or at rest) is consistent with exercise-induced myocardial ischemia. Areas of scar characteristically show no uptake, either initially or during later redistribution. In addition to the uniformity of isotopic uptake, ventricular cavity size, myocardial wall thickness, and occurrence of pulmonary accumulation can be observed.

Planar Th-201 imaging provides average sensitivity and specificity of 83% and 88%, respectively. More recently, advances in radionuclide imaging such as quantification of radionuclide data, tomographic imaging technique, and single photon emission computed tomography (SPECT) have enhanced sensitivity and specificity beyond that provided by planar imaging. A review of studies using SPECT analysis indicated overall sensitivity of 89% and specificity of 76%. Positron emission tomography (PET), a newer and significantly more costly image acquisition technology, appears to provide accuracy comparable to SPECT in diagnosing and predicting the severity of CAD. PET may be superior in obese patients or in those with equivocal thallium SPECT studies. Sensitivity and specificity for PET range from 78%-100% and 87%-97%, respectively (26).

Newer technetium-99m (Tc-99m) based radiopharmaceuticals may potentially provide diagnostic benefits on the basis of variable biological attributes. Tc-99m sestamibi has a shorter half-life than Th-201. This allows administration of a larger dose thereby providing superior images. Thus far, studies demonstrate similar sensitivity and specificity for Th-201 and Tc-99m sestamibi scintigraphy (26).

When diagnostic testing is required in patients who are unable to exercise, potent selective coronary vasodilators, such as dipyridamole and adenosine, and isotopes, such as Th-201, Tc-99m sestamibi or rubidium-82, are used with SPECT and PET (27). A typical hemodynamic response to these agents is decreased blood pressure due to vasodilation with a slight reflex increase in heart rate. These techniques have proven efficacy and are especially important for subjects who are incapable of exercise, unable to achieve appropriate heart rates via exercise, or are in the early post-uncomplicated acute myocardial infarction period and require a more definitive diagnostic study. Minor side effects are experienced in 50% of patients receiving dipyridamole and 80% of patient receiving adenosine. Mean sensitivity and specificity using with dipyridamole SPECT imaging and either Th-201 or sestamibi, averages 90% and 70%, respectively, while use of adenosine averages 85% and 90%, respectively (26).

No test is clearly superior to others in every clinical circumstance (28). Moreover, none have been shown to provide sensitivity and specificity above 90% consistently (25). Therefore, the use of radionuclide imaging for diagnostic purposes in populations with a lower prevalence of disease is of only moderate value. However, for the assessment of patients with moderate pretest probability of disease, functional significance of CAD, or prognosis in patients with ischemic heart disease, the addition of these noninvasive imaging modalities to exercise testing is of great value.

Ventriculography

The diagnosis of CAD can also be aided by performing multiple gated acquisition study (MUGA), or a **first pass** study, during exercise. This allows assessment and comparison of resting and exercise cardiac function including systolic and diastolic function, right and left ventricular ejection fraction, cardiac output, and regional wall motion.

An increase in left and right ventricular ejection fraction of 5% or more is a normal response to exercise. Failure to increase or a decrease in ejection fraction during exercise may be an indicator of failing ventricular function due to ischemia. This is further confirmed by observing abnormal ECG changes and/or segmental wall motion abnormalities during exercise that would indicate compromised coronary flow. Abnormal left ventricular ejection fraction response to exercise is sensitive, but not specific to CAD.

EXERCISE ECHOCARDIOGRAPHY

Exercise echocardiography combines surface echocardiography and exercise ECG testing (29). Echocardiographic images are viewed using side-by-side digital display of resting and exercise echocardiograms. Exercise echocardiographic images can be obtained during exercise, using cycle ergometry, or within the immediate post-exercise period using a treadmill. Acquisition of immediate post-exercise images must be complete within 1–2 minutes of test termination. Both techniques require superior sonographic skill.

Like radionuclide ventriculography, exercise echocardiography allows assessment of cardiac function including wall motion abnormality, ejection fraction, and systolic and diastolic function. In one study, exercise echocardiography significantly improved sensitivity of stress testing (80% vs. 42%, $p < 0.0001$) even after exclusion of negative exercise ECGs with submaximal stress and all nondiagnostic exercise ECGs (87% vs. 63% for ECG, $p = 0.001$) (30). In a population with very high prevalence of symptomatic CAD (77%), a higher sensitivity (97% vs 51% for ECG, $p < 0.0001$) has been observed (31). Specificity is enhanced by exercise echocardiography as well. Specificity in normal tests is 93%, 82% after exclusion of non-diagnostic tests, compared to 77% for ECG (30). Stress echocardiography is useful in women and in those with concurrent valvular or primary myocardial disease. Stress echo is less optimal in patients with multiple myocardial infarctions, complex wall motion abnormality, or a poor imaging window (e.g., obese patients). In patients who are unable to exercise, intravenous dobutamine, a beta adrenergic stimulating agent, offers a pharmacologic alternative. Infusion of an incremental dose of dobutamine provokes a positive inotropic response, a less significant chronotropic response, and increased contractility. Unlike dipyridamole and adenosine, dobutamine more closely parallels the "exercise" response by creating an oxygen supply and demand imbalance.

The most significant limitation in performing stress echocardiography is the learning curve associated with image acquisition and interpretation. High quality images are required within 1–2 minutes of termination of exercise. Interpretation of exercise echocardiographic images is highly subjective, limited in part by current imaging technology and lack of algorithms for quantification and enhancement of data. Physicians require significant training before diagnostic reliability is achieved (32).

CORONARY ANGIOGRAPHY

Coronary angiography involves the selective opacification of the coronary arteries during x-ray exposure. This produces a contrast image defining the internal diameter of a visualized artery. For many years, it comprised the "gold standard" for diagnosis of the presence and extent of coronary atherosclerosis and it remains the most sensitive, readily available test for this purpose. Findings at catheterization correlate well with clinical coronary events over an extended period of time (33). The technique does not provide extensive information about the wall of the artery, nor does it address the presence of ischemia, the "bottom line" of atherosclerotic disease.

Selective coronary angiography is generally combined with a contrast left ventriculogram. With the widespread availability of radionuclide and echocardiographic imaging, the left ventriculogram during catheterization is not as important as in previous years. The measurement of left and right ventricular hemodynamics and pressures is rarely performed today. Echo-Doppler is generally determined to be satisfactory for this purpose.

Coronary angiography is clearly indicated in patients with intractable or unstable angina to determine whether they are appropriate candidates for interventional or surgical revascularization. In patients with established disease who are stable, coronary arteriography may be indicated, particularly in those who demonstrate non-invasive indicators forecasting a poor prognosis. Randomized studies show improved survival rates following revascularization in patients with three-vessel CAD, or its equivalent, and in those with two-vessel disease when the proximal portion of the left anterior descending coronary artery is critically obstructed (34, 35). In addition, patients with acute myocardial infarction with recurrent chest pain due to myocardial ischemia despite intensive medical therapy or those who have structural complications of acute infarction, require coronary arteriography.

While angiography reflects luminal distortion of the atherosclerotic coronary plaque, intravascular ultrasound directly demonstrates the compositional and structural anatomy of plaque invading the coronary arterial wall. However, the current major use of intravascular ultrasound is as a research tool and for specialized applications by the interventional cardiologist (36).

▶ SUMMARY

The diagnosis of CAD begins with careful consideration of signs, symptoms, resting ECG, and risk factor profile. The determination of pretest probability of having CAD assists in determining the need for additional diagnostic studies. Patients with low pre-test probability may not require further testing. Patients with low to intermediate pre-test probability may undergo exercise ECG testing for further risk stratification. Patients with intermediate pre-test probability receive clear benefit from exercise ECG testing. The decision to use an imaging or non-imaging modality is based on clinical factors. For detection of the presence of CAD, patients with high pre-test probability receive little diagnostic advantage from noninvasive testing. Patients with a high pretest probablility are most likely to be assessed using coronary angiography and may require subsequent noninvasive diagnostics for localization of ischemia and determination of prognosis.

References

1. Pashkow FJ. Contemporary considerations in exercise ECG testing. *Cleve Clin J Med* 59:231–232, 1992.
2. American College of Sports Medicine. *ACSM's Guidelines for Exercise Testing and Prescription.* 5th ed. Baltimore: Williams & Wilkins, 1995:42, 86, 97.
3. Hanson P. Clinical Exercise Testing. In: *ACSM Resource Manual for Guidelines for Exercise Testing and Prescription.* Philadelphia: Lea & Febiger, 1988:219–221.
4. Weiner D, Ryan T, McCabe C, et al. Correlations among history of angina, ST-segment response and prevalence of coronary artery disease in the Coronary Artery Surgery Study (CASS). *N Engl J Med* 301:230–235, 1979.
5. Patterson RE, Eng C, Horowitz SF, et al. Bayesian comparison of cost-effectiveness of different clinical approaches to diagnose coronary artery disease. *J Am Coll Cardiol* 4:278–289, 1984.
6. Hung J, Chaitman BR, Lam J, et al. A logistic regression analysis of multiple noninvasive tests for the prediction of the presence and extent of coronary artery disease in men. *Am Heart J* 110:460–469, 1985.
7. Morise AP, Duval RD. Comparison of three Bayesian methods to estimate posttest probability in patients undergoing exercise stress testing. *Am J Cardiol* 64:1117–1122, 1989.

8. Fuller T, Movahed A. Current review of exercise testing: application and interpretation. *Clin Cardiol* 10:189–200, 1987.
9. Detrano R, Froelicher VF. Exercise testing: uses and limitations considering recent studies. *Prog Cardiovasc Dis* 31: 173–204, 1988.
10. Sox H Jr, Littenberg B, Garber AM. The role of exercise testing in screening for coronary artery disease [see comments]. *Ann Intern Med* 110:456–469, 1989.
11. Froelicher V. Diagnostic Applications of Exercise Testing. In: *Manual of Exercise Testing.* 2nd ed. St Louis: Mosby, 1994:90–102.
12. Detrano R, Froelicher V. A logical approach to screening for coronary artery disease. *Ann Intern Med* 106:846–852, 1987.
13. Sheffield L. Exercise stress testing for coronary artery disease. In: Braunwald E, ed. *Heart Disease. A Textbook of Cardiovascular Medicine.* 3rd ed. Philadelphia: W.B. Saunders, 1988:223–241.
14. Patterson RE, Horowitz SF. Importance of epidemiology and biostatistics in deciding clinical strategies for using diagnostic tests: a simplified approach using examples from coronary artery disease. *J Am Coll Cardiol* 13:1653–1665, 1989.
15. Ribisl P, Morris C, Kawaguchi T. Angiographic patterns and severe coronary artery disease. *Arch Intern Med* 152:1618–1624, 1992.
16. McNeer J, Margolis J, Lee K. The role of the exercise test in the evaluation of patients for ischemic heart disease. *Circulation* 57:64–70, 1978.
17. Weiner D, McCabe C, Ryan T. Identification of patients with left main and three vessel coronary disease with clinical and exercise test variables. *Am J Cardiol* 46:21–27, 1980.
18. Froelicher V, Duarte G, Oakes D, et al. The prognostic value of the exercise test. *Dis Mon* 34:677–735, 1988.
19. DeBusk RF. Specialized testing after recent acute myocardial infarction. *Ann Intern Med* 110:470–481, 1989.
20. Bogaty P, Dagenais GR, Cantin B, et al. Prognosis in patients with a strongly positive exercise electrocardiogram. *Am J Cardiol* 64:1284–1288, 1989.
21. Nielsen JR, Mickley H, Damsgaard EM, et al. Predischarge maximal exercise test identifies risk for cardiac death in patients with acute myocardial infarction. *Am J Cardiol* 65: 149–153, 1990.
22. Brener S, Pashkow F, Harvey S, et al. Chronotropic response to exercise predicts angiographic severity in patients with suspected or stable coronary artery disease. *Am J Cardiol* 76:1228–1232, 1995.
23. Bruce RA, Fisher LD, Hossack KF. Validation of exercise-enhanced risk assessment of coronary heart disease events: longitudinal changes in incidence in Seattle community practice. *J Am Coll Cardiol* 5:875–881, 1985.
24. Morise AP, Duval RD. Accuracy of ST/heart rate index in the diagnosis of coronary artery disease. *Am J Cardiol* 69: 603–606, 1992.
25. Crawford MH. Overview: diagnosis of ischemic heart disease by noninvasive techniques. *Circulation* 84:I50–I51, 1991.
26. Ritchie J, et al. Guidelines for Clinical Use of Cardiac Radionuclide Imaging; Report of the ACC/AHA Task Force on Assessment of Diagnostic and Therapeutic Cardiovascular Procedures, Developed in Collaboration with the American Society of Nuclear Cardiology. *Am J Cardiol* 25: 521–547, 1995.
27. Marwick T. Application of noninvasive cardiac imaging modalities to post MI rehabilitation; tests of left ventricular function, perfusion and metabolism. In: Pashkow F, Dafoe W, eds. *Clinical Cardiac Rehabilitation: A Cardiologist's Guide.* Baltimore: Williams & Wilkins, 1992:102–114.
28. Kotler TS, Diamond GA. Exercise thallium-201 scintigraphy in the diagnosis and prognosis of coronary artery disease. *Ann Intern Med* 113:684–702, 1990.
29. Ryan T, Feigenbaum H. Exercise echocardiography. *Am J Cardiol* 69:82H–89H, 1992.
30. Marwick TH, Nemec JJ, Pashkow FJ, et al. Accuracy and limitations of exercise echocardiography in a routine clinical setting. *J Am Coll Cardiol* 19:74–81, 1992.
31. Crouse LJ, Harbrecht JJ, Vacek JL, et al. Exercise echocardiography as a screening test for coronary artery disease and correlation with coronary arteriography. *Am J Cardiol* 67:1213–1218, 1991.
32. Orlandini A, Picano E, Lattanzi F, et al. Stress echocardiography and the human factor: the importance of being an expert. *J Am Coll Cardiol* 15:52a, 1990.
33. Ellis SG. Role of Coronary Angiography. In: Fuster V, Ross R, Topol EJ, eds. *Atherosclerosis and Coronary Artery Disease.* Philadelphia: Lippincott-Raven Publishers, 1996:1433–1435.
34. Weiner DA, Ryan TJ, McCabe CH, et al. Value of exercise testing in determining the risk classification and the response to coronary artery bypass grafting in three-vessel coronary artery disease: a report from the Coronary Artery Surgery Study (CASS) registry. *Am J Cardiol* 60:262–266, 1987.
35. Ringqvist I, Fisher LD, Mock M, et al. Prognostic value of angiographic indices of coronary artery disease from the Coronary Artery Surgery Study (CASS). *J Clin Invest* 71: 1854–1866, 1983.
36. DeFranco AC, Tuzcu EM, Brenner S, et al. Interventional Applications of Coronary Intravascular Ultrasound, Angioscopy, and Doppler Flow. In: Fuster V, Ross R, Topol EJ, eds. *Atherosclerosis and Coronary Artery Disease.* Philadelphia: Lippincott-Raven Publishers, 1996:1451–1453.

Suggested Readings

AHA Medical/Scientific Statement Special Report. Exercise Standards; A Statement for Healthcare Professionals From the AHA. American Heart Association Publication 1995.

Ellestad MH. *Stress Testing: Principles and Practice.* 4th ed. Philadelphia: FA Davis Co, 1996

Froelicher VF. *Manual of Exercise Testing.* 2nd ed. St Louis: Mosby, 1994.

Pashkow FJ, Dafoe WA. *Clinical Cardiac Rehabilitation: A Cardiologist's Guide.* Baltimore: Williams & Wilkins, 1993.

Report of the ACC/AHA Task Force on Assessment of Cardiovascular Procedures. Guidelines on Exercise Testing. *Am J Cardiol* 8:725–738, 1986.

Report of the ACC/AHA Task Force on Assessment of Diagnostic and Therapeutic Cardiovascular Procedures. Guidelines for Clinical Use of Cardiac Radionuclide Imaging. *Am J Cardiol* 25:521–547, 1995.

Schlant RC, Alexander RW, et al. *Hurst's The Heart.* 8th ed. New York: McGraw-Hill, Inc., 1994.

365, 366, 367, 368 351, 353, 355, 356

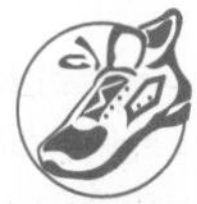

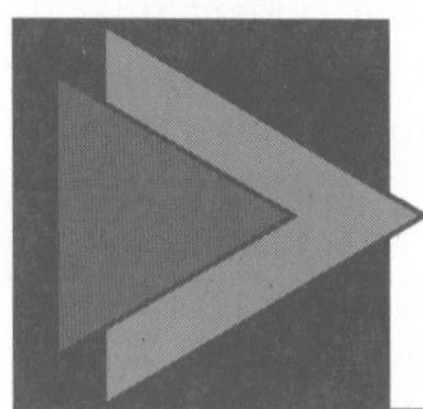

CHAPTER 29
MEDICAL AND INVASIVE INTERVENTIONS IN THE TREATMENT OF CORONARY ARTERY DISEASE

Sorin J. Brener and Fredric J. Pashkow

Cholesterol deposition in the arterial wall begins as early as the second decade of life and progresses throughout the ensuing 20–40 years (1, 2). Initially, the coronary artery remodels by increasing its outer dimensions, accommodating the plaque burden without limiting blood flow (3). Gradually, this adaptive mechanism is exhausted and progressive encroachment of the lumen develops. The ability of the coronary tree to supply augmented blood flow necessitated by increasing physiological demand becomes impaired, leading to symptomatic coronary artery disease (CAD).

In general, those with obstructive CAD present in equal frequency with either chronic effort-induced stable angina pectoris or unstable coronary syndromes and, more rarely (10–15%), sudden cardiac death. The transition from chronic stable angina to unstable syndromes relates to plaque fissuring and thrombus formation with significant reduction in effective lumen dimensions (4, 5). The presence of a lipid-rich plaque with a thin cap and platelet deposition on thrombogenic ruptured plaque play an important role in the cascade of events leading to acute myocardial infarction, or sudden death. These pathophysiologic aspects bear importantly on therapy of CAD.

MEDICAL INTERVENTION IN CAD

Once the diagnosis of CAD is established, or strongly suspected, there are a number of therapeutic challenges. They are to:

1. Identify and modify risk factors leading to the progression of disease.
2. Provide symptomatic relief in order to enhance quality of life.
3. Consider the necessary diagnostic steps for risk stratification.
4. Institute therapy that may prolong life, or prevent significant morbidity.

The following sections provide a scaffold for an integrative approach to treat CAD, with special emphasis on pharmacological and mechanical aspects of therapy. Where appropriate, the reader is referred to more extensive reviews of certain topics.

Risk Factor Modification

The following recommendations are a prudent course for persons with clinically diagnosed CAD. Patients should be encouraged to follow the American Heart Association Diet step II to maintain adequate body weight and lower cholesterol intake. Hypertension should be controlled and strict control of diabetes mellitus must be implemented (6, 7). Physical activity is beneficial once initial symptoms are mediated. In addition, patients with premature appearance of symptomatic CAD should undergo detailed evaluation of genetic and other rare predisposing factors for atherosclerosis, especially as it pertains to transmission of these traits to offspring. A detailed discussion of these issues can be found elsewhere (8).

Once the risk factors have been identified and addressed, the mainstay of therapy rests on antiplatelet, cholesterol-lowering, and anti-anginal agents. Mechanical revascularization via percutaneous transluminal coronary angioplasty (PTCA) or coronary artery bypass grafing (CABG) is reserved for those with unremitting symptoms, inability to tolerate pharmacological therapy, or certain clinical and angiographic characteristics associated with poor survival. Mechanical revascularization should serve as an adjunct to the other interventions, not as a substitute.

Pharmacological Therapy

Platelet-inhibitor Agents

Platelets play a key role in the development of unstable coronary syndromes. Circulating platelets adhere to the site of endothelial injury and promote further platelet aggregation and activation of the coagulation system, a process that leads to vessel occlusion. The mechanism of platelet inhibition varies among commonly used agents. Aspirin inhibits the cyclooxygenase pathway, reducing levels of thromboxane A2 secreted by platelets (9). Overall, the anti-aggregatory effect of aspirin is weak because many other stimuli can bypass the thromboxane pathway and directly activate the glycoprotein receptor IIb/IIIa, which aggregates platelets by cross-linking with fibrinogen.

The other commonly used platelet inhibitor is ticlopidine, but the mechanism of action is less well understood. Ticlopidine appears to change the configuration of the platelet membrane in a way that reduces interaction with fibrinogen and von Wilebrandt factor. Recently, an intravenous compound (ReoPro®, Eli Lilly, Indianapolis) that directly inhibits the glycoprotein receptor for fibrinogen responsible for platelet aggregation has been approved by the FDA for use during high risk coronary angioplasty (10).

Importantly, platelet inhibition is associated with significant clinical benefit. The treatment of unstable angina centers around anti-platelet and antithrombotic therapy. Aspirin alone reduced mortality by 50–70% in patients with unstable angina, with a persistent benefit up to 1-year of follow-up, as demonstrated by the VA Cooperative Study and the Canadian Multicenter Study (11, 12). In acute myocardial infarction, the ISIS 2 study showed that aspirin alone reduced mortality by 23%, similar to the effect of streptokinase alone (13). A doubling of the effect was noted when both agents were administered. Following the acute phase of myocardial infarction, aspirin reduces risk of vascular death by 13%, nonfatal reinfarction by 31%, nonfatal stroke by 42%, and all vascular events by 25% (14). Finally, either aspirin or ticlopidine decrease the risk of acute thrombotic occlusion following angioplasty, as well as maintaining patency of saphenous vein grafts (15). Sulfinpyrazone and dipyridamole have not been shown to have additional benefit. This conclusive evidence led to the recommendation that a daily dose of aspirin (81–325 mg/day) be administered to patients with all forms of CAD.

Cholesterol-lowering Therapy

The pathophysiology of atherosclerosis is intimately related to lipid metabolism, therefore it is logical that reductions in serum lipids result in clinical benefit. This hypothesis has been tested in numerous trials with both angiographic and clinical endpoints. A detailed description of these studies and the drugs used can be found elsewhere (16). In general, it has been demonstrated that lowering total and low-density lipoprotein cholesterol leads to minimal regression of existent luminal narrowing and to significant increase in the number of lesions that do not progress. Despite these modest angiographic improvements, the clinical benefit is rewarding. The 4S Trial addressed secondary prevention of CAD in patients with previous myocardial infarction or angina pectoris (17). Simvastatin, administered over a 5.4 year interval, reduced total mortality by 30% and coronary mortality by 42%. Important reductions were observed in rate of recurrent infarction and stroke across all age groups and in both genders.

The apparent disparity between angiographic and clinical endpoints can be explained by the mechanism of reduction in clinical events. The lipid-rich plaques, prone to fissuring, become quiescent after cholesterol reduction. Fibrotic material in plaque increases in parallel with cholesterol depletion, further stabilizing the atheroma (18).

These data are the basis for the recent enthusiasm among practitioners for aggressive lipid-lowering. Various classes of cholesterol lowering drugs and expected effects on blood lipid constituents are shown in Table 29.1.

Anti-ischemic Agents

Three classes of anti-ischemic agents are in common use for relief of symptoms in patients with symptomatic CAD. **Beta adrenergic blockers** moderate both the chronotropic (rate) and inotropic (force) response of the myocardium to exercise and activity, preventing imbalance between oxygen supply and demand that may occur during exertion. Patients can increase duration of exercise and reinfarction in survivors of myocardial infarction is reduced by 26–36% (19, 20). Beta-blockers also reduce the propensity for malignant ventricular arrhythmia during ischemia and, when used in the setting of acute myocardial infarction, diminish incidence of cardiac rupture.

Calcium channel blockers share some of the properties of beta adrenergic blockers. They decrease myocardial contractility and reduce cardiac workload via improved afterload profile. These agents are extremely

Table 29.1. **Lipid-lowering Agents and Their Expected Effect**

DRUG	TC	LDL-C	HDL-C	TG
Bile-acid resins	↓20%	↓20–25%	↑35%	Neutral or ↑
Nicotinic acid	↓25%	↓25%	↑15–30%	↓20–50%
Fibric acid derivatives	↓10–20%	↓5–25%	↑10–30%	↓20–60%
Probucol	↓25%	↓10–15%	↓20–30%	Neutral
Reductase inhibitors	↓15–30%	↓20–35%	↑2–12%	↓10–25%

TC = Total cholesterol, LDL-C = Low-density lipoprotein cholesterol, HDL-C = High-density lipoprotein cholesterol, TG = Triglycerides, ↓ = Decreases, ↑ = Increases.

(Adapted from Farmer JA, Gotto AM Jr. Lipid abnormalities—Management. In: Fuster V, Ross R, Topel EJ, eds. *Atherosclerosis and Coronary Artery Disease.* Philadelphia: Lippincott-Raven, 1996.

effective in reducing ischemia, both at rest and during exertion, but have not been demonstrated to reduce mortality in large randomized trials. Due to increasing concerns of blood flow redistribution in non-ischemic areas and reflex tachycardia related to vasodilatation, they should be used in addition to beta blockers, when symptoms cannot be sufficiently controlled.

Nitrates are the third important tool in the arsenal of anti-ischemic agents. They cause vasodilatation in large arterial and venous conduits. Their anti-ischemic effect is mediated by enhanced coronary circulation and reduced preload. They are efficacious for relief of angina, as both prophylactic or post-hoc agents. There are no convincing data indicating mortality benefit either in the chronic phase of CAD, or during acute myocardial infarction. Two large trials—GISSI 3 and ISIS 4—did not demonstrate significant reduction in 30-day mortality for patients treated with oral, or intravenous nitrates in addition to thrombolytic therapy, aspirin, and angiotensin converting inhibitors (21, 22).

Additional medications are used in the management of selected patients. Anticoagulation is essential in acute coronary syndrome, as well as in the context of severe ischemic cardiomyopathy. Thrombolytic therapy is the standard of care for acute myocardial infarction. Magnesium replacement may have a role in preventing arrhythmia and reperfusion injury during acute restoration of flow and angiotensin converting inhibitors have been established as the therapy of choice for left ventricular systolic dysfunction (23). This armamentarium of adjunctive therapies has led to significant improvement in the outcome of acute myocardial infarction, unstable angina, and chronic CAD.

INVASIVE TREATMENT OF CAD

Despite important advancements in pharmacological therapy, a large number of patients with CAD require mechanical revascularization. Relief of symptoms, prevention of (re)infarction, and prolongation of life are principal indications for implementation of this therapy. Once coronary arteries were visualized, restoration of normal lumen dimensions was a logical step. First CABG (1967) and, later, PTCA (1979) were introduced and quickly accepted as cornerstones in the treatment of obstructive CAD. While the former strategy diverts blood flow to healthier arterial segments beyond critical obstructions, the latter approach acutely remodels the arterial wall and atheroma, such that laminar flow ensues in the diseased portion of the vessel. Each strategy will be discussed separately, followed by a comparison of the two for various clinical scenarios.

Coronary Bypass Surgery

Coronary artery bypass grafting (CABG) uses arterial or venous conduits to circumvent obstructions in proximal epicardial arteries. Initially, reversed saphenous veins were connected to proximal aorta and to distal coronary segments during cardiopulmonary bypass. In the past 15 years, arterial conduits, in situ or as free grafts, have become increasingly popular. Despite anti-platelet and cholesterol-lowering therapy, 40–60% of venous bypasses become dysfunctional by 10 years after implantation, causing a significant number of myocardial infarctions and leading to ventricular dysfunction. In contrast, arterial conduits maintain a patency rate of approximately 90% at 10 years. The pathophysiology of saphenous venous graft disease differs with the interval from surgery.

In the first year, thrombosis in situ and surgical imperfections at anastomotic sites predominate as the cause for graft malfunction. During the next 2 years, intimal hyperplasia assumes the principal role for vein obstruction. Subsequently, atherosclerosis similar to that encountered in native coronary vessels afflicts these conduits and leads to dysfunction. For unclear reasons, all three mechanisms seem to be less applicable to arterial conduits, whether internal thoracic, radial, gastroepiploic, or hypogastric arteries. As the technique of cardiac surgery improves, more arterial conduits are used per patient, thus increasing the odds of durable revascularization.

The landmark trials of the late 1970s have established the main indications for CABG in those with chronic stable angina pectoris. Compared to medical therapy alone, surgical revascularization leads to significantly improved longevity and less angina in patients with involvement of all three epicardial vessels, in those with left main stenosis, and in subjects with left ventricular dysfunction.

A meta-analysis of the VA Study, The European Coronary Surgery Study and the Coronary Artery Surgery Study indicated that surgery confers a survival benefit over medical therapy up to 7 years. This advantage disappears after 10 years. Moreover, relief of angina was excellent in the first 10 years after surgery. Subsequently, attrition of grafts led to recurrent angina, such that only 3% of patients were free of angina at 15 years, similar to the medically treated group (24). There was no difference in the rate of new Q-wave myocardial infarction between surgically and medically treated groups.

These studies also highlight the relentless progression of CAD, typified by a high rate of crossover to CABG among patients assigned initially to medical therapy (40% at 10 years and 62% at 18 years). It is reasonable to conclude that, as important as these studies are in defining the natural history and progression of CAD, they do not reflect current common practice. For example, only 50% of patients received aspirin and only 6% were treated with lipid-lowering drugs. The use of pharmacological interventions has significantly increased in current clinical practice.

The use of CABG in patients with unstable angina was tested in a large VA study in the early 1980s. Patients

(N = 823) were randomly allocated to surgery or medical therapy. The results were similar to the chronic stable angina trials detailed above. Two years from randomization, mortality was reduced in surgically treated patients with impaired ventricular function, without significant differences in incidence of Q-wave infarctions. At 5-year follow-up, all patient groups with three-vessel disease assigned to CABG demonstrated survival rates superior to those in medical groups, regardless of degree of ventricular impairment.

Improved methods of myocardial and graft preservation and increased use of arterial bypasses are promising. Pretreatment of saphenous vein grafts with nitroglycerin and verapamil leads to more rapid endothelial coverage, potentially improving long term outcome. Preliminary reports indicate that transmyocardial laser revascularization may be useful in relieving angina in patients with severe, distal, and diffuse CAD. Moreover, renewed interest in minimally invasive CABG has led to placement of internal thoracic artery grafts to the left anterior and right coronary arteries via anterior or lateral small thoracotomy with minor morbidity. This technique may be extended in the future to patients with previous CABG.

Percutaneous Transluminal Coronary Angioplasty

The field of percutaneous coronary angioplasty (PTCA) has expanded significantly since the original report by Gruntzig in 1979 (25). Balloon angioplasty (Fig. 29.1) was initially designed for treatment of a discrete, single stenosis in a straight segment of a proximal coronary artery. As equipment improved, more difficult lesions were tackled with increasing rates of angiographic and clinical success. Similar to CABG, continuous improvements in technique and periprocedural care have paved the way to an exponentially increasing number of percutaneous coronary interventions.

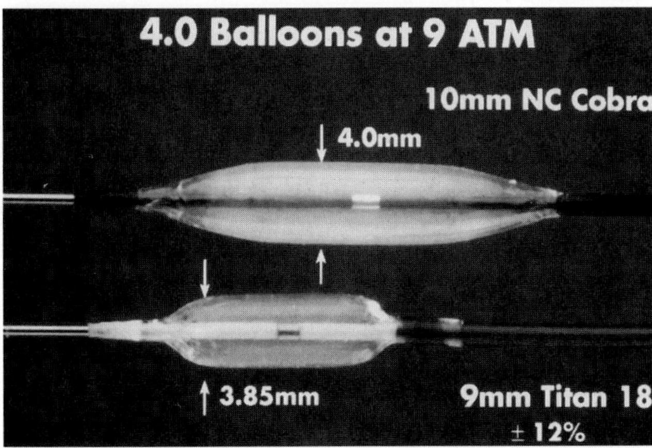

Figure 29.1. Percutaneous transluminal coronary angioplasty (PTCA) devices are manufactured in various sizes and from materials with different levels of compliance.

The only study comparing medical therapy to PTCA for patients with chronic stable angina is the Veterans Affairs Angioplasty Compared to Medicine (ACME) trial (26). Two hundred twelve patients were randomly assigned to PTCA or medical therapy. After 6 months, PTCA patients had a significantly greater increase in exercise tolerance (primary endpoint), compared with medically treated patients. Furthermore, 64% of patients treated with PTCA were free of angina, compared with only 46% in the medical group. This advantage diminished with time and was achieved at higher cost and complications related to the procedure. This trial provided the first evidence that angioplasty improves symptoms in patients with stable CAD.

In contrast, the application of PTCA in the setting of acute myocardial infarction has been studied in greater detail. In general, direct angioplasty can be expected to restore adequate blood flow in an infarct-related artery in 90% of cases, compared with 50–60% of thrombolysis subjects. In a meta-analysis of major trials of direct angioplasty versus thrombolysis, O'Neal, et al. found a 60% reduction in mortality (2.5% vs. 6.4%) and 75% reduction in reinfarction (2% vs. 7.9%) during initial hospitalization in patients treated with angioplasty. Recurrent ischemia, reinfarction, and need for future revascularization were all reduced in the angioplasty group at 6–12 months of follow-up, despite the occurrence of restenosis in 35–45% in these patients.

Obviously, the use of angioplasty for patients with acute myocardial infarction is limited by availability of 24-hour, fully staffed catheterization laboratories. It follows that thrombolytic therapy remains the mainstay of treatment in acute myocardial infarction in most institutions. Numerous studies indicate that routine angioplasty performed after administration of thrombolysis is deleterious. Patients manifesting spontaneous, or inducible ischemia, should undergo coronary angiography, followed by revascularization if indicated. These recommendations may be altered in patients with documented significant left ventricular dysfunction, or with previous myocardial infarction, in whom delineation of coronary anatomy may be instrumental in leading to revascularization, even in the absence of post infarction ischemia.

The main limitation of balloon angioplasty is the incidence of restenosis in the dilated segment. This process is intimately related to arterial injury occurring during balloon dilatation. The intima is fractured to allow plaque shifting from the lumen and the whole arterial circumference is stretched to accommodate the displacement. It appears that restenosis occurs as a two-pronged event. First, there is recoil of the artery toward the initial dimension. Second, smooth muscle cells located in the media undergo activation and a hyperplastic response ensues. Consequently, lumen dimensions decrease over 3–6 months leading to angiographically demonstrable restenosis in 30–50% of patients.

Clinically, half of the patients with angiographic restenosis require repeat revascularization. The important predictors of restenosis are diabetes mellitus, unstable angina at the time of angioplasty, continued smoking, and a high degree of residual stenosis. Despite 15 years of intense research, the ideal treatment for restenosis has not been found. Two avenues have been explored: a mechanical approach (attempts to design a better device), and pharmacological agents capable of inhibiting exuberant neointimal proliferation which follows balloon injury.

New mechanical devices have been designed to attempt to minimize arterial injury and post-procedural residual stenosis. Most of the new devices are designed to ablate atheroma by various means. The Simpson atherectomy catheter (Fig. 29.2) "shaves" plaque, while the Rotational atherectomy device (Fig. 29.3) uses a high-speed rotating metal burr coated with diamonds to pulverize plaque. The laser catheter delivers laser energy through an array of fibers to an obstructing lesion. Finally, the extraction atherectomy catheter (TEC) (Fig. 29.4) dislodges and suctions plaque into a reservoir. None of the randomized trials comparing balloon angioplasty to these newer devices have shown consistent reduction in the incidence of restenosis (27). Nevertheless, it should be noted that the ablation catheters

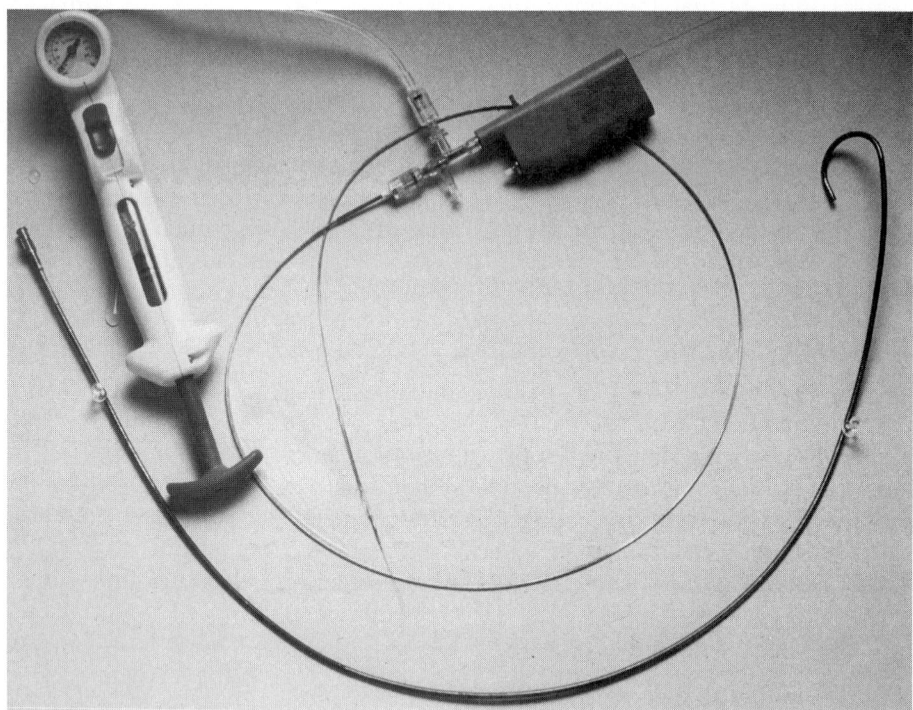

Figure 29.2. Directional coronary atherectomy (DCA) consists of a motor unit, spinning at ~2,000 rpm, and a cutter that travels inside a chamber. The large bore guiding catheter needed for device insertion is shown as well.

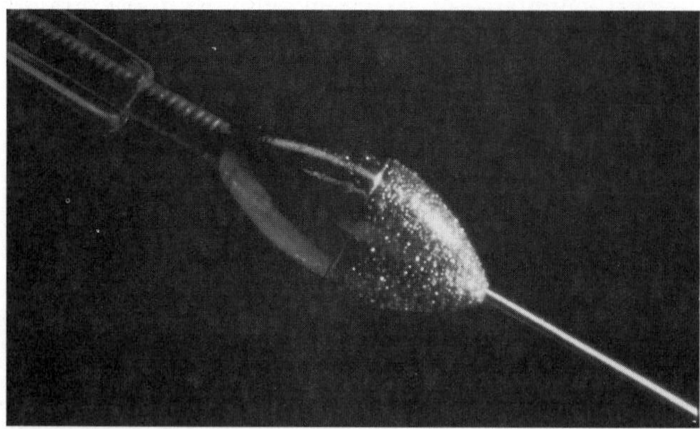

Figure 29.3. Rotational atherectomy burr, which is diamond-coated, spins at ~200,000 rpm and preferentially ablates calcified or fibrotic plaque material.

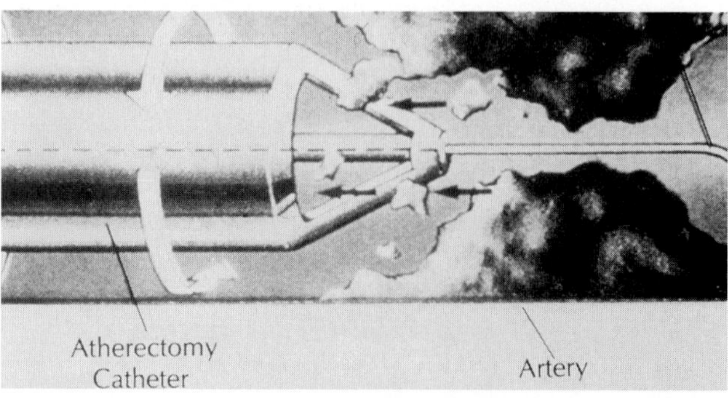

Figure 29.4. The Transluminal Extraction Catheter (TEC) consists of a suction device connected to a high-flow flush jet, and is particularly useful in the treatment of thrombus-laden arteries or bypass grafts.

achieve better angiographic results than balloon angioplasty and allow treatment of lesions not approachable with dilatation therapy.

The only mechanical device shown to affect restenosis is the endoluminal prosthesis known as "coronary stent." The stent serves as a scaffold that buttresses the arterial lumen. The stent undergoes endothelialization soon after its deployment. In selected patients and lesions, coronary stenting reduces restenosis by 30%, with promising long term outcome. Designed as slotted stainless steel tubes (Fig. 29.5) or coil springs, stents virtually eliminate arterial recoil and are effective in treating diseased saphenous vein grafts and restenotic lesions. The main drawbacks are the potential, albeit very low risk, for sub-acute thrombosis (< 1%) and higher cost.

Pharmacological interventions designed to reduce the incidence of restenosis focus on inhibition of smooth muscle proliferation. This response to arterial wall injury occurs universally in all species and determines whether restenosis causes impairment of flow. Experiments in animals demonstrate that heparin, cholesterol-lowering drugs, colchicine, angiotensin converting enzyme inhibitors, angiopeptin, and others can suppress healing, and thus reduce restenosis. These results have not been reproduced in humans.

A number of explanations have been proposed to reconcile the contradictory outcome observed in animal and human restenosis trials. Importantly, the concentrations of drugs applied to animal arterial wall were considerably higher than those in humans, despite the introduction of local delivery systems. Moreover, intravascular ultrasound examination performed serially in patients undergoing angioplasty highlighted the importance of recoil in the process of arterial lumen diminishment after dilatation. Intravascular ultrasound also made it possible to measure neointima formation after using different devices and it is apparent that arterial response to injury is proportional to luminal gain.

Recently, the clinical application of platelet fibrinogen receptor (IIB/IIIA) inhibitors has been shown to be a promising pharmacological intervention that can inhibit smooth muscle cell proliferation and reduce restenosis. The combination of these agents with stents may be even more effective in the treatment of angioplasty-induced restenosis. Elimination, or even halving of this process, will produce substantial economic benefit.

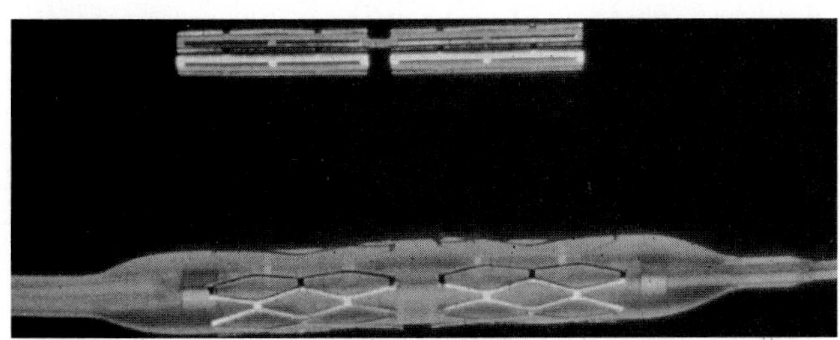

Figure 29.5. The coronary stent, tubular-slotted stainless-steel design manufactured by Johnson & Johnson, is shown in the compacted (top) and expanded (bottom) forms.

Comparison of Bypass Surgery and Angioplasty

Rigorous examination of relative efficacy of PTCA and CABG for primary revascularization in patients with symptomatic CAD has been undertaken in randomized trials (28–33). All studies reported similar outcomes with respect to in-hospital and 1–5 year event rate in over 4,500 patients (Table 29.2). In-hospital death was 0.8–1.7% in PTCA patients and 0.9–4.6% in a CABG cohort, while myocardial infarction was diagnosed in 2.3–6.3% of angioplasty patients and in 2.4–10.3% of CABG patients. In contrast, all studies conclusively indicated a higher rate of repeat revascularization in the patients assigned to PTCA (2.5–22 times) compared with

Table 29.2. Primary Revascularization Trials: CABG vs. PTCA

VARIABLE	RITA		ERACI		GABI		CABRI		EAST		BARI	
F/U (YR)	2.5		1		1		1		3		5	
	PTCA	CABG	PTCA	CABG	PTCA	CABG	PTCA	CABG	PTCA	CABG	PTCA	CABG
n	510	501	63	64	182	177	541	513	198	194	915	914
Death	3.1	3.6	4.8	4.6	2.2	5.1	3.9	2.1	7.1	6.21	13.7	10.7
MI	6.7	5.2	9.5	7.8	3.8	7.3	2.9	3.3	14.6	19.6	21.1	19.6
PTCA*	18.2	0.8	14.2	3.3	27.5	1.1	20.1	7.2	40	13	30.3	5.4
CABG*	18.8	3.2	17.5	0	22.5	4.0	20.2	1.4	21.2	0.5	27.2	0.9

Data are presented as percentage of groups.
F/U = Follow-up period, RITA = The Randomized Intervention Treatment of Angina Study, ERACI = Argentine Randomized Trial of Percutaneous Transluminal Coronary Angioplasty vs. Bypass Surgery Investigation, GABI = German Angioplasty vs. Bypass-Surgery Investigation, CABRI = Coronary Angioplasty vs. Bypass Revascularization Investigation, EAST = Emory Angioplasty Surgery Trial, BARI = Bypass Angioplasty Revascularization Investigation, MI = Myocardial infarction, * 4 years of follow-up for the BARI trial.

those receiving CABG. In addition, there was a trend toward more freedom from angina in CABG patients.

▶ SUMMARY

CAD continues to exact a toll despite significant advances in understanding of diagnosis, pathophysiology, natural history, prognosis, and treatment. Patients present either with typical effort-related angina pectoris, unstable coronary syndromes, or sudden death in approximately equal proportions. Once diagnosis of symptomatic CAD is made or strongly suspected, medical care providers should secure active participation of the patient in a comprehensive treatment program to minimize the impact of previous events and prevent new events.

The process begins with assessment of predisposing risk factors for development of CAD and the steps required to favorably modify them. Special attention directed toward adequate control of hypertension, diabetes mellitus, hypercholesterolemia, as well as immediate and lasting cessation of smoking is necessary.

The presence of unstable angina mandates judicious pharmacological intervention until stabilization. With few exceptions, patients with CAD should be treated indefinitely with aspirin, 81–325 mg/day. Pharmacological cholesterol-lowering therapy is recommended in all patients in whom the recommendations of the National Cholesterol Education Program II guidelines can not be met with dietary modification alone. Survivors of complete or incomplete Q-wave myocardial infarction should receive beta-adrenergic inhibitors. Angiotensin converting enzyme inhibitors should be added if systolic dysfunction exists.

Mechanical revascularization via angioplasty or bypass surgery is reserved for patients with significant left ventricular systolic dysfunction, angiographic features associated with poor prognosis on medical therapy alone, or in those with unacceptable symptomatology despite aggressive pharmacological therapy. Mechanical restoration of flow should not replace other interventions, but rather complement them in selected patients.

References

1. National Center for Health Statistics. Vital statistics of the United States, 1988. Vol. II, Part A. Washington: USDHHS; 1991.
2. Strong JP, McGill HC Jr. The natural history of atherosclerosis. *Am J Pathol* 40:37, 1962.
3. Glagov S, Zarins CK, Giddens DP, et al. Hemodynamic and atherosclerosis. Insights and perspectives gained from studies of human arteries. *Arch Pathol Lab Med* 112:1018, 1988.
4. Fuster V, Badimon L, Badimon JJ, et al. The pathogenesis of coronary artery disease and the acute coronary syndromes. *N Engl J Med* 326:242, 1992.
5. Fuster V, Badimon L, Badimon JJ, et al. The pathogenesis of coronary artery disease and the acute coronary syndromes (part II). *N Engl J Med* 326:310, 1992.
6. National Cholesterol Education Program. Second report of the Expert Panel on Detection, Evaluation, and Treatment of High Blood Cholesterol in Adults (Adult Treatment Panel II). *Circulation* 89:1329, 1994.
7. Joint National Committee on Detection, Evaluation, and Treatment of High Blood Pressure. The fifth report of the Joint National Committee on Detection, Evaluation, and Treatment of High Blood Pressure (JNC V). *Arch Int Med* 153:154, 1993.
8. Brewer HB Jr, Santamarina-Fojo SM, Hoeg JM. Genetic dyslipoproteinemias. In: Fuster V, Ross R, Topol EJ, eds. *Atherosclerosis and Coronary Artery Disease.* Philadelphia: Lippincott-Raven, 1996.
9. Hirsh J, Dalen J, Fuster V, et al. Aspirin and other platelet active drugs: the relationship between dose, effectiveness, and side effects. *Chest* 102(Suppl):327S, 1992.
10. The EPIC Investigators. Use of a monoclonal antibody directed against the platelet glycoprotein IIb/IIIa receptor in high-risk coronary angioplasty. *N Engl J Med* 330:956, 1994.
11. Lewis HD, Davis JW, Archibald GD, et al. Protective effect of aspirin against acute myocardial infarction and death in men with unstable angina. *N Engl J Med* 309:396, 1983.
12. Cairns JA, Gent M, Singer J, et al. Aspirin, sulfinpyrazone, or both in unstable angina. Results of a Canadian multicenter trial. *N Engl J Med* 313:1369, 1985.
13. ISIS-2 (Second International Study of Infarct Survival) Collaborative Group. Randomized trial of intravenous streptokinase, oral aspirin, both, or neither among 17,187 cases of suspected acute myocardial infarction: ISIS-2. *Lancet* 2:349, 1988.
14. Antiplatelet Trialists' Collaboration. Secondary prevention of vascular disease by prolonged antiplatelet treatment. *Br Med J* 296:320, 1988.
15. Limet R, David JL, Magotteaux P, et al. Prevention of aorta-coronary bypass graft occlusion. *J Thorac Cardiovasc Surg* 94:773, 1987.
16. Farmer JA, Gotto AM Jr. Lipid Abnormalities—Management. In: Fuster V, Ross R, Topol EJ, eds. *Atherosclerosis and Coronary Artery Disease.* Philadelphia: Lippincott-Raven, 1996.
17. Scandinavian Simvastatin Survival Study Group. Randomised trial of cholesterol lowering in 4444 patients with coronary heart disease: the Scandinavian Simvastatin Survival Study (4S). *Lancet* 344:1383, 1994.
18. Brown BG, Zhao XQ, Sacco DE, et al. Lipid lowering and plaque regression. New insights into prevention of plaque disruption and clinical events in CAD. *Circulation* 87:1781, 1993.
19. Beta-Blocker Heart Attack Trial Research Group. A randomized trial of propranolol in patients with acute myocardial infarction. *JAMA* 247:1707, 1981.
20. Norwegian Multicenter Study Group. Timolol-induced reduction in mortality and reinfarction surviving acute myocardial infarction. *N Engl J Med* 304:801, 1981.
21. Grouppo Italiano per lo Studio della Sopravivenza nell'Infarcto miocardico. GISSI-3: Effects of lisinopril and

transdermal glyceryl trinitrate singly and together on 6-week mortality and ventricular function after acute myocardial infarction. *Lancet* 343:1115, 1994.

22. ISIS-4 (Fourth International Study of Infarct Survival) Collaborative Group. ISIS-4: A randomized trial assessing early oral captopril, oral mononitrate, and intravenous magnesium sulphate in 58050 patients with suspected acute myocardial infarction. *Lancet* 345:669, 1995.
23. Pfeffer MA, Braunwald E, Moye LA, et al. Effect of captopril on mortality and morbidity in patients with left ventricular dysfunction after myocardial infarction. *N Engl J Med* 327: 669, 1992.
24. Coronary Artery Bypass Surgery Trialists Collaboration. Effect of coronary artery bypass surgery on survival: overview of 10-year results from randomized trials. *Lancet* 344:563, 1994.
25. Gruentzig AR, Senning A, Siegenthaler WE. Non-operative dilatation of coronary artery stenosis: Percutaneous Transluminal Coronary Angioplasty. *N Engl J Med* 301:61, 1979.
26. Parisi EF, Folland ED, Hartigan P, et al. A comparison of angioplasty with medical therapy in the treatment of single-vessel coronary disease. *N Engl J Med* 326:10, 1992.
27. Moliterno DJ, Topol EJ: Clinical evaluation of restenosis. In: Fuster V, Ross R, Topol EJ, eds. *Atherosclerosis and Coronary Artery Disease.* Philadelphia: Lippincott-Raven, 1996.
28. RITA Trial Participants. Coronary angioplasty versus coronary artery bypass surgery: The Randomized Intervention Treatment of Angina (RITA) trial. *Lancet* 341:573, 1993.
29. Rodriguez A, Boullon F, Perez-Balino L, et al. Argentine randomized trial of percutaneous transluminal coronary angioplasty versus coronary artery bypass surgery in multivessel disease (ERACI): in-hospital results and 1-year follow-up. *J Am Coll Cardiol* 22:1060, 1993.
30. Hamm CW, Reimers J, Ischinger T, et al. A randomized study of coronary angioplasty compared with bypass surgery in patients with symptomatic multivessel coronary disease. German Angioplasty Bypass Surgery Investigation (GABI). *N Engl J Med* 331:1037, 1994.
31. CABRI Investigators. First year results of CABRI. *Lancet* 346: 1179, 1995.
32. King SB III, Lembo NJ, Weintraub WS, et al. A randomized trial comparing coronary angioplasty with coronary bypass surgery. *N Engl J Med* 331:1044, 1994.
33. BARI Investigators. Comparison of coronary bypass surgery with angioplasty in patients with multivessel disease. The Bypass Angioplasty Revascularization Investigation. *N Engl J Med* 335:217, 1996.

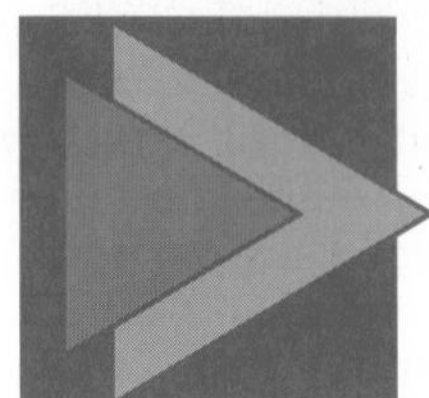

CHAPTER 30

COMPREHENSIVE CARDIOVASCULAR RISK REDUCTION IN PATIENTS WITH CORONARY ARTERY DISEASE

Neil F. Gordon and Tom LaFontaine

Despite a 24.5% decline in the death rate from cardiovascular disease during the past decade in the United States, cardiovascular disease remains the leading cause of morbidity and mortality. In particular, coronary artery disease (CAD) causes approximately 500,000 deaths/year and over 11 million Americans have established CAD (1). More than $50 billion is spent annually on the treatment of these individuals, yet fewer than 17% initiate comprehensive therapy aimed at cardiovascular risk reduction and continue it for more than 6 months (2). Current evidence provides a strong rationale for long term aggressive control of CAD risk factors as essential strategy to:

- Normalize coronary artery endothelial function
- Halt or reverse the progression of coronary atherosclerosis
- Prevent the instability, rupture, and thrombosis of atherosclerotic plaques
- Reduce mortality, recurrent hospitalization, and ongoing cost of medical care.

Existing barriers to effective implementation of comprehensive cardiovascular risk reduction strategies and recent expert guidelines for clinical practice will be summarized in this chapter.

PROGRESSION/REGRESSION OF ATHEROSCLEROSIS

Atherosclerotic coronary artery occlusions are estimated to progress at a "natural" rate causing a 1.5% reduction in artery diameter per year (3). Rate of progression is reported to be 3–6 times greater in grafted versus ungrafted vessels (3). Recent arteriographic secondary prevention clinical trials have convincingly demonstrated that while progression of coronary atherosclerosis is common when CAD patients receive usual medical care, aggressive modification of risk factors may slow the atherosclerosis progression rate or induce partial regression. This section summarizes key findings of these studies.

The NHLBI Type II Coronary Intervention Study first suggested that lipid lowering using dietary therapy and cholestyramine could retard progression of atherosclerosis in patients with hyperlipidemia (4). In the Cholesterol Lowering Atherosclerosis Study (CLAS), 162 male post-coronary artery bypass surgery patients were randomly assigned to diet therapy plus placebo or diet therapy plus colestipol and niacin (5). After 2 years of intervention, assessment of arteriographic change revealed significantly more regression in the drug treated group compared with the placebo group (16.2% vs. 2.4%). After 4 years of intervention, nonprogression of atherosclerosis occurred more often in the drug treated group compared with the placebo group (52% vs. 15%), as did regression (18% vs. 6%) (6).

These initial trials prompted a series of arteriographic secondary prevention trials to evaluate the impact of CAD risk factor modification by pharmacologic, lifestyle, and surgical strategies on underlying atherosclerosis process (Tables 30.1, 30.2, and 30.3). Differences in methodology preclude meaningful comparison of the amount of regression observed. However, analysis of arteriographic data from the study in which the greatest magnitude of regression occurred, namely the Lifestyle Heart Trial, is of interest since it provides insight into the degree to which the underlying atherosclerosis process can be affected. In this study, the average stenosis regressed from 40.0% to 37.8 % with 1 year of intensive lifestyle intervention and progressed from 42.7% to 46.1% with 1 year of usual medical care. When occlusions greater than 50% were analyzed, the average stenosis regressed from 61.1% to 55.8% in the intervention group and progressed from 61.7% to 64.4% in the usual care group (7).

Several important observations have emerged from existing arteriographic secondary prevention clinical trials including the following:

Table 30.1. Percentage of Patients Experiencing Progression or Regression of Atherosclerosis in Arteriographic Secondary Prevention Trials Involving Lifestyle Intervention Alone or in Combination With Drug Treatment

Study (Year Published)	Subjects	Intervention	Design	Duration (yrs)	Progression (% Patients)		Regression (% Patients)	
					Intervention Group	Control Group	Intervention Group	Control Group
Lifestyle Heart Trial (1990)	Male: n = 36 Female: n = 5 Age = 35–75 yrs	Multiple lifestyle intervention	Randomized	1	18	53	82	42
STARS (1992)	Male: n = 50 Female: n = 0 Age < 66 yrs	Diet	Randomized	3.25	15	46	38	4
	Male: n = 48 Female: n = 0 Age < 66 yrs	Diet + cholestyramine	Randomized	3.25	12	46	33	4
Heidelberg (1992)	Male: n = 113 Female: n = 0 Age = 35–68 yrs	Exercise + diet	Randomized	1	23	48	32	17
SCRIP (1994)	Male: n = 259 Female: n =41 Age < 75 yrs	Multiple lifestyle intervention + lipid lowering drugs if indicated	Randomized	4	50	50	20	10

Abbreviations: STARS = St. Thomas' Atherosclerosis Regression Study (*Lancet* 339: 563–569, 1992; Heidelberg = Schuler et al. (see reference 8); SCRIP = Stanford Coronary Risk Intervention Project (see reference 14). For Lifestyle Heart Trial, see reference 7.

1. Progression of atherosclerosis can be expected to occur when CAD patients receive usual medical care.
2. Non-progression and regression of coronary atherosclerosis occurs significantly more often in patients who aggressively modify CAD risk factors compared with those receiving usual medical care.
3. The magnitude of regression is modest at best and usually on the order of 1–10% of the original stenosis.
4. The underlying atherosclerosis process can be favorably affected by single or multiple interventions and by pharmacologic, lifestyle, or surgical modulation of CAD risk factors.

In addition, it is evident from these studies that effective interventions are usually well-tolerated and acceptable.

MYOCARDIAL PERFUSION AND CLINICAL EVENTS

Though modest changes in anatomic severity of coronary artery stenoses ensue after aggressive CAD risk factor modification, the precise value of such therapy might be questioned. More important than anatomic arteriographic improvement, however, is the impact of risk factor intervention on myocardial perfusion and clinical cardiac events.

According to the Poiseuille equation, resistance to flow is inversely proportional to the radius raised to the fourth power. Therefore, even minor improvements in percent diameter stenosis can be expected to produce proportionately greater improvements in myocardial perfusion. In this respect, Schuler et al. documented a reduction in exercise-induced myocardial ischemia, assessed by thallium scintigraphy, in patients with stable angina pectoris who participated in 12 months of exercise training combined with a low fat diet (8). More recently, Gould et al. evaluated changes in size and severity of myocardial perfusion abnormalities by positron emission tomography in patients with CAD randomized to 5 years of intensive risk factor modification or to usual care as part of the Lifestyle Heart Trial (9). Risk factor modification consisted of a very low-fat, low-cholesterol, vegetarian diet, smoking cessation, the practice of stress management techniques for 82 minutes daily, and participation in mild to moderate aerobic exercise for over 4 hours/week. The study demonstrated that the size and severity of myocardial perfusion abnormalities at rest and after dipyridamole stress improve in patients undergoing intense risk factor modification, while patients treated with usual therapy demonstrated increasing perfusion abnormalities. The relative magnitude of change in size and severity of perfusion abnormalities was comparable to changes in stenosis.

Improvements in myocardial perfusion with aggressive risk factor modification are thought to be related to improved endothelial-mediated coronary artery and arteriolar vasomotor function (10, 11). Animal and human studies document improvement in myocardial per-

Table 30.2. Percentage of Patients Experiencing Progression or Regression of Atherosclerosis in Arteriographic Secondary Prevention Trials Involving Single Drug Therapy or Ileal Bypass Surgery

Study (Year published)	Subjects	Intervention	Design	Duration (yrs)	Progression (% Patients)		Regression (% Patients)	
					Intervention Group	Control Group	Intervention Group	Control Group
NHLBI Type II Coronary Intervention Study (1984)	Male: n = 94 Female: n = 22 Age = 21–55 yrs	Cholestyramine	Randomized, double-blind, placebo-controlled	5	32	49	7	7
MARS (1993)	Male: n = 247 Female: n = 23 Age = 37–67 yrs	Lovastatin	Randomized, double-blind, placebo-controlled	2	29	41	23	12
CCAIT (1994)	Male: n = 269 Female: n = 62 Age = 27–70 yrs	Lovastatin	Randomized, double-blind, placebo-controlled	2	33	50	10	7
MAAS (1994)	Male: n = 336 Female: n = 45 Age = 30–67 yrs	Simvastatin	Randomized, double-blind, placebo-controlled	4	3	4	4	4
REGRESS (1995)	Male: n = 885 Female: n = 0 Age < 70 yrs	Pravastatin	Randomized, double-blind, placebo-controlled	2	22	28	8	5
POSCH (1990)	Male: n = 760 Female: n = 78 Age = 30–64 yrs	Partial ileal bypass surgery	Randomized	9.7	55	85	6	4

Abbreviations: MARS = Monitored Atherosclerosis Regression Study (*Ann Intern Med* 119: 969–976, 1993); CCAIT = Canadian Coronary Atherosclerosis Intervention Trial (*Circulation* 89: 959–968, 1994); MAAS = Multicent Anti-Atheroma Study (*Lancet* 344: 633–638, 1994); REGRESS = Regression Growth Evaluation Statin Study (*Circulation* 91: 2528–2540, 1995); POSCH = Program on the Surgical Control of the Hyperlipidemias (*N Engl J Med* 323: 946–955, 1990). For NHLBI Type II Coronary Intervention Study, see reference 4.

Table 30.3. Percentage of Patients Experiencing Progression or Regression of Atherosclerosis in Arteriographic Secondary Prevention Trials Involving Multiple Drug Therapy

					Progression (% Patients)		Regression (% Patients)	
Study (Year Published)	Subjects	Intervention	Design	Duration (yrs)	Intervention Group	Control Group	Intervention Group	Control Group
CLASS-1 (1987)	Male: n = 162 Female: n = 0 Age = 40–59 yrs	Colestipol + niacin	Randomized, double-blind, placebo-controlled	2	39	61	16	2
FATS (1990)	Male: n = 82 Female: n = 0 Age < 63 yrs	Colestipol + niacin	Randomized, double-blind, placebo-controlled	2.5	25	46	39	11
	Male: n = 84 Female: n = 0 Age < 63 yrs	Colestipol + lovastatin	Randomized, double-blind, placebo-controlled	2.5	21	46	32	11
SCOR (1990)	Male: n = 31 Female: n = 41 Age = 19–72 yrs	Colestipol + niacin + lovastatin	Randomized	2.17	20	41	33	13
CLASS-11 (1990)	Male: n = 103 Female: n = 0 Age = 40–59 yrs	Colestipol + niacin	Randomized, double-blind, placebo-controlled	4	30	79	18	6
HARP (1994)	Male: n = 70 Female: n = 9 Age = 30–75 yrs	Intensive drugs (1–4 lipid drugs)	Randomized, single-blind, placebo-controlled	2.5	33	38	13	15

Abbreviations: CLASS = Cholesterol-Lowering Atherosclerosis Study (see references 5, 6); FATS = Familial Atherosclerosis Treatment Study (*N Engl J Med* 323: 1289–1298, 1990); SCOR = University of California, San Francisco, Arteriosclerosis Specialized Center of Research Intervention Trial (*JAMA* 264: 3007–3012, 1990); HARP = Harvard Atherosclerosis Reversibility Project (*Lancet* 344: 1182–1186, 1994.)

fusion within weeks to months after vigorous cholesterol lowering by fat restriction and/or drugs, before the occurrence of anatomic regression (11–13).

Recent arteriographic secondary prevention trials were specifically designed to assess impact of risk factor modification on atherosclerotic progression or regression. A significant reduction in major clinical cardiac events including sudden cardiac death, nonfatal myocardial infarction, new onset angina pectoris, and need for primary revascularization procedures, has been documented (Table 30.4).

Of the investigations performed to date, the Stanford Coronary Risk Intervention Project (SCRIP) is perhaps of greatest practical significance (14). SCRIP used aggressive modification of multiple risk factors via lifestyle intervention and medication. Moreover, SCRIP employed a physician-supervised, nurse case-manager model with consultation from other health professionals that can potentially be implemented in other health care settings. SCRIP studied 300 men and women with arteriographically defined CAD. They were randomly assigned to usual care or multifactor risk reduction for the 4-year study period. Patients assigned to risk reduction were provided individualized programs involving a low-fat, low-cholesterol diet, exercise, weight loss, smoking cessation, and medications to favorably alter lipoprotein profiles. Intensive cardiovascular risk reduction resulted in significant improvements in various CAD risk factors, including low-density lipoprotein (LDL) cholesterol and apolipoprotien B, high-density lipoprotein (HDL) cholesterol, plasma triglycerides, body weight, exercise capacity, and intake of dietary fat and cholesterol, compared with relatively small changes in the usual care group. Progression of atherosclerosis in the risk reduction group was 47% less than for the usual care group. In addition, there were 25 hospitalizations in the risk reduction group initiated by clinical cardiac events compared with 44 in the usual care group. Interestingly, during the final 3 years of the study, risk reduction patients were hospitalized for clinical cardiac events only 8 times compared with 35 times for the usual care patients.

Cholesterol lowering has caused some concern because the observed reduction of cardiac deaths appears to be offset by an increase in noncardiac mortality, particularly due to cancer and violent death. In the Scandinavian Simvastatin Survival Study (4S), a landmark secondary prevention study, 4,444 patients with angina pectoris or previous myocardial infarction and high serum cholesterol were randomized to double-blind treatment with simvastatin or placebo (15). Over the 5.4 year follow-up period, treatment resulted in a 42% reduction in cardiac deaths, a 37% reduction in risk of undergoing revascularization procedures, and a 30% reduction in all-cause mortality. This improvement in survival was

Table 30.4. Reduction in Clinical Cardiac Events With Risk Factor Modification in Recent Secondary Prevention Trials

Study (Year Published)	Duration (Yrs)	Cardiac Events	Intervention	Reduction in Cardiac Events
POSCH (1990)	9.7	CAD death + MI + CABG	Partial ileal bypass surgery	49%, $p \le 0.05$
FATS (1990)	2.5	CVD death + MI + revascularization	Colestipol + niacin	78%, $p \le 0.05$
			Colestipol + lovastatin	66%, $p \le 0.05$
STARS (1992)	3.25	CVD death + MI + CABG + PTCA	Diet	69%, $p \le 0.05$
			Diet + cholestyramine	89%, $p \le 0.05$
MARS (1993)	2	CAD death + MI + CABG + PTCA + unstable angina	Lovastatin	28%, p = NS
CCAIT (1994)	2	CAD death + MI + unstable angina	Lovastatin	22%, p = NS
SCRIP (1994)	4	CVD death + MI + CABG + primary PTCA	Multiple lifestyle intervention + lipid lowering drugs if indicated	39%, $p \le 0.05$
MAAS (1994)	4	CAD death + MI + CABG + PTCA	Simvastatin	24%, p = NS
PLAC-II (1994)	3	CAD death + MI	Pravastatin	60%*
HARP (1994)	2.5	CAD death + MI + CHF + CABG + PTCA + unstable angina	Intensive drugs (1–4 lipid drugs)	33%, p = NS
4S (1994)	5.4	CAD death + MI + resuscitated cardiac arrest	Simvastatin	34%, $p \le 0.05$
REGRESS (1995)	2	CAD death + MI	Pravastatin	38%*
PLAC-I (1995)	3	CAD death + MI	Pravastatin	53%*
CARE (1996)		CAD death + MI	Pravastatin	24%, $p \le 0.05$

Abbreviations: See Tables 30.1, 30.2, 30.3. PLAC-I = Pravastatin Limitation of Atherosclerosis in the Coronary Arteries Trial (see reference 18); 4S = Scandinavian Simvastatin Survival Study (see reference 15); PLAC-II = Pravastatin, Lipids, and Atherosclerosis in the Carotid Arteries Trial (see reference 18); CARE = Cholesterol and Recurrent Events study (see reference 19). CAD = coronary artery disease; CVD = cardiovascular disease.

* Statistical significance not provided—when data from these 3 trials are combined with data from Kuopio Atherosclerosis Prevention Study (KAPS), $p \le 0.05$ for reduction in CAD death + MI (51% reduction; see reference 18).

achieved without an increase in non-CAD mortality. The beneficial impact of simvastatin on CAD risk appeared to begin after about 1 year of therapy and increased steadily thereafter, a finding consistent with several angiographic studies (16).

Recent similar findings have been reported in patients treated with diet, lovastatin, and cholestyramine following coronary artery bypass surgery (17). Aggressive lowering of LDL cholesterol to < 100 mg/dl was associated with a 31% reduction in per-patient percentage of grafts showing progression of atherosclerosis. It was concluded that these findings were consistent with the recommendation of the National Cholesterol Education program that the LDL-cholesterol level should be reduced to < 100 mg/dl in patients with documented CAD. These findings have been corroborated by the West of Scotland Coronary Prevention Study and the Pravastatin Atherosclerosis and MI Reduction Analysis, which represents a combined analysis of clinical event data from four independent secondary prevention studies (PLAC 1, PLAC II, REGRESS, and KAPS) (18–20).

Most recently, data from the Cholesterol and Recurrent Events (CARE) study of 4,159 patients who survived a myocardial infarction, but did not have elevated cholesterol levels (total cholesterol = 180–239 mg/dl) have been published (21). In this trial, treatment with pravastatin resulted in a reduction of nonfatal myocardial infarction or CAD deaths (24%) and a reduction in the need for revascularization procedures (27%).

MECHANISM OF REDUCTION IN CARDIAC EVENTS

Based on recent advances in understanding pathophysiology of atherosclerosis and acute cardiac syndromes, the paradoxical observation of a significant reduction in clinical cardiac events despite modest arteriographic benefits following aggressive risk factor modification is evolving (22, 23):

1. Less severe atherosclerotic plaques may rapidly progress to severe stenoses or total coronary artery occlusions and may account for up to two-thirds of patients in whom unstable angina pectoris or acute myocardial infarction develops.
2. Rupture of a vulnerable plaque with resultant thrombus formation may be the most important mechanism underlying rapid progression.
3. Most ruptures occur at the periphery of the fibrous cap covering the lipid-rich core of the plaque—sites where the cap is usually thinnest and most heavily infiltrated by macrophage foam cells.
4. Vulnerability to plaque rupture depends on composition rather than size or volume. Although hard collagenous tissue usually constitutes the largest component, soft lipid-rich core and cap weakening (perhaps macrophage-related) are predisposed to plaque rupture and determine vulnerability.
5. The plaque components responsible for vulnerability (soft lipid and probably macrophages) appear to be more mobile with greater potential to regress than more voluminous collagenous components. Aggressive risk factor modification may stabilize plaques, leaving them less vulnerable, though not necessarily less voluminous.
6. Aggressive risk factor modification may further stabilize plaques in the absence of atherosclerotic regression by normalizing endothelial function; endothelium can profoundly affect vascular tone by releasing contracting factors, such as endothelin-1, and relaxing factors, such as prostacyclin and endothelium-derived relaxing factor (EDRF, now known to be nitric oxide).

Possibilities other than plaque stabilization that are likely to further contribute to reduced clinical cardiac events with aggressive risk factor modification include a favorable impact on thrombogenic propensity and on factors that trigger plaque rupture (e.g., reduced blood pressure and/or heart rate) (21, 22).

COST-EFFECTIVENESS

Health care costs in the United States exceed one trillion dollars annually and consume 14% of gross domestic product. In 1994, approximately 850,000 coronary revascularizations together with charges for hospitalization, medical personnel, health care facilities, and medications resulting from treatment of CAD are estimated to have cost over $50 billion.

Strategies targeted at secondary prevention of CAD can be expected to reduce the economic toll. The public health approach to CAD prevention, targeting the entire population to modify risk factors, is the least expensive method for accomplishing this. To identify individuals with CAD and aggressively manage risk factors complements public health strategies, but is more expensive. While the benefits of the clinical approach in reduced cardiac events is well documented, economic considerations dictate that such benefits be weighed against the costs to produce them.

Cost-effectiveness analysis is a method of considering the effectiveness and the cost of an intervention. In cost-effectiveness analysis, costs are expressed in monetary terms, whereas effectiveness is expressed as a health benefit (typically, years of life saved or quality-adjusted years of life saved). Cost-effective analysis constitutes a useful method for expressing potential benefit from a particular investment. It has been proposed that if the cost per year of life saved (or quality-adjusted year of life saved) is less than $20,000, the intervention should be considered

Table 30.5. Coronary Artery Disease Cost-Effectiveness Overview

INTERVENTION	CONDITION	PATIENTS	$/YLS OR $/QALY*
Lovastatin (20 mg/dl)	Hyperlipidemia	CAD, chol ≥ 250 mg/dl, men 45–54 yrs	Saves $ and lives
Enalapril	HF	Ejection fraction ≤ 0.35	Saves $ and lives
Nurse counseling manual	Smoking	Post-myocardial infarction	250
Beta-blocker	Post-myocardial infarction	High risk	3600
Lovastatin (20 mg/dl)	Hyperlipidemia	CAD, chol ≥ 250 mg/dl, women 45–54 yrs	4700
PTCA	Chronic CAD	Severe angina, 1 vessel disease	8700–10200*
CABG	Chronic CAD	Severe angina, left main disease	9200*
Cardiac rehabilitation	Post-myocardial infarction	Depressed patients	9200*
CABG	Chronic CAD	Mild angina, 3 vessel disease	18200*
Beta-blocker	Post-myocardial infarction	Low risk	20200
CABG	Chronic CAD	Severe angina, 2 vessel disease	42500*
CABG	Chronic CAD	Severe angina, 1 vessel disease	72900*
PTCA	Chronic CAD	Mild angina, 1 vessel disease	91500*

Abbreviations: * Values with an asterisk are in dollars per quality-adjusted life years ($/QALY) and those without an asterisk are in dollars per year of life saved ($/YLS); CAD = coronary artery disease; chol = cholesterol; HF = heart failure; PTCA = percutaneous transluminal coronary angioplasty; CABG = coronary artery bypass grafting. Values are in 1993 dollars. (Adapted from Fuster V, Gotto AM, Libby P, et al. Task Force I. Pathogenesis of coronary disease: the biological role of risk factors. *J Am Coll Cardiol* 27: 964–976, 1996.)

very cost-effective, whereas if it is greater than $75,000, the intervention should be considered very expensive (24).

Published cost-effectiveness analyses are available for a variety of strategies for modifying CAD risk factors, including smoking cessation, lipid management, blood pressure control, and cardiac rehabilitation exercise training (Table 30.5). Generally, these data support the cost-effectiveness of risk factor modification in CAD patients. The cost-effectiveness of aggressive modification of multiple-risk factors (as compared to single-risk factors) in patients with CAD has not been examined as rigorously or extensively as the clinical benefits. However, in view of the reduction in clinical cardiac events that can be expected with such approaches (22–89%), there is little doubt that they are both clinically effective and cost-effective.

Table 30.6. Estimates of Levels of Risk Factor Management in Patients Surviving Myocardial Infarction

Referral to cardiac rehabilitation program*	< 5%
Smoking cessation counseling†	20%
Lipid-lowering drug therapy‡	25%
Beta-blocker therapy†	40%
ACE inhibitor therapy (reduced LV ejection fraction)†	60%
Aspirin†	70%

* Coronary Artery Surgery Study (CASS): a randomized trial of coronary artery bypass surgery. Quality of life in patients randomly assigned to treatment groups. Circulation 1983;68:951–960. † Vogel RA. Risk factor intervention and coronary artery disease: clinical strategies. Coronary Artery Dis 1995;6:466–471. ‡ Pearson TA. personal communication, September 1995. ACE = angiotensin-converting enzyme; LV = left ventricular. (Reprinted with permission from Goldman L, Garber AM, Grover SA, et al. Task Force 6. Cost-effectiveness of assessment and management of risk factors. *J Am Coll Cardiol* 27:1020–1030, 1996.)

BARRIERS TO IMPLEMENTATION

There is now overwhelming evidence as to the clinical benefits of aggressive risk factor modification in patients with established CAD. In fact, there are more published trials showing decreased cardiac events by aggressive risk factor modification than reports on decreased cardiac events by elective percutaneous transluminal coronary angioplasty or coronary artery bypass surgery in patients with stable CAD (11). Despite this, it is clear that long term management of CAD patients is fragmented (and usually unsatisfactory) and that the proportion of patients receiving appropriate care is alarmingly low (Table 30.6) (25). The failure of the current status of medical management of CAD to reflect recent advances in knowledge of risk factors and effective modification undoubtedly results in avoidable death, disability, and financial expenditure.

A variety of barriers to successful implementation of effective services for the secondary prevention of CAD have been identified (Table 30.7) (26). These include barriers at the level of the patient, physician, health care setting, community, and society. Strategies to overcome these barriers include:

1. Development of clinical practice guidelines for cardiovascular risk reduction.
2. Implementation of model programs for cardiovascular risk reduction proven to be effective.
3. Inclusion of risk factor management as a key indicator of quality of care in quality assurance programs.

Table 30.7. Barriers to Implementation of Preventive Services

Patient
- Lack of knowledge and motivation
- Lack of access to care
- Cultural factors
- Social factors

Physician
- Problem-based focus
- Feedback on prevention is negative or neutral
- Time constraints
- Lack of incentives, including reimbursement
- Lack of training
  - Poor knowledge of benefits
  - Perceived ineffectiveness
  - Lack of skills
- Lack of specialist-generalist communication
- Lack of perceived legitimacy

Health care settings (hospitals, practices, etc.)
- Acute care priority
- Lack of resources and facilities
- Lack of systems for preventive services
- Time and economic constraints
- Poor communication between specialty and primary care providers
- Lack of policies and standards

Community/society
- Lack of policies and standards
- Lack of reimbursement

Reprinted with permission from Goldman L, Garber AM, Grover SA, et al. Task Force 6. Cost-effectiveness of assessment and management of risk factors. *J Am Coll Cardiol* 27:1060–1070, 1996.

4. Adequate insurance reimbursement for effective risk reduction strategies.
5. Requirement of expertise in risk factor management in training and credentialing programs.

It is clear that an appropriate level of care cannot be provided by health care personnel not knowledgeable of the pathogenesis of atherosclerosis and the multiple factors that comprise safe and effective implementation of cardiovascular risk reduction (27).

An American College of Cardiology task force has recently recommended use of "**optimal medical management**" rather than "secondary prevention" when referring to cardiovascular risk reduction in patients with established disease (27). Reasons for this are:

1. In addition to lifestyle modification, comprehensive cardiovascular risk reduction includes appropriate use of cardioactive, vasoactive, lipid-lowering, and other drugs.
2. The qualifier "secondary" implies lesser importance to patient and provider.
3. "Preventive" care services may not be compensated in insurance and managed care programs.

GUIDELINES FOR CLINICAL PRACTICE

Compelling scientific and clinical evidence supports aggressive management of risk factors as an integral part of optimal care of patients with established CAD (28, 29). The rationale for aggressive risk factor modification extends to patients with other types of documented atherosclerotic vascular disease including transient ischemic attack, stroke, or aortic or peripheral vascular disease (26). A guide to comprehensive risk reduction has been developed by the American Heart Association and endorsed by the American College of Cardiology (28, 29).

Recent expert guidelines for comprehensive cardiovascular risk reduction emphasize individualization of risk factor management for each patient, the requirement for lifelong management of risk, and use of a team approach to ensure provision of optimal care (28–30). Physicians, nurses, exercise physiologists, dietitians, behavioral scientists, and other health professionals should collaborate in a structured fashion to manage risk reduction via follow-up techniques including office or clinic visits, attendance of cardiac rehabilitation sessions, and mail/telephone contact.

Although the precise approach varies depending on a variety of factors, such as health care setting, patient population, and available resources, implementation of model programs for risk factor management shown to be effective is recommended. Such approaches should include the following fundamental components:

1. Initial evaluation and risk assessment.
2. Identification of specific goals for each CAD risk factor.
3. Formulation and implementation of an individualized treatment plan that includes lifestyle and pharmacologic interventions for accomplishing specific risk factor goals.
4. Effective long-term follow-up to enhance compliance and revise the treatment plan as indicated.
5. Mechanism for outcomes-based long term assessment of each patient.

The American Heart Association has urged that every effort be made throughout the spectrum of medical care to promote effective strategies for comprehensive cardiovascular risk reduction in all eligible patients (2).

ROLE OF CARDIAC REHABILITATION

Comprehensive cardiac rehabilitation combines prescriptive exercise training with risk factor modification (31). The goals of cardiac rehabilitation are to improve functional capacity, alleviate or lessen activity-related symptoms, reduce disability, and identify and modify CAD risk factors in an effort to reduce subsequent cardiovascular-related morbidity and mortality. A recent extensive review of existing scientific literature by the Agency for Health Care Policy and Research has substantiated the efficacy of traditional cardiac rehabilitation in accomplishing many of these goals (32). Moreover, it has been estimated that participation in cardiac rehabilitation by as few as 25–30% of eligible patients would translate into a savings of $31.4–62.8 million in direct medical and non-medical costs after 21 months (32).

Cardiac rehabilitation programs and health professionals are ideally positioned to assume a pivotal role in rendering comprehensive cardiovascular risk reduction. In particular, lifestyle intervention, patient education, compliance, patient tracking and on-going follow-up, and outcomes assessment are primary areas for targeting. However, the extent to which traditional cardiac rehabilitation programs can successfully deliver key components of comprehensive cardiovascular risk reduction is limited by several fundamental deficiencies, including:

1. It is estimated that 11–38% of eligible patients participate in cardiac rehabilitation.
2. Most cardiac rehabilitation programs are 12 weeks in duration with little structured follow-up; a life long approach is required if optimal results are to be achieved.
3. Cardiac rehabilitation services are generally not closely integrated with other aspects of medical care.

▶ SUMMARY

Increasing evidence supports aggressive risk factor modification in the medical treatment of CAD. Endothelial stabilization and decreased progression or regression of atherosclerotic plaque lead to decreased mortality and morbidity in populations with (and without) CAD. This treatment is cost-effective and safe and, although barriers to this type of treatment exist, current programs and trained health care professionals are able to provide this type of care.

References

1. American Heart Association. Heart and Stroke Facts: 1995 Statistical Supplement. Dallas, Texas. American Heart Association 1994.
2. Smith SC. AHA President's letter. *Circulation* 92:1, 1995.
3. Superko HR, Krauss RM. Coronary artery disease regression. Convincing evidence for the benefit of aggressive lipoprotein management. *Circulation* 90:1056–1069, 1994.
4. Brensike JF, Levy RI, Kelsey SF, et al. Effects of therapy with cholestyramine on progression of coronary arteriosclerosis: results of the NHLBI Type II Coronary Intervention Study. *Circulation* 69:313–324, 1984.
5. Blankenhorn DH, Nessim SA, Johnson RL, et al. Beneficial effects of combined colestipol-niacin therapy on coronary atherosclerosis and coronary venous bypass grafts. *JAMA* 257:3233–3240, 1987.
6. Cashin-Hemphill L, Mack WG, Pagoda JM, et al. Beneficial effects of colestipol-niacin on coronary atherosclerosis: a 4-year follow-up. *JAMA* 264:3013–3017, 1990.
7. Ornish D, Brown SE, Scherwitz LW, et al. Can lifestyle changes reverse coronary heart disease? The Lifestyle Heart Trial. *Lancet* 336:129–133, 1990.
8. Schuler G, Hambrecht R, Schlierf G, et al. Regular physical exercise and low-fat diet. Effects on progression of coronary artery disease. *Circulation* 86:1–11, 1992.
9. Gould KL, Ornish D, Scherwitz L, et al. Changes in myocardial perfusion abnormalities by positron emission tomography after long-term, intense risk factor modification. *JAMA* 274:894–901, 1995.
10. Hornig B, Maier V, Drexter H. Physical training improves endothelial function in patients with chronic heart failure. *Circulation* 93:210–214, 1996.
11. Gould KL. Reversal of coronary atherosclerosis. Clinical promise as the basis for noninvasive management of coronary artery disease. *Circulation* 90:1558–1571, 1994.
12. Gould KL, Martucci JP, Goldberg DL, et al. Short-term cholesterol lowering decreases size and severity of perfusion abnormalities by positron emission tomography after dipyridamole in patients with coronary artery disease: a potential noninvasive marker of healing coronary endothelium. *Circulation* 89:1530–1538,1994.
13. Benzuly KH, Padget RC, Kaul S, et al. Functional improvement precedes structural regression of atherosclerosis. *Circulation* 89:1810–1818, 1994.
14. Haskell WL, Alderman EL, Fair JM, et al. Effects of intensive multiple risk factor reduction on coronary atherosclerosis and clinical cardiac events in men and women with coronary artery disease. The Stanford Coronary Risk Intervention Project (SCRIP). *Circulation* 89:975–990, 1994.
15. Scandinavian Simvastatin Survival Group. Randomized trial of cholesterol lowering in 4,444 patients with coronary heart disease: the Scandinavian Simvastatin Survival Study (4S). *Lancet* 344:1383–1389, 1994.
16. Brown BG, Zhao XQ, Sacco DE, et al. Arteriographic view of treatment to achieve regression of coronary atherosclerosis and to prevent plaque disruption and clinical cardiovascular events. *Br Heart J* 69 (Suppl):S48–S53, 1993.
17. The Post Coronary Artery Bypass Graft Trial Investigators. The effect of aggressive lowering of low-density lipoprotein cholesterol levels and low-dose anticoagulation on obstructive changes in saphenous vein coronary artery bypass grafts. *N Engl J Med* 336:153–162, 1997.
18. Shepard J, Cobbe SM, Ford I, et al. Prevention of coronary heart disease with pravastatin in men with hypercholesterolemia. *N Engl J Med* 333:1301–1307, 1995.
19. The West of Scotland Coronary Prevention Study Group. Baseline risk factors and their association with outcome in the West of Scotland Coronary Prevention Study. *Am J Cardiol* 79:756–762, 1997.
20. Byington RP, Jukema JW, Salonen JT. Reduction in cardiovascular events during pravastatin therapy. Pooled analysis of clinical events of the pravastatin atherosclerosis program. *Circulation* 92:2419–2425, 1995.
21. Sacks FM, Pfeffer MA, Moye LA, et al. The effect of pravastatin on coronary events after myocardial infarction in patients with average cholesterol levels. *N Engl J Med* 335: 1001–1009, 1996.

22. Fuster V, Gotto AM, Libby P, et al. Task Force I. Pathogenesis of coronary disease: the biological role of risk factors. *J Am Coll Cardiol* 27:964–976, 1996.
23. Falk E. Why do plaques rupture? *Circulation* 86(Suppl III): 111-30–111-42, 1992.
24. Goldman L, Garber AM, Grover SA, et al. Task Force 6. Cost-effectiveness of assessment and management of risk factors. *J Am Coll Cardiol* 27:1020–1030, 1996.
25. Swan HJC, Brown J, Davidson MH, et al. ACC policy statement. Preventive cardiology and atherosclerotic disease. *J Am Coll Cardiol* 24:838, 1994.
26. Pearson TA, McBride PE, Houston-Miller N, et al. Task Force 8. Organization of preventive cardiology service. *J Am Coll Cardiol* 27:1039–1047, 1996.
27. Swan HJ, Gerch BJ, Graboys TB, et al. Task Force 7. Evaluation and management of risk factors for the individual patient (case management). *J Am Coll Cardiol* 27:1030–1039, 1996.
28. Smith SC, Blair SN, Criqui MH, et al. AHA consensus panel statement. Preventing heart attack and death in patients with coronary disease. Circulation 92:2–4, 1995.
29. Pearson TA, Fuster V. 27th Bethesda Conference. Executive summary. *J Am Coll Cardiol* 27:961–963, 1996.
30. Pearson T, Rapaport E, Cricqui M, et al. Optimal risk factor management in the patient after coronary revascularization. *Circulation* 90:3125–3133, 1994.
31. Balady GJ, Fletcher BJ, Froelicher ES, et al. AHA position statement. Cardiac rehabilitation programs. A statement for health care professionals from the American Heart Association. *Circulation* 90:1602–1610, 1994.
32. Wenger NK, Froelicher ES, Smith LK, et al. Cardiac rehabilitation. Clinical Practice Guidelines No 17. Rockville, MD: U.S. Department of Health and Human Services, Public Health Service, Agency for Health Care Policy and Research and the National Heart, Lung, and Blood Institute. AHCPR Publication No. 96–0672. October 1995.

SECTION SIX

OTHER CHRONIC DISEASE

SECTION EDITOR: *Tom LaFontaine, PhD, FACSM*

74 85, 86, 88 343, 344 357, 363

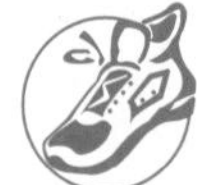
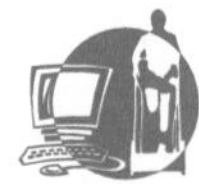

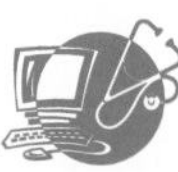

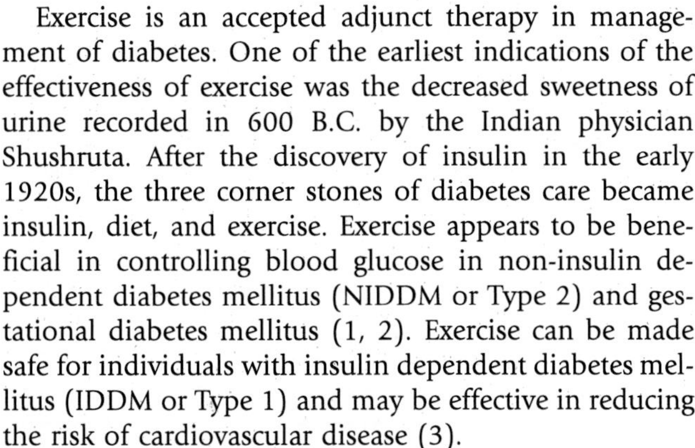

CHAPTER 31
EXERCISE AND DIABETES MELLITUS

Barbara N. Campaigne

Exercise is an accepted adjunct therapy in management of diabetes. One of the earliest indications of the effectiveness of exercise was the decreased sweetness of urine recorded in 600 B.C. by the Indian physician Shushruta. After the discovery of insulin in the early 1920s, the three corner stones of diabetes care became insulin, diet, and exercise. Exercise appears to be beneficial in controlling blood glucose in non-insulin dependent diabetes mellitus (NIDDM or Type 2) and gestational diabetes mellitus (1, 2). Exercise can be made safe for individuals with insulin dependent diabetes mellitus (IDDM or Type 1) and may be effective in reducing the risk of cardiovascular disease (3).

This chapter describes exercise recommendations for managing patients with diabetes. Although background information is given individually for Types 1 and 2 diabetes mellitus, issues relevant to both are discussed in greater detail. Both have distinct hereditary and environmental components and are separate diseases. Both cultural and geographic factors have roles in the cause of each disease. In Type 1 diabetes, the primary abnormality is insulin deficiency with insulin resistance as a secondary factor. In Type 2 diabetes, a series of events caused by insulin resistance leads to stages of disease including further insulin resistance and insulin and glucose abnormalities. Many complications are common to both Type 1 and 2 diabetes. Chronic neurologic and cardiovascular complications are brought about by long term, elevated levels of blood glucose and insulin. Short term hypoglycemic and hyperglycemic responses result in acute complications. The complications of diabetes and use of exercise are described. The major characteristics of Type 1 and 2 diabetes are presented in Table 31.1.

INSULIN DEPENDENT DIABETES MELLITUS

That exercise improves glycemic control in Type 1 diabetes is not well-documented, perhaps because increased caloric consumption or decreased insulin treatment are used to prevent exercise-associated hypoglycemia. Regular exercise does result in improvements in insulin sensitivity, glucose metabolism, and cardiovascular disease (CVD) risk factors. Exercise recommendations should be designed to assist individuals to exercise safely and to decrease their risk of CVD. Depending on duration and intensity, exercise is characterized by endocrine and neural responses. The availability and use of metabolic fuel is largely controlled by the balance of insulin, glucagon, and catecholamines (epinephrine and norepinephrine). Other factors that may have significant influence on fuel metabolism during exercise in Type 1 diabetes include the central nervous system, glycemic state, and general metabolic profile (4–6). Accordingly, this chapter focuses on diverse aspects of the physiological environment of diabetes that influence response to exercise and, conversely, how acute exercise may affect the physiological environment. Table 31.2 gives the benefits of exercise for individuals with Type 1 diabetes. Table 31.3 presents general recommendations for regular exercise in relatively healthy individuals with Type 1 diabetes.

Blood Glucose Regulation

Because acute exercise results in increased glucose use, increased glucose production is necessary to maintain normal blood glucose levels. In the diabetic state, increased glucose production is sometimes compromised by presence of insulin and/or inability to increase glucose because of abnormal hormonal responses. Therefore, it is important to understand the effects of insulin on blood glucose when planning insulin use in conjunction with exercise. Figure 31.1 illustrates the powerful effects of circulating insulin on blood glucose in diabetes. If treatment with intravenous insulin infusion (insulin pump) brings about normal portal insulin levels, production of glucose equals that of glucose use and normal circulating glucose status can be maintained. In

Table 31.1. Major Characteristics of Type 1 and Type 2 Diabetes

FACTOR	TYPE 1	TYPE 2
Age of onset	Usually early, but may occur at any age	Usually over age 30, but may occur at any age
Type of onset	Usually abrupt	Insidious
Genetic susceptibility	HLA-related DR3, DR4, and others	Frequent genetic background, not HLA-related
Environmental factors	Virus, toxins, autoimmune stimulation	Obesity, nutrition
Islet-cell antibody	Present at onset	Not observed
Endogenous insulin	Minimal or absent	Stimulated response is either adequate but delayed secretion or reduced but not absent; insulin resistance present
Nutritional status	Thin, catabolic state	Obese or may be normal
Symptoms	Thirst, polyuria, polyphagia, fatigue	Mild or frequently none
Ketosis	Prone; at onset or during insulin deficiency	Resistant; except during infection or stress
Control of diabetes	Often difficult with wide glucose fluctuation	Variable; helped by dietary adherence, weight loss, and exercise
Dietary management	Essential	Essential; may suffice for glycemic control
Insulin	Required for all	Required for 20% to 30%
Oral hypoglycemics	Not effective	Effective
Vascular and neurologic complications	Seen in majority after 5 or more years of diabetes	Frequent

Adapted from Shulman CR. Diabetes Mellitus: definition, classification, and diagnosis. In: Galloway JA, Potvin JH, Shulman CR, eds. *Diabetes Mellitus,* 9th ed. Indianapolis, IN: Lilly Research Laboratories. Copyright 1988 by Eli Lilly and Company. Adapted by permission.

Table 31.2. Benefits of Exercise for Insulin Dependent Diabetes Mellitus

1. Improved insulin sensitivity
2. Improved blood lipids and liporoteins
3. Increased caloric expenditure resulting in reduction or maintenance of body weight, reduction in body fat and preservation of lean body mass
4. Improved physical fitness
5. Improved flexibility and strength
6. Decreased blood pressure in hypertensives
7. Decreased risk of cardiovascular disease
8. Improved psychological well being including; enhanced quality of life, improved self esteem

the case of insulin deficiency, glucose utilization may not take place with exercise which, in combination with exercise-induced increase in liver glucose production, may bring about hyperglycemia. In the third scenario, if insulin absorption is enhanced with pre-exercise insulin (over-insulinization) as shown in Figure 31.1, inhibition of glucose production may occur. In conjunction with increased glucose utilization, over-insulinization may lead to hypoglycemia.

Table 31.4 shows recommendations for adapting insulin in Type 1 diabetes patients who are participating in exercise programs. In addition, other recommendations include avoiding intramuscular injection, perpendicular injection into a skinfold, and use of needles less than 8.0 mm in length.

Table 31.3. General Exercise Recommendations for Relatively Healthy Type 1 Diabetes

COMPONENT	RECOMMENDATION[a]
Type	[b]Aerobic: walking, jogging, cycling, stair climbing, cross country skiing, etc. Strength (moderate level resistance training): circuit programs using light weights with 10–15 repetitions
Intensity	60–90% maximum heart rate or 50–85% $\dot{V}O_2$-max
Duration	20–60 minutes plus 5–10 minute warm up and cool-down period
Frequency	Daily in order to ensure optimal blood glucose control
Timing	The timing of exercise is particularly important for individuals with IDDM. Both insulin therapy and blood glucose level at the time of exercise need to be considered. Avoid exercise at time of peak insulin action.

[a] A bracelet or shoe tag identifying the individual has diabetes and other relevant medical information should be worn at all times.
[b] Performed in ways that do not traumatize the feet.

Timing and Mode of Insulin Treatment

To optimize blood glucose control, the majority of individuals with Type 1 diabetes use subcutaneous injections consisting of a mixed insulin, split dose regimen. This includes administration of a mixture of short-acting insulin and longer-acting (sustained release) insulin in morning and afternoon doses. Carbohydrate and caloric intake should be matched to insulin therapy. Optimal

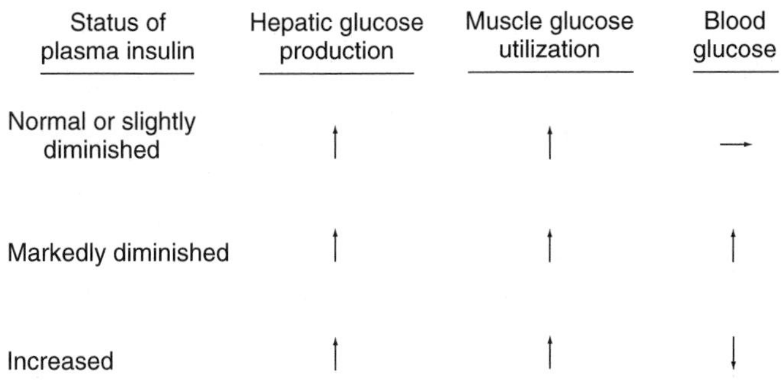

Status of plasma insulin	Hepatic glucose production	Muscle glucose utilization	Blood glucose
Normal or slightly diminished	↑	↑	→
Markedly diminished	↑	↑	↑
Increased	↑	↑	↓

Figure 31.1. The influence of plasma insulin on blood glucose levels of individuals with IDDM. (With permission from Campaigne BN, Lampman RL. *Exercise in the Clinical Management of Diabetes Mellitus.* Champaign, IL: Human Kinetics Publishers, 1994.)

Table 31.4. General Guidelines for Avoiding Hypoglycemia During and After Exercise

Blood Glucose Monitoring

1. Monitor blood glucose immediately before, during (if possible every 30 minutes) and 15 minutes after exercise.
2. Delay exercise if blood glucose is > 250 mg/dl and ketones are present in the urine or if > 300 mg/dl.[a]
3. Consume carbohydrates if blood glucose is ≤ 100 mg/dl.
4. Learn individual glucose response to different types of exercise.
5. Avoid exercising late at night.

Insulin

1. Decrease insulin dose:
   a. Intermediate-acting insulin—decrease by 30–35% on the day of exercise.
   b. Intermediate and short-acting insulin—omit dose of short-acting insulin that precedes exercise.
   c. Multiple doses of short-acting insulin—reduce the dose prior to exercise by 30–35% and supplement carbohydrates.
   d. Continuous subcutaneous infusion—eliminate meal time bolus or increment that precedes or immediately follows exercise.
2. Avoid exercising muscle underlying injections of short-acting insulin for one hour after injection.
3. Do not exercise at the time of peak insulin action. (see Table 31.1)

Adapted from Vitug A, Schneider SH, Ruderman NB. Exercise and Type I diabetes mellitus. *Exerc Sport Sci Rev* 16:285–304, 1988.

[a] ACSM Guidelines state that 200–400 mg/dl requires medical supervision and that > 400 mg/dl contraindicates exercise. The above guideline is taken from a recent ACSM position statement (Diabetes Mellitus and Exercise).

exercise times vary and general recommendations include avoiding exercise at peak time of insulin action or altering insulin dose to prevent peak effect at the time of exercise. Exercise is recommended at times when insulin effects are least and blood glucose is rising. To prevent hypoglycemia when exercise is unplanned, a rapidly assimilated carbohydrate snack can be consumed prior to exercise. Exercising before insulin administration and breakfast may decrease need for short-acting insulin. Once an exercise routine is established, insulin dose and caloric intake can be adjusted. Table 31.5 gives a summary of action of various insulin preparations.

NON-INSULIN DEPENDENT DIABETES MELLITUS

The treatment of Type 2 diabetes usually includes weight loss and oral hypoglycemic agents to help restore peripheral insulin receptor sensitivity and stimulate pancreatic insulin release. The benefits of regular exercise for individuals with Type 2 diabetes have been clearly documented (1, 3) Table 31.6). Regular physical activity for individuals with Type 2 diabetes is a current recommendation of the American Diabetes Association (ADA) (7). Regular exercise results in improved daily blood glucose control and, therefore, a decrease in glycosylated hemoglobin. Exercise training improves insulin sensitivity and may be responsible for increased insulin receptor affinity (8). Reductions in blood pressure in individuals with hypertension and improvements in blood lipid profile resulting from regular exercise lowers CVD risk. Lipid and lipoprotein changes include decreased triglycerides, very-

Table 31.5. Activity Characteristics of Insulin[a]

	Onset (hrs)	Peak (hrs)	Duration (hr)
Rapid Acting			
Regular	½–1	2–4	6–8
Intermediate Acting			
Lente or NPH	1–3	6–12	18–26
Long Acting			
Ultralente or Human	4–8	12–18	24–28

[a] Onset, peak, and duration of action vary considerably and may depend upon the individual patient, injection site, vascularity, and temperature.

Table 31.6. Benefits of Exercise for Type 2 Diabetes

1. Reduced blood glucose and glycosylated hemoglobin levels
2. Improved glucose tolerance
3. Improved insulin response to oral glucose stimulus
4. Improved peripheral and hepatic insulin sensitivity
5. Improved blood lipid and lipoprotein levels
6. Decreased blood pressure in hypertensives
7. Decreased risk of cardiovascular disease
8. Improved physical fitness
9. Increased caloric expenditure resulting in reduction or maintenance of body weight, reductions in body fat, and preservation of lean body mass
10. Improved psychological well-being including enhanced quality of life and increased self esteem
11. Improved flexibility and strength

low density lipoprotein, and increased high-density lipoprotein (HDL). Decreases in systolic and diastolic blood pressure have been reported in mild to moderate hypertension and may be associated with effects of lowered insulin levels on renal sodium retention (1). An important effect of regular exercise for Type 2 diabetes is weight loss in conjunction with dietary intervention and preservation of lean tissue (9).

Table 31.7. General Exercise Recommendations for Relatively Healthy Type 2 Diabetes

Component	Recommendation
Type	Aerobic: walking, jogging, cycling, stair climbing, cross country skiing, etc. Strength (moderate level resistance training): circuit programs using light weights with 10–15 repetitions
Intensity	60–90% maximum heart rate or 50–85% $\dot{V}O_2$-max
Duration	20–60 minutes plus 5–10 minute warm up and cool-down period
Frequency	3–5 times per weekly: daily if on insulin therapy

Modified from Campaigne BN, Lampman RL. Exercise in the Clinical Management of Diabetes Mellitus. Champaign IL: Human Kinetics Pubs, Inc., 1994.

Comparisons of rural and urban cultures provide evidence of lower prevalence of Type 2 diabetes among active rural populations (10). Some data, available from cross sectional studies, show that glucose intolerance and diabetes occur more often in sedentary compared to active individuals (11). These findings are independent of body mass and age. Physical activity has been recommended as an important approach to preventing Type 2 diabetes in men and women (12, 13). In a prospective cohort of 87,253 women aged 34–59 years, Manson et al. reported that women who exercised vigorously at least once per week had significantly lower risk of Type 2 diabetes compared to women who did not participate in weekly exercise (13). Statistical adjustment for family history of diabetes, age, body mass index, and other variables does not change the effects of exercise on diabetes risk. Epidemiological evidence indicates physical activity does have a potential role in preventing Type 2 diabetes (14). Table 31.7 presents recommendations for exercise in relatively healthy individuals with Type 2 diabetes.

DIABETES MEDICATION OTHER THAN INSULIN

Available evidence shows no effect of hypoglycemic agents on electrocardiograms, blood pressure, or heart rate. Because of other underlying medical conditions, in-

Table 31.8. Possible Glucose Altering Effects of Common Medications

	Mechanism of Action		
	Insulin Secretion	Glucose Disposal	Comments
Potentially increases blood glucose			
Diuretics (thiazides, chlorthalidone, furosemide, metolazone)	↓	↓	K^+ depletion, other effects
β-adrenergic antagonists (propranolol, nadolol, timolol)	0, ↓	0, ↓	More likely with noncardioselective agents
Ca^{2+} channel blockers (dihydropyridine derivatives)	0	0, ↓	Effect rarely significant
Glucocorticoids	↑	↓	Cause marked insulin resistance
Anabolic steroids	0	↓	Cause major lipid altering effects
Growth hormone	↑	↓	A major insulin antagonist
Niacin	↑	↓	Particularly with high dosage
Cyclosporine	↓	↓	Often used with glucocorticoids
Potentially decreases blood glucose			
α-adrenergic antagonists (prazosin, doxazosin, terazosin)	0, ↑	0, ↑	Rarely significant
ACE inhibitors	0	0, ↑	
β-adrenergic antagonists (propranolol, nadolol, timolol)			May prevent proper recovery from hypoglycemia
Salicylates	0, ↑	0	With high dosage
Alcohol	0, ↑	↑	May cause hyperglycemia with the long term use
Pentamidine	↑	0	May cause hyperglycemia with the long term use
Quinine	↑	0, ↑	May cause severe hypoglycemia

Modified from Ganda OP. Patients on various drug therapies. In: Ruderman N, Devlin JT, eds. The Health Professionals Guide to Diabetes and Exercise. Alexandria, VA: American Diabetes Association, 1995:236.

dividuals with diabetes may be treated with a variety of medications. To prescribed exercise safely and effectively, it is important to be aware of all medications and their effects on blood glucose. Table 31.8 shows the possible glucose altering effects of various medications.

GESTATIONAL DIABETES

There are three significant factors that influence development of gestational diabetes (GDM): a genetic predisposition, a decrease in insulin action, and impaired Beta cell function (1). During pregnancy development of insulin resistance depends on several factors including:

- The hormonal environment
- Genetic predisposition
- Age
- Excess body weight
- Physical activity level

It is documented that glucose tolerance worsens during gestation. The effects of exercise on insulin secretion, insulin sensitivity, and glucose metabolism make it reasonable that regular exercise may be effective in preventing or treating GDM, although, little data are available (15). Research indicates that exercise training improves glucose tolerance in women with GDM (16). Hyperglycemia, occurring with gestational diabetes, can be prevented by arm ergometry (17). In contrast, diet management alone produces no significant improvement in glucose control (16). These results suggest insulin administration may be avoided in some women with GDM by the safe application of regular exercise. Further research is needed in this area.

COMPLICATIONS OF DIABETES

Exercise is routinely recommended for patients with diabetes, but when secondary complications of diabetes occur, exercise is often neglected. Inactivity can not only affect the complications of diabetes, the complications can affect ability to tolerate exercise. The complications of diabetes combined with inactivity may lead to increased disability (17).

An understanding of diabetic complications is required to recommend clinically sound exercise for patients with diabetes. The screening process should reveal complications that would influence recommendations for exercise. Some unique concerns for individuals with diabetes that warrant attention include autonomic and peripheral (sensory) neuropathy, retinopathy, and nephropathy. Most patients with diabetes develop some neuropathy after 2–3 years. Neuropathy is associated with poor glucose control, therefore individuals in poor control are more likely to develop neuropathy. Clinical manifestations of neuropathy include both sensory and motor deficits. Table 31.9 shows precautions for patients with specific complications.

Recommendations for Specific Complications

Autonomic Neuropathy

Exercise associated with change in position or high intensity activity should be avoided because of the risk of hypotension, especially after vigorous activity. Exercise in hot or cold environments should be avoided because

Table 31.9. Special Precautions When Recommending Exercise for Patients with Complications of Diabetes

Complication	Precaution
Retinopathy[a,b]	With proliferative and severe stages of retinopathy, avoid strenuous, high intensity activities that involve breath holding (e.g., weight lifting and isometrics). Avoid activities which lower the head (e.g., yoga, gymnastics) or that risk jarring the head. Consult opthalmologist for specific weight restrictions and limitations.
Hypertension	Avoid heavy weight lifting or breath holding. Perform primarily dynamic exercise using large muscle groups, such as walking and cycling at a moderate intensity.
Autonomic Neuropathy[b]	Likelihood of hypoglycemia and hypertension. Elevated resting heart rate and reduced maximal heart rate. Use of RPE[c] recommended. Prone to dehydration and hypothermia.
Peripheral Neuropathy	Avoid exercise that may cause trauma to the feet (e.g., prolonged hiking, jogging or walking on uneven surfaces). Non weight bearing activities most appropriate (e.g., cycling and swimming). Swimming not recommended if active ulcers are present. Regular assessment of the feet recommended. The feet should be kept clean and dry. Careful choice of shoes for proper fit. Activities requiring a great deal of balance should be avoided.
Nephropathy	Avoid exercise that raises blood pressure (e.g., weight lifting, high intensity "aerobic" exercises and breath holding).
All Patients	Carry identification with diabetes information. Rehydrate carefully (drink fluids; before, during, and after exercise). Avoid exercise in the heat of the day and in direct sunlight (wear hat and sunscreen when in sun).

[a] If proliferative retinopathy present and patient has recently undergone photocoagulation or surgical treatment or is not properly treated, exercise is contraindicated.

[b] Submaximal exercise testing recommended for patients with proliferative retinopathy and autonomic neuropathy.

[c] RPE = rate of perceived exertion.

With permission from Campaigne BN, Lampman RL. Exercise in the Clinical Management of Diabetes Mellitus. Champaign, IL: Human Kinetic Publishers, 1994.

of the risk of dehydration and poor cold tolerance. Such patients are prone to hypoglycemia and should be monitored carefully.

Additional recommendations include:

1. Use of submaximal testing and rate of perceived exertion (RPE) to determine exercise intensity (avoid high intensity activity).
2. Use of water activities or stationary cycling (maintain blood pressure).
3. Careful glucose monitoring.
4. Avoid extreme environments.

Peripheral Neuropathy

Complications from peripheral neuropathy include ulceration of the feet and decreased healing ability. Severe neuropathy can result in multiple fractures and dislocation of bones of the feet and ankle. Patients may or may not be aware of these problems because of loss of sensation in the periphery. Although exercise does not reverse occurrence of peripheral neuropathy, it may be beneficial in preventing further deterioration of functional capacity associated with disuse. Range of motion activities for the major joints (i.e., ankle, knee, hip, trunk, shoulder, elbow and wrist) should be performed on a daily basis to prevent or minimize contracture. Additional recommendations include:

1. Use of RPE to determine exercise intensity.
2. Use of non-weight-bearing activities (swimming, cycling, arm exercise).
3. Use of activities to improve balance.
4. Proper foot care and footwear.
5. Gentle, pain free stretching.

Retinopathy

Patients with **background retinopathy** do not require the same monitoring as those with proliferative retinopathy. Low impact activities that do not significantly increase blood pressure (>180 mmHg) are most suitable. Strenuous upper extremity exercise (e.g., arm ergometry) should be avoided due to increased peripheral resistance, resulting in increased blood pressure. Exercise is contraindicated with recent retinal photocoagulation or eye surgery. Additional recommendations include:

1. Use of heart rate and RPE based on blood pressure response to determine intensity.
2. Maintain systolic blood pressure < 170 mm Hg during exercise.
3. Avoid Valsalva maneuvers.
4. Avoid heavy weight lifting, breath holding, high intensity exercise (see Table 31.10 for greater detail on retinopathy).

Nephropathy

Renal patients often present with multi-system disease and should be fully evaluated before exercise is prescribed. Exercise should not be initiated until the patient has been stabilized on medication, dialysis (when indicated) and diet. Fluid replacement is essential because of the effects of fluid balance changes on blood pressure. It

Table 31.10. Considerations for Activity Limitation in Diabetic Retinopathy

Level of DR	Acceptable Activities	Discouraged Activities	Ocular and Activity Reevaluation
No DR	Dictated by medical status	Dictated by medical status	12 Months
Mild NPDR	Dictated by medical status	Dictated by medical status	6–12 Months
Moderate NPDR	Dictated by medical status	Activities that dramatically elevate blood pressure: Power lifting Heavy Valsalva maneuvers	
Severe NPDR and very severe NPDR	Dictated by medical status	Limit systolic blood pressure, Valsalva maneuvers, and active jarring: Boxing Heavy competitive sports	2–4 Months (may require laser surgery)
PDR	Low impact cardiovascular conditioning: Swimming (not diving) Walking Low-impact aerobics Stationary cycling Endurance exercises	Strenuous activity, Valsalva maneuvers, pounding or jarring: Weight lifting Jogging High-impact aerobics Racquet sports Strenuous trumpet playing	1–2 Months (may require laser surgery)

With permission from Aiello LM, Cavellerno J, Aiello LP, et al. Retinopathy. In: Ruderman N, Devlin JT, eds. The Health Professionals Guide to Diabetes and Exercise. Alexandria, VA: American Diabetes Association, 1995:163–174.

DR = Diabetic Retinopathy, NPDR = non proliferative diabetic retinopathy, PDR = proliferative diabetic retinopathy is unclear whether exercise accelerates nephropathy, however, sustained elevations in blood pressure do accelerate diabetic nephropathy. It is prudent to avoid activities that involve sustained elevation in blood pressure. Additional recommendations include:

1. Dynamic, weight bearing, low impact activities.
2. Submaximal weight lifting or isometrics when blood pressure is controlled and left ventricular function is normal.
3. Avoid intense aerobic activities and Valsalva maneuvers.
4. Use cushioned shoes (e.g., gel, air).
5. Special attention to maintain hydration.

The importance and clinical significance of careful screening for underlying complications is evident. When complications are present specific considerations and precautions should be considered.

EXERCISE RECOMMENDATIONS AND SPECIAL CLINICAL CONSIDERATIONS

Since it is not clear that exercise improves glycemic control in IDDM, but does have specific health benefits, exercise programs should be designed to educate people with IDDM to exercise safely and decrease risk for CVD. The benefits of regular exercise in patients with Type 2 diabetes are well established, but until recently, information has not been readily available to exercise professionals for planning and carrying out individualized exercise prescription for patients with diabetes.

Screening is required prior to recommending individual exercise programs. Glycemic control must be monitored closely and modifications in diet and insulin therapy may be required frequently. Specific recommendations for type of exercise and precautions for patients with neuropathy, retinopathy, and nephropathy should be given. The specifics of exercise programs, including follow-up and risks and benefits should be addressed to ensure the greatest chance of adherence. Table 31.11 gives specific recommendations for screening patients with diabetes for exercise programs. Absolute contraindications for vigorous exercise include:

1. Poor glycemic control (Type 1, >250 mg/dl and presence of ketones in urine or Type 2, > 300 mg/dl).
2. Proliferative retinopathy.
3. Microangiopathy.
4. Severe neuropathy.
5. Nephropathy.
6. Evidence of underlying cardiovascular disease.

Table 31.11. Recommended Screening Procedures Before Beginning Exercise in Patients with Diabetes

History and Physical Examination
(for those newly diagnosed or without up to date records)
Review all systems
Identification of medical problems (e.g., asthma, arthritis, orthopaedic limitations)
Diabetes Evaluation
Glycosylated hemoglobin (HbA_1)
Ophthalmoscopic exam (retinopathy)
Neurologic exam (neuropathy)
Nephrologic evaluation (microalbumin or protein in urine)
Nutritional status evaluation (underweight/overweight)
Cardiovascular Evaluation
Blood pressure
Peripheral pulses
Bruits
12-lead electrocardiogram
Serum lipid profile (total cholesterol, triglycerides, HDL and LDL cholesterol)
Exercise ECG in patients with known or suspected CAD (for IDDM, those over 30 years of age or diabetes of longer than 15 years duration; for NIDDM, those over 35 years of age)

Modified from Campaigne BN, Lampman RL. Exercise in the Clinical Management of Diabetes Mellitus. Champaigne, IL: Human Kinetic Publishers, 1994.

Abbreviations: HDL = high density lipoprotein, LDL = low density lipoprotein, CAD = coronary artery disease.

▶ SUMMARY

Regular physical activity is an important part of management for individuals with diabetes, particularly those with NIDDM. Regular physical activity reduces risk of many diseases to which individuals with diabetes are predisposed including hypertension, coronary heart disease, and obesity. A comprehensive approach to diabetes management including diet, insulin, other medications, and exercise can facilitate optimal blood glucose and lipid levels, assist in weight management, and prevent exacerbation of underlying complications.

References

1. Horton ES. Exercise in the treatment of NIDDM: Applications for GDM? *Diabetes* 40 (Suppl 2):175–178, 1991.
2. Bung P, Atral R, Khodiguian N, et al. Exercise in gestational diabetes: an optional therapeutic approach? *Diabetes* 40(Suppl 2):182–185, 1991.
3. Campaigne BN, Lampman RL. *Exercise in the Clinical Management of Diabetes Mellitus.* Champaign, IL: Human Kinetics Publishers, 1994.
4. Kjaer M, Secher NH, Bach FW, et al. Role of motor center activity for hormonal changes and substrate mobilization in humans. *Am J Physiol* 253:R687–R695, 1987.
5. Jenkins AB, Furler SM, Chisholm DJ, et al. Regulation of hepatic glucose output during exercise by circulating glu-

cose and insulin in humans. *Am J Physiol* 250:R411–R417, 1986.

6. Katz A, Broberg S, Sahlin K, et al. Leg glucose uptake during maximal dynamic exercise in humans. *Am J Physiol* 251:E65–E70, 1986.
7. American Diabetes Association. Technical Review on Diabetes and Exercise. *Diabetes Care,* 17:924–937, 1994.
8. Denoria JT, Heishman M, Horton EL, et al. Enhanced peripheral and splanchnic insulin sensitivity in NIDDM after single bout of exercise. *Diabetalogia* 365:434–439, 1987.
9. Lampman RM, Schteingart DE, Santinga JT, et al. The influence of physical training on glucose tolerance, insulin sensitivity, and lipid and lipoprotein concentrations in middle aged hypertriglyceridemic and carbohydrate intolerant men. *Diabetologia* 30:380–385, 1987.
10. Zimmet P, Dowse G, Finch C, et al. The epidemiology and natural history of NIDDM-lessons from the South Pacific. *Diabetic Metab Rev* 6:1–124, 1990.
11. Dowse GK, Zimmet PZ, Gareeboo H, et al. Abdominal obesity and physical inactivity as risk factors for NIDDM and impaired glucose tolerance in Indians, Creole, and Chinese Mauritians. *Diabetes Care* 14:271–282, 1991.
12. Helmrich SP, Raglund DR, Leung RW, et al. Physical activity and reduced occurrence of non-insulin dependent diabetes mellitus. *N Engl J Med* 325:147–152, 1991.
13. Manson JE, Rimm EB, Stampfer MJ, et al. Physical activity and incidence of non-insulin-dependent diabetes mellitus in women. *Lancet* 338:774–778, 1991.
14. Kriska AM, Blair SN, Pereira MA. The potential role of physical activity in the prevention of non-insulin dependent diabetes mellitus: epidemiological evidence. *Exerc Sport Sci Rev* 22:121–143, 1994.
15. Jovanovic-Peterson L, Durak EP, Peterson CM. Randomized trial of diet versus diet plus cardiovascular conditioning on glucose levels in gestational diabetes. *Am J Obstet Gynecol* 161:415–419, 1989.
16. Jovanovic-Peterson L, Peterson CM. Dietary manipulation as a primary treatment strategy for pregnancies complicated by diabetes. *J Am Coll Nutr* 9:320–325, 1990.
17. Graham C, Lasko-McCarthey P. Exercise options for persons with diabetic complications. *Diabetes Educator* 16: 212–220, 1990.

Suggested Reading

American College of Sports Medicine. *ACSM's Exercise Management for Persons with Chronic Disease and Disabilities.* Champaign, IL: Human Kinetics Publishers, 1997.

American Diabetes Association: Technical Review on Diabetes and Exercise. *Diabetes Care* 17:924–937, 1994

Campaigne BN, Lampman RL. *Exercise in the Clinical Management of Diabetes Mellitus.* Champaign, IL: Human Kinetics Publishers, Inc, 1994

Diabetes Mellitus and Exercise: A joint position statement of the American College of Sports Medicine and The American Diabetes Association. *Med Sci Sport Exerc* 29:1–5, 1997.

Report of the Expert Committee on the Diagnosis and Classification of Diabetes Mellitus. *Diabetes Care* 20:1183–1197, 1997.

Ruderman N, Devlin JT, eds. *The Health Professionals Guide to Diabetes and Exercise.* Alexandria, VA: American Diabetes Association, Inc., 1995.

159 54 85, 86 424 363

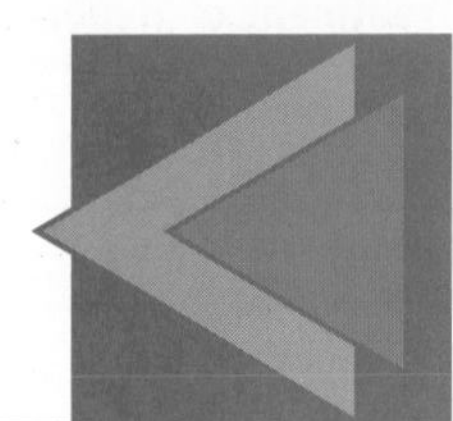

CHAPTER 32

Exercise and Hypertension

Kerry J. Stewart

OVERVIEW OF THE DISEASE

Approximately 50 million adults in the United States have systolic blood pressure (SBP) ≥ 140 mm Hg and/or diastolic blood pressure (DBP) ≥ 90 mm Hg (1). African Americans are more likely to have hypertension than Caucasians, although the specific reasons for this difference are not known. Hypertension is a primary risk factor for cardiovascular disease such as stroke, heart failure, angina, renal failure, and myocardial infarction at all ages and in both genders. While the highest risk is for stroke and heart failure, coronary heart disease is the most common disease outcome of hypertension (2).

Epidemiological data suggest that coronary heart disease risk in hypertensive patients is highest in those with a high total cholesterol:high-density lipoprotein (HDL)-cholesterol ratio, impaired glucose tolerance, high fibrinogen, electrocardiogram abnormalities, and cigarette smokers (3). Stroke risk in hypertensive, persons is highest in those with cardiovascular disease, diabetes, atrial fibrillation, left ventricular hypertrophy, and cigarette smoking. Because of the health risks of hypertension, treatment (including exercise) is essential to improved patient outcome. One advantage of exercise as a treatment for hypertension is its positive affect on other cardiac risk factors.

DEFINITION, CAUSES, EPIDEMIOLOGY, AND DIAGNOSIS

The 1993 Joint National Commission on Detection, Evaluation, and Treatment of Hypertension (JNC V) reclassified the risk categories for hypertension as shown in Table 32.1. The Third National Health and Nutrition Examination reported that two-thirds of those with hypertension were aware of the diagnosis and 53% were taking prescribed medication (4). However, 33% of Hispanics with hypertension were receiving treatment and 14% achieved control in contrast to 25% and 24% of non-Hispanic black and non-Hispanic white populations with hypertension, respectively (Fig. 32.1).

Increased blood pressure has a positive and continuous association with vascular events (5). Within the DBP range of 70–110 mm Hg, there is no threshold below which lower blood pressure does not reduce stroke and coronary artery disease risk. Among individuals treated for hypertension, an average 15/6 mm Hg reduction in blood pressure reduced stroke by 34% and coronary heart disease by 19% over 4.7 years (6). The absolute benefits in older subjects were more than twice those in younger subjects. Hypertension may be a stronger independent risk factor for mortality from coronary heart disease among elderly women than among elderly men (7).

PATHOPHYSIOLOGY AND IMPLICATIONS FOR EXERCISE TESTING AND TRAINING

Essential hypertension is the most common classification of hypotension. It is characterized by increased DBP and is related to generalized arteriolar vasoconstriction which increases SBP. While there is no single cause of essential hypertension, blood pressure is primarily determined by cardiac output and total peripheral resistance. Population factors associated with hypertension are obesity, high sodium intake, low potassium intake, physical inactivity, heavy alcohol consumption, and psychosocial stress (8). Recent studies suggest that accumulation of intra-abdominal visceral fat and hyperinsulinemia play a role in the pathogenesis of hypertension (9–11). For these reasons, lifestyle changes that favorably modify these factors are a substantial part of treatment for hypertension. Potential interactions between these lifestyle factors and genetic predisposition is also likely to contribute to the disorder.

Hypertension imposes an afterload on the heart, resulting in increased left ventricular wall thickness (concentric hypertrophy) and reduced early diastolic filling (12, 13). Aging also alters left ventricular mass and di-

Table 32.1. Classification of Blood Pressure: Joint National Commission on Detection, Evaluation, and Treatment of Hypertension Recommendation

Blood Pressure Category	Systolic (mm Hg)	Diastolic (mm Hg)
Normal	< 130	< 85
High Normal	130–139	85–89
Hypertension		
Stage 1 (Mild)	140–159	90–99
Stage 2 (Moderate)	160–179	100–109
Stage 3 (Severe)	180–209	110–119
Stage 4 (Very Severe)	> 210	> 120

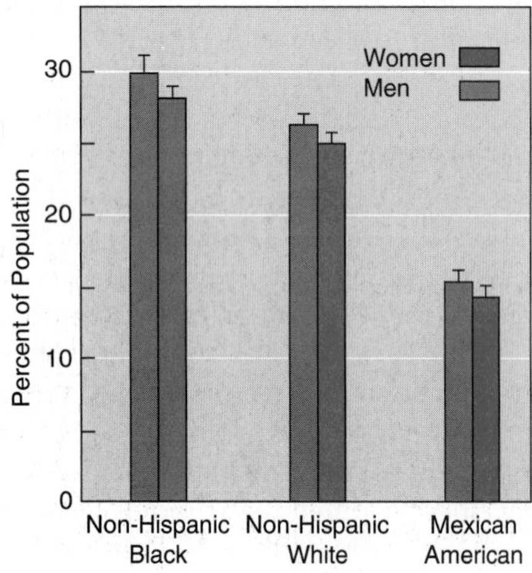

Figure 32.1. Prevalence of hypertension in the United States adult population by race/ethnic groups.

astolic filling and the combination of hypertension and advancing age markedly raises risk for coronary heart disease and heart failure (14). The strong correlation of left ventricular mass with cardiovascular disease emphasizes the importance of classifying patients by this risk factor. In the Framingham study the predictive value of left ventricular mass on cardiovascular disease outcomes was independent of all other risk factors. Although several antihypertensive agents are capable of inducing regression of left ventricular hypertrophy, the long term clinical benefits of reducing left ventricular mass have yet to be documented (15).

Recent data also suggest that hypertension and, in particular, the duration of hypertension promotes the presence and extent of coronary calcium, itself a potential predictor of sudden death (in parallel with the extent of peripheral atherosclerosis) (16). Hypertension is also associated with subclinical changes in the brain (e.g., impaired cognitive function) and thickening and stiffening of medium and small blood vessels. Hypertension may also lead to retinopathy and nephropathy.

ACUTE BLOOD PRESSURE RESPONSES TO EXERCISE

The typical blood pressure response to acute bouts of aerobic exercise is a gradual increase in SBP and gradual decrease or no change in DBP. The expected peak blood pressure during maximal exercise is between 180–210/60–85 mm Hg for most individuals. Age, gender, and body weight often cause variation in these responses. Along with resting blood pressure, excessive SBP response to exercise may also predict future hypertension. The CARDIA study explored this relationship in normotensive black and white young adults undergoing treadmill testing (17). Those with an exaggerated blood pressure response to exercise at baseline were 1.7 times more likely to develop hypertension than persons with a normal response. After adjustment for many variables, exaggerated exercise blood pressure was associated with >2 mm Hg increase in SBP after 5 years. Although the increase in SBP was only 1–3 mm Hg, this increment sustained over time could lead to increased occurrence of hypertension and hypertension-related pathological complications.

Exercise blood pressure may also predict coronary disease events. In apparently healthy men followed for an average of 16 years, exercise blood pressure at baseline was more strongly related to both morbidity and mortality from myocardial infarction than mildly elevated resting blood pressure (18). This suggests that exercise blood pressure may distinguish between severe and less severe hypertension.

Another study compared cardiovascular response to exercise in normotensive men at high risk for hypertension compared to those at low risk of hypertension (19). During exercise, high-risk men with exaggerated blood pressure responses (230/100 mm Hg) had blunted response in peripheral resistance decline. This suggests impaired capacity for exercise-induced vasodilation as a mechanism for future hypertension.

POSSIBLE MECHANISMS BY WHICH EXERCISE MAY REDUCE HYPERTENSION

There are several possible mechanisms by which exercise may lower blood pressure. Lowering of both cardiac output and peripheral vascular resistance at rest and at any given level of work after exercise training is one theory. Lowered cardiac output may be primarily due to reduced heart rate. Other potential exercise training induced mechanisms are reduced serum catecholamines and reduced plasma renin activity (20).

Lack of consistent association between exercise-induced changes in blood pressure and changes in body weight or body composition suggest that anthropomorphic parameters may not be primary mechanisms in causing hypertension. Recent attention has focused on body fat distribution. It was recently shown in subjects with and without a parental history of hypertension that offspring of hypertensive parents had more central obesity (9). However, there were no differences in fitness or physical activity based on parental hypertension, suggesting a role for central obesity in the etiology of primary hypertension.

Another study examined changes in blood pressure and fat distribution after a 12-week low calorie diet in obese, hypertensive women (10). Subjects lost a mean of 9.4 ±4.1 kg, and mean blood pressure fell from an average of 112 ±9 to 101 ±12 mm Hg ($p < .001$). Change in blood pressure was not correlated with change in body weight or body mass index, but was correlated with a reduction in visceral fat and in the ratio of visceral fat to subcutaneous fat. Thus, a decrease in visceral fat, rather than simply body weight, may reduce blood pressure in obese subjects.

Because increased fitness or physical activity may also reduce central fat deposition, it may be through this mechanism that exercise decreases blood pressure (21–23).

MEDICAL THERAPY AND IMPLICATIONS FOR EXERCISE

Because the relationship between blood pressure and vascular disease is continuous, the level of hypertension at which to initiate medical treatment is arbitrary. However, effective pharmacologic and nonpharmacologic management of hypertension can significantly reduce mortality for all patients (1).

Medical management is often complicated by concomitant hyperlipidemia, hyperinsulinemia, glucose intolerance, reduced arterial compliance, sympathetic overactivity, and obesity found in hypertensive patients. These additional disorders compound the risk of hypertension. This clustering of risk factors (Table 32.2) has been called the metabolic cardiovascular syndrome or "hypertension syndrome" (24, 25).

Age, race, sex, and the presence of other risk factors should be considered in determining treatment strategies. Subtle abnormalities in insulin resistance and hyperinsulinemia may cause systemic hypertension through multiple mechanisms (11). Insulin has a sodium-retaining effect in the kidney, augments catecholamine release, increases vascular sensitivity to vasoconstrictor substances, and decreases vascular sensitivity to vasodilator substances. In addition, insulin increases production of tissue growth factors and facilitates retention of cellular sodium and calcium. Insulin resistance, like hypertension, can be treated with regular aerobic exercise, weight reduction, high fiber diet, and/or medications. To provide maximal protection against cardiovascular complications, hypertension should be managed to reduce total cardiovascular risk burden (Table 32.3) (26).

Another consideration is that some antihypertensive agents adversely affect other risk factors, whereas exercise, diet, and weight loss improve multiple risk factors. JNC V recommendations regarding pharmacologic agents are flexible but controversial (3). Because of potential cardioprotective effects, angiotensin-converting enzyme inhibitors, calcium channel blockers, alpha-blockers, and alpha-beta-blockers have gained favor over diuretics and beta-blockers in the United States (1). In a recent study of the use of antihypertensive drugs, diuretics accounted for 56% of antihypertensive drugs in 1982, but only 27% in 1993 (27). Use of beta-blockers and central agents also declined whereas the use of calcium antagonists and angiotensin-converting enzyme inhibitors increased. Although the use of newer agents has increased markedly, the large-scale clinical trials of antihypertensive drugs that have demonstrated a reduction in morbidity and mortality from cardiovascular disease used diuretics and beta-blockers (27, 28).

Patient adherence to antihypertensive medication is often a problem, particularly for active adults or individuals for whom exercise is encouraged (29). In many cases, exercise training may reduce or eliminate the need for antihypertensive medications in patients with mild or severe hypertension (30, 31).

Table 32.2. Prevalence of Other Risk Factors in Patients with Hypertension

Risk Factor	Percent
Smoking	35
Hypercholesterolemia > 240 mg/dL	40
Decreased HDL cholesterol < 40 mg/dL	25
Obesity	40
Diabetes	15
Hyperinsulinemia	50
Sedentary lifestyle	> 50

Adapted from Kaplan NM. Management of hypertension. *Dis Mon* 38: 769–838, 1992.

Table 32.3. Five Steps to Minimize the Total Cardiovascular Risk Burden

1. Carefully monitor blood pressure in response to therapy.
2. Assess concomitant cardiovascular risk factors.
3. Institute lifestyle changes to help control hypertension and other risk factors.
4. Use antihypertensive drugs, chosen to best manage the overall risk burden in a way that will lower blood pressure gradually while avoiding adverse reactions.
5. Identify the goal of therapy: blood pressure levels that are neither too high to avoid increased risks for cerebral and renal damage nor too low to avoid increased risks for coronary ischemia.

Adapted from Kaplan NM. Management of hypertension. *Dis Mon* 38: 769–838, 1992.

AEROBIC EXERCISE AND THE TREATMENT OF HYPERTENSION

Both the JNC V and the ACSM recommend aerobic exercise to lower blood pressure (3, 32). The JNC V treatment guidelines for high normal blood pressure emphasize lifestyle modification including diet, weight loss, and exercise; 3–6 months of lifestyle change is recommended for stage 1 hypertension prior to initiating medication. Furthermore, lifestyle change including exercise may be used for stage 2 if hypertension is the only risk factor. Stages 3 and 4 usually require medication and adequate blood pressure control before vigorous exercise is initiated. Nevertheless, dietary and other nonpharmacologic strategies have not been shown to reduce clinical events even when blood pressure is reduced (25).

In a study of adult men and women, subjects performing 4 months of aerobic exercise did not attain greater reductions in blood pressure than controls (33). A review from the same investigator concludes that, although exercise and weight loss may be effective in treatment of hypertension, the available research is inconclusive, the mechanism unknown, and further research is needed to clarify the issue (34). Yet, several studies using moderate intensity exercise demonstrate decreased blood pressure by an average 7/ 7 mm Hg (35, 36). As shown in Figure 32.2, a meta-analysis of nine randomized controlled exercise trials representing 245 subjects found decreased resting SBP and DBP of approximately 7 ± 5 and 6 ± 2 mm Hg, respectively, in treatment groups (36).

A recent review summarized 47 studies concerned with endurance exercise training in individuals with hypertension (37). Over 70% of the groups in these studies decreased resting SBP and DBP with exercise training by an average of 10.5/8.6 mm Hg from an initial mean of 154/98 mm Hg. This review concluded that beneficial blood pressure responses associated with exercise are significantly more prevalent than negative or equivocal responses. Less consistent were reductions in ambulatory blood pressure with exercise training.

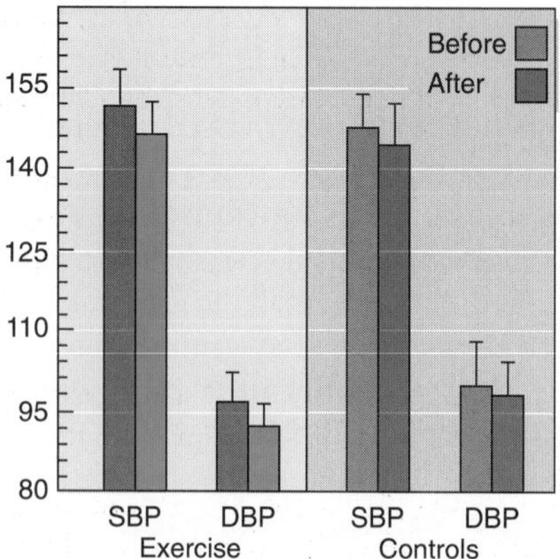

Figure 32.2. Blood pressure results from nine randomized studies of aerobic exercise in hypertension. (SBP = systolic blood pressure, DBP = diastolic blood pressure.)

EXERCISE GUIDELINES

Aerobic Exercise

The ACSM recommends endurance exercise for mild hypertension (32). The recommended mode (large muscle exercises), frequency (3–5 days/week), duration (20–60 minutes), and intensity (50–85% of maximal oxygen uptake) recommended are generally the same as those for healthy adults. For individuals with markedly elevated blood pressure, exercise training at somewhat lower intensities (40–70%) is recommended after initiated pharmacologic therapy.

The effectiveness of exercise training as a complement to pharmacologic therapy was demonstrated recently in adult black men with severe hypertension (SBP > 180 mm Hg or DBP > 110 mm Hg) (31). After antihypertensive medications were administered in a stepped approach, subjects were divided into exercise group and sedentary groups. Endurance exercise for 3 days a week, 45 minutes/day at 75% of maximum heart rate for 16–32 weeks was the training program. By week 16 the exercise group lowered SBP and DBP and reduced left ventricular mass. These effects persisted through 32 weeks, even after a reduction in antihypertensive medication. Thus, moderate aerobic exercise may reduce blood pressure, left ventricular hypertrophy, and the number of antihypertensive medications required to control blood pressure.

Weight Training

Isometric exercise or weight lifting results in increased SBP and an associated increase in DBP. Static exercise, however, results in a smaller increase in heart rate compared to aerobic exercise. In many instances, the myocardial oxygen demand (directly related to the heart rate × SBP often called "**rate pressure product**") may be lower during resistive exercise rather than aerobic exercise if performed at the same level of total body energy demand. This response was demonstrated in two studies of hypertensive men performing weight training and walking/jogging (29, 30). Heart rate was higher during walking/jogging, while blood pressure was higher during weight training. The rate pressure product was similar during both. However, it is important to note that blood pressure response to aerobic or resistive exercise is variable and blood pressure at rest does not provide independent prognostic information about exercise response. Therefore, exercise testing that includes assessment of blood pressure to static forms of exercise (e.g., handgrip or isometrics) should be considered for subjects with hypertension.

Most studies have focused on endurance training for reducing blood pressure, but few studies investigate weight training in hypertensive patients. Circuit weight training has been shown to result in a modest drop in DBP and no change in SBP (38). Another study examined the effects of circuit weight training combined with aerobic exercise in patients randomly assigned to either antihypertensive medications or placebo (29, 30). After 12 weeks of training, resting blood pressure decreased significantly (Fig. 32.1). The most striking finding was that resting blood pressure fell similarly in both groups; that is, there appeared to be no added benefit of the medication if subjects exercised regularly. Further research is needed to more clearly define the role of weight training as part of the exercise prescription for reducing blood pressure.

SCREENING AND TESTING

The Guide to Clinical Preventive Services states that blood pressure should be measured regularly in all persons aged three and above (39). The optimal interval for screening has not been determined and is left to clinical discretion. Current opinion is that blood pressure should be assessed once every 2 years if a previous DBP and/or SBP were < 85 mm Hg and 140 mm Hg, respectively, or annually if the previous DBP was 85–89 mm Hg. Hypertension should not be diagnosed from a single measurement, but confirmed from readings at each of three separate visits.

The ACSM does not recommend mass exercise testing to specifically determine blood pressure responses to exercise for prognosis of hypertension (40). Exercise testing before participation in moderate to vigorous exercise should be made according to usual risk stratification guidelines. However, because hypertension often clusters with other risk factors such as hyperlipidemia, hyperinsulemia, and obesity, individuals with hypertension are likely to be candidates for exercise testing before exercise training.

SUMMARY

Hypertension is a common, chronic problem and adequate treatment is likely to reduce cardiovascular morbidity and mortality, particularly in the elderly. Physical activity has an important therapeutic role in treatment of hypertension. Based on cross-sectional and experimental findings, regular physical activity and exercise training appear to lower blood pressure. However, the specific mechanisms underlying this relationship are not entirely clear. Some major exercise-induced physiological changes from exercise that may account for the antihypertensive effects include decreased heart rate resulting from increased vagal tone and associated reductions in plasma catecholamine and plasma renin levels. Although there are no consistent relationships between reduced body weight or improved body composition and decreased blood pressure, recent data suggest that increased abdominal visceral fat, along with insulin and glucose intolerance, play a role in the pathogenesis of hypertension. These risk factors, which are also independent risk factors for coronary heart disease, can be improved substantially with physical activity.

Exercise prescription for hypertension should be based on medical history and risk factor status. Because resting blood pressure alone is often an inadequate prognostic indicator for risk of hypertension, exercise testing may help to identify exaggerated blood pressure response to exercise and underlying latent ischemic heart disease. The exercise prescription should also be adapted to antihypertensive medications that may affect exercise heart rate and blood pressure. Finally, although much of the exercise literature has focused on aerobic exercise for subjects with hypertension, there is growing evidence that incorporating resistive training into the exercise prescription may be of value for controlling blood pressure.

References

1. Sutherland J, Castle C, Friedman R. Hypertension: current management strategies. *J Am Board Fam Pract* 7:202–217, 1994.
2. Kannel WB. Potency of vascular risk factors as the basis for antihypertensive therapy. *Eur Heart J* 13:34–42, 1992.
3. The fifth report of the Joint National Committee on Detection, Evaluation, and Treatment of High Blood Pressure (JNC V). *Arch Intern Med* 153:154–183, 1993.
4. Burt VL, Whelton P, Roccella EJ, et al. Prevalence of hypertension in the US adult population. Results from the Third National Health and Nutrition Examination Survey, 1988–1991. *Hypertension* 25:305–313, 1995.
5. MacMahon S, Peto R, Cutler J, et al. Blood pressure, stroke, and coronary heart disease. Part 1, Prolonged differences in blood pressure: prospective observational studies corrected for the regression dilution bias. *Lancet* 335:765–774, 1990.
6. MacMahon S, Rodgers A. The effects of blood pressure reduction in older patients: an overview of five randomized controlled trials in elderly hypertensives. *Clin Exp Hypertens* 15:967–978, 1993.
7. Weijenberg MP, Feskens EJ, Bowles CH, Kromhout D. Serum total cholesterol and systolic blood pressure as risk factors for mortality from ischemic heart disease among elderly men and women. *J Clin Epidemiol* 47:197–205, 1994.
8. Perry IJ, Whincup PH, Shaper AG. Environmental factors in the development of essential hypertension. *Br Med Bull* 50:246–259, 1994.
9. de Visser DC, van Hooft IM, van Doornen LJ, et al. Anthropometric measures, fitness and habitual physical activity in offspring of hypertensive parents. Dutch Hypertension and Offspring Study. *Am J Hypertens* 7:242–248, 1994.
10. Kanai H, Tokunaga K, Fujioka S, Yamashita S, Kameda-Takemura K, Matsuzawa Y. Decrease in intra-abdominal

visceral fat may reduce blood pressure in obese hypertensive women. *Hypertension* 27:125–129, 1996.

11. Mediratta S, Fozailoff A, Frishman W. Insulin resistance in systemic hypertension—Pharmoacotherapeutic implications. *J Clin Pharmacol* 35:943–956, 1995.
12. Liebson PR, Grandits G, Prineas R, et al. Echocardiographic correlates of left ventricular structure among 844 mildly hypertensive men and women in the Treatment of Mild Hypertension Study (TOMHS). *Circulation* 87:476–486, 1993.
13. Missault LH, Duprez DA, Brandt AA, et al. Exercise performance and diastolic filling in essential hypertension. *Blood Press* 2:284–288, 1993.
14. Messerli FH, Ketelhut R. Left ventricular hypertrophy: a pressure-independent cardiovascular risk factor. *J Cardiovasc Pharmacol* 22:S7–13, 1993.
15. Eselin JA, Carter BL. Hypertension and left ventricular hypertrophy: is drug therapy beneficial? *Pharmacotherapy* 14: 60–88, 1994.
16. Megnien JL, Simon A, Lemariey M, et al. Hypertension promotes coronary calcium deposit in asymptomatic men. *Hypertension* 27:949–954, 1996.
17. Manolio TA, Burke GL, Savage PJ, et al. Exercise blood pressure response and 5-year risk of elevated blood pressure in a cohort of young adults: the CARDIA study. *Am J Hypertens* 7:234–241, 1994.
18. Mundal R, Kjeldsen SE, Sandvik L, et al. Exercise blood pressure predicts mortality from myocardial infarction. *Hypertension* 27:324–329, 1996.
19. Wilson MF, Sung BH, Pincomb GA, et al. Exaggerated pressure response to exercise in men at risk for systemic hypertension. *Am J Cardiol* 66:731–736, 1990.
20. Dubbert PM, Martin JE, Cushman WC, et al. Endurance exercise in mild hypertension: effects on blood pressure and associated metabolic and quality of life variables. *J Hum Hypertens* 8:265–272, 1994.
21. Despres JP, Pouliot MC, Moorjani S, et al. Loss of abdominal fat and metabolic response to exercise training in obese women. *Am J Physiol* 261:E159–E167, 1991.
22. Schwartz RS, Shuman WP, Larson V, et al. The effect of intensive endurance exercise training on body fat distribution in young and older men. *Metabolism* 40:545–551, 1991.
23. Schwartz RS, Cain KC, Shuman WP, et al. Effect of intensive endurance training on lipoprotein profiles in young and older men. *Metabolism* 41:649–654, 1992.
24. Westheim A, Os I. Physical activity and the metabolic cardiovascular syndrome. *J Cardiovasc Pharmacol* 20:S49–S53, 1992.
25. Weber MA. Controversies in the diagnosis and treatment of hypertension: a personal review of JNC V. *Am J Cardiol* 72:3H–9H, 1993.
26. Kaplan NM. Management of hypertension. *Dis Mon* 38: 769–838, 1992.
27. Manolio TA, Cutler JA, Furberg CD, et al. Trends in pharmacologic management of hypertension in the United States. *Arch Intern Med* 155:829–837, 1995.
28. Rutan GH, Cushman WC. Relative benefits of different antihypertensive drugs in the prevention of vascular complications. *Curr Opin Nephrol Hypertens* 4:240–244, 1995.
29. Stewart KJ, Effron MB, Valenti SA, et al. Effects of diltiazem or propranolol during exercise training of hypertensive men. *Med Sci Sports Exerc* 22:171–177, 1990.
30. Kelemen MH, Effron MB, Valenti SA, et al. Exercise training combined with antihypertensive drug therapy. Effects on lipids, blood pressure, and left ventricular mass. *JAMA* 263:2766–2771, 1990.
31. Kokkinos P, Narayan P, Colleran J, et al. Effects of regular exercise on blood pressure and left ventricular hypertrophy in African-American men with severe hypertension. *N Engl J Med* 333:1462–1467, 1995.
32. American College of Sports Medicine. Position Stand. Physical activity, physical fitness, and hypertension. *Med Sci Sports Exerc* 25:i–x, 1993.
33. Blumenthal JA, Siegel WC, Appelbaum M. Failure of exercise to reduce blood pressure in patients with mild hypertension. Results of a randomized controlled trial. *JAMA* 266:2098–2104, 1991.
34. Blumenthal JA, Thyrum ET, Gullette ED, et al. Do exercise and weight loss reduce blood pressure in patients with mild hypertension? *N C Med J* 56:92–95, 1995.
35. Arroll B, Beaglehole R. Does physical activity lower blood pressure: a critical review of the clinical trials. *J Clin Epidemiol* 45:439–447, 1992.
36. Kelley G, McClellan P. Antihypertensive effects of aerobic exercise. A brief meta-analytic review of randomized controlled trials. *Am J Hypertens* 7:115–119, 1994.
37. Hagberg JM. Physical Activity, Physical Fitness, and Blood Pressure. NIH Consensus Development Conference: Physical Activity and Cardiovascular Health. Bethesda, MD: Office of the Director National Institutes of Health; 1995:69–71.
38. Harris KA, Holly RG. Physiological responses to circuit weight training in borderline hypertensive subjects. *Med Sci Sports Exerc* 19:246–252, 1987.
39. U.S. Preventive Services Task Force Guide to Clinical Preventative Services. 2 ed. Baltimore: Williams & Wilkins, 1995.
40. ACSM's Guidelines for Exercise Testing and Prescription. Baltimore: Williams & Wilkins, 1995:373.

357, 363, 365 342, 424

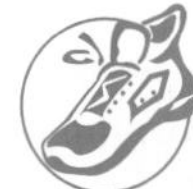

CHAPTER 33

Exercise in the Management of Peripheral Arterial Disease

Judith G. Regensteiner and William G. Hiatt

Peripheral arterial disease (PAD) is a common manifestation of atherosclerosis. The prevalence of PAD increases with age and the disease affects about 12% of the general population, but up to 20% of older individuals (1, 2). Patients with PAD have similar cardiovascular risk factors to patients with coronary artery disease. In addition, since persons with PAD have systemic atherosclerosis, there is an associated increase in morbidity and mortality from other cardiovascular diseases (3).

PAD produces exercise-induced muscle aching or cramping (intermittent claudication) secondary to ischemia in the calf, thighs, or buttocks (Table 33.1). In patients with claudication, this symptom only occurs during walking, but in more severe forms of the disease, pain in the limb at rest, ischemic ulceration, gangrene, and ultimately the need for amputation may exist. There is a relatively stable natural history of symptoms of intermittent claudication such that the ability to walk may not worsen over intervals of up to several years (4). However, there is almost never spontaneous improvement in walking ability in the absence of intervention.

PAD has profound detrimental effects on functional status (5, 6). Clinically, PAD is an important cause of impaired functional ability because symptomatic patients are typically able to walk less than one to three blocks before rest is required. Peak oxygen consumption ($\dot{V}O_2$peak) ranges from 10–16 ml/kg/min, equivalent to Class C on the Weber Scale of heart failure (7). Limited ability to walk leads to disability which may prevent performance of personal, social, or occupational activities of daily living. For example, occupational activities that require walking short distances, shopping, and outdoor recreational activities may be limited. Thus, a major goal of therapy in PAD is to relieve symptoms of intermittent claudication and disability and to restore functional status.

Risk factors for PAD include diabetes mellitus, cigarette smoking, hypertension, hyperlipidemia (particularly disorders in the metabolism of triglycerides and high-density lipoprotein cholesterol), abnormalities of hemostatic function and hemorheology, lipoprotein (a), and abnormalities of homocysteine metabolism (8–15). Aggressive treatment of risk factors may slow or stabilize the atherosclerotic disease process and may positively influence cardiac mortality, but does not, for the most part, improve exercise performance. In fact, of the risk factors, only smoking cessation has been shown to improve claudication symptoms (16). Helping patients to quit smoking and to normalize lipids is beneficial for preventing the progression of PAD.

AVAILABLE SURGICAL AND PHARMACOLOGIC TREATMENTS

Interventional Treatments

Surgery or angioplasty may be necessary for the relief of symptoms, and/or limb preservation in patients with severe forms of the disease. In patients with claudication, interventional therapy is associated with improvements in ability to walk, but there is higher morbidity and mortality, as well as higher costs for both surgery and angioplasty than for noninvasive treatments (17–21). In most cases, claudication can be treated with alternative methods.

Pharmacology

The only approved drug for treating intermittent claudication is pentoxifylline, a hemorheologic agent that decreases blood viscosity. This drug is associated with a 22% improvement over placebo in pain-free walking distance and 12% improvement in walking distance (22). Thus, the clinical benefits are relatively modest. Currently, there is interest in the development of new drugs for claudication. Examples of drugs being tested include antiplatelet and anticoagulant drugs, hemorheologic drugs, novel vasodilators, prostaglandins, and drugs that alter muscle metabolism. Results are pending for these studies.

Table 33.1. Pathophysiology of Peripheral Arterial Disease

Acute:	Muscle blood flow supply/demand mismatch
Chronic:	Deconditioning and Denervation + Impaired Oxidative Metabolism
	Claudication during walking limits ability to carry out normal daily activities.

Interventional and pharmacologic therapies are used to treat claudication and improve walking ability. The development of new pharmacologic therapies is growing, but it is unknown which agents will emerge as efficacious.

METHODS OF EVALUATION

Assessment Procedures

Programs using exercise rehabilitation or other therapies for claudication must have appropriate evaluation procedures to assess hemodynamic and functional status of each patient before and after treatment. In this way, information about effectiveness can be provided to both the program director and the patient for purposes of feedback.

Screening

Prior to initiating an exercise rehabilitation program for a patient with PAD, cardiovascular screening should be performed due to the increased prevalence of coronary atherosclerosis in persons with PAD. Screening should include a history and physical exam, as well as resting and exercise electrocardiograms during the initial exercise test. If clinically significant coronary artery disease is present, the patient should be referred for treatment.

Hemodynamic Assessment

The peripheral circulation is commonly assessed by measuring resting and post-exercise systolic blood pressures in the ankle and arm using Doppler ultrasound. At rest, the ratio of ankle-to-arm systolic blood pressure (ankle/brachial index [ABI]) is used to measure the severity of the underlying vascular disease (23). Using a large population of controls and diabetics, abnormal ABI has been defined as less than 0.90 at rest and a 20% decrease after exercise (23).

Before the ABI is measured, patients should rest for 10–15 minutes. Blood pressure measurements in the dorsalis pedis, posterior tibial, and brachial arteries are duplicated for greater accuracy. These tests are practical because they are easy to perform, well-tolerated by patients, require simple equipment, and are relatively inexpensive. ABI measurements are important for assessing change in severity of PAD. However, the hemodynamic severity of vascular disease defined by ABI is not well correlated to treadmill exercise performance and therefore, this measurement should not be used to test the functional effects of intervention (24).

Treadmill Testing in PAD

Treadmill testing, on entry to an exercise rehabilitation program as well as after completion of the program, is an objective means of assessing changes in performance. Importantly, in contrast to treadmill testing in healthy people, the protocol used in PAD patients must be much less strenuous given the severe limitations. Slower speed and less rapidly increasing grade than other treadmill protocols is used. **Claudication-free walking time or distance** (initial claudication distance [ICD]) and **maximal, claudication-limited walking time or distance** (absolute claudication distance [ACD]) are the most commonly used criteria to evaluate performance. Until recently, the most common type of treadmill protocol was a constant-load test, conducted at a speed of 1.5–2 mph, with a fixed grade of 8–12% (25). Despite the constant work load, most (but not all) persons reach maximum claudication pain, at which point walking is discontinued. Constant-load protocol tests are easy to administer and require simple equipment, but have several potential serious problems limiting reproducibility and sensitivity to change (24, 26).

Graded treadmill protocols have been developed to test patients with PAD (24, 26). Two widely used graded protocols maintain a walking speed of 2.0 mph. One protocol increases grade 3.5% every 3 minutes while the other, uses 2.0% grade increments every 2 minutes (24, 26). All patients limited by claudication are reproducibly brought to maximal levels of discomfort using either protocol. The graded protocol is highly reproducible (coefficient of variation = 0.88) and sensitive to change (24). The use of a graded treadmill protocol is therefore, to evaluate change in exercise performance.

Measurement of Oxygen Consumption

Peak oxygen consumption ($\dot{V}O_2$peak) may be used to assess cardiopulmonary fitness in a PAD patient. $\dot{V}O_2$peak measurements are reproducible in the PAD population and can be modified with exercise training (24, 27, 28). However, obtaining $\dot{V}O_2$peak measurements requires expensive equipment, specially trained personnel, and it is not commonly available in most clinical settings.

Functional Status Measures

Laboratory-based tests, such as treadmill tests, and questionnaires, should be used to comprehensively evaluate functional status of PAD patients (Table 33.2). The Walking Impairment Questionnaire (WIQ) assesses de-

Table 33.2. Questionnaires Used to Assess the Functional Status of Patients with Peripheral Arterial Disease

Questionnaire	Walking Impairment Questionnaire	Physical Activity Recall	Medical Outcomes Study (SF-36)
Domain(s) evaluated	Ability to walk distances, speeds, stair-climbing ability, claudication severity	Habitual physical activity level (work, housework, leisure)	Physical, role, social functioning, bodily pain, mental health, vitality, general health perception
Mode of administration	Interviewer	Interviewer	Self or Interviewer
Time required for administration and scoring	6–8 minutes	6–8 minutes	5–7 minutes
Scoring	Four scores, 0–100% scale	One score MET/hrs or kcals per week	Eight scores 0–100% scale
Validation	PAD population	PAD population Diabetes population Healthy sedentary adults	Numerous healthy and diseased populations (including PAD)

MET-metabolic equivalent
For a complete review of the questionnaires, refer to Regensteiner JG, Hiatt WR. Exercise rehabilitation for patients with peripheral arterial disease. *Exerc Sports Sci Rev* 23:1–4, 1995.

fined walking distances, speeds, stair climbing ability, and claudication severity in the PAD population (5, 6). The WIQ has been used to evaluate changes in walking ability resulting from an exercise training program as well as from peripheral bypass surgery (5, 6).

The Physical Activity Recall questionnaire provides a general measure of habitual physical activity in patients with PAD. This questionnaire has been modified from the original Stanford Physical Activity Recall for use in sedentary and diseased populations (6, 29). Energy expenditure in the home, at work, and during leisure time is measured (6).

The Medical Outcomes Study questionnaire evaluates physical, social, and role functioning as well as perception of general health and well-being. This questionnaire has been used to evaluate functional status in a number of disease states (including cardiac) as well as in healthy persons (30).

Questionnaires, such as the ones discussed above, are easily used to evaluate the impact of exercise rehabilitation on functional status in the PAD patient with claudication. The information provided is a valuable adjunct to laboratory-based measures. It is not recommended that the questionnaires replace treadmill testing in clinical trials given the valuable information obtained from more objective tests. However, in settings where treadmill testing is not available, the questionnaires are useful in providing some outcome information.

EXERCISE REHABILITATION

A supervised exercise rehabilitation program has been shown to be highly effective in treating claudication (Table 33.3) (27, 28, 31–35). Repetitive of such programs, most often consisting of treadmill walking, are associated with improvements in both treadmill exercise performance and walking ability in patients with claudication. Therefore, exercise rehabilitation has been recommended in varying forms for nearly 50 years to improve walking ability in PAD.

Table 33.3. Improvements in Exercise Performance After Exercise Rehabilitation

- Improved treadmill exercise performance
  - Two- to threefold increase in walking distance
- 15–30% increase in oxygen consumption
- Improved walking ability
  - increased speed, duration
  - less claudication pain
- Improved perception of physical functioning
- Increased level of habitual physical activity

Of the many exercise rehabilitation studies on PAD performed to date, relatively few have been randomized or controlled (27, 28, 31–35). However, all studies of exercise conditioning in persons with PAD report increased maximal claudication time, as well as initial (pain-free) walking time during exercise. In randomized, controlled trials, it has been observed that both exercise performance (by treadmill) and functional status (by questionnaire) are improved after 12 weeks and 24 weeks (Table 33.4) (17, 27, 28, 31–36). Exercise performance prior to exercise conditioning is lower than that of normal, sedentary individuals. It is especially notable that VO_2peak is reduced in PAD by about 50% (27, 28). This finding reflects the extreme disability imposed by intermittent claudication.

Exercise Training-specific Methods

Exercise rehabilitation should begin after entry screening and assessment of exercise performance and func-

Table 33.4. Summary of Randomized Controlled Trials Evaluating the Efficacy of Exercise Rehabilitation for Patients with Peripheral Arterial Disease

Author	Group	N	Intervention	Treadmill Test	Duration of Program	Functional Assessment	Change in ICD	Change in ACD
Larsen 1966 (33)	T	7	Daily walks	Constant-load	6 months	No	106%*	183%*
	C	7	Placebo pill				−11%	−6%
Holm 1973 (34)	T	6	Dynamic leg exercise	Constant-load	4 months	No	220%*	133%*
	C	6	Placebo pill				No change	No change
Dahllof 1974 (31)	T	23	Dynamic leg exercise	Constant-load	6 months	No	150%*	117%*
	C	11	Placebo pill				No change	No change
Dahllof 1976 (32)	T	10	Dynamic leg exercise	Constant-load	4 months	No	170%*	135%*
	C	8	Placebo pill				120%*	75%*
Mannarino 1991 (35)	T1	10	Dynamic leg exercise + daily walks	Constant-load	6 months	No	90%*	86%*
	T2	10	Exercise + antiplatelet				120%*	105%*
	T3	10	Antiplatelet				35%*	38%*
Lundgren 1989 (36)	T1	25	Dynamic leg exercise	Constant-load	6 months	No	179%*	151%*
	T2	25	Surgery + dynamic leg exercise				698%*	263%*
	T3	25	Surgery				376%*	173%*
Creasy 1990 (17)	T1	20	Exercise	Constant-load	6 months treatment (follow-up of 12 months)	No	296%*	442%*
	T2	13	Angioplasty				21%	57%
Hiatt 1990 (27)	T	10	Walking exercise	Graded	3 months	Yes	165%*	123%*
	C	9	Non-exercising control				6%	20%*
Hiatt (28)	T	10	Walking exercise	Graded	6 months	Yes	209%*	128%*
	C	8	Non-exercising control		3 months		−18%	−1%

T = Treat and C = Control; Functional Assessment = Use of questionnaire to evaluate community-based functional status; "No change" = A finding of no improvement is stated but the data are not given. For the Creasy study, the data given are for the 12 month follow-up time point. * = $P < 0.05$ compared to baseline. Numbers in parentheses are reference numbers.

tional status (as described previously) (5, 6, 27, 28). Exercise sessions should be held three times a week for 1 hour each for 3 months (Table 33.5). Telemetry monitoring can be used to evaluate heart rate response, or may be required in the case of existent cardiovascular disease in addition to PAD. Warm-up should precede exercise and cool-down should follow to minimize risk of injury (Table 33.5). The initial training load is determined from a symptom limited maximal treadmill test, such that the intensity of the exercise causes claudication pain. In subsequent visits, the speed or grade is increased if the patient is able to walk 8–10 minutes, or longer, at the lower work load without moderate claudication pain.

The goal of the initial training session is for the patient to spend 10–15 minutes on the treadmill, exclusive of the warm-up and cool-down, with subsequent increases of 5 minutes each session until 35 minutes of treadmill walking in a 50 minute exercise session is accomplished. During exercise sessions, rest periods (induced by claudication) are interspersed between bouts of walking. The patient walks until mild to moderate claudication pain is perceived (3–4 on a 1 to 5 scale); at

Table 33.5. Specific Methods of Exercise Training

Warm-up period and Cool-down period (5 minutes each should precede and end the 1 hour session)

Training Intensity

- Initial
  - Set by results of peak treadmill
  - Starting exercise work load brings on claudication pain
- Subsequent
  - Speed or grade increased if patient walks ≥ 10 minutes
    - Grade increased first if speed ≥ 2 mph
    - Speed increased first if < 2 mph

Duration

- Initial
  - 35 minutes (intermittent walking)
- Subsequent
  - Add 5 minutes every session until 50 minutes (intermittent walking) is possible
- Total time period
  - 3 months (36 sessions)

Frequency

- Three to five times per week[a]

Specificity of activity

- Treadmill walking is the recommended exercise

[a] ACSM Guidelines specify daily; literature supports the beneficial effects of 3 to 5 times per week.

that point, the patient sits and rests until the pain abates. The patient resumes walking until a mild or moderate level of pain is reached again, followed by another rest period. This process is repeated until the 50 minute exercise period has elapsed. Generally, after some conditioning, walking comprises about 35 minutes and rest periods total about 15 minutes of the total 50 minute period (27, 28).

Resistive Training

The benefits of resistive training in PAD are less well-known than walking. In one randomized controlled trial, 12 weeks of strength training alone was less effective than 12 weeks of supervised treadmill walking for improving walking ability (28). In addition, sequential use of strength training followed by exercise or concomitant walking and strength training had no incremental effect on walking ability. Since, in claudication, the main deficit is ability to walk and given the principle of specificity of training, it is not surprising that walking results in greater benefit.

Assessment of Gait

Preliminary data suggest that gait is affected by PAD. Step length and steps per minute are reduced in PAD patients compared to controls (Scherer, unpublished data). Changes in walking speed, step frequency, and other aspects of gait have not been measured in training studies, yet it is possible that inefficient gait may be a factor increasing the difficulty of walking. Rehabilitation physicians may be consulted if evaluation of gait abnormalities is desired.

Home-based Walking Program

Home-based exercise programs have been evaluated for PAD patients (37). Results are variable, but generally suggest that a hospital-based program has greater efficacy. Clearly, where a home-based program is mandated, feedback and evaluation remains important.

Exercise Precautions and Special Considerations

For the most part, patients tolerate exercise training well. However, the potential for adverse events exists in any exercise program. There are two types of potential problems, cardiovascular and musculoskeletal. A cardiovascular problem is possible in PAD patients since they have high prevalence of cardiac disease as well as PAD. To promote safety, all patients with clinical evidence of co-morbid coronary disease are telemetry monitored during exercise sessions to evaluate heart rate and rhythm. Blood pressure is recorded before and after each training session. In our experience, to date, of treadmill training in over 100 patients, no patient has experienced cardiovascular complication (serious arrhythmia, myocardial infarction, or stroke) during rehabilitation. Six patients have reported exacerbation of existing musculoskeletal problems (i.e., knee stiffness).

EXERCISE REHABILITATION: POTENTIAL MECHANISMS OF IMPROVEMENT

The mechanism(s) by which an exercise rehabilitation program benefits persons with PAD remains incompletely delineated. Potential mechanisms for improvement include adaptations in peripheral blood flow or distribution of flow and changes in muscle metabolism.

Peripheral Blood Flow

Although various studies demonstrate increased peripheral blood flow with exercise training, more commonly, lack of increased peripheral blood flow has been observed (27, 32–36). Increased blood flow, when reported, is not correlated with changes in exercise performance. In addition to increased flow per se, other modifications of flow may occur which could improve oxygen delivery to skeletal muscle. For example, decreased blood viscosity (38), or increased capillary density may alter exchange of oxygen and substrate at the capillary/muscle fiber interface.

Muscle Metabolism

In healthy subjects, exercise training is associated with improved oxidative metabolism of skeletal muscle (39). These changes are associated with improved extraction of oxygen and substrate during exercise. It has been postulated that chronic arterial insufficiency in PAD is associated with adaptive changes in the metabolic state of muscle (40). However, results have been variable. Increased oxidative enzyme activity in skeletal muscle is not always present in PAD (41). In addition, enzyme activities do not correlate with exercise performance and one study demonstrated no change in citrate synthase after 12 weeks of rehabilitation (42).

In healthy individuals, carnitine is required for transportation of long-chain fatty acyl groups into mitochondria. Under abnormal metabolic conditions, such as muscle ischemia, carnitine interacts with the cellular acyl-CoA pool to form acylcarnitines, which remove a variety of acyl groups derived from the corresponding acyl-CoA intermediates (43). In these circumstances, the formation of acylcarnitines reflects the underlying metabolic state of the cellular acyl-CoA pool and, by removing potentially toxic acyl groups, may serve to maintain normal metabolism (44, 45).

Claudication pain experienced during exercise is associated with (among other factors) an increased muscle concentration of acylcarnitines, reflecting the abnormal metabolic state of ischemic muscle (46). Exercise training reduces the plasma concentration of short-chain acylcarnitines. Additionally, subjects who improved most from training also had the greatest reduction in plasma short-chain acylcarnitine concentration (27). It has recently been reported that training-induced changes in muscle carnitine metabolism are associated with improved functional status in the patient with claudication (42).

Changes in Walking Efficiency

It is possible that improvement in walking ability may be related to a change in gait or pain threshold. The effects of exercise training on aspects of gait such as step length and steps per minute have not been assessed in PAD. However, it has been shown that oxygen consumption for a given constant work load decreases after exercise training (27). If the onset of claudication is due to mismatched oxygen delivery and oxygen demand, lower oxygen consumption per work load may be associated with ability to walk longer after exercise training. This observation suggests that a change in the biomechanics of walking with training improves walking efficiency and decreases energy requirements of a given work load.

SUMMARY

Intermittent claudication, resulting from PAD, impairs functional status. Reducing disability is, therefore, an important goal of treatment. To evaluate the efficacy of an intervention designed to improve functional status requires appropriate outcome measures. Such outcome measures include graded treadmill intervention (exercise rehabilitation). Importantly, exercise therapy has been shown to be efficacious and well-tolerated. Patients improve both walking ability (in the laboratory) and functional status. Because of the efficacy of this treatment, in addition to the low associated morbidity, exercise therapy is recommended as a major treatment option for persons with intermittent claudication due to PAD.

References

1. Criqui MH, Fronek A, Barrett-Connor E, et al. The prevalence of peripheral arterial disease in a defined population. *Circulation* 71:510–515, 1985.
2. Hiatt WR, Marshall JA, Baxter J, et al. Diagnostic methods for peripheral arterial disease in the San Luis Valley Diabetes Study. *J Clin Epidemiol* 43:597–606, 1990.
3. Criqui MH, Coughlin SS, Fronek A. Noninvasively diagnosed peripheral arterial disease as a predictor of mortality: Results from a prospective study. *Circulation* 72:768–773, 1985.
4. Lassila R, Lepantalo M, Lindfors O. Peripheral arterial disease-natural outcome. *Acta Med Scand* 220:295–301, 1986.
5. Regensteiner JG, Steiner JF, Panzer RJ, et al. Evaluation of walking impairment by questionnaire in patients with peripheral arterial disease. *J Vasc Med Biol* 2:142–152, 1990.
6. Regensteiner JG, Steiner JF, Hiatt WR. Exercise training improves functional status in patients with peripheral arterial disease. *J Vasc Surg* 1996:23;104–115.
7. Weber KT, Janicki JS. *Cardiopulmonary Exercise Testing: Physiologic Principles and Clinical Applications.* Philadelphia: WB Saunders, 1986.
8. Brand FN, Abbott RD, Kannel WB. Diabetes, intermittent claudication, and risk of cardiovascular events. *Diabetes* 38: 504–509, 1989.
9. Coleridge-Smith PD, Thomas P, Scurr JH, et al. Causes of venous ulceration: A new hypothesis. *Br Med J* 296:1726–1727, 1988.
10. Dormandy JA, Hoare E, Khattab AH, et al. Prognostic significance of rheological and biochemical findings in patients with intermittent claudication. *Br Med J* 4:581–583, 1973.
11. Kannel WB, McGee DL. Diabetes and cardiovascular disease. The Framingham Study. *JAMA* 241:2035–2038, 1979.
12. Pomrehn P, Duncan B, Weissfeld L, et al. The association of dyslipoproteinemia with symptoms and signs of peripheral arterial disease. The lipids research clinics program prevalence study. *Circulation* 73 (Suppl I):I100–I107, 1986.
13. Kannel WB, McGee DL. Update on some epidemiologic features of intermittent claudication: The Framingham Study. *J Am Geriatr Soc* 33:13–18, 1985.
14. Taylor LM, DeFrang RD, Harris EJ, et al. The association of elevated plasma homocyst(e)ine with progression of symptomatic peripheral arterial disease. *J Vasc Surg* 13: 128–136, 1991.
15. Cantin B, Moorjani S, Dagenais GR, et al. Lipoprotein(a) distribution in a French Canadian population and its relation to intermittent claudication (The Quebec Cardiovascular Study). *Am J Cardiol* 75:1224–1228, 1995
16. Quick CR, Cotton LT. The measured effect of stopping smoking on intermittent claudication. *Br J Surg* 69 (Suppl): S24–S26, 1982.
17. Creasy TS, McMillan PJ, Fletcher EW, et al. Is percutaneous transluminal angioplasty better than exercise for claudication? Preliminary results from a prospective randomised trial. *Eur J Vasc Surg* 4:135–140, 1990.
18. Regensteiner JG, Hargarten ME, Rutherford RB, et al. Functional benefits of peripheral vascular bypass surgery for patients with intermittent claudication. *Angiology* 44:1–10, 1993.
19. Doubilet P, Abrams HL. The cost of underutilization. Percutaneous transluminal angioplasty for peripheral vascular disease. *N Engl J Med* 310:95–102, 1984.
20. Jeans WD, Danton RM, Baird RN, et al. A comparison of the costs of vascular surgery and balloon dilatation in lower limb ischaemic disease. *Br J Radiol* 59:453–456, 1986.
21. Tunis SR, Bass EB, Steinberg EP. The use of angioplasty, bypass surgery, and amputation in the management of peripheral vascular disease. *N Engl J Med* 325:556–562, 1991.
22. Porter JM, Cutler BS, Lee BY, et al. Pentoxifylline efficacy in the treatment of intermittent claudication: Multicenter controlled double-blind trial with objective assessment of chronic occlusive arterial disease patients. *Am Heart J* 104: 66–72, 1982.
23. Orchard TJ, Strandness DE, Cavanaugh PR, et al., Assessment of peripheral vascular disease in diabetes. Report and recommendations of an international workshop. *Circulation* 1993;88:819–828.

24. Hiatt WR, Nawaz D, Regensteiner JG, et al. The evaluation of exercise performance in patients with peripheral vascular disease. *J Cardiopulm Rehab* 12:525–532, 1988.
25. Patterson JA, Naughton J, Pietras RJ, et al. Treadmill exercise in assessment of the functional capacity of patients with cardiac disease. *Am J Cardiol* 30:757–762, 1972.
26. Gardner AW, Skinner JS, Cantwell BW, et al. Progressive vs single-stage treadmill tests for evaluation of claudication. *Med Sci Sports Exerc* 23:402–408, 1991.
27. Hiatt WR, Regensteiner JG, Hargarten ME, et al. Benefit of exercise conditioning for patients with peripheral arterial disease. *Circulation* 81:602–609, 1990.
28. Hiatt WR, Wolfel EE, Meier RH, et al. Superiority of treadmill walking exercise vs. strength training for patients with peripheral arterial disease. Implications for the mechanism of the training response. *Circulation* 90:1866–1874, 1994.
29. Sallis JF, Haskell WL, Wood PD, et al. Physical activity assessment methodology in the five-city project. *Am J Epidemiol* 121:91–106, 1985.
30. Tarlov AR, Ware JE, Greenfield S, et al. The medical outcomes study. An application of methods for monitoring the results of medical care. *JAMA* 262:925–930, 1989.
31. Dahllof A, Bjorntorp P, Holm J, et al. Metabolic activity of skeletal muscle in patients with peripheral arterial insufficiency. Effect of physical training. *Eur J Clin Invest* 4:9–15, 1974.
32. Dahllof A, Holm J, Schersten T, et al. Peripheral arterial insufficiency. Effect of physical training on walking tolerance, calf blood flow, and blood flow resistance. *Scand J Rehab Med* 8:19–26, 1976.
33. Larsen OA, Lassen NA. Effect of daily muscular exercise in patients with intermittent claudication. *Lancet* 2:1093–1096, 1966.
34. Holm J, Dahllof A, Bjorntorp P, et al. Enzyme studies in muscles of patients with intermittent claudication. Effect of training. *Scand J Clin Lab Invest* 31(Suppl 128):201–205, 1973.
35. Mannarino E, Pasqualini L, Innocente S, et al. Physical training and antiplatelet treatment in stage II peripheral arterial occlusive disease: Alone or combined? *Angiology* 42:513–521, 1991.
36. Lundgren F, Dahllof A, Lundholm K, et al. Intermittent claudication–surgical reconstruction or physical training? A prospective randomized trial of treatment efficiency. *Ann Surg* 209:346–355, 1989.
37. Regensteiner JG, Meyer T, Krupski W, et al. Comparison of home vs. hospital based rehabilitation for patients with peripheral arterial disease. *Angiology* 48:291–300, 1997.
38. Ernst EE, Matrai A. Intermittent claudication, exercise, and blood rheology. *Circulation* 76:1110–1114, 1987.
39. Holloszy JO, Coyle EF. Adaptations of skeletal muscle to endurance exercise and their metabolic consequences. *J Appl Physiol* 56:831–838, 1984.
40. Jansson E, Johansson J, Sylven C, et al. Calf muscle adaptation in intermittent claudication. Side-differences in muscle metabolic characteristics in patients with unilateral arterial disease. *Clin Physiol* 8:17–29, 1988.
41. Regensteiner JG, Wolfel EE, Brass EP, et al. Chronic changes in skeletal muscle histology and function in peripheral arterial disease. *Circulation* 87:413–421, 1993.
42. Hiatt WR, Regensteiner JG, Carry M, et al. Brass. Effect of exercise training on skeletal muscle histology and metabolism in peripheral arterial disease. *J Appl Physiol* 81:780–788, 1996.
43. Bieber LL, Emaus R, Valkner K, et al. Possible functions of short-chain and medium-chain carnitine acyltransferases. *Fed Proc* 41:2858–2862, 1982.
44. Brass EP, Hoppel CL. Relationship between acid-soluble carnitine and coenzyme A pools in vivo. *Biochem J* 190: 495–504, 1980.
45. Brass EP, Fennessey PV, Miller LV. Inhibition of oxidative metabolism by propionic acid and its reversal by carnitine in isolated rat hepatocytes. *Biochem J* 236:131–136, 1986.
46. Hiatt WR, Wolfel EE, Regensteiner JG, et al. Skeletal muscle carnitine metabolism in patients with unilateral peripheral arterial disease. *J Appl Physiol* 73:346–353, 1992.

Suggested Readings

Ernst E, Fialka V. A review of the clinical effectiveness of exercise therapy for intermittent claudication. *Arch Intern Med* 153:2357–2360, 1993.

Gardner AW, Poehlman ET. Exercise rehabilitation programs for the treatment of claudication pain. A meta-analysis. *JAMA* 274:975–980, 1995.

Regensteiner JG, Hiatt WR. Exercise rehabilitation for patients with peripheral arterial disease. *Exerc Sports Sci Rev* 23:1–24, 1995.

59 424, 427

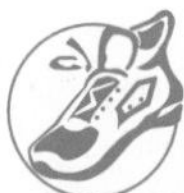

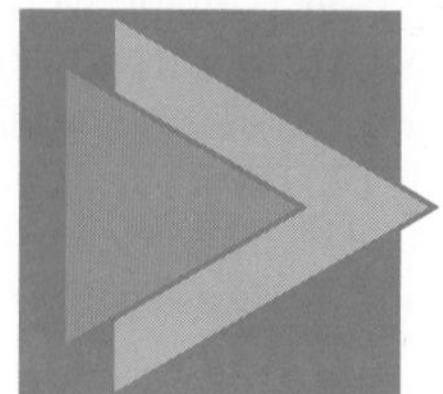

CHAPTER 34
EXERCISE FOR SKELETAL HEALTH AND OSTEOPOROSIS PREVENTION

Janet M. Shaw and Kara A. Witzke

Osteoporosis is a systemic skeletal disease characterized by low bone mass and microarchetectural deterioration of bone tissue leading to bone fragility and increased risk of fracture. It is estimated that over 1.5 million fractures occur annually which clearly establishes osteoporosis as a major public health care concern. Common fracture sites include the wrist, spine, and hip. Estimates of direct health care costs associated with these three types of fractures in Caucasian women over the age of 45 have been projected to be $45.2 billion over the next 10 years (1). Hip fractures account for the majority of these expenses and are the most devastating with respect to personal consequence; that being loss of independence, prolonged immobility, and death due to multi-system failure. As with other chronic disease, preventing osteoporotic fracture is the focus of much research and debate. Preventive measures include altering lifestyle, such as nutrition and exercise, as well as administration of pharmacological agents (e.g., hormone replacement, amino bisphosphonates). This chapter presents a brief overview of skeletal physiology, research findings to define the role of exercise in decreasing risk for osteoporotic fractures, and practical applications for developing an appropriate exercise prescription for skeletal health.

PURPOSE AND ORGANIZATION OF THE SKELETON

There are three primary purposes of the skeleton:

- To provide support for loads against gravity and to aid in locomotion by providing sites for muscular attachment
- To provide a protective barrier for vital organs and bone marrow
- To serve as a mineral reservoir able to support blood levels of calcium and phosphorus when required

The skeleton can be divided into appendicular (peripheral) and axial (central) compartments. The appendicular skeleton comprises approximately 80% of total skeletal mass and consists primarily of cortical ("compact") bone. The concentric orientation of lamellae deposited around a central nutrient canal in cortical bone forms very dense tissue. Eighty to ninety percent of the total volume of cortical bone is calcified. In contrast, the axial skeleton has a high percentage of trabecular ("spongy") bone, in which lamellae are arranged along a flat surface. Only 15–25% of trabecular bone volume is calcified. The remaining volume is occupied by bone marrow, fat, and blood vessels. Trabecular bone has a high surface area-to-volume ratio and is in close proximity to hematopoietic activity of red marrow in the adult skeleton. Thus, trabecular bone is more metabolically active than cortical bone and consequently exhibits a greater rate of turnover.

BONE REMODELING

In the mature skeleton, bone is subjected to a dynamic process of breakdown and renewal termed **remodeling.** The purpose of remodeling is to maintain mechanical integrity of tissue by replacing fatigue-damaged, older bone with new bone. Multinucleated osteoclasts erode portions of the bone surface creating resorptive cavities. Osteoblasts secrete a collagen matrix within the cavity which becomes mineralized. The events in a typical remodeling cycle are depicted in Figure 34.1. Under normal conditions, remodeling is a coupled process (i.e., formation follows resorption). However, it is suspected that this process is inefficient and that small deficits in formation remain at the completion of a remodeling cycle. The accumulation of these formation deficits is thought to be partially responsible for age-related losses in bone mass. Thus, bone that experiences the greatest number of remodeling cycles will be at highest risk for age-related losses in mass. Due to its metabolic activity and amount of surface area exposed, the relatively high rate of turnover in trabecular bone predis-

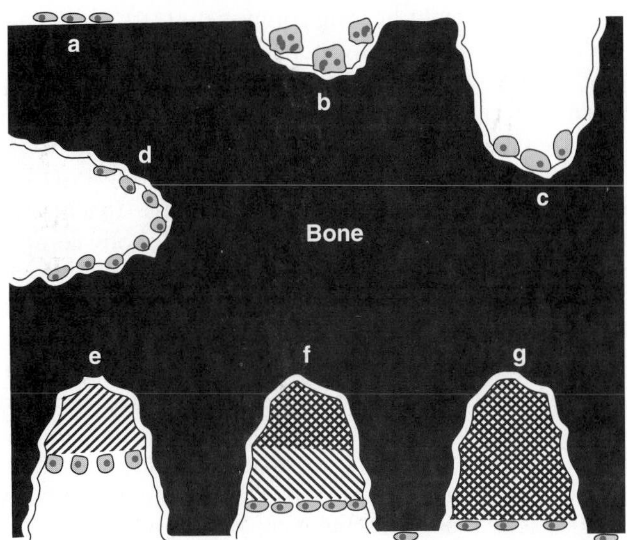

Figure 34.1. **a,** Resting trabecular surface. **b,** Multinucleated osteoclasts dig a cavity of approximately 20 Tm. **c,** Completion of resorption to 60 Tm by mononuclear phagocytes. **d,** Recruitment of osteoblast precursors to the base of the resorptive cavity. **e,** Secretion of new matrix by osteoblasts. **f,** Continued secretion of matrix, with initiation of calcification. **g,** Completion of mineralization of new matrix. Bone has returned to a quiescent state, but a small deficit in bone mass persists. (Reprinted with permission from Marcus R. Normal and abnormal bone remodelling in man. *Adv Int Med* 38:129–141, 1987.)

poses it to age-related losses and hence, fractures. In contrast to the mature skeleton, **modeling**, or new bone formation **not** preceded by resorption, is the dominant activity in growing bones. Modeling is the process by which bones experience net gains in mass as well as modifications in shape.

Reproductive hormones, calcium intake, and mechanical loading are three primary factors that regulate remodeling. When reproductive hormone status is compromised, such as in young, amenorrheic or estrogen-deplete, postmenopausal women, reductions in bone mineral density (BMD) are observed. Hypoestrogenism, characterized by increased resorption, is typically reversed with hormone replacement therapy (HRT). Hence HRT is considered **anti-resorptive,** effectively arresting bone loss in most postmenopausal women. The connection between bone metabolism and testosterone levels is not as clear; however, in some cases, levels of testosterone in men have been weakly associated with BMD (2). Although the mechanism of action is poorly understood, androgens are thought to be important for skeletal health.

Remodeling activity is increased when dietary calcium intake is insufficient. This effect, mediated by the parathyroid hormone (PTH), provides an important means of maintaining adequate blood levels of calcium. Calcium intake during growth is critical in order to supply the raw materials necessary for optimal bone mineral accretion. However, older individuals, particularly estrogen-deplete postmenopausal women, may have impaired intestinal absorption of calcium and therefore calcium requirements are higher in this group. Calcium supplementation in this group may reduce rate of bone loss, although supplementation is not as effective as hormone replacement. Hence, adequate calcium nutriture reduces the likelihood of PTH hypersecretion, and thus, increased bone turnover. Attention to calcium intake is most important during maturation and in older adults whose compensatory mechanisms for regulation of circulating calcium is less robust than in younger adults.

Lastly, bone responds to alterations in mechanical forces and regulation of bone strength is a function of skeletal load. In the absence of mechanical forces (space flight or prolonged bedrest) urinary calcium excretion increases and BMD decreases (3, 4). This probably results from increased resorption and reduction in new bone formation. Mechanical stimuli are important for maintaining bone mass and may be the only type of stimuli capable of inducing modeling in mature bone. Mechanical force magnitude has been shown to be more important for skeletal modeling than the number of force repetitions or load cycles (5). Although this has been demonstrated in animal models, the ideal exercise prescription that replicates these loading characteristics and effectively increases bone mass in humans has yet to be defined.

BONE MASS ASSESSMENT

Technological advances over the past 10 years have enabled researchers to noninvasively assess bone mass at important fracture sites (distal radius, proximal femur (hip), and lumbar spine) with great precision. The assessment technique commonly used (dual-energy x-ray absorptiometry [DXA]) quantifies mineral content per unit area of bone. Outcome variables include bone mineral content (BMC in grams) and BMD (in g/cm^2). The latter is sometimes termed "apparent" or "areal" density, since it is expressed per unit area, and is therefore not a true volumetric measure. Nonetheless, it is abbreviated BMD and in this chapter will be used synonymously with bone mass.

BONE MASS CHANGES WITH AGE

Changes in BMC across the lifespan of females are depicted in Figure 34.2. Periods of growth are dominated by modeling and rapid increases in bone mass. Peak bone mass is attained at the conclusion of longitudinal growth, after which a plateau in BMD is observed in the second to third decades of life. Bone loss probably begins somewhere between the end of the second to the

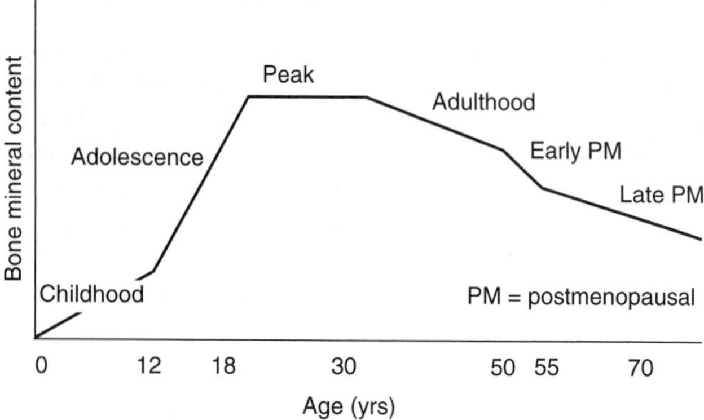

Figure 34.2. Model of bone mineral content changes with age in women. (Reprinted with permission from Snow-Harter C. Exercise, calcium and estrogen: Primary regulators of bone mass. *Contemp Nutr* 17(4), 1992.)

start of the third decade, notably at sites with a high percentage of trabecular bone, at a rate of 0.5–1% per year (6). This gradual rate of loss continues throughout adult years, but is interrupted by menopause. Secondary to estrogen deficiency, women not on HRT exhibit accelerated rate of loss in the first 5–7 years of menopause [early post-menopausal (PM)]. Bone loss returns to a slower rate once adaptation to hormone deficiency has occurred (late PM).

Bone mass changes across the lifespan of males are similar to those observed in females with a few exceptions. Rate of loss in men may not be as great as in women and losses may begin later in life (7). Testosterone levels decline with age, however, hormonal changes are not as uniform in men nor are they as strongly correlated with reductions in BMD as that observed in postmenopausal women.

EXERCISE AND BONE MASS

Physical activity transmits mechanical loads to the skeleton via gravitational forces and muscular pull at sites of attachment. Support for exercise as a preventive measure for osteoporosis is provided by observations that physically active individuals and athletes typically have higher bone mass than sedentary controls. Within athletic groups, those active in sports with unilateral activity, such as tennis, demonstrate higher BMD in the dominant arm than in the nondominant arm (8). Attempts to further delineate types of loading associated with highest bone mass have resulted in more specific athletic group comparisons. Recent cross-sectional research suggests that athletes involved in activities requiring high power output and high impact loads have higher bone mass than those involved in endurance training (9). Further, activities characterized by substantial muscular involvement without gravitational forces (e.g., swimming) are associated with lower BMD than those with a weight-bearing component (10). This is not to de-emphasize the many benefits of nonweight-bearing modes of exercise, but rather to emphasize the importance of weight-bearing in achieving optimal stimulus for skeletal development.

In addition to athletic group comparisons, BMD has been correlated with parameters of fitness. Specifically, maximal oxygen consumption ($\dot{V}O_2max$), body composition, and muscle strength are associated with bone mass in various age groups. The relationship between $\dot{V}O_2$ max and bone mass is probably a function of loading patterns experienced by subjects tested in those studies (i.e., running, aerobic dance). Some have observed associations between fat mass and BMD although this relationship is not well understood. Adiposity affords additional loading, albeit nonspecific, by increasing body weight. It is plausible that increased adiposity benefits the skeleton by increasing circulating levels of estrogens. Muscle strength has been found to be an important determinant of BMD in children, and in young and older adults, and this association appears to be site-specific. For example, muscle strength of the hip abductors, which attach at the greater trochanter, is the best predictor of hip (femoral neck) BMD in both pre- and postmenopausal women (11). Moreover, the relationship between muscle mass and BMD is well-established.

The associations between muscle strength, mass, and BMD suggest that weight training is a promising avenue for increasing or maintaining bone mass. Potential selection bias warrants caution in interpretation of these results. These data have been used, however, as a spring board for designing longitudinal interventions to determine the extent to which physical training affects bone mass.

LONGITUDINAL STUDIES AND PRINCIPLES OF TRAINING

Longitudinal data demonstrate equivocal findings in studies that induce mechanical loads through exercise intervention. With few exceptions, changes from small increases (1–2%) in, or maintenance of BMD (no change) to decrements in bone density have been demonstrated. The improvements in BMD are much smaller than expected from the cross-sectional literature. Any successful exercise program must adhere to principles of training to produce beneficial effects in a target tissue or system. Drinkwater has emphasized the importance of including training principles in exercise intervention programs for bone (12). To date, many studies neglect one or more of these principles which may be the reason for minimal to no training effects on bone. The application of these principles to the skeletal system is outlined in Table 34.1.

The exact physiological mechanism causing bone to sense and respond to alterations in mechanical loads is unclear, however, adaptations appear to be site-specific.

Table 34.1. Principles of Training

Specificity	Overload	Reversibility	Initial Values	Diminishing Returns
The impact of the training should be at the bone site of interest since loading seems to have a localized effect.	The training stimulus must include forces much greater than that afforded by habitual activity.	In the absence of the training stimulus, the positive effect on bone will be lost.	Individuals with low BMD will have the greatest potential to gain from increased mechanical loading.	Each individual's biological ceiling determines the extent of adaptation to the training.

Adapted from Drinkwater BL. 1994 C.H. McCloy research lecture: Does physical activity play a role in preventing osteoporosis? *Res Q Exerc Sport* 65:197–206, 1994.

Weight training may be a plausible stimulus for specific sites and young male weight lifters exhibit high bone mass, especially at the hip and spine (13). However, most lower body exercises on weight machines are performed while seated, a position that effectively reduces forces at the hip. This may partially explain why machine-based resistance training regimens have difficulty in achieving increases in hip BMD. Conversely, the spine is sufficiently loaded while seated. Forces at the lumbar spine during weight training are estimated to be 5–6 times body weight and increased spine BMD has been demonstrated in this type of training (14). This evidence is supported by dramatically reduced hip BMD associated with spinal cord injury in those confined to a wheelchair. In contrast, spine BMD in this population appears to be similar to able-bodied people (15).

Appropriate overload in a program for improving bone mass must induce forces greater than those experienced by activities of daily living and, in effect, stimulate bone to respond and reorganize because of increased load. Optimal overload is difficult to define, given the scarcity of data on load quantification at specific skeletal sites during various activities. Weight-bearing modes of training are considered best for the skeleton, however, intensity of the activity deserves attention. Walking is an excellent mode of training for improving cardiovascular fitness, however the ability to produce sufficient stimulus for bone to adapt is questionable, especially in the able-bodied and ambulatory. Limited data suggest that walking results in forces approximately 1 times the body weight at the lumbar spine. Walking alone has not been shown to be effective in arresting bone loss in postmenopausal women (16).

With respect to appropriate overload, gymnasts have exhibited increases in spine and hip BMD after 9 months of training (17). Forces on the skeleton during gymnastics training are quite high. The ground reaction forces during landings are estimated to be 10–12 times body weight. However, bone mass appears to return to baseline values in gymnasts during periods of detraining when high-impact loads are withdrawn. Jumping may be a plausible exercise mimicking forces experienced during gymnastics training. Increased hip BMD has been observed in premenopausal women who performed 50 two-footed jumps, 3 days per week over a period of 6 months (18). Jumping may provide an adequate stimulus for bone, and appears to be safe and appropriate in older, **non-osteoporotic** women as well (19).

The principle of reversibility states that once the osteogenic stimulus is removed, positive effects on bone will be lost. Improvements in spinal BMD were demonstrated in postmenopausal women with a program consisting of vigorous, progressive exercises including walking, jogging, stair climbing, and rowing (20). Discontinued participation in the exercise program was associated with reversal in bone mass, thus confirming that the benefits of training persist only as long as the stimulus is present. The prospective increased bone mass in collegiate gymnasts during training and subsequent declines during de-training provide another example of reversibility.

Initial values play a role in expected skeletal response to increased mechanical loads. Individuals with low initial values are more likely to respond to exercise training. Once a training habit is established and maintained, further responses require longer to achieve and magnitude of change is less (diminishing returns). The time course for training response to plateau has not been established and is difficult to determine. The bone response to an appropriate training stimulus may also depend on age. It has been proposed that young bone responds to increased mechanical stimuli more favorably than older bone. The aforementioned changes in gymnasts provide support for this since they demonstrated improvement despite having high initial values.

In addition to the principles of training, it is important to emphasize the time necessary to produce changes in bone mass. The time course of a trabecular remodeling cycle is approximately 3–4 months. About 9 months to 1 year of follow-up are required to detect significant change in bone mass. In contrast to the muscular system, in which magnitude of change is great (20–200%, depending on initial values) over a relatively short period of time (8–16 weeks), a $>$ 1% increase in bone mass over 9 months is meaningful, especially given that average rate of loss is 0.5–1% per year.

SPECIAL CONSIDERATIONS

Amenorrheic and Postmenopausal Women

From puberty and into adulthood, reproductive hormones assume a critical role in maintenance of optimal bone health. This is especially evident in young women with menstrual cycle dysfunction and those in early postmenopause (21). These groups experience accelerated loss in bone mineral associated with hypoestrogenism. It has been proposed that reproductive hormones play a permissive role in the ability of mechanical loading to increase bone mass. It is not likely that additional loading from exercise counteracts the negative effects of hypoestrogenism observed in amenorrhea and early menopause. Low caloric intake and generally poor nutrition, low body weight and body fat, and high-volume physical training are probably contributing factors to exercise amenorrhea. The negative influence of amenorrhea on bone mass is well-documented and there is little evidence that bone loss with amenorrhea can be recovered with resumption of menses. Therefore, maintaining normal reproductive endocrine function should be a high priority in young women. Exercise should be considered an adjunct to HRT in early postmenopausal women.

Fall Risk

Muscle strength, mass, and power all decline with age and it is established that these factors are important for maintaining optimal function in older populations. Falls in older, nonclinical, community-dwelling adults are associated with lower extremity muscular weakness, reductions in reaction time and postural instability. The majority of hip fractures and some vertebral fractures occur in a fall. Hence, fall risk, in addition to BMD, is a major consideration in the prevention of fractures in older adults. One intervention demonstrated improvements in muscle strength, muscle mass, bone mass, and dynamic balance in estrogen-deplete, postmenopausal women (22). This regimen included dynamic resistance training 2 days/week on pneumatic machines. Earlier reports confirmed via muscle biopsies that older men and women exhibit muscle hypertrophy in response to weight training and that this type of program is well-tolerated in older adults.

Although falls are a leading cause of injury in older adults, most do not result in hip fracture. Closer examination of fall characteristics reveals impact area and fall velocity are important determinants of fracture (23). Falls to the side where the impact is absorbed directly at the hip are more likely to result in fracture (24). Results of a recent intervention using a weighted vest and jumping exercises in postmenopausal women suggest potential for decreasing risk of falls to the side (25). Improvements in lower body muscle strength, power, and mass in addition to lateral postural stability were demonstrated after 9 months of training using weight-bearing exercises such as squats, lunges, chair raises, and jumping. The intervention encouraged power development in hip abductors and leg extensors, both of which are related to improvement in indices of lateral stability. Incorporation of activities that increase muscle strength, power, and mass and also promote improvements in dynamic balance should be encouraged in older adults.

SUMMARY AND PRACTICAL IMPLICATIONS

As an osteoporosis prevention strategy, exercise has three main applications:

- To **increase** bone mass during and just after periods of growth, thus improving upon peak bone mass
- To **maintain** bone mass or **decrease** the rate of loss in adulthood
- To **decrease** indices of fall propensity in older adults.

In light of the research and in consideration of principles of training, weight bearing modes of exercise emphasizing high load and encouraging muscular development of strength and power are recommended. Deciding upon an exercise modality requires consideration of the age and/or physical limitations. Certainly, adolescents and younger individuals can perform more intense loading activities such as jumping than the frail elderly, but modifications to optimize the effects of a program for older adults are possible. For example, younger individuals are likely to benefit from increased acceleration by jumping from various heights as in plyometric training. However, older individuals can attain higher forces using added mass (such as with free weights or weighted vests). Jumping in place is appropriate in nonosteoporotic, old patients (60–75 years), but the intensity should be lower in this group than in adolescents and young adults.

Young bone is likely to respond more favorably to mechanical loading than old bone and, therefore, introduction of high mechanical loads during this stage of life may elicit the best skeletal response. Achieving optimal peak bone mass at the end of longitudinal growth affords skeletal protection by delaying critical reduction in BMD and the point at which fractures are more likely. Calcium intake and self-reported physical activity are important contributors to increased spine bone mass in young women in the third decade, a time when bone mass may plateau (26). Thus, it is at this time that a window of opportunity for improving BMD through increased mechanical load may exist.

Once age-related losses begin, it is unlikely that significantly increased bone mass is attainable. However, small improvements in, or maintenance of bone mass could affect the fracture risk profile. Resistance training appears to best mimic loading patterns that demonstrate skeletal benefits in animals (i.e., high force magnitude, low repetitions) and it provides additional protection in older adults by reducing key indices of fall risk. Weight training programs are recommended for middle-aged and older adults. The number of load cycles should be relatively low initially (i.e., one set of 5–8 exercises) with an emphasis on lower body development. It is difficult to recommend a specific intensity, however, 1–3 sets at 10–15 repetition maximum (RM) are appropriate for initial levels with gradual progression to 3–4 sets at 6–10 RM. Frequency of training should be 2–3 days per week (minimum). A simple jumping protocol (50 two-footed jumps, 3 days/wk) may complement resistance training in healthy, premenopausal women (18). The effectiveness and practicality of such a protocol in older adults is not clear and should only be considered in those without osteoporosis.

References

1. Chrischilles C, Sherman T, Wallace R. Cost and health effects of osteoporotic fractures. *Bone* 15:377–386, 1994.
2. Kelly PJ, Pocock NA, Sambrook PN, et al. Dietary calcium, sex hormones, and bone mineral density in men. *Br Med J* 300:1361–1364, 1990.
3. Mack PB, LaChance PA, Vose GP, et al. Bone demineralization of foot and hand of Gemini-Titan IV, V and VII astronauts during orbital flight. *AJR* 100:503–511, 1967.
4. Nishimura H, Fukuoka M, Kiriyama M, et al. Bone turnover and calcium metabolism during 20 days bed rest in young healthy males and females. *Acta Physiol Scand* 150: Suppl 616:27–35, 1994.
5. Rubin CT, Lanyon LE. Osteoregulatory nature of mechanical stimuli: Function as a determinant for adaptive remodeling in bone. *J Orthop Res* 5:300–310, 1987.
6. Marcus R, Kosek J, Pfefferbaum A, et al. Age-related loss of trabecular bone in premenopausal women: A biopsy study. *Calcif Tiss Int* 35:406–409, 1983..
7. Orwoll ES, Klein RF. Osteoporosis in men. *Endocrine Rev* 16:87–116, 1995.
8. Kannus P, Haapasalo H, Sievanen H, et al. The site-specific effects of long-term unilateral activity on bone mineral density and content. *Bone* 15:279–284, 1994.
9. Robinson TL, Snow-Harter C, Taaffe DR, et al. Gymnasts exhibit higher bone mass than runners despite similar prevalence of amenorrhea and oligomenorrhea. *J Bone Miner Res* 10:26–35, 1995.
10. Taaffe DR, Snow-Harter C, Connolly DA, et al. Differential effects of swimming versus weight-bearing activity on bone mineral status of eumenorrheic athletes. *J Bone Miner Res* 10:586–593, 1995.
11. Snow-Harter C, Robinson T, Shaw J, et al. Determinants of femoral neck mineral density in pre- and postmenopausal women. *Med Sci Sports Exerc* 25:Suppl S153, 1993.
12. Drinkwater BL. 1994 C.H. McCloy research lecture: Does physical activity play a role in preventing osteoporosis? *Res Q Exerc Sport* 65:197–206, 1994.
13. Conroy BP, Kraemer WJ, Maresh CM, et al. Bone mineral density in elite junior Olympic weightlifters. *Med Sci Sports Exerc* 25:1103–1109, 1993.
14. Granhad H, Jonson R, Hansson T. The loads on the lumbar spine during extreme weight lifting. *Spine* 12:146–149, 1987.
15. Biering-Sorensen F, Bohr H, Schaadt O. Longitudinal study of bone mineral content in the lumbar spine, the forearm and the lower extremities after spinal cord injury. *Eur J Clin Invest* 20:330–335, 1990.
16. Cavanaugh DJ, Cann CE. Brisk walking does not stop bone loss in postmenopausal women. *Bone* 9:201–204, 1988.
17. LaRiviere J, Snow-Harter C, Robinson TL. Bone mass changes in female competitive gymnasts over two training seasons. *Med Sci Sports Exerc* 27(Suppl):S68, 1995.
18. Bassey EJ, Ramsdale SJ. Increase in femoral bone density in young women following high-impact exercise. *Osteoporosis Int* 4:72–75, 1994.
19. Shaw JM, Snow CM, Protiva K. Effects of lower body resistance training on lean mass and power in older women, *Med Sci Sports Exerc* 27Suppl:S233, 1995.
20. Dalsky GP, Stocke KS, Eshani AA. Weight-bearing exercise training and lumbar bone mineral content in postmenopausal women. *Ann Int Med* 108:824–828, 1988.
21. Drinkwater BL, Milson K, Chestnut CH III. Bone mineral content of amenorrheic and eumenorrheic athletes. *N Engl J Med* 311:277–281, 1984.
22. Nelson ME, Fiatarone MA, Morganti CM, et al. Effects of high-intensity strength training on multiple risk factors for osteoporotic fractures. *JAMA* 272:1909–1914, 1994.
23. Hayes WC, Myers ER, Morris JN, et al. Impact near the hip dominates fracture risk in elderly nursing home residents who fall. *Calcif Tiss Int* 52:192–198, 1993.
24. Greenspan SL, Myers ER, Maitland LA, et al. Fall severity and bone mineral density as risk factors for hip fracture in ambulatory elderly. *JAMA* 271:128–133, 1994.
25. Shaw JM, Snow CM. Weighted vest exercise improves indices of hip fracture risk in older women. (under review), 1996.
26. Recker RR, Davies KM, Hinders SM, et al. Bone gain in young adult women. *JAMA* 268:2403–2408, 1992.

Suggested Readings

ACSM. ACSM position stand on osteoporosis and exercise. *Med Sci Sports Exerc* 27(4):i–vii, 1995.

Drinkwater BL. 1994 C.H. McCloy research lecture: Does physical activity play a role in preventing osteoporosis? *Res Q Exerc Sport* 65:197–206, 1994.

Marcus R, Feldman D, Kelsey J, eds. *Osteoporosis.* San Diego: Academic Press, 1996.

Snow-Harter C, Marcus R. Exercise, bone density, and osteoporosis. *Exerc Sport Sci Rev* 19:351–388, 1991.

204 83, 85 344, 424 359, 363

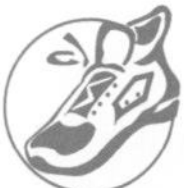   

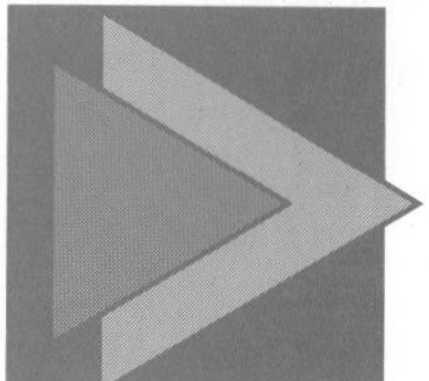

CHAPTER 35
EXERCISE AND LIPOPROTEINS

Tom R. Thomas and Tom LaFontaine

Cardiovascular disease (CVD) is the leading cause of death in the United States (2). Atherosclerosis, the primary etiology of CVD, is an accumulation of cholesterol, smooth muscle, and other material in the arterial wall. Since fat and fat-like substances are found in atherosclerotic plaque, research has focused on the transportation of fat and cholesterol as lipoprotein in the blood. Understanding this process may help in developing lifestyle prescriptions and drug therapies to prevent or reverse the disease.

OVERVIEW OF LIPOPROTEINS

Lipoproteins are large molecules which consist primarily of lipid and protein (apolipoprotein-apo), but also contain various amounts of phospholipids, carbohydrate, and cholesterol. There are five classes of lipoproteins, each with several subclasses. The largest lipoprotein is the chylomicron which transports digested fat post-prandially, primarily triglycerides (TG), to various tissues and to other lipoproteins (Fig. 35.1). Very low-density lipoprotein (VLDL) receives much of its lipid content from chylomicrons, and VLDL is the major transporter of TG in the blood. Low-density lipoprotein (LDL) contains large amounts of esterified and non-esterified (free) cholesterol. It is the cholesterol associated with LDL that is believed to be taken up by the arterial wall to eventually become a part of the atherosclerotic process (19). The cholesterol carried in the LDL subfraction, LDL-III, appears to have the highest association with atherosclerosis. Lipoprotein(a) shares many characteristics with LDL and has been linked to atherosclerosis. In addition, lipoprotein(a) may be associated with cardiovascular disease due to the ability to inhibit thrombolytic reactions in the blood. This effect would cause a greater tendency to form a thrombus (clot) which could get trapped in a narrowed artery. Cholesterol from LDL and peripheral tissues can be transferred to high density lipoprotein (HDL) and taken to the liver for degradation and excretion in feces. This "reverse cholesterol transport process" is believed to be helpful in preventing or reversing atherosclerosis. HDL also may hinder progression of atherosclerosis by diminishing the potential oxidation of LDL-cholesterol, by limiting LDL uptake by the scavenger system, and/or by serving as an oxidization substrate itself (34).

Although the lipid components of lipoproteins have received the most attention from those studying CVD, the proteins also are important to consider in the prevention or cause of the disease. Apolipoprotein B (Apo B) has been shown to be associated with obstructive coronary artery disease (19). It is the part of the LDL molecule that binds to the LDL receptor which is responsible for clearing most of the cholesterol from blood. Both LDL and chylomicrons contain Apo B protein. Once taken up by the cell at the LDL receptor, some cholesterol is stored in cells via the enzyme acyl-CoA acyltransferase (ACAT). The increased cholesterol content reduces cellular synthesis of cholesterol by inhibiting the enzyme HMG-CoA reductase. In addition, the elevated cholesterol concentration causes a down regulation of LDL receptors which, in turn, decreases cellular uptake of cholesterol (28). Although all of these effects may be beneficial, uptake of cholesterol by either the LDL receptor or the unregulated scavenger system may allow for free radical attack and subsequent cholesterol oxidation, one of the initiating steps in the atherosclerotic process (19).

Another important apoprotein is Apo A-I, the major protein of HDL. This protein activates lecithin cholesterol acyl transferase (LCAT), an enzyme important in attaching cholesterol to HDL for eventual deposition in the liver. Apo C-I and C-II, components of HDL and VLDL, also activate anti-atherogenic enzymes LCAT and lipoprotein lipase, respectively. Apo E, found in VLDL, HDL, and chylomicrons, is another protein that interacts with the LDL receptor as well as another receptor in the liver for VLDL remnants (28).

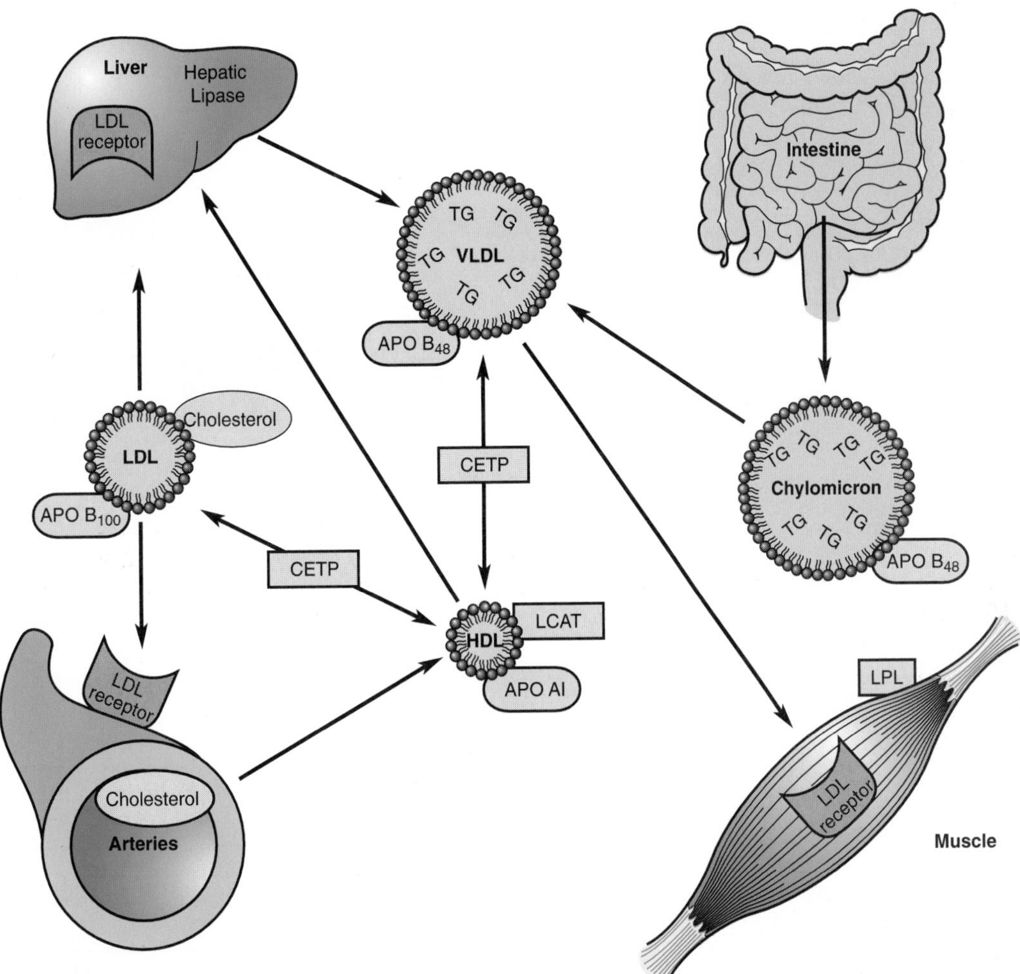

Figure 35.1. Interactions of lipoproteins. Many tissues play a role in lipoprotein synthesis, uptake, and degradation. Most of the transfer of particles between lipoproteins occurs in the blood. (VLDL = very low density lipoprotein, LDL = low density lipoprotein, HDL = high density lipoprotein, apo = apolipoprotein, CETP = cholesterol ester transfer protein, LCAT = lecithin cholesterol acyltransferase, LPL = lipoprotein lipase, rec = receptor, TG = triglycerides.)

The action of the lipoproteins is intimately tied to the activity of a variety of enzymes. Some of these enzymes are associated with atherogenesis. HMG-CoA reductase is the rate limiting enzyme of cellular synthesis of cholesterol. Many lipid lowering drugs inhibit this enzyme and, thus, decrease blood cholesterol. Another enzyme believed to be associated with atherogenesis is hepatic lipase, which is involved in the conversion of HDL_2 to HDL_3 in the liver (Fig. 35.1). HDL_2 appears to be the HDL subfraction that is protective against CVD.

Other anti-atherogenic enzymes have been studied and reviewed in the scientific literature. LCAT stimulates the attachment (esterification) of cholesterol to HDL (Fig. 35.1). This is a key step in the reverse cholesterol transport system. LCAT is also involved in the conversion of HDL_3 to HDL_2. Lipoprotein lipase, an enzyme located in the endothelium of capillaries, is also involved in conversion of chylomicrons and VLDL remnants to HDL and HDL_3 to HDL_2 (Fig. 35.2). LPL degrades VLDL-TG which allows the uptake of TG by cells for use as energy in the working muscle. Other products of this reaction are called VLDL remnants. These proteins and lipids can be transferred to other lipoproteins or be transported to the liver where they serve as precursors to lipoproteins including HDL (Fig. 35.2), especially during recovery from exercise (6). Triglyceride lipase (or hormone sensitive lipase) stimulates the degradation of TG to free fatty acids (FFAs) and glycerol and is found in adipose tissue and muscle. FFAs can be metabolized for energy while glycerol is released into the blood. The use of FFAs by muscle stimulates LPL to degrade more VLDL-TG. Cholesterol ester transfer protein (CETP) is believed to cause the transfer of triglycerides to HDL in exchange for cholesterol (Fig. 35.1). This transfer may decrease the ability of HDL to promote excretion of cholesterol.

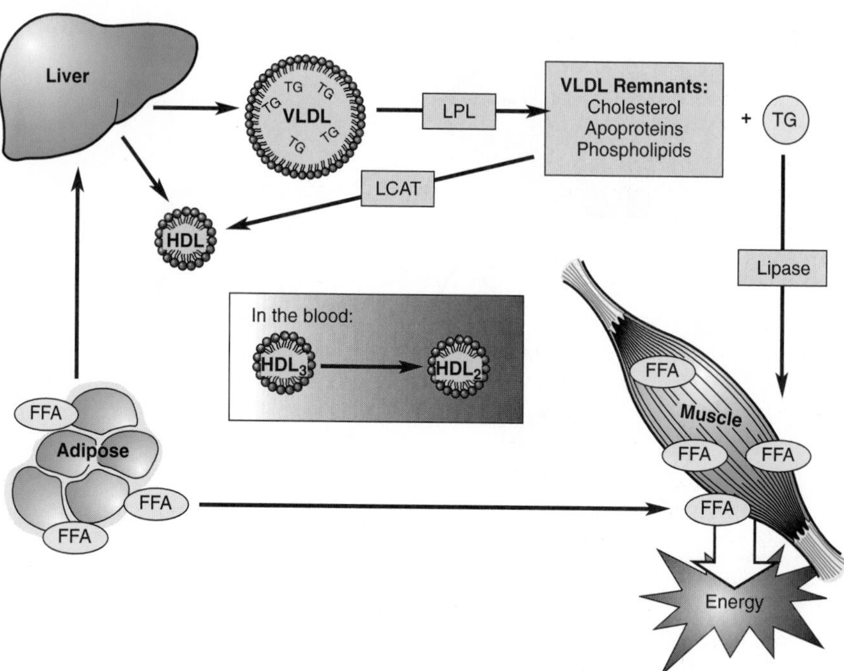

Figure 35.2. Proposed mechanism of exercise effect on HDL synthesis. The use of fat as energy by working muscles initiates a cascade of reactions which stimulates HDL production in the liver and HDL_2 conversion in blood. (Abbreviations: VLDL = very low density lipoprotein, HDL = high density lipoprotein, FFA free fatty acids, LCAT = lecithin cholesterol acyltransferase, TG = triglycerides).

Other enzymes important to the atherogenic process are involved with cholesterol oxidation. Several reactions generate free radicals which subsequently react with cell structures. Oxidative metabolism during exercise increases free radical production. This process may cause cholesterol to be more reactive and cause endothelial injury. Both processes have been associated with atherosclerosis (19). Fortunately, exercise training also increases antioxidant systems, including superoxide dismutase (SOD) and glutathione peroxidase (GPX) enzymes which inhibit free radical reactions within the cell. Antioxidant nutrients such as vitamin E, vitamin C, beta-carotene (a form of vitamin A), and selenium, which may help inhibit oxidation of cholesterol by free radicals.

NORMAL AND RECOMMENDED VALUES FOR LIPIDS

In 1988, the National Heart Lung and Blood Institute (NHLBI) established the National Cholesterol Education Program (NCEP) (30). The basis for this initiative was twofold:

1. Cholesterol is an independent risk factor for the progression and development of atherosclerosis.
2. Lowering cholesterol, particularly LDLs, results in a decreased rate of atherosclerotic events (heart attack, stroke, coronary artery bypass surgery, etc.).

Large population studies suggest that, for each 1% reduction in blood cholesterol level, there is a 2–3% reduction in incidence of cardiovascular events (31).

Table 35.1. Target Lipid Levels in Adults Over 19 Years of Age and Adolescents

Category	Total Cholesterol (mg/dL)	LDI Cholesterol (mg/dL)	HDL Cholesterol (mg/dL)
Without documented CVD 20+ yrs of age	< 200	< 130	> 35[a,b]
With documented CVD 20+ yrs of age	< 200	< 100	> 35[a,b]
Youth 13–19 yrs of age	< 170	< 100	no recommendation

[a] It is the opinion of the authors that HDL should be > 45 mg/dl in females with or without CVD.
[b] An HDL > 60 mg/dl is considered a negative risk factor.

In 1993, the NCEP guidelines (NCEP II) were updated (37). Table 35.1 summarizes target values for adults over 19 years old with and without documented atherosclerosis and for youth 13–19 years old. There is no consensus regarding target values for youth under 13 years. However, it seems reasonable to strive for a cholesterol below 170 mg/dl in all children under age 13. The NCEP II advises that both total cholesterol and HDL be assessed on initial screening.

EXERCISE TRAINING AND LIPOPROTEINS

One of the most beneficial results of regular exercise may be the long term effects on lipid metabolism. Many adaptions to exercise occur concurrent with a single vigorous or prolonged session of exercise. Decreased plasma TG is a consistent effect of acute aerobic exercise; however, the decrease may be delayed for several hours after which TG may remain depressed for 24–48 hours (14). Increased LPL activity induced by exercise may stimulate decreased TG through breaking the VLDL-TG bond and increasing the potential for TG uptake and use by skeletal muscle. The resulting increase in VLDL remnants may also stimulate the synthesis of HDL. Cholesterol and LDL-cholesterol may decrease in the 24 hr period following vigorous aerobic exercise, but this is not consistent and the physiological importance of this is unknown (23).

Although many lipoprotein changes occur with a single bout of exercise, these adaptations are transient and may not become chronic until the exercise program is maintained for several months. HDL cholesterol normally increases as a result of chronic exercise training. This is due to the increase in HDL_2 cholesterol believed beneficial because of the potential for increasing cholesterol excretion by the liver (13). Total TG are decreased with exercise training. The effects on total cholesterol and LDL cholesterol are more controversial. These lipoproteins usually do not change with exercise unless caloric restriction and weight loss also occur (45). However, exercise training alone may lower total and LDL cholesterol under certain conditions (41).

Changes in LDL subfractions may also occur with aerobic exercise training. Cross-sectional studies indicate that endurance trained individuals have higher levels of large LDL subfractions (LDL_1) and lower levels of small, dense LDL subfraction (LDL_3) than sedentary individuals (6). Others have reported that overweight individuals who lose body mass due to diet or exercise decrease dense LDL (43). Elevated LDL_3 levels have been observed in individuals with coronary artery disease (CAD). This subfraction has been associated with increased plasma levels of TG, Apo B, and total cholesterol (5).

Enzyme changes have also been associated with chronic aerobic exercise training. LPL, LCAT, and TG lipase increase, while hepatic lipase generally decreases. It is possible that LDL receptors may be up-regulated as the result of an aerobic training program. Lp(a) may be resistant to exercise training, but CETP has been shown to decrease or increase with exercise training (6, 18, 36). Antioxidant enzymes appear to increase and cellular oxidation decrease with chronic aerobic exercise (1, 22).

The precise exercise intensity and duration necessary to produce the multitude of lipoprotein changes is unknown. It appears that the total quantity of aerobic exercise (i.e., total caloric expenditure) is the major determinant related to the beneficial changes. Many of the lipoprotein changes may require several months to become permanent (40). However, after a brief training period (8–16 weeks), the changes reverse rapidly if exercise training ceases.

The effects of resistance training on lipoprotein metabolism are equivocal. Investigators who observed lipoprotein changes have used circuit resistance training which closely parallels the exercise intensity and duration of aerobic exercise and it is unknown whether heavy resistance training influences lipoprotein metabolism (20, 21). It is known that individuals involved in heavy resistance training over several years have similar lipoprotein profiles to untrained individuals. However, body builders tend to have better lipoprotein profiles than power lifters (20).

The mechanisms of these effects of exercise are unknown. Figure 35.2 illustrates one hypothesis, whereby exercise stimulates muscle oxidative processes which increase the uptake of TG, stimulating the release of FFA from adipose tissue. The resulting chain of events increases lipid metabolism by muscle and elevated HDL levels. Ironically, much of this beneficial cascade of reactions may occur in recovery when lipid metabolism is high even if carbohydrate is the primary energy source (38). Some investigators speculate that total energy expenditure is the key to lipoprotein changes rather than the specific metabolism of lipids. However, athletes undergoing vigorous anaerobic training programs generally do not have similar lipoprotein patterns as aerobic endurance athletes (39).

STRATEGIES TO IMPROVE BLOOD LIPIDS

There are three primary nonpharmacological strategies for improving blood lipids: diet, exercise training, and body weight and fat loss. These are discussed below and guidelines for optimal nonpharmacologic management of blood lipids are summarized.

Dietary Therapy

Several dietary factors influence lipoprotein levels. Studies in primates show that a diet high in saturated fat and cholesterol results in progression of atherosclerosis from fatty streaks to advanced fibrous plaques within 5 months after the onset of hyperlipidemia. There is a direct relationship between the level of dietary saturated fat and cholesterol and blood cholesterol (29). Changes in saturated fat intake explain 60% of the change in blood cholesterol (29). Table 35.2 summarizes these findings.

Restriction of dietary fat, saturated fat, and cholesterol reduces blood cholesterol (8, 32). However, there is wide variability in responsiveness to diet therapy. In 1984, the American Heart Association (AHA) recommended a three step approach to dietary management, but conspicuously deleted Step III (Table 35.3) (30). Subse-

Table 35.2. Estimated Blood Cholesterol Lowering Based on Dietary Fat, Saturated Fat, and Cholesterol Intake

	Total Fat (% calories)	Saturated Fat (% calories)	Cholesterol (mg/day)	Change in Blood Cholesterol (mg/dL)
Traditional diet	40	15	500	Baseline
Phase I diet	30–35	12–14	< 350	−18
Phase II diet	25	8	< 200	−39
Phase III diet	< 20	< 5	< 100	−53

Modified from Connor WE, Connor S. The dietary prevention and treatment of coronary heart disease. In: Connor WE, Bristow JD, eds. *Coronary Heart Disease: Prevention, Complications, and Treatment*. Philadelphia: J.B. Lippincott, 1985: 43–64.

Table 35.3. American Heart Association Dietary Therapy Recommendations for Treating Abnormal Lipids

Step	% Fat Cals	% Sat Fat Cals	% Protein	% Carbohydrates	mg/day Cholesterol
I	< 30	10	15	55	300 or less
II	< 25	8	15	60	200–250 or less
III	< 20	< 7	15	65	100–150 or less

With permission from American Heart Association. Recommendations for Treatment of Hyperlipidemia in Adults. *Am Heart J* 69:1065A–1084A, 1984.

quently, NCEP I and II included recommendations for the dietary treatment of abnormal lipids (16, 37).

There are reports that lowering fat and increasing carbohydrate intake may increase triglycerides and decrease HDL cholesterol (15, 17, 42). However, others report regression, or lack of progression, of atherosclerosis in response to a very low fat diet (as well as exercise and stress management) in spite of a slight decrease in HDL cholesterol (32). Others suggest that combining a low fat diet with moderate exercise to produce weight loss results in increased HDL cholesterol and decreased in LDL and VLDL cholesterol (3, 46).

The following dietary factors also are known to positively influence blood lipids:

1. Two ounces of oat bran (11 g of total, 6 g soluble fiber) (34).
2. Replacing animal sources of protein with soy protein (47 g/day) (4).
3. A large dose of omega-3 fatty acids, however, the dose is costly and contributes significantly to total fat and calorie intake which may not be desirable (9).
4. 400 mg/day of folic acid (due to a decrease in blood homocysteine levels) (7).

Table 35.4 summarizes an optimal diet for improving blood lipids.

Exercise Therapy

The primary effects of exercise on lipoproteins are decreased TG and increase HDL. Forty-five minutes of daily aerobic exercise substantially lowers TG. The minimal weekly threshold for caloric expenditure to increase HDL is 1000–1200 kcals. Several studies report a dose-response relationship between fitness and/or weekly caloric expenditure and increase in HDL (25, 29, 44). Simultaneous weight and fat loss results in a greater HDL increase (35, 46). The lower the initial level of HDL, the greater the increase; it often takes several months of regular weekly caloric expenditure >1000 before becoming apparent. See Table 35.5 for exercise recommendations.

Weight Loss

The importance of weight loss is often overlooked in the control of blood lipids. A significant relationship exists between body mass index and cholesterol in men and women between 20 and 74 years of age (10, 11). A recent trial demonstrated a significantly greater decrease in TG and LDL and greater increase in HDL through weight loss by diet only compared with exercise (24). A second study in men and women with LDL levels > 130 mg/dl demonstrated reduction in LDL cholesterol and no change in cholesterol/HDL cholesterol ratio when

Table 35.4. Optimal Diet for Improving Blood Lipids

Dietary Component	Recommendation
Total Calories	Adequate to support nutritional needs but low enough (not < 1500 calories) to allow a 10% loss of weight if indicated
Total Fat Intake	20% of calories or less
Saturated Fat Intake	7% of calories or less
Cholesterol intake	100–150 mg/day or less
Fiber Intake	25–40 g/day
Soluble Fiber Intake	10–15 g/day
Protein	15% of calories (0.50–0.55 g/lb bdw in active persons) with an increase in vegetable and decrease in animal protein
Carbohydrate	65% of calories (55% complex)

bdw = body weight

Table 35.5. Target Exercise Guidelines for Improving Lipids[a]

Type	Intensity (%VO_2max)	Frequency (d/wk)	Duration (min/session)	Minimum (kcals/wk)	Optimum (kcals/wk)	Time (months)	% Responding
Aerobic	50–85%	3.5–7	30–60	1000–1200	2000–3500	9–12	90% HDL 70% TG

[a] These guidelines may require modification for sedentary, obese individuals, and patients with chronic disease such as diabetes, high blood pressure, and coronary heart disease. For more information on special populations, see ACSM Guidelines for Exercise Testing and Prescription, 5th ed. Baltimore: Williams & Wilkins, 1995.
HDL, High-density lipoprotein; TG, Triglycerides.

subjects consumed an ad libitum 15% fat calorie diet resulting in weight loss (35). In contrast, after 5–6 weeks of consuming the same diet while maintaining weight, there was a reduction in LDL cholesterol and an increase in the cholesterol/HDL cholesterol ratio.

Numerous studies suggest that weight loss through exercise and modest dietary restriction of total and fat calories is key to improving blood levels of lipoproteins. Despres and Lamarche suggest that if the energy expenditure is sufficient (60 minutes daily), exercise intensities between 50 and 80% should produce similar improvements in "metabolic fitness"(12). In conclusion, the dietary guidelines suggested in Table 35.4 and exercise guidelines in Table 35.5 should be effective in inducing significant weight loss.

SUMMARY

The metabolism of lipoproteins is intimately related to cardiovascular health and disease. Both the lipid and protein components of lipoprotein play roles in prevention (and cause) of atherosclerosis. HDL_2, Apo A-I, and LCAT play significant roles in clearing cholesterol from cells. LPL and TG lipase are important in clearing fat from blood and initiating a complex series of reactions that increase HDL. Elevated LDL cholesterol, Apo B_{100}, and hepatic lipase are associated with increased prevalence of atherosclerosis. The oxidation of free radical-induced oxidation of LDL cholesterol may lead to an inflammatory process and the formation of foam cells and fatty streaks from which plaque is eventually formed.

The NCEP was developed with specific goals for blood lipid levels to reduce prevalence of CVD. The most notable goal is for all American adults to achieve plasma cholesterol levels below 200 mg/dL. The NCEP also proposed goals for LDL and HDL. The reduction of saturated fat in the diet has been one of the most successful strategies for lowering plasma cholesterol.

Exercise training of sufficient intensity, duration, and longevity favorably impacts lipoprotein metabolism. The most predictable changes occur in plasma HDL and HDL_2 and TG. The effects on total cholesterol and LDL are less remarkable and may be linked to weight loss. The antioxidant effect of exercise training may also be a major benefit, but evidence for this effect is not consistent. Aerobic training appears to produce more consistent changes in lipoproteins than resistance training. The combination of exercise training and diet may be the most effective means of altering blood lipids.

References

1. Alessio HM, Goldfarb AH. Lipid peroxidation and scavenger enzymes during exercise: adaptive response to training. *J Appl Physiol* 64:1333–1336, 1988.
2. American Heart Association Heart and Stroke Facts: 1995 Statistical Supplement. American Heart Association. Dallas, Texas, 1995.
3. Anderson SA, Haaland A, Hjermann I, et al. Oslo Diet and Exercise Study: a one-year randomized intervention trial. Effect on hemostatic variables and coronary risk factors. *Nutr Metab Cardiovasc Dis* 5:189–200, 1995.
4. Anderson JW, Johnstone BM, Cook-Newell ME. Meta-analysis of the effects of soy protein intake on serum lipids. *N Engl J Med* 333:276–282, 1995.
5. Austin MA, Hokanson JE. Epidemiology of triglycerides, small dense low-density lipoproteins, and lipoprotein (a) as risk factors for coronary heart disease. *Med Clin North Am* 78:99–115, 1994.
6. Berg A, Frey I, Baumstark MW, et al. Physical activity and lipoprotein lipid disorders. *Sports Med* 17:6–21, 1994.
7. Boushey CJ, Beresford SA, Omenn GS, et al. A quantitative assessment of plasma homocysteine as a risk factor for vascular disease: Probable benefits of increasing folic acid intakes. *JAMA* 274:1049–1057, 1995.
8. Connor WE, Conner S. The dietary prevention and treatment of coronary heart disease. In: Connor WE, Bristow JD, eds. *Coronary Heart Disease: Prevention, Complications, and Treatment.* Philadelphia: JB Lippincott, 1985:43–64.
9. Davidson MH, Hurns JH, Subbaiah PV, et al. Marine oil capsule therapy for the treatment of hyperlipidemia. *Arch Intern Med* 151:1732–1740, 1991.
10. Denke MA, Sempos CT, Grundy SM. Excess bodyweight: an underrecognized contributor to high blood cholesterol

levels in White American Men. *Arch Intern Med* 153:1093–1103, 1993.

11. Denke MA, Sempos CT, Grundy SM. Excess bodyweight: an underrecognized contributor to dyslipidemia in white American women. *Arch Intern Med* 154:401–410, 1994.
12. Despres JP, Lamarche B. Low-intensity endurance exercise training, plasma lipoproteins and risk of coronary heart disease. *J Intern Med* 236:7–22, 1994.
13. Despres JP, Pouliot MC, Moorjani S, et al. Loss of abdominal fat and metabolic response to exercise training in obese women. *Am J Physiol* 261:E159–E167, 1991.
14. Dufaux B, Order U, Muller R, et al. Delayed effects of prolonged exercise on serum lipoproteins. *Metabolism* 35:105–109, 1986.
15. Ginsberg H, Olefsky JM, Kimmerling G, et al. Induction of hypertriglyceridemia by a low fat diet. *J Clin Endocrinol Metab* 42:729–735, 1976.
16. Gotto AM, Bierman EL, Connor WE, et al. Recommendations for treatment of hyperlipidemia in Adults. *Circulation* 69:1065A–1084A, 1984.
17. Grundy SM, Nix D, Whelan MF, et al. Comparison of three cholesterol-lowering diets in normolipidemic men. *JAMA* 256:2351–2355, 1986.
18. Gupta AK, Ross EA, Myers JN, et al. Increased reverse cholesterol transport in athletes. *Metabolism* 42:684–690, 1993.
19. Hensrud DD, Heimburger DC. Antioxidant status, fatty acids, and cardiovascular disease. *Nutrition* 10:170–175, 1994.
20. Hurley BF. Effects of resistive training on lipoprotein-lipid profiles: a comparison to aerobic exercise training. *Med Sci Sports Exerc* 21:689–693, 1989.
21. Hurley BF, Hagberg JM, Goldberg AP, et al. Resistive training can reduce coronary risk factors without altering VO2max or percent body fat. *Med Sci Sports Exerc* 20:150–154, 1988.
22. Ji LL. Exercise and oxidative stress: role of cellular antioxidant systems. *Exerc Sport Sci Rev* 23:135–166, 1995.
23. Kantor MA, Cullinane EM, Sady SP, et al. Exercise acutely increases high density lipoprotein-cholesterol and lipoprotein lipase activity in trained and untrained men. *Metabolism* 36:188–192, 1987.
24. Katzel LI, Bleecker ER, Colman EG, et al. Effects of weight loss vs aerobic exercise training on risk factors for coronary disease in healthy, obese, middle-aged, and older men. *JAMA* 274:1915–1921, 1995.
25. Ketelhut RG, Ketelhut K, Messerli FH, et al. Fitness in the fit: does physical conditioning affect cardiovascular risk factors in middle-aged marathon runners? *Eur Heart J* 17:199–203, 1996.
26. Keys A, Anderson JT, Grande F. Prediction of serum-cholesterol responses of man to changes in fats in the diet. *Lancet* 1:966, 1957.
27. Kokkinos PF, Holland JC, Narayan P, et al. Miles run per week and high-density lipoprotein cholesterol levels in healthy, middle-aged men. *Arch Intern Med* 155:415–420, 1995.
28. Mayes PA. Cholesterol synthesis, transport, and excretion. In: Murray RK, Granner DK, Mayes PA, et al., eds. *Harper's Biochemistry.* Englewood Cliffs: Appleton & Lange, 1988: 249–260.
29. Messenick RP, Katan MB. Effect of dietary fatty acids on serum lipids and lipoproteins: a meta-analysis of 27 trials. *Arterioscler Thromb* 12:911–919, 1992.
30. National Cholesterol Edcuation Program, Report of the Expert Panel on Population Stratetgies for Blood Cholesterol Redcuction. National Heart,Lung, and Blood Institute, National Institutes of Health. *Arch Intern Med* 148:36–69, 1988.
31. National Cholesterol Education Program. Report of the Expert Panel on Blood Cholesterol Levels in Children and Adolescents. U.S. Department of Health and Human Services, Public Health Service, National Institutes of Health, National Heart Lung and Blood Institure. September, 1991, NIH Pub. No. 91–2732.
32. Ornish DM, Brown SE, Scherwitz LW, et al. Can lifestyle changes reverse coronary artery disease? The Lifestyle Heart Trial. *Lancet* 336:129–133, 1990.
33. Parthasarathy S, Barnett J, Fong LG. High-density lipoprotein inhibits the oxidative modification of low-density lipoprotein. *Biochem Biophys Acta* 1044:275–283, 1990.
34. Ripsin CM, Keenan JM, Jacobs DR, et al. Oat products and lipid lowering: A meta-analysis. *JAMA* 267:3317–3325, 1992.
35. Schaefer EJ, Lichtenstein AH, Lamon-Fava S, et al. Bodyweight and low-density lipoprotein cholesterol changes after consumption of a low-fat ad libitum diet. *JAMA* 274:1450–1455, 1995.
36. Seip RL, Moulin P, Cocke T, et al. Exercise training decreases plasma cholesteryl ester transfer protein. *Arterioscler Thromb* 13:1359–1367, 1993.
37. Summary of the Second Report of the National Cholesterol Education Program (NCEP) Expert Panel on Detection, Evaluation, and Treatment of High Blood Cholesterol in Adults (Adult Treatment Panel II). *JAMA* 269:3015–3021, 1993.
38. Thomas TR. Prolonged recovery from eccentric versus concentric exercise. *Can J Appl Physiol* 19:441–450, 1994.
39. Thomas TR, Etheridge GL. The effect of track and field training cardiovascular fitness. *Phys Sportsmed* 9:49–61, 1981.
40. Thompson CE, Thompson TR, Thomas J, et al. Response of HDL cholesterol, apoprotein A-I, and LCAT to exercise withdrawal. *Atheroscler Thromb* 54:65–73, 1985.
41. Tran V, Weltman A, Glass GV, et al. The effects of exercise on blood lipids and lipoproteins: a meta-analysis of studies. *Med Sci Sports Exerc* 15:393–402, 1983.
42. Tuswell AS. Food carbohydrates and plasma lipids: an update. *Am J Clin Nutr* 59(Suppl):710S–718S, 1994.
43. Williams PT, Krauss RM, Vranizan DM, et al. Changes in lipoprotein subfractions during diet-induced and exercise-induced weight loss in moderately overweight men.*Circulation* 81:1293–1304, 1990.
44. Williams PT. High density lipoprotein cholesterol and other risk factors for coronary heart disease in female runners. *N Engl J Med* 1996;334:1298–1303.
45. Wood PD, Stefanick ML, Dreon DM, et al. Changes in plasma lipids and lipoproteins in overweight men during weight loss through dieting as compared with exercise. *N Engl J Med* 319:1173–1179, 1988.
46. Wood PD, Stefanick ML, Williams PT, et al. The effects on plasma lipids of a prudent weight-reducing diet with or

withiout exercise in overweight men and women. *New Engl J Med* 325:461–466, 1991.

Suggested Readings

Durstine JL, Haskell WL. Effects of exercise training on plasma lipids and lipoproteins. *Exerc Sports Sci Rev* 22:477–521, 1994.

Kanter MM. Free radicals, exercise, and antioxidant supplementation. *Intl J Sport Nutr* 4:205–220, 1994.

Superko HR. Advances in lipoprotein Metabolism: applications in the cardiac rehabilitation setting. In: Pashkow FJ, Dafoe WA, eds. *Clinical Cardiac Rehabilitation: A Cardiologist's Guide.* Baltimore: Williams & Wilkins, 1993:196–226.

SECTION SEVEN

CHRONIC LUNG DISEASE

SECTION EDITOR: *Moira Kelsey, RN, MS*

73 41, 49, 54 86 301, 302, 338 307, 341 357, 360

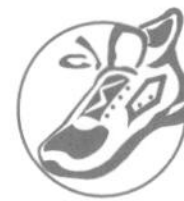

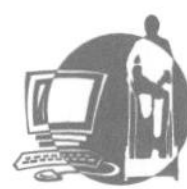
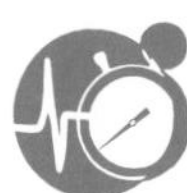

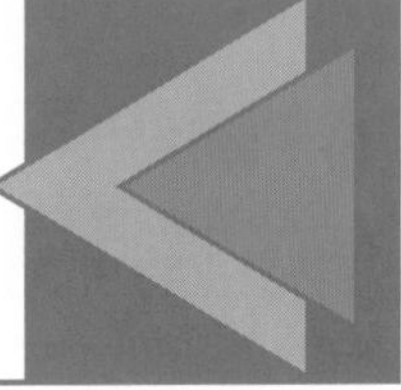

CHAPTER **36**

PULMONARY ADAPTATIONS TO DYNAMIC EXERCISE

Kenneth C. Beck and Bruce D. Johnson

Key to Pulmonary Physiology Abbreviations

A-a D_{O2}	Alveolar-arterial oxygen difference
C_L	Lung compliance
EELV	End-expiratory lung volume
EILV	End-inspiratory lung volume
f_b	Breathing frequency
FEV_1	Forced expiratory volume in 1 second
$F_{I,O2}$	Fractional concentration of oxygen in inspired gas
LT	Lactate threshold
MEFV	Maximal expiratory flow-volume (curve)
MIFV	Maximal inspiratory flow-volume (curve)
MVV	Maximal voluntary ventilation
$P_{a,CO2}$	Partial pressure of carbon dioxide in arterial blood
$P_{A,CO2}$	Partial pressure of carbon dioxide in alveolar gas
$P_{a,O2}$	Partial pressure of oxygen in arterial blood
$P_{A,O2}$	Partial pressure of oxygen in alveolar gas
P_{CO2}	Partial pressure of carbon dioxide
$P_{I,O2}$	Partial pressure of oxygen in inspired gas
$P_{max,E}$	Maximal expiratory pressure
P_{O2}	Partial pressure of oxygen
P_{pa}	Pulmonary artery pressure
P_{pw}	Pulmonary artery wedge pressure
$\dot{Q}$	Cardiac output (total pulmonary blood flow)
RER	Respiratory exchange ratio
T_E	Expiratory time
T_I	Inspiratory time
$\dot{V}_A$	Minute alveolar ventilation
$\dot{V}CO_2$	Carbon dioxide production
V_D	Dead space of the lungs
$\dot{V}_E$	Expired minute ventilation
$\dot{V}O_2$	Oxygen consumption
$\dot{V}O_2max$	Maximal oxygen consumption
V_T	Tidal volume
VT	Ventilatory threshold

Increasing levels of exercise require acute adaptations in the cardiorespiratory system to maintain homeostasis (1). As tissues increase oxygen uptake ($\dot{V}O_2$) and CO_2 output ($\dot{V}CO_2$), cardiac output increases to deliver more oxygen to the tissues and transport more CO_2 away. Likewise, the ventilation must increase to meet the demand for oxygen and eliminate the CO_2. Without these adaptations, tissue hypoxia, hypercarbia, and acidosis result, compromising cellular function. This review focuses on adaptations in the pulmonary system that occur to meet increasing metabolic demands during exercise. The lungs, chest wall, and respiratory centers of the central nervous system meet this demand under most circumstances. However, while muscular and cardiovascular capacity chronically adapt to the demands of training, the capacity of the pulmonary system remains, for the most part, fixed. Chronically increased demands on the pulmonary system may eventually reach limits of the ventilatory mechanism. The normal pulmonary adaptations to exercise and definitions of the limits of the pulmonary response are discussed.

COUPLING OF INTERNAL TO EXTERNAL RESPIRATION

Internal respiration refers to the cellular exchange of O_2 and CO_2. **External respiration** refers to the exchange of O_2 and CO_2 between organ systems, facilitated by the cardiac, circulatory, and pulmonary systems. Increased $\dot{V}O_2$ and $\dot{V}CO_2$ production raises the required level of ventilation to maintain adequate tissue oxygenation and acid-base balance. The magnitudes of $\dot{V}O_2$ and $\dot{V}CO_2$ are related to the external work load.

As the tissues consume O_2, they produce CO_2 at a rate dependent on the metabolic fuel being used and the amount of anaerobic metabolism. CO_2 must be eliminated by the lungs to maintain proper acid-base balance in the tissues. The ratio of $\dot{V}CO_2/\dot{V}O_2$, termed respiratory exchange ratio (RER), steadily increases from about 0.7–0.8 at lower exercise intensity to 1.0 at moderate intensities and finally 1.1–1.3 near maximum. This increase is due to a shift from predominately fat metabolism to carbohydrate and finally to anaerobic metabolism. Although anaerobic metabolism neither consumes O_2 nor produces CO_2, a shift to anaerobic metabolism increases RER secondary to buffering of lactic acid. Buffering releases CO_2 stored in blood and tissues through the combination of bicarbonate (HCO_3^-) with hydrogen ions (H^+). The additional CO_2 excretion due to buffering can be substantial (2).

The Ventilatory (Anaerobic) Threshold

Pulmonary ventilation in a healthy person is generally adequate to support tissue oxygenation. The ventilatory demand imposed solely by the $\dot{V}O_2$ is nearly linear with increases in external work. Because of the need to eliminate CO_2 to maintain constant partial pressure of arterial CO_2 ($P_{a,CO2}$) during exercise of moderate to high intensity, pulmonary ventilation increases out of proportion to the increased $\dot{V}O_2$. $\dot{V}CO_2$, therefore, becomes proportionately greater than $\dot{V}O_2$. These relationships are demonstrated in Figure 36.1 which illustrates exercise-associated changes in minute ventilation ($\dot{V}_E$), $\dot{V}O_2$ and $\dot{V}CO_2$ with increased work rate. Below *arrow A*, metabolism is predominantly aerobic and RER < 1.0. Above *arrow A*, a significant portion of total metabolic rate becomes progressively anaerobic. During anaerobic metabolism, additional CO_2 is transported to and eliminated by the lungs (see above), and RER > 1.0. Between *arrow A* and *B*, $\dot{V}_E$ keeps pace with increasing $\dot{V}CO_2$. At *arrow B*, minute ventilation begins to increase out of proportion to increases in $\dot{V}CO_2$. Some of the increase may be related to hydrogen ion stimulation of peripheral chemoreceptors (3, 4).

The events shown in Figure 36.1 can be expressed mathematically. Within the lungs, mass balance relationships lead to the following equation which relates metabolic CO_2 production to minute ventilation at the alveolar level:

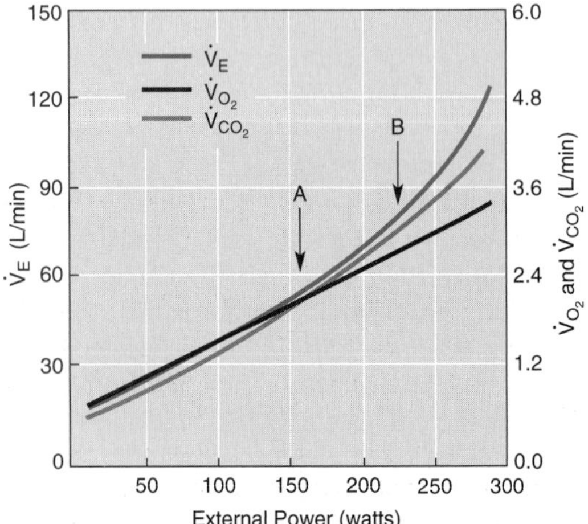

Figure 36.1. The relationship of minute ventilation ($\dot{V}_E$) to $\dot{V}CO_2$ and $\dot{V}O_2$ during progressive exercise. Note the parallel relationship observed between $\dot{V}_E$ and $\dot{V}CO_2$ (up to point B) during the majority of exercise until the higher intensities (beyond point B).

$$\dot{V}_A = \frac{0.863 \times \dot{V}CO_2}{P_{a,CO2}}$$

where: $\dot{V}_A$ = minute alveolar ventilation (converted to BTPS conditions),
$\dot{V}CO_2$ = metabolic CO_2 production (measured at the lungs, expressed in STPD conditions), and
$P_{a,CO2}$ = arterial partial pressure of CO_2.

The constant (0.863) is the factor required to transform fractional gas concentration to partial pressure and to express gas volumes at body temperature and pressure saturated with water vapor. $\dot{V}_A$ cannot be measured directly, but is inferred from measurement of total minute ventilation measured at the mouth and the physiological dead space:

$$\dot{V}_A = \dot{V}_E \times (1 - V_D / V_T)$$

where: $\dot{V}_E$ is total minute ventilation (converted to BTPS conditions) and V_D / V_T is the ratio of physiological dead space to tidal volume (discussed below). Combining equations 1 and 2 gives:

$$\dot{V}_E = \frac{K \times \dot{V}CO_2}{P_{a,CO2} \times (1 - V_D/V_T)}$$

From this equation, it is apparent that $\dot{V}_E$ is proportional to $\dot{V}CO_2$ and inversely proportional to the $P_{a,CO2}$. In addition, increasing the V_D/V_T must result in an increase in $\dot{V}_E$, in order for $P_{a,CO2}$ to remain constant.

Use of the third equation and understanding cellular metabolism forms the basis for non-invasive methods to detect the so-called **anaerobic threshold,** which roughly corresponds to the point at which lactic acid begins to build up in the blood. Noninvasive detection of blood lactate acidosis relies on measurements of gas exchange ($\dot{V}O_2$, $\dot{V}CO_2$) and ventilation ($\dot{V}_E$), referred to as the ventilatory threshold (VT). This distinguishes noninvasive determination from analysis of blood lactate, the lactate threshold (LT) and from the determination of anaerobic energy use at the cellular level, the anaerobic threshold. Though there is general agreement between VT and LT in most but not all studies, a cause-effect relationship between the two should not be inferred (5, 6).

There is not clear consensus in the literature for defining invasively determined LT from blood lactate versus $\dot{V}O_2$ curves. Some of the criteria that have been applied are listed in Table 36.1. Despite the lack of consensus for determining LT, it is clear that there is an exercise intensity in all healthy individuals above which exercise becomes increasingly difficult to sustain, probably due to a nonsteady state accumulation of lactic acid (7, 8). This point occurs somewhere between 40–80% of maximal oxygen consumption depending, in part, on fitness level (9). Using methods to define this point from noninvasive criteria or invasively by one of the methods

Table 36.1. Methods for Determining Lactate Threshold

	Criterion	References
1	The $\dot{V}O_2$ or external power output at which blood lactate shows a "systematic" increase	12, 5
2	The $\dot{V}O_2$ or external power output at which blood lactate increases by 1 mM above value obtained at rest.	
3	A "clear change" in slope of lactate plotted against either $\dot{V}O_2$ or external power output (this includes log-log transformations to enhance the change in slope)	6
4	The $\dot{V}O_2$ or external power output at which blood lactate exceeds a fixed value such as 2.0 or 4.0 mM/l	11
5	The $\dot{V}O_2$ at which the slope of the lactate (mM/l) versus $\dot{V}O_2$ (l/min) curve equals 1.0	

in Table 36.1, it has been demonstrated that $\dot{V}O_2$ at LT correlates better with exercise performance in predominately aerobic tasks than maximum oxygen consumption ($\dot{V}O_2max$) (10, 11). Furthermore, exercise training raises $\dot{V}O_2max$ more effectively if training is performed at or just above LT (12).

Determination of the VT identifies the increase in $\dot{V}CO_2$ associated with buffering of lactic acid and the relative increase in $\dot{V}_E$ signaling the start of hyperventilation. In earlier studies, VT was determined from the point beyond which the RER exceeded 1.0. However, RER can be affected by hyperventilation, which transiently increases $\dot{V}CO_2$ measured at the mouth. A more sensitive method involves using the "ventilatory equivalents" for O_2 and CO_2. To understand the utility of these two indices, the third equation can be rearranged:

$$\frac{\dot{V}_E}{\dot{V}CO_2} = \frac{K}{P_{a,CO_2} \times (1 - V_D/V_T)}$$

$$\frac{\dot{V}_E}{\dot{V}O_2} = \frac{K \times RER}{P_{a,CO_2} \times (1 - V_D/V_T)}$$

The ventilatory equivalents for CO_2 (top equation) normally decrease with progressively increasing exercise intensity as V_D/V_T falls, reflecting improved gas exchange efficiency. Ventilatory equivalents for CO_2 increase near LT as ventilation is driven to the point that P_{a,CO_2} (and end-tidal PCO_2) begins to decrease. Similarly, ventilatory equivalents for O_2 decreases initially, but begins to increase sooner than the increase in ventilatory equivalents for CO_2 because of increased RER.

The commonly accepted definition of the VT using ventilatory equivalents is as follows: when following an exercise protocol with incrementally increasing exercise intensity, the VT is the $\dot{V}O_2$ at which there is:

- a rise in ventilatory equivalents for O_2,
- a steady or slowly falling ventilatory equivalents for CO_2,
- constant or slowly rising end-tidal partial pressure of carbon dioxide (P_{CO_2}) (13).

The final two criteria are included to avoid assigning VT to a point where simple hyperventilation is occurring, since hyperventilation can cause ventilatory equivalents for CO_2 to rise prematurely. In a normal response, the point at which the ventilatory equivalents for CO_2 rises and end-tidal P_{CO_2} begins to decline should occur later than the point at which ventilatory equivalents for O_2 rise, marking the beginning of relative hyperventilation and the end of isocapnic buffering.

In order to apply this method, data for $\dot{V}_E$, $\dot{V}O_2$, and $\dot{V}CO_2$, and end-tidal P_{CO_2} should be obtained in relatively short intervals using progressively increasing exercise intensity to volitional fatigue. There are no studies that investigate the "optimal" sampling interval for obtaining $\dot{V}_E$, $\dot{V}O_2$, and $\dot{V}CO_2$. The interval should be long enough to smooth breath-to-breath variations, but not so long that changes marking VT are obscured. An interval of 20–30 seconds is probably ideal. Thus, breath-by-breath data acquisition with 20–30 second averaging or a mixing chamber system with chamber size about 30–50% of the minute ventilation is sufficient.

A recent modification of the method for determining VT involves plotting the $\dot{V}CO_2$ against $\dot{V}O_2$ to locate a breakpoint in the relationship (14). The breakpoint identifies the $\dot{V}O_2$ at which the $\dot{V}CO_2$ rises disproportionately due to buffering.

The determination of VT is useful in many clinical and research settings. However, it should be stressed that the identification of VT and the relationship to blood lactate acidosis are strongly dependent on a normal breathing response to exercise. A certain proportion of individuals do not have an identifiable VT by any method due to deviations in breathing pattern (CO_2 retention or hyperventilation).

The Ventilatory Response to Exercise

The mechanisms by which $\dot{V}_E$ is closely coupled to metabolism during exercise are unclear. During exercise, P_{a,CO_2} is maintained near resting level until very heavy exercise when it begins to decrease. Decreased P_{a,CO_2} is thought to result from acidosis stimulating chemoreceptors. Chemoreceptors are found in the brain and appear to be responsive to hydrogen ions and dissolved CO_2 primarily within the cerebrospinal fluid (CSF), but are also influenced by local blood flow and metabolism (3). There are also peripheral chemoreceptors located in the carotid bodies and aortic arch that respond to decreased arterial pH and P_{a,O_2} and increased P_{a,CO_2}, serum K^+, and norepinephrine (15).

Nerve centers (nuclei) in the brainstem that drive motor neurons of the respiratory muscles control the periodic nature of inspiration and expiration. These centers are probably influenced by afferent sensory inputs from the respiratory system and, perhaps, working muscles (3, 16). Lung stretch receptors may play a role in terminating a breath and in regulating end inspiratory lung volume. However, studies in heart-lung transplant patients devoid of stretch receptor feedback demonstrate only small differences in breathing pattern from normal subjects and only at low levels of exercise. Lung irritant receptors are thought to lie between epithelial cells within the airways and appear to play a role during the bronchoconstriction of asthma in response to released histamine or bradykinin. Juxta-capillary receptors (J-receptors) are found in the alveolar walls and respond to chemicals in the pulmonary circulation. Stimulation of these receptors causes rapid shallow breathing. Increased interstitial fluid volume of the alveolar walls may activate these receptors. They may play a role in the dyspnea associated with congestive heart failure. They have also been implicated in the rapid shallow breathing noted after heavy exercise (17). Additional receptors are found in the nose and upper airways which respond to both mechanical and chemical stimulants. Respiratory muscles also contain muscle spindles, golgi tendon organs and nerve endings which may respond to length changes, rate of change, load or metabolites produced with muscle fatigue.

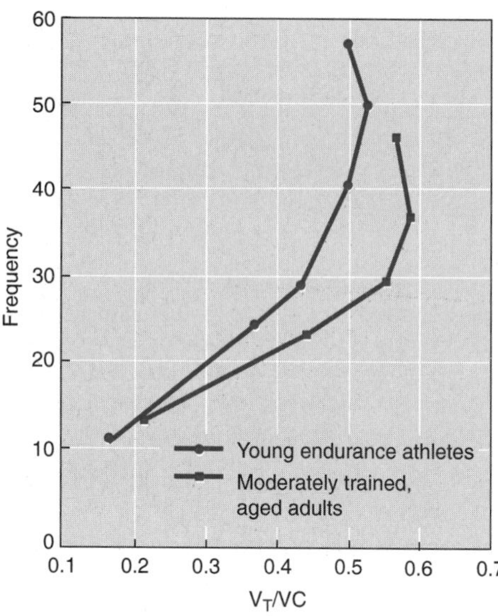

Figure 36.2. Frequency and tidal volume (V_T) relationship normalized for vital capacity (VC) during progressive exercise in young endurance athletes (*circles*) and moderately trained aged adults (*squares*). (Adapted from Johnson BD, Badr MS, Dempsey JA. Impact of the aging pulmonary system on the response to exercise. *Clin Chest Med* 15:229, 1994.)

BREATHING MECHANICS

The processes of increasing $\dot{V}_E$ through integration and recruitment of respiratory muscles and the alterations of airway diameter is known as breathing mechanics. The study of breathing mechanics includes the study of airway function, of breathing pattern (respiratory rate and tidal volume), and of work of breathing and the oxygen cost of doing the work.

Breathing Pattern

Light exercise is generally associated with both increased depth, tidal volume (V_T) and frequency of breathing (f_b) (Fig. 36.2). V_T and f_b increase until about 70–80% of peak exercise after which increased frequency becomes the primary response (18). V_T usually plateaus at 50–60% of vital capacity (19). Breathing frequency increases one- to threefold in most subjects, but in more fit athletes may be increased six- to sevenfold at high levels of $\dot{V}_E$. In some subjects at extremely high ventilatory demands, V_T may decrease as f_b increases. Figure 36.2 shows average changes in breathing pattern with progressive exercise in a group of young highly fit subjects and a group of older active individuals (20).

Increased V_T is due to both decreased end-expiratory lung volume (EELV) and increased end-inspiratory lung volume (EILV). Decreased EELV is thought to optimize inspiratory muscle length (for force development) and to help reduce the inspiratory work by allowing breathing to occur at a lower average lung volume, therefore lowering average lung recoil pressure. In addition, the energy stored in the abdominal wall because of active expiration may provide some passive recoil at the initiation of the ensuing inspiration. In endurance athletes at high ventilatory demands (>150 L/min), EELV may begin to increase, perhaps secondary to expiratory airflow limitation (18).

Increased f_b with exercise is associated with decreased inspiratory (T_I) and expiratory time (T_E). At moderate to high ventilatory demands, T_E decreases more than T_I (17). Due to the greater decrease in T_E, the increase in mean expiratory flow is greater than the increase in mean inspiratory flow.

Airflow and Pressure-volume Responses

The maximal expiratory flow versus volume (MEFV) curve produced by routine spirometry represents the maximal flow the lungs can sustain. Thus, the degree to which expiratory flows during exercise come close to the MEFV curve indicates the approach to a ventilatory limitation during exercise (see below). The maximal inspiratory flow versus volume (MIFV) curve represents the dynamic capacity of the inspiratory muscles, since the lungs do not limit inspiratory flows (Fig. 36.3).

Inspiratory pressure generation gradually increases (becomes more negative) as ventilatory demand increases. Peak inspiratory pressure reaches only 50% of

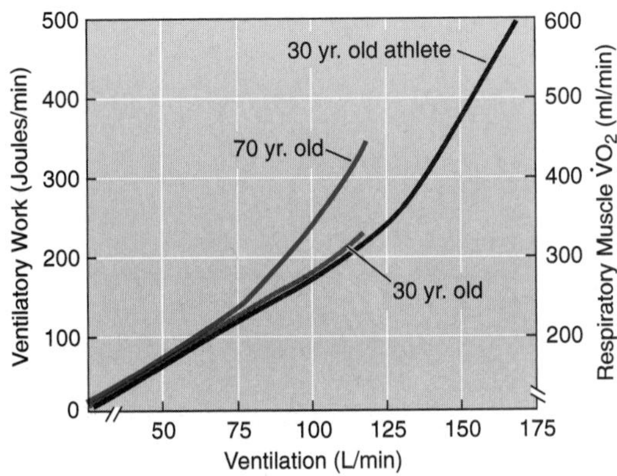

Figure 36.3. Ventilatory work and the oxygen cost of breathing during progressive exercise in 30-year-old untrained adults, 30-year-old athletes, and 70-year-old moderately fit older adults.

the dynamic capacity of the inspiratory muscles for pressure production (21). Peak expiratory pressures become positive only with heavy exercise and only near EELV. Thus, expiratory pressures for a given lung volume are well below the maximum pleural expiratory pressure ($P_{max,E}$) even in heavy exercise (18, 22).

Airway Function and Pulmonary Resistance

The lungs are largely passive structures, and gas exchange occurs as respiratory muscles cause lung expansion and contraction to move air in and out of alveoli. The muscles must work against the static recoil of the lungs and the resistance to movement of air in the pulmonary airways. Airway function is therefore an important parameter for normal lung function and can be assessed in two ways: through direct measurement of pulmonary resistance (R_L) with assistance of an esophageal balloon, or using MEFV curves.

The change in airway function during exercise is somewhat controversial. In normal individuals, airways are thought to dilate slightly during exercise, probably mediated by a change in vagus nerve activity. In individuals with asthma, airway function is more variable and can show this variability with changes in exercise intensity (26). After exercise, asthmatics can show marked deterioration in airway function, probably related to heat and water exchange in the airway during exercise.

The work that must be expended to more airflow can be estimated and the oxygen cost of the work of breathing is thought to be < 5% of the total $\dot{V}O_2$ at rest and during mild to moderate exercise. During heavy exercise in athletes, however, the work of breathing and the oxygen cost of the work can approach 20% of the $\dot{V}O_2$ (23). In pulmonary diseases, the oxygen cost of work that is related to increased airway resistance can also be substantial.

Nasal Breathing vs. Mouth Breathing

Though variable, the majority of individuals nose breathe at rest (24). This occurs despite the fact that nasal airflow resistance is greater than mouth airflow resistance. The switch from primarily nasal breathing to oronasal breathing with exercise appears to occur at a ventilation of 22–44 L/min (24). The proportion of nasal to total ventilation has been found to vary between 26–64% during low level activity and to progressively decrease to 25–30% during exercise at 90% of peak power (24, 25).

Exercise has been shown to decrease nasal airflow resistance presumably by dilation of the alai nasi muscles (26). Resistance to airflow can be decreased by 30% with the activation of these muscles (27). Despite this active dilation, airflow resistance is approximately 4 times greater through the nose at rest and 9 times greater during exercise (24).

Indices of Ventilatory Constraint

Normal individuals, who are not elite athletes, generally do not have pulmonary limits to exercise. Pulmonary limitation can be defined in a number of ways. There is a mechanical limit to the amount of pressure the respiratory muscles can generate and the amount of inspiratory or expiratory flow the lungs can support. Maximal voluntary ventilation (MVV) is a crude index of maximal ventilation of the lungs and respiratory muscles. Calculated over 12–15 seconds, it may overestimate true maximal sustainable ventilation, but represents an upper limit to the capacity of the pulmonary system. If an MVV is not measured, it can be estimated:

$$MVV = FEV_1 \times 37 \text{ (or 40)}$$

where: FEV_1 = spirometrically measured forced expiratory volume in 1 second. There are other methods for measuring mechanical limitation (28).

Endurance athletes may approach both flow-volume and pressure generating capacity near maximum exercise. As a result of increased lung volume at which peak inspiratory pressures occur, the demand for high flows (velocity of shortening) and the large pressures, peak inspiratory pressures approach a greater percent of the maximum available pressure (mean peak inspiratory pressure averaged 90% of the maximal available pressures) (18). An attempt to further stimulate ventilation by the addition of hypercapnic and hypoxic gases to inspired air near peak exercise results in little increase in ventilation (18). A likely explanation for the limitation to further increase ventilation is that despite the chemical stimulus to increase minute ventilation, the increased work and cost of breathing and demand for blood flow competing with the locomotor muscles is too much for the system to effect a ventilatory response. The oxygen cost of breathing has been estimated to be, on average, 10–15% of total body $\dot{V}O_2$ in more fit subjects. This requires a substantial percent of the available cardiac output to be diverted to respiratory muscles (18).

GAS EXCHANGE

Adequate delivery of oxygen to and removal of carbon dioxide from working muscles depends on efficiency of gas exchange in the lungs. Oxygen delivery to the tissues is the product of blood oxygen content and cardiac output. In situations where oxygen delivery is compromised, exercise may be limited by the ability to deliver oxygen to the tissues. Maintenance of partial pressure of oxygen in arterial blood ($P_{a,O2}$) is critical to exercise performance and is dependent on the efficiency of gas exchange in the lungs. The lungs are efficient gas exchangers at rest and become more efficient at CO_2 removal during exercise. However, the efficiency of oxygenation deteriorates somewhat, requiring compensation through enhanced ventilatory response.

Not all gas exchanging units of the lung (acini) have the same amount of ventilation ($\dot{V}_A$) or perfusion, leading to inhomogeneity of gas exchange. An acinus that is well perfused has lower $P_{a,O2}$ and higher $P_{a,CO2}$ compared with a poorly perfused, but adequately ventilated acinus.

A crude index of degree of $\dot{V}_A/\dot{Q}$ mismatching is the V_D/V_T ratio ($\dot{Q}$ = cardiac output), which is obtained by comparing $P_{a,CO2}$ to mixed expired P_{CO2} ($P_{E,CO2}$, obtained by collecting expired air in a large bag or by digital integration of expiratory flow and P_{CO2} signals):

$$\frac{V_D}{V_T} = \frac{P_{a,CO2} - P_{E,CO2}}{P_{a,CO2}}$$

where $P_{a,CO2}$ is obtained from an arterial blood gas sample. The V_D/V_T ratio should decrease to less than 30% at maximal exercise (20, 29). However, normal range for exercise V_D/V_T increases with age (20). It is tempting to substitute end-tidal P_{CO2} (P_{ETCO2}) measurements for $P_{a,CO2}$ in the V_D/V_T equation. However, P_{ETCO2} may not equate to $P_{a,CO2}$, especially during exercise, so the "non-invasive" V_D/V_T should be used cautiously in diagnostic testing.

Oxygenation during exercise, as indicated by the $P_{a,O2}$, is generally well maintained, though reduced oxygenation has been noted in elite athletes (4, 18). An example of arterial blood gases obtained during exercise in a highly fit group of young endurance athletes relative to average fit young subjects and fit older adults is shown in Figure 36.4. There is conflicting data concerning the effect of age on arterial oxygenation near maximal exercise. In one study, there was no age effect, though others suggest a deterioration in oxygenation with age (20, 29). However, it should be noted that there is a progressive decrease in $\dot{V}O_2$max with age and older athletes who can

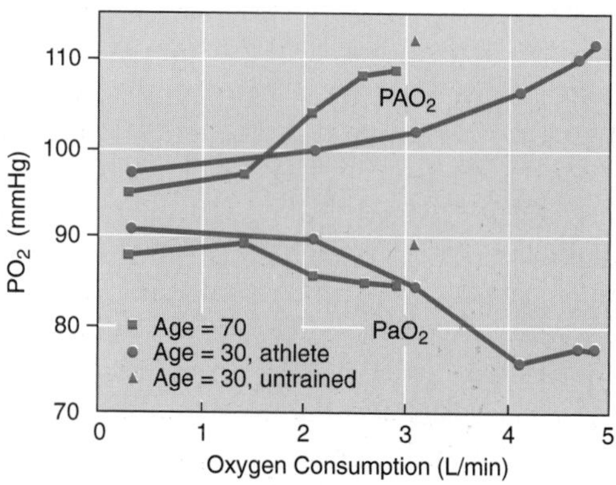

Figure 36.4. Alveolar and arterial partial pressures during incremental exercise in an average fit group of subjects (*diamonds*, peak exercise only, $\dot{V}O_2$max, = 42 ml/kg/min) relative to that found in a group of endurance athletes (*open circles*, n = 8, peak $\dot{V}O_2$max = 73 ml/kg/min) and a group of relatively fit older adults (*circles*, n = 19, $\dot{V}O_2$max = 42 ml/kg/min). P_{A},O_2 = Partial pressure of alveolar oxygen; Pa,O_2 = Partial pressure of arterial oxygen. (With permission from Johnson BD, Badr MS, Dempsey JA. Impact of the aging pulmonary system on the response to exercise. *Clin Chest Med* 15:229, 1994.)

work at greater metabolic demands than sedentary individuals (near those achieved in the average fit young adult), may become hypoxemic for reasons similar to the elite young endurance athlete.

The alveolar arterial oxygen gradient (A-a D_{O2}) is a useful index of gas exchange efficiency. The average alveolar PO_2 ($P_{A,O2}$) is lowered by reduced inspired oxygen ($P_{I,O2}$, e.g., altitude) and by increased alveolar and $P_{a,CO2}$ (hypoventilation).

$$P_{A,O2} = P_{I,O2} - P_{a,CO2}\left[F_{I,O2} - \frac{1 - F_{I,O2}}{RER}\right]$$

where: $P_{I,O2}$ = inspiratory partial pressure;
$F_{I,O2}$ = fractional concentration of oxygen in inspired gas, and
$RER = \dfrac{\dot{V}CO_2}{\dot{V}O_2}$

Hypoxemia (reduced $P_{a,O2}$) is caused by:

- Decreased alveolar ventilation relative to CO_2 output, which increases $P_{a,CO2}$ (A-aD_{O2} is normal),
- Diffusion limitation related to reduction in time the red blood cell is exposed to alveolar gas,
- An increase in $\dot{V}_A/\dot{Q}$ mismatching, and
- Increased shunted blood (4, 30, 31).

PULMONARY HEMODYNAMICS

Pulmonary Circulation

The role of the pulmonary circulation is to provide for efficient gas exchange between mixed venous blood entering the pulmonary capillaries and alveolar air. This is achieved by an extremely thin interface between the capillaries and the alveoli and by a large network of capillary-alveolar interactions (see gas exchange section). The perfusion of capillaries is thought to depend on body position (gravity) and the driving pressures through the pulmonary capillaries. Recent studies suggest there may also be inherent regional differences in vascular resistance dictating a gravity independent anatomical distribution of blood flow (32). The driving pressure for pulmonary blood flow is determined by the difference between the pulmonary artery pressures (P_{pa}) and the left atrial pressure or pulmonary artery wedge pressure (P_{pw}). The resting driving pressure through the pulmonary circulation is 7–8 mm Hg.

With moderate exercise ($\dot{V}O_2$ = 1.5–2.0 L/min), the driving pressure increases to 11–12 mm Hg which, though small, probably increases the number of perfused capillaries and increases distention in already perfused capillaries. With heavy exercise ($\dot{V}O_2$ = 3.0–4.0 L/min), the driving pressure may increase up to 10–15 mm Hg. Studies performed on older subjects note increased P_{pa} relative to younger individuals at a given $\dot{V}O_2$, however, the P_{pw} is also elevated so that the driving pressures remain essentially unchanged (33). It is thought in older adults, that mild diastolic dysfunction may contribute to the elevated P_{pw}.

Bronchial Circulation

In addition to the pulmonary circulation, the lung has a second vascular source provided by the bronchial circulation. This vascular supply originates from branches of the aorta such as the intercostal, internal mammary, and subclavian arteries and supplies the bronchi, branching with the airways as far as the terminal bronchioles (34). This circulation may play a role in temperature regulation and may be involved in lung fluid balance as implied by its close proximity to the lymphatic circulation. Previous studies note marked increases in bronchial blood flow during exercise and during exposure to dry air (e.g., hyperventilation) (35). Under extremely adverse conditions, the bronchial circulation may play a role in gas exchange and in preventing pulmonary hypertension (34). Typically, however, it combines with Thebesian vessels of the heart and contributes to a physiological veno-arterial shunt (4, 34).

The bronchial circulation has been estimated to account for approximately 1–1.5% of total cardiac output at rest and during exercise. At the very high energy expenditures achieved by some endurance athletes, shunt would be expected to contribute proportionately more to increased widening in the A-a DO_2 because the mixed venous oxygen content is probably reduced to < 5 ml O_2/100 ml blood. It is unlikely, however, that shunt accounts for all or even a major portion of the severe exercise induced hypoxemia observed in some athletes because mild hyperoxia during heavy exercise causes proportionate increases in alveolar and arterial PO_2 and PaO_2 is normal, even in those subjects who are the most hypoxemic (4).

AIRWAY FLUID BALANCE

The lumen side of the airway is complex tissue, composed of epithelial cells protected by the mucosal surface layer, secretory glands, nerves, smooth muscle, and cells of the immune system including mast cells and macrophages. In disease states, there may be more inflammatory cells populating the airway, including eosinophils and neutrophils. As is true with mast cells, the ionic milieu of the lumenal surface may affect functioning of these cell types (36).

The amount of fluid present and the concentration of ions in the mucosa reflects a dynamic balance between fluid production by glandular structures, fluid transport from alveoli, fluid resorption by airway cells and fluid evaporation (37). Most of the fluid evaporation probably occurs in the upper airway (oro and naso-pharynx) (38, 39). Although there are no studies in humans, animal research suggests that increased ventilation causes increased ionic concentration in the airway fluid layer of larger airways presumably due to evaporative water loss (40). Modeling studies suggest that water loss occurs in smaller airways (38, 39). The ionic milieu may be affected in important ways during exercise as evaporative water loss upsets the normal homeostatic balance. There are both passive and active compensatory mechanisms that activate to restore the ionic milieu. The passive compensations include increased fluid or ion fluxes across the airway secondary to changes in concentration gradients for ions or water as water evaporates from the airways. Active mechanisms include neural and humoral control of both glandular secretion and resorption mechanisms (37). Mechanical stresses associated with increased ventilation may cause increased production of mediators, such as nitrous oxide and prostaglandins, that influence airway fluid balance (37). The study of airway fluid balance in humans is in its infancy. Recent studies suggest that control of airway fluid balance may be different in normal versus asthmatic individuals (41).

▶ SUMMARY

As exercise intensity increases, oxygen consumption and CO_2 production by working muscles increases dramatically. The cardio-respiratory system is required to deliver oxygen to and transport CO_2 from these tissues in an attempt to maintain cellular homeostasis. The central nervous system responds by increasing neural ventilatory and cardiac drive, resulting in increased activity of cardiac and respiratory muscles. The lungs are largely passive and the increased ventilatory and cardiac drives result in increasing blood and airflow and increased rate of transfer of oxygen and CO_2 across the gas exchanging surfaces of the alveoli. However, there are limits to the degree to which increased airflow and blood flow can be supported, which can lead to pulmonary limitations to exercise, either from mechanical ventilatory constraints, or compromised gas exchange. These limitations are generally not manifested in healthy individuals except in elite or older athletes.

References

1. Wagner PD. Central and peripheral aspects of oxygen transport and adaptations with exercise. *Sports Med* 11: 133–142, 1991.
2. Whipp BJ. The bioenergetic and gas exchange basis of exercise testing. *Clin Chest Med* 15:173–192, 1994.
3. Dempsey JA, Vidruk EH, Mitchell GH. Pulmonary control systems in exercise: update. *Fed Proc* 44:2260–2270, 1985.
4. Dempsey JA, Hanson PG, Henderson KS. Exercise-induced arterial hypoxemia in healthy human subjects at sea level. *J Physiol* 355:161, 1984.
5. Powers SK, et al. Precision of ventilatory and gas exchange alterations as a predictor of the anaerobic threshold. *Eur J Physiol* 52:173–177, 1984.
6. Wasserman K, et al. Gas exchange theory and the lactic acidosis (anaerobic) threshold. *Circulation* 81(suppl II): II14-II30, 1990.
7. Ribeiro JP, et al. Metabolic and ventilatory responses to steady state exercise relative to lactate thresholds. *Eur J Appl Physiol* 55:215–221, 1986.
8. Roston WL, et al. Oxygen uptake kinetics and lactate concentration during exercise in humans. *Am Rev Resp Dis* 135: 1080–1084, 1987.
9. Wasserman K, et al, eds. Normal Values. In: *Principles of exercise testing and interpretation.* Philadelphia: Lea & Febiger, 1987:72–86.
10. Kumagai S, et al. Relationships of the anaerobic threshold with the 5 km, 10 km and 10 mile races. *Eur J Appl Physiol* 49:13–23, 1982.
11. Weltman A, et al. Prediction of lactate threshold and fixed blood lactate concentrations from 3200-m running performance in male runners. *Intl J Sports Med* 8:401–406, 1987.
12. Henritze J, et al. Effects of training at and above the lactate threshold on the lactate threshold and maximal oxygen uptake. *Eur J Physiol* 54:84–88, 1985.
13. Wasserman K. The anaerobic threshold measurement to evaluate exercise performance. *Am Rev Resp Dis* 129(Suppl):S35–S40, 1984.
14. Beaver WL, et al. A new method for detecting anaerobic threshold by gas exchange. *J Appl Physiol* 60:2020–2027, 1986.
15. Busse M, Maassen N, Konrad H. Relation between plasma K+ and ventilation during incremental exercise after glycogen depletion and repletion in man. *J Physiol* 443:469–76, 1991.
16. Duffin J. Neural drives to breathing during exercise. *Can J Appl Physiol* 19:289–304, 1994.
17. Syabbalo NC, Krishnan B, Zintel T, et al. Differential ventilatory control during constant work rate and incremental exercise. *Respir Physiol* 97:175–187, 1994.
18. Johnson BD, Saupe KW, Dempsey JA. Mechanical constraints on exercise hyperpnea in endurance athletes. *J Appl Physiol* 73:874–886, 1992.
19. Blackie SP, et al. Normal values and ranges for ventilation and breathing pattern at maximal exercise. *Chest* 100:136–142, 1991.
20. Johnson BD, Badr MS, Dempsey JA. Impact of the aging pulmonary system on the response to exercise. *Clin Chest Med* 15:229, 1994.
21. Leblanc P, Summers E, Inman MD, et al. Inspiratory muscles during exercise: a problem of supply and demand. *J Appl Physiol* 64:2482–2489, 1988.
22. Olafsson S, Hyatt RE. Ventilatory mechanics and expiratory flow limitation during exercise in normal subjects. *J Clin Invest* 48:564–573, 1969.
23. Aaron EA, Seow KC, Johnson BD, et al. Oxygen cost of exercise hyperpnea: implications for performance. *J Appl Physiol* 72:1818–1825, 1992.
24. Wheatley JR, Amis TC, Engel LA. Oronasal partitioning of ventilation during exercise. *J Appl Physiol* 71:546–551, 1991.
25. Fregossi RF, Lansing RW. Neural drive to nasal dilator muscles. Influence of exercise intensity and oronasal flow partitioning. *J Appl Physiol* 79:1330–1337, 1995.
26. Syabbalo NC, Bundgaard A, Widdicombe JG. Effects of exercise on nasal airflow resistance in healthy subjects and in patients with asthma and rhinitis. *Bull Eur Physiopathol Respir* 21:507–513, 1985.
27. Strohl EP, O'Cain CF, Slutsky AS. Alae nasi activation and nasal resistance in healthy subjects. *J Appl Physiol* 52:1432–1437, 1982.
28. Johnson BD, Scanlon PD, Beck KC. Regulation of ventilatory capacity during exercise in asthmatics. *J Appl Physiol* 79:892–901, 1995.
29. Malmberg P, Hedenström H, Fridriksson HV. Reference values for gas exchange during exercise in healthy nonsmoking and smoking men. *Bull Eur Physiopathol Respir* 23: 131, 1987.
30. Hammond MD, Gale GE, Kapitan KS, et al. Pulmonary gas exchange in humans during exercise at sea level. *J Appl Physiol* 60:1590, 1986.
31. Wagner PD. Ventilation-perfusion matching during exercise. *Chest* 101(Suppl):192S, 1992.
32. Beck KC, Rehder K. Factors determining pulmonary blood flow and gas distribution: new insights. *Curr Op Anaesthesiol* 7:536–542, 1994.
33. Reeves JT, Dempsey JA, Grover RF. Pulmonary circulation during exercise. In: Weirand EK, Reeves JT, eds. *Pulmonary Vascular Physiology and Pathophysiology.* New York: Marcel Dekker, Inc., 1989:107–133.
34. Tobin CE. The bronchial arteries and their connections with other vessels in the human lung. *Surg Gyn Ob* 95: 741–750, 1952.
35. Manohar M. Blood flow to the respiratory and limb muscles and to abdominal organs during maximal exertion in ponies. *J Physiol* 377:25–35, 1986.
36. Pearce FL, Flint KC, Leung KB, et al. Some studies on human pulmonary mast cells obtained by bronchoalveolar lavage and by enzymatic dissociation of whole lung tissue. *Intl Arch Allergy Appl Immunol* 82:507–512, 1987.
37. Al-Bazzaz FJ. Regulation of salt and water transport across airway mucosa. *Clin Chest Med* 7:259–272, 1986.

38. Gilbert IA, Fouke JM, McFadden ER. Heat and water flux in the intrathoracic airways and exercise-induced asthma. *J Appl Physiol* 63:1681–1691, 1987.
39. Hanna LM, Scherer PW. A theoretical model of localized heat and water vapor transport in the human respiratory tract. *J Biomech Eng* 108:19–27, 1986.
40. Boucher RC, Stutts MJ, Bromberg PA, et al. Regional differences in airway surface liquid composition. *J Appl Physiol* 50:613–620, 1981.
41. Daviskas E, Anderson SD, Gonda I, et al. Changes in mucociliary clearance during and after isocapnic hyperventilation in asthmatic and healthy subjects. *Eur Resp J* 8:742–751, 1995.

85, 86, 88 302, 330, 338 341, 353 357, 360

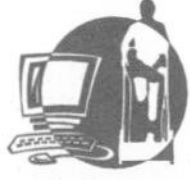 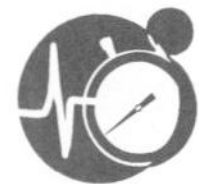 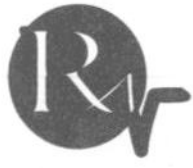 

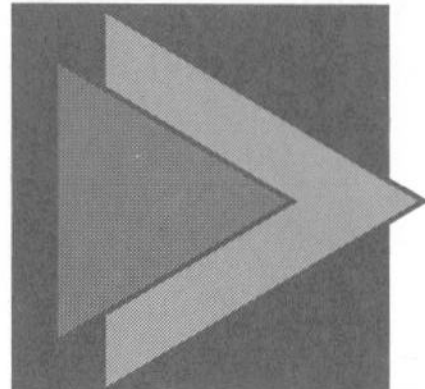

CHAPTER 37
PATHOPHYSIOLOGY OF LUNG DISEASE

Connie C.W. Hsia

Key to Pulmonary Physiology Abbreviations

A-a D_{O2}	Alveolar-arterial oxygen difference
COPD	Chronic obstructive pulmonary disease
CPAP	Continuous positive airway pressure
D_L	Lung diffusing capacity
$D_L/\dot{Q}$	Ratio of diffusion conductance of the alveolar tissue to perfusion of pulmonary vasculature
D_LO_2	Diffusing capacity of oxygen
FEF_{25-75}	Forced expiratory flow at mid-range (25%-75%)
FEV_1	Forced expiratory volume in 1 second
FVC	Forced vital capacity
MSV	Maximum sustained ventilation
MVV	Maximal voluntary ventilation
$P_{a,CO2}$	Partial pressure of carbon dioxide in arterial blood
$P_{a,O2}$	Partial pressure of oxygen in arterial blood
RV	Residual volume
RV/TLC	Ratio of residual volume to total lung capacity
TLC	Total lung capacity
$\dot{V}_A/\dot{Q}$	Ventilation to perfusion ratio (ventilation/cardiac output)

Diseases of the respiratory tract can be classified according to mechanisms of derangement:

- Obstructive airway disease
- Restrictive disease involving lung parenchyma, pleura, thorax, or respiratory muscles
- Pulmonary vascular disease
- Hypoventilation syndromes

This chapter reviews the general pathophysiological patterns of lung disease and the fundamental concepts of how lung disease limits aerobic capacity. Exogenous causes of lung disease (infection, trauma, neoplasm, and congenital abnormalities) are not discussed.

NORMAL VENTILATORY MECHANICS

During inspiration the diaphragm contracts and descends, while the rib cage moves upward and outward. These actions generate a negative pressure inside the thorax, relative to pressure at the mouth, causing air flow into the lungs. During expiration the diaphragm relaxes and moves upward, while the rib cage moves inward. At rest, expiration is a passive process requiring no active muscular contraction. Lung tissue possesses intrinsic elasticity and a natural tendency to recoil inward which forces air out of the lung. However, during exercise expiration is aided by active contraction of the abdominal and thoracic expiratory muscles which further pushes the abdominal contents upward and the rib cage inward. These muscular actions generate positive pressure inside the thorax pushing air out of the lungs.

Large airways are supported by cartilage in the walls and the dimensions are less affected by thoracic pressure changes. Small airways contain progressively less cartilage, until the final branches where there is none. They are tethered to the surrounding alveolar mesh by radial traction and are influenced by intra-thoracic pressure changes. Negative intra-thoracic pressure increases lung volume, stretches the alveolar mesh, increases radial traction and pulls airways open. Positive intrathoracic pressure reduces lung volume and radial traction; hence, airway caliber is larger during inspiration than expiration (Fig. 37.1). The potential energy stored in radial traction of airways and alveoli at a given lung volume is known as elastic recoil pressure; this pressure determines the diameter of small airways and resistance to flow. Elastic recoil pressure is greatest at higher lung volumes and decreases as lung volume decreases.

During expiration there is a progressive loss of elastic recoil resulting in airway closure as lung volume decreases. The maximum expiratory flow that can be generated is related to intrathoracic pressure (determined by muscular effort at very high lung volumes and by chest wall and lung elastic recoil at lower lung volumes) and resistance of the airways (determined by airway diameter and geometry). Flow rates are reduced when there is neuromuscular weakness (polyneuropathy, polio), loss of

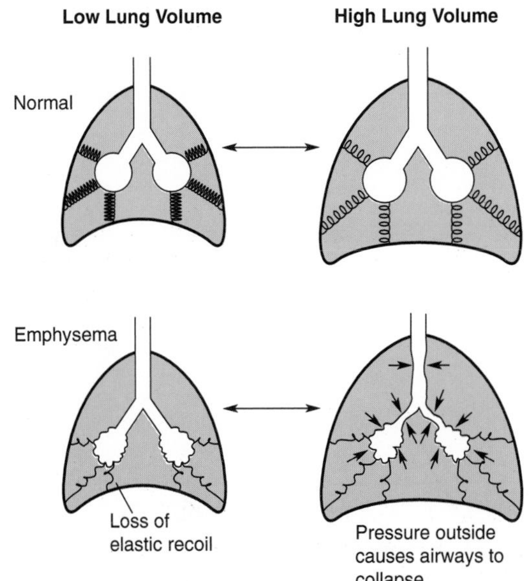

Figure 37.1. Intrathoracic airways are tethered open by radial traction. Their caliber depends on recoil of the lung which is greater at a high lung volume; hence airway caliber is also greater at a high lung volume. In diseases where elastic recoil is lost, these airways are prone to dynamic collapse when pressure outside the airway becomes more positive.

elastic recoil (emphysema), and narrowing of airways (asthma, chronic bronchitis). Others provide a more detailed discussion of the mechanics of breathing (1, 2).

OBSTRUCTIVE AIRWAY DISEASES

Obstructive airway diseases result from a narrowing of airways and can be caused by intraluminal, intramural, or extramural lesions. Airway narrowing within the lung increases resistance to air flow resulting in uneven distribution of ventilation. Obstruction of extrathoracic airways causes a prominent reduction in inspiratory flow rates (3). Obstruction of intrathoracic airways causes a prominent expiratory flow limitation, shown by a disproportionate reduction in forced expiratory flow rates relative to lung volume, that is, low ratio of forced expiratory volume in 1 second to forced vital capacity, (FEV_1/FVC), or low forced expiratory flow rate at the mid-range (25%-75%) of vital capacity, (FEF_{25-75}). The pattern of large, intrathoracic airway obstruction is distinct from obstruction distal to the trachea and mainstem bronchi.

In diffuse obstructive airway disease associated with a loss of lung elastic recoil, airways begin to close at an abnormally high lung volume above the resting end-expiratory volume, resulting in increased residual volume (RV) at the end of a forced exhalation. The increase in RV is known as "air-trapping." Total lung capacity (TLC) and the ratio RV/TLC both increase in obstructive airway disease. Air-trapping displaces the diaphragm downward, causing the muscle to lose its normal dome-like configuration (Fig. 37.2). Flattening of the diaphragm places the muscle at a mechanical disadvantage, reduces the efficiency of contraction and increases the oxygen cost of breathing. Airway involvement is usually not uniform, hence regional distribution of ventilation becomes nonuniform, resulting in regional mismatch of ventilation to perfusion ($\dot{V}_A/\dot{Q}$ ratio) which impairs the efficiency of gas exchange between alveolar air and blood (4).

Chronic Obstructive Pulmonary Disease

Chronic obstructive pulmonary disease (COPD) is a common disorder characterized by progressive expiratory flow obstruction, dyspnea on exertion, and some degree of reversible airway hyperreactivity (Fig. 37.3) (5). Symptoms develop insidiously over years to decades. Patients are often chronic cigarette smokers. There are two main clinical-pathophysiological syndromes: chronic bronchitis and emphysema. A third syndrome, small airway disease, is sometimes designated separately to indicate obstruction of small airways. However, there are often overlapping features of all three.

Chronic Bronchitis

Chronic bronchitis is characterized by a chronic cough and excessive sputum production. The histological hallmark of chronic bronchitis is enlargement and overabundance of mucous glands in the walls of large bronchi. The airway wall becomes thickened and the surface, irregular. There may be bronchial and peribronchial inflammation reducing luminal diameter. These changes are exacerbated by bacterial colonization of the airway associated with episodes of acute bronchitis.

Narrowing of large bronchi produces a marked increase in air flow resistance, while intrathoracic pressure generated by muscular effort and lung elastic recoil are normal. Expiratory flow rates may improve after inhaled bronchodilator therapy, but usually cannot be completely normalized. Lung units with high airway resistance receive less ventilation, while pulmonary blood flow either decreases or remains unchanged and are, therefore, underventilated and over-perfused (i.e., low $\dot{V}_A/\dot{Q}$ ratio) leading to arterial hypoxemia. Hypoxemia is a potent stimulus of smooth muscle constriction in pulmonary arterioles and venules, leading to increased pulmonary vascular resistance, pulmonary arterial hypertension, and right ventricular strain.

In chronic severe disease, secondary right heart failure (**cor pulmonale**) eventually develops. Hypoxemia stimulates the production of erythropoietin resulting in excessively increased blood volume, hemoglobin concentration and hematocrit (**secondary polycythemia**). Polycythemia may lead to high blood viscosity increas-

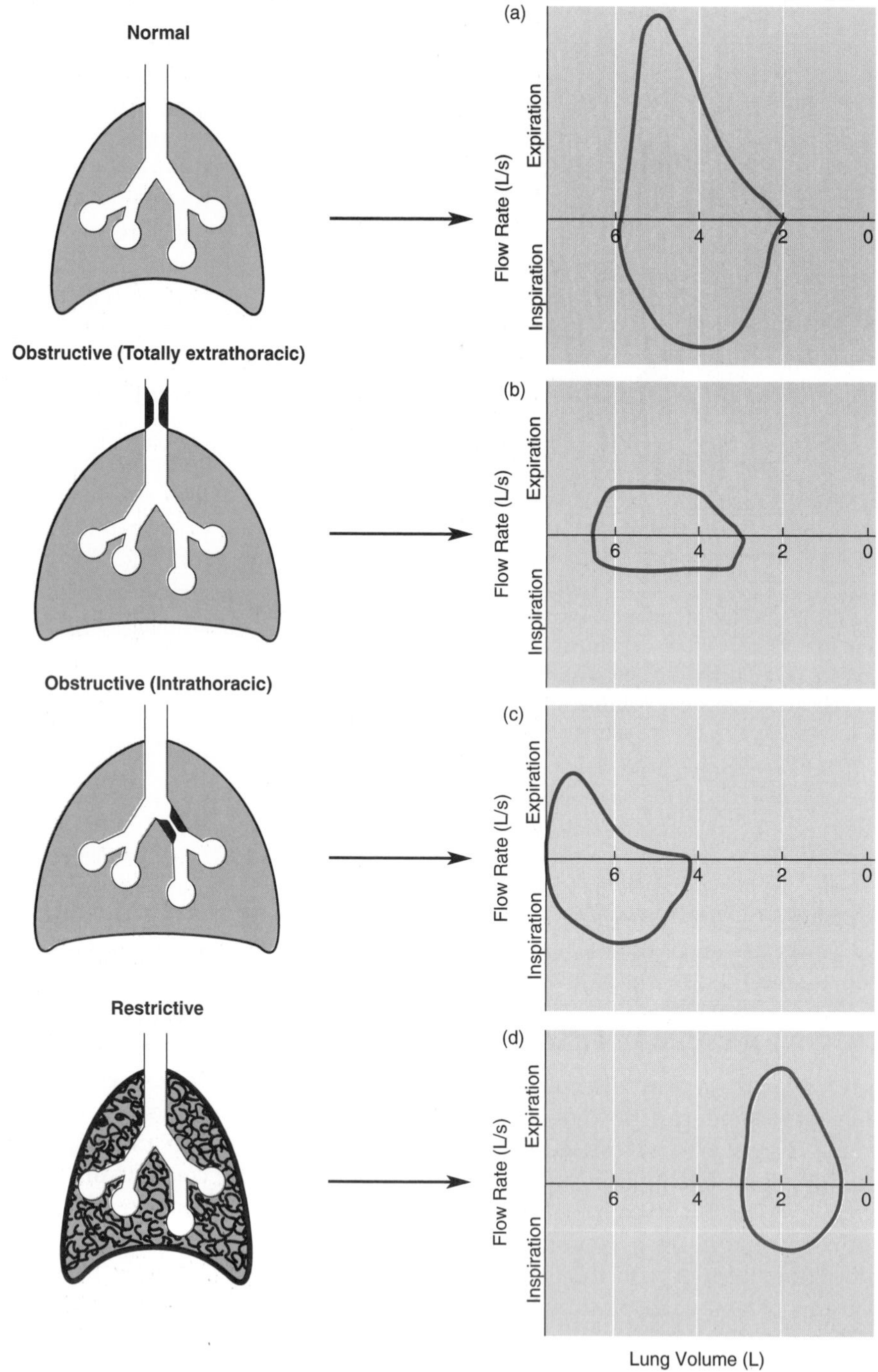

Figure 37.2. Maximal flow-volume curves in normal subject, extra-thoracic airway obstruction, intrathoracic airway obstruction, and restrictive lung disease.

ing flow resistance in blood vessels and potentially compromising blood flow in small vessels of the brain and heart.

The typical patient with severe chronic bronchitis is known as a "**blue bloater**" because they exhibit a stocky habitus with central and peripheral cyanosis. Reduced air flow rate is associated with only mildly increased lung volumes and a relatively normal rate of oxygen transfer across the alveolar-capillary barrier (lung diffusing capacity or D_L). Secondary derangement in ventilatory control may develop and patients with chronic bronchitis tend to maintain a low minute ventilation which may further decline during sleep resulting in nocturnal hypoxemia. They may also develop daytime hypoxemia and CO_2 retention. The clinical progression of chronic bronchitis is shown in Figure 37.4.

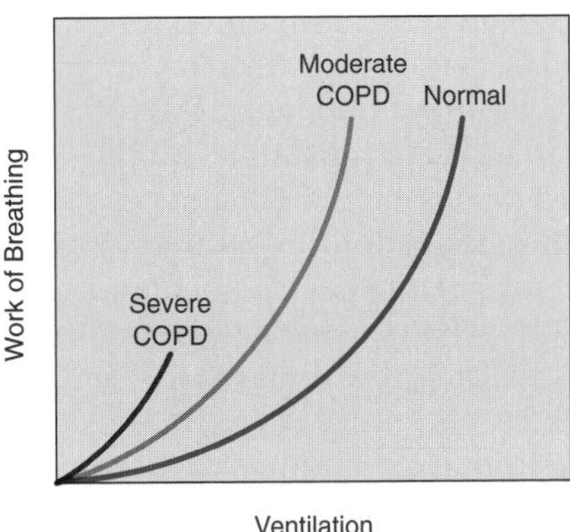

Figure 37.3. Work of respiratory muscles increases as ventilation increases. In moderate COPD work of breathing is greater than normal at any given level of ventilation. In severe COPD with the onset of respiratory muscle fatigue, work of breathing is further increased; in addition, the maximum work that can be generated by respiratory muscle is diminished.

Chronic cough and sputum production

↓

Expiratory airflow limitation
Progressive dyspnea on exertion

↓

Progressive $\dot{V}_A/\dot{Q}$ mismatch
↓arterial pO_2
↓arterial pCO_2

↓

Pulmonary hypertension
Right heart strain
Polycythemia

↓

Right heart failure

Figure 37.4. Progression of Chronic Bronchitis.

Emphysema

Emphysema is technically a disease of the lung parenchyma secondarily affecting small airways (6). The pathology includes abnormal permanent enlargement of airspaces accompanied by destruction of alveolar walls.

The biochemical basis of the disease is an imbalance in the protease versus anti-protease equilibrium. Elastin is a major connective tissue component of the alveolar wall. Proteases promote degradation of elastin and anti-proteases inhibit degradation. Destruction of lung tissue results either from increased protease activity or a deficient anti-protease activity. Smokers demonstrate significantly increased pulmonary proteolytic activities, possibly related to accumulation of inflammatory cells (neutrophils, macrophages) containing a high concentration of protease enzymes (7). On the other hand, those with a genetic deficiency of alpha-1-antitrypsin, a potent anti-protease, are prone to develop severe emphysema at an early age even in the absence of a smoking history.

The hallmark of emphysema is loss of lung elasticity and reduction of elastic recoil pressure due to accelerated alveolar destruction. Small airways lose radial traction to the surrounding alveolar walls and become easily collapsible during expiration because intra-thoracic pressure becomes more positive (Fig. 37.1). Patients with emphysema can expel a larger volume during a slow exhalation than during a maximal forced exhalation because intra-thoracic pressure is less positive and airway compression is minimized during a slow exhalation.

Expiratory flow limitation in emphysema is unresponsive to bronchodilator therapy because the basis of obstruction is related to mechanical properties of the lung tissue. Patients can minimize air-trapping and dyspnea by "purse lip breathing" (the lips are puckered during exhalation) (8). Pursing the lips creates external resistance to flow and maintains a more positive intra-airway pressure during exhalation retarding small airway compression. Since loss of elastic recoil primarily affects airway resistance during forced expiration, airway resistance during quiet breathing may be relatively normal. However, even with normal airway resistance, the loss of elastic recoil as a driving force leads to a reduction in expiratory flow rate.

Distribution of ventilation is also not uniform in emphysema and lung units that are not well ventilated tend to receive less perfusion due to destruction of the capillary bed. Some ventilation goes to lung units containing no capillaries and dead space is increased. This physiological pattern is distinct from that seen in chronic bronchitis.

To overcome high physiological dead space, patients must chronically sustain high minute ventilation, therefore the typical patient with severe emphysema is known as the "pink puffer." Patients with emphysema are barrel-chested because of marked air-trapping. They are thin with generalized muscle wasting, attributed to malnutrition, secondary to the excessive energy cost of breathing. Malnutrition impairs respiratory muscle strength and makes it more difficult to sustain high ventilatory demands. Patients are not usually cyanotic and have little cough or sputum production. In addition to reduced lung elasticity (i.e., high lung compliance), lung diffusing capacity is reduced due to loss of alveolar-capillary units. Ventilatory control is normal.

In moderate emphysema arterial oxygen and carbon dioxide pressures ($P_{a,O2}$ and $P_{a,CO2}$) are generally well maintained. With severe end-stage disease, respiratory muscle fatigue sets in and $P_{a,CO2}$ rises, while $P_{a,O2}$ drops. Progressive destruction of alveolar-capillary units leads to elevated pulmonary vascular resistance, right heart strain and eventually right heart failure. Disease progression is outlined in Figure 37.5.

Small Airway Disease

Small airway disease is an early manifestation of the same pathological processes that eventually lead to chronic bronchitis and/or emphysema. Inflammation around small airways (< 2 mm in diameter) occurs in response to irritant exposure and is associated with reduced forced expiratory flow rates in the mid-range of lung volume (FEF_{25-75}), while maximal expiratory flow rates at high lung volumes (peak flow rate or FEV_1) may be minimally affected. Cigarette smoking increases risk of small airway flow obstruction and loss of elastic recoil in a dose-dependent fashion. Objective abnormalities in small airway flow pattern can be demonstrated within 1–5 years of smoking; in early stages, such abnormalities are largely reversible with cessation of smoking. Subjective symptoms are usually mild in the absence of large airway or parenchymal involvement.

Management

The management of patients with these types of COPD generally includes the following strategies:

1. Identify and eliminate sources of bronchopulmonary inflammation (i.e., cigarette smoking, inhaled irritants, recurrent respiratory infections).
2. Identify and treat reversible airway narrowing with inhaled or oral bronchodilators and corticosteroids.
3. Prevent exacerbations by routine vaccination against infectious agents such as pneumococcus and influenza, by adequate respiratory hygiene and, in selected patients, by prophylactic administration of antibiotics.
4. Establish individualized rehabilitation programs for stable patients.

Rehabilitation programs generally have some component of moderate physical and breathing exercises. Maximal oxygen uptake may improve if significant deconditioning is present. Selective respiratory muscle training can improve ventilatory capacity in patients with lung disease and exercise performance may also improve in some patients (9). Neither cardiovascular nor selective respiratory muscle training significantly improves mechanical lung function or alveolar gas exchange. However, exercise training improves oxygen delivery and extraction; hence overall efficiency of oxygen use is

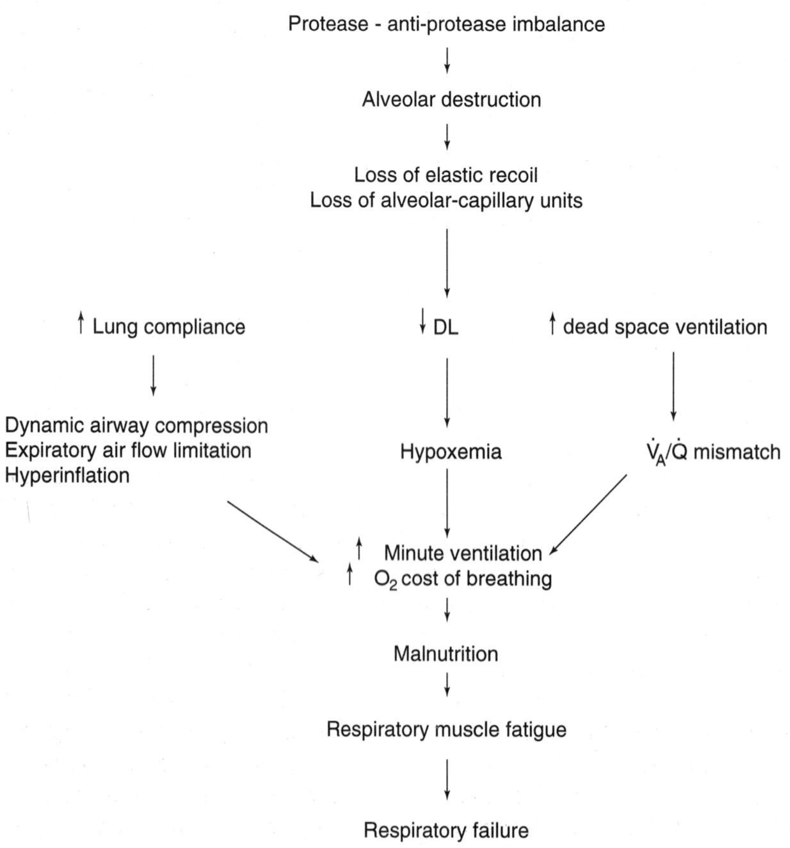

Figure 37.5. Progression of Emphysema.

enhanced and endurance for submaximal exercise is improved (5).

Chronic home oxygen therapy is indicated for patients in respiratory failure whose $P_{a,O2}$ remains below 55 mmHg despite optimal medical therapy. The goal is to alleviate hypoxemia, minimize hypoxic pulmonary vasoconstriction, reduce pulmonary vascular resistance and, ultimately, prevent right heart failure. The dose of oxygen must be determined individually. In the presence of chronic CO_2 retention, ventilatory response to CO_2 is blunted and hypoxemia becomes the predominant stimulus to ventilation. Excessive oxygen administration can abolish the hypoxic ventilatory drive and potentially lead to apnea.

Asthma

Asthma affects about 5% of the general population. It is characterized by increased airway reactivity to various stimuli, resulting in widespread, reversible narrowing of airways (10, 11). The episodic nature and reversibility of the narrowing are important features. It is sometimes possible to identify specific agents that precipitate attacks (allergic asthma), such as pollens, dust mites, animal dander, drugs, foods, wine, exposure to fumes and chemicals. Asthma attacks may also be induced by non-specific stimuli, such as emotional stress, exercise, exposure to cold or a viral respiratory infection. Often no precipitating factors can be identified (perennial asthma). Asthma may be associated with allergic rhinitis, nasal polyps, and aspirin sensitivity. There is a strong tendency for familial clustering.

The classical mechanism triggering an attack is coupling of an antigen to IgE antibodies present on the surface of sensitized mast cells, leading to release of various biochemical mediators causing airway smooth muscle constriction (bronchospasm). The antigen-antibody interaction may also stimulate vagal neural reflexes directly to cause bronchoconstriction. Physical stimuli such as cooling and fluid evaporation across airway epithelium during exercise or cold air exposure may directly stimulate the release of chemical mediators (12).

Prolonged bronchospasm leads to secondary mucosal edema and mucus accumulation. These secondary processes must be aggressively prevented and treated since they reduce the physiological response to bronchodilator therapy and further contribute to air flow obstruction, hyperinflation and $\dot{V}_A/\dot{Q}$ mismatch.

The diagnosis is made by demonstrating airflow obstruction (reduced maximal expiratory flow rates, increased inspiratory and expiratory air flow resistance, elevated RV, TLC and the ratio of RV/TLC) which is abolished by the administration of a bronchodilator or by a challenge test using inhaled methacholine which causes bronchoconstriction in individuals with heightened airway reactivity (13). Patients with exercise-induced asthma may demonstrate normal airway function at rest, but bronchospasm may develop during or after exercise. This can be relieved by administration of inhaled bronchodilator. Since exercise-induced asthma is thought to be related to physical stimuli directly causing mast cell degranulation, prophylactic use of an inhaled bronchodilator or a mast cell stabilizing drug such as cromolyn sodium before exercise is often effective in preventing attacks.

During an acute asthmatic attack lung units distal to constricted bronchi are underventilated and regions of low $\dot{V}_A/\dot{Q}$ ratio develop (14, 15). Patients typically hyperventilate initially, maintaining a normal $P_{a,O2}$ while $P_{a,CO2}$ drops. As the attack worsens, the distribution of $\dot{V}_A/\dot{Q}$ becomes more abnormal and $P_{a,O2}$ declines despite persistent hyperventilation. Severe or prolonged attacks unresponsive to therapy (i.e., status asthmaticus) may lead to respiratory failure with hypoxemia and hypercapnia.

Management

Management of asthmatic patients generally includes the following strategies:

1. Identification and elimination of precipitating agents.
2. Preventing and minimizing attacks through patient education to improve compliance with medication. Pharmacological prophylaxis can be achieved by using inhaled corticosteroid preparations to reduce airway inflammation and inhaled cromolyn sodium to stabilize mast cells.
3. Optimizing inhaled or oral bronchodilator therapy to achieve the maximal possible flow rates and maximal exercise tolerance.

RESTRICTIVE LUNG DISEASES

This term denotes a restriction of lung volume by diseases involving the thorax or the lung parenchyma, including diseases of the rib cage and spine (kyphoscoliosis, ankylosing spondylitis, pectus excavatum), respiratory muscles and nerves (spinal cord injury, neuropathy, myopathy, diaphragm paralysis), pleura (effusion, pleuritis, fibrothorax, mesothelioma) and alveolar septum (interstitial fibrosis, alveolitis). Morbid obesity can also produce restrictions of the thorax and respiratory muscles. Restriction of the rib cage or pleura, from any cause, leads to low lung volume and reduced excursion of lung volume during exercise. Chronic restriction also leads to secondary atelectasis of some alveolar units. Functional surface of air-tissue interface decreases, eventually resulting in impaired gas exchange.

There are over 200 potential causes of diffuse interstitial and alveolar lung disease including (16):

- Infection (tuberculosis, fungal and viral)
- Neoplastic disease (lymphoma, metastatic cancer)
- Thromboembolism
- Toxic inhaled organic and inorganic substances (farmer's lung, bird-fancier's disease, silicosis, asbestosis)
- Drugs (chemotherapeutic agents, amiodarone)
- Pulmonary edema
- Systemic immunologic disease (rheumatoid arthritis, lupus erythematosus, sarcoidosis)
- Radiation injury
- Idiopathic interstitial lung disease (cause unknown)

The histological hallmark of many, but not all types of restrictive lung disease, is inflammation of the interstitium and alveolar tissue with varying degrees of fibrosis. These changes directly reduce lung compliance leading to non-uniform distribution of ventilation, increased work of breathing and respiratory muscle oxygen demand, and increased airway size and expiratory flow rates.

A stiff lung requires more energy to stretch and a greater transpulmonary pressure is required to achieve a given tidal volume. At the same time, maximal tidal volume is restricted. Hence, ventilation must be increased, primarily via increased respiratory rate. This pattern of rapid, shallow breathing leads to alveolar hyperventilation and decreased $P_{a,O2}$. Interstitial and alveolar inflammation eventually causes normal alveolar-capillary membrane to be replaced with fibrous tissue, leading to reduced rate of oxygen uptake by blood; therefore both mechanical and gas exchange functions are impaired.

PULMONARY VASCULAR DISEASE

The most common pulmonary vascular disease is thromboembolism in which a blood clot occludes a pulmonary blood vessel. A clot may originate within a pulmonary vessel (thrombus), or be dislodged from elsewhere in the venous system (embolus). Conditions that predispose to peripheral venous thrombosis include:

- Prolonged bed rest
- Postoperative period
- Pregnancy
- Chronic cardiac or pulmonary disease
- Peripheral venous insufficiency
- Injury to the lower extremities
- Disorders of the clotting system

Occasionally other forms of emboli may develop, such as infected clots from intravenous drug use or indwelling vascular catheters, fat droplets following fracture of long bones, or amniotic fluid components following obstetrical procedures. The size of the embolus determines the site of occlusion and the functional consequences. A large embolus obstructing a main pulmonary artery may be immediately fatal; a smaller one obstructing a peripheral pulmonary arteriole may not cause symptoms. Since lung tissue is normally well supplied with oxygen from inspired air, as well as bronchial arterial circulation, pulmonary infarction (where lung tissue distal to an embolus dies from ischemia) is uncommon. Usually, lung tissue remains perfused from the bronchial circulation. In time the embolus is either dissolved by endogenous fibrinolytic processes or exogenously administered drugs, or becomes organized into a firm adherent lump and distal perfusion is partially restored. In patients with preexisting cardiopulmonary disease, the impact of an embolus is greatly exaggerated.

The obstruction of a pulmonary artery does not, in itself, cause hypoxemia. Ventilation reaching alveoli distal to the obstructed vessel is wasted, so dead space ventilation increases. Lung compliance is reduced and local irritant receptors are activated leading to tachypnea, hyperventilation and a drop in $P_{a,CO2}$. Secondary smooth muscle constriction develops in small airways, both in embolized lung units and adjacent normal units, causing redistribution of ventilation away from affected regions. Widespread airway constriction leads to distal atelectasis and shunting of blood through the under-ventilated lung units (17). These secondary processes are responsible for the arterial hypoxemia and high alveolar-arterial oxygen tension gradient (A-a D_{O2}) associated with pulmonary embolism.

Since total effective vascular bed available for gas exchange is reduced, there is also a reduction in lung diffusing capacity. In addition, local inflammatory reaction may develop, disrupting the integrity of alveolar-capillary membrane and causing fluid leakage into the interstitium to further aggravate $\dot{V}_A/\dot{Q}$ mismatch and diffusion impairment. Hemodynamically, pulmonary vascular resistance increases and pulmonary arterial hypertension may develop. However, capacitance of the pulmonary vascular bed is sufficiently large that redistribution of pulmonary blood flow, after an embolic event, can often be accommodated without a rise in vascular pressure. Almost 40% of the vascular bed must be occluded in a normal subject before there is significant rise in resting pulmonary artery pressure (18). In less extensive occlusions, pulmonary artery pressure may be normal at rest, but rises abnormally during exercise. In order to maintain a normal cardiac output against a high pulmonary resistance, right ventricular strain may develop.

Treatment consists of supportive measures (oxygen, fluids) and administration of anticoagulants (heparin and warfarin) to prevent further peripheral clot formation. Thrombolytic agents that promote dissolution of the clot are given to patients with massive pulmonary embolism who develop vascular collapse. In patients susceptible to recurrent embolization or patients who are already hemodynamically compromised, prophylactic insertion of a filter device into the inferior vena cava may effectively trap dislodged clots from the lower extremities and prevent further episodes of embolism.

HYPOVENTILATION SYNDROMES

The neural drive to breathe may be blunted by drugs (narcotics), diseases of the central nervous system (stroke, tumor, encephalitis), sleep apnea syndromes, primary idiopathic disorders involving the respiratory control center (rarely). Sleep apnea syndromes are characterized by periodic cessation of breathing during sleep. Three pathophysiological patterns can be distinguished:

1. Obstructive apnea, associated with oronasal blockage of air flow even though breathing efforts continue.
2. Central apnea, associated with cessation of respiratory muscle contraction.
3. Mixed apnea, associated with features of both obstructive and central apnea.

Obstructive Sleep Apnea

The patency of the upper airway is normally maintained by contractions of muscles of the pharynx, tongue and neck. In obstructive sleep apnea, these muscles lose tone during deep sleep, causing soft tissues of the posterior pharynx to collapse and obstruct air flow, while the diaphragm and abdominal muscles continue to contract against the occluded airway. The highest incidence of obstructive sleep apnea is seen in obese, middle aged males. Patients often exhibit small nasal and oral passages, hypertrophied tonsils or anatomical abnormalities of the jaw that predispose upper airway obstruction.

Partial obstruction within the pharynx gives rise to snoring. Complete obstruction may lead to arterial hypoxemia and bradycardia. Eventually, there is momentary arousal, muscular tone returns, the obstruction is abolished and gas exchange and hemodynamics normalize. The same pattern repeats itself hundreds of times each night. Since patients cannot sleep restfully at night, they awake with a headache and may become somnolent during the day. In the early stages of disease, physiological function during waking hours is normal. With chronic sleep deprivation and nocturnal hypoxemia, a gradual change in personality and intellect may become apparent. Pulmonary and systemic arterial hypertension, secondary polycythemia and a variety of cardiac arrhythmias may develop.

Diagnosis is made by the constellation of clinical symptoms and signs, or documented by a sleep study demonstrating cessation of air flow accompanied by continued respiratory muscle effort (19). Effective treatment includes administration of continuous positive airway pressure (CPAP) via tight face mask to prevent upper airway closure during sleep as well as weight reduction. Both treatment measures require considerable motivation and persistence, hence patient compliance is generally poor. Any anatomical abnormalities of the upper airway should be corrected, but surgical treatment by indiscriminately removing excessive soft tissue from the pharynx (uvulopalatopharyngoplasty) has demonstrated mixed results and is not generally recommended.

Obesity-hypoventilation Syndrome

The most common form of central hypoventilation, also known as "Pickwickian syndrome," occurs in association with morbid obesity. The causal relationship between obesity and hypoventilation is incompletely understood. In addition to mechanical effects of morbid obesity (reduced chest wall compliance and restriction of lung volume) described previously, severe obesity is also associated with impaired ability to augment ventilation in response to the usual stimuli such as hypoxia or CO_2 inhalation. During deep sleep, patients develop periods of apnea with cessation of both air flow and respiratory muscle effort. Secondary upper airway obstruction may develop due to the loss of pharyngeal muscle tone. Clinical manifestations are similar to those in patients with obstructive apnea. Weight reduction and careful administration of respiratory stimulants are effective in producing improvement in these abnormalities.

EXERCISE LIMITATION IN LUNG DISEASE

The following are general mechanisms by which lung disease limits exercise:

- Blunting of ventilatory response
- Mechanical limitation of air flow and respiratory muscle function
- Impairment of gas exchange by $\dot{V}_A/\dot{Q}$ mismatch, shunting and diffusion limitation

Blunting of Ventilatory Response

In hypoventilation syndromes related to morbid obesity, neuromuscular disease or respiratory depressant drugs, the respiratory center fails to respond appropriately to the normal metabolic and neural ventilatory stimuli during exercise (lactic acid and CO_2 accumulation and mechanoreceptor input from working muscles). Hypoxia is normally a secondary stimulus to ventilation, but can assume greater importance in patients with significant lung disease who develop chronic CO_2 retention. Inadequate ventilatory response to CO_2 may be detected by a lower than normal relationship between ventilation and inhaled CO_2 concentration (Fig. 37.6). Similarly, inadequate ventilatory response to hypoxia may be detected by lower than normal relationship between ventilation and inhaled oxygen concentration (Fig. 37.6). With significant ventilatory suppression, CO_2 is not adequately eliminated from the blood; P_{a,CO_2} in-

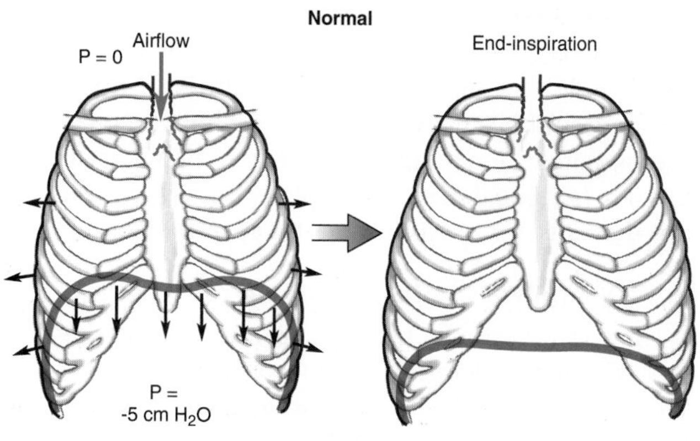

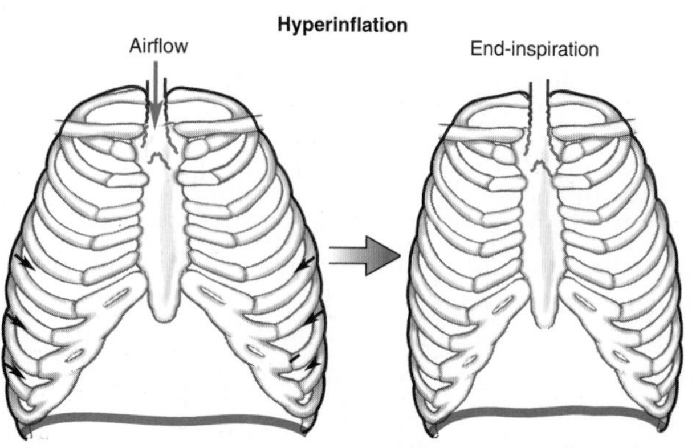

Figure 37.6. Top panel: Normally, contraction of the dome-shaped diaphragm causes the muscle to shorten and descend, leading to obligatory outward movement of the rib cage (*arrows*). These actions generate a negative pressure inside the thorax causing air flow into the lungs. Bottom panel: In hyperinflation the diaphragm loses its dome shape and the ability to expand lung volume. Upon contraction the diaphragm cannot descend and it causes an obligatory inward movement of the rib cage (*arrows*).

creases causing a corresponding decline in $P_{a,O2}$ and pH. The hypoxemia of hypoventilation is readily corrected by the administration of 100% oxygen.

Mechanical Ventilatory Limitation

Patients with obstructive lung disease and skeletal or neuromuscular disease of the thorax are primarily restricted by abnormal mechanics of breathing, manifested by derangement in the following:

- Respiratory pattern
- Maximal air flow rates
- Respiratory muscle energy balance upon exercise

At rest, ventilatory capacity assessed by maximal voluntary ventilation (MVV) for 15 seconds and maximal sustained ventilation (MSV) for 4 minutes are reduced. Dead space ventilation is increased, while tidal volume is reduced, hence breathing pattern consists of rapid shallow breaths at a high end-expiratory lung volume. This pattern is very inefficient resulting in a high energy cost of breathing. In patients with airway flow obstruction, expiratory flow rate during exercise quickly reaches the limit of maximum flow and cannot be further increased. Bronchospasm may be induced or exaggerated on exercise. High transpulmonary pressure must be generated to overcome partial airway obstruction with each breath, further increasing respiratory muscle work and energy cost of breathing (Fig. 37.7).

Increased energy demand and oxygen cost of breathing may limit exercise by diverting a greater fraction of the available oxygen delivery away from exercising locomotive muscles (20). If a significant fraction of total body oxygen supply is required by respiratory muscles to sustain ventilation, locomotive muscles must rely more heavily on anaerobic metabolism; muscle production of lactate increases, producing more CO_2 and further stimulating ventilation which increases oxygen demand by respiratory muscles. The only way to mitigate the excessive rise in ventilatory oxygen demand is to blunt the ventilatory response to exercise, allowing $P_{a,CO2}$ to rise. This response further compromises oxygen uptake. Further, if right heart strain develops as a result of chronic lung disease, cardiac output and oxygen de-

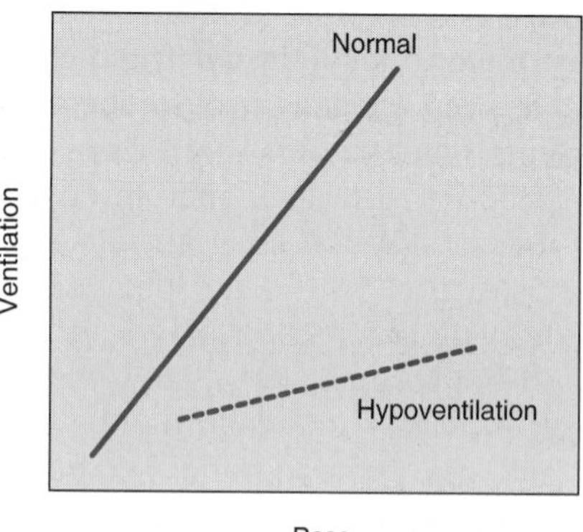

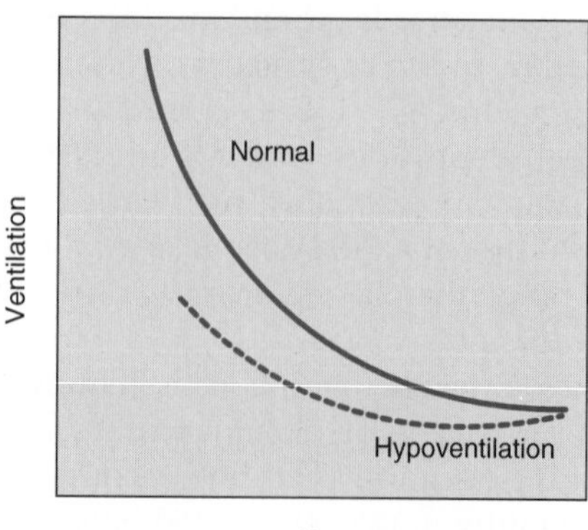

Figure 37.7. Ventilatory responses to high P_{CO_2} and low P_{O_2} are blunted in patients with hypoventilation syndromes.

livery are reduced, intensifying the competition for oxygen between respiratory and non-respiratory muscle (21). Eventually exercise must be discontinued either because locomotive muscles do not receive enough oxygen or because ventilatory capacity is exceeded.

Patients with neuromuscular or skeletal disease of the thorax are primarily limited by poor respiratory muscle strength and endurance. In neuromuscular disease, the mass of functioning respiratory muscle is diminished, indicated by low maximal inspiratory pressure. In addition, chronic thoracic disease may be associated with secondary atelectasis or fibrosis of the lung parenchyma reducing lung compliance, increasing ventilatory work and impairing gas exchange.

Gas Exchange Limitation

Impairment of gas exchange can be due to $\dot{V}_A/\dot{Q}$ mismatch, shunting or diffusion limitation. Each is marked by incomplete oxygenation of blood leaving the lung, resulting in arterial hypoxemia and abnormally high A-a D_{O2}. Abnormalities are accentuated during exercise.

$\dot{V}_A/\dot{Q}$ Mismatch

$\dot{V}_A/\dot{Q}$ mismatch occurs when ventilation and blood flow are not evenly distributed in different regions of the lung (4). In an ideal homogeneous lung, the $\dot{V}_A/\dot{Q}$ ratio should be 1:0; in regions with $\dot{V}_A/\dot{Q}$ mismatch, the ratio is either higher or lower than 1:0. Mismatch of $\dot{V}_A/\dot{Q}$ is the most common gas exchange derangement, although it should be noted that only low $\dot{V}_A/\dot{Q}$ ratios can cause hypoxemia. Mismatch may develop in any disease that disturbs the distribution of ventilation (chronic bronchitis, asthma) or the distribution of pulmonary blood flow (pulmonary hypertension, thromboembolism). $\dot{V}_A/\dot{Q}$ mismatch impairs efficiency of gas exchange because blood flow through low $\dot{V}_A/\dot{Q}$ regions remains hypoxic, while blood flow through high $\dot{V}_A/\dot{Q}$ regions cannot be more than 100% saturated with oxygen; hence the final mixture of blood leaving lung still has a lower pO_2 than mixed alveolar gas, i.e., the A-a D_{O2} is elevated.

In normal subjects a small degree of $\dot{V}_A/\dot{Q}$ mismatch normally exists. $\dot{V}_A/\dot{Q}$ mismatch is exaggerated in lung disease, but may improve from rest to exercise. Anatomic distribution of $\dot{V}_A$ can be grossly assessed by ventilation and perfusion scans with inhaled or injected tracers, respectively. Hypoxemia related to lung regions characterized by low $\dot{V}_A/\dot{Q}$ ratio may be distinguished from hypoxemia due to shunt by application of 100% oxygen, which corrects the former, but not the latter. Precise quantification of physiological distribution of $\dot{V}_A/\dot{Q}$ ratios requires invasive measurements such as the multiple inert gas elimination technique.

Shunting

Shunting develops when venous blood enters the arterial system without oxygenation. Shunts are classified by anatomic location and can be include the following:

- Intracardiac (right-to-left heart)
- Intrapulmonary
- Postpulmonary (venous return emptying directly into the left ventricle)

Intrapulmonary shunts can be viewed as an extreme form of $\dot{V}_A/\dot{Q}$ mismatch described above. Hypoxemia due to shunting worsens during exercise as blood flow through a shunted region increases and mixed venous pO_2 decreases; hypoxemia due to shunt cannot be corrected by the administration of 100% O_2. $P_{a,CO2}$ is usually not increased if chemoreceptor control of ventilation is normal.

Diffusion Limitation

The rate of O_2 transfer from alveolar air to blood and combination with hemoglobin is known as the diffusing capacity (D_L). The magnitude of D_L is determined by the alveolar-capillary surface available for gas exchange, oxygen carrying capacity of blood and pulmonary capillary blood volume. Normally, the diffusing capacity of oxygen (D_LO_2) increases by 40%–100% from rest to exercise. Increased D_L is the combined result of increased tidal volume which opens partially collapsed alveoli and exposes more alveolar surface to inspired gas, increased pulmonary blood flow which opens previously collapsed capillaries and increases capillary volume and surface for diffusion, and changes in red blood cell flow pattern so the regional distribution of red blood cells within and among capillaries becomes more uniform.

Diffusion limitation develops when blood traverses and leaves the pulmonary capillary bed without fully equilibrating with alveolar pO_2 ($P_{A,O2}$), resulting in a low $P_{a,O2}$ and high A-a D_{O2}. On average blood requires < 1 second to traverse the lung. Upon exposure to oxygen, deoxygenated red cells require about 0.25 seconds to become fully oxygenated. Normally, red blood cells have sufficient time to equilibrate with alveolar oxygen before exiting the lung. Complete oxygenation of blood flowing across the alveolar-capillary bed is determined by the ratio of diffusion conductance of the alveolar blood-tissue barrier to the perfusion of the pulmonary vascular bed, expressed by the ratio $D_L/\dot{Q}$, where $\dot{Q}$ = pulmonary blood flow (22).

From rest to exercise the rate of increase in $\dot{Q}$ is greater than D_L; hence the ratio $D_L/\dot{Q}$ progressively declines as exercise intensity increases. In the average subject during maximal exercise at sea level, maximal $\dot{Q}$ is reached before the ratio of $D_L/\dot{Q}$ declines to a level causing a significant drop in arterial oxygen saturation. Therefore, in the average subject, maximal exercise at sea level is primarily limited by cardiovascular oxygen delivery and peripheral extraction, not by pulmonary uptake of oxygen. Pulmonary diffusion limitation develops under two conditions:

1. When the increase in $\dot{Q}$ is so great that the ratio of $D_L/\dot{Q}$ falls below a critical threshold for complete oxygenation of red cells;
2. When a significant portion of the alveolar-capillary membrane is destroyed or is ineffective for oxygen transfer, D_L cannot increase and the ratio of $D_L/\dot{Q}$ falls.

The first condition may occur in elite athletes whose maximum $\dot{Q}$ is significantly increased through physical training. A lower ratio of $D_L/\dot{Q}$ at maximum exercise is achieved, hence blood may not be fully oxygenated upon leaving the pulmonary capillary bed. In achieving maximum performance, the elite athlete may exhibit a significant drop in arterial oxygen saturation (23).

The second condition occurs in pulmonary fibrosis, emphysema or pulmonary embolism. Because of the presence of large physiological reserves in D_L, more than 50% of total alveolar-capillary membrane must be destroyed before diffusion becomes the primary source of exercise limitation (24). Impaired diffusion may be detected by a reduction in D_L at a given cardiac output or by a failure of D_L to increase appropriately from rest to exercise (25–27). Since diffusion is a passive transport process, arterial hypoxemia, due to a low D_L, can be overcome by increasing the driving pressure, i.e., increasing $P_{A,O2}$ by the administration of 100% oxygen.

▶ SUMMARY

In a normal subject of average fitness, exercise capacity is usually limited by cardiovascular, not pulmonary, factors, because oxygen transport capacity of the lungs exceeds that of the heart. However, when capacity of the heart is enhanced to match the lungs (as in elite athletes), or when capacity of the lungs is reduced by lung disease, then pulmonary factors may significantly limit exercise. In most patients with lung disease, a combination of mechanisms is responsible for exercise limitation, including derangement of ventilatory control, lung and chest wall mechanics or alveolar-capillary gas exchange. Progressive pulmonary disease eventually leads to increased ventilatory work and respiratory muscle fatigue as well as right heart strain and impaired cardiac output. Understanding these mechanisms and the associated consequences allows the exercise professional to rationally evaluate functional disability and appropriately direct therapy.

ACKNOWLEDGMENT

This work was supported by an American Heart Association Established Investigator Award.

References

1. Tisi GM. *Pulmonary physiology in clinical medicine.* 2nd ed. Baltimore: Williams & Wilkins, 1985.
2. West JB. *Respiratory physiology—the essentials.* 3rd ed. Baltimore, MD: Williams & Wilkins, 1985.
3. Kryger M, Bode F, Antic R, et al. Diagnosis of obstruction of the upper and central airways [Review]. *Am J Med* 61:85–93, 1976.
4. West JB. Ventilation-perfusion relationships [State of the art]. *Am Rev Respir Dis* 116:919–943, 1977.
5. American Thoracic Society. Standards for the diagnosis and care of patients with chronic obstructive pulmonary disease. *Am J Resp Crit Care Med* 152:S77–S120, 1995.
6. Robins AG. Pathophysiology of emphysema [Review]. Clinics in Chest Medicine. 4:413–420, 1983.
7. Evans MD, Pryor WA. Cigarette smoking, emphysema, and damage to alpha 1-proteinase inhibitor [Review]. *Am J Physiol* 266(6 Pt 1):L593–611, 1995. (published errata appear in *Am J Physiol* 268(1 Pt 1):section L, 1995; and 268(6 Pt 3):section L, 1995).
8. Faling LJ. Pulmonary rehabilitation—physical modalities. [Review]. *Clin Chest Med* 7:599–618, 1986.
9. Pardy RL, Rivington RN, Despas PJ, et al. The effects of inspiratory muscle training on exercise performance in chronic airflow limitation. *Am Rev Respir Dis* 123:426–433, 1981.
10. Tattersfield AE. The site of the defect in asthma. Neurohumoral, mediator or smooth muscle? [Review]. *Chest* 91(6 Suppl):184S–189S, 1987.
11. Hargreave FE, Dolovich J, O'Byrne PM, et al. The origin of airway hyperresponsiveness [Review]. *J Allergy Clin Immunol* 78(5 Pt 1):825–832, 1986.
12. McFadden ER Jr. Exercise-induced asthma. Assessment of current etiologic concepts [Review]. *Chest* 91(6 Suppl): 151S–157S, 1987.
13. de Benedictis FM, Canny GJ, MacLusky IB, et al. Comparison of airway reactivity induced by cold air and methacholine challenges in asthmatic children. *Pediat Pulmonol* 19:326–329, 1995.
14. Roca J, Ramis L, Rodriguez RR, et al. Serial relationships between ventilation-perfusion inequality and spirometry in acute severe asthma requiring hospitalization. *Am Rev Respir Dis* 137:1055–1061, 1988.
15. Ballester E, Reyes A, Roca J, et al. Ventilation-perfusion mismatching in acute severe asthma: effects of salbutamol and 100% oxygen *Thorax* 44:258–267, 1989 [published erratum appears in *Thorax* 44:833, 1989].
16. Reynolds HY, Matthay RA. Diffuse interstitial and alveolar inflammatory disease. In: George RB, Light RW, Matthay MA, et al, eds. *Chest Medicine, Essentials of Pulmonary and Critical Care Medicine.* Baltimore: Williams & Wilkins, 1990:209–248.
17. Kapitan KS, Buchbinder M, Wagner PD, et al. Mechanisms of hypoxemia in chronic thromboembolic pulmonary hypertension. *Am Rev Respir Dis* 139:1149–1154, 1989.
18. Moser KM, ed. *Pulmonary Vascular Disease. Lung Biology in Health and Disease.* Vol. 14. New York: Marcel Dekker, 1979.
19. American Thoracic Society. Indications and standards for cardiopulmonary sleep studies. *Am Rev Respir Dis* 139:559–568, 1988.
20. Otis AB. The work of breathing. In: Fenn WO, Rahn H, eds. *The Handbook of Physiology.* Washington DC: American Physiological Society, 1964:463–476.

21. Hsia CC, Ramanathan M, Estrera AS. Recruitment of diffusing capacity with exercise in patients after pneumonectomy. *Am Rev Respir Dis* 145:811–816, 1992.
22. Piiper J, Scheid P. Comparison of diffusion and perfusion limitations in alveolar gas exchange. *Respir Physiol* 51:287–290, 1983.
23. Dempsey JA. Exercise-induced arterial hypoxemia in healthy human subjects at sea level. *J Physiol* 355:161–175, 1984.
24. Johnson RL Jr. Exercise testing in lung disease. In: Sackner MA, ed. *Diagnostic Techniques in Pulmonary Disease, Part I.* New York: Marcel Dekker, 1980:473–501.
25. American Thoracic Society. Single breath carbon monoxide diffusing capacity (transfer factor): Recommendations for a standard technique. *Am Rev Respir Dis* 136:1299–1307, 1987.
26. Hsia CC, McBrayer DG, Ramanathan M. Reference values of pulmonary diffusing capacity during exercise by a rebreathing technique. *Am J Resp Crit Care Med* 152:658–665, 1995.
27. Hughes JM, Lockwood DN, Jones HA, et al. DLCO/Q and diffusion limitation at rest and on exercise in patients with interstitial fibrosis. *Respir Physiol* 83:155–166, 1991.

86 338, 378, 380 341, 353 365

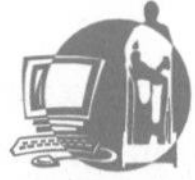
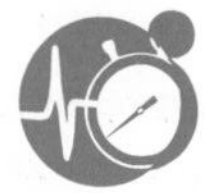

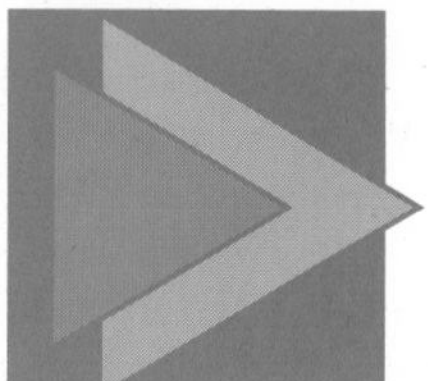

CHAPTER 38
PULMONARY ASSESSMENT

Tony G. Babb

Index to Pulmonary Physiology Abbreviations

A-a D_{O2}	Alveolar-arterial oxygen difference
AT	Anaerobic threshold
DL_{CO}	Lung diffusing capacity of carbon monoxide
EELV	End-expiratory lung volume
EILV	End-inspiratory lung volume
FEV_1	Forced expiratory volume in 1 second
FRC	Functional residual capacity
FVC	Forced vital capacity
IC	Inspiratory capacity
MVV	Maximal voluntary ventilation
$P_{a,CO2}$	Partial pressure of carbon dioxide in arterial blood
$P_{a,O2}$	Partial pressure of oxygen in arterial blood
P_{eCO2}	Pressure of expired carbon dioxide
P_{ETCO2}	Partial pressure of end tidal carbon dioxide
RER	Respiratory exchange ratio
RPB	Rating of perceived breathlessness
RV	Residual volume
SaO_2	Saturation of oxygen in arterial blood
TLC	Total lung capacity
$\dot{V}CO_2$	Carbon dioxide production
V_D/V_T	Ratio of ventilatory dead space to tidal volume
$\dot{V}_E$	Expired minute ventilation
$\dot{V}O_2$	Oxygen consumption
$\dot{V}O_2max$	Maximal oxygen consumption
VT	Ventilatory threshold

The purpose of cardiopulmonary exercise (CPX) testing in the pulmonary patient is to determine whether exercise tolerance is limited and to help identify and/or distinguish between various physiological factors contributing to the limitation. Distinguishing among these factors depends on recognition of normal and abnormal response patterns including:

- Oxygen ($\dot{V}O_2$) uptake
- Carbon dioxide ($\dot{V}CO_2$) production
- Pulmonary gas exchange
- Ventilation ($\dot{V}_E$)
- Breathing pattern
- Metabolic demands
- Cardiovascular function
- Various combinations of these responses during incremental exercise

Even in known pulmonary disease, the factors responsible for exercise limitation are not always apparent. Therefore, attention cannot be limited to the respiratory system during CPX testing in the pulmonary patient.

This discussion is divided into areas of assessment of pulmonary function and CPX testing for pulmonary patients. Although this material emphasizes assessment of known pulmonary disease, it is also applicable to CPX testing, especially in patients with unexplained shortness of breath upon exertion.

PRELIMINARY INFORMATION

Pulmonary Function Testing

In the patient with known or suspected pulmonary disease, basic pulmonary function including spirometry, lung volume, and diffusing capacity should be assessed. Information on pulmonary function provides the basis for determining the type of pulmonary disease, as well as the following:

1. The level of impairment (1, 2).
2. Type of exercise protocol that is appropriate.
3. The potential causes of exercise-related limitations.
4. Indications of potential exercise end-points.

Based on pulmonary function testing, patients usually fall into three broad categories:

- Obstructive lung disease
- Restrictive lung disease
- Pulmonary vascular disease

The purpose of spirometry is to assess airway patency and the volume of air that can be moved in and out of the lungs in one breath (3). Spirometry includes measures of forced vital capacity (FVC), forced expiratory flow rates, such as the forced expiratory volume in 1 second (FEV_1), and FEV_1/FVC ratio, and flow-volume loops. Maximum ventilatory volume (MVV) is sometimes included in pulmonary function assessment and is helpful in estimating maximal ventilatory capacity, but it can be estimated from other measures of pulmonary function as well.

Lung volumes are also commonly measured in pretest assessment and include measures of functional residual capacity (FRC), total lung capacity (TLC) and residual volume (RV). Diffusing capacity of the lung for carbon monoxide (DL_{CO}) indicates the rate at which carbon monoxide can enter the blood per driving pressure of the gas. These assessments assist in evaluating the mechanical properties of the lungs and chest wall, as well as inspiratory muscle strength. When indicated, measurements of arterial blood gases, bronchoprovocation testing, and/or maximal inspiratory and expiratory pressures may also be helpful in the interpretation of pulmonary impairment.

TEST MODE

CPX testing generally begins at low work rates (even unloaded pedaling in patients with severe limitations) and continues with regular, progressive increases in work rate. The cycle ergometer is used most often for testing pulmonary patients for the following reasons:

1. Ease of use.
2. Accuracy of work rate determination.
3. Independence of body weight on determining work rate.
4. The skill of cycling is relatively easy for most patients.
5. Ease of performing invasive measurements during exercise.
6. Ability to begin an incremental test at low work rates.
7. Ability to make small adjustments in work rate.
8. Availability of normal predictive values for cycle ergometry (4, 5).

Although a treadmill may be used, quantifying and incrementing work rate is more difficult. In addition, many treadmills do not run at sufficiently slow speeds for pulmonary patients. Treadmill testing may be appropriate in patients who use this as a training mode.

Predicting End Points

Selecting a protocol for CPX testing should be individualized so that the test lasts 8–12 minutes. Predicting the maximum work rate can be accomplished in a number of ways. Predicted maximal oxygen uptake ($\dot{V}O_2max$) can be used as a target end point, but appropriate norms applicable to both patient population and mode of testing must be used (4–6). Comparing observed heart rate (HR) to predicted maximal HR may also be helpful for determining the relative intensity during each test stage and for targeting maximum exercise capacity.

Since respiratory function is likely to be the limiting factor in exercise for pulmonary patients, it may be helpful to estimate a mechanical ventilatory ceiling (7–9). Using the method of Carter and others where $FEV_1 \times 37.5$ estimates the maximal exercise $\dot{V}_E$, a patient with an FEV_1 of 1.0 L has an estimated mechanical ventilatory ceiling of 37.5 L (8). Using this as the estimated mechanical ventilatory ceiling, and estimating the relationship between $\dot{V}O_2$ and $\dot{V}_E$ ($\dot{V}_E$ = 29.28), a 70 kg patient approaches the mechanical ventilatory ceiling at a $\dot{V}O_2$ of approximately 1184 ml/min ($\approx$80 W $\times$ [1184 – 3.5 $\times$ KG $\div$ 2] $\div$ 6) (10).

Although these are rough estimates, they may be helpful in estimating mechanical ventilatory limitations for patients, which is helpful in selecting an individualized exercise protocol. Starting at 0 W with increments of 10 W, for example, may yield up to nine increments for data collection prior to the termination of the test because of mechanical ventilatory limitations. While a patient may obviously terminate for other respiratory or nonrespiratory reasons, this is also useful information. That is, that the test required termination before estimated mechanical ventilatory limitation, indicating a reason for exercise limitation other than mechanical ventilatory limitation.

Variables

Assessment can determine the variables measured during CPX testing. Variables can be noninvasive or invasive, simple or complex. In general, all exercise tests in pulmonary patients require monitoring of the electrocardiogram (ECG), HR, blood pressure (BP), oxygen saturation (SaO_2) by pulse oximetry, ratings of perceived exertion (RPE), ratings of perceived breathlessness (RPB), and discomfort, symptoms, and/or fatigue. These measurements are required to assess safety of exercise and for safety of the CPX test. In addition, measurement of $\dot{V}O_2$, $\dot{V}CO_2$, anaerobic threshold (AT), $\dot{V}_E$, and work rate establish physiological response, abnormal respiratory and/or cardiovascular function, acid-base status, ventilatory demand, neuromuscular function, and/or maximum exercise tolerance. Measurement of flow-volume characteristics helps to determine the mechanical ventilatory limitation while arterial blood gases determine the effectiveness and efficiency of pulmonary gas exchange. With or without arterial blood gases, monitoring of end-tidal CO_2 (P_{ETCO2}) yields valuable information regarding gas exchange (5).

Without proper presentation of results, the most sophisticated measurements are of little value to the exercise professional or the attending physician. It is important to present physiological responses so that each variable, or combination of variables, contributes to determining whether the patient is exercise limited and the factors most likely to be responsible. A standard, general presentation format is useful in this regard, as is normative data to compare responses. Further details on the display format of exercise test data and interpretation can be found in other sources (5, 6, 11).

MAXIMAL EXERCISE TOLERANCE

Although the primary objective of CPX testing is to determine the source of the limitation, there are other reasons for CPX testing in pulmonary patients including:

- Determining treatment strategies for improving respiratory mechanics or dyspnea
- Distinguishing other organ involvement
- Determining therapeutic strategy
- Determining appropriate exercise intensity
- Determining functional capacity after exercise training, and/or
- Determining whether changes in exercise tolerance are related to new causes
- Recently, evaluating candidates for lung transplant and lung volume reduction surgery are newer indications for CPX testing in pulmonary patients.

Predicted Maximum

The amount of exercise intolerance is determined by comparing predicted exercise capacity to measured exercise capacity. Predicted $\dot{V}O_2$max or predicted maximal work rate can be used to quantify maximal exercise capacity. In Figure 38.1A, both of these variables are used (6).

Comparing $\dot{V}O_2$max to predicted $\dot{V}O_2$max requires caution, especially if 100% predicted $\dot{V}O_2$max is obtained at a work rate significantly lower than predicted (i.e., normal cardiopulmonary functional capacity, but low exercise tolerance) (Fig. 38.1B). This result can be associated with obesity or increased work of breathing (increased ventilatory demand, airways resistance, or respiratory elastance) (6). However, in severely limited pulmonary patients $\dot{V}O_2$max is not normally obtained. If predicted $\dot{V}O_2$max is based on actual body weight, it may be overestimated in overweight patients, thus underestimating cardiorespiratory capacity. Estimating relative peak $\dot{V}O_2$ (ml/kg/min) is also useful for determining which activities of daily living are within patient capacity (12).

Maximal Effort

It is important to assure that a "maximal" exercise test is obtained when determining whether exercise tolerance is normal (6). There are several ways to determine whether maximal exercise is obtained including determining whether:

- Predicted $\dot{V}O_2$max is reached
- 90%, or greater, of predicted maximal HR is obtained
- A respiratory exchange ratio (RER) of > 1.1 is achieved
- $\dot{V}_E$ is near or greater than MVV
- Marked desaturation occurs
- Blood lactate > 8 mMol/L, and/or

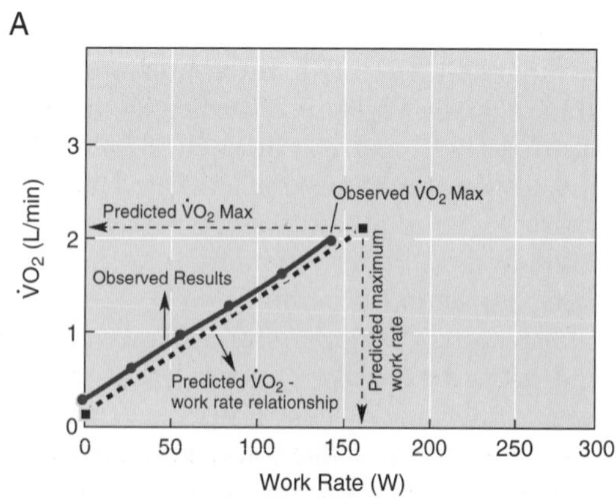

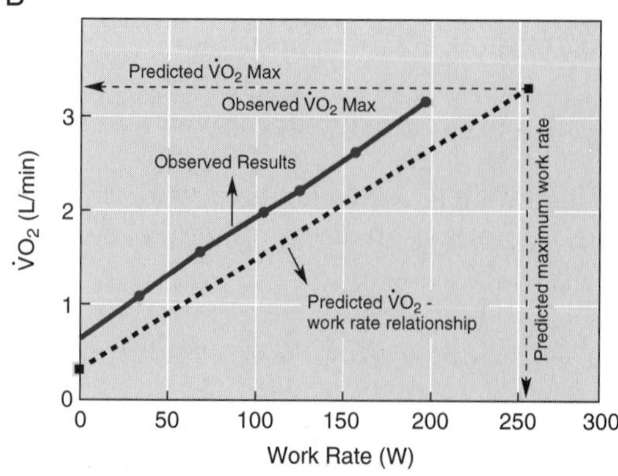

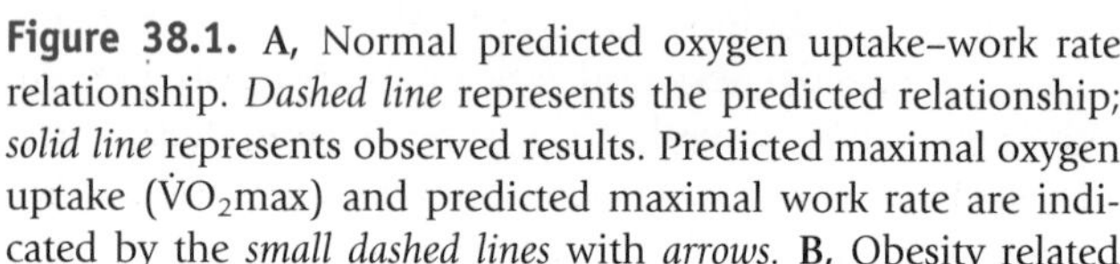
Figure 38.1. **A,** Normal predicted oxygen uptake–work rate relationship. *Dashed line* represents the predicted relationship; *solid line* represents observed results. Predicted maximal oxygen uptake ($\dot{V}O_2$max) and predicted maximal work rate are indicated by the *small dashed lines* with *arrows*. **B,** Obesity related increase in oxygen uptake–work rate relationship. *Dashed line* represents predicted relationship; *solid line* represents observed results. (Adapted from Younes M, Kivinen G. Respiratory mechanics and breathing pattern during and following maximal exercise. *J Appl Physiol* 57:1773–1782, 1984.)

- The test is limited by discomfort or symptoms (e.g., dyspnea or termination of test because of ECG abnormality) (6).

However, attaining one of the above criteria does not always indicate that it is the limiting factor (6). For example, when $\dot{V}_E$ matches or exceeds MVV, it does not necessarily indicate that ventilatory limitation is the primary cause of reduced exercise tolerance. If ventilatory demand is increased because of lactic acidosis then ventilatory limitation may be the reason to discontinue exercise, but cardiovascular disease may cause the limitation. In practice it may be difficult to make these distinctions.

VENTILATORY LIMITATIONS

Mechanical Ventilatory Limitation

In determining possible causes for exercise limitation in pulmonary patients, it is important to determine the presence and extent of mechanical ventilatory limitations. Mechanical ventilatory limitation occurs when ventilatory requirement reaches or exceeds ventilatory capacity. Currently there is no generally accepted, objective method to quantify the magnitude of mechanical ventilatory limitation. However, there are measures that assist with this determination.

The $\dot{V}_E$/MVV ratio is often used as an index of mechanical ventilatory limitation. $\dot{V}_E$ at maximal exercise ($\dot{V}_E$max) is expressed as a percentage of the MVV ($\dot{V}_E$/MVV). A ratio of 60–70% is normal, though the accepted range may vary with population (6, 13). Ventilatory limitation is not expected in individuals without pulmonary disease, but in patients with obstructive pulmonary disease, both MVV and ventilatory reserve are decreased. Reaching or exceeding the normal range for $\dot{V}_E$/MVV may be an indication of the presence of a mechanical ventilatory limitation (6). However, it has been shown that patients with mild-to-moderate chronic obstructive pulmonary disease (COPD) with a ratio between 60–70%, may have significant mechanical ventilatory limitation, but only sightly reduced exercise capacity (14). Therefore, elevated $\dot{V}_E$/MVV is helpful, but not definitive. The difference between $\dot{V}_E$max and MVV, termed "ventilatory reserve," may also be used as an index of mechanical ventilatory limitation. A reserve of 20–50% of the MVV is normal (5).

Tidal flow-volume loops measured at each increment of exercise or at maximal exercise can also be used to assess mechanical ventilatory limitation. The loops are compared to the maximal flow-volume loop measured at rest before exercise, or immediately after exercise (7, 14). The post-exercise maximal flow-volume loop should be used if there is suspected bronchodilation during exercise, otherwise using the pre-exercise loop may result in estimating more ventilatory limitation than is actually present. Additionally, it is sometimes helpful to use the maximal flow-volume loop measured in a pressure-compensated volume-displacement body plethysmograph (flow box), which corrects volume for the gas compression artifact. To compare the exercise tidal flow-volume loops to the maximal flow-volume loop, the loops must be placed properly within the maximal flow-volume loop. By viewing the tidal flow-volume loops relative to the maximal flow-volume loop, it is easily apparent when the maximal flow-volume loop over a large percentage of tidal volume is reached (over 40–60% of tidal volume, expiratory flow meets maximal expiratory flow). However, by separate visual inspection of the flow-volume loops, it is difficult to quantify the magnitude of mechanical ventilatory limitation. More recently, techniques that more easily quantify mechanical ventilatory limitation have been developed, but they have not been validated for clinical use (7).

Calculating dynamic lung volumes estimated during exercise from inspiratory capacity (IC)—end-expiratory lung volume (EELV) and end-inspiratory lung volume (EILV)—can be used to assess mechanical ventilatory limitation. EELV and EILV, compared to resting lung volumes, indicate the degree of hyperinflation during exercise, which occurs with tidal expiratory limitation (14). When EELV $\geq$ resting FRC, and/or EILV $>$ 90% of TLC, expiratory airflow limitation may be a factor in mechanical ventilatory limitation.

Ventilatory Response Limitations

The normal exercise response of $\dot{V}_E$ is linear up to approximately 50% of peak exercise. Beyond this, $\dot{V}_E$ becomes nonlinear with $\dot{V}O_2$ or work rate. It is important to determine whether $\dot{V}_E$ is appropriate or excessive for the external work rate during the linear portion of the relationship. Increased ventilatory requirement increases ventilatory load on the respiratory system, which may already be limited. Increased demand also increases the likelihood of obtaining a "ventilatory ceiling" earlier during exertion. Identification of the cause of increased ventilatory demand (acidosis, hypoxemia, hyperventilation, dead space ventilation, etc.) is important because, in some cases, demand can be lowered therapeutically. If demand can be decreased, increased exercise function may be achieved (6).

Comparison to norms or normal data collected in your own laboratory can help determine the appropriateness of $\dot{V}_E$ per work rate (5, 6, 10). Figure 38.2 illustrates $\dot{V}_E$ displayed for interpretation. Note that the axes are expressed in relative units ($\dot{V}_E$ as a percentage of predicted MVV and $\dot{V}O_2$ as a percentage of predicted $\dot{V}O_2$max) making individual comparison easier (6). In addition, maximal and tidal flow-volume loops are shown. This type of representation may be helpful in determining whether $\dot{V}_E$ is within normal range.

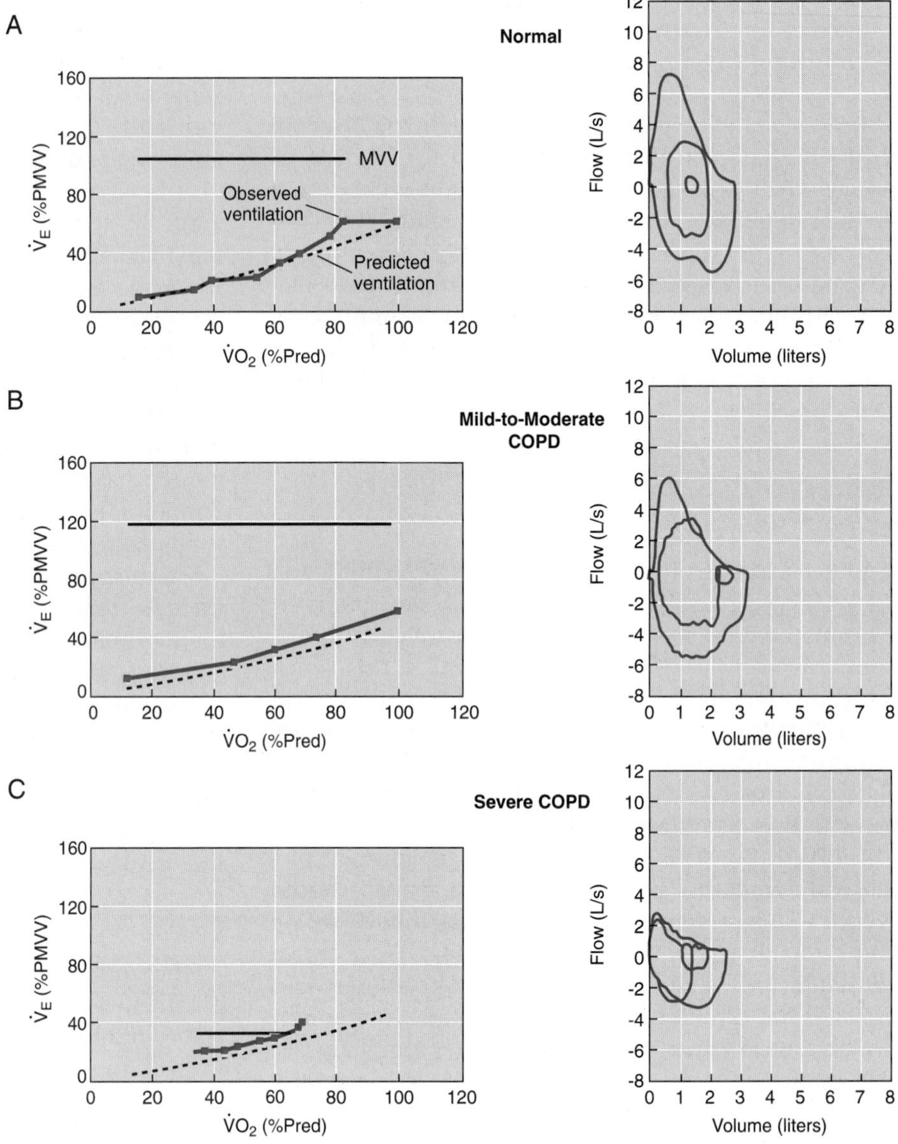

Figure 38.2. A, Determination of mechanical ventilatory limitation from ventilation-% predicted maximal voluntary ventilation ($\dot{V}_E$/%PMVV) ratio plotted against oxygen uptake ($\dot{V}O_2$, % predicted) and maximal and tidal flow-volume loops for individual with normal lung function. **B**, Mild-to-moderate chronic obstructive lung disease. **C**, Severe chronic obstructive lung disease. *Solid line* is observed results; *dotted line* is predicted relationship. Side Panels: Maximal flow-volume loop (large loop), tidal flow-volume loop at rest (smallest loop), and tidal flow-volume loop during maximal exercise (large loop inside maximal loop).

Another method for determining whether ventilatory demand is elevated is to determine ventilatory equivalents for oxygen and CO_2 ($\dot{V}_E/\dot{V}O_2$, and $\dot{V}_E/\dot{V}CO_2$, respectively). Normal $\dot{V}_E/\dot{V}O_2$ ratio is 20–30 up to an intensity of approximately 50–60% $\dot{V}O_2$max, after which it increases (5, 15). Normal $\dot{V}_E/\dot{V}CO_2$ is between 25–35; it does not increase significantly until near maximum. When ventilatory requirement is increased, these ratios may be near normal at rest, but increase disproportionately during exercise. In other cases, the ratios may be elevated at rest and decrease during exercise, though remaining above normal. Ventilatory equivalents may be elevated at rest because of hyperventilation which can be assessed by a respiratory exchange ratio (RER) near or exceeding 1.00. During exercise, ventilatory equivalents return to normal if the hyperventilation is secondary to anxiety or use of a mouthpiece.

The "break point" in the ventilatory response during exercise is referred to as the ventilatory threshold (VT) if it is determined from ventilatory variables. The VT may or may not be present in the pulmonary patient (16, 17). Absence of VT may be due to inability to exercise at an intensity sufficient to accumulate lactic acid or inability to hyperventilate. The most appropriate technique for determining VT in the pulmonary patient remains controversial (16–18).

In summary, it is important to know whether there is increased requirement for $\dot{V}_E$ and whether mechanical ventilatory limitation is reached. In addition, it is important to distinguish between mechanical ventilatory limitation during exercise and exercise limited by ventilation.

Breathing Pattern

Pattern of breathing is important because of the association with dead space ventilation (V_D/V_T) and economy of breathing. Increased $\dot{V}_E$ during low level exercise occurs primarily by increased V_T. During heavy exercise, increased breathing frequency (f_b) contributes more to increased $\dot{V}_E$. V_T at maximum exercise is approximately 50–60% of vital capacity. Breathing frequency is generally 35–50/minute and usually < 60/minute (19). Variations in breathing pattern, in combination with other exercise variables ($\dot{V}_E$ and gas exchange) can provide insight into the reason for the limitation (6, 20).

PULMONARY GAS EXCHANGE

Adequacy and efficiency of $\dot{V}_E$ is determined by pulmonary gas exchange. Any abnormality related to hypoventilation, the matching of $\dot{V}_E$ and perfusion in the lungs (maldistribution of $\dot{V}_E$ or perfusion), diffusion limitation in the lung, or right-to-left shunt alters gas exchange variables and is indicative of pulmonary disease. Hypoxemia can be caused by any of the four above abnormalities. Hypercapnia can be caused by hypoventilation and ventilation-perfusion mismatch and the presence of either at rest, or during exercise, indicates inadequate gas exchange (21). Several reviews on CPX testing or gas exchange in pulmonary patients discuss these abnormalities in the context of disease (5, 6, 11, 21–23).

To assess gas exchange, such measures as SaO_2, P_{ETCO2}, diffusing capacity (at rest), V_D/V_T using P_{ETCO2}, average expired CO_2 (P_{eCO2}), partial pressure of oxygen in arterial blood ($P_{a,O2}$), partial pressure of carbon dioxide in arterial blood ($P_{a,CO2}$), and A-a D_{O2} (with calculation of V_D/V_T) are all useful. When using these variables note rest abnormalities and exertional changes in the exercise test summary.

Saturation

SaO_2 can be determined noninvasively by pulse oximetry which, in most cases, is adequate during exercise. SaO_2 is generally stable during exercise at a value similar to the resting SaO_2 which varies with age (24). A saturation < 90% indicates significant hypoxemia. Assessment of SaO_2 during exercise on room air and, if desaturation occurs, with supplemental oxygen can determine appropriate level of supplemental oxygen.

End-Tidal CO_2

P_{ETCO2} is helpful in determining the adequacy of gas exchange (hypercapnia). Normal resting P_{ETCO2} is 36–42 mm Hg; it increases by 3–8 mm Hg during submaximal exercise, but decreases during heavy exercise. While P_{ETCO2} is not always accurate when compared with $P_{a,CO2}$, especially in pulmonary patients, the trend can be assessed with incremental exercise. If P_{ETCO2} changes, $P_{a,CO2}$ is also likely to be changed. Inadequate gas exchange may be one reason (5).

Arterial Blood Gases

Sampling arterial blood gases during exercise may be important to assess the accuracy of noninvasive measures such as SaO_2 or P_{ETCO2}. Multiple blood gas samples during incremental or constant load exercise are important for determining the adequacy of gas exchange. There is little change in $P_{a,O2}$ during exercise (± 10 mm Hg), but a significant decrease in $P_{a,O2}$ (> 20 mmHg) is associated with interstitial lung disease or pulmonary vascular disease. $P_{a,CO2}$ is usually stable up to 50–60% of maximal exercise capacity (36–42 mm Hg), but decreases progressively thereafter.

Alveolar-Arterial Oxygen Difference

A greater A-a D_{O2} results from decreased SaO_2 ($P_{a,O2}$), which is indicative of ventilation-perfusion mismatch, diffusion limitation, or right-to-left shunt. A-a D_{O2} is normally approximately 10 mm Hg (± 5 mm Hg) at rest and increases to about 20 mm Hg (±10 mm Hg) during exercise (24). In some patients with ventilation-perfusion mismatch (pulmonary fibrosis or pulmonary vascular disease), $P_{a,O2}$ decreases progressively as exercise intensity increases. However, if $P_{a,O2}$ decreases and A-a D_{O2} does not widen, desaturation usually indicates hypoventilation ($P_{a,CO2}$ may increase as well), which could result from mechanical ventilatory limitation.

Dead Space Ventilation

When blood gases are measured, it is possible to calculate V_D/V_T, an indicator of physiological dead space (21, 24). V_D/V_T is normally about 40% at rest and progressively declines (to about 20%) during exercise. It decreases with age (30% at rest) (5). In the pulmonary patient, V_D/V_T increases at rest and may not decrease during exercise (22). This increases ventilatory demand in the pulmonary patient, who already has reduced ventilatory capacity. It is caused by ventilation-perfusion mismatch or by abnormal breathing pattern (shallow breathing). It is important to determine the proportion of wasted $\dot{V}_E$ that must be overcome.

CARDIOVASCULAR RESPONSES TO EXERCISE

In most CPX testing, HR, ECG, and blood pressure should be monitored. HR and O_2 are strong indicators of cardiovascular function which may be limiting in known lung disease (11).

Maximum Heart Rate

Maximum heart rate (HR_{MAX}) is not normally attained by pulmonary patients because of ventilatory limitations or leg discomfort. HR_{MAX}, expressed as a percent of predicted maximum, is lower in pulmonary patients than in age matched individuals with normal pulmonary function (25). In contrast, $\dot{V}_E$/MVV ratio is higher (at a lower exercise intensity) than in normals. Although, HR is usually lower than normal at maximum exercise in severe pulmonary patients, it may be normal, or near normal, in patients with mild-to-moderate obstructive disease (26).

Oxygen Uptake-Work Rate Relationship

The $\dot{V}O_2$/work rate slope has been suggested as an indicator of cardiovascular status (11). In the absence of impaired cardiovascular status, HR-$\dot{V}O_2$ relationship is usually normal in pulmonary patients (26).

Hemodynamics

Although hemodynamic measurements may be difficult to obtain during exercise, they may be useful since changes may occur as a result of lung disease. Pulmonary patients usually have a normal cardiac output-$\dot{V}O_2$ relationship during exercise, but discontinue exercise at a lower level of cardiac output and $\dot{V}O_2$ than normal individuals (27). Although cardiac output is normal, stroke volume is lower and HR is higher in pulmonary patients at the same $\dot{V}O_2$. Pulmonary artery pressure may be normal or slightly increased at rest, though during exercise it is usually inappropriately high for the level of cardiac output. Thus, pulmonary patients have increased vascular resistance given a normal cardiac output response (26, 27). This increases the incidence of right ventricular dysfunction during exercise in pulmonary patients; severity of this dysfunction depends upon the acuity of the pulmonary disease. Pulmonary hypertension may be present at rest and worsen with exercise secondary to airflow limitation and decreased arterial blood gases. A minority of pulmonary patients demonstrate left ventricular dysfunction during exercise, although it is unclear whether this is related to concomitant coronary artery disease (27). Hypoxemia, acidosis, bulging of the intraventricular septum in the left ventricular cavity, alterations in intrathoracic pressure, as well as the markedly negative swings in pleural pressure during exercise have been proposed to contribute to the possibility of left ventricular function during exercise in pulmonary patients (27).

SHORTNESS OF BREATH

It is important to note the influence of distress and discomfort during CPX testing. In the pulmonary patient, it is particularly important to note the effect shortness of breath or breathlessness on exercise tolerance (6). The complaint of breathlessness during exercise may be the primary reason pulmonary patients seek medical attention and may also be the variable most often responsible for discontinuing exercise. Pulmonary patients may also be limited by leg fatigue (25). Furthermore, RPB and leg fatigue at peak exercise are similar between pulmonary patients and normals, although pulmonary patients are limited by breathlessness more frequently and at a significantly lower exercise capacity (25). It is important to assess perception of breathlessness throughout exercise (28). There appears to be some desensitization to the RPB with regular exercise training in pulmonary patients (28).

The Borg 0–10 scale and visual analog scale are commonly used to quantify breathlessness (25). These are valid, reliable, and responsive indicators (25, 28).

END OF TEST

Reasons for test termination are important to interpretation. The test summary should note the reason for termination, whether the test was a maximal test, whether the patient experienced distress or symptoms, who was responsible for stopping the test (i.e., patient, technician, or physician), and the maximum work load achieved.

▶ SUMMARY–INTERPRETATION

The interpretation of CPX testing should clearly indicate the following whether exercise tolerance was limited and the factors most likely involved in the limitation. If the reasons for limitations are unclear, then information from the CPX test may suggest appropriate clinical tests for follow-up. The interpretation of CPX testing is an art requiring an understanding of exercise physiology, integrative physiology, and clinical physiology.

References

1. American Thoracic Society. Evaluation of impairment/disability secondary to respiratory disorders. *Am Rev Respir Dis* 133:1205–1209, 1986.
2. American Thoracic Society. Lung function testing: Selection of reference values and interpretive strategies. *Am Rev Respir Dis* 144:1202–1218, 1991.
3. Enright PL, Hyatt RE. *Office Spirometry: A Practical Guide to the Selection and Use of Spirometers.* Philadelphia: Lea & Febiger, 1987:1–253.
4. Jones NL. *Clinical Exercise Testing.* Philadelphia: W.B. Saunders, 1988.
5. Wasserman K, Hansen JE, Sue DY, et al. *Principles of Exercise Testing and Interpretation.* Philadelphia: Lea & Febiger, 1987:261.
6. Younes M. Interpretation of clinical exercise testing in respiratory disease. *Clin Chest Med* 5:189–206, 1984.

7. Babb TG, Rodarte JR. Estimation of ventilatory capacity during submaximal exercise. *J Appl Physiol* 74:2016–2022, 1993.
8. Carter R, Peavler M, Zinkgraf S, et al. Predicting maximal exercise ventilation in patients with chronic obstructive pulmonary disease. *Chest* 92:253–259, 1987.
9. Dillard TA, Piantadosi S, Rajagopal KR. Prediction of ventilation at maximal exercise in chronic air-flow obstruction. *Am Rev Respir Dis* 132:230–235, 1985.
10. Levison H, Cherniack RM. Ventilatory cost of exercise in chronic obstructive pulmonary disease. *J Appl Physiol* 25: 21–27, 1968.
11. Sue DY, Wasserman K. Impact of integrative cardiopulmonary exercise testing on clinical decision making [Review]. *Chest* 99:981–992, 1991.
12. Becklake MR, Rodarte JR, Kalica AR, et al. Scientific issues in the assessment of respiratory impairment. *Am Rev Respir Dis* 137:1505–1510, 1988.
13. Dillard TA, Hnatiuk OW, McCumber TR. Maximum voluntary ventilation. Spirometric determinants in chronic obstructive pulmonary disease patients and normal subjects. *Am Rev Respir Dis* 147:870–875, 1993.
14. Babb TG, Viggiano R, Hurley B, et al. Effect of mild to moderate airflow limitation on exercise capacity. *J Appl Physiol* 70:223–230, 1991.
15. Ruppel GE. *Manual of Pulmonary Function Testing.* St Louis: Stamathis, 1994:1–505.
16. Patessio A, Casaburi R, Carone M, et al. Comparison of gas exchange, lactate, and lactic acidosis thresholds in patients with chronic obstructive pulmonary disease. *Am Rev Respir Dis* 148:622–626, 1993.
17. Sue DY, Wasserman K, Moricca RB, et al. Metabolic acidosis during exercise in patients with chronic obstructive pulmonary disease. Use of the V-slope method for anaerobic threshold determination. *Chest* 94:931–938, 1988.
18. Belman MJ, Epstein LJ, Doornbos D, et al. Noninvasive determinations of the anaerobic threshold. Reliability and validity in patients with COPD. *Chest* 102:1028–1034, 1992.
19. Blackie SP, Fairbarn MS, McElvaney MG, et al. Normal values and ranges for ventilation and breathing pattern at maximal exercise. *Chest* 100:136–142, 1991.
20. Gallagher CG, Younes M. Breathing pattern during and after maximal exercise in patients with chronic obstructive lung disease, interstitial lung disease, and cardiac disease, and in normal subjects. *Am Rev Respir Dis* 133:581–586, 1986.
21. West JB. Assessing pulmonary gas exchange [editorial]. *N Engl J Med* 316:1336–1338, 1987.
22. Jones NL, Berman LB. Gas exchange in chronic air-flow obstruction. *Am Rev Respir Dis* 129:S81–S83, 1984.
23. Wagner PD, Rodriguez-Roisin R. Clinical advances in pulmonary gas exchange. *Am Rev Respir Dis* 143:883–888, 1991.
24. Jones NL. Normal values for pulmonary gas exchange during exercise. *Am Rev Respir Dis* 129:S44–S46, 1984.
25. Killian KJ, Leblanc P, Martin DH, et al. Exercise capacity and ventilatory, circulatory, and symptom limitation in patients with chronic airflow limitation. *Am Rev Respir Dis* 146:935–940, 1992.
26. Gallagher CG. Exercise and chronic obstructive pulmonary disease. *Med Clin North Am* 74:619–641, 1990.
27. Macnee W. Pathophysiology of core pulmonale in chronic obstructive pulmonary disease: Part One. *Am J Respir Crit Care Med* 150:833–852, 1994.
28. Mahler DA, Horowitz MB. Perception of breathlessness during exercise in patients with respiratory disease. *Med Sci Sports Exerc* 26:1078–1081, 1994.

Suggested Readings

Johnson BD, Scanlon PD, Beck KC. Regulation of ventilatory capacity during exercise in asthmatics. *J Appl Physiol* 79:892–901, 1995.

Jones NL, Robertson DG, Kane JW. Difference between end-tidal and arterial PCO_2 in exercise. *J Appl Physiol* 47:954–960, 1979.

Macnee W. Pathophysiology of core pulmonale in chronic obstructive pulmonary disease: Part One. *Am J Respir Crit Care Med* 150:833–852, 1994.

Mahler DA, Horowitz MB. Perception of breathlessness during exercise in patients with respiratory disease. *Med Sci Sports Exerc* 26:1078–1081, 1994.

Marciniuk DD, Sridhar G, Clemens RE, et al. Lung volumes and expiratory flow limitation during exercise in interstitial lung disease. *J Appl Physiol* 77:963–973, 1994.

Younes M, Kivinen G. Respiratory mechanics and breathing pattern during and following maximal exercise. *J Appl Physiol* 57:1773–1782, 1984.

54 86 427, 433 357, 363

 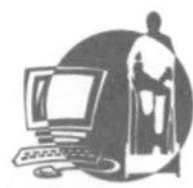  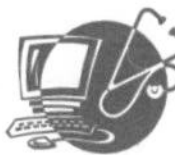

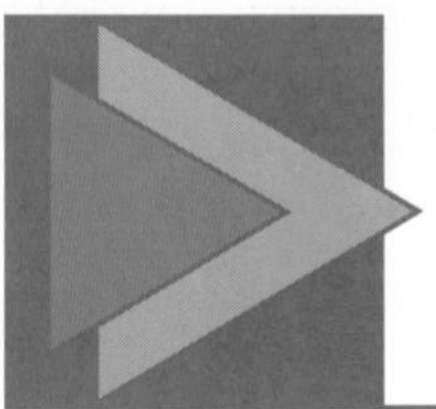

CHAPTER 39

Special Considerations for Exercise Training in Chronic Lung Disease

Richard Casaburi

Key to Pulmonary Physiology Abbreviations

COPD	Chronic obstructive pulmonary disease
$P_{a,CO2}$	Partial pressure of carbon dioxide in arterial blood
$P_{a,O2}$	Partial pressure of oxygen in arterial blood
$\dot{V}CO_2$	Rate of carbon dioxide production
V_D/V_T	Ratio of ventilatory dead space to tidal volume
$\dot{V}_E$	Expired minute ventilation

Before the 1950s, the general consensus was that patients with chronic, symptomatic lung disease should avoid physical activity. For these patients, exercise elicits dyspnea, a sensation of uncomfortable shortness of breath. However, unlike other unpleasant sensations (e.g., cardiac angina), dyspnea does not signal tissue damage. Beginning with the pioneering work of Alvan Barach, it has been demonstrated that patients with chronic lung disease benefit from physical activity (1).

The tendency of most patients with lung disease is to gradually decrease activity level. By the time they present for medical attention, patients are often sedentary and capable of only low level activity (2). For these patients, an organized exercise program is often of great benefit. Knowledge regarding exercise benefits and the prescription of exercise in patients with chronic lung disease has accumulated rapidly in recent years. However, most research concerns a single disease entity: chronic obstructive pulmonary disease (COPD). This chapter focuses on exercise training in COPD. In addition, the final section presents what is known regarding other chronic lung diseases.

THE PULMONARY REHABILITATION PROGRAM MODEL

Though an exercise program may be prescribed as an isolated intervention, most commonly a coordinated program of pulmonary rehabilitation is prescribed. Table 39.1 lists components usually included in such a program. This therapy is administered by a multidisciplinary team often including a pulmonary physician, a nurse coordinator, physical, occupational and respiratory therapists, a dietician and an exercise specialist. Comprehensive pulmonary rehabilitation programs are generally 4–6 weeks in duration with half-day sessions held three times per week. As exercise programs are acknowledged to be of central importance, it is common to have 1–1.5 hours devoted to exercise in each rehabilitation session.

PSYCHOLOGICAL BENEFITS OF EXERCISE PROGRAMS

Two distinct strategies, physiological and psychological, have been defined for improving exercise tolerance in patients with lung disease. The psychological approach posits that patients can be desensitized to the symptom of exertional dyspnea (3). To date, the most effective method to achieve this desensitization is a program of regular exercise. The desensitizing effects of exercise have been explained in several ways (4):

- The antidepressant hypothesis holds that patients successfully participating in an exercise program gain positive feedback from mastering something perceived as being difficult.
- The social interaction hypothesis implies that progressive exercise in a supervised program with others having similar debilities calms unrealistic fears. This explanation is consistent with the generally inferior results obtained from home exercise programs.
- The distraction hypothesis theorizes that dyspneic stimuli are perceived as less intense when attention is focused on non-dyspneic stimuli. Thus listening to music or exercising with a group of people distracts patients from dyspneic sensations.

Psychological benefits from an exercise program can be substantial, though there are few established guidelines to define the most efficient exercise program parameters to achieve this goal. Intuitively, the setting, the exercise partners and an experienced and dedicated rehabilitation staff are important. Precise frequency, duration and intensity targets may be of lesser importance.

Table 39.1. Components of a Pulmonary Rehabilitation Program

Assessment
Education
Optimization of medical therapy
Psychosocial support
Exercise training
Chest physical therapy
Controlled breathing techniques
Nutritional therapy
Continuing care programs

PHYSIOLOGICAL FACTORS LIMITING EXERCISE TOLERANCE IN COPD

Patients with COPD of moderate or greater severity are often **ventilatory limited** in exercise tolerance (exercise terminates because pulmonary ventilation cannot be increased to meet physiological demand). Several physiological abnormalities conspire to yield reduced exercise tolerance. Breathing reserve is the difference between the maximal pulmonary ventilation that can be sustained and peak ventilation achieved during a maximal exercise test. In healthy subjects, breathing reserve is high, whereas in COPD patients it is low. Breathing reserve is low both because the ability to ventilate the lung is low and the ventilatory requirement for a given level of exercise is high. Amelioration of either abnormality predictably improves exercise tolerance. COPD is associated with four physiological deficits that impair exercise tolerance:

1. *Impaired Lung Mechanics.* Airways resistance is high during expiration leading to high work of breathing. Further, airways tend to close as expiration proceeds and progressive hyperinflation ensues. This puts the respiratory muscles (especially the diaphragm) at a mechanical disadvantage. As a result, the respiratory muscles tend to fatigue at relatively low levels of exercise.
2. *Inefficient Pulmonary Gas Exchange.* The factors dictating the level of ventilation ($\dot{V}_E$) required for a given level of exercise can be understood by considering the alveolar mass balance equation for CO_2 (5):

$$\dot{V}_E = \frac{k\,\dot{V}CO_2}{P_{a,CO2}\,(1 - V_D/V_T)}$$

where: $\dot{V}CO_2$ = rate of CO_2 output
$P_{a,CO2}$ = partial pressure of arterial CO_2
V_D/V_T = fraction of the tidal volume (V_T) that is not effective in expelling CO_2 from the lung k is a constant.

In COPD, V_D/V_T is often high during exercise because emphysematous airspaces are ventilated, but poorly perfused (alveolar dead space). If the patient experiences clinically significant hypoxemia during exercise ($P_{a,O2}$ < approximately 60 torr), the carotid bodies are stimulated resulting in increased ventilatory drive (and lower $P_{a,CO2}$). Note, however, that many patients with COPD employ a compensatory mechanism which reduces ventilatory requirement at a given level of exercise. Rather than maintaining a constant $P_{a,CO2}$, it drifts upward with exercise (CO_2 retention) allowing a lower level of ventilation, albeit at a cost of a lower arterial pH (6).

3. *Pulmonary Vascular Insufficiency.* In COPD patients with extensive alveolar destruction, pulmonary vasculature is also destroyed. Rather than recruiting pulmonary capillaries during exercise, resulting in decreased pulmonary vascular resistance, recruitment is limited and pulmonary artery pressure rises resulting in increased right heart work. If the right heart is unable respond adequately, cardiac output is inappropriately low and oxygen delivery to exercising muscle is sacrificed. Whether this is an important mechanism of exercise intolerance in COPD is unclear; most studies demonstrate that COPD patients do not have an abnormally low cardiac output response for a given level of exercise (7).
4. *Abnormal Skeletal Muscle Metabolism.* Increasing evidence shows that part of exercise intolerance experienced by COPD patients may be due to abnormalities in exercising muscle. Several potential mechanisms of muscle dysfunction are present. COPD patients lead a sedentary life, therefore **deconditioning** is a likely factor (2). It has been posited that **malnutrition** contributes to muscle wasting that is frequently documented (8). **Low levels of anabolic hormones** are observed in ambulatory COPD patients (9). Both the growth hormone axis and the sex steroid axis seem to be abnormal; the resultant failure to provide anabolic stimuli to the muscle may result in decreased muscle mass. Finally, it is plausible that there is a primary **skeletal muscle myopathy** associated with chronic lung disease. Oral corticosteroid therapy and perhaps chronic hypoxemia may result in maladaptive changes in muscle structure and function (10).

DESIGN OF EXERCISE TRAINING PROGRAMS FOR COPD PATIENTS

Substantial literature reports the results of exercise programs for COPD patients including a comprehensive review (11, 12). Three conclusions can be drawn from these studies:

1. Patients completing an exercise program generally feel that exercise tolerance has increased.
2. On effort-dependent measures of exercise endurance, performance is generally better.

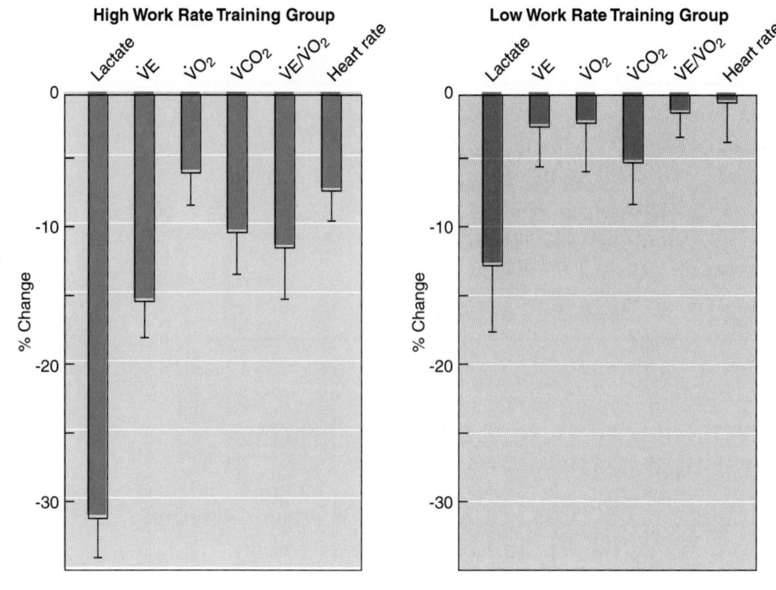

Figure 39.1. Changes in the physiological responses to an identical exercise task (a constant work rate test at a high exercise intensity) produced by two exercise training strategies in patients with COPD. The left panel shows the changes of responses in a group (N = 11) who trained at a high work rate; the right panel presents responses of a similar group (N = 8) who trained at a lower intensity but for a longer session duration so that total work per session was identical irrespective of group assignment. Vertical bars are 1 SEM. Decreases in blood lactate, ventilation, O_2 uptake, CO_2 output, ventilatory equivalent for O_2 and heart rate are observed for both training regimens, but decreases are appreciably greater for the high work rate training group. (Reproduced with permission from Casaburi R, Patessio A, Ioli F, et al. Reduction in exercise lactic acidosis and ventilation as a result of exercise training in obstructive lung disease. Am Rev Respir Dis 143:9, 1991.)

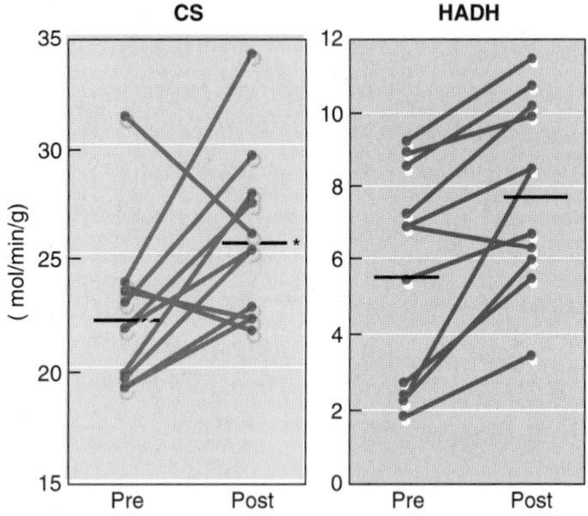

Figure 39.2. Eleven patients with severe COPD underwent a rigorous program of exercise training. Before and after training, patients underwent percutaneous biopsy of the vastus lateralis muscle. The activity of the oxidative enzymes citrate synthase (CS) and 3-hyroxyacyl-CoA dehydrogenase (HADH) increased significantly as a result of training (*$p<0.05$, †$p<0.01$). The activity of three glycolytic enzymes did not change significantly. These results show that skeletal muscle oxidative capacity of COPD patients improves after a rigorous exercise program. (Reproduced with permission from Maltais F, LeBlanc P, Simard C, et al. Skeletal muscle adaptations to endurance training in patients with COPD. Am J Resp Crit Care Med 154:442–447, 1996.)

3. These benefits cannot be traced to improvements in disease severity; lung function is not improved.

However, a careful examination of this literature shows that there are few controlled studies, the design of exercise programs varies widely, and the adequacy of the program is difficult to evaluate (12). In particular, exercise was performed on non-calibrated devices and intensity was "increased as tolerated." Moreover, outcome measures in most studies have been effort dependent (e.g., timed walking tests) (13). As a result, most published literature cannot be used to determine the parameters of an exercise program that are effective in improving the physiological ability to exercise.

More recently, however, several studies confirm that COPD patients can, indeed, achieve a physiological training effect from a well-designed program of exercise training. Casaburi et al. demonstrated that patients with predominantly moderate COPD respond to a program of high intensity training with reduced levels of blood lactate and pulmonary ventilation at a given heavy work rate (Fig. 39.1) (14). The same group demonstrated that a vigorous training program for patients with severe COPD results in improved exercise tolerance and evidence of improved muscle function (including more rapid oxygen uptake kinetics following onset of exercise) (15). Maltais et al. recently demonstrated increased aerobic enzyme concentrations (with muscle biopsy) as a result of vigorous training (Fig. 39.2) (16).

SAFETY CONSIDERATIONS

Patients with chronic lung disease, are often elderly and may have high co-existing impairment of other organ systems. This is especially true of patients with COPD. Such patients require systematic assessment before assuming the safety of an exercise program. An evaluation by a physician including medical history, physical examination, basic blood tests (hematology and chemistry), chest x-ray, and a resting electrocardiogram (ECG) is prudent. A recent pulmonary function test and arterial blood gas analysis can serve as objective evidence of disease severity. Patients should be in a stable phase of the disease and pharmacological therapy should be maximized. Since cigarette smoking is self-destructive behavior and may subvert the therapeutic environment of the group, most programs do not accept participants who have not stopped smoking. Referral to a smoking cessation program, prior to undertaking an exercise program, is appropriate.

A cardiopulmonary exercise test is appropriate in a preprogram evaluation (17). Serial 12-lead ECGs allow detection of cardiac arrhythmias or ischemia that might contraindicate vigorous exercise. Pulse oximetry can detect exercise induced hypoxemia. If arterial oxygen saturation drops below approximately 90%, supplemental oxygen (via nasal cannula) should be prescribed during exercise. However, pulse oximetry is not always accurate and it is sometimes advisable to sample arterial blood during exercise. If arterial oxygen falls below 55 torr during exercise, supplemental oxygen should be prescribed. Some authorities give supplemental oxygen to patients with lesser degrees of hypoxemia in the hope that exercise tolerance will be improved and the training program will be more effective; however this strategy has not been validated. Cardiopulmonary exercise testing can also be used to establish an exercise intensity prescription (see below). If testing is repeated after exercise training, an objective measure of improvement is available.

CHARACTERISTICS OF AN EFFECTIVE TRAINING PROGRAM

Empiric evidence concerning the optimal characteristics of an exercise training program in patients with lung disease is not available. However, certain extrapolations from the response of healthy subjects seem warranted. An aerobic training response can only be expected if the training modality involves large muscle groups. Walking, cycling, stair climbing and swimming, for example, are likely to be effective modalities. Although upper extremity exercise involves a smaller muscle mass, upper extremity training may assist patients in performing activities of daily living (e.g., hair combing) and may also improve function of accessory muscles of respiration (18, 19). Training the muscles of respiration (e.g., by breathing against a resistance) has been extensively investigated, but has not generally been demonstrated to improve exercise capacity (20).

It seems reasonable to include 3–5 sessions per week with at least 30 minutes of exercise per session, since these parameters are effective in healthy subjects. Programs should last at least 5 weeks, preferably longer. Once an aerobic training effect has been achieved, it is necessary to pursue a maintenance program or the benefits are lost within a few weeks.

THE SPECIAL PROBLEM OF EXERCISE INTENSITY PRESCRIPTION

Intensity prescriptions suitable for healthy elderly subjects or even patients with other chronic diseases cannot be used for patients with chronic lung disease. Criteria based on heart rate or oxygen uptake are especially problematic. Since patients with chronic lung disease are usually ventilatory limited, peak effort is associated with a heart rate and $\dot{V}O_2$ less than predicted levels. Standard criteria that dictate exercise intensity (e.g., 70% of **predicted** maximum heart rate or $\dot{V}O_2$) may well be above peak exercise tolerance. On the other hand, a prescription based on a similar percentage of the **observed** peak heart rate or $\dot{V}O_2$ may lead to unreasonably low intensity targets (e.g., below unloaded pedaling requirements). Calculating heart rate reserve may not be appropriate since resting heart rate is often increased and varies considerably day-to-day.

Casaburi et al. proposed using the lactic acidosis threshold for establishing a minimum training intensity target in patients with COPD (21). However, an appreciable number of patients with severe COPD do not manifest elevated blood lactate levels at the highest tolerable work rate. Recently, however, it has been demonstrated that vigorous exercise elicits evidence of a physiological training effect in these patients (15).

A more practical approach was suggested by Ries and coworkers (22, 23). Patients with COPD are able to tolerate high fractions of peak exercise tolerance for prolonged periods of time. A reasonable procedure is to perform an incremental exercise test on a calibrated ergometer prior to initiating a training program. The target work rate can be selected as 85% of the peak work rate observed in the incremental test. If exercise is not to be performed on a calibrated cycle ergometer, the heart rate associated with a work rate equal to 85% of the peak work rate during the incremental test is noted and this is used as the heart rate target. Occasionally, this initial target may require adjustment, up or down, by the rehabilitation therapist at the onset of the exercise program. Further, it may be appropriate to allow the patient to break the exercise session into two or more portions during the initial few sessions.

It is common practice in some rehabilitation programs to prescribe exercise intensity strictly on rating of perceived exertion. It seems unlikely that such a subjective criterion can reliably result in an exercise stimulus sufficient to elicit a physiological training effect. If physiological benefits are the goal of the training program, perceived exertion is not an adequate yardstick for exercise intensity.

STRENGTH VERSUS ENDURANCE TRAINING

Most research investigating the benefits of exercise for patients with lung disease uses cardiovascular endurance training, despite the fact that many rehabilitative exercise programs include a strength training component. The rationale usually given for emphasizing endurance activity is that impaired endurance severely decreases quality of life (e.g., inability to walk in the park). However, decreased strength may lead to significant disability as well. Deceased leg strength is associated with falls in the elderly, which frequently lead to broken bones and substantial morbidity (24). Further study is required before specific recommendations for strength training in patients with lung disease can be presented.

CONSIDERATIONS IN PATIENTS WITH LUNG DISEASE OTHER THAN COPD

Patients with chronic restrictive lung diseases, such as those with chest wall deformity, pneumoconiosis or rheumatological lung disease, often receive rehabilitative exercise training alongside the COPD patients. Though patients with restrictive lung disease may benefit from different training strategies, little research is available to define optimal therapeutic programs for this diverse patient group (25).

Other groups of patients with lung disease are generally treated in separate rehabilitative settings. Cystic fibrosis patients are generally young and various exercise modalities has been reported successful, although secretion clearance and infection management are continuing concerns (26). Asthmatics are often asymptomatic (or minimally symptomatic) between exacerbations providing an opportunity for a vigorous exercise training (27). Lung and heart-lung transplantation (and, more recently, lung volume reduction surgery) has led to the design of exercise programs for the preoperative and postoperative period (2, 28). Occasionally, exercise training is so effective that transplantation is no longer indicated. Finally, facilities have been established to care for patients dependent on mechanical ventilation. Exercise programs are a part of therapy designed to improve quality of life and decrease reliance on ventilatory support (29).

▶ SUMMARY

Exercise training is an established component of pulmonary rehabilitation programs. Exercise training is an effective modality for increasing functional capacity in patients with lung disease, particularly COPD, and physiological adaptation to exercise training has been demonstrated as a result of these programs. In addition, psychological adaptation may play a significant role in the process. Although the intensity of exercise prescription is not easily established, the safety of exercise training in COPD can be determined through proper evaluation and assessment. While the effects of exercise training in other types of lung disease are not as well established, it appears that exercise may be beneficial in these patients as well.

References

1. Barach AL, HA Bickerman, G Beck. Advances in the treatment of non-tuberculous pulmonary disease. *Bull NY Acad Med* 28:353, 1952.
2. Casaburi R: Deconditioning. In: Fishman AP, ed. *Pulmonary Rehabilitation. Lung Biology in Health and Disease Series.* New York: Marcel Dekker, 1996:213.
3. O'Donnell DE, McGuire M, Samis L, et al. The impact of exercise reconditioning on breathlessness in severe chronic airflow limitation. *Am J Respir Crit Care Med* 152:2005, 1995.
4. Haas F, Salazar-Schicchi J, Axen R. Desensitization to dyspnea in chronic obstructive pulmonary disease. In: Casaburi R, Petty TL, eds. *Principles and Practice of Pulmonary Rehabilitation.* Philadelphia: Saunders, 1993:241.
5. Casaburi R. Mechanisms of the reduced ventilatory requirement as a result of exercise training. *Eur Respir Rev* 4: 42, 1995.
6. Barstow TJ, Casaburi R. Ventilatory control in lung disease. In: Casaburi R, Petty TL, eds. *Principles and Practice of Pulmonary Rehabilitation.* Philadelphia: Saunders, 1993:50.
7. Morrison DA, Zuckerman BD. Cardiovascular consequences of chronic obstructive pulmonary disease. In: Casaburi R, Petty TL, eds. *Principles and Practice of Pulmonary Rehabilitation.* Philadelphia: Saunders, 1993:50.
8. Schols AM, Soeters PB, Dingemans AM, et al. Prevalence and characteristics of nutritional depletion in patients with stable COPD eligible for pulmonary rehabilitation. *Am Rev Respir Dis* 147:1151, 1993.
9. Casaburi R, Goren S, Bhasin S. Substantial prevalence of low anabolic hormone levels in COPD patients undergoing rehabilitation. *Am J Respir Crit Care Med* 153:A128, 1996.
10. Decramer M, Lacquet LM, Fagard R, et al. Corticosteroids contribute to muscle weakness in chronic airflow obstruction. *Am J Respir Crit Care Med* 150:11, 1994.
11. Ries AL. The scientific basis of pulmonary rehabilitation. *J Cardiopulm Rehabil* 10:418, 1990.
12. Casaburi R. Exercise training in chronic obstructive lung disease. In: Casaburi R, Petty TL, eds. *Principles and Practice of Pulmonary Rehabilitation.* Philadelphia: Saunders, 1993: 204.
13. Steele B. Timed walking tests of exercise capacity in chronic cardiopulmonary illness. *J Cardiopulm Rehabil* 16:25, 1996.
14. Casaburi R, Patessio A, Ioli F, et al. Reduction in exercise lactic acidosis and ventilation as a result of exercise training in obstructive lung disease. *Am Rev Respir Dis* 143:9, 1991.
15. Casaburi R, Porszasz J, Burns MR, et al. Physiologic benefits of exercise training in rehabilitation of severe COPD patients. *Am J Respir Crit Care Med* 155:1541–1551, 1996.
16. Maltais F, LeBlanc P, Simard C, et al. Skeletal muscle adaptation to endurance training in patients with COPD. *Am J Respir Crit Care Med* 42–447.

SECTION EIGHT

HEALTH AND FITNESS

SECTION EDITOR: *Moira Kelsey, RN, MS*

103 111, 113, 115 371

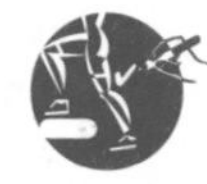

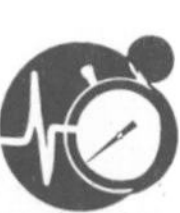

CHAPTER **40**

Pre-participation Health Appraisal in the Nonmedical Setting

Neil F. Gordon

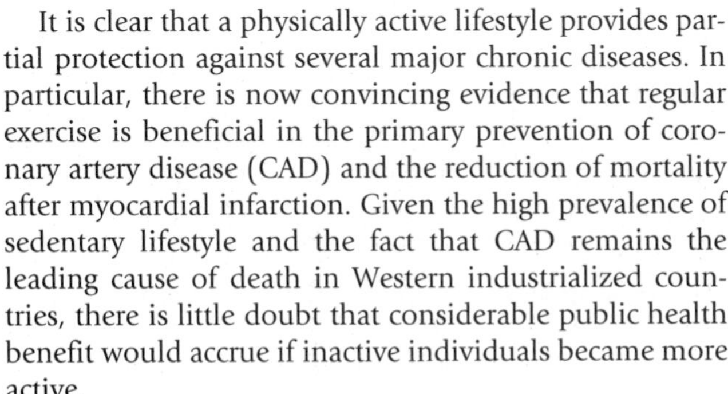

It is clear that a physically active lifestyle provides partial protection against several major chronic diseases. In particular, there is now convincing evidence that regular exercise is beneficial in the primary prevention of coronary artery disease (CAD) and the reduction of mortality after myocardial infarction. Given the high prevalence of sedentary lifestyle and the fact that CAD remains the leading cause of death in Western industrialized countries, there is little doubt that considerable public health benefit would accrue if inactive individuals became more active.

The many health-related benefits of a physically active lifestyle are well documented. However, it is essential to realize that to be most efficacious, regular exercise must be combined with other positive lifestyle interventions and, where applicable, with appropriate medical therapy. Furthermore, although exercise is extremely safe for most individuals, it is prudent to take certain precautions to optimize the benefit-to-risk ratio.

To ensure an optimal benefit-to-risk ratio, the exercise professional should incorporate some form of health appraisal before performing fitness testing or initiating an exercise program. The purpose of such an appraisal is to provide information relevant to the safety of fitness testing before beginning exercise training, to identify known diseases and risk factors for CAD and other potentially preventable chronic diseases so that appropriate lifestyle interventions can be initiated, and to identify additional factors that require special consideration when developing an appropriate exercise prescription and programming that optimize adherence, minimize risks, and maximize benefits.

It is essential that the pre-participation health appraisal be both cost-effective and time-efficient so that unnecessary barriers to exercise can be avoided. The precise nature and extent of the appraisal should be determined by the age, sex, and perceived health status characteristics of the participants, as well as the available economic, personnel and equipment resources. Health appraisals can range from a short questionnaire to interviews and sophisticated computerized evaluations.

This chapter presents information that may be incorporated into a health appraisal for

- Safety of exercise
- Health behaviors and risk factors
- Other special considerations for exercise prescription and programming

SAFETY OF EXERCISE

Most prospective participants in exercise programs conducted in nonmedical settings are apparently healthy individuals whose goals are to enhance fitness and well-being, reduce weight, and reduce risk for chronic disease. For such individuals, the primary safety goal of a pre-participation health appraisal is to identify individuals who should receive further medical evaluation to determine whether there are contraindications to exercise testing or training, or whether referral to a medically supervised exercise program is necessary.

According to ACSM guidelines, asymptomatic, apparently healthy men under age 40 and women under age 50, with fewer than two CAD risk factors, do not require medical evaluation by a physician before initiating a program of vigorous exercise training (i.e., exercise intensity $> 60\%$ $\dot{V}O_2max$) (1). It is also considered unnecessary for asymptomatic apparently healthy men and women, irrespective of age or CAD risk factor status, to have a medical evaluation by a physician before embarking on a program of moderate exercise training (i.e., exercise intensity 40–60% $\dot{V}O_2max$) (1). For such individuals, pre-participation screening can be accomplished using validated self-administered questionnaires, such as the Physical Activity Readiness Questionnaire (PAR-Q).

Although there are many questionnaires available for pre-exercise screening, the PAR-Q is well developed and has a sensitivity of nearly 100% and specificity of ap-

Table 40.1. Physical Activity Readiness Questionnaire: Matching Questions of Original and Revised Versions

Original	Revised
1. Has your doctor ever said you have heart trouble?	1. Has your doctor ever said that you have a heart condition and that you should only do physical activity recommended by a doctor?
2. Do you frequently have pains in your heart and chest?	2. Do you feel pain in your chest when you do physical activity?
3. Do you often feel faint or have spells of severe dizziness?	4. Do you lose your balance because of dizziness or do you ever lose consciousness?
4. Has a doctor ever said your blood pressure was too high?	6. Is your doctor currently prescribing drugs (for example, water pills) for your blood pressure or heart condition?
5. Has your doctor ever told you that you have a bone or joint problem such as arthritis that has been aggravated by exercise or might be made worse with exercise?	5. Do you have a bone or joint problem that could be made worse by a change in your physical activity?
6. Is there a good physical reason not mentioned here why you should not follow an activity program even if you wanted to?	7. Do you know of any other reason why you should not do physical activity?
7. Are you over 65 and not accustomed to vigorous exercise?	(No matching question. Introductory comments state: If you are over 69 years of age, and you are not used to being very active, check with your doctor.)
(No matching question)	3. In the past month, have you had chest pain when you were not doing physical activity?

proximately 80% for detecting medical contraindications to exercise (2). (When used in this context, **sensitivity** refers to the percent of persons with medical contraindications to exercise who answer "yes" to one or more questions; **specificity** refers to the percent of persons without medical contraindications to exercise who answer "no" to all questions.) The PAR-Q is only one example of a pre-exercise screening questionnaire; limitations of this questionnaire are discussed below. The responsibility of adding to or modifying the pre-exercise screening tool lies with the director of the exercise program and should be determined primarily by the population served.

Despite the obvious ease of use and cost-effectiveness of the PAR-Q, several important limitations exist when it is used in the original format. These limitations, which should be kept in mind, include:

1. The less than desirable specificity for detecting contraindications to exercise.
2. Limited sensitivity (approximately 35%) and specificity (approximately 80%) for predicting subsequent exercise electrocardiogram (ECG) abnormalities.
3. Inability to screen out persons with two or more major CAD risk factors (who require a medical examination before participation in vigorous exercise).
4. Automatic referral for medical evaluation by a physician of asymptomatic, apparently healthy individuals over age 65, even if participation in moderate exercise is the goal.
5. Inability to identify medications that may affect exercise safety.
6. Inability to identify pregnant women, for whom special safety precautions may be required.
7. From an overall health perspective, the absence of questions aimed at the identification of adverse health behaviors other than a sedentary lifestyle.

Recognition of such limitations of the PAR-Q has led to several revisions of the questionnaire (1–3). The original and newest revision of the PAR-Q are shown in Table 40.1. The significance/clarification of each of the question in the new version of the PAR-Q is outlined in Table 40.2. This revised version enhances the specificity for detecting contraindications to exercise and thereby minimizes unnecessary medical referrals (3). It is important to note differences in phrasing of questions, so customized questionnaires may be developed within various settings that meet the needs of individual programs. Customized questionnaires can be developed to address the limited capability of the PAR-Q, to obtain information about risk factors, personal history, health behaviors, and to obtain other information that may warrant special considerations.

PERSONAL HEALTH HISTORY AND CAD RISK FACTORS

In addition to readiness/safety of exercise, it is important for exercise professionals to assess other aspects of personal health history and risk factors for chronic diseases, in particular, CAD (which constitutes the leading cause of death in Western industrialized countries, including exertion-related sudden death). Because several risk factors for CAD (discussed elsewhere in this book) and other chronic diseases are behavior-dependent, health behaviors of participants should be assessed. The PAR-Q touches on several risk factors for CAD; however, it is designed to determine the safety of exercise, not the overall risk for CAD. The following includes additional information on aspects of the personal health history and risk factors that should be identified to further clarify the risk for events during exercise, prioritize interventions, and encourage changes in lifestyle to re-

Table 40.2. Physical Activity Readiness Questionnaire (PAR-Q)

For most people, physical activity should not pose any problem or hazard. PAR-Q has been designed to identify the small number of adults for whom physical activity might be inappropriate or those who should have medical advice concerning the type of activity most suitable.

1. Has a doctor ever said that you have a heart condition *and* that you should only do physical activity recommended by a doctor?
   (**Significance/Clarification:** Persons with known heart disease are at increased risk for cardiac complications during exercise. They should consult a physician and undergo exercise testing before starting an exercise program. The exercise prescription should be formulated in accordance with standard guidelines for cardiac patients. Medical supervision may be required during exercise training.)
2. Do you feel pain in your chest when you do physical activity?
3. In the past month, have you had chest pain when you were not doing physical activity?
   (**Significance/Clarification:** A physician should be consulted to identify the cause of the chest pain, whether it occurs at rest or with exertion. If ischemic in origin, the condition should be stabilized before starting an exercise program. Exercise testing should be performed with the patient on his or her usual medication and the exercise prescription formulated in accordance with standard guidelines for cardiac patients. Medical supervision may be required during exercise training.)
4. Do you lose your balance because of dizziness or do you ever lose consciousness?
   (**Significance/Clarification:** A physician should be consulted to establish the cause of these symptoms which may be related to potentially life-threatening medical conditions. Exercise training should not be undertaken until serious cardiac disorders have been excluded.)
5. Do you have a bone or joint problem that could be made worse by a change in your physical activity?
   (**Significance/Clarification:** Existing musculoskeletal disorders may be exacerbated by inappropriate exercise training. Persons with forms of arthritis known to be associated with a systemic component (for example, rheumatoid arthritis) may be at an increased risk for exercise-related medical complications. A physician should be consulted to determine whether any special precautions are required during exercise training.)
6. Is your doctor currently prescribing drugs (for example, water pills) for your blood pressure or heart condition?
   (**Significance/Clarification:** See question 1. Medication effects should be considered when formulating the exercise prescription. The exercise prescription should be formulated in accorance with guidelines for the specific cardiovascular disease for which medications are being used. A physician should be consulted to determine whether the condition/factor requires special precautions during exercise training or contraindicates exercise training.)
7. Do you know of any other reason why you should not do physical activity?
   (**Significance/Clarification:** The exercise prescription may need to be modified in accordance with the specific reason provided. Depending on the specific reason, a physician may need to be consulted.)

If a person answers yes to any question, vigorous exercise or exercise testing may need to be postponed. Medical clearance may be necessary.

duce disease risk. The information may also be important in developing or modifying the exercise program.

Personal History

A personal health history can be quite extensive and may require medically trained professionals for interpretation. As a part of an overall health risk appraisal, personal history should be tailored to emphasize specific factors that help categorize an individual in regard to several broad areas. The most important areas are those of **known diseases** and **manifestation of symptoms** (symptomatic or asymptomatic). Beyond this stratification is documentation concerning whether a symptom-free individual is at **high risk for the future development of disease.** Some of this information is identified on the PAR-Q, however, in certain instances, more information may be beneficial.

Evidence of **known cardiovascular disease** or of **symptoms of cardiovascular disease,** such as angina pectoris, must be documented. Symptoms of peripheral vascular disease, particularly discomfort in one or both legs with walking, should also be determined and documented. A history of **respiratory disease** should be determined as well. Seasonal difficulties with breathing or breathing discomfort brought on by physical or emotional stress warrant particular attention.

Diabetes is an independent contributor to the risk of cardiovascular disease development, with the relative risk being higher in women than men (4). This excessive risk includes CAD, peripheral vascular disease, and congestive heart failure. Diabetes is a metabolic disease which requires specific diet and exercise therapy alone or in combination with prescribed medications (see Chapter 10 of *ACSM's Guidelines for Exercise Testing and Prescription*).

Obesity is a common problem and is an independent risk factor for the development of CAD and is frequently a predecessor of Type 2 diabetes (5). Body composition measurement is thoroughly discussed elsewhere in this book. The exercise professional must be able to identify the individual who is at risk for weight-related problems and appropriately intervene (or refer) for weight management.

Elevated blood pressure is associated with stroke, heart failure and myocardial infarction. Exercise professionals are strongly encouraged to measure blood pressure during each patient visit (6). Blood pressure measurement and categorization of blood pressure elevations have been standardized. National guidelines for the follow-up and management of persons with high blood pressure are also available and individuals with hypertension should be under medical care (6). Exercise training and dietary modifications are an important part of medical management of hypertension.

Abnormal blood lipid levels are known to be the basis of the atherosclerotic process. Serum total cholesterol and high density lipoprotein (HDL) cholesterol should be measured in all adults 20 years of age and older (7). Triglyceride levels should be measured in patients with CAD, diabetes, peripheral vascular disease, hypertension, chronic renal disease, and familial hyperlipidemic disorders. Individuals with abnormal lipid profiles are encouraged to modify diet to reduce, in particular, intake of saturated fat and cholesterol. These individuals should be identified and encouraged to maintain control of dietary fat and cholesterol intake, in addition to participation in regular exercise.

Heart disease tends to be familial. The development of heart disease is independently associated with a positive **family history** (8). This history goes beyond measured risk factors such as cigarette smoking, excess weight, nutritional factors, and physical inactivity. Therefore, genetic predisposition to the development of CAD is important. The family history should identify any first-degree relatives (parents, siblings, and children). The risk of developing a myocardial infarction is particularly high when the family history documents myocardial infarction or sudden death before 55 years of age in a male first-degree relative, or before 65 years of age in a female first-degree relative. Family history of other diseases, specifically diabetes mellitus and certain types of cancer, may be important in emphasizing dietary change in certain individuals.

Health Behaviors

There is a clear link between **dietary habits** and the development of several disease states. Most clear is a link between dietary saturated fat and cholesterol and the development of atherosclerosis. Diets high in cholesterol and saturated fat must be modified to decrease the risk of progressive atherosclerosis (9). Diets high in sodium can lead to persistent elevation of systemic blood pressure, or more importantly, worsening of heart failure. Diets deficient in complex carbohydrates and fiber have been linked with excessive rates of development of carcinomas of the gastrointestinal tract.

Ideally, diet appraisal should include documentation and analysis of usual dietary choices, specifically total caloric intake, saturated fat, cholesterol, sodium, and types of carbohydrates. Appraisal of dietary intake can range from a simple evaluation of dietary preferences to computer-scored instruments that analyze 24-hour dietary patterns, 3-day food records, and even 7-day food records.

Relating dietary analysis to objective measures of health (e.g., excessive calories in overweight individuals, excess sodium and weight in hypertensive individuals) can be an excellent starting point for changing dietary patterns to improve health status.

Identification of past **exercise habits** assists the practitioner in developing appropriate prescriptions and programming with realistic goals, optimal adherence, and safety for the individual. The appraisal of exercise habits should include a history of vigorous physical activity, current physical activity habits (both leisure and vocational), and documentation of symptoms associated with activity, particularly chest discomfort, lightheadedness, and/or disproportionate shortness of breath related to physical activity. Any muscle or joint discomfort associated with, or aggravated by exercise should be identified.

Cigarette smoking is one of the most well-established risk factors (10). The adverse impact of cigarette smoking is most dramatic in the areas of cardiovascular disease and lung cancer (the disease is attributable to smoking in 90% of persons with lung carcinoma). The rate of smoking in young women and adolescents is increasing. In addition to increased risk for developing CAD, risk of sudden death (defined as death within 1 hour in an apparently clinically stable or asymptomatic individual) occurs five times more commonly among pack-per-day smokers compared to nonsmokers.

Such bleak statistics are counterbalanced by the encouraging and well-documented benefits of smoking cessation. Within 2 years of stopping cigarette smoking, the excess risk of cardiovascular disease drops dramatically. This decline in cardiovascular risk is a dose-response

Table 40.3. Pathological Conditions Possibly Associated with Sudden Cardiac Death During Exercise

Conditions Resulting in Myocardial Ischemia
Atherosclerotic coronary artery disease
Coronary artery spasm
De novo coronary artery thrombus
Myocardial bridging
Hypoplastic coronary arteries
Anomalous coronary arteries
Structural Abnormalities
Hypertrophic cardiomyopathy
Idiopathic concentric left ventricular hypertrophy
Right ventricular hypertrophy
Mitral valve prolapse
Other valvular heart disease
Marfan's syndrome
Congenital defects
Conduction Abnormalities
Wolff-Parkinson White syndrome
Lown-Ganong-Levine syndrome
QT interval prolongation syndrome
Miscellaneous
Heat stroke
Myocarditis
Sarcoidosis

With permission from Sadaniantz A, Thompson PD. The problem of sudden death in athletes as illustrated by case studies. *Sports Med* 9:199, 1990; Kohl HW, Powell KE, Gordon NF, et al. Physical activity, physical fitness and sudden cardiac death. *Epidemiol Rev* 14:37, 1992.

phenomenon; the heavier the prior habit, the more dramatic the benefits. The rate of progression of atherosclerosis is likely to decline in the ex-smoker as well. Every effort should be made to provide smoking participants with clear and persuasive information regarding risks associated with continuing smoking and benefits of cessation.

The **type A behavior pattern** is believed to contribute to the overall risk of developing CAD (11). The original description and identification of type A behavior requires a difficult and elaborate technique of structured interview. Subsequent means of evaluating type A behavior are more objective and streamlined. One of these methods may be included as a component of an appraisal of health behavior. Identification of participants whose behavior pattern places them at high risk for myocardial infarction is important and counseling should be provided to lower that risk.

OTHER FACTORS REQUIRING SPECIAL CONSIDERATION

The PAR-Q has been recommended as a minimum pre-exercise screening standard for entry into low to moderate intensity physical activity program. (1) Once an individual has been provided with medical clearance to participate in an exercise program (by virtue of either the PAR-Q or a more comprehensive health appraisal), it is important for the exercise professional to determine whether there are any additional health-related factors that require special consideration. Although a variety of potential risks are associated with exercise participation,

Table 40.4. Health-Related Factors that can Potentially Affect the Exercise Prescription

Factor: Alcohol and other substance abuse.
Implications/Significance: Alcohol intake may elevate heart rate response to submaximal effort, impair exercise tolerance, promote dehydration, and increase risk for heat injury. Habit-forming drugs, such as cocaine, may accentuate risk for cardiac complications during exercise.

Factor: Cigarette smoking.
Implications/Significance: Acute cigarette smoking may elevate heart rate, respiration, and blood pressure response to exercise, increase susceptibility toward ventricular arrhythmias, increase platelet aggregability (and risk for thrombosis), and predispose to coronary artery spasm. Chronically, cigarette smoking accentuates the risk for atherosclerosis.

Factor: Diet/nutrition.
Implications/Significance: Dietary content, especially total fat, saturated fat and cholesterol intake, affects serum lipids and lipoproteins and, thus, the risk for coronary artery disease. Individuals on a calorie-restricted diet should take care to consume adequate carbohydrates to replenish muscle glycogen stores that may be depleted during exercise. Resistance training may be of particular benefit for preservation of lean body mass and minimizing a decline in resting metabolic rate during dieting.

Factor: Diseases.
Implications/Significance: Chronic diseases, such as coronary artery disease, diabetes mellitus, hypertension, cerebrovascular disease, AIDS, cancer, osteoporosis, renal disease, arthritis, and COPD, require special consideration when devising an exercise prescription. For patients with such conditions, the exercise prescription should be individualized in accordance with standard guidelines.

Factor: Eating disorders, such as anorexia nervosa.
Implications/Significance: Care should be taken to de-emphasize weight loss and, possibly, high caloric expenditure exercise, where appropriate. To preserve lean body mass, resistance training should be emphasized.

Factor: Environmental considerations.
Implications/Significance: The environment in which the individual exercise will occur must be considered when devising an exercise prescription; in particular, weather (heat, humidity, cold), altitude, and air pollution (carbon monoxide, ozone), should be factored into the design of the exercise prescription.

Factor: Family history.
Implications/Significance: Family history of premature cardiovascular disease increases risk for such diseases in a given individual.

Factor: Medications.
Implications/Significance: Certain medications may alter heart rate and/or blood pressure response to exercise, evoke electrocardiographic abnormalities, and alter exercise capacity.

Factor: Obesity.
Implications/Significance: Place emphasis on increasing caloric expenditure and minimizing risk for muscle soreness, orthopedic injury, or other discomfort, initially, lower-intensity exercise of longer duration should be emphasized.

Factor: Past and present exercise history.
Implications/Significance: Previous history of exercise experiences, specifically exertion-related orthopedic injuries and reason for noncompliance, should be considered. Present exercise participation is of importance when decisions are made about the type, frequency, intensity, and duration at which exercise training should be initiated.

Factor: Personality/behavior pattern.
Implications/Significance: May influence compliance with exercise guidelines and decisions regarding individual or group training.

Factor: Pregnancy and breast feeding.
Implications/Significance: Exercise should be prescribed in accordance with accepted guidelines for pregnant and lactating women. Women who already participate in a regular exercise program generally can continue during pregnancy. Other women are advised to obtain physician approval and begin exercising with low (or non-) impact activities, such as walking and swimming.

With permission from Sadaniantz A, Thompson PD. The problem of sudden death in athletes as illustrated by case studies. *Sports Med* 9:199, 1990; Kohl HW, Powell KE, Gordon NF, et al. Physical activity, physical fitness and sudden cardiac death. *Epidemiol Rev* 14:37, 1992.

the most important is precipitation of sudden cardiac death. Several studies clearly demonstrate that the transiently increased risk of cardiac arrest occurring during vigorous exercise results largely from the presence of preexisting cardiac abnormalities, in particular CAD (Table 40.3).

Other health-related conditions that may affect exercise prescription (or program) are discussed in Table 40.4. The significance and clarification in exercise prescription and programming are also presented in the table. The factors presented should be viewed as "red flags" because they may indicate adaptation of type, frequency, intensity, duration, and/or progression of the exercise to make it most appropriate for the individual.

▶ SUMMARY

It is essential that the exercise professional obtain as much information as possible about a participant to optimize the benefit-to-risk ratio. A regular re-evaluation of health status and health behaviors via a health appraisal should be incorporated into long-term programs to update prescriptions and programming according to changing needs.

References

1. American College of Sports Medicine. *Guidelines for Exercise Testing and Prescription*, 5th ed. Baltimore: Williams & Williams, 1995.
2. Shephard RJ, Thomas S, Weller I. The Canadian home fitness test. 1991 Update. *Sports Med* 11:358, 1991.
3. Cardinal BJ, Esters J, Cardinal MK. Evaluation of the revised Physical Activity Readiness Questionnaire in older adults. *Med Sci Sports Exer* 28:468, 1996.
4. Kannel WB, McGee DL. Diabetes and cardiovascular disease: The Framingham study. *JAMA* 241:2035, 1979.
5. Kannel WB, et al. Obesity as an independent risk factor for cardiovascular disease; A 26-year follow-up of participants in the Framingham Heart Study. *Circulation* 67:968, 1983.
6. National High Blood Pressure Education Program. The fifth report of the Joint National Committee on Detection, Evaluation, and Treatment of High Blood Pressure (JNC V). *Arch Int Med* 153:54–183, 1993.
7. National Institutes of Health. Summary of the second report of the National Cholesterol Education Program (NCEP) Expert Panel on Detection, Evaluation, and Treatment of High Blood Cholesterol in Adults (Adult Treatment Panel II). *JAMA* 269:3015, 1993.
8. Snowden CB, et al. Predicting coronary disease in siblings–a multivariate assessment: The Framingham Heart Study. *Am J Epidemiol* 115:217, 1982.
9. Forrester JS, Merz NB, Bush TL, et al. Task Force 4. Efficacy of Risk Factor Management. *J Am Coll Cardiol* 27:991, 1996.
10. Fielding JE. Smoking: Health effects and control. *N Engl J Med* 313:491, 1985.
11. Haynes SG, Feinleib M, Kannel WB. The relationship of psychosocial factors to coronary heart disease in the Framingham study III. *Am J Epidemiol* 111:37, 1980.

103, 107, 108

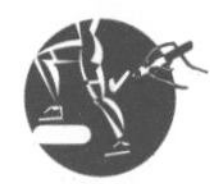

111, 112, 115, 120, 122, 124, 126

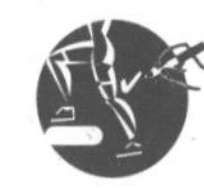

369, 372, 377, 381, 382, 386

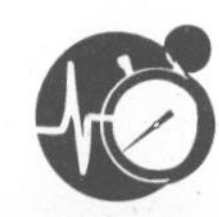

CHAPTER 41

Cardiorespiratory Assessment of Apparently Healthy Populations

Timothy R. McConnell

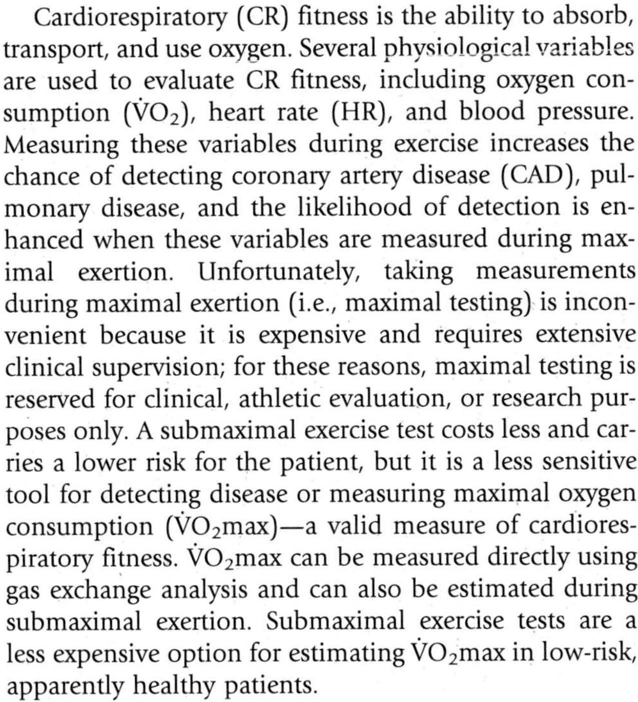

Cardiorespiratory (CR) fitness is the ability to absorb, transport, and use oxygen. Several physiological variables are used to evaluate CR fitness, including oxygen consumption ($\dot{V}O_2$), heart rate (HR), and blood pressure. Measuring these variables during exercise increases the chance of detecting coronary artery disease (CAD), pulmonary disease, and the likelihood of detection is enhanced when these variables are measured during maximal exertion. Unfortunately, taking measurements during maximal exertion (i.e., maximal testing) is inconvenient because it is expensive and requires extensive clinical supervision; for these reasons, maximal testing is reserved for clinical, athletic evaluation, or research purposes only. A submaximal exercise test costs less and carries a lower risk for the patient, but it is a less sensitive tool for detecting disease or measuring maximal oxygen consumption ($\dot{V}O_2max$)—a valid measure of cardiorespiratory fitness. $\dot{V}O_2max$ can be measured directly using gas exchange analysis and can also be estimated during submaximal exertion. Submaximal exercise tests are a less expensive option for estimating $\dot{V}O_2max$ in low-risk, apparently healthy patients.

PRETEST SCREENING

Pretest health screening can help determine whether submaximal exercise testing is appropriate and whether additional clinical testing and supervision is required (5). A medical referral should be obtained prior to testing when there is any concern about the appropriateness of the test. Pretest screening can be used to identify the following:

1. Medical contraindications to exercise.
2. Symptoms suggesting cardiac or pulmonary disease.
3. Angina or other forms of discomfort at rest or during exercise.
4. Unusual shortness of breath at rest or during light exercise.
5. Dizziness or lightheadedness.
6. Orthopedic complications that may prevent adequate effort or compromise the validity of test results.
7. Other unusual signs or symptoms that may preclude testing.
8. Multiple risk factors for coronary heart disease.
9. History of major cardiorespiratory events.

The Participant Activity Readiness Questionnaire (PAR-Q) should be completed as part of the pre-test health screen, and informed consent must be obtained (5).

SUBMAXIMAL EXERCISE TESTING

Heart rate varies linearly with $\dot{V}O_2$; thus, maximal testing is not necessary to estimate $\dot{V}O_2max$. In submaximal testing, predetermined workloads are used to elicit a steady state of exertion. The heart rate at each work level is displayed graphically and extrapolated to $\dot{V}O_2$ at the age-predicted maximal heart rate (HR = 220 − age) (Fig. 41.1). $\dot{V}O_2max$ can also be estimated from values in commonly used protocols (e.g., the Bruce, Balke, and Naughton protocols) or calculated using prediction equations (5).

Some basic assumptions about submaximal protocols include the following:

1. Workloads are reproducible.
2. A steady-state heart rate is obtained during each stage of the test.
3. The maximal heart rate for a given age is uniform (HR = 220 − age), although the error of prediction is 10% to 15%.
4. A linear relationship exists between heart rate and $\dot{V}O_2$ over a wide range of values; thus, the slope of HR/$\dot{V}O_2$ regression can be extrapolated to an assumed maximum HR.
5. Mechanical efficiency (i.e., $\dot{V}O_2$ at a given work rate) is consistent.

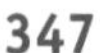

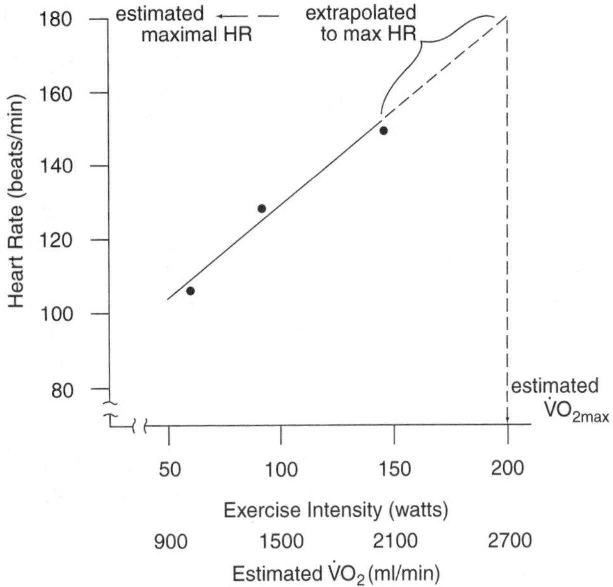

Figure 41.1. Heart rate (HR) obtained from at least two (more are preferable) submaximal exercise intensities may be extrapolated to the age-predicted maximal HR. A vertical line to the intensity scale estimates maximal exercise intensity from which an estimated $\dot{V}O_2$max can be calculated. (With permission from Kenney WL. ACSM's Guidelines for Exercise Testing and Prescription, 5th ed. Baltimore: Williams & Wilkins, 1995.)

The objectives of cardiorespiratory fitness assessments in the apparently healthy population are to:

1. Determine the level of CR fitness and establish fitness program goals, objectives and a safe, effective exercise prescription.
2. Document improvements in CR fitness (or other treatment effects) as a result of exercise training.
3. Motivate individuals to initiate an exercise program or comply with an established program.
4. Provide information concerning health status (2–4).

Considerations with Submaximal Exercise Testing

Test Selection

The selection of a method of evaluating cardiorespiratory fitness is based on a number of practical and theoretical factors, some of which are discussed below.

Safety

When the participant is familiar with the testing modality, the risk of emotional and physical trauma is minimized. An additional safety measure involves identifying orthopedic or other limitations that preclude a particular modality during pretest screening.

Staffing

The staff administering the tests should be ACSM-certified and academically trained in exercise science, or at least have a basic knowledge of exercise physiology and exercise testing. Staff members should be able to

1. Establish a rapport with the patient and make him or her feel comfortable.
2. Identify acute and chronic responses to exercise.
3. Recognize abnormal signs and symptoms during exercise.
4. Provide Basic Life Support measures competently.
5. Adhere to established procedures and protocols.
6. Explain test results to the patient in an understandable manner.

Budget

Financial considerations of exercise testing include

- Equipment costs
- Staff-to-patient ratio
- Procedures for interpreting and reporting test results
- Space requirements
- Paper, forms, and other office supplies
- Other indirect costs

Table 41.1 provides a comparison of the costs of various modalities of submaximal exercise testing.

Equipment

Testing equipment is a major expense. Treadmills comprise the most expensive modality. Bicycle ergometers, which are less expensive than treadmills and require less space, may be the most commonly used modality. With the exception of field tests, stepping benches are, perhaps, the least expensive option. They can be constructed or purchased for individual-station or multiple-station testing. The use of a standard 8-inch step eliminates the need for different step heights. Field tests may be performed in any measured walking area, such as a track, parking lot, or gym area, and can usually be conducted at minimal or no cost.

Table 41.1. Cost Comparison of Submaximal Testing Modalities

Costs	Treadmill	Cycle	Step	Field
Equipment	+ + +	+ +	+	+
Staff Needs	+ + +	+ + +	+	+
Interpretation	+ +	+ +	+ +	+ +
Space	+ + +	+ +	+ +	+
Paper/Forms	+ +	+ +	+ +	+ +
Other Indirects	+ + +	+ + +	+ +	+

+ + + - greater expense; + - lesser expense
(With permission from Kenney WL, ed. ACSM's Guidelines for Exercise Testing and Prescription. 5th ed. Baltimore: Williams & Wilkins, 1995: 113–118.)

Other equipment and supplies necessary for test administration include blood pressure cuffs, stethoscopes, clocks or stopwatches, test interpretation software, paper forms, and other office supplies. These additional costs vary with the protocol of the institution, but may not differ significantly between test types.

Space

The type of testing also affects space requirements. Field tests may be performed at a school track or in any large area where distance can be measured. Treadmills occupy more floor space than cycle ergometers and are difficult to relocate; that space, therefore, may not be available when the treadmill is in use. Cycle ergometers require less space than treadmills and can be moved easily. Most stepping benches do not require much space (unless they are designed for multiple stations) and are relatively easy to move.

Table 41.2. Financial Considerations of Submaximal Testing

	Least Expensive	Most Expensive
Patient Volumes	Group testing	One client at a time
Space	Field or gym area	Allocated testing room
Equipment	Indoor or outdoor track	Treadmill
Staff	Multiple client per staff	One on one testing

With permission from Kenney WL, ed. ACSM's Guidelines for Exercise Testing and Prescription. 5th ed. Baltimore: Williams & Wilkins, 1995: 25.

Other space considerations include changing areas, locker rooms, showers, and waiting areas. The same equipment can be used for testing and exercise programs to reduce the need for duplicate facilities and equipment and, perhaps, help decrease costs.

Patient Volumes

The volume of tests to be performed influences several administrative decisions. Although group testing has financial advantages, it may not be desirable for patient care and customer satisfaction. The volume of tests can also influence staffing patterns. Group testing requires a staff-to-patient ratio that ensures safe and appropriate care as well as the accurate acquisition of data. If one-on-one testing is performed, a reasonable time period for the efficient use of staff and to ensure appropriate patient care should be allotted. Table 41.2 compares the cost of several options for submaximal testing.

Test Type

Procedural guidelines for several submaximal testing protocols are provided in the *ACSM Guidelines for Exercise Testing and Prescription* (Fig 41.2) (5).

Treadmill Tests

Treadmill tests are not commonly used for submaximal exercise testing because the equipment is expensive, the space requirement is high, the test volume is limited. The prediction error for $\dot{V}O_2$max is reported to be up to 17.5% (6–9), because patients are not familiar with equipment, handrail support is used, and the amount of time required to bring the patient to a steady state varies (9–11).

FUNCTIONAL CLASS	CLINICAL STATUS	O_2 COST ml/kg/min	METS	BICYCLE ERGOMETER	TREADMILL PROTOCOLS: BRUCE (3 MIN STAGES) MPH	BRUCE \GR	KATTUS MPH	KATTUS \GR
				1 WATT = 6 KP; FOR 70 KG BODY WEIGHT KP	5.5	20		
NORMAL AND I	HEALTHY, DEPENDENT ON AGE, ACTIVITY	56.0	16		5.0	18		
		52.5	15					
		49.0	14				4	22
		45.5	13	1500	4.2	16		
		42.0	12	1350			4	18
	SEDENTARY HEALTHY	38.5	11	1200			4	14
		35.0	10	1050	3.4	14		
		31.5	9	900			4	10
		28.0	8					
	LIMITED	24.5	7	750	2.5	12	3	10
	SYMPTOMATIC	21.0	6	600				
II		17.5	5	450	1.7	10	2	10
		14.0	4	300	1.7	5		
III		10.5	3	150				
		7.0	2		1.7	0		
IV		3.5	1					

TREADMILL PROTOCOLS: BALKE-WARE (\GRADE AT 3.3 MPH, 1-MIN STAGES)	ELLESTAD (3/2/3 MIN STAGES) MPH	ELLESTAD % GR	USAFSAM MPH	USAFSAM % GR	"SLOW" USAFSAM MPH	"SLOW" USAFSAM % GR	McHENRY MPH	McHENRY % GR	STANFORD % GRADE AT 3 MPH	STANFORD % GRADE AT 2 MPH	METS
26 25 24 23 22 21 20 19 18 17 16 15 14 13 12 11 10 9 8 7 6 5 4 3 2 1											16
	6	15									15
			3.3	25							14
	5	15					3.3	21			13
			3.3	20			3.3	18	22.5		12
							3.3	15	20.0		11
	5	10	3.3	15	2	25			17.5		10
									15.0		9
	4	10	3.3	10	2	20	3.3	12	12.5		8
	3	10			2	15			10.0	17.5	7
			3.3	5	2	10	3.3	9	7.5	14	6
	1.7	10					3.3	6	5.0	10.5	5
			3.3	0	2	5			2.5	7	4
							2.0	3	0.0	3.5	3
			2.0	0	2	0					2
											1

Figure 41.2. Common exercise protocols and estimated $\dot{V}O_2$ values for each work stage. (With permission from Kenney WL. ACSM's Guidelines for Exercise Testing and Prescription, 5th ed. Baltimore: Williams & Wilkins, 1995.)

Cycle Protocols

Cycle ergometers are the most common modality used for submaximal exercise testing. They offer the advantages of the following:

- A lower expense
- Portable equipment
- Smaller space requirements
- Ease of use by both clients and exercise professionals
- Heart rate and $\dot{V}O_2$ responses that are reproducible at standardized workloads
- A lower rate of prediction errors (approximately 10%) (12–16).

Frequently used cycle protocols include the YMCA protocol and the Astrand/Rhyming protocol. Both tests have norms and predict $\dot{V}O_2max$ reliably (23).

Stepping Protocols

Stepping protocols are less expensive, in terms of equipment and staffing needs, because they allow concurrent, multiple testing. Most step-testing requires an established time and place. After the step test is completed, the heart rate is counted for a fixed time interval, according to the protocol selected.

The primary physiological assumption of this test is that the rate of recovery indicates the of level of CR endurance (1). The mean prediction error for step-testing is 12.4%, and a 95% confidence interval of 16% has been demonstrated (18, 19). Step tests are easily administered and follow guidelines similar to those used by the YMCA (17).

Field Tests

Field tests are being used more frequently. They offer the advantages of easy administration, the ability to perform them in any measured space, the possibility of concurrent administration of multiple tests, and a reliability in predicting $\dot{V}O_2max$, with prediction errors of approximately 12% (20). In walking tests, the participant is usually required to cover a fixed distance as quickly as possible or to walk as far as possible within a fixed time interval. Participants should be told that test accuracy relies on their cooperation and willingness to make a good effort. The accuracy of the test may be improved with a pilot test or by having the participant perform the test two or three times and using the best score (21, 22).

Cureton, et al. developed and cross-validated the following multiple regression equation for predicting peak oxygen consumption ($\dot{V}O_2peak$) from mile-run or mile-walk time for males and females (23):

$$\dot{V}O_2peak = -8.41(MRW) + .34(MRW)^2 + .21(Age \times Gender) - .84(BMI) + 108.94$$

where:

MRW = mile run/walk time in minutes
Age = years
Gender = 0 for females/1 for males
BMI = body mass index (kg/m^2)
($R = .72$; $SEE = 4.9$ ml/kg/min)

Another commonly used field test is the Cooper 12 minute run/walk. The objective of this test is to walk or run the maximum distance possible in 12 minutes. This test can be easily performed on any measured area using a single staff member to time the test. The test results are used to estimate $\dot{V}O_2max$ as follows (5, 24):

$$\dot{V}O_2max\ (ml/kg/min) = 3.126 \times (\text{meters covered in 12 minutes}) - 11.3$$

SOME CAVEATS FOR TEST TYPE AND PROTOCOL SELECTION

Although institutions may standardize procedures and use specific tests, some flexibility in test and protocol selection is required. Orthopedic limitations due to injury, arthritis, deconditioning, or specific muscle group weakness may prevent the use of specific protocols or modalities. For example, some patients may perform better on a nonweight-bearing modality (cycle versus treadmill) while others may not have the required range of motion in the hip or knee to pedal and would perform better on the treadmill.

Specific protocols may also require modification. For patients who are deconditioned, weak, or elderly, it may be necessary to start the test at a lower work level and increase the work load in smaller increments. Also, field tests may not be appropriate for individuals who require much supervision during testing, who do not understand the concept of pacing, or who may not put forth a good effort. More consistent results may be obtained by testing young children, for example, in a laboratory setting, which is more controlled.

PATIENT MONITORING AND ABNORMAL RESPONSES

Submaximal exercise tests allow the exercise professional to obtain data on patients at varying levels of fitness. For those at higher risk and who require greater supervision, individual testing in a laboratory may be more appropriate than field testing. During treadmill or cycle ergometer tests, heart rate, electrocardiogram, blood pressure, rate of perceived exertion, and signs or symptoms can be recorded easily. Vital signs should be assessed prior to the test, at each workload, and during recovery, for a total of at least 4–8 minutes.

Field or group testing may be appropriate for lower-risk individuals. Under field testing conditions, it may be possible to record only time or distance during the test and heart rate at the completion of the test. Furthermore, it may only be possible to monitor for visible signs of distress rather than measurable signs and symptoms. However, monitoring is crucial. Participants should be assessed carefully prior to the test. Throughout the testing and recovery periods, supervisors should position themselves so that they can maintain visual contact with each participant.

Although individuals may be thoroughly screened prior to testing, evidence of occult disease may arise at any time during the testing and recovery periods. For this reason, the following variables should be monitored throughout the testing period:

- Rating of perceived exertion (RPE) (Table 41.3).
- Signs or symptoms of cardiac or pulmonary distress or signs of overexertion including chest pain or other discomfort, shortness of breath, dizziness or lightheadedness, or profuse sweating.
- Heart rate and rhythm.
- Blood pressure.

Submaximal tests should be terminated according to ACSM or other accepted guidelines (Table 41.4) (5). In the event of an abnormal response, the test should be terminated, the Medical Director and the primary care physician notified, and all specified follow-up procedures performed. Tests should also be terminated if monitoring capabilities are compromised.

Table 41.3. Original and Revised Scales for Ratings of Perceived Exertion (RPE)*

ORIGINAL SCALE		REVISED SCALE	
6		0	Nothing at all
7	Very, very light	0.5	Very, very weak
8		1	Very weak
9	Very light	2	Weak
10		3	Moderate
11	Fairly light	4	Somewhat strong
12		5	Strong
13	Somewhat hard	6	
14		7	Very strong
15	Hard	8	
16		9	
17	Very hard	10	Very, very strong
18		•	Maximal
19	Very, very hard		
20			

(With permission from Kenney WL, ed. ACSM Guidelines for Exercise Testing and Prescription, 5th ed. Williams & Wilkins, 1995;68. *Noble BJ, Borg GAV, Jacobs I, Ceci R, Kaiser P: A category-ratio perceived exertion scale: Relationship to blood and muscle lactates and HR. Med Sci Sports Exerc 15:523–528, 1983.)

Table 41.4. General Indications for Stopping an Exercise Test in Apparently Healthy Adults*

1. Onset of angina or angina-like symptoms
2. Significant drop (20 mm Hg) in systolic blood pressure or a failure of the systolic blood pressure to rise with an increase in exercise intensity
3. Excessive rise in blood pressure: systolic pressure >260 mm Hg or diastolic pressure >115 mm Hg
4. Signs of poor perfusion: lightheadedness, confusion, ataxia, pallor, cyanosis, nausea, or cold and clammy skin
5. Failure of heart rate to increase with increased exercise intensity
6. Noticeable change in heart rhythm
7. Subject requests to stop
8. Physical or verbal manifestations of severe fatigue
9. Failure of the testing equipment

* Assumes that testing is nondiagnostic and is being performed without direct physician involvement or electrocardiographic monitoring.
(With permission from Kenney WL, ed. ACSM's Guidelines for Exercise Testing and Prescription, 5th ed. Williams & Wilkins, 1995:78.)

Procedures for the most common emergencies that occur during exercise (e.g., angina, myocardial infarction, dysrhythmia, hypoglycemia, dizziness, and cardiac arrest) should be clearly posted in the testing area, known by every staff member, and practiced frequently. All professional exercise staff members should have appropriate ACSM and Basic Life Support (BLS) certification.

CONSIDERATIONS FOR ACCURACY

The ability to obtain valid and reproducible results is essential in testing. It should be ensured that any differences between pre- and post-treatment test results are due to exercise training or variables other than the test itself. Inconsistencies that are inherent in test results may increase variability. These include:

1. Submaximal heart rate, which may vary daily and which is influenced by factors such as time of day, eating, smoking, and familiarization with test procedures (25).
2. Prediction equations for estimating $\dot{V}O_2$max, which may overestimate trained individuals and underestimate untrained individuals (26).
3. The efficiency of motion during walking, running, and cycling.
4. Cardiac output and $\dot{V}O_2$, which can vary by 3–4% during repeat testing (27, 28).
5. Psychological factors, such as pre-test anxiety, which may influence the heart rate, especially at rates of less than 120 beats per minute and at lower workloads. It is not unusual for the heart rate and/or blood pressure to be higher at rest than during the initial stages of exercise in these cases (29).

Factors that can cause variation in the heart rate response to testing include:

- Dehydration
- Prolonged heavy exercise prior to testing
- Environmental conditions (heat, humidity, ventilation, etc.)
- Fever
- Use of alcohol, tobacco, or caffeine 2 to 3 hours prior to testing.

Because of inherent inconsistencies, the standardized procedures for each test must be followed strictly. These procedures may include the following:

1. Standardizing testing protocol
   - The same testing modality and protocol must be used for repeat testing
   - Constant pedal speed is required throughout cycle ergometer testing (32)
   - Cycle seat height must be properly adjusted, recorded, and standard for each test
   - If possible, the time of day for repeat testing should be consistent
   - Data should be collected in the same way throughout each test.
2. Test conditions should be standard, subjects should be free of infection and in normal sinus rhythm.
3. Prior to the test, subjects should not engage in intense or prolonged exercise for 24 hours, smoke for 2 to 3 hours, consume caffeine for 3 hours, or consume a heavy meal for 3 hours.
4. Room temperature should be at 18°C to 20°C and air movement should be provided.

▶ SUMMARY

Cardiorespiratory endurance ($\dot{V}O_2max$) can be predicted accurately from submaximal exercise test results in individuals who do not require maximal testing. Test accuracy is enhanced by adhering to standardized protocols; selecting an appropriate test modality; and standardizing data collection methods, testing conditions and procedures, and subject conditions. Cardiorespiratory endurance status is an important component of overall health status, since it indicates the capacity to perform routine activities of daily living, required occupational tasks, and recreational endeavors, and, thus, the patient's quality of life.

References

1. Blomqvist CG. Cardiovascular adaptations to physical training. *Ann Rev Physiol* 1983;45:169–189.
2. Blair SN, Kohl HW, Paffenbarger RS, et al. Physical fitness and all-cause mortality: A prospective study of healthy men and women. *JAMA* 1989;262:2395–2401.
3. Pate RR, Pratt M, Blair SN, et al. Physical activity and public health: A recommendation from the Centers for Disease Control and Prevention and the American College of Sports Medicine. *JAMA* 1995;273:402–407.
4. Paffenbarger RS, Hyde RT, Wing AL, et al. The association of changes in physical activity and other lifestyle characteristics with mortality among men. *N Engl J Med* 1993;328:538–545.
5. Kenney WL, ed. *ACSM's Guidelines for Exercise Testing and Prescription*, 5th ed. Baltimore: Williams & Wilkins, 1995.
6. Ragg KE, Murray TF, Karbonit LM, Jump DA. Errors in predicting functional capacity from a treadmill exercise stress test. *Am Heart J* 1980;100:581–583.
7. Haskell WL, Savin W, Oldridge N, et al. Factors influencing estimated oxygen uptake during exercise testing soon after myocardial infarction. *Am J Cardiol* 1982;50:299–304.
8. Foster C, Jackson AS, Pollock ML, et al. Generalized equations for predicting functional capacity from treadmill performance. *Am Heart J* 1984;107:1229–1234.
9. Workman JM, Armstrong BW. A nomogram for predicting treadmill-walking oxygen consumption. *J Appl Physiol* 1964;19:150–151.
10. McConnell TR, Clark BA. Prediction of maximal oxygen consumption during handrail-supported treadmill exercise. *J Cardiopulm Rehab* 1987;7:324–331.
11. Roberts JM, Sullivan M, Froelicher VF, et al. Predicting oxygen uptake from treadmill testing in normal subjects and coronary artery disease patients. *Am Heart J* 1984;108:1454–1460.
12. Astrand PO, Rhyming I. A nomogram for calculation of aerobic capacity (physical fitness) from pulse rate during submaximal work. *J Appl Physiol* 1954;7:218–221.
13. deVries H, Klafs C. Predicting maximal oxygen intake from submaximal tests. *J Sports Med* 1965;4:207.
14. Patton JF, Vogel JA, Mello RP. Evaluation of a maximal predictive cycle ergometer test of aerobic power. *Eur J Appl Physiol* 1982;49:131–140.
15. Davies CTM. Limitations to the prediction of maximum oxygen intake from cardiac frequency measurements. *J Appl Physiol* 1968;24:700–706.
16. Wilmore JH, Roby FB, Stanforth PR, et al. Ratings of perceived exertion, heart rate, and power output in predicting maximal oxygen uptake during submaximal cycle ergometry. *Phys Sports Med* 1986;14:133–143.
17. Golding LA, Myers CR, Sinning WE, eds. *The Y's Way to Physical Fitness.* Rosemont IL: YMCA of the USA, 1982: 88–101.
18. Brouha L. The step test: a simple method of measuring physical fitness for muscular work in young men. *Res Q Exerc Sport* 1943;14:31–35.
19. McArdle WD, Katch FI, Katch VL. *Exercise Physiology: Energy, Nutrition, and Human Performance.* Philadelphia: Lea & Febiger, 1991:226.
20. Kline GM, Porcari JP, Hintermeister R, et al. Estimation of $\dot{V}O_2max$ from a one-mile track walk: gender, age, and body weight. *Med Sci Sports Exerc* 1987;19:253–259.
21. Butland RJA, Pang J, Gross ER, et al. Two-, 6-, and 12-minute walking tests in respiratory disease. *Br Med J* 1982;284:1607–1608.
22. Guyatt GH, Thompson PJ, Berman LB, et al. How should we measure function in patients with chronic heart and lung disease. *J Chron Dis* 1985;38:517–524.

23. Cureton KJ, Sloniger MA, O'Bannon JP, et al. A generalized equation for prediction of $\dot{V}O_2$peak from 1-mile run/walk performance. *Med Sci Sports Exerc* 1995;27:445–451.
24. Cooper K. A means of assessing maximal oxygen intake. Correlation between field testing and treadmill testing. *JAMA* 1968;203:201–204.
25. Taylor HL, Wang Y, Rowell L, et al. The standardization and interpretation of submaximal and maximal tests of working capacity. *Pediatrics* 1963;32:703–722.
26. Wyndham CH. Submaximal tests for estimating maximal oxygen intake. *Can Med Assoc J* 1967;96:736–742.
27. McArdle WD, Katch FI, Katch VL. *Exercise Physiology: Energy, Nutrition, and Human Performance.* Philadelphia: Lea & Febiger, 1991:177.
28. Faulkner JA, Heigenhauser GF, Schork MA. The cardiac output–oxygen uptake relationship of men during graded bicycle ergometry. *Med Sci Sports Exerc* 1977;9:148–154.
29. Astrand PO. Aerobic work capacity in men and women with special reference to age. *Acta Physiol Scand* 1960;49:S169.
30. Jessup GT. Validity of the W170 test for predicting maximal oxygen intake. *Eur J Appl Physiol* 1977;37:191–196.

103, 107

112, 113, 115, 120, 122, 124, 126

335, 369, 371, 372, 374, 376, 378, 379, 380, 381, 382, 386

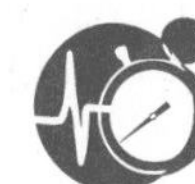

303, 306, 348, 350, 393

361, 362, 365, 366, 409, 413

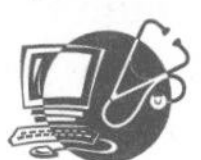

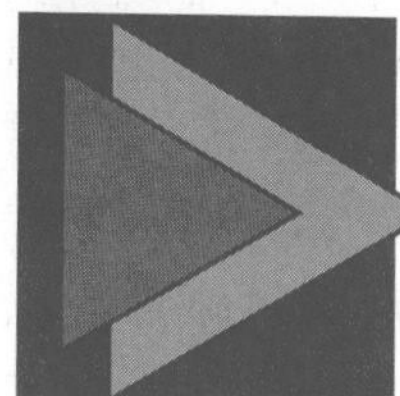

CHAPTER 42

Cardiorespiratory Assessment of High Risk or Diseased Populations

Peter H. Brubaker

Of the many advances in the diagnosis of coronary artery disease (CAD), exercise testing remains an indispensable tool. When performed appropriately, exercise testing yields valuable diagnostic, prognostic, functional, and therapeutic information at a relatively low cost and with minimal risk. Data from several studies indicate that exercise testing is safe, even in high risk patients, with no more than one death, four myocardial infarctions, and approximately five hospital admissions per 10,000 exercise tests (1). To minimize the risk to the patient, the exercise professional must follow guidelines established by professional fitness organizations, including the American College of Sports Medicine (ACSM), the American Association of Cardiovascular and Pulmonary Rehabilitation (AACVPR), and the American Heart Association (AHA) (2–4). This chapter describes these guidelines and other important considerations in test administration.

PRE-TEST CONSIDERATIONS

Prior to an exercise test, a complete medical history and a physical examination to identify contraindications for exercise testing should be standard practice (2). The history should include any past and current medical problems, symptoms, and medications, as well as findings from previous physical examinations and laboratory tests. Physical activity patterns and vocational activity requirements should be assessed, as well as any family history of cardiopulmonary and metabolic disorders. When any absolute contraindications to exercise are identified, the patient should be referred to a primary physician for further medical management. Patients with relative contraindications may be tested after careful evaluation of the risk–benefit ratio for the exercise test. Major CAD risk factors and signs and symptoms of cardiopulmonary disease should be used to stratify patient risk and to determine the appropriate level of medical supervision (2).

The patient should be advised prior to the test to refrain from food, alcohol, caffeine, or tobacco within 3 hours of testing. Patients should be well rested for the exercise test; therefore, they should also be advised to, avoid vigorous activity on the day of testing. Patients should continue any prescribed medical regimens, unless instructed otherwise by a physician. For example, test sensitivity may increase if patients taper their beta blocker intake or discontinue anti-anginal medications for several days prior to testing.

The exercise professional should explain the potential risks and discomforts associated with exercise testing to the patient as thoroughly as possible. Specific steps should be taken to ensure patient safety during the test, such as a demonstration of the safe use of the treadmill. Steps should also be taken to reduce patient anxiety, such as answering questions and describing expectations (reporting symptoms, level of exertion expected, test endpoints, etc.). Informed consent should be obtained, as it has important ethical and legal implications and ensures the patient is aware of the purposes and risks associated with test.

To ensure patient comfort during the testing procedure, patients should be advised to wear clothing that is comfortable and that provides freedom of movement. Suggestions should be made regarding clothing that allows the tester to place electrocardiogram (ECG) electrodes and the blood pressure cuff appropriately. Proper fitting shoes with rubber soles should also be recommended to ensure good traction, particularly for treadmill testing.

EXERCISE TEST SELECTION

The specific exercise test should be selected on the basis of the purpose of the test, the health and fitness status of the client, the most appropriate exercise modality, and the selected exercise protocol. In many exercise laboratories, these issues are determined by the availability of equipment and by custom, each of which can have a profound effect on the response to the exercise test.

Modes

The purpose of exercise testing is to increase total-body and myocardial oxygen demand at safe increments within a reasonable time period. This requires dynamic exercise that uses major muscle groups, permitting a large increase in cardiac output, oxygen delivery, and gas exchange (Fig. 42.1). The modalities used for diagnostic testing include cycle ergometers, treadmills, arm ergometers, steps, and, recently, chemical stressors.

Pharmacologic Testing

Pharmacologic stress is a relatively new consideration in exercise testing, with important applications for echo and nuclear techniques. Dipyridamole (Persantine), a platelet adhesion inhibitor that was developed to prevent thromboembolic complications in patients with cardiac valve replacements, is commonly used in such tests. The mode of action for dipyridamole is not known, although it is believed to block the uptake of adenosine (a substance that modules excitatory neurotransmitter activity), which suggests a hypotensive effect; this hypothesis is supported by the fact that an overdose of dipyridamole results in transient hypotension. When compared with standard exercise testing, dipyridamole demonstrates similar or slightly better diagnostic accuracy (5, 6).

Pharmacologic stress techniques are advantageous for patients who are unable to exercise at an acceptable level, including patients with peripheral vascular disease or neurologic or musculoskeletal disorders. The disadvantages of dipyridamole stress testing include side effects (40%–50%) and lack of a cardiovascular response (10%) (7, 8).

Bicycle Ergometer

The bicycle ergometer and treadmill are the most commonly used exercise testing modalities. A bicycle is generally less expensive, occupies less space, and is less noisy. During cycling, upper body motion is decreased, making blood pressure and ECG recording easier. The workload on simple, mechanically braked bicycle ergometers is not always accurate however, and is dependent upon pedaling speed, which may vary. This variation in workload can be overcome by using electronically braked bicycle ergometers, which maintain a constant workload over a wide range of pedaling speeds. In either case, bicycle ergometer work may be expressed in kilogram meters per minute (kgm/min), or watts.

Treadmill

The treadmill is used mainly in North America (9). It is more expensive than a cycle ergometer, is relatively immobile, and noisier. Researchers comparing treadmill and bicycle ergometry report that maximal oxygen uptake is 10% to 20% higher (range, 6%–25%) and maximal heart rate is 5% to 20% higher on the treadmill (10–12). Increased reports of ST segment changes and angina have been reported during treadmill testing (11–13). Exercise-induced myocardial ischemia identified by thallium scintigraphy was recently reported to be greater after treadmill testing than after cycle ergometry (12). Although most of the differences between the two modalities are minor, the treadmill is preferred when the major goals of the test are to assess functional limits and to identify ischemia.

Protocols

The selection of an exercise protocol is influenced by the purpose of the exercise test. For example, a maximal, symptom-limited test using a relatively demanding protocol is not appropriate (or informative) for a severely limited patient, just as a gradual protocol may not be useful for an apparently healthy, active individual. Thus, the testing goals help to determine whether submaximal testing is appropriate and such specific protocol-related issues as the mode of exercise, the method by which oxygen uptake is to be measured during exercise, and the need for physician supervision.

Submaximal Testing

Submaximal exercise testing is appropriate clinically for predischarge evaluations, especially in patients who have suffered an acute myocardial infarction (MI). Testing has been shown to be effective for risk stratification, activity recommendations, assessment of medical therapy, or to determine the need for further intervention (14). Submaximal testing is also appropriate for patients with a high risk for complex dysrhythmias. A submaximal, predischarge test seems to predict future events as well as a symptom-limited test within a month following an MI. The end-points for submaximal testing are traditionally arbitrary, but should always be based on sound clinical judgment. A heart rate limit of 140 beats per minute (bpm) and 7 METs (metabolic equivalents) are often used in patients younger than 40 years of age; 130 bpm and 5 METs are often used for patients over 40 years of age. The rating of perceived exertion (RPE) is used in patients taking beta-blockers; "hard" exercise is a conservative endpoint. Maximal testing is more appropriate when conducted at least 1 month after an MI occurs. It is used safely for risk stratification.

A 1980 survey suggests that roughly two-thirds of practitioners in North America use the Bruce protocol for exercise testing (9). Since that time, the use of more gradual, individualized protocols has increased (10, 11, 15–19). Large, unequal work increments result in less accurate estimates of exercise capacity, particularly in pa-

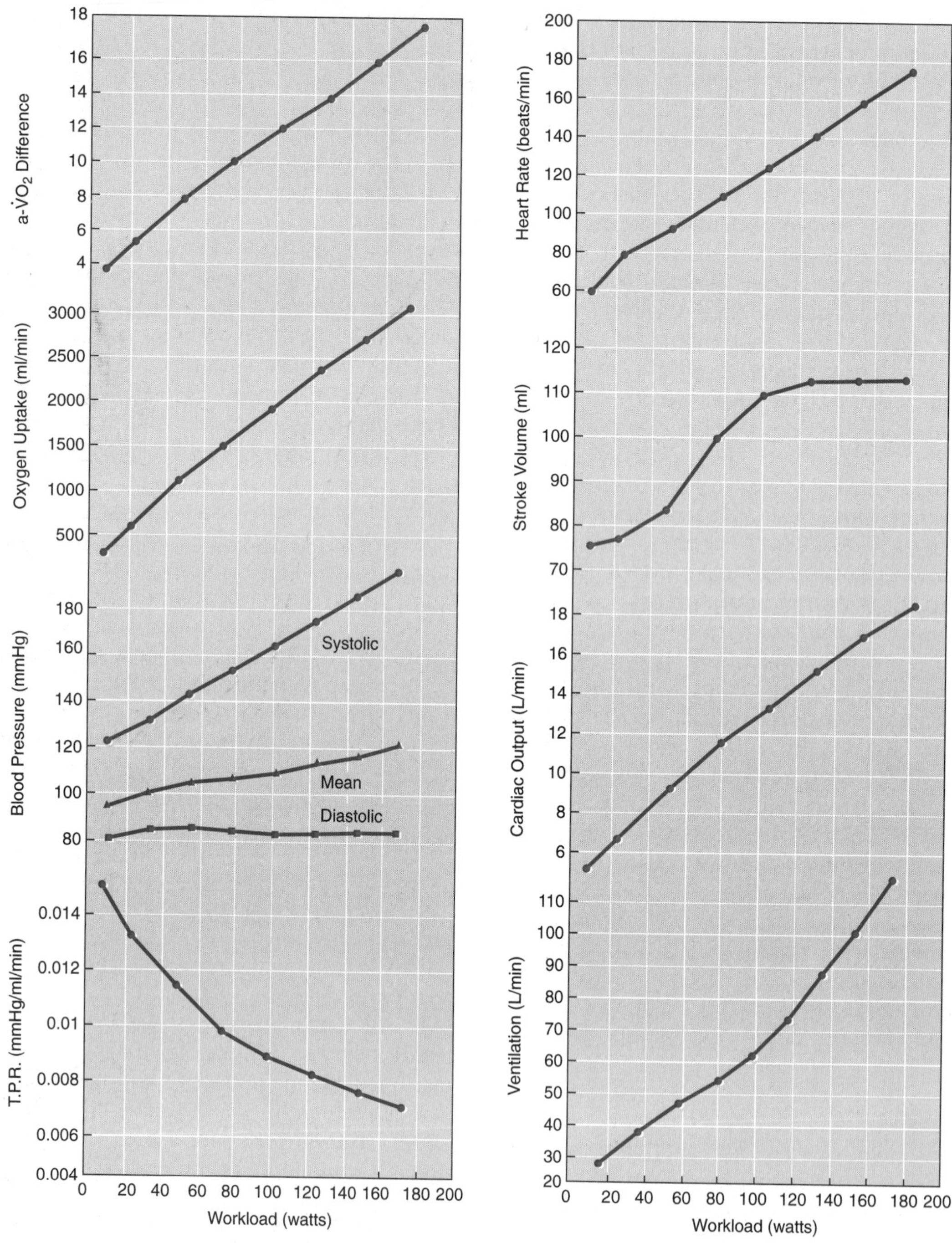

Figure 42.1. Response of basic hemodynamic and metabolic variables from rest to a moderately high level of exercise in the upright position. (Adapted from Myers J. The physiology of exercise testing. *Primary Care* 21(3): 415–437, 1994.

tients with CAD. Recent investigations demonstrate that excessive or rapid increments in rate of work result in

- An overestimate of exercise capacity
- A less reliable assessment of the effects of therapy
- Reduced accuracy for detecting CAD (19).

Individualized protocols offer several advantages for cardiopulmonary assessment. Protocols should begin with a low-intensity warm-up phase followed by progressive, continuous exercise in which oxygen demand is elevated to its maximum level within 8 to 12 minutes. It is important to report exercise capacity in METs rather than treadmill time, so that uniform measures of exercise capacity can be compared. Modifications of the Balke Ware protocol are often used with a constant treadmill speed of 2.0 to 3.3 miles per hour and equal increments in grade (2.5 or 5.0%) every 2 minutes.

A ramp test can overcome some of the limitations of incremental protocols. A ramp protocol uses a constant and continuous increase in metabolic demand instead of the "staging" used in conventional tests. The uniform increase in work results in a steady rise in physiological response and permits a more accurate estimation of oxygen uptake (11, 14). A Bruce ramp protocol has been developed to reduce problems encountered with large increments of work (20).

A key issue emphasized in recent literature is individualization, a process designed to optimize the information yield and permit the use of test that take the recommended 8 to 12 minutes to complete. This duration has been justified on the basis of convenience, evaluation response, and limits of the cardiorespiratory system, as well as for its ability to predict exercise capacity.

MEASUREMENT TECHNIQUES AND SEQUENCES

Electrocardiography

The ECG remains an integral part of cardiopulmonary assessment. However, it must be performed correctly to ensure patient safety. Proper skin preparation techniques and precise electrode placement are critical to obtaining an accurate electrocardiograph. Skin preparation decreases resistance at the skin–electrode interface and improves the signal-to-noise ratio. Hair should be removed from the general areas where the electrodes will be placed. Each placement site should be rubbed vigorously with alcohol to remove skin oil. The skin should then be abraded with abrasive pads, gels, or similar products to reduce resistance further. Finally, each electrode should be carefully placed in the proper location to ensure good contact with both the conducting gel and the adhesive surfaces of the electrode.

In clinical settings, the 12-lead Mason–Likar placement (Fig. 42.2) is generally used because it produces fewer artifacts and restricts movement less than the standard limb placement procedure. However, the Mason–Likar placement can result in differences in the amplitude and axis of the ECG wave form (22). Because these shifts may be misinterpreted as diagnostic change, a resting supine ECG should be recorded using standard limb lead placement. However, it should be noted that position changes may also alter the ECG. The majority (probably more than 90%) of ST changes occur in lateral precordial leads (23). Miranda recently studied 178 men to evaluate the diagnostic value of ST depression in the inferior leads. The results suggested that lead V5 has better sensitivity and specificity than lead II, and that ST depression frequently represents a false-positive response.

During the exercise test, at least 3 ECG leads (representing lateral, inferior, and anterior views) should be monitored continuously. 12-Lead ECGs should be recorded in the later part of each stage, more often if an abnormal reading or clinical or symptoms are observed.

"Serious" dysrhythmias during exercise are indications to terminate the test. Serious dysrhythmias may be overt (e.g., ventricular tachycardia), or more subtle (e.g., unifocal premature ventricular contractions [PVCs] or supraventricular tachycardia). Second-degree or third-degree heart block and ventricular tachycardia of any duration are reasons for immediate termination. If there is any doubt about the nature or origin of the dysrhythmia, the test should be terminated. Isolated PVCs, even when frequent, are not ominous signs. Recent studies demon-

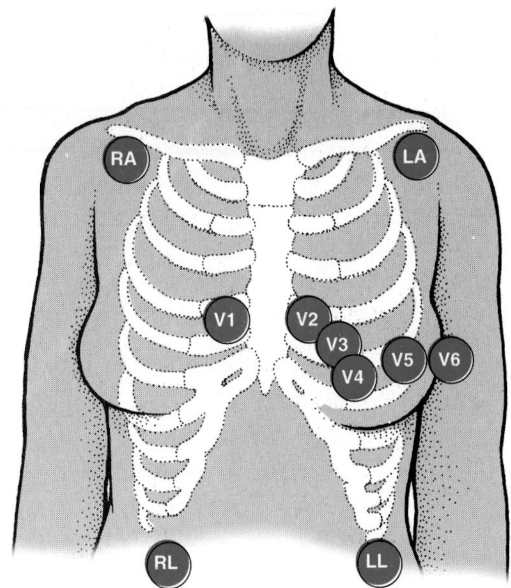

Figure 42.2. The Mason–Likar simulated 12-lead ECG electrode placement for exercise testing.

strate that PVCs during an exercise test are minimally prognostic (24). Therefore, PVCs should be interpreted within the context of the patient's medical history along with current hemodynamics and/or associated symptoms.

Patients referred for exercise testing are likely to be taking medications that can have profound effects on heart rate response. The most common medications are beta blockers and calcium channel blocking agents, which attenuate heart rate at rest and during exercise. Nitrates, which are commonly prescribed, can increase heart rate (2). Because of the effects of these medications, age-predicted maximal heart rate should not be used as a test end-point.

Blood Pressure

The systolic and diastolic blood pressures (SBP and DBP) should be taken at rest and during exercise to ensure patient safety and to obtain important diagnostic and prognostic information. Properly trained personnel can obtain an accurate and reliable blood pressure using auscultatory techniques (25, 26). Blood pressure should be measured at rest prior to the exercise test in supine and standing positions to assess postural hypotension. The resting blood pressure may be elevated due to pre-test anxiety. Persistent, pre-test hypertension is a relative contraindication to exercise testing (2). However, anxiety-related elevations in blood pressure are not uncommon. The blood pressure may decrease slightly during the initial stages of exercise. However, a fall in SBP below baseline carries a poor prognosis (27).

SBP and DBP should be assessed during the last minute of each stage of testing, more frequently if hypotension or hypertension is apparent. Normally, SBP increases with increased workload. Values exceeding 200 mm Hg are not uncommon. However, when the SBP exceeds 260 mm Hg, the test should be terminated (2). The DBP normally stays the same or increases slightly during exercise. The fifth korotkov sound is frequently heard to 0 mm Hg in young, healthy individuals. When the DBP exceeds 115 mm Hg , the test should be terminated (2). When the SBP falls with increased workload the blood pressure should be taken again; if symptoms are also present, the test should be terminated.

Measuring Oxygen Consumption ($\dot{V}O_2$)

The oxygen consumption ($\dot{V}O_2$) and ventilatory variables provide important information about cardiopulmonary function. The measurement of these variables requires careful attention to detail and a working knowledge of the measuring equipment and basic exercise physiology. Maximal oxygen consumption ($\dot{V}O_2$max) is the most common and generally the most useful measurement derived from gas exchange data during an exercise test. $\dot{V}O_2$max defines the upper limits of the cardiorespiratory function (i.e., the ability to increase heart rate, stroke volume, and oxygen extraction by active muscles). The clinical importance of an objective and accurate measurement of exercise capacity is underscored by studies on the prognosis in patients with heart disease. In a recent review, exercise capacity was selected most frequently as a significant determinant of survival (28). In congestive heart failure, peak oxygen consumption ($\dot{V}O_2$peak) is one of the best predictors of survival and is widely used to determine the timing of cardiac transplantation. In one study of patients awaiting cardiac transplantation, a $\dot{V}O_2$peak of at least 14 ml/kg/min was associated with a 1-year survival of 94%; with a $\dot{V}O_2$peak below 14 ml/kg/min, the 1-year survival was 47% (29).

Although $\dot{V}O_2$peak is most accurately determined by measuring expired gases directly, the technology to do so is not always available. Equations that can be used to predict $\dot{V}O_2$peak for walking, running, arm and leg ergometry, as well as stair stepping have been described (2). These equations were developed from experiments that used primarily young, healthy subjects; therefore, their use in other populations may result in significant error of prediction. Many factors such as age, functional capacity, disease status, medications, and use of handrail support, can affect the accuracy of prediction equations. Recently published equations can predict $\dot{V}O_2$peak in clinical populations with greater accuracy (30, 31).

Ventilatory and gas exchange variables should be monitored continuously during exercise, since they may be useful for determining maximum exertion and end-points of testing. Symptoms, deconditioning, and/or unwillingness to tolerate fatigue may prevent the patient from reaching maximal levels; when these factors arise, it may be more appropriate to use $\dot{V}O_2$peak. Although breath-by-breath measurements of $\dot{V}O_2$ and other gas exchange parameters is possible, reported peak exercise values should be based 30-second averages (19).

Subjective Assessments

Symptoms and perception of effort should be assessed during exercise to help ensure patient safety and yield valuable diagnostic information. In order to make a valid assessment of subjective variables during exercise, the exercise professional must explain the scoring scale thoroughly prior to testing. For example, angina and dyspnea (the most common symptoms elicited during exercise testing) are each usually evaluated on a 4-point scale (2).

Patients should be encouraged to report all symptoms. In addition, they should be evaluated by the exercise professional at least once during each stage of the exercise test for the presence of cardiopulmonary symptoms, such as angina and dyspnea. Signs and symptoms can be reported while expired gases are being measured through the use of hand signals (Fig. 42.3) or by having the patient point at charts.

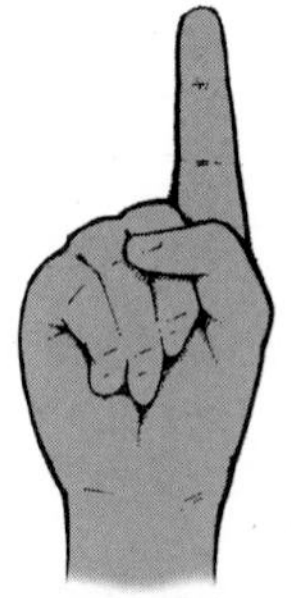
1 ONSET OF DISCOMFORT
You notice chest sensation.

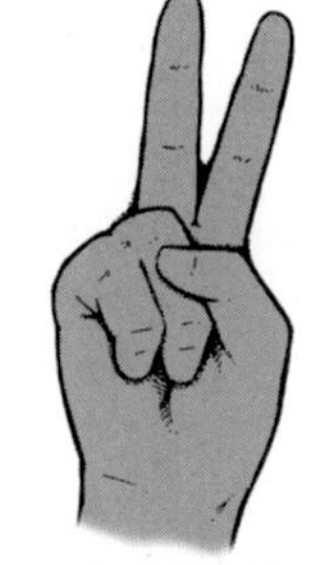
2 MODERATE DISCOMFORT
You feel the pain increasing.

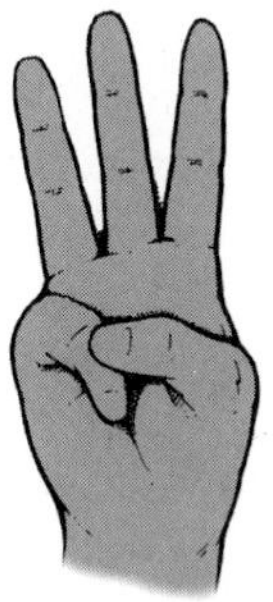
3 MODERATELY SEVERE
The discomfort would cause
you to rest or take nitroglycerin.

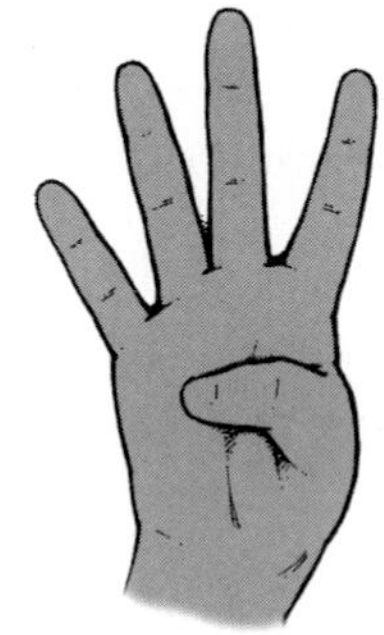
4 SEVERE DISCOMFORT

Figure 42.3. Rating scale for exertional chest discomfort. The scale is particularly useful when using gas exchange techniques, as chest discomfort can be expressed nonverbally using hand signals. A rating of 3 is the appropriate endpoint.

Typical vs Atypical Angina

Typical angina is pain that is consistent in presentation and location, is brought on by physical or emotional stress, and is relieved by rest or nitroglycerin. **Atypical angina** refers to long-term pain in an unusual location, with inconsistent precipitating factors. It is usually unresponsive to nitroglycerin. Exercise-induced chest discomfort resembling typical angina confirms the presence of CAD better than any other test response. A combination of typical angina and abnormal ST response is 98% predictive of significant CAD. Moderately severe angina (grade III) or pain that would normally cause cessation of daily activities and/or nitroglycerin administration is an indication to terminate exercise (32).

Dyspnea

Dyspnea can be the predominant symptom in some patients with CAD, but it is more often associated with reduced left ventricular function or chronic obstructive pulmonary disease. In the former, it is usually accompanied by poor exercise capacity and can occur with impaired SBP response. Dyspnea is appropriately quantified using a 4-point scale (2).

Rate of Perceived Exertion

The rate of perceived exertion (RPE), when properly assessed during exercise, can be used to identify the endpoint of maximum effort. The Borg perceived exertion scale provides reproducible measures of effort and is generally not affected by medications, such as beta blockers (2). An RPE should be obtained at least once during each stage of the exercise test.

TEST TERMINATION

The overall goal of the exercise test in individuals known or suspected of having cardiovascular disease is to obtain a near maximum level of exertion to evaluate the cardiopulmonary response. Determining the endpoint of a clinical exercise test may be difficult, as it requires the integration of objective physiological data and termination criteria with subjective judgement based on clinical experience. Furthermore, patients may be unable or unwilling to exercise to an adequate level. A symptom-limited, maximal test is generally useful when assessing cardiorespiratory response in someone with known or suspected disease. Patients should be instructed to exercise to the point which they can no longer continue because of fatigue, dyspnea, or other symptoms. They should be informed that the test will be terminated if clinical evidence indicates. Patients should be encouraged to exercise as long as possible, but they should not be pushed beyond capacity. Furthermore, any patient request to stop the test should be honored. When the exercise professional is unable to monitor the patient's responses fully, the test should be terminated immediately.

POST-TEST CONSIDERATIONS

One of the purposes of the exercise test is to determine recovery protocol. Whether post-exercise activities should be active or passive is a controversial issue. For diagnostic purposes, the supine position may be the most valuable position immediately after exercise because it increases venous return, thereby increasing ventricular volume, myocardial wall stress, and, consequently, myocardial oxygen consumption. Several studies have shown that ST segment abnormalities are enhanced in the supine position and that active recovery may attenuate these changes (33). ST segments observed 3 to 4 minutes into recovery may be helpful in detecting ischemia. Patients with symptom-limiting angina or dyspnea may have greater discomfort in the supine position and should be placed in a seated or semi-recumbent position during recovery. A passive recovery in the standing position should be avoided due to potential complications associated with venous pooling. For a nondiagnostic test, an active recovery, at low workloads, may be safer and more comfortable. Active recovery decreases the risk of hypotension and minimizes the risk of dysrhythmia secondary to elevated catecholamines.

Regardless of the protocol, the recovery period should be monitored for at least 5 minutes. Blood pressure, ECG, and symptoms should be monitored and recorded at 1-2 minute intervals. The recovery period should be extended to resolve symptoms or abnormal hemodynamic and/or electrocardiograph responses.

At the end of the recovery period, patients should be told to avoid long, hot showers or baths immediately afterward. They should also be warned that fatigue and muscle soreness may occur and instructed to avoid heavy exertion that day. Patients should also be advised to report any pain or discomfort experienced the day after the test to the physician immediately.

Table 42.1. Terms Used to Demonstrate the Diagnostic Value of a Test

Sensitivity =	$\frac{TP}{TP + FN} \times 100$
Specificity =	$\frac{TN}{TN + FP} \times 100$
Positive Predictive Value =	$\frac{TP}{TP + FP} \times 100$
Negative Predictive Value =	$\frac{TN}{TN + FN} \times 100$

TP = true positives, or those with abnormal test results and with disease.
FN = false negatives, or those with normal test results and with disease.
FP = false positives, or those with abnormal test results and no disease.
TN = true negatives, or those with normal test results and no disease.

DATA INTERPRETATION

The majority of patients sent for exercise testing are referred for an evaluation of chest pain, most commonly to make a diagnosis of CAD. Thus, the exercise test serves as a screen for further evaluation. Any screening test must be evaluated for its sensitivity and specificity for the condition being evaluated. **Sensitivity** is the percentage of tests that correctly identify that condition; in this case, CAD. **Specificity** is the percentage of tests that identify individuals without CAD. Sensitivity and specificity are inversely related. Furthermore, they vary with the population tested, the definition of the disease, and the criteria used for an abnormal test. For example, if the population being tested is at risk for severe forms of CAD (e.g., triple vessel disease or left main coronary disease), the test will have a higher sensitivity. Alternatively, the specificity of the test will be lower in low-risk populations, such as a group of young, healthy subjects.

The diagnostic value of a test can be determined by its **predictive value**. A **positive predictive value** is the percentage of persons with an abnormal test who also have the disease. A **negative predictive value** is the percentage of persons with a normal test who do not have disease. The predictive value of a test cannot be determined directly from sensitivity and specificity; rather, it is strongly associated with the prevalence of disease in the population being tested. The calculations used to determine sensitivity, specificity, and predictive value are presented in Table 42.1.

False-Positive and False-Negative Responses

A **false-positive** test (an abnormal response in an individual without disease) can decrease specificity. A **false-negative** test (a normal response in an individual with disease) may indicate the need for an alternative diagnostic procedure; in the case of CAD, for example, an echocardiogram or radionuclide test may be indicated. Factors associated with a false positive or false negative response have been documented, and should be considered prior to testing (2).

Prognosis

Exercise testing is valuable for determining the prognosis, or outcome of disease, in patients with CAD (34). A prognosis should be established because it provides information that can be useful for planning vocational and recreational activity and making important financial decisions. It is also useful for identifying additional interventions that may improve the outcome of therapy. An accurate estimation of risk can be obtaining by using any of a number of techniques to "score" exercise tests (14).

Supplementary Diagnostic Tests

Radionuclide imaging complements the exercise ECG in known or suspected cases of CAD. It is particularly helpful with equivocal exercise ECG or in patients who are likely to exhibit false-positive or false-negative responses. Nuclear imaging can be used to clarify the meaning of an abnormal ST segment response in asymptomatic individuals or the cause of chest discomfort. Patients with a positive exercise ECG and a positive radionuclide scan are 2.6 times more likely to have a subsequent event than patients with negative results (35).

Nuclear imaging of the coronary vessels is somewhat more sensitive and specific for CAD than the exercise ECG. The literature suggests that sensitivity and specificity of exercise thallium scintigraphy are 84% and 87%, respectively (35). This modality also permits localization of ischemia, which is not possible with an ECG, and permits differentiation between fixed defects (representing myocardial infarction) and reversible defects (representing ischemia).

Echocardiography is being used more often during exercise and pharmacologic testing. The diagnostic accuracy of echocardiography depends primarily on the methodology and as well as the clinical experience of the interpreter. The sensitivity and specificity of this technique are approximately 85% each (36).

SUMMARY

The exercise test continues to be useful in evaluating and managing patients known or suspected of having CAD. The exercise test is a primary "gatekeeper" to more costly and invasive procedures, as it is the most accessible tool for evaluating medical therapy, quantifying exercise tolerance, helping to determine prognosis, and developing an exercise prescription. The exercise test is relatively inexpensive and safe. The most reliable information is obtained through careful attention to methodology and by interpretation of data by technicians who have a thorough understanding of the basic physiology of exercise and test safety issues, experience interpreting ECGs and hemodynamic responses, and, finally, familiarity with various professional guidelines.

References

1. Thompson P. The safety of exercise testing and participation. In: *Guidelines for Exercise Testing and Prescription.* 2nd ed. Philadelphia: Lea & Febiger; 1993:359–363.
2. American College of Sports Medicine. *Guidelines for Exercise Testing and Exercise Prescription.* 5th ed. Baltimore: Williams & Wilkins, 1995.
3. American Association of Cardiovascular and Pulmonary Rehabilitation. *Guidelines for Cardiac Rehabilitation Programs.* 2nd ed. Champaign: Human Kinetics, 1995.
4. Fletcher GF, Froelicher VF, Hartley LH, et al. Exercise standards: a statement for health professionals from the American Heart Association 1995;91:580–615.
5. Severi S, Picano E, Michelassi C, et al. Diagnostic and prognostic value of dipyridamole echocardiography in patients with suspected coronary artery disease: comparison with exercise electrocardiography. *Circulation* 1994;89: 1160–1173.
6. Bolognese L, Sarasso G, Aralda D, et al. High dose dipyridamole echocardiography early after uncomplicated acute myocardial infarction: correlation with exercise testing and coronary angiography. *J Am Coll Cardiol* 1989;14:357–363.
7. Ranhosky A, Kempthorne-Rawson J. The safety of intravenous dipyridamole thallium myocardial perfusion imaging. *Circulation* 1990;81:1205–1209.
8. Wilson RF, Laughlin DE, Ackell PH, et al. Transluminal, subselective measurement of coronary artery blood flow velocity and vasodilator reserve in man. *Circulation* 1985;72(1):82–92.
9. Stuart RJ, Ellestad MH. National survey of exercise stress testing facilities. *Chest* 1980;77:94–97
10. Buchfuhrer MJ, Hansen JE, Robinson TE, et al. Optimizing the exercise protocol for cardiopulmonary assessment. *J Appl Physiol* 1983;55:1558–1564.
11. Myers J, Buchanan N, Walsh D, et al. Comparison of the ramp versus standard exercise protocols. *J Am Coll Cardiol* 1991;17:1334–1342.
12. Hambrecht R, Schuler GC, Muth T, et al. Greater diagnostic sensitivity of treadmill versus cycle exercise testing of asymptomatic men with coronary artery disease. *Am J Cardiol* 1992;70:141–146.
13. Wicks JR, Sutton JR, Oldridge NB, et al. Comparison of the electrocardiographic changes induced by maximum exercise testing with treadmill and cycle ergometer. *Circulation* 1978;57:1066–1069.
14. Froelicher VF. *Manual of Exercise Testing.* St. Louis: CV Mosby, 1994.
15. Haskell W, Savin W, Oldrige N, et al. Factors influencing estimated oxygen uptake during exercise testing soon after myocardial infarction. *Am J Cardiol* 1982;50:299–304.
16. Webster MWI, Sharpe DN. Exercise testing in angina pectoris: The importance of protocol design in clinical trials. *Am Heart J* 1989;117:505–508.
17. Tamesis B, Stelken A, Byers S, et al. Comparison of the asymptomatic cardiac ischemia pilot versus Bruce and Cornell exercise protocols. *Am J Cardiol* 1993;72:715–720.
18. Panza J, Quyyumi AA, Diodati JG, et al. Prediction of the frequency and duration of ambulatory myocardial ischemia in patients with stable coronary artery disease by determination of the ischemia threshold from exercise testing: Importance of the exercise protocol. *J Am Coll Cardiol* 1991;17:657–663.
19. Myers J. *Essentials of Cardiopulmonary Exercise Testing.* Champaign, IL: Human Kinetics, 1996.
20. Kaminsky LA, Roeker MS, Whaley MH, et al. Evaluation of the BSU/Bruce Ramp Protocol. Med Sci Sports Exerc 3;25: S13.
21. Reference deleted.
22. Gamble P, McManus H, Jensen D, et al. A comparison of the standard 12-lead electrocardiogram to exercise electrode placement. *Chest* 1984;85:616–622.
23. Miranda CP, Liu J, Kadar A, et al. Usefulness of exercise-induced ST-segment depression in the inferior leads during exercise testing as a marker for coronary artery disease. *Am J Cardiol* 1992;69:303–307.
24. Yang JC, Wesley RC, Froelicher VF. Ventricular tachycardia during routine treadmill testing: risk and prognosis. *Arch Intern Med* 1991;151:349–353.
25. Bailey RH, Bauer JH. A review of common errors in the indirect measurement of blood pressure. *Arch Intern Med* 1993;153:2741–2748.
26. Iyriboz Y, Hearon CM. Blood pressure measurement at rest and during exercise: controversies, guidelines, and procedures. *J Cardiopulm Rehab* 1992;12:277–287.
27. Mazzotta G, Scopinaro G, Falcidieno M, et al. Significance of abnormal blood pressure during exercise-induced myocardial dysfunction after recent acute myocardial infarction. *Am J Cardiol* 1987;59:1256–1260.
28. Morris CK, Ueshima K, Kawaguchi T, et al. The prognostic value of exercise capacity: a review of the literature. *Am Heart J* 1991;122:1423–1431.
29. Mancini DM, Eisen H, Kussmaul W, et al. Value of peak exercise oxygen consumption for optimal timing of cardiac

transplantation in ambulatory patients with heart failure. *Circulation* 1991;83:778–786
30. Berry MJ, Brubaker PH, O'Toole ML, et al. Estimation of $\dot{V}O_2$ in older individuals with osteoarthritis of the knee and cardiovascular disease. *Med Sci Sports Exerc* 1996;28: 808–814.
31. Foster C, Crowe AJ, Daines E, et al. Predicting functional capacity during treadmill testing independent of exercise protocol. *Med Sci Sports Exerc* 1996;28:752–756.
32. Myers JN. Perception of chest pain during exercise testing in patients with coronary artery disease. *Med Sci Sports Exerc* 1994;26:1082–1086.
33. Lachterman B, Lehmann KG, Abrahamson D, et al. "Recovery only" ST segment depression and the predictive accuracy of the exercise test. *Ann Intern Med* 1990;112: 11–16.
34. Chang JA, Froelicher VF. Clinical and exercise test markers of prognosis in patients with stable coronary artery disease. *Curr Prob Cardiol* 1994;19:533–588.
35. Kotler TS, Diamond GA. Exercise thallium-201 scintigraphy in the diagnosis and prognosis of coronary artery disease. *Ann Intern Med* 1990;113:684–702.
36. Greco CA, Salustri A, Seccareccia F, et al. Prognostic value of dobutamine echocardiography early after uncomplicated acute myocardial infarction: a comparison with exercise electrocardiography. *J Am Coll Cardiol* 1997;29: 267–271.

107 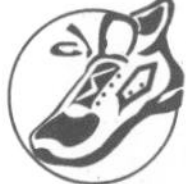

111, 118 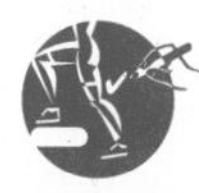

CHAPTER 43
ASSESSMENT OF MUSCULAR STRENGTH AND ENDURANCE

James E. Graves, Michael L. Pollock, and Cedric X. Bryant

Muscular fitness is one of the primary components of physical health. It includes two basic physiological components: muscular strength and muscular endurance.

Muscular strength refers to the ability to generate force at a given speed (velocity) of movement (1). Muscular endurance refers to the ability to persist in physical activity or to resist muscular fatigue (2). Muscular strength and endurance are developed by placing an overload on the targeted muscle or muscle groups. Through adaptation, the muscle groups become stronger or better able to sustain muscular activity.

The process of overloading the muscular system is referred to as resistance training. **Resistance training,** in this chapter, refers to all types of "strength" or "weight" training, including free weights, isokinetic training, variable resistance, and static (isometric) training. Resistance training not only develops muscular strength and endurance, it also improves the ability of the muscles to recover from physical activity. In addition, properly performed resistance training can induce an increase in muscle mass, bone mineral density, and the strength and integrity of connective tissue (3).

Research demonstrates that physical fitness declines with age; however, many of the detrimental, age-related changes in physiological function are due to decreased physical activity and can be attenuated or even reversed with proper exercise training. Just as aerobic training is required to develop and maintain cardiorespiratory fitness, resistance training is required to develop and maintain muscular fitness.

The importance of resistance training for maintaining muscle mass has been demonstrated in a study of master athletes (4). The investigators measured the aerobic capacity and body composition of 24 master track athletes, 50 to 82 years of age, over a 10-year period. The results of the study demonstrate that cardiorespiratory fitness remains unchanged but body fat increases during aerobic training. The change in body composition was attributed to reduced fat-free weight (i.e., muscle mass), specifically in the upper body, and not increased fat weight. Three athletes who supplemented aerobic training with either resistance training or cross-country skiing were able to maintain upper body muscle mass.

Recognizing the need for a well-rounded training program to develop and maintain muscular as well as cardiorespiratory fitness, the American College of Sports Medicine (ACSM) has revised its original Position Stand on "The Recommended Quantity and Quality of Exercise for Developing and Maintaining Fitness in Healthy Adults" to include resistance training (5). The ACSM recommends that resistance training of a moderate to high intensity, sufficient to develop and maintain muscle mass, become an an integral part of fitness programs. One set of 8 to 12 repetitions consisting of 8 to 10 exercises with major muscle groups at least 2 days per week is the recommended minimum.

The adaptations that follow resistance training are beneficial for middle-aged and older adults, especially postmenopausal women, who lose bone mineral density rapidly. Research has also demonstrated the following health benefits associated with resistance training:

- Modest improvements in cardiorespiratory fitness (6)
- Reductions in body fat (7)
- Modest reductions in blood pressure (8)
- Reduced glucose-stimulated plasma insulin concentrations (9)
- Improved blood lipid–lipoprotein profiles (9)

These health benefits are most often associated with **circuit weight training,** a method of resistance training in which a series of exercises are performed in succession with a minimal amount of rest between exercises.

Muscular fitness is required for successful performance in most sports. Thus, resistance training is common among both recreational and professional athletes who wish to enhance athletic performance. Resistance training is also prescribed in rehabilitation programs designed to facilitate recovery from accidents and sport-related injuries. The effectiveness of resistance training exercises in clinical rehabilitation is well documented (10).

An important benefit associated with resistance training is a reduction in the risk of orthopedic injury. Strong muscles and connective tissue support and help protect underlying joints. Inadequate levels of muscular strength can lead to serious musculoskeletal disorders, resulting in pain and discomfort, as well as loss of income due to disability and premature retirement. The overall strengthening of the musculoskeletal system (muscle, bone and connective tissue) resulting from resistance training reduces the risk of elbow and shoulder injuries in tennis players and swimmers (11). Resistance training may have an even greater importance for individuals participating in contact sports and in reducing the risk of injury due to accidents. Low back pain is a major health problem in all industrialized societies. Increasing muscular strength may reduce the risk of developing low back pain as well as minimizing pain in patients with low back disorders (12, 13). Thus, the adaptations to resistance training increase the potential to enhance the quality of life. This chapter addresses methods of assessing muscular strength and endurance.

SPECIFICITY OF TRAINING

The increase in strength resulting from resistance training is specific to the type of contraction used in training, the range of motion (ROM) through which training occurs, the velocity of contraction during training, and whether exercises are performed unilaterally or bilaterally. These examples of specificity of training are at least partially attributed to neural adaptation; however, for specificity of contraction, and type and velocity of contraction, evidence suggests that resistance training also has specific effects on the contractile properties of the muscle. Each of these examples of specificity of resistance training will be discussed briefly.

There are two basic types of muscle activity: static and dynamic. In **static muscular activity,** the muscle attempts to shorten against a fixed or immovable resistance. Thus, there is no skeletal movement, and the muscle neither shortens nor lengthens forcibly. **Dynamic muscle action** involves movement, which may be concentric (i.e., h the force produced by the muscle is sufficient to overcome resistance and muscle shortening occurs) or eccentric (i.e., the muscle exerts force, lengthens, and is overcome by the resistance).

Training a muscle group with dynamic actions (e.g., lifting weights) produces a relatively large increase in dynamic muscle strength but only small increases in isometric strength. Isometric training, on the other hand, improves isometric strength more than dynamic strength (14). Similar improvements in isometric strength at various positions through an ROM are noted following both isometric and dynamic training, when dynamic training involves slow, controlled repetitions (15). In addition to specificity in the isometric and dynamic modes of training, lifting weights improves weight-lifting strength to a greater extent than isokinetic (constant velocity), concentric muscular strength.

Increases in voluntary strength are specific to the ROM that is trained for both isometric and dynamic resistance training. A significant transfer of isometric strength within 20° of the training angle occurs following an isometric strength training program (16). At positions beyond 20° from the training angle, little transfer of isometric strength occurs. Thus, when isometric exercises are used to improve muscular strength, training should occur at multiple positions throughout the ROM. When training consists of dynamic muscle actions performed through a limited ROM, strength gains have been noted up to 50° away from the ROM used for training (17). However, improvements in the untrained ROM have been significantly less than those in the ROM in which training was conducted.

Strength training at slow speeds results in relatively large increases in the ability of the muscle to generate force at slow speeds, but relatively small increases during contractions at faster speeds. The carry-over of strength from high speed training to slow speed testing is also reduced (18). An intermediate training velocity is best for increasing strength at all velocities of movement. Thus, for individuals interested in general fitness, an intermediate training velocity is recommended (11).

REDUCED TRAINING

Muscle strength and muscle mass are decreased when resistance training is discontinued. How much resistance training is required for long-term maintenance of muscular strength and endurance, as well as the exact effects of periodic reduction of either frequency or intensity on strength is unknown. Several studies indicate that if training intensity is maintained, training frequency can be reduced to as little as one day per week for up to 12 weeks without significant loss in strength (19, 20). It is important to note that the subjects in these studies were initially untrained and that the duration of training was 12 to 18 weeks. Whether highly trained athletes can similarly reduce training frequency or whether reduced training can be carried out for more than 12 weeks without loss of strength has not been determined. Available evidence suggests that an occasional missed session does not adversely affect muscular fitness. It is important not to discontinue training altogether.

MEASUREMENT DEVICES

The cable tensiometer is an instrument used to measure static strength by recording the tension applied to a steel cable. This instrument was originally designed to measure aircraft cable tension, was adapted and later refined to measure the strength of various muscle groups. One end of the cable is attached to a fixed object (e.g., a wall or the floor) and the other end is fitted with a device to which force can be applied. In order for the measurement to accurately reflect muscle force production, the cable must be in the plane of movement and must make a 90° angle at its point of attachment to the body or body part. The tensiometer, which is placed along the length of the cable, measures cable tension when the subject applies force to the cable.

Because the force generating capacity varies through a ROM, establishing the proper angle of measurement is critical. A goniometer is used to set the joint angle for testing. The cable tensiometer strength test can accurately measure the static strength of virtually all major muscle groups. The device is highly reliable when used on normal subjects under standardized conditions. However, the cable and attachments often stretch during testing making positional standardization difficult.

The dynamometer is an instrument used to measure static strength by recording the amount of force exerted. Two portable types of dynamometers are widely available, one for hand grip and one for back and leg strength. The most common type is the hand or grip dynamometer. Grip strength is measured as kilograms of force exerted by squeezing the hand dynamometer as hard as possible.

Dynamometers are popular for testing large numbers of people because they are easy to use and portable. Cumbersome set-up procedures that often accompany other types of muscle performance measurements are not required. However, dynamometers can be used to measure only a few muscle groups and their reliability is not well established. In addition, isolation of specific muscle groups is not accomplished which makes standardization difficult.

Strain-gauge devices can be employed to measure static and dynamic muscle force for a variety of muscle groups. Strain gauges are made of electroconductive material that is usually applied to the surfaces of finely machined metal parts. When a load (from a muscle contraction) is placed on the metal parts, the metal and the strain gauge attached to it, deforms. The deformation of the strain gauge causes change in the electrical resistance current passed through it. The change in voltage is related to the load and can be recorded on a strip chart, digital display, or volt meter. In most instances, strain gauges are used to measure static strain or compression by pushing or pulling on the device. Applications of strain gauges for dynamic strength measures, however, are commercially available (e.g., isokinetic machines). Strain gauge measurements are reliable, but they have the same limitations as the cable tensiometer.

One repetition maximum (1-RM) tests measure the greatest amount of weight that can be lifted one time for a specific weight-lifting exercise. These tests are usually limited to the amount of weight that can be lifted at the weakest position in the ROM and, therefore, do not assess muscle performance through a full ROM. Generally, the test begins with an amount of weight that can be easily lifted. After a successful trial, a 2–3 minute rest period is allowed. The weight is increased by 5–10 pounds (or more depending on the difficulty of the previous lift) and another trial is attempted. The 1-RM is the amount of weight for the last trial that can be successfully completed with good form and can usually be obtained in 4–6 trials. The 1-RM provides a measure of dynamic strength that can be applied to almost any weight lifting exercise. 1-RM tests are commonly used because they are easy to administer and can often be performed with the same equipment used for training. They are highly reliable although they do involve a skill factor and subsequent tests may yield greater results due to practice. Thus, 1-RM tests may not be specific for muscle force production.

The application of computer technology and advancements in machine design have improved the accuracy and standardization of muscular strength testing. Electromechanical dynamometers have been developed for both static and dynamic measures of muscular strength and some are capable of both static and dynamic strength measurements. Many electromechanical dynamometers employ a load cell to measure static strength. This method may be considered the electronic equivalent of the cable tensiometer. A major advantage of machines that use load cells, however, is the ease of making multiple measurements through a ROM. Cable tensiometer systems are usually cumbersome to adjust and, therefore, are usually used to provide a measure of static strength at only a single joint angle. Because strength varies through a ROM based on the biomechanical arrangement of the muscles and bony levers of the skeletal system, single joint angle measures do not provide an indication of how strength varies through the ROM. Multiple joint–angle isometric tests are often employed to quantify full ROM static strength. Multiple joint–angle isometric tests have been shown to be highly reliable for a variety of muscle groups.

Some electromechanical instruments have been designed to measure dynamic muscular strength at a preset movement speed. In theory, these constant velocity (isokinetic) dynamometers are thought to measure the maximum force that can be applied throughout the constant velocity movement. Because a period of acceleration is required to reach the pre-selected velocity of movement, and a period of deceleration is required at the end of the movement, isokinetic dynamometers cannot measure force production through a full ROM. In addition, oscillation in observed forces, called torque overshoot, can limit the accuracy of these devices. Torque overshoot represents impact forces between the moving body part and the measurement device. Manufacturers have attempted to overcome these measurement errors by various software controlled averaging systems (called dampening mechanisms) with limited success. While data averaging may be effective at presenting smooth force curves, it cannot eliminate potentially dangerous impact forces. Measurement error associated with the isokinetic dynamometer has been discussed in detail (21). Unfortunately, in spite of the shortcomings, isokinetic dynamometers are a common method of strength assessment in many clinical and research settings.

MEASUREMENT OF MUSCULAR STRENGTH

The primary function of skeletal muscle is to generate force. In most instances, forces generated by skeletal muscles are used to produce movement or for anatomical stabilization. The measurement of muscle force production is used for the following purposes:

- To assess muscular fitness
- To identify weakness
- To monitor progress in rehabilitation programs
- To measure the effectiveness of resistance training

The maximum amount of force that a muscle or group of muscles generates can be measured by a variety of methods including, a cable tensiometer, dynamometer, strain-gauge device, a 1-RM test, or computer assisted force and work output determination. Each of these methods is briefly described.

Regardless of the method chosen to assess muscular strength, certain conditions are required for accurate and reliable measurement of muscle force output. Body position must be stabilized to allow only the desired movement. In the case of measuring muscle force generation during an isometric contraction, the involved joint or joints at which movement would occur must be isolated. An example of the need for stabilization to isolate a specific group of muscles for functional assessment occurs during the measurement of lumbar extensor torque production. The lumbar extensors work in conjunction with the larger, more powerful, gluteus and hamstring muscles to extend the trunk. If the pelvis is free to move during lumbar extension, the pelvis will rotate as the gluteus and hamstring muscles contract. Pelvic rotation would then contribute to the observed torque. Thus, pelvic stabilization is required to accurately assess isolated lumbar extensor function.

Muscle force production varies throughout the range of motion (ROM). The most descriptive measures of muscle function account for this. The term "strength curve" describes a plot of the resultant force exerted versus an appropriate measure of the joint configuration. Because of acceleration at the initiation and deceleration at the termination of all movements and because dynamic strength is influenced by the speed of movement, dynamic strength tests are not appropriate for the quantification of muscle function through a ROM. In addition, if dynamic muscle actions are performed at fast speeds, kinetic forces may be recorded that give an inaccurate measure of true force production. Depending on the specific movement, these kinetic forces are potentially dangerous, especially for populations with orthopedic problems because of the impact that occurs upon rapid deceleration. Isometric tests can safely and accurately quantify muscle force production throughout the ROM if multiple joint angles are measured.

A final consideration required for the accurate assessment of muscle force production is whether the mass of the involved body part influences the measurement. For example, if the force generated by the quadriceps muscles during knee extension does not equal or exceed the mass of the lower leg, no measurable force is observed. Thus, the mass of the lower leg detracts from observed force production of the quadriceps muscles during knee extension testing. This mass must be accounted for to accurately quantify force. Although there is some controversy concerning the need for correction of the influence of gravitational forces during testing because most bodily actions are not "corrected" for gravity, the actual force generated by specific muscles in certain positions may be significantly influenced by body mass (22). Thus, although one cannot neglect the fact that in normal daily activities muscles are influenced by body mass, standardization of testing position and correction for gravitational forces are required for accurate quantification of muscle force production. The need for stabilization, positional standardization, compensation for gravitational influences and measurement through a ROM have been recently discussed by Pollock, et al. (12).

MEASUREMENT OF MUSCULAR ENDURANCE

Almost all of the devices for measuring strength can also be used for assessing muscular endurance. Tests of muscular endurance should be designed to evaluate the ability of a muscle group to produce submaximal force for repeated contractions. More specifically, the length of time a muscle contraction can be held or the number of repeated submaximal contractions a muscle group can make should be determined. Accordingly, similar to strength, muscular endurance can be assessed either statically or dynamically.

Measuring Muscle Endurance Statically

Two basic methods exist for assessing static muscular endurance. One method involves performing a maximal static contraction and sustaining that level of contraction for 60 seconds. The force being exerted by the muscle should be recorded at 10-second intervals. Accordingly, individuals who experience a slower rate of decline in force production are exhibiting a greater level of muscle endurance for that specific muscle group than those whose level of recorded force falls at a faster rate. A second method for assessing static muscular endurance is to determine the length of time a given percentage of a maximum voluntary contraction strength can be sustained.

Measuring Muscle Endurance Dynamically

Several ways exist to determine dynamic muscular endurance. One way dynamic muscle endurance is assessed is to perform the maximum number of repetitions possible using a set weight, a given percentage of maximum strength (e.g., of 1-RM), or some set percentage of body weight. The endurance of a muscle group can be determined isokinetically through the performance of successive maximal repetitions. Isokinetic muscular endurance is measured as the number of repetitions completed before the torque production drops below 50% of the maximal torque value. Perhaps the most commonly used method for evaluating muscular endurance is calisthenic-type (e.g., sit-ups, push-ups, pull-ups, etc.) exercise testing. During such tests, the maximum number of times one can lift their body weight is used as the measure of endurance. For persons of below-average muscular fitness or above-average body weight, however, calisthenic-type exercises often involve more of a measure of muscular strength than muscular endurance.

▶ SUMMARY

Resistance training is an important part of a fitness program and is recommended by the ACSM. Chronic resistance training stimulates many positive changes in physiology and, while much athletic competition requires strength, the benefits derived are particularly advantageous to adults and, especially, post-menopausal women. The measurement of muscular strength and endurance requires knowledge of the specificity of training as well as common measurement devices and advantages/disadvantages of each.

References

1. Knuttgen HG, Kraemer WJ. Terminology and measurement in exercise performance. *J Appl Sport Sci Res* 1987;1(1): 1–10.
2. Baumgartner TA, Jackson AS. *Measurement for Evaluation in Physical Education and Exercise Science.* Dubuque, IA: William C. Brown Publishers, 1987.
3. Stone MH. Connective tissue and bone response to strength training. In: Komi PV, ed. *Strength and Power in Sport.* Oxford: Blackwell Scientific, 1992:279–290.
4. Pollock ML, Foster C, Knapp D, et al. Effect of age and training on aerobic capacity and body composition of master athletes. *J Appl Physiol* 1987;62:725–731.
5. American College of Sports Medicine. Position stand: the recommended quantity and quality of exercise for developing and maintaining cardiorespiratory and muscular fitness in healthy adults. *Med Sci Sports Exerc* 1990;22: 265–274.
6. Fleck SJ. Cardiovascular adaptations to resistance training. *Med Sci Sports Exerc* 1988;20:S146–151.
7. Wilmore JH. Alterations in strength, body composition, and anthropometric measurement consequence to a ten-week weight training program. *Med Sci Sports Exerc* 1974;6: 133–38.
8. Goldberg L, Elliott DL, Kuehl, KS. A comparison of the cardiovascular effects of running and weight training. *J Strength Condition Res* 1994;8(4):219–224.
9. Hurley BF, Hagberg JM, Goldberg AP, et al. Resistive training can reduce coronary risk factors without altering VO_2 max or percent body fat. *Med Sci Sports Exerc* 1988;20(2): 150–154.
10. Grimby G. Progressive resistance exercise for injury rehabilitation. *Sports Med* 1985;2:309–315.
11. Fleck SJ, Kraemer WJ. *Designing Resistance Training Programs,* 2nd ed. Champaign, IL: Human Kinetics Publishers, 1997.
12. Pollock ML, Graves JE, Carpenter DM, et al. Muscle. In: Hockshuler SH, Colter HB, Colter RD, et al, eds. *Rehabilitation of the Spine: Science and Practice.* St. Louis, MO: Mosby, 1993:263–284.
13. Risch SV, Norvell NK, Pollock ML, et al. Lumbar strengthening in chronic low back pain patients. *Spine* 1993;18(2): 232–238.
14. Amusa LO, Obajuluwa VA. Static versus dynamic training programs for muscular strength using the knee-extensors in healthy young men. *J Ortho Sports Phys Ther* 1986;8: 243–247.
15. Graves JE, Pollock ML, Foster D, et al. Effect of training frequency and specificity on isometric lumbar extension strength. *Spine* 1990;15(6):504–509.
16. Knapik JJ, Mawdsley RH, Ramos NU. Angular specificity and test mode specificity of isometric and isokinetic strength training. *J Orthop Sports Phys Ther* 1983;5:58–65.
17. Graves JE, Pollock ML, Jones AE, et al. Specificity of limited range of motion variable resistance training. *Med Sci Sports Exerc* 1989;21(1):84–89.
18. Kanehisa H, Miyashita M. Specificity of velocity in strength training. *Eur J Appl Physiol* 1983;52:104–106.
19. Graves JE, Pollock ML, Leggett SH, et al. Effect of reduced training frequency on muscular strength. *Intl J Sports Med* 1988;9(5):316–319.
20. Tucci JT, Carpenter DM, Pollock ML, et al. Effect of reduced frequency of training and detraining on lumbar extension strength. *Spine* 1992;17:1497–1501.
21. Winter DA, Wells RT, Orr GW. Errors in the use of isokinetic dynamometers. *Eur J Appl Physiol* 1981;46:397–408.
22. Ford WJ, Bailey SD, Babich K, et al. Effect of hip position on gravity effect torque. *Med Sci Sports Exerc* 1994;26(2): 230–234.

4, 105, 107 12, 13, 37, 118

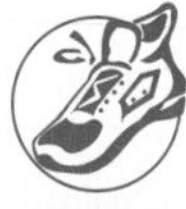

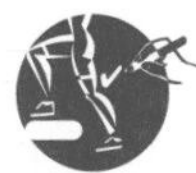

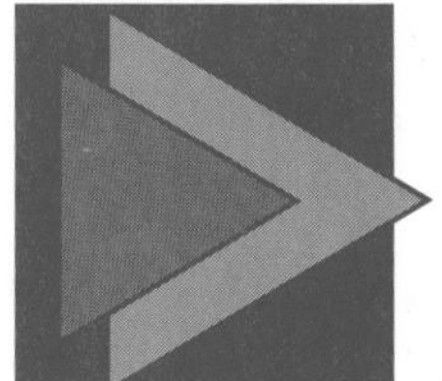

CHAPTER 44 FLEXIBILITY AND RANGE OF MOTION

Elizabeth J. Protas

Joint flexibility is an important component of movement. The range of motion (ROM) of various joints is measured as a part of any evaluation of fitness or work capacity, as well as a clinical assessment of joint function. Consequently, ROM is measured in screening and intervention programs and listed among clinical outcomes and impairment ratings (1). In rehabilitation settings, ROM measures are used to:

- Assess current status
- Describe any change in status
- Establish short-term and long-term treatment goals
- Explain performance
- Predict outcomes
- Motivate patients (2).

FACTORS THAT INFLUENCE RANGE OF MOTION

Joint ROM is the result of a combination of factors. The structure of the joint determines the degree of freedom of movement. For example, the elbow joint allows flexion and extension, but the articulation of its bony surfaces limits extension. In contrast, the shoulder allows movement in all planes; the loose fit between the head of the humerus and the acromion process offers less bony restriction to movement than in the elbow. Some movements are possible only when the joint is in a particular position. When bony surface areas are in maximum contact, the joint is in the "close-packed" position, (i.e., it is in a stable position and resists separation by distractive force) (3). The knee in full extension is an example of the close-packed position. All other joint positions are "loose packed." Spin, roll, and gliding motions occur in the loose-packed position.

The rigidity of ligaments helps stabilize and protect joints from excess motion during dynamic movements. For example, the anterior cruciate ligament of the knee limits the movement of the tibia on the femoral heads. Intracapsular structures, such as articular cartilage and synovial membranes, facilitate smoothness of movement while maintaining integrity of the joint. The extensibility of periarticular soft tissue, such as the joint capsule and surrounding muscle and tendon, also influence movement. One of the most common examples is the limitation imposed upon straight leg-raising by "tight" knee flexors (hamstrings). Some important, functional ROMs are not limited to a single joint, but result from a combination of movements by multiple joints. The ability to bend and pick up an object requires adequate ROM in trunk, hip, and shoulder; similarly, complete ROM in shoulder abduction requires both glenohumeral and scapulothoracic motions (4).

Table 44.1 shows the normative ROM for each of the major joints (5–7). These values vary with age: Children generally have larger ROMs than adults, whereas adults more than 40 years of age have a gradual decline in ROM in many joints (Fig. 44.1) (8–10). Roach and Miles, using hip and knee ROM data from adults aged 25 to 74 years, in the United States found evidence suggesting that the difference in ROM in younger and older age groups is small and not clinically significant (11). The exception is a 20% decrease in hip extension with age. Additionally, older African-American women exhibited significantly less hip flexion; this may be attributable to a larger body mass index. ROM may vary by gender in some joints, as girls tend to have greater hip joint ROM than boys. Women aged 60 to 84 years tend to have a greater ROM than men in the shoulder and elbow, and in medial hip rotation and ankle plantar flexion (8, 9).

The published values for normal ROMs vary. For example, values for normal knee flexion vary from 130° to 150° and for hip flexion from 115° to 125° (11). Many sources do not categorize ROM by age, gender, or body type. Roach and Miles suggest that a difference in active ROM of less than 10% (of the expected norm) may not be significant, but may relate more to variability among individuals and measurement error (11). Even within the same individual, asymmetrical differences in ROM can

Table 44.1. Range of Motion of the Major Joints

Joint	Motion	Average Ranges (degrees)
Spinal		
Cervical	Flexion	0–60
	Extension	0–75
	Lateral flexion	0–45
	Rotation	0–80
Thoracic	Flexion	0–50
	Rotation	0–30
Lumbar	Flexion	0–60
	Extension	0–25
	Lateral flexion	0–25
Upper Extremity		
Shoulder	Flexion	0–180
	Extension	0–50
	Abduction	0–180
	Adduction	0–50
	Internal rotation	0–90
	External rotation	0–90
Elbow	Flexion	0–140
Forearm	Supination	0–80
	Pronation	0–80
Wrist	Flexion	0–60
	Extension	0–60
	Ulnar deviation	0–30
	Radial deviation	0–20
Thumb	Abduction	0–60
	Flexion	
	Carpal-metacarpal	0–15
	Metacarpal-phalangeal	0–50
	Inter-phalangeal	0–80
	Extension	
	Carpal-metacarpal	0–20
	Metacarpal-phalangeal	0–5
	Interphalangeal	0–20
Fingers	Flexion	
	Metacarpal-phalangeal	0–90
	Proximal Interphalangeal	0–100
	Distal Interphalangeal	0–80
	Extension	
	Metacarpal-phalangeal	0–45
Lower Extremity		
Hip	Flexion	0–100
	Extension	0–30
	Abduction	0–40
	Adduction	0–20
	Internal rotation	0–40
	External rotation	0–50
Knee	Flexion	0–150
Ankle	Dorsiflexion	0–20
	Plantar flexion	0–40
Subtalar	Inversion	0–30
	Eversion	0–20

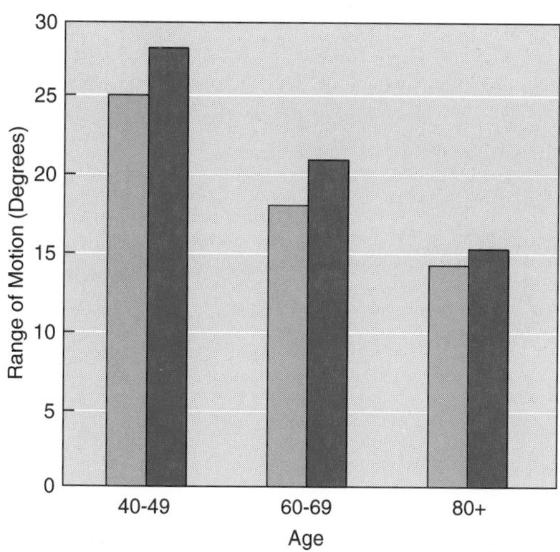

Figure 44.1. Changes in thoracic flexion with age for men and women. (With permission from Olson S. Reliability and validity of trunk range of motion with age. Unpublished data, 1996.)

occur as a result of joint use and/or limb dominance (Fig. 44.2).

NATURE OF MOVEMENTS IN MAJOR JOINTS

Movements occurring in the trunk and the upper and lower extremities are listed in Table 44.1. Flexion and extension occur in the sagittal plane. **Flexion** is an anterior movement for the head, trunk, upper extremity, and hip, but a posterior movement for the knee, ankle (plantar flexion), and toes (12). **Extension** usually occurs in the opposite direction of flexion. **Hyperextension** refers to excessive movement in the direction of extension.

Abduction is movement away from the midline of the body; **adduction** is movement toward the midline in the coronal plane. Exceptions to this are the abduction and adduction of fingers and toes. The midline of the hand or foot rather than the body is the reference for these movements.

Rotation is movement in the transverse plane for the cervical and thoracic spine, the pelvis (right and left rotation), shoulder, and hip (internal and external rotation). Some movements combine other motions, such as the subtalar and forefoot movements of inversion (supination, plantar flexion, and adduction) and eversion (pronation, abduction, and dorsiflexion).

The scapula has several additional motions as it moves on the thorax. **Scapular elevation** (shrugging) and **depression** (caudal movement) are upward and downward movements in the coronal plane. **Scapular protraction** is the position with shoulders slumped forward, whereas **retraction** is the position of the scapula in erect posture. Upward rotation of the scapula accom-

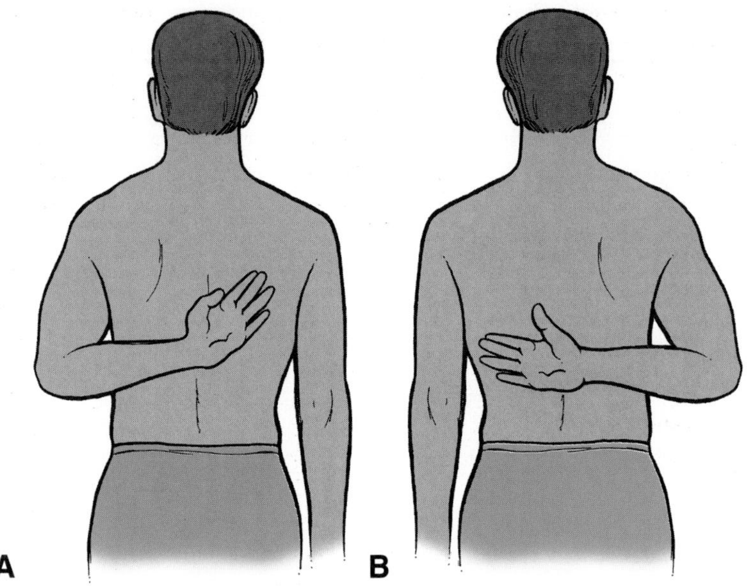

Figure 44.2. Difference in combined shoulder internal rotation and extension between left (A) and right (B) extremities. The individual is a right-handed water polo player. Muscle development on the right limits range of motion.

panies shoulder flexion, and downward rotation accompanies shoulder extension. Additional pelvic motions include the **anterior pelvic tilt**, which accompanies increased lumbar lordosis, and **posterior pelvic tilt**, which occurs with bilateral hip flexion and flattening of lumbar lordosis.

FLEXIBILITY EVALUATION

There are many methods for evaluating joint ROM. Visual estimates and/or measurements are made, often with a special instrument. Movement may be produced actively or passively. Differences in technique vary from the use of warm-up exercises prior to measurement to changing the starting position. Measurement technique may vary, depending upon the joint and motion. Differences in methodology suggest accuracy and consistency can be achieved by following procedural principles. Furthermore, precision in assessment techniques enhances both accuracy and reliability.

Visual Estimate vs. Measured ROM

Visual estimates of ROM have been shown to be inaccurate for both extremity and spinal movements (1, 13). Gross or visual estimates of movement may, however, be useful for fitness screenings, group evaluations, and field testing, which are discussed below.

Active vs. Passive Movement

Although ROM measurements are commonly taken for both passive and active movements, it is more difficult to obtain an accurate measurement during passive ROM (13). Passive joint movement can exert variable forces which may alter the ROM. When the individual is unable to move an extremity actively, e.g., due to paralysis or primary muscle disease, passive ROM can be measured reliably. Pandya found high intratester reliability with repeated measurements of seven common passive upper and lower extremity ROMs in children with Duchenne muscular dystrophy (14). Passive, goniometric measurement of ankle dorsiflexion in children with cerebral palsy has also been reliable (15).

Technique

Technique can have significant effect on accuracy. Improper identification of anatomical landmarks is a source of error in the trunk and extremities (1, 13). Use of surface markings and standardized bony landmarks increases reliability, as does the correct positioning of the individual and the proximal joint segment (1, 16). Using a standard position that stabilizes the proximal segment and allows full range of movement in the distal segment improves reliability (1, 13, 17). It is not clear whether a single measure or multiple measures of a single movement improves reliability. Measurement of a simple hinge joint movement (e.g., elbow flexion) is more accurate than the measurement of a complex movement (e.g., ankle inversion). Repeated trials of passive straight–leg-raising can increase the ROM as a result of moving the limb to the extremes of the ROM (18). When possible, measurements should be taken starting with the limb in an anatomically neutral position to increase reliability; this is particularly important when edema or contracture is present. Placement and stabilization of the measuring device can affect measurement reliability (1).

Intratester vs. Intertester

Intratester reliability is greater than intertester reliability, regardless of the joint or method of measurement (1, 13). Intratester reliability is also higher for upper extremity joints (19). Rothstein reported correlation coefficients of 0.86 to 0.99 for repeated measures of elbow and knee ROM by the same tester using three different goniometers (20). The error of repeated measures for the same tester is usually up to 5%; between testers variability increases up to 10% (13). A single tester should conduct repeated measures on the same subject over time to reduce measurement error.

MEASUREMENT DEVICES

Range of motion is most often measured by goniometers, inclinometers, tape measures, and flexible rules. The selection of the device may depend upon the joint being measured.

Goniometers

Goniometers are the most commonly used measuring device for ROM because they are inexpensive and portable. The **universal goniometer** consists of two arms, a stationary arm that is stabilized on the proximal portion of the joint and a moving arm aligned with the distal portion of the joint which is moved through the arc of motion during measurement. There are also dorsal and pendular goniometers (flexometers).

The reliability of goniometers is high if standard techniques are utilized. Rothstein compared three different types of universal goniometer for elbow and knee ROM and found high interdevice reliability ($r > 0.91$) (20). Goniometry may be inaccurate in spinal and complex movements (1).

Inclinometers

Inclinometers are handheld, electronic, or mechanical devices that use gravity to track the arc of motion during movement of the head, trunk or extremity. One type of inclinometer is a fluid filled device, similar to a carpenter's level, attached to a compass. Good to excellent intratester and intertester reliability has been reported with inclinometers in the lumbar and cervical spines (except during lumbar extension) (21, 22). Both single and double inclinometer techniques have been described. Rondinelli reports that a double inclinometer technique resulted in greater error (10.5°) than a single inclinometer technique (8.5°) when measuring lumbar flexion (23). Inclinometers are acceptable for measuring complex movements when standardized techniques are used.

Tape Measures

Tape measures can be used to measure spinal and finger movements. The skin distraction technique can be used to measure trunk flexion and lateral trunk flexion by comparing differences in position of two marks placed appropriately on the skin prior to and after movement (21). Variation for this were 6% to 10%. Tape measure techniques may be more reliable for lumbar flexion and lateral trunk flexion than inclinometry. Measurement of fingertip-to-floor distance using tape measure is unreliable (21).

Tape measures can also assess loss of ROM in the carpometacarpal and interphalangeal joints. These techniques are useful only if the individual cannot make a fist.

Flexible Rule

The flexible rule can be used to measure spinal movements. The tangent of an arc described by applying the rule to the contours of the back during movement is the measure. Although the flexible rule is reliable, it is not widely used (1).

GROUP AND FIELD FLEXIBILITY SCREENING

Group or field assessment of flexibility is most appropriate when highly accurate measures of ROM are not required. Field testing is commonly used to observe postural alignment (malalignment may make an individual prone to injury). The most common field tests are shown in Figures 44.3 through 44.6. Tests that isolate trunk flexibility (Fig. 44.4C) from hamstring flexibility (Fig. 44.6**D**) are recommended because of the relationship to back injury. Figure 44.7 illustrates postural assessment.

FLEXIBILITY AND FITNESS

The relationship between level of fitness and flexibility is still being studied. It may be especially important in older adults who usually exhibit a decline in movement capability. Walker found that physical activity, as measured by the Physical Activity Questionnaire, was not related to specific changes in ROM in men and women aged 60 to 84 years (9). Jette, Branch, and Berlin, however, studied community-dwelling elders and found a relationship between decreased lower extremity ROM and functional impairments such as the ability to use public transportation or shop (24). There is limited evidence to support the assumption that flexibility is related to fitness level in older adults.

The relationship between flexibility and injury is another pertinent issue. Reid examined the correlation between lower extremity flexibility and hip and knee injuries in classical ballet dancers (25). Unbalanced flexibility, along with decreased ROM in hip adduction and internal rotation, was associated with increased incidence of lateral knee and anterior hip pain. Waddell found that reduced mobility in trunk flexion, lateral flexion, and extension, and decreased straight leg-raising is frequently associated with chronic low back pain (26). However, decreased ROM is not always associated with injury. In a prospective study, men with increased lumbar mobility were more likely to experience an acute episode of low back pain within one year of the flexibility examination (27).

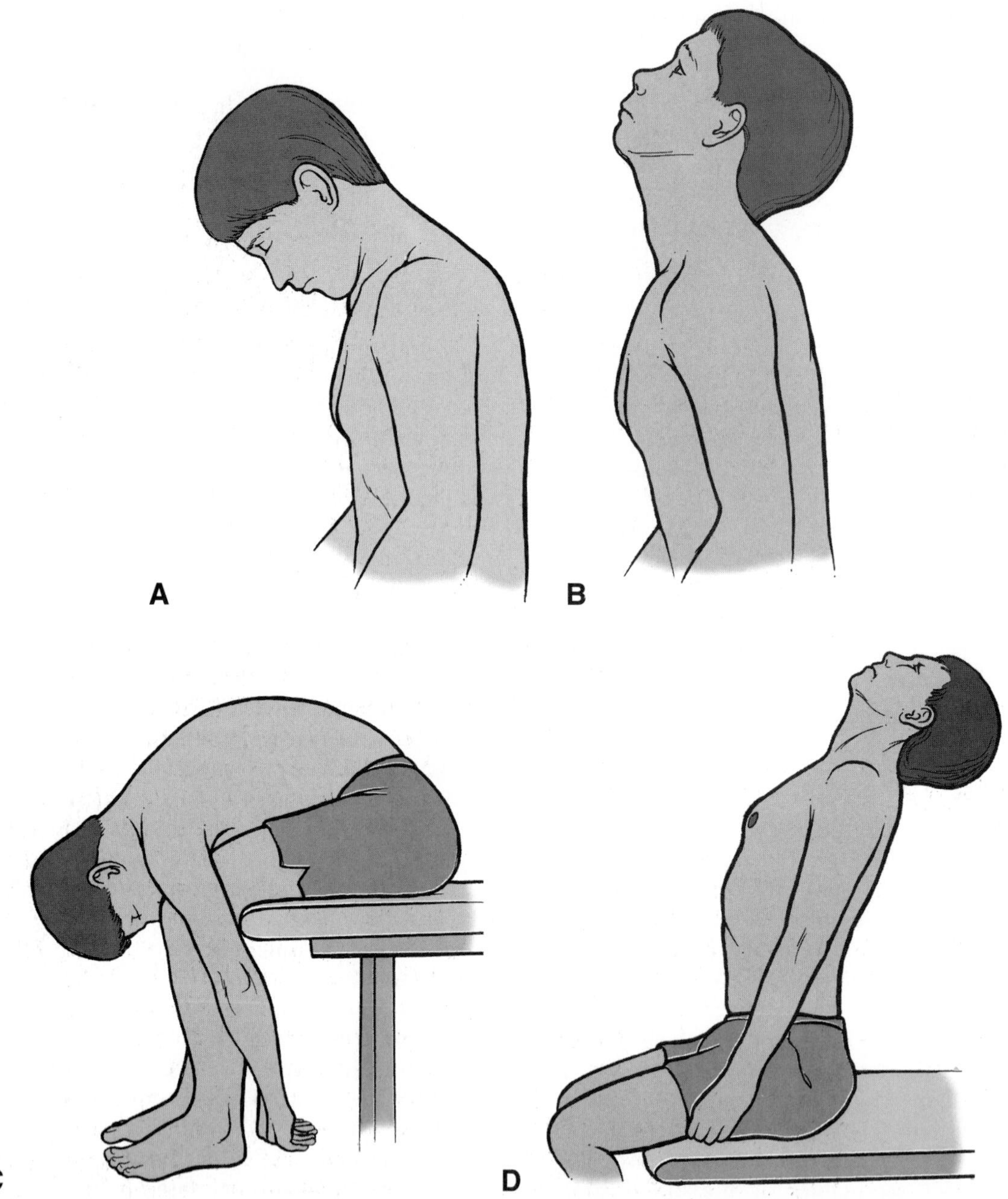

Figure 44.3. Neck and trunk flexibility screening. **A,** Cervical flexion—the chin should touch the chest. **B,** Cervical extension—the head should bend as far as possible posteriorly. **C,** Vertebral flexion, with the hips and knees bent, the trunk should touch the anterior thighs. **D,** Vertebral extension, backward movement of the trunk as far posterior as possible without hip extension.

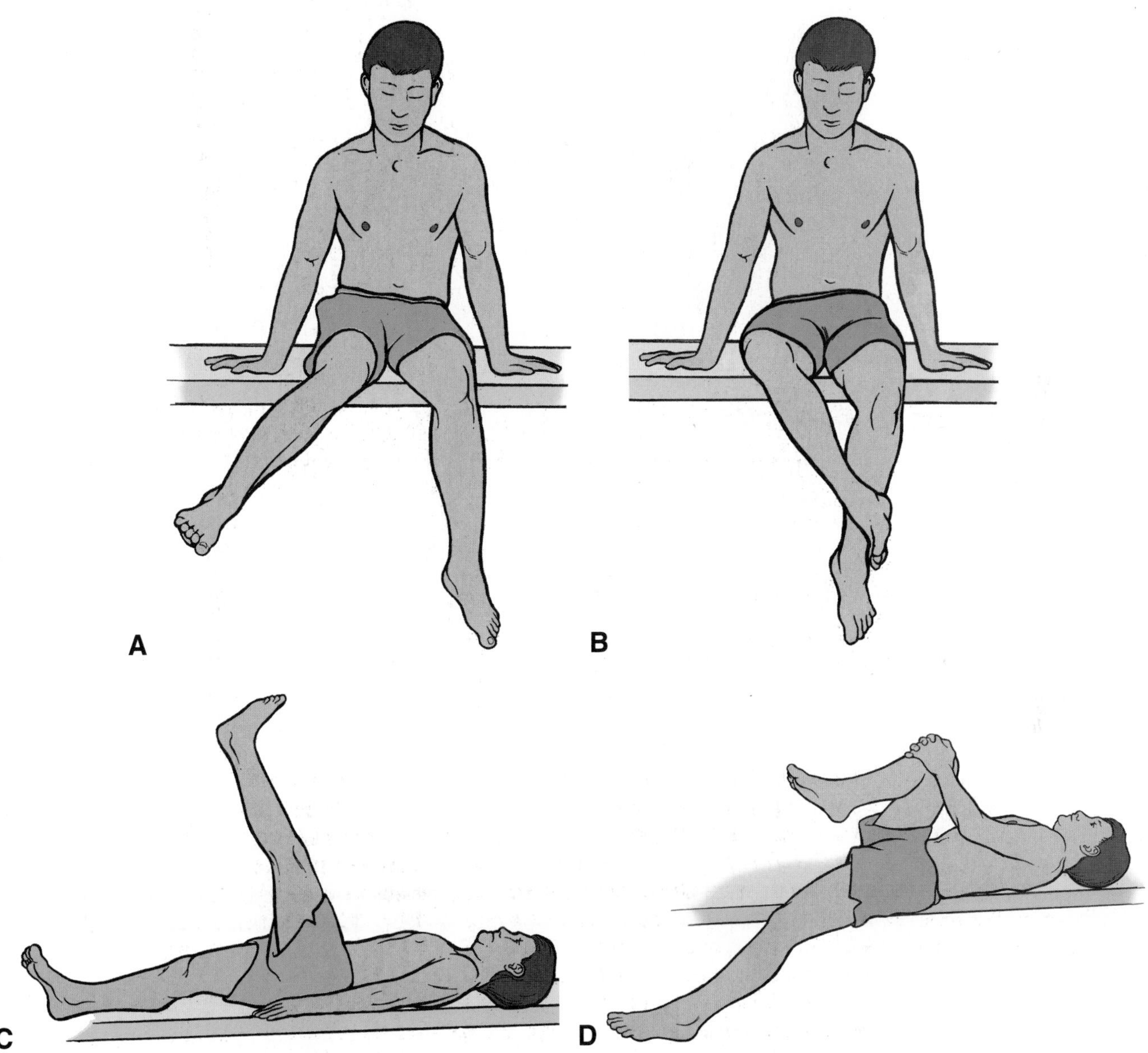

Figure 44.4. Hip flexibility screening. **A,** Internal rotation—with the hip and knee flexed, move the leg as far to the side as possible by rolling the thigh. **B,** External rotation moving the leg as far as possible past the midline by rolling the thigh outward. **C,** Straight leg raising keeping the contralateral lower extremity in full extension while lifting the other extremity without bending the knee. Note limited hamstring flexibility. **D,** Combined test of hip flexion on the right by bringing the bent hip and knee as close to the chest as possible with a Thomas Test for hip extension on the left by allowing the limb to drop over the edge of the table into extension.

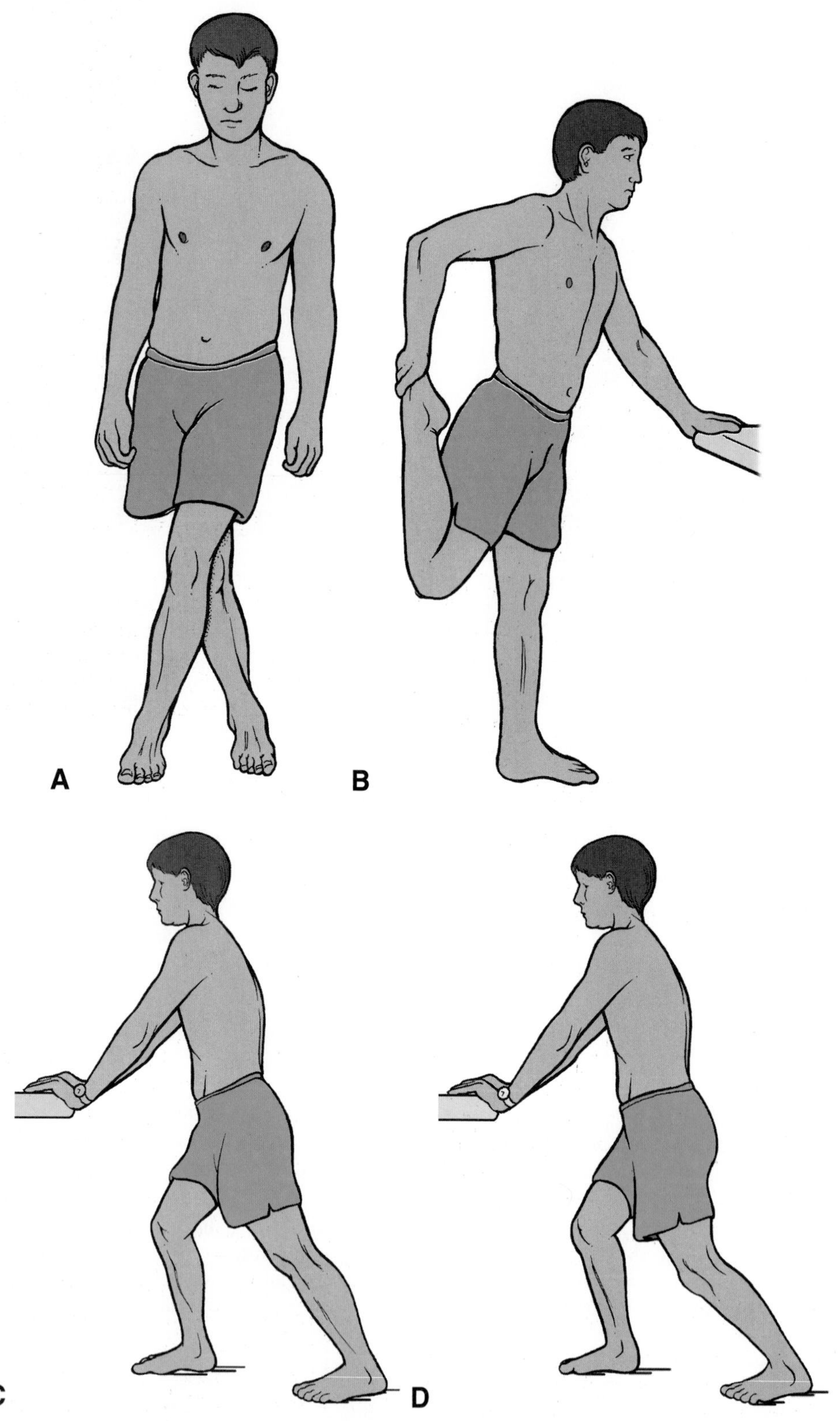

Figure 44.5. Lower extremity flexibility. **A,** Iliotibial band tightness—while standing cross the lower extremity in front of the other limb and rotate the hip internally. **B,** Rectus femoris length; with full hip extension, the leg should almost touch the buttocks. **C,** Gastrocnemius ROM; with knee straight and limb placed as far posteriorly as possible, the heel remains flat on the floor. **D,** Soleus ROM; same position as gastrocnemius except with bent knee. Heel remains on the floor.

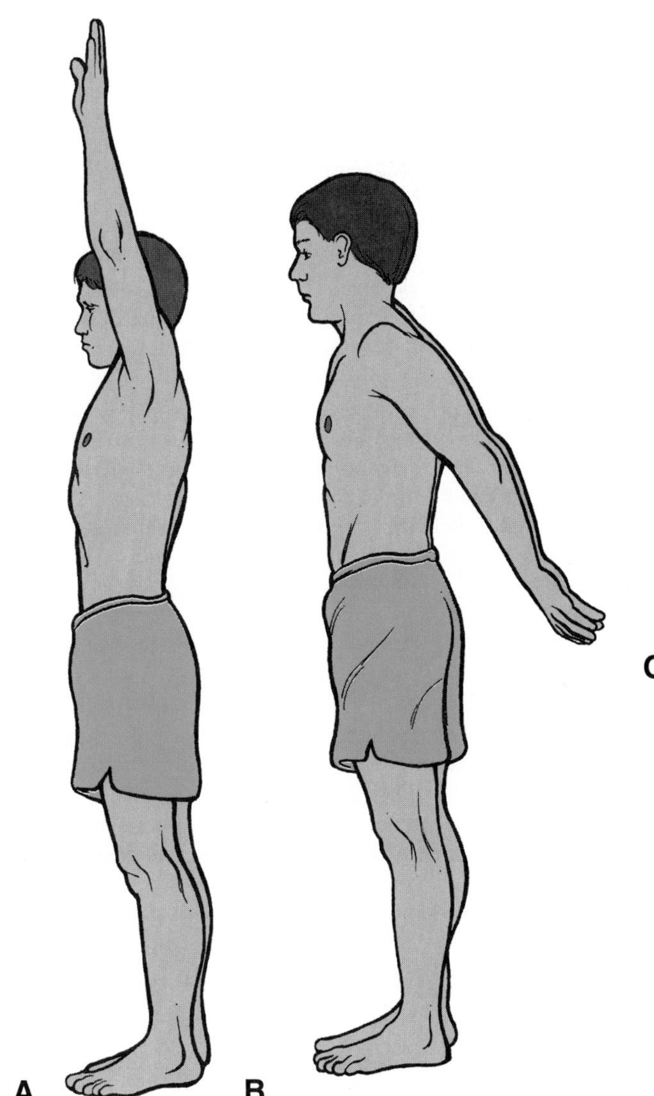

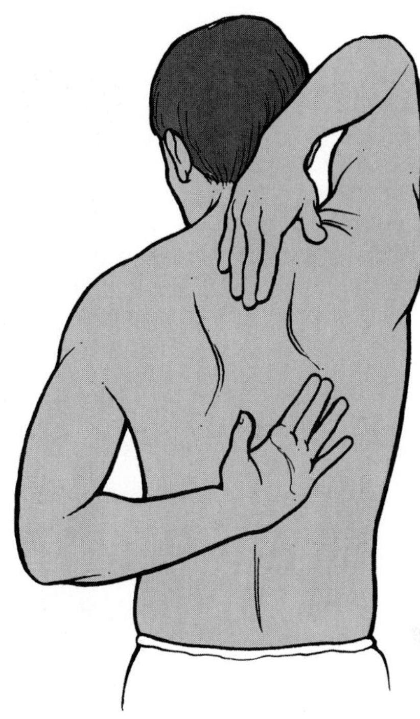

Figure 44.6. Shoulder flexibility. **A,** Flexion; reach forward and upward as far as possible, the humerus will be parallel to the ear. **B,** Extension; reach as far backwards as possible. **C,** Combined bilateral should rotation and elbow flexion; normally fingertips should almost touch.

Mobility is an important element in performing physical activities, but the ROM required may be specific to the activity. For example, a baseball player requires more dynamic shoulder flexibility than a soccer player. Flexibility assessment is often included in pre-season evaluation as a means of preventing injuries, but the relationship between flexibility and injury remains unclear (28).

IDENTIFYING RISK FACTORS FOR ACTIVITY

Exercise professionals should be able to identify client conditions that require additional consultation before they begin an exercise program. An accurate and complete health history can elicit significant information. Persistent or recurrent joint pain may identify possibly arthritic joints. Medical consultation is advisable if pain, swelling, and/or heat in a joint or multiple joints is reported. A change in physical activity is not recommended during an acute arthritic episode. Likewise, if these symptoms occur with activity and persist, the client should be referred to a physician to rule out joint injury, osteoarthritis, and early rheumatoid arthritis.

Individuals sometimes report a "trick" knee or ankle, which suggests that the extremity may spontaneously collapse during weight-bearing activity. This is often accompanied by reports of an injury. It is important to determine whether a medical diagnosis was made.

An individual who reports either recent, acute back pain or a history of chronic back pain should be referred to a physician. Back pain is one of the most common and costly musculoskeletal problems in middle-aged adults. Although individuals with back pain are commonly able to participate in exercise programs, they should be referred to a physician and/or a physical therapist for an evaluation. Early intervention may reduce pain and decrease the likelihood that an acute problem

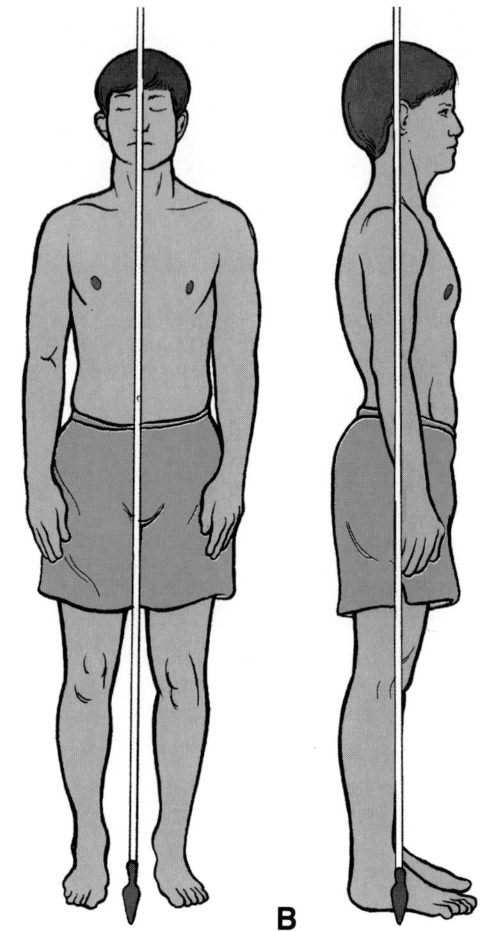

Figure 44.7 Postural assessment with a plumb line. **A**, Anterior; observe for symmetry and knee position. **B**, Lateral; observe alignment of head, shoulders, hips, knees, and ankles.

will become chronic. This is consistent with the guidelines for management of acute back pain recently published by the Health Care Financing Administration (29). The chronicity of the problem negatively impacts fitness by reducing activity during exacerbation of pain. An individualized exercise program for persons with chronic back pain, supervised by a physical therapist, may improve function, decrease disability, and reduce pain (30).

Complaints of musculoskeletal pain persisting and/or increasing with exercise is a primary reason for seeking a medical consultation. Understanding the underlying cause of pain and the effect of exercise are important considerations for the exercise professional in planning exercise programs.

References

1. Lea RD. Current concepts review: range of motion measurements. *J Bone Joint Surg* 1995;77A:784.
2. Gilliam J, Barstow A. Assessment of joint range of motion. In: van Deusen K, Brunt D, eds. *Assessment in Occupational and Physical Therapy.* New York: WB Saunders, in press.
3. Soderberg GL. *Kinesiology: Application to Pathological Motion.* Baltimore, MD: Williams & Wilkins, 1986:58.
4. Rowe CR. Joint measurement in disability evaluation. *Clin Orthop* 1992;32:43.
5. American Academy of Orthopedic Surgeons Committee for the Study of Joint Morton. Joint motion: method of measuring and recording. Chicago: The American Academy of Orthopedic Surgeons, 1965.
6. Boone DC, Azen SP. Normal range of motion of joints in male subjects. *J Bone Joint Surg* 1979;61A:756.
7. Greene WR, Heckman JD (eds). *The Clinical Measurement of Joint Motion.* Rosemont, IL: The American Academy of Orthopedic Surgeon, 1994.
8. Svenningsen S, Terjesen T, Auflem M, et al. Hip motion related to age and sex. *Acta Orthoped Scand* 1989;60:97.
9. Walker JM, Sue D, Miles-Elkousey N, et al. Active mobility of the extremities in older subjects. *Phys Ther* 1984;64:919.
10. Olson S. Reliability and validity of trunk range of motion with age. Unpublished data, 1996.
11. Roach KE, Miles TP. Normal hip and knee active range of motion: the relationship to age. *Phys Ther* 1991;71:656.
12. Kendall HO, Kendall FP, Wadsworth GE. *Muscle: Testing and Function.* 2nd ed. Baltimore: MD: Williams & Wilkins, 1971:21.
13. Gajdosik RL, Bohannon RW. Clinical measurement of range of motion: Review of goniometry emphasizing reliability and validity. *Phys Ther* 1987;67:1867.
14. Pandya S, Florence J, King W, et al. Reliability of goniometric measurements in patients with Duchenne muscular dystrophy. *Phys Ther* 1985;65:1339.
15. Tardieu C, de la Tour H, Bret MD, et al. Muscle hypoextensiblity in children with cerebral palsy: I. Clinical and experimental observations. *Arch Phys Med Rehabil* 1982;63:97.
16. Keeley J, Mayer TG, Cox R, et al. Quantification of lumbar function. Part 5: Reliability of range-of-motion measures in the sagittal plane and an in vivo torso rotation measurement technique. *Spine* 1986;11:31.
17. Watkins MA, Riddle DL, Lamb RL, et al. Reliability of goniometric measurements and visual estimates of knee range of motion obtained in a clinical setting. *Phys Ther* 1991;71:90.
18. Atha J, Wheatley DW. The mobilising effects of repeated measurements of hip flexion. *Br J Sports Med* 1976;10:22.
19. Boone DC, Azen SP, Lin CM, et al. Reliability of goniometric measurements. *Phys Ther* 1978;58:1355.
20. Rothstein JM, Miller PJ, Roettger RF. Goniometric reliability in a clinical setting. *Phys Ther* 1983;63:1611.
21. Merritt JL, McLean TJ, Erickson RP. Measurement of trunk flexibility in normal subjects: reproducibility of three clinical methods. *Mayo Clin Proc* 1986;61:192.
22. Youdas JW, Carey JR, Garrett TR. Reliability of Measurements of cervical spine range of motion: comparison of three methods. *Phys Ther* 1991;71:198.
23. Rondinelli R, Murphy J, Esler A, et al. Estimation of normal lumbar flexion with surface inclinometry. *Am J Phys Med Rehabil* 1992;71:219.
24. Jette AM, Branch LG, Berlin J. Musculoskeletal impairments and physical disablement among the aged. *J Gerontol* 1990;45:M203.

25. Reid DC, Burnham RS, Saboe LA, et al. Lower extremity flexibility patterns in classical ballet dancers and their correlation to lateral hip and knee injuries. *Am J Sports Med* 1987;15:347.
26. Waddell G, Somerville D, Henderson I, et al. Objective clinical evaluation of physical impairment in chronic low back pain. *Spine* 1992;17:617.
27. Biering-Sorensen F. Physical measurements as risk indicators for low-back trouble over a one-year period. *Spine* 1984;2:106.
28. Knapik JJ, Bauman CL, Jones BH, et al. Pre-season strength and flexibility imbalances associated with athletic injuries in female collegiate athletes. *Am J Sports Med* 1991;19:76.
29. Agency of Health Care Policy and Research. Clinical practice guidelines: acute low back problems in adults. Washington, DC: US Department of Health and Human Services, Public Health Service #14, 1995.
30. Beekman CE, Axtell L. Ambulation, activity level, and pain: outcomes of a program for spinal pain. *Phys Ther* 1985;65:1649.

106, 107 119

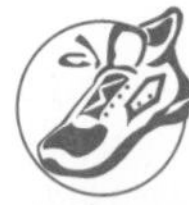

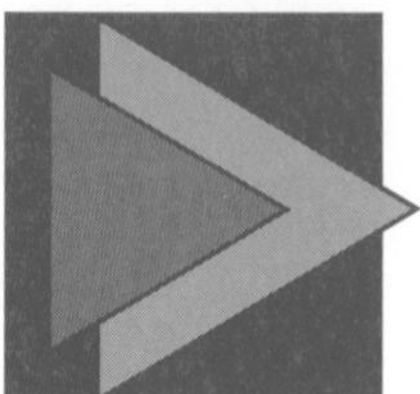

CHAPTER 45
Body Composition

Scott Going and Rebecca Davis

Body composition refers to the absolute and relative amounts of the body constituents. Using current technology, body composition can be assessed on elemental (atomic), chemical, cellular, and tissue/system levels (1). It is possible to measure over thirty components of human composition (2). Comprehensive descriptions of the technical aspects of most methods are available in several recent publications, although many methods are not applicable outside of laboratory situations (3–5). Nevertheless, some familiarity with the principles underlying the more common laboratory methods is useful since they provide the foundation upon which simpler field methods are developed.

There are many reasons to assess body composition. The strong association between obesity, especially excess intra-abdominal (visceral) fat and increased risk of coronary artery disease, non-insulin dependent diabetes, hypertension and certain types of cancer, have received considerable attention in recent years. An excessively low level of fat is also detrimental, as evidenced by the physiological dysfunction of individuals who are chronically undernourished. In addition, assessment of body composition is useful to establish optimal weight for health and performance in athletes, to formulate dietary guidelines and exercise prescriptions for modifying body composition and evaluating efficacy, and to monitor changes in composition with growth, maturation, and aging to distinguish "normal" changes from pathology.

Although body fat is often the focus of assessment, lean tissue mass and its components (fluid, muscle, and bone) are equally, if not more important. Low levels of lean mass and loss of lean tissue contribute directly to metabolic complications, as well as indirectly through impaired functional capacity, reduced physical activity, and energy expenditure, and, thus, a greater risk of fat gain. Low bone mass and density are primary predictors of osteoporotic fracture risk. The muscle wasting that occurs with certain diseases and with aging not only decreases muscle strength and the capacity for even routine activities, but is also a strong correlate of mortality. Recently there has been increased emphasis on the development of interventions to increase lean tissue mass in healthy aging and clinical populations, as well as in athletes. Assessment of lean mass is a crucial aspect of evaluating success towards that goal.

Exercise professionals generally use field techniques to assess body composition. Although the distinction between laboratory and field techniques is arbitrary, field techniques generally require less complex and more portable equipment, are less costly, and can be applied outside of controlled laboratory conditions. Anthropometric assessment using skinfolds and circumferences continues to be the most common approach, although newer techniques, such as bioelectric impedance analysis (BIA), are useful. There are now well over 100 different anthropometric and BIA equations for estimating body composition. As a result, one of the most difficult problems practitioners face is the selection of the most suitable method and equation.

To evaluate the usefulness of and choose the appropriate methods and equations for clients, exercise professionals must be familiar with the development of those methods. Validation procedures are followed when a new method or equation is developed. Cross-validation occurs when the method or equation is tested in another sample from the same or a different population. An understanding of these procedures requires a basic knowledge of criterion methods, the models, and the assumptions. Understanding the statistical criteria used to evaluate the outcomes of validation and cross-validation studies is also important. Thus, this discussion will address these areas and provide practitioners with information needed to evaluate current, as well as future methods so the most accurate method may be selected.

HIERARCHY OF METHODOLOGY

Although more detailed taxonomies have been proposed, body composition methods can be categorized as being direct, indirect, or doubly indirect (6, 7). In vivo assessment is done using indirect or doubly indirect methods. Direct methods, such as dissection and chemical analysis of isolated tissues to whole cadavers, are not suitable for in vivo assessment. Nonetheless, they are central to in vivo assessment because they provide basic data that is the foundation from which indirect techniques are developed.

Indirect methods can be either property- or component-based (2). Property-based methods are based on measurement of specific properties, such as body volume, decay properties of specific isotopes, or electrical resistance. The development of in vivo neutron activation analysis, for example, has made possible nondestructive chemical analysis by measuring the radiation given off during the decay of excited atoms (8). An example of a more common property-based method is the estimation of total body water (TBW) from tritium dilution (9).

Component-based methods depend on well-established models that usually represent ratios of measurable quantities to components that are assumed constant both within and between individuals. With component-based methods, the measured quantity is first assessed using a property-based method and the component is then estimated by application of the model. Thus, fat free mass (FFM), a component of the two component model described below, can be estimated from body water by using tritium dilution to measure TBW which is then converted to FFM based on the relationship between TBW and FFM ($1.37 \times \text{TBW} = \text{FFM}$).

Two types of mathematical functions are used when estimating composition with property and component-based methods. The model approach, which depends on knowing the relationship (ratio) between a particular constituent and the component of interest is illustrated above. In the second approach, regression analysis is used with experimental data to derive an equation which relates a measured property or component to an "unknown" (estimated) component. Typically, the equation is developed by measuring the unknown component and the known component in the same subjects. Regression analysis is then used to derive the equation relating the known component to the unknown component. Equations for estimating body fat from skinfold thicknesses or bioelectrical resistance are developed in this manner. Because they generally depend on a combination of methods then used to estimate an unknown component, they are considered to be doubly indirect methods.

It is clear from the preceding discussion that a hierarchy of methods exists. Direct methods represent the most fundamental approach to assessment, property-based methods are one step removed, and component-based methods are two steps removed. Assessment methods are structured in a way such that measurement errors or inaccurate assumptions are propagated from one level to the next. Thus, doubly indirect methods, farthest removed from direct methods, are most susceptible to inaccuracies unless precautions are taken to minimize errors.

MODELS

Many models have been proposed for characterizing the human body on different levels of analysis. A common feature of all useful models is that the sum of the components closely approximates body weight. Molecular level models are generally the most accessible with current technology and have been used in most validation studies of field methods. The usefulness of a model depends primarily on its validity for a given population and on the availability of the required technology. Simple models require fewer measurements and are generally more accessible. However, simple models that combine constituents require more assumptions and are not as generalized.

The TBW, total body potassium and hydrodensitometry methods are three common laboratory methods for estimating fat and fat-free masses (8–10). Measurement errors and inaccuracies due to invalid assumptions are propagated from one step to the next and contribute to the total error in estimates of fat and FFM.

As noted above, models represent the conceptual basis from which the mathematical functions for estimating composition are derived. Thus, TBW and total body potassium can be converted to FFM based on the respective concentrations in the FFM determined through direct (chemical) analysis of human cadavers. In an analogous way, body density from hydrodensitometry can be converted to percent fat based on the relationship between whole body density and the proportions and densities of the components (10). Many different equations can be derived. For example, the Siri equation ($f = 4.95/D_B—4.50$), one of the most common two component (2C) equations, was derived using the assumed densities for reference man from direct chemical analyses of cadavers (11, 12). It follows that equations reflect the models from which they are derived.

CRITERION REFERENCE METHODS

A criterion reference method predicts the unknown component by a regression equation. Reference methods are also used to derive the conversion constant which relates an unknown body component (e.g., FFM) to one of its constituents (e.g., TBW). It is essential that criterion estimates of composition be as accurate as possible since error in the criterion measurement is propagated and contributes to the total error in the new equation.

Laboratory methods, such as the TBW, total body potassium, and hydrodensitometry methods, based on the 2C model, are the most common reference methods.

Each is based on an assumption of chemical constancy (i.e., that the composition and density of the FFM is similar and constant in all individuals). This approach is accurate for all individuals for whom the model is valid. Error (model error) is introduced when the actual composition of the individual is different from that assumed by the model. Higher order models (3C and 4C models) require fewer assumptions about the composition of the FFM. For this reason, the higher order models are valid for more people and should give more accurate results. However, their application requires more measurements and the gain in less model error can be lost to increased technical error (measurement or method error) unless all measurements are made accurately.

The Siri equation generally gives accurate estimates of fat and FFM in young to middle-aged Caucasian men. In contrast, systematic differences in children, different racial/ethnic groups, athletes, and elderly men and women, related to differences in maturation, race/ethnicity, training, and aging lead to error in estimation of body fat and invalidates the Siri equation in these groups. The choice of an appropriate model depends on the component of FFM that is expected to vary the most. For example, young children have proportionately less mineral and more water than adults. Thus, a 4C model which adjusts for variability in both water and mineral is useful, although good results can be achieved with a 3C model which adjusts for TBW. A 3C model that adjusts for differences in mineral is useful in African-American men and women, in the elderly, and in many athletes since racial-, training-, and aging-related differences are due primarily to systematic variation in bone mineral mass and density. A more comprehensive review of the application of different models can be found elsewhere (2, 10).

In situations where instrumentation is limited and 3C and 4C models are not possible, population-specific equations which are adjusted for systematic differences in the composition of the FFM can be used to improve accuracy. Population-specific equations appropriate for children and older adults, various racial and ethnic groups, and some clinical populations have been reviewed (3, 13, 14). Though inaccuracy is always a factor, adjusted equations are more valid and give more accurate estimates since they are based on population-specific data.

METHOD SELECTION

Selection of an appropriate method is based on the relative precision, reliability, and accuracy of available methods, the availability of appropriate equations, and affordability (Table 45.1). Percent body fat and FFM can be estimated with field techniques with errors of ≥3% and ≥2.5–3.0 kg, respectively. Generally, they are adequate for screening and for following moderate changes in composition over time. When greater precision and accuracy is needed, laboratory techniques must be used.

Anthropometry

Weight for height indices and measurements of skinfold thicknesses, limb and trunk circumferences, and skeletal dimensions all have been used to estimate body composition. Generally, skinfolds give more accurate estimates of percent fat and FFM since they are direct measurements of subcutaneous fat. Circumferences are affected by both fat and muscle and do not provide accurate estimates of fatness in the general population. However, in obese persons, where skinfold measurements can be difficult to obtain, circumferences can give useful estimates of fatness. Circumferences may also work well in athletic populations to estimate FFM since athletes tend to vary more in muscularity than body fat.

Skinfolds and circumferences are also useful for assessing fat pattern and, indirectly, distribution. The ratio of subscapular to triceps skinfolds, for example, has been used to reflect a central versus peripheral fat pattern, and the ratio of waist to hip circumferences (WHR) is a common index of upper versus lower body fat distribution. Epidemiological studies identify WHR as a predictor of chronic disease risk and standards are available (Table 45.2). The assessment of fat pattern and distribution in combination with an estimate of total body fat is an important aspect of the assessment of disease risk.

Table 45.1. Ratings of the Validity and Objectivity of Body Composition Methods

METHOD	PRECISION	OBJECTIVITY	ACCURACY	VALID EQUATIONS	OVERALL
Body Mass Index	1	1	4,5	4,5	4
Near-Infrared Interactance	1	1,2	4	4	3.5
Skinfolds	2	2,3	2,3	2,3	2.5
Bioelectric Impedance	2	2	2,3	2,3	2.5
Circumferences	2	2	2,3	2,4	3.0

1 = Excellent, 2 = Very Good, 3 = Good, 4 = Fair, 5 = Unacceptable
Precision = reliability within investigators; Objectivity = reliability between investigators; Accuracy = comparable to a criterion method; Valid equations = equations are cross validated.

Table 45.2. Waist-To-Hip Circumference Ratio (WHR) Standards for Men and Women

		Risk			
	Age	Low	Moderate	High	Very High
Men	20–29	< 0.83	0.83–0.88	0.89–0.94	> 0.94
	30–39	< 0.84	0.84–0.91	0.92–0.96	> 0.96
	40–49	< 0.88	0.88–0.95	0.96–1.00	> 1.00
	50–59	< 0.90	0.90–0.96	0.97–1.02	> 1.02
	60–69	< 0.91	0.91–0.98	0.99–1.03	> 1.03
Women	20–29	< 0.71	0.71–0.77	0.78–0.82	> 0.82
	30–39	< 0.72	0.72–0.78	0.79–0.84	> 0.84
	40–49	< 0.73	0.73–0.79	0.80–0.87	> 0.87
	50–59	< 0.74	0.74–0.81	0.82–0.88	> 0.88
	60–69	< 0.76	0.76–0.83	0.84–0.90	> 0.90

(With permission from Heyward VH, Stolarcyzk LM. Appied Body Composition Assessment. Champaign, IL: Human Kinetics, 1996:82.)

Table 45.3. Body Mass Index (Kg/M^2) Standards for Men and Women

Classification	Men	Women
Normal	24–27	23–26
Moderately obese	28–31	27–32
Severely obese	> 31	> 32

(Data from Department of Health and Human Services. The Surgeon General's report on nutrition and health (DHHS [PHS] Publication 88-50210). Washington D.C.: U.S. Government Printing Office 1998.)

The body mass index (BMI), a weight for height ratio widely used in epidemiological studies is calculated as weight in kilograms divided by height in meters squared. Obesity standards (Table 45.3) based on BMI have been developed and increased BMI is associated with increased risk of chronic disease. Ironically, BMI is a poor predictor of percent body fat and often misclassifies individuals as obese if they have above average muscularity and skeletal mass rather than excess fat. In children and the elderly, for whom the muscle and bone to height relationship is changing, BMI is especially misleading. Although the BMI may be useful when no other method is available, the results must be interpreted cautiously, and a follow-up exam with a more accurate method should be sought for persons for whom interventions are considered.

The reliability and validity of skinfolds and anthropometric methods are affected by

- Skill of the measurer
- Type of caliper (due to pressure differences) or tape measure (if calibration is lost)
- Subject factors related to skinfold compressibility, edema, and variability in fat pattern and distribution
- The prediction equation used to estimate fatness.

Failure to properly locate and measure the site is a major source of technical error in the skinfold method. To avoid these errors, technicians must be trained and certified against an expert, and all measurements should be made according to standard techniques (15). Equipment error can be controlled by regular calibration (using vernier calipers or a meter stick).

The skinfold method assumes that the distribution of subcutaneous and internal fat is the same for all individuals in whom a particular equation is applied. Moreover, it is assumed that the sites included in a particular equation adequately represent the subcutaneous fat pattern of the individual in whom it is applied. For example, an equation that includes only limb sites underestimates fatness in a person with a predominantly truncal fat. Similarly, fatness is underestimated if an equation which includes only upper body sites is applied in a person with a predominantly lower body fat pattern. Equation error can be reduced by selecting prediction equations based on the age, sex, race and level of physical activity in the population being assessed.

Bioelectrical Impedance Analysis

Bioelectrical impedance analysis (BIA) is a rapid, noninvasive, and relatively inexpensive method for estimating fat and FFM. Although the relative prediction accuracy is similar to the skinfold method, BIA may be preferable in some settings because it does not require a high degree of technician skill and is generally more comfortable, requires minimal cooperation, and intrudes less on privacy. For an excellent overview of BIA, the reader is referred to papers by Baumgartner and Kushner (16, 17).

In the most common application of BIA, a single frequency (50 kHz), low-level excitation current (500 μA to 800 μA) is used to measure whole body impedance. Unlike lower frequency current, which flows through the extracellular fluid, higher frequencies penetrate the cell membranes and flows through both the intracellular and extracellular fluid. Given that the FFM contains large amounts of water (~73%) and electrolytes, it is a good conductor, unlike fat which is anhydrous and a poor conductor of electrical current. Thus, total body impedance at the constant frequency of 50 kHz primarily reflects the volumes of water (intra- and extracellular fluid) and muscle compartments comprising the FFM.

As with anthropometry, the accuracy and precision of the BIA method is affected by instrumentation, subject factors, technician skill, and the prediction equation used to estimate FFM (17). Research has shown that whole body resistance measured by different single frequency analyzers can differ as much as 36 ohms (18). To control this error, analyzers must be calibrated prior to measurement, the same instrument should be used when following changes in composition, and, ideally, the same brand of analyzer should be used as was used to develop the equation. Factors such as eating, drinking, and exercising must be controlled since hydration status is an important source of error in resistance measurements. Technician error is minor provided that standard procedures for electrode positioning and subject positioning are followed. Finally, as with skinfolds, equation error can be reduced by selecting prediction equations based on age, sex, race, and level of physical activity.

Recent research suggests that with multiple frequency bioelectrical impedance analysis (MFBIA) it may be possible to estimate extracellular and intracellular water compartments along with TBW (16). As a result, MFBIA may be less affected by hydration status and, thus, provide better estimates of FFM. MFBIA may also enhance the clinical application of BIA to assess changes and shifts between intra- and extracellular fluid compartments associated with certain diseases.

EQUATION SELECTION

Prediction equations are either population-specific or generalized. Population-specific equations are derived for use in a specific homogeneous population (e.g., prepubescent Caucasian males or elderly African-American females). Thus, they are likely to systematically under- or over-estimate body composition if applied to individuals from other populations. In contrast, generalized equations can be applied to individuals who differ greatly in physical characteristics. Generalized equations are developed from diverse, heterogenous samples and account for differences in age, sex, race, ethnicity and other characteristics by including these variables as predictors in the equation.

To develop prediction equations, a representative sample of the specific population is selected. The predictor variables (e.g., height and weight, age, race, skinfolds or BIA) and the criterion estimates of body composition (percent fat or FFM) are measured in the same subjects and the equation is statistically developed. The usefulness of the equation depends on the strength of association between the variables and the accuracy which the dependent variable is estimated. Useful equations give estimates of percent fat or FFM that are significantly correlated ($R \geq 0.80$) with criterion measurements. Moreover, the means and standard deviations of the estimated and criterion scores should be nearly equal and the standard error of estimate (SEEs) for predicting the criterion measurements from the estimated values should be approximately 2.5–3.5% for percent fat and 2.5–3.5 kg for FFM.

To select the most appropriate equation, it is important to evaluate the relative merit of the various methods and equations. The following questions should be considered (3):

1. *To whom is the equation applicable?* The answer to this questions lies in a careful examination of the characteristics of the population used to derive the equation. Factors such as age, race, sex, physical activity level, and level of body fatness need to be examined carefully. Unless the equation has been shown to generalize to other groups, it should not applied in groups with different characteristics.
2. *Was an appropriate reference method used to develop the equation?* Error in the reference measure is propagated and contributes to the total error in the equation. Multiple component models require fewer assumptions and give more accurate reference measurements than methods based on the 2C model. Equations derived from reference measurements based on 3C and 4C models should be used in populations in which the assumptions underlying the 2C model are not valid. Alternatively, population-specific conversion formulas should be used to derive reference estimates of FFM and percent fat.
3. *Was a representative sample of the population studied?* Large, randomly selected samples (100–400 subjects) are needed to ensure the sample is representative. If random sampling is not possible and convenience samples are used, the procedure is acceptable as long as a sufficient numbers of subjects are studied. With an appropriate sample size, a more stable, valid, and generalizable equation will be derived.
4. *How were the predictor variables measured?* When applying any equation, it is important that the predictor variables be measured as they were measured by the investigators who developed the equation. Although it is recommended that standard procedures and sites be used this is not always done and errors are larger if the original procedures are not followed (5).
5. *Was the equation cross-validated in another sample of the population?* Because of investigator- and laboratory-specific procedural differences, equations that give accurate validation results may not be as accurate when used in different laboratory or by a different investigator and the equation should be tested in other samples of the same population. Sometimes, this is done by dividing the original sample into validation and cross-validation groups and tested in both groups. Although this approach is reasonable, it does not demonstrate whether the equation can be truly generalized outside of the laboratory where it was developed. It is preferable to test the equation in samples in a different laboratory to determine its validity and ability to be generalized. In addition, cross-validation studies in different populations are necessary to determine the accuracy in different groups.

6. *Does the equation give accurate estimates of composition?* In validation studies, the multiple correlation between the variables should be ≥0.80 and SEEs should range from 2.5–3.5% when estimating percent fat and 2.5–3.5 kg when estimating FFM. In addition, the prediction equation should yield a comparable average and distribution (range and standard deviation) of scores, and the total error should not be much larger than the SEE (13).

RECOMMENDED EQUATIONS

The task of equation selection was recently made easier by Heyward and Stolarczyk who reviewed the available equations and developed "decision trees" for selecting the most useful equations (Fig. 45.1 and 45.2) (3). Decision trees can be used to find appropriate equations for African-American, Caucasian, and Hispanic males and females. The mathematical formulas for each equation are given in Tables 45.4 and 45.5. Equations for other minority groups and athletes are also available (3). These equations do not meet all criteria outlined above, however, they are the most useful to date.

BODY FAT STANDARDS

There are no accepted percent body fat standards for all ages. Most body composition studies use small

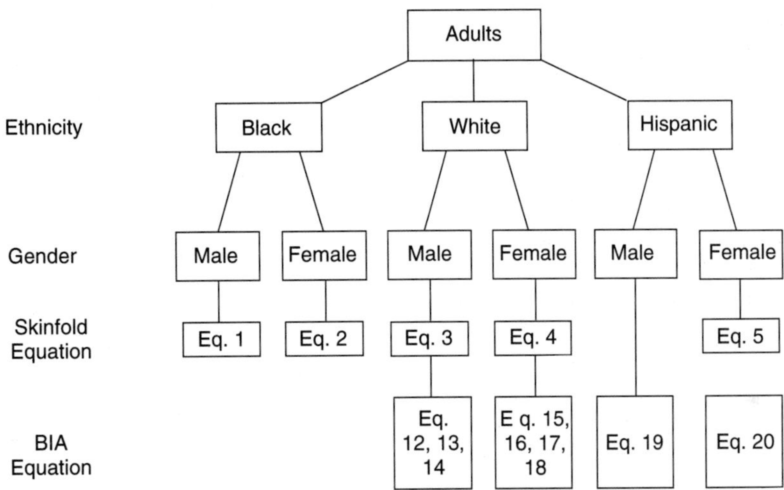

Figure 45.1. Skinfold and bioelectrical impedance analysis (BIA) equation finder for adults. (Adapted from Heyward VH, Stolarzcsyk LM. *Applied Body Composition Assessment.* Champaign, IL: Human Kinetics, 1996:165–168.)

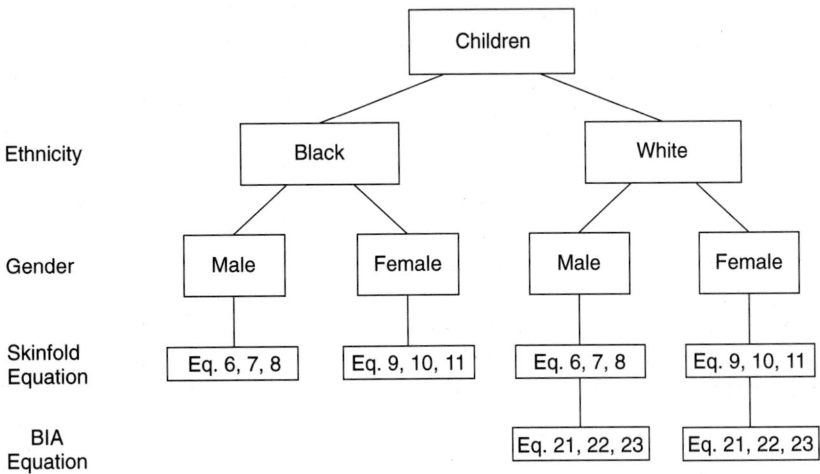

Figure 45.2. Skinfold and bioelectrical impedance analysis (BIA) equation finder for children. (Adapted from Heyward VH, Stolarzcsyk LM. *Applied Body Composition Assessment.* Champaign, IL: Human Kinetics, 1996:165–168.)

Table 45.4. Skinfold Prediction Equations

	ETHNICITY	GENDER	AGE	EQUATION	
1	black	males	18–61	Db (g/cc) = 1.1120 − 0.00043499 (Σ 7SKF chest, abdomen, thigh, triceps, subscapular, suprailiac, midaxillary) + 0.00000055 (Σ 7SKF)^2 − 0.00028826 (age).	Jackson & Pollock (1978).
2	black	females	18–55	Db (g/cc) = 1.0970 − 0.00046971 (Σ 7SKF chest, abdomen, thigh, triceps, subscapular, suprailiac, midaxillary) + 0.00000056 (Σ 7SKF)^2 − 0.00012828 (age).	Jackson et al. (1980).
3	white	males	18–61	Db (g/cc) = 1.109380 − 0.0008267 (Σ 3SKF chest, abdomen, thigh) + 0.0000016 (Σ 3SKF)^2 − 0.0002574 (age).	Jackson & Pollock (1978).
4	white	females	18–55	Db (g/cc) = 1.0994921 − 0.0009929 (Σ 3SKF triceps, suprailiac, thigh) + 0.0000023 (Σ 3SKF)^2 − 0.0001392 (age).	Jackson et al. (1980).
5	hispanic	females	20–40	Db (g/cc) = 1.0970 − 0.00046971 (Σ 3SKF chest, abdomen, thigh, triceps, subscapular, suprailiac, midaxillary) + 0.00000056 (Σ 7SKF)^2 − 0.00012828 (age).	Jackson et al. (1980).
6	black & white	males	≤ 18	%BF = 0.735 (Σ 2SKF triceps, calf) + 1.0	Slaughter et al. (1988).
7	black & white	males (SKF > 35 mm)	≤ 18	%BF = 0.735 (Σ 2SKF triceps, subscapular) + 1.6	Slaughter et al. (1988).
8	black & white	males (SKF > 35 mm)	≤ 18	%BF = 0.783 (Σ 2SKF triceps, subscapular) − 0,008 (Σ 2SKF)^2 + 1*.	Slaughter et al. (1988).
9	black & white	females	≤ 18	%BF = 0.610 (2SKF triceps, calf) + 5.1	Slaughter et al. (1988).
10	black & white	females (SKF > 35 mm)	≤ 18	%BF = 0.546 (Σ 2SKF triceps, subscapular) + 9.7	Slaughter et al. (1988).
11	black & white	females (SKF > 35 mm)	≤ 18	%BF = 1.33 (Σ 2SKF triceps, subscapular) − 0.013 (Σ 2SKF)^2 − 2.5.	Slaughter et al. (1988).

(Adapted from Heyward VH, Stolarcyzk LM. Applied Body Composition Assessment. Champaign IL: Human Kinetics, 1996:173–185.)
* = intercept substitutions based on maturation and ethnicity for boys:

age	black	white
prepubescent	−3.2	−1.7
pubescent	−5.2	−3.4
postpubescent	−6.8	−5.5

groups who are usually young adults. These studies demonstrate that body fat typically ranges between 10–20% for men and between 20–30% for women. Based on these studies, recommendations of 15% for men and 25% for women have been made. These "standards" essentially represent the average percent fat for young adults. Their usefulness in other groups has not been established.

National data for describing percent fat for the U.S. population are not available. However, there are skinfold data from the National Health and Nutrition Examination Survey (NHANES) on a large (20,000) representative sample of U.S. men and women. Despite the limitations of skinfolds, these national data provide a better basis for developing standards than convenience samples. Conversion of the NHANES skinfold data (triceps and subscapular skinfolds) to percent fat using published equations shows the average (50th percentile) percent fats for 20–34 year old men and women are 12% and 28%, respectively (19, 20). The percent fats corresponding to the 15th (low) and 85th percentiles (high) are 5% and 22%, respectively, for young men, and 22% and 39% for young women. It is clear that the percent fats corresponding with the median and low and high skinfold percentiles vary with age as well as sex. It is possible that standards should also vary with age, although typically the young adult values are applied to all ages.

Using this approach, new percent fat health standards have been recently proposed (Fig. 45.3) (15). Some increase in percent fat with age was allowed. This was done in consideration of recent studies showing that lower body fat or reduced body fat in middle-age women is associated with a lower bone mineral content putting those women at risk for osteoporosis and bone fractures. Thus, the emphasis on lower percent fat to prevent heart disease, especially in women, must be balanced against the increased risk of bone fractures, especially if bone mineral content is already low.

Standards for active men and women have also been developed (Table 45.6). These standards are not necessarily associated with better health but may be associated with improved physical performance.

Table 45.5. Bioelectric Impedance Analysis (BIA) Prediction Equations

	Ethnicity	Gender	Age	Equation	
12	white	males	18–29	FFM (kg) = 0.485 (HT²/r) + 0.338 (BW) + 5.32	Lohman (1992)
13	white	males (<20% BF)	17–62	FFM (kg) = 0.00066360 (HT²) − 0.02117 (R) + 0.62854 (BW) − 0.12380 (age + 9.33285)	Segal et al. (1988)
14	white	males (≥20% BG)	17–62	FFM (kg) = 0.00088580 (HT²) − 0.02999 + 0.42688 (BW) − 0.07002 (age) + 14.52435	Segal et al. (1988)
15	white	females	18–29	FFM (kg) = 0.476 (HT²/r) + 0.295 (BW) + 5.49	Lohman (1992)
16	white	females	30–49	FFM (kg) = 0.493 (HT²/r) + 0.141 (BW) + 11.59	Lohman (1992)
17	white	females	50–70	FFM (kg) = 0.474 (HT²/r) + 0.180 (BW) + 7.3	Lohman (1992)
18	white	females	22–74	FFM (kg) = 0.00151 (HT²) − 0.0344 (R) + 0.140 (BW) − 0.158 (age) + 20.387	Gray et al. (1989)
19	Hispanic	males	19–59	FFM (kg) = 13.74 + 0.34 (HT²/r) + 0.33 (BW) − 0.14 + (age) + 6.18	Rising et al. (1991)
20	Hispanic	females	20–40	FFM (kg) = 0.00151 (HT²) − 0.0344 (R) + 0.140 (BW) − 0.158 (age) + 20.387	Gray et al. (1989)
21	white	males and females	6–10	TBW (L) = 0.593 (HT²/r) + 0.65 (BW) + 0.04	Kushner (1992)
22	white	males and females	10–19	FFM (kg) = 0.61 (HT²/r) + 0.25 (BW) + 1.31	Houtkooper et al. (1992)
23	white	males and females	8–15	FFM (kg) = 0.62 (HT²/r) + 0.21 (BW) + 0.10 (Σc) + 4.2	Lohman (1992)

Adapted from Heyward YH, Stolarczyk LM. Applied Body Composition Assessment. Champaign IL: Human Kinetics, 1996:173–185.
HT = height (cm), BW = body weight (kg), R = resistance (Ω), Σ_c = reactance (Ω), TBW = total body water (L)
To convert TBW to FFM, use the following hydration constants:

Boys		Girls	
	5–6 yr FFM (kg) = TBW/0.77		5–6 yr FFM (kg) = TBW/0.78
	7–8 yr FFM (kg) = TBW/0.768		7–8 yr FFM (kg) = TBW/0.776
	9–10 yr FFM (kg) = TBW/0.762		9–10 yr FFM (kg) = TBW/0.77

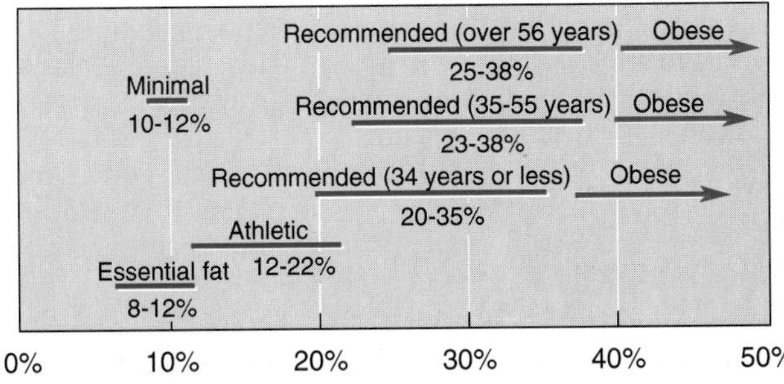

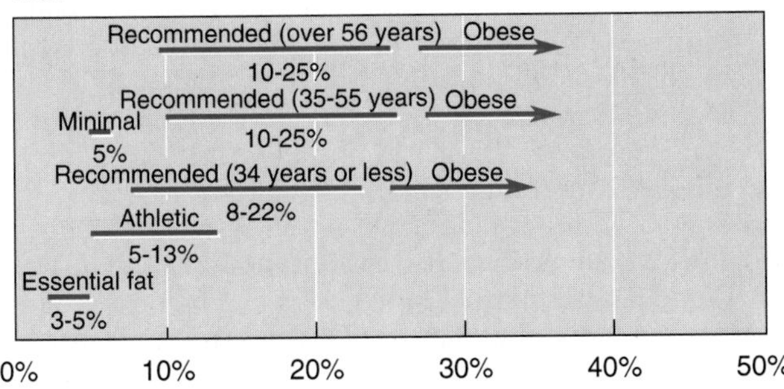

Figure 45.3. Percent fat standards for men and women.

Table 45.6. Percent Fat Standards for Active Men and Women

	Not Recommended	Recommended Body Fat Levels (%) Low	Mid	Upper
Men				
young adult	< 5	5	10	15
middle adult	< 7	7	11	18
elderly	< 9	9	12	18
Women				
young adult	< 16	16	23	28
middle adult	< 20	20	27	33
elderly	< 20	20	27	33

(Adapted from Lohman TG, Houtkooper LB, Going SB. Body composition assessment: body fat standards and methods in the field of exercise and sports medicine. ACSM Health Fitness J (in press).)

Recently, a unique approach to derive percent fat standards for children and adolescents has been reported (21). In this study, the authors sought to develop criterion-referenced standards by assessing risk for high levels of blood pressure, total cholesterol, and low-density lipoprotein and low levels of high-density lipoprotein in males and females aged 6–18 years at different levels of body fatness. No excess risk was found until percent fat exceeded 25% in males and 30% in females. Age and race were not significant predictors of risk in this age group. Thus, >25% fat in males and >30% fat in females have been proposed as useful health standards for African-American and Caucasian males and females aged 6–18 years. A similar criterion-referenced approach would be useful in adults to determine whether risk varies with age and percent fat, or whether one standard is valid for all ages.

RESOURCES FOR BODY COMPOSITION ASSESSMENT

A number of excellent resources are available with additional information on both laboratory and field methods for assessing body composition. For a comprehensive review of laboratory techniques the reader is referred to the monograph by Lohman, *Advances in Body Composition Assessment,* and the recent book by Roche, Heymsfield, and Lohman, *Human Body Composition* (5, 13). For information on field techniques, the monograph by Heyward and Stolarcyzk, *Applied Body Composition Assessment,* is particularly helpful, as is the *Anthropometric Standardization Reference Manual* from the Arlie conference which describes the recommended standard techniques for anthropometry (3, 4). There are also video tapes, manuals, and software packages available from Human Kinetics Publishers (Champaign, IL) for training and standardizing procedures and for simplifying calculations and reporting results.

References

1. Wang ZM, Pierson RN, Heymsfield SB. The five level model: a new approach to organizing body composition research. *Am J Clin Nutr* 56:19–28, 1992.
2. Heymsfield SB, Wang ZM, Withers RT. Multicomponent molecular level models of body composition. In: Roche AF, Heymsfield SB, Lohman TG, eds. *Human Body Composition.* Champaign, IL: Human Kinetics, 1996:129–147.
3. Heyward VH, Stolarzcsyk LM. *Applied Body Composition Assessment.* Champaign, IL: Human Kinetics, 1996.
4. Lohman TG, Roche AF, Martorell R, eds. *Anthropometric Standardization Reference Manual.* Champaign, IL: Human Kinetics, 1988.
5. Roche AF, Heymsfield SB, Lohman TG, eds. *Human Body Composition.* Champaign, IL: Human Kinetics, 1996.
6. Wang ZM, Heshka S, Pierson RN, et al. Systematic organization of body composition methodology: An overview with emphasis on component-based methods. *Am J Clin* Nutr 61:457–465, 1995.
7. Heymsfield SB, Wang J, Lichtman S, et al. Body composition in elderly subjects: a critical appraisal of clinical methodology. *Am J Clin Nutr* 50:1167–1175, 1989.
8. Ellis, KJ. Whole-body counting and neutron activation analysis. In: Roche AF, Heymsfield SB, Lohman TG, eds. *Human Body Composition.* Champaign, IL: Human Kinetics, 1996:45–61.
9. Schoeller DA. Hydrometry. In: Roche AF, Heymsfield SB, Lohman TG, eds. *Human Body Composition.* Champaign, IL: Human Kinetics, 1996:25–43.
10. Going SB. Densitometry. In: Roche AF, Heymsfield SB, Lohman TG, eds. *Human Body Composition.* Champaign, IL: Human Kinetics, 1996:3-23.
11. Brozek J, Grande F, Anderson JT, et al. Densitometric analysis of body composition: Revision of some quantitative assumptions. *Ann NY Acad Sci* 110:113–140, 1963.
12. Siri WE. The gross composition of the body. *Adv Biol Med Physiol* 4:239–280, 1956.
13. Lohman TG. *Advances in Body Composition Assessment.* Champaign, IL: Human Kinetics, 1992.
14. Going SB, Williams DP, Lohman, TG. Aging and body composition: biological changes and methodological issues. *Exerc Sport Sci Rev* 23:411–458, 1995.
15. Lohman TG, Houtkooper LB, Going SB. Body composition assessment: body fat standards and methods in the field of exercise and sports medicine. *ACSM Health Fitness J* 1: 30–35, 1997.
16. Baumgartner RN. Electrical impedance and total body electrical conductivity. In: Roche AF, Heymsfield SB, Lohman TG, eds. *Human Body Composition.* Champaign, IL: Human Kinetics, 1996:79–107.
17. Kushner RF. Bioelectrical impedance analysis: A review of principles and applications. *J Am Coll Nutr* 11:199–209, 1992.
18. Graves JE, Pollock ML, Colvin AB, et al. Comparison of different bioelectrical impedance analyzers in the prediction of body composition. *Am J Hum Biol* 1:603–611, 1989.
19. Jackson AS, Pollock ML. Generalized equations for predicting body density of men. *Br J Nutr* 61:497–504, 1978.
20. Jackson AS, Pollock ML, Ward A. Generalized equations for predicting body density of women. *Med Sci Sports Exerc* 12:175–182, 1980.
21. Williams DP, Going SB, Lohman TG, et al. Body fatness and risk for elevated blood pressure, total cholesterol, and serum lipoprotein ratios in children and adolescents. *Am J Public Health* 82:358–363, 1992.
22. Department of Health and Human Services. The Surgeon General's report on nutrition and health (DHHS [PHS] Publication 88–50210). Washington, DC: U.S. Government Printing Office, 1988.
23. Slaughter MH, Lohman TG, Boileau RA, et al. Skinfold equations for estimation of body fatness in children and youth. *Human Biol* 60:709–723, 1988.
24. Segal KR, Van Loan M, Fitzgerald PI, et al. Lean body mass estimation by bioelectrical impedance analysis: a four site cross-validation study. *Am J Clin Nutr* 47:7–14, 1988.
25. Gray DS, Bray GA, Bauer M, et al. Effect of obesity on bioelectric impedance. *Am J Clin Nutr* 50:255–260, 1989.
26. Rising R, Swinburn B, Larson K, et al. Body composition in Pima Indians: validation of bioelectrical resistance. *Am J Clin Nutr* 53:594–598, 1992.
27. Houtkooper LB, Going SB, Lohman TG, et al. Bioelectrical impedance estimation of fat-free body mass in children and youth: a cross-validation study. *J Appl Physiol* 72: 366–373, 1992.

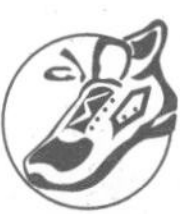

CHAPTER 46
NUTRITION

Donna Israel

Nutrition assessment is a broad-based method of determining the nutritional status and nutrient requirements of individuals. The assessment is designed to be completed by a Registered Dietitian (14). The American Dietetic Association defines nutrition assessment further as "the evaluation of nutrition needs of individuals based upon appropriate biochemical, anthropometric measurements, and laboratory data (1)." Thus, four types of data are evaluated in a nutrition assessment:

- Dietary
- Biochemical
- Anthropometric
- Physical.

Information on which dietary data are based is typically subjective and includes appetite, food habits, exercise habits, special diets, bowel function, and food allergies. In contrast, biochemical data are based on objective values, such as laboratory values for urine, blood, and other tissues, as are anthropometric data, which include height, weight, skinfold, and body circumferences. Physical data are based on an examination of the patient for clinical signs of nutrient deficiency or excess. Physical data can be obtained through observation of the patient's skin, face, lips, nails, hair, teeth, eyes, and musculature. The musculoskeletal systems require functional assessments. Functional evaluations may be necessary in other systems, also, to rule out impairments (1, 33).

The assessment often includes data from other health or clinical settings, and follows a model similar to the following:

- Identification and screening
- Planning
- Implementation
- Evaluation and monitoring.

TOOLS FOR NUTRITION ASSESSMENT

Nutrition Screening

Nutrition screening is the "process of identifying characteristics known to be associated with nutrition problems. Its purpose is to pinpoint individuals who are malnourished or at nutritional risk (1)." The screening process should:

- Work in any setting
- Compliment the process of promoting early intervention
- Include data on risk factors and interpret them correctly to facilitate treatment
- Determine the need for nutrition assessment
- Be cost effective

24-Hour Recall

The purpose of the 24-hour recall is to evaluate food choices within the past 24 hours. It is a method of estimating food intake that limits the risk of the patient reporting food habits inaccurately. To enhance the accuracy of this tool, it should be based on a recent 24-hour period. The tool may be self-administered, but it is usually more accurate when a nutritionist uses it to interview the patient, asking open-ended questions designed to encourage the patient to report all foods and beverages consumed, usually in chronological order. This form of assessment is most appropriate when unhealthy eating habits are suspected or in an initial session.

Three-Day Diet Records

A three-day diet record adds insight and accuracy to the assessment of eating patterns. The disadvantage of diet records is that patients often underestimate portion size. This can be overcome through proper instruction concerning estimating portion size. With a three-day record, the patient may use food models, measure food, or even observe measuring cups and spoons to visualize portion size. Forms specifying time, location, food type (include brand name), portion size, method of preparation, and, perhaps, emotional state should be used. The patient is instructed to record each food and beverage consumed, including water, gum, and candy, over the course of the recording period (usually two weekdays and one weekend day). Three-day diet records are useful in tracking frequent eating patterns, analyzing diets for a deficiency or excess of nutrients, and as a teaching tool to demonstrate healthy alternatives to inappropriate food choices.

Diet History

A diet history is used to determine the patient's normal intake over a period of time. Questions such as, "What do you typically eat for breakfast?" or "What do you usually eat first when you awaken?" are often included in the interview. Responses to these questions may be cross-checked with a food frequency form (Fig 46.1), although such forms may not be appropriate when dietary patterns vary.

This tool differs somewhat from the food frequency method, described below, in that the diet history is used to determine overall intake and prevalence of certain foods in the diet rather than to identify food intake patterns. Unlike the food frequency method, the diet history method also requires significant interviewing skills to obtain accurate data.

Food Frequency Questionnaire

A food frequency questionnaire is useful for monitoring patterns of food intake. The questionnaire can be used to identify specific foods or types of foods that are consumed in excessive or insufficient amounts. Underestimation of portion size is a common problem with this tool, although food models and/or measuring devices may be used during the interview to indicate portion sizes as accurately as possible.

A French model recently challenged the reliability of information gained by using the food frequency questionnaire (34). When used to assess the quality of food intake by French adults, the food frequency form revealed that the French diet failed to meet some of the USDA dietary guidelines (e.g., those summarized in the Food Pyramid and US Dietary Guidelines). However, a modified diet quality index (DQI), a dietary diversity (DD) score, and a dietary variety score (DVS) indicated that the French diet was more diverse than the standard American diet. This implies that the "French paradox"—the lower-than-expected mortality from coronary heart disease in a society where the diet is rich in fat, especially saturated fat—may be linked to overall diet quality rather than with specific foods.

Physical Examination

Clinical examination of a patient is an essential component of a thorough assessment. Even a gross examination of the eyes, hair, face, teeth, skin, nails, and lips can provide key information regarding the patient's nutritional status. Functional evaluation of the musculoskeletal, cardiovascular, and gastrointestinal systems can yield additional information.

ANTHROPOMETRIC DATA

Anthropometric data are based on measurements of the following:

- Height
- Weight
- Body mass index (BMI)
- Body composition
- Waist-to-hip ratio

These measurements are compared to norms that consider age, gender, body frame, and ethnicity. Anthropometry has many advantages. These measurements are usually less expensive and easier to obtain than clinical data. They are also safer for the patient because they can be obtained noninvasively. Anthropometric measurements may be obtained in the field as well as in clinical settings. and can be taken by individuals with minimal training. Field work presents a few disadvantages, however: the measurements may be less accurate when taken by untrained or poorly trained individuals. In addition, measurements may be affected by the testing environment (1). Another concern in anthropometry in general is that the equipment used for assessment must be properly maintained and calibrated regularly for accurate results. To ensure the most accurate measures possible, the same technician should assess the patient on each visit.

Height

It is usually more important to measure height in children than in adults. However, periodic measurements in adults (every 3 to years) is recommended. Unfortunately, height is often self-reported by adults and, thus, may be inaccurate. An inaccurate measurement may make it difficult to assess body weight.

A stadiometer is often used to measure height. Height can be measured indirectly through knee height and arm span. Knee height is measured from the heel to the anterior surface of the thigh while the knee is flexed 90°. This may be useful in individuals with spinal deformities, or with patients on bedrest or who are unable to stand (1). Knee height can be extrapolated to total height by means of a regression equation (4). **Arm span** may also be measured to estimate skeletal length. Arm span is the distance from the longest fingertip of one hand to the longest fingertip of the opposite hand when the arms are fully abducted at shoulder level (1).

Weight

Weight is most commonly measured using a platform balance scale. Weight without shoes, without objects in

FOOD INTAKE RECORD

Please indicate which foods you eat.

	Less than once a week	Not daily but at least once a week	Daily
Milk, yogurt			
Cheese			
Red meat			
Poultry			
Fish			
Eggs			
Mixed dishes			
Dried beans, legumes			
Peanut butter			
Nuts			
Breads, cereal			
Potatoes, pasta, rice			
Fruits, juices			
Vegetables			
Margarine, butter			
Cooking oil			
Sour cream, salad dressing			
Ice cream			
Cookies, cake, pie			
Candy			
Soft drink			
Coffee			
Tea, iced tea			
Alcohol			

Describe your usual daily eating pattern (include amount eaten).

Time	Meal	Food/method of preparation	Amount eaten	Calculations (for RD)
	Breakfast			
	Snack			
	Lunch			
	Dinner			
	Snack			

Medical Nutrition Therapy Across the Continuum of Care

Figure 46.1. Food intake record.

pockets, and while wearing light clothing is standard. If a change in weight is crucial for a diagnosis or selecting a treatment, it should be measured at least 2 hours after food or liquid intake and while wearing light clothing (1).

A weight history may help the health care professional determine patterns of nutrition and exercise behavior. Typical questions regarding weight history include highest and lowest adult weight, preferred weight, usual weight, and weight change during the past 6 to 12 months (1).

The Metropolitan Life Insurance Company introduced normative tables for weight in 1959. More recently, higher norms were introduced due to increased weight in the general population. Because of this, the 1959 tables are no longer used (5, 6).

Hamwi presents an alternative method for determining ideal body weight (7):

Women: Ideal Body Weight
= *100 lbs for the first 5 feet + 5 lbs for each inch over 5 feet*

Men: Ideal Body Weight
= *106 lbs for the first 5 feet + 6 lbs for each inch over 5 feet*

Body Mass Index (BMI)

BMI is a ratio of weight to height in adults that indicates body composition (10). BMI can be used to define the degree of adiposity without accounting for body frame size. It is calculated by the Quetelet equation (8).

$$BMI = weight\ (kg)/[height\ (m)]^2$$

The BMI correlates the least with body height and the most with independent measures of body fatness in adults, including the elderly. A BMI score of 20 to 25 is associated with the lowest risk for excessive or deficient adipose tissue. Obesity is divided into three grades:

- Grade I = 25.0–29.9
- Grade II = 30–40
- Grade III = 40+

A BMI of at least 27 indicates obesity and increased health risk. BMI increases with age; therefore, age-specific guidelines for interpreting the BMI in the elderly have been recommended.

Body Composition

Percent body fat can be used to stratify the risk for cardiovascular disease (CAD) in patients. The amount of body fat can be estimated by underwater weighing, skinfold thickness measurements, circumferences, bioelectric impedance, and dual x-ray absorptiometry.

Waist-to-Hip Ratio

The waist-to-hip (W:H) ratio is used to estimate the risk for coronary artery disease (CAD). Values of >0.8 for women and >0.9 for men indicate an increased risk for cardiovascular disease and diabetes mellitus. A W:H value greater than 1.0 indicates a significantly increased risk for CAD. For lean and normal-weight individuals, the most accurate method of estimating the risk for CAD may be to combine the W:H ratio and BMI (1).

SUBJECTIVE GLOBAL ASSESSMENT

Subjective global assessment (SGA) includes a physical examination and medical evaluation. The medical evaluation assesses changes in weight and dietary intake; gastrointestinal (GI) symptoms, such as nausea, diarrhea, and vomiting; systemic function; metabolic demands; and environmental factors, such as stress and illness (1). The physical examination should include a measurement of subcutaneous fat to identify muscle wasting, edema, or ascites (1).

ADDITIONAL TOOLS FOR A COMPLETE ASSESSMENT

A complete medical history is the basis of a thorough and accurate nutrition assessment. The most pertinent components of that history are

1. Family history, including a history of diabetes mellitus, stroke, cancer, cardiovascular disease, hypertension, and GI or orthopedic problems which may require nutrition intervention.
2. Personal medical history, including past and current illnesses and surgeries that may indicate nutritional status and intervention requirements.
3. Prescription medications, to rule out the possibility of drug-nutrient interactions, especially in elderly patients, who are 2 to 3 times more susceptible than younger patients (1) (Table 46.1). Common interactions include:
   - Reduced drug efficacy, due to the effects of food on gastric motility or pH
   - Nutrient deficiencies, caused by appetite suppression or emesis (e.g., due to chemotherapy) or increased mineral loss
   - Nutrient excess, caused by appetite stimulation (e.g., due to steroids or tranquilizers)
   - Allergic reactions
4. Alcohol, smoking, and illicit drug use, that may alter caloric requirements and caloric intake, resulting in nutrient deficiencies.
5. Weight history, which may include patterns of change that may indicate a positive or negative energy balance and may provide a reason for signs of nutrient deficiency or excess.
6. Exercise and activity, which may indicate total energy expenditure and can be used to estimate the basal metabolic rate (BMR). BMR can be estimated by the Harris-Benedict equation and then multiplied by an activity factor (below) to yield caloric requirements.

   Formula for Calculation of BMR

   Men: BMR
   = *66 + 13.8(weight in kg) + 5(height in cm) − 6.8 (age)*

   Women: BMR
   = *655 + 9.6 (weight in kg) + 1.8(height in cm) − 4.7 (age)*

   Activity factors
   - 1.2 Bedrest
   - 1.3 Sedentary
   - 1.4 Active
   - 1.5 Very active
7. Stress, which can increase metabolic and micronutrient requirements (11–15).

Table 46.1. **Drug-Food Interactions**

MEDICATION: BRAND NAME (GENERIC NAME) [FUNCTION]	NUTRITIONAL IMPLICATIONS
Cardiovascular agents:	
Inderal (Propanolol HCL) [β-Blocker]	Take with food to enhance absorption (may cause constipation, nausea)
Lanoxin (Digoxin) [Glycoside]	Take on an empty stomach (may cause anorexia, nausea)
Lasix (Furosemide) [Diuretic]	Take with food or milk (may cause nausea, diarrhea, potassium loss)
Procardia (Nifedipine) [Ca^{++} Blocker]	Take with food or milk (may cause diarrhea, constipation)
Anti-Infectives:	
Amoxicillin [Antibiotic]	Take tablet or liquid forms without regard to meals (may cause diarrhea, nausea, vomiting)
Ceclor (Cefaclor) [Antibiotic]	Take without regard to meals (may cause nausea, vomiting, diarrhea)
Erythromycin [Antibiotic]	Take with meals (not milk) to prevent GI distress
Tetracycline [Antibiotic]	Take on an empty stomach. Do not give with dairy products or medical nutritional products
Flagyl (Metronidazole) [Anti-fungal]	Take with food (may cause nausea, vomiting, diarrhea, GI distress)
Analgesics:	
Tylenol (Acetaminophen) [Analgesic]	Take with food to prevent GI distress
Aspirin (Acetylsalicylic acid) [Analgesic]	Take with food to prevent GI distress
Motrin, Advil (Ibuprofen) [Analgesic]	Take with food to prevent GI distress
Codeine [Analgesic, antitussive, narcotic]	Take with food or water to prevent GI distress
Antidepressants:	
Tofranil (Imipramine) [Antidepressant]	Take with food to prevent GI distress (may cause diarrhea, nausea, vomiting)
Nardil (Phenelzine) [MAOI Antidepressant]*	Avoid foods high in tyramine. Limit caffeine-containing foods and beverages.

LABORATORY DATA

The following laboratory data are often used in the nutritional assessment (9):

1. Blood nutrient levels.
2. Urinary excretion rates for nutrients.
3. Urinary nutrient metabolite levels.
4. Abnormal metabolic byproducts in blood.
5. Changes in blood components or enzyme activities related to nutrient intake.
6. Response to a loading, saturation, or isotopic test.

Pertinent laboratory data include albumin, creatinine, cholesterol (blood lipids), triglycerides, glucose, white blood cell (WBC) count, transferrin, hemoglobin, hematocrit, potassium, sodium, chloride, calcium, phosphorus, and carbon dioxide content. Diagnoses are not usually made on the basis of laboratory values alone.

ASSESSMENT THROUGHOUT THE LIFE CYCLE

Protocols for nutrition assessments taken during a specific stage of life should address risk factors common to that age group (16–26). Several of these are discussed below.

Pediatric Population

One of the best indicators of nutritional status in children may be physical growth. Length or stature and weight are commonly used to assess growth. Physical examination of the teeth, gums, and tongue is also helpful in determining the nutritional status of children (1). However, the fact that their eating habits may be affected by a myriad of factors—including flavor acceptance, and the physiological development of taste, as well as habits, ethnicity, social interaction, food availability and convenience, family economic status, emotions, the physical appearance of food, current or prior nutritional status—must be taken into consideration in the development of nutrition interventions.

Anthropometric measures commonly used in this population include the weight-for-height index, height-for-age index, weight-for-age index, head circumference, mid-upper-arm circumference, and triceps skinfold thickness. These indexes can be plotted on standardized forms. The mid-upper-arm circumference and triceps skinfold thickness can help identify wasting since these measures correlate with lean body mass (2, 3). The triceps skinfold can help determine whether excess weight is due to excess fat or excess lean tissue (e.g., muscle hypertrophy in athletes); however, this measurement is not the most reliable measure of body composition (1).

Assessments in the pediatric population should also consider activity level. The Harris-Benedict equation can be used to estimate the caloric requirements.

Adolescent Population

The pediatric patient is considered an adolescent on reaching puberty. Up to 20% of adult height and 50% of weight may be gained during this period. Both body fat and lean muscle mass increase. Females generally experience larger increases in body fat than males, and males usually experience larger increases in lean tissue (31). It is important to use age-specific norms in assessing this population.

Nutrient needs increase significantly during adolescence to accommodate rapid growth. Adolescents are less likely to obtain adequate amounts of vitamins and minerals due to a sudden increase in requirements and generally poor food choices. Nutritional assessment should include an evaluation of the patient's nutritional environment—including parental, peer, school, cultural, personal, and lifestyle factors—as well as attitude toward food and nutrition in general (31). Growth rate as well as exercise habits should be considered when determining the nutritional requirements of adolescents. The development of body image concerns during adolescence may lead to a desire to change the growth rate or body proportions with further dietary manipulation and often has negative consequences. Consequently, a variety of eating disorders may develop during this period (27, 29). Use of tobacco, alcohol, marijuana, and other drugs can also affect the patient's nutritional status.

Adult Population

When the epiphyseal plates close, (about at age 18), adolescents may be considered "adults" for the purposes of nutrition assessment. Weight is particularly useful in assessing the nutritional status of adults. Height and weight should both be measured, as adults commonly overestimate height and underestimate weight. Weight loss reflects an acute inability to meet nutritional requirements and may indicate a nutritional risk factor or illness (31). The use of the Metropolitan Life Insurance table and/or the BMI can help determine appropriate body weight (10). The previously mentioned methods of assessing body composition may also be used to determine nutritional status. Assessments for adults should consider activity and exercise levels. The Harris-Benedict equation can be used to estimate caloric requirements.

Elderly Population

Aging is marked by a progressive loss of lean body mass and increased body fat, and is accompanied by changes in most physiological systems (31). Lean body mass in the healthy elderly is 30% to 40% less than in young adults. This represents the loss of both muscular and visceral protein and leads to functional and metabolic changes. Basal metabolic rate and, therefore, energy requirements decrease by 20% between the ages of 30 and 90, mainly because of decreased lean body mass (31). The Harris-Benedict equation can be used to estimate caloric requirements in this population.

Nutrition assessment of older adults should take into consideration the activity level and the possible existence of chronic disease. Physical activity helps maintain bone and muscle mass and functional capacity in this population and also helps maintain a normal metabolic rate. When caloric requirements fall below 1,800 calories a day in the elderly, inadequate amounts of protein, calcium, iron, and vitamins may be consumed. For this reason, the metabolic rate should be maintained to ensure an adequate nutritional status (31). Most older adults maintain eating habits that they established at younger ages (31). This may present a challenge to the dietitian who may have to help them alter eating habits to meet current needs.

Causes of malnutrition in the elderly include ignorance of appropriate nutrition, financial restrictions, physical disabilities that interfere with the purchase and preparation of food, social isolation, mental disorders, loss of vision, chewing and swallowing difficulties, and changes in taste acuity (31). Other causes of malnutrition include malabsorption, anorexia, alcohol abuse, and long-term use of certain therapeutic drugs.

Approximately 5% of persons aged 65 years and older are institutionalized. Nutrition care of institutionalized elderly is directed at meeting their physiological and psychological needs. The nutrition assessment of elderly patients should consider the current nutritional status, as well as recent illnesses and surgeries, changes in appetite, bowel function and weight. Excellent sources of information regarding the clinical nutrition assessment of elderly individuals with chronic disease are available (13, 32, 35).

▶ SUMMARY

Nutritional assessment is an important tool for evaluating health behavior. In the hands of a good interviewer, this assessment can be used to identify specific factors, such as lifestyle, taste, cultural background, disease, economic status, ability to process food, that affect food intake, and use the information to help the patient achieve a positive behavior change (30).

Five of the leading causes of death in the United States are related to food practices; therefore, changes in these practices may have a significant, effect on the health of the nation. By combining expertise in food and nutrition with a strong background in medical care and behavior modification techniques, medical nutrition therapy provided by a Registered Dietitian, can help prevent or delay the development of disease.

References

1. Simko MD, Cowell C, and Gilbride JA. *Nutrition Assessment: a Comprehensive Guide for Planning Intervention.* Gaithersburg, MD: Aspen Publishers, 1995.
2. Trowbridge FL, Hiney CD, Robertson AD. Arm muscle indicators and creatinine excretion in children. *Am J Clin Nutr* 1982;36:691–696.
3. Chen LC, et al. Anthropometric assessment of energy-protein malnutrition and subsequent risk of mortality among preschool aged children. *Am J Clin Nutr* 1980;33:1836–1845.
4. Chumlea WC, Roche AF, Mukherjee D. *Nutritional Assessment of the Elderly Through Anthropometry.* Columbus, OH: Ross Laboratories, 1987.
5. Metropolitan Life Insurance Company. New weight standards for men and women. *Stat Bull* 1959;40:1–4.
6. Metropolitan Life Foundation. 1983 Metropolitan height and weight tables. *Stat Bull* 1983;64:2–9.
7. Dikovics A. *Nutritional Assessment: Case Study Methods.* Philadelphia, PA: George F. Stickley Co, 1987.

8. Kuskowska-Wolk A, Bergstrom R, Bostrom G. Relationship between questionnaire data and medical records of height, weight, and body mass index. *Intl J Obesity* 1992;16:1–9.
9. King JW, Faulkner WR, eds. *Critical Reviews in Clinical Laboratory Science.* Cleveland, OH: CRC Press, 1973.
10. Fidanza F. *Nutritional Status Assessment: a Manual for Population Studies.* New York, NY: Chapman & Hall, 1991.
11. Snetselaar LG. *Nutrition Counseling Skills: Assessment, Treatment, and Evaluation.* Gaithersburg, MD: Aspen Publishers, 1989.
12. Israel DA, Moores S, eds. *Beyond Nutrition Counseling.* Chicago, IL: American Dietetic Association, 1996.
13. American Dietetic Association. *Medical Nutrition Therapy Across the Continuum of Care: Patient Protocols.* Smyrna, GA: Morrison Health Care, Inc, 1996.
14. Posthauer RD, et al. Identifying patients at risk: ADA's definitions for nutrition screening and nutrition assessment. *J Am Diet Assoc* 1994;94(8):838–839.
15. Gates G. Clinical reasoning: an essential component of dietetic practice. *Top Clin Nutr* 1992;7(3):74–80.
16. American Dietetic Association Public Health Nutrition Dietetic Practice Group. Quality assurance criteria for nutritional care of prenatal women and adolescents. Atlanta, GA: US Dept of Agriculture, Public Health Service, Centers for Disease Control and Prevention, Division of Nutrition, 1993.
17. Dietetics in Developmental and Psychiatric Disorders Dietetic Practice Group. *Clinical Criteria and Indicators for Nutrition Services in Developmental Disabilities, Psychiatric Disorders, and Substance Abuse.* Chicago, IL: American Dietetic Association, 1993.
18. Dietitians in Pediatric Practice Dietetic Practice Group. *Quality Assurance Criteria for Pediatric Nutrition Conditions.* Chicago, IL: American Dietetic Association, 1988.
19. Dwyer JT. *Screening Older Americans' Nutritional Health: Current Practices and Future Possibilities.* Washington, DC: Nutrition Screening Initiative, 1991.
20. Franz MJ. Practice guidelines for nutrition care by dietetics practitioners for outpatients with non-insulin-dependent diabetes mellitus: consensus statement. *J Am Diet Assoc* 1992:92:1136.
21. Gerwick C, ed. *Consultant Dietitians in Health Care Facilities Dietetic Practice Group. Nutrition Care in Nursing Facilities.* Chicago, IL: American Dietetic Association, 1992.
22. *Minimum Data Set (MDS) Manual.* Natick, MA: Eliot Press, 1993.
23. Nutrition Services Payment Systems Committee. *Reimbursement and Insurance Coverage for Nutrition Services.* Chicago, IL: American Dietetic Association, 1991.
24. Queen P, Caldwell M, Balogun L. Clinical indicators for oncology, cardiovascular and surgical patients: report of the ADA Council on practice quality management committee. *J Am Diet Assoc* 1993;93:338.
25. Wilkins K, Schiro K, eds. *Renal Dietitians Dietetic Practice Group. Suggested Guidelines for Nutrition Care of Renal Patients.* 2nd ed. Chicago, IL: American Dietetic Association, 1992.
26. Winkler M, Lysen L, eds. *Dietitians in Nutrition Support Dietetic Practice Group. Suggested Guidelines for Nutrition and Metabolic Management of Adult Patients Receiving Nutrition Support.* Chicago, IL: American Dietetic Association, 1993.
27. American Dietetic Association. Nutrition intervention in the treatment of anorexia nervosa, bulimia nervosa, and binge eating. *J Am Diet Assoc* 1994;94(8):902–907.
28. Reiff D, Reiff KL. *Eating Disorders: Nutrition Therapy in the Recovery Process.* Gaithersburg, MD: Aspen Publishers, 1992.
29. Berg F. Health risks of weight loss. Hennings, SD: Health Weight Journal, 1994.
30. Helm KK, Klawitter, B, eds. *Nutrition Therapy: Advanced Counseling Skills.* Lake Dallas, TX: Helm Seminars, 1995.
31. Mahan KL, Arlin M. *Krause's Food Nutrition and Diet Therapy,* 8th ed. Philadelphia, PA: WB Saunders, 1992.
32. *Dietitian's Patient Education Manual.* Gaithersburg, MD: Aspen Publishers, 1995.
33. Detsky AS. Is this patient malnourished? *JAMA* 1994; z.27(1):54–57.
34. Drewnowski A, et al. Diet quality and dietary diversity in France: implications for the French paradox. *J Am Diet Assoc* 1996;96(7):663–669.
35. Shils ME, Young VR. *Modern Nutrition in Health and Disease* 8th Ed. Philadelphia, PA: Lea & Febiger, 1993.

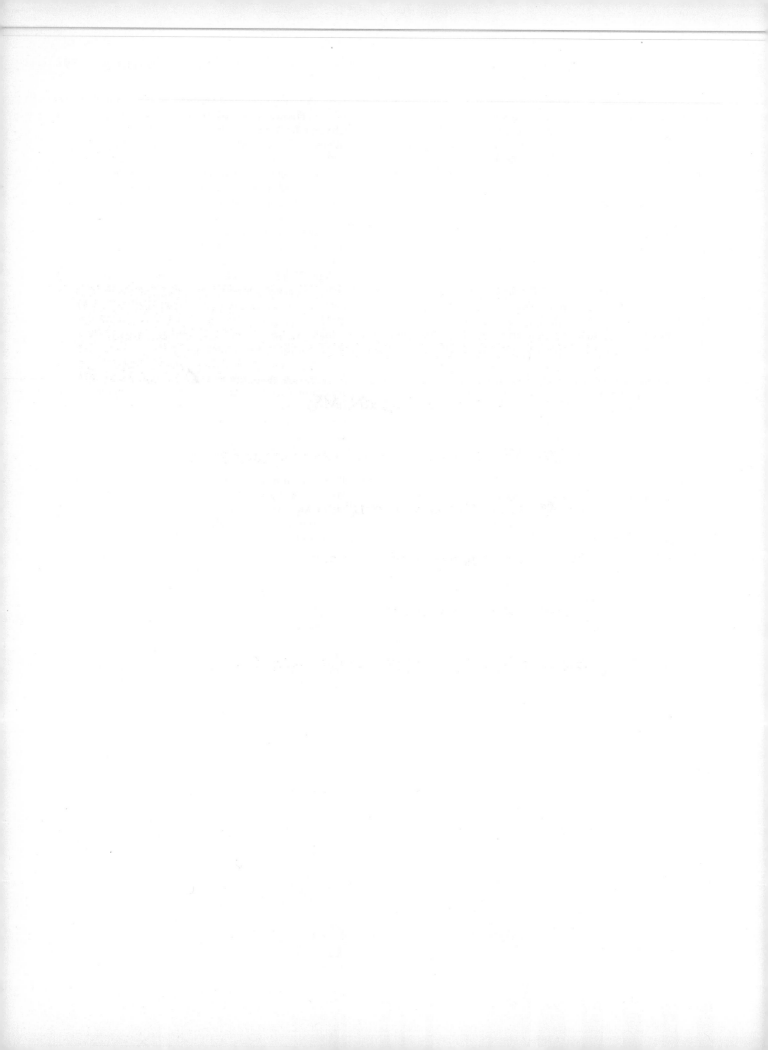

SECTION 9

ELECTROCARDIOGRAPHY

SECTION EDITOR: *Moira Kelsey, RN, MS*

286, 287, 395 400

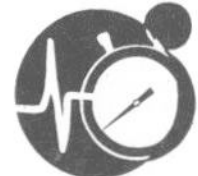

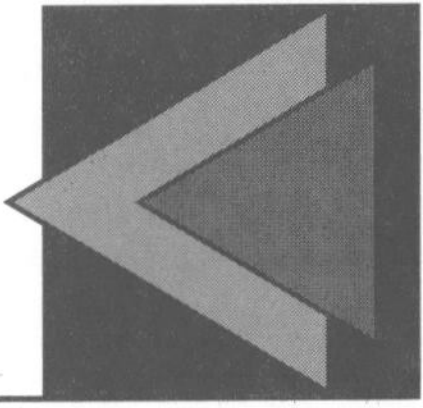

CHAPTER 47
BASIC PRINCIPLES OF ELECTROCARDIOGRAPHY

John A. Larry and Stephen F. Schaal

Electrocardiography (ECG) is the study of the electrical events which occur in the heart. Despite the development of newer modalities that assist clinicians in evaluating cardiac disorders, the ECG has remained an invaluable diagnostic tool. By careful assessment of the ECG tracing, one may obtain information about the heart rate and rhythm, the presence of chamber enlargement and conduction derangements, evidence of acute or previous myocardial infarctions, myocardial ischemia, drug and metabolic effects, and much more. The monitoring of the ECG during exercise is a valuable means of evaluating patients with chest pain.

Although much information can be obtained from electrocardiography, there are limitations. A patient may have electrocardiographic abnormalities and have no underlying heart disease or exhibit a normal ECG in the setting of significant cardiac disease. It is therefore important to interpret the ECG in the context of the history and physical examination findings. This chapter provides an introductory discussion of electrocardiography.

ACTION POTENTIALS

Electrical events occur due to the movement of ions across the membrane of the cell. In the resting phase, cardiac myocytes have a greater number of negatively charged ions within the cell which results in a voltage difference across the cell membrane. This difference is called the transmembrane potential and is approximately −80 to −90 mV. When the cell is stimulated, channels in the cell membrane open and allow positively charged sodium ions to enter the cell, causing depolarization (Fig. 47.1). The changes in membrane potential over time can be depicted as in Figure 47.2, a diagram of the action potential. Depolarization occurs during Phase 0 of the action potential. The depolarization of one cell leads to the depolarization of neighboring cells; in this fashion an impulse (Phase I) is propagated through the heart. Once a cell depolarizes it may not depolarize again until repolarization has occurred. The time interval during which the cell cannot depolarize is termed the refractory period. Repolarization is the restoration of transmembrane potential and occurs during Phases 2 and 3 of the action potential. Phase 4 is a quiescent phase for most cardiac cells. However, in certain cells, such as those at the sinus node, ions travel across the membrane during Phase 4 resulting in a gradual decrease of the membrane potential. Once the voltage reaches a threshold level, depolarization occurs. Cells which possess this property of automaticity include the sinus node, AV node, and His-Purkinje fibers. The sinus node possesses the most rapid Phase 4 depolarization causing it to depolarize first and, thereby, function as the pacemaker of the heart. The rate of Phase 4 depolarization may be delayed by certain classes of medications, namely beta blockers and some calcium channel antagonists, resulting in a slowing of the heart rate. Exercise, via enhanced sympathetic nervous system stimulation and elevated circulating catecholamines, increases the Phase 4 depolarization rate, thereby elevating the heart rate.

Electrocardiography measures the summation of the action potentials of the cardiac cells. The P wave recorded is the summation of atrial action potentials, while the QRS complex recorded is an aggregation of depolarization of the ventricular cells. Each depolarization can be thought of as a vector, a force which has both direction and magnitude. By placing recording leads at different locations on the chest wall, a variety of views of these electrical forces can be obtained. If the recording lead is parallel with the vector of depolarization, the maximum voltage will be recorded. Conversely, if the recording lead is perpendicular to the vector, less displacement of the recording electrode will take place. By definition, electrical depolarization moving toward a positive lead produces an upright deflection on the ECG.

ELECTROCARDIOGRAPHIC LEADS

The standard ECG records the cardiac impulse using 12 leads. **Bipolar limb leads,** which were introduced by Einthoven, record the changes in voltage potentials occurring in the frontal plane. Lead I records the differences in potential between the left arm and the right arm, lead II between the left leg and the right arm, and lead III between the left leg and left arm. By definition, the right arm is the negative pole and the left arm is the positive pole for lead I, the right arm is negative and the left leg is positive for lead II, while the left arm is negative and the left leg is positive for lead III. Figure 47.3 depicts the locations and directions of the standard limb leads and illustrates Einthoven's triangle. Einthoven's law states

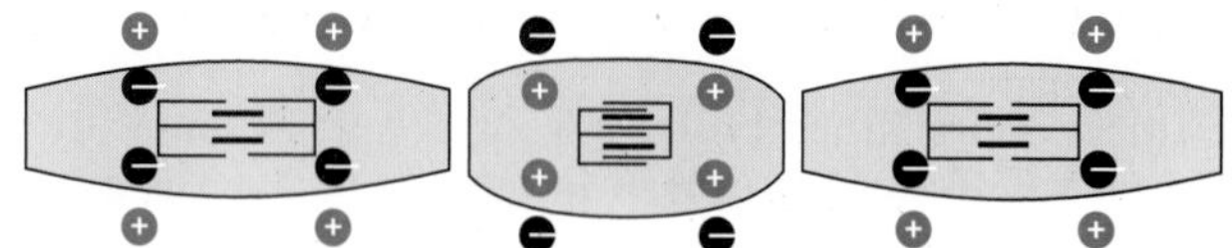

Figure 47.1. When the cell is stimulated, channels in the cell membrane open and allow positively charged sodium ions to enter the cell, causing depolarization.

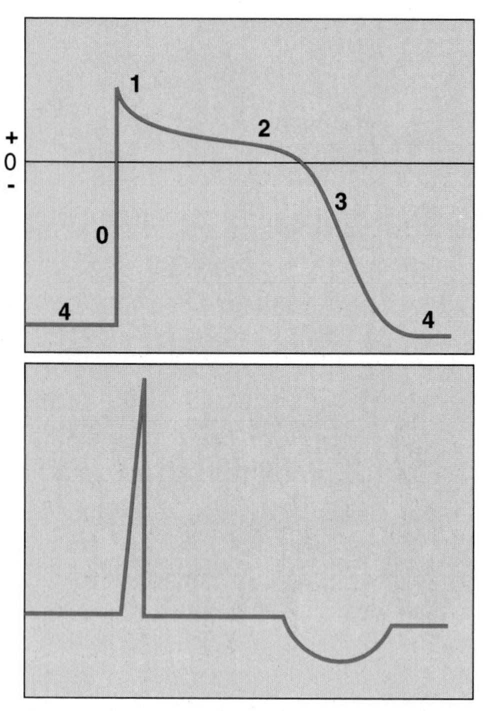

Figure 47.2. Changes in membrane potential over time.

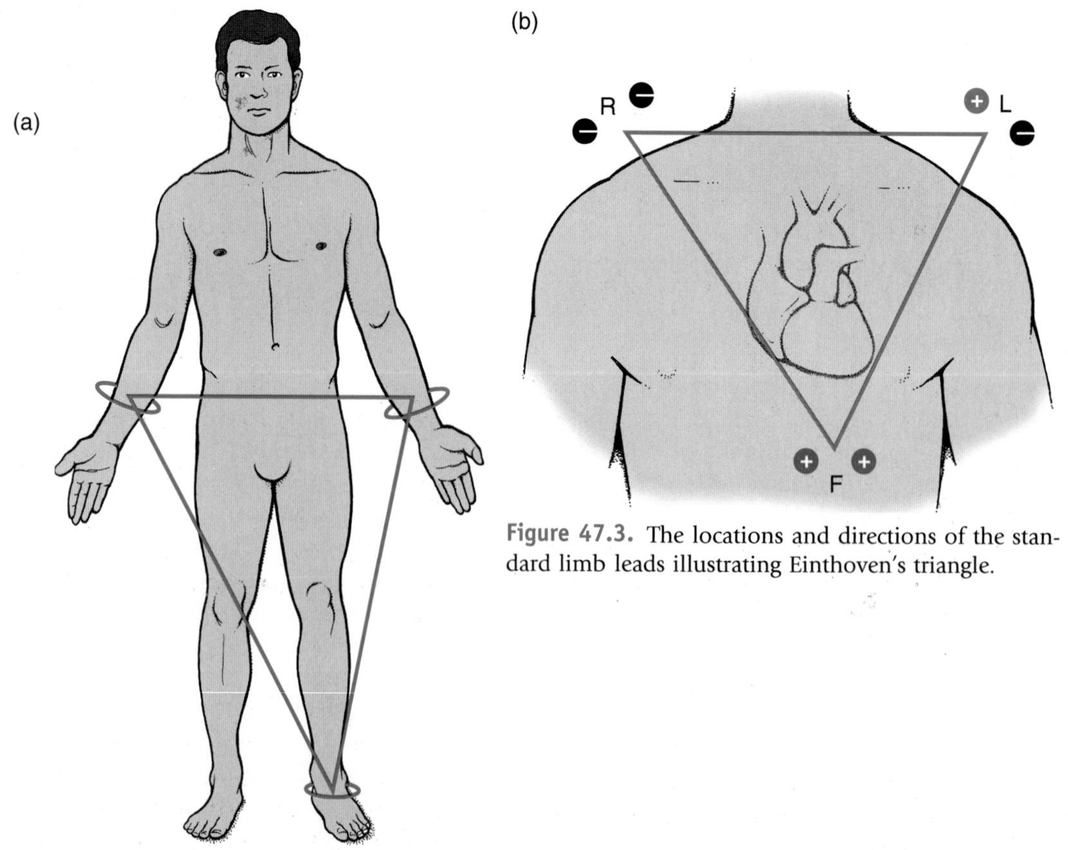

Figure 47.3. The locations and directions of the standard limb leads illustrating Einthoven's triangle.

that the sum of the complexes in leads I and III is equal to the complex in lead II.

Lead I + Lead III = Lead II

This rule is helpful in detecting situations of lead malposition or transposition.

The **unipolar limb leads** are created by connecting all three limb electrodes through a resistance of 5000 ohms to form a central terminal which, for practical purposes, is considered to have a zero potential (Fig. 47.4). The central terminal can be connected to an exploring electrode (designated by the letter V) where the potential difference recorded is dominated by local events. Potentials are recorded from the right arm (R), the left arm (L), and the left leg (F). Since this voltage recorded is quite low, the central terminal is disconnected from the location of the exploring electrode, thus augmenting the voltage recorded. These leads consequently are named aVR, aVL, and aVF.

Figure 47.5 depicts the location and direction of each lead in the frontal plane. Each lead has a positive and a negative pole. Leads I and aVL are considered the high lateral leads, while II, III, and aVF are the inferior or diaphragmatic leads. The positive directions of the limb leads are illustrated in Figure 47.5. Leads V1 through V6 are known as the precordial leads, and record electrical potentials in the transverse plane of the body. The exploring electrode is placed at various locations on the chest wall which allows evaluation of the anteroseptal, anterior, and anterolateral walls of the left ventricle. The positive direction of these leads are shown in Figure 47.6.

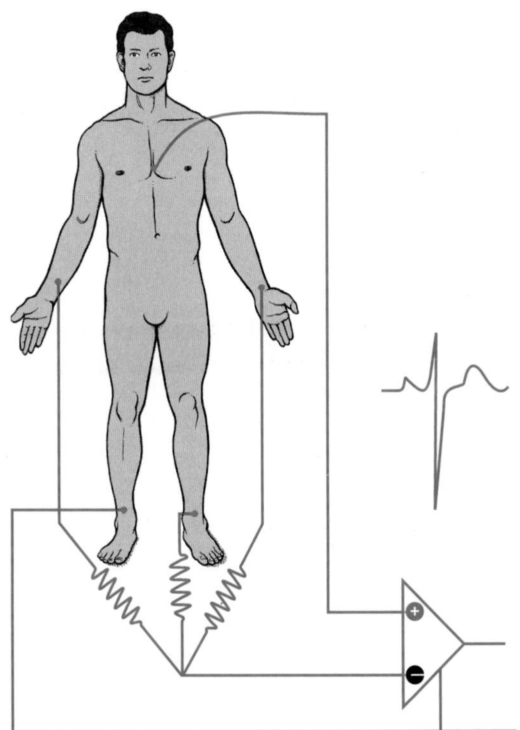

Figure 47.4. The unipolar limb leads are created by connecting all three limb electrodes through a resistance of 5000 ohms to form a central terminal which, for practical purposes, is considered to have a zero potential.

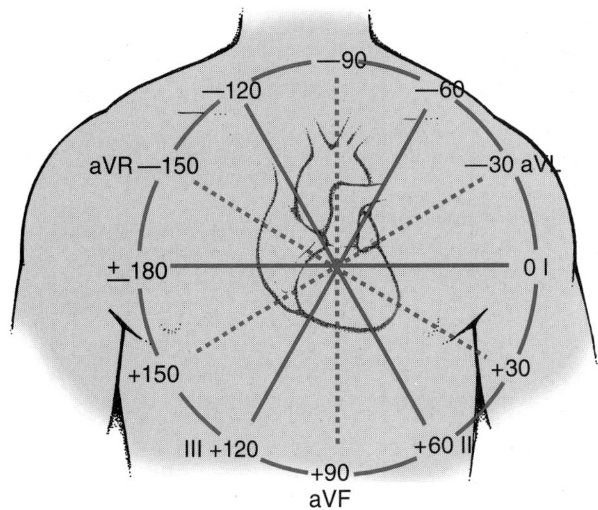

Figure 47.5. The location and direction of each lead in the frontal plane.

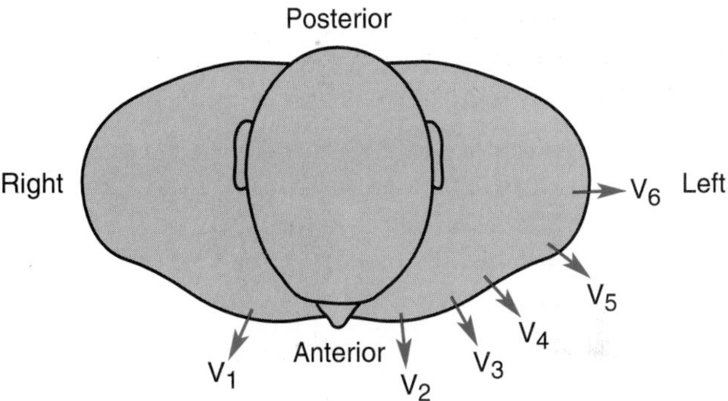

Figure 47.6. The exploring electrode is placed at various locations on the chest wall which allow us to evaluate the anteroseptal, anterior, and anterolateral walls of the left ventricle. The positive direction of these leads are shown here.

PERFORMANCE OF AN ECG

The location of the recording leads is very important since minor variations in lead placement can significantly affect the ECG recording. The limb electrodes are attached to the appropriate wrists and ankles. The electrode attached to the right leg serves as a ground. There are important landmarks on the chest wall which are vital to correct precordial lead placement. These include:

1. The sternal angle (i.e., the junction between the manubrium and the sternum which is located at the level of the second rib).
2. The midclavicular line, half way between the sternoclavicular and acromioclavicular joints.
3. The anterior axillary line, an imaginary vertical line down the anterior fold of the axilla.
4. The mid-axillary line, an imaginary vertical line down the midportion of the axilla.

The standard placement of the unipolar precordial leads is depicted in Figure 47.7. The patient should be in the supine position to achieve proper lead placement. Lead V1 is located in the fourth intercostal space to the right of the sternum. Lead V2 is placed to the left of the sternum also in the fourth intercostal space. Lead V4 should be located in the midclavicular line in the fifth intercostal space, with lead V3 half way between leads V2 and V4. Leads V5 and V6 are aligned with the anterior axillary line and mid-axillary line respectively at the level of lead V4.

The apposition of the ECG leads to the patient is quite important so as to ensure a technically good tracing and minimize artifacts. In some cases, it may be necessary to shave the chest. Relative quiet is necessary in order to minimize skeletal muscle twitching and reduce the likelihood of recording artifact. The skin where the leads will be placed can be cleaned with alcohol and in some cases abraded gently with fine sandpaper or gauze after the alcohol evaporates in order to remove the top layer of skin. This improves the electrical conductance between the patient and the recording electrode.

The standard ECG paper is designed with horizontal and vertical lines at 1 mm intervals (Fig. 47.8). At each 5 mm interval, the line on the grid is accentuated. The ECG is recorded at a speed of 25 mm/sec such that a 5 mm distance represents 0.2 seconds (200 msec). A 1 mm interval (each small box) is equivalent to 0.04 seconds or 40 msec. A 1 second interval is defined by 5 bold lines or large boxes.

The ECG is calibrated such that 1.0 mV of voltage recorded is represented by 10 mm of vertical deflection on the grid. In only rare instances, when the voltage is not totally recorded on the paper or too great to be displayed without merging with the lead above, should this be altered. All modern ECG recorders display a calibration signal (Fig. 47.8). The vertical height is the standardization of a 1.0 mV signal. The calibration signal is 0.2 seconds in duration and documents the paper speed. A 5 mm width of the calibration signal confirms a paper speed of 25 mm/sec.

Different ECG recorders display the standard 12 leads in varying formats. The most common layout is shown in Figure 47.8. In this format, three leads are recorded simultaneously. The initial group consists of leads I, II, and III, followed by leads aVR, aVL, and aVF, then V1, V2, and V3, and finally V4, V5, and V6. In addition to recording a 12-lead ECG, a rhythm strip (not shown

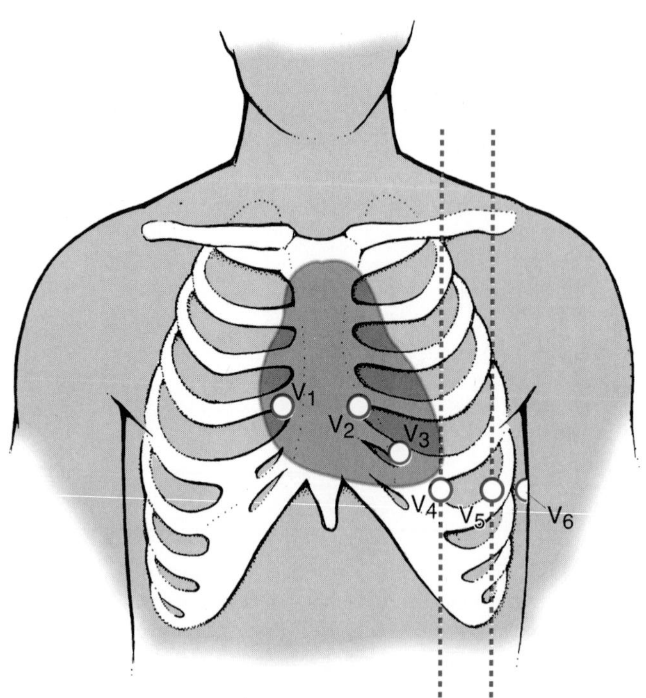

Figure 47.7. The standard placement of the unipolar precordial leads.

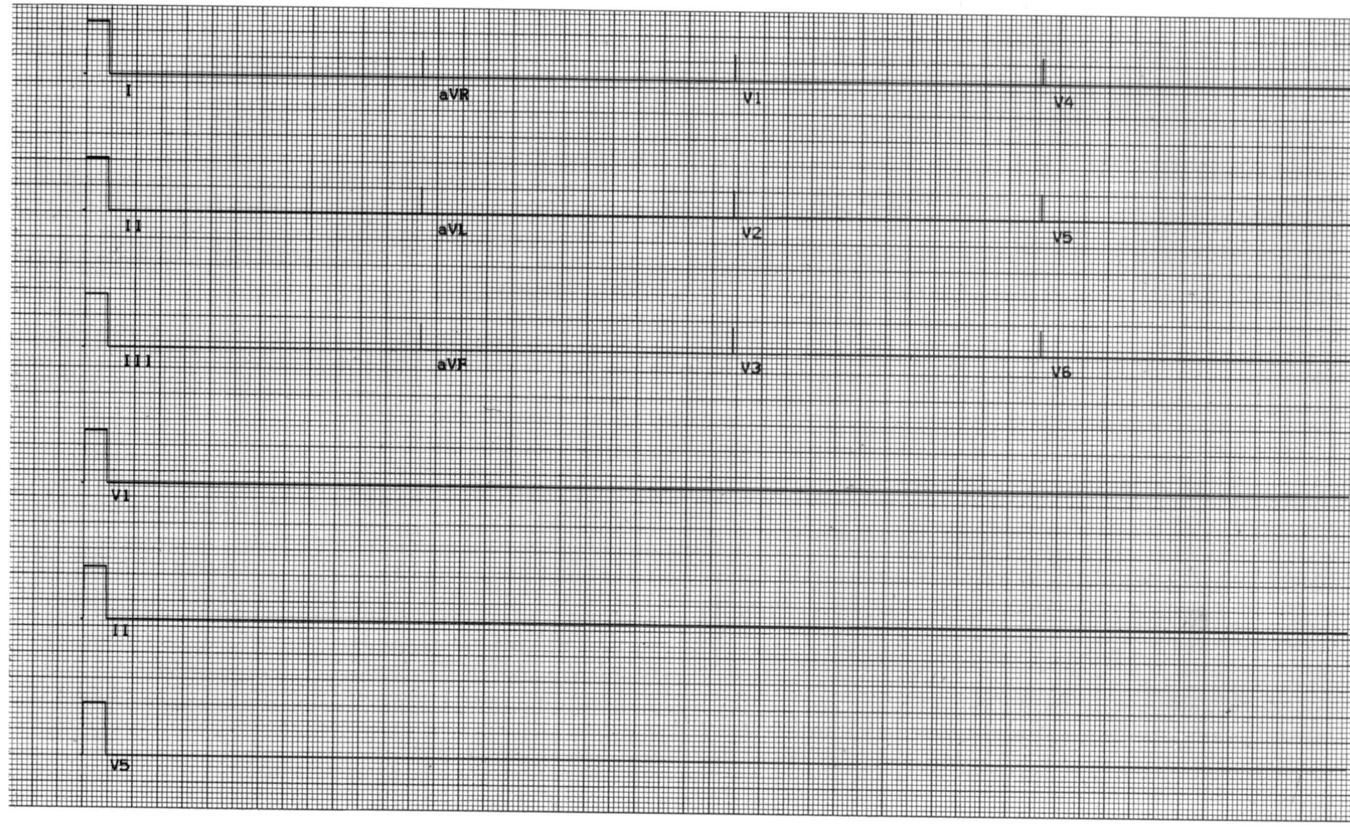

Figure 47.8. The standard ECG paper is designed with horizontal and vertical lines at 1 mm intervals.

here) can be recorded. A rhythm strip is a recording of a single lead, or three leads simultaneously, usually leads V1, II, and V5, and may be useful when a rhythm is unclear on the standard 12-lead ECG.

▶ SUMMARY

Proper technique is vital to obtain a high quality 12-lead ECG recording. The patient must be supine, the leads correctly placed with good contact to the chest wall and limbs, and the correct standardization of settings on the recorder must be employed. The standard 12-lead ECG is comprised of the standard limb leads (I, II, and III), the augmented limb leads (aVR, aVL, and aVF), and the precordial leads (V1 through V6). These leads record the summation of the electrical forces or vectors which are generated by depolarization of the myocardial cells.

Suggested Readings

Braunwald E. Heart Disease: A textbook of cardiovascular medicine, 5th ed. Philadelphia: W.B. Saunder Company, 1997.

Wagner GS. Marriott's Practical Electrocardiography. 9th ed. Baltimore: Williams & Wilkins, 1994.

394, 395, 396, 398 399, 402

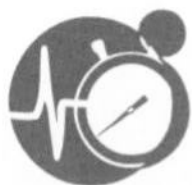

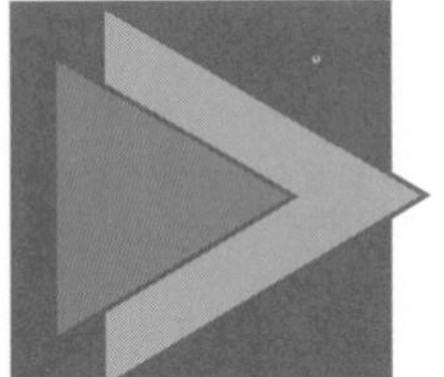

CHAPTER 48
NORMAL ELECTROCARDIOGRAMS

John A. Larry and Stephen F. Schaal

ANATOMY OF THE CONDUCTION SYSTEM

The anatomy of the conduction system is depicted in Fig. 48.1. The impulse that drives electrical depolarization of the heart originates in the sinoatrial (SA) or sinus node. This area is located in the right atrium near the superior vena cava. The wave of activity initially spreads in a radial fashion through the right atrium and subsequently the left atrium. The impulse reaches the atrioventricular (AV) node, an ovoid structure that lies at the base of the intra-atrial septum. The impulse takes approximately 100 msec to traverse the AV node and depolarize the bundle of His. In the normal heart, the AV node and the His bundle are the only point of connection between the atria and ventricles. The bundle of His extends through the fibrous skeleton of the heart into the superior portion of the intraventricular septum and divides into right and left bundles. The right bundle is quite discrete and travels down the right side of the interventricular septum and through a structure known as the moderator band, beyond which it branches into the right ventricle. The left bundle divides into anterior and posterior divisions; in reality, these divisions are more complex and diffuse as they fan out into the left ventricle. The bundle branches terminate in Purkinje fibers (specialized cells that spread the electrical activity rapidly through the myocardium). The depolarization wave stimulates myocardial cells to contract by initiating a series of events referred to as excitation-contraction coupling.

ELECTROCARDIOGRAM NOMENCLATURE: THE NORMAL DEPOLARIZATION AND REPOLARIZATION SEQUENCE

A normal rhythm strip is depicted in Figure 48.2 with the correlation between the electrical events and their electrocardiogram (ECG) manifestations illustrated in Table 48.1. The electrical activity recorded during atrial depolarization is termed the P wave. Following the inscription of the P wave, the impulse travels through the AV node, the His bundle and the Purkinje system. These structures are electrically silent on the surface ECG and are depolarized during the PR interval. The delay of the impulse through the AV node permits optimal contribution of atrial contraction to ventricular filling.

Depolarization of the myocardial cells of the ventricles generates the QRS complex. By definition, the initial downstroke of the QRS complex is designated the Q wave. The initial upstroke is termed R wave. Depending on the lead and the underlying cardiac disease, the initial deflection from the baseline may be a Q wave or an R wave. The negative deflection which follows the R wave is termed an S wave.

The ST segment and the T wave are the surface correlates of repolarization of the cardiac myocytes (Phases 2 and 3 of the action potential). The ST segment begins at the J point, the point separating the termination of the QRS complex from the ST segment. The J point is important to identify because criteria established to evaluate ST segment changes during exercise testing (indicative of myocardial ischemia) use the J point as a reference. The T wave represents the completion of repolarization. During or shortly after repolarization, the myocardial cells will not depolarize again if presented with another stimulus. This time period is called the refractory period.

Certain patients exhibit a U wave. The exact cause of this wave is not clearly defined, but investigators have suggested it may represent repolarization of the papillary muscles, or the Purkinje fibers, or special cells in the ventricle known as M cells.

VECTORS RESPONSIBLE FOR THE NORMAL ECG

The P wave exhibits certain characteristics when the depolarization originates in the sinus node. Because the sinus node is located in the right superior portion of the right atrium, the initial atrial depolarization wave is directed leftward, inferiorly and anteriorly. This results in

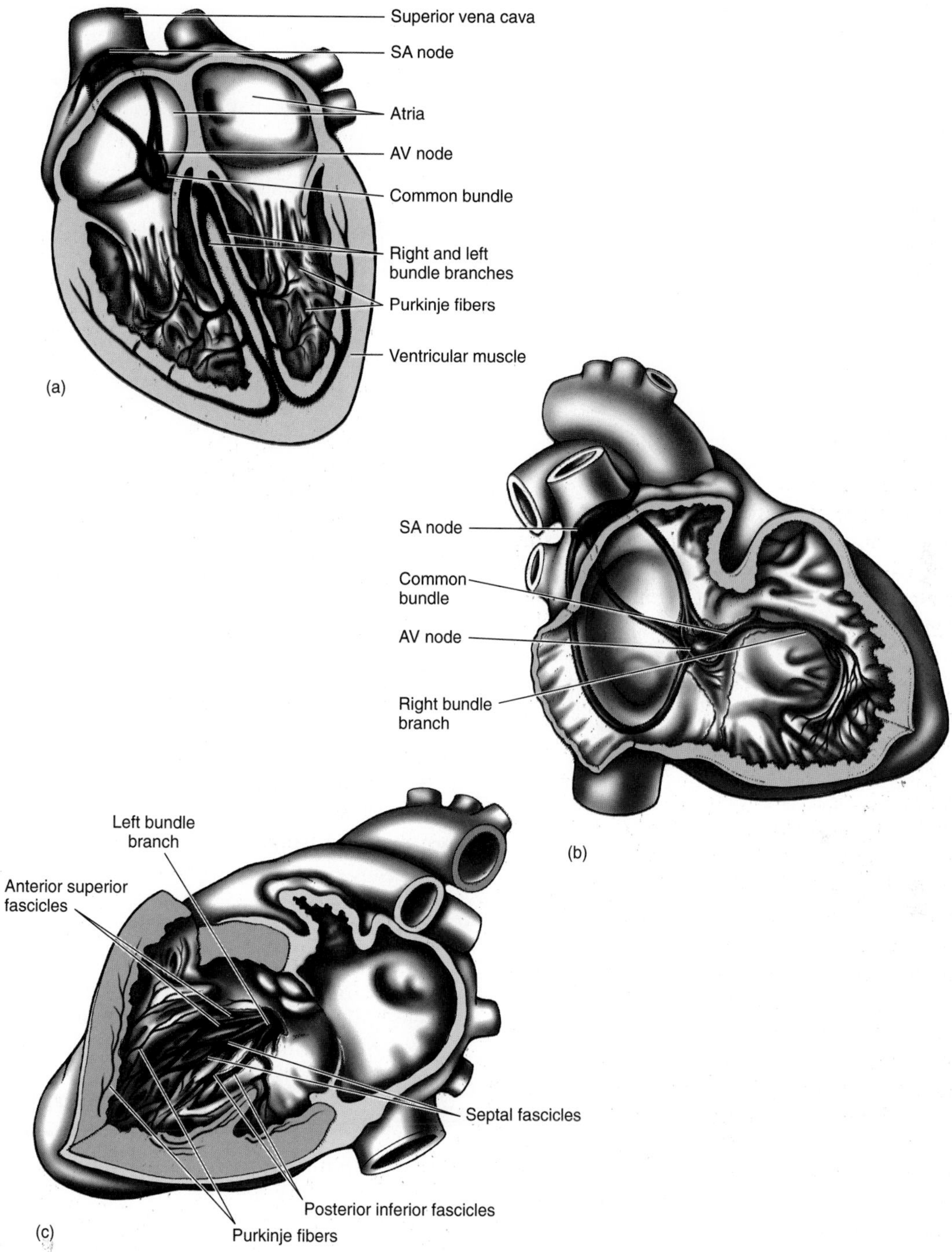

Figure 48.1. The anatomy of the conduction system.

an upright P wave in leads I, II, and aVL and an initial upright deflection in lead V1 (Fig. 48.3). Depolarization vectors moving toward the positive pole of a lead result in an upright deflection (see Chapter 46). As the impulse spreads to the left atrium, the mean vector of depolarization rotates posteriorly (the left atrium is located posterior to the right atrium), thus causing the P wave in lead V1 to become inverted. Consequently, a biphasic P-wave is recorded in lead V1 in sinus rhythm with upright P waves in leads I, II, aVL, V5, and V6. Other leads may exhibit some variability in P wave morphology.

The vectors that generate the normal QRS complex are more complex than those responsible for the P wave. After the AV node and the Bundle of His are depolarized, the impulse traverses the left and right bundle branches. The left bundle branch gives off branches to the septum

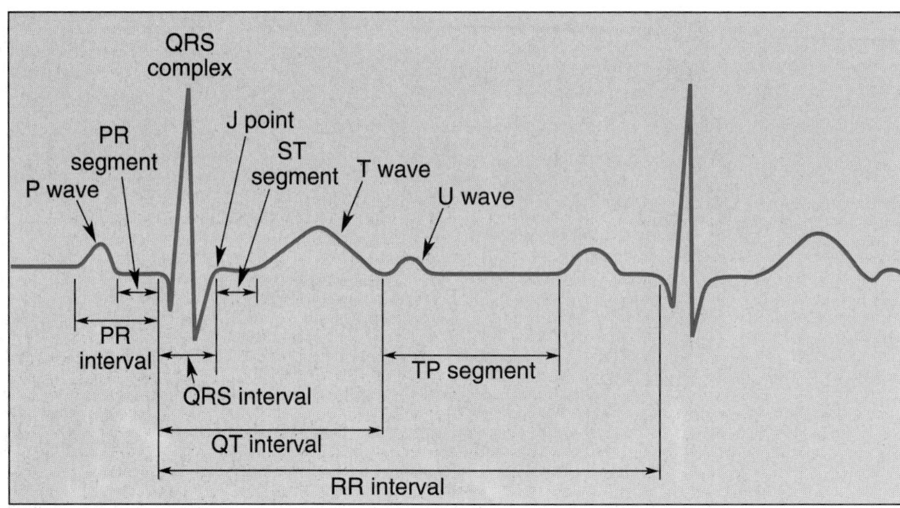

Figure 48.2. A normal rhythm strip.

Table 48.1. Normal Sequence of Depolarization and the ECG Correlation

Sinoatrial node	Silent
Atrial depolarization	P wave
Atrioventricular node	PR interval
His bundle	PR interval
Purkinje fibers	PR interval
Ventricular muscle depolarization	QRS complex
Ventricular isoelectric period	ST segment
Ventricular muscle repolarization	T wave

first; thus the left side of the septum depolarizes earliest. Consequently, the impulse travels across the intraventricular septum from left to right, causing an initial vector directed superiorly, rightwardly, and anteriorly. This yields an initial force on the ECG depicted as small upright R waves in leads V1 and V2 and small, narrow Q waves may be noted in leads I, aVL, II, III, aVF, V5, and V6 (Fig. 48.3). Subsequently, the impulse travels through the right and left ventricles nearly simultaneously. Since the left ventricle has a much greater mass than the right ventricle, the resulting electrical activity generated by the left ventricle overwhelms that of the right ventricle. This generates a vector directed leftward, posteriorly and inferiorly. This inscribes an upright R wave in leads I, II, aVL, the precordial leads, with variable morphology in lead III, and a downgoing complex in lead aVR.

Repolarization is the regeneration of the membrane potential of the cardiac cells. The repolarization of the atrium occurs during depolarization of the ventricle and is, therefore, not seen on the ECG. Ventricular muscle repolarization generates the T wave. The ventricle depolarizes from endocardium to epicardium, but repolarizes from epicardium to endocardium, thus resulting in a T wave vector that generally follows the QRS vector. Consequently, the T wave is typically upright when the QRS is upright and usually downwardly deflected when the QRS is downward (Fig. 48.3).

BASIC INTERPRETATION STRATEGY

Many recording systems provide a computer interpretation of the ECG, but they can be inaccurate and should not be relied upon as a final diagnostic tool. A systematic approach is necessary when interpreting ECGs.

Initial Assessment

Before beginning to interpret the ECG, it is necessary to check the name of the patient and the date and time the ECG was performed. It is obviously useless to render an interpretation on the wrong patient; attributing findings to the wrong patient may have serious consequences. Once you are certain the tracing is the correct one, check the calibration signal to determine the paper speed is 25 mm/sec and that the amplitude of the signal is such that 1 mV is represented by 10 mm. The calibration signal displays 1 mV for 0.2 seconds. Consistency with Einthoven's law should be assured (see Chapter 46).

Rate

The first step is to determine the ventricular rate in beats per minute (bpm). There are several methods for achieving this. One strategy is to mark off a 6 second time period (30 heavy lines on the ECG grid), count the number of QRS complexes in that interval and multiply by 10. This method is not efficient, but can be useful and should be used when the heart rate is irregular. A second method that can be used when the rhythm is regular requires dividing 60,000 (the number of milli-

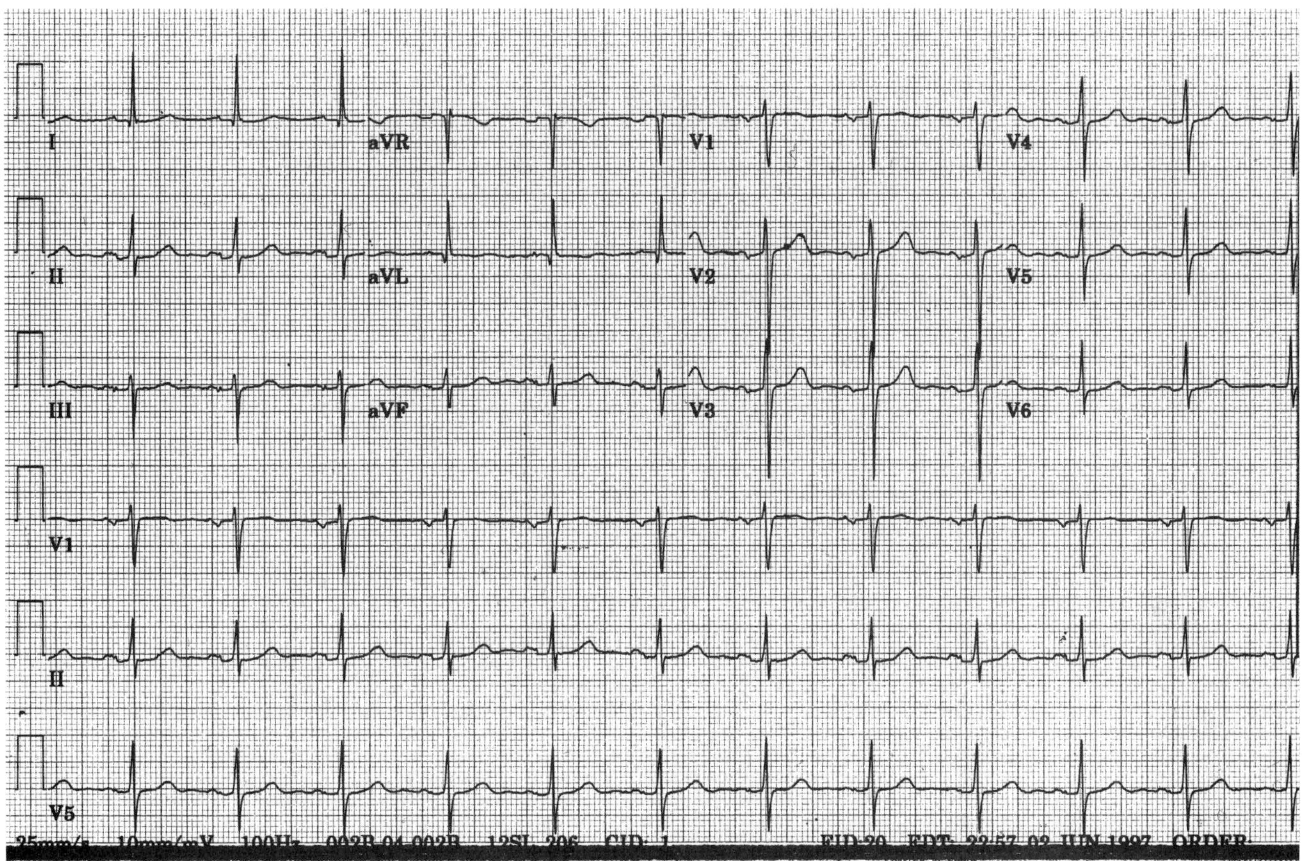

Figure 48.3. An upright P wave in leads I, II, and aVL and an initial upright deflection in lead V1.

seconds in one minute) by the milliseconds between QRS complexes. This calculation yields beats per minute.

$$BPM = \frac{60{,}000 \ msec/minute}{msec/beat}$$

In addition, applying this principle for derivation of a rapid approach to estimate the heart rate is possible. If a complex occurs at every heavy line (i.e., one beat every 0.2 seconds) the rate would be 300 bpm. If a complex occurs every second large box, the rate would be one-half of 300, or 150 bpm. Frequent use of this method can allow rapid quantification of the heart rate by identifying the number of heavy lines between QRS complexes (Fig. 48.3). In Figure 48.3, the ventricular rate is 80 bpm. A normal heart rate is between 60 and 100 bpm.

Rhythm

The second step, evaluation of the rhythm, is performed after the ventricular rate is ascertained. To assess the rhythm, one must identify the P waves and QRS complexes and determine the relationship between them. In the example of normal sinus rhythm (Fig. 48.3), a single P wave responsible for generating a single QRS complex. Furthermore, the P wave exhibits a normal vector. The P wave is upright in leads I and II, V5 and V6 and is biphasic in lead V1 with an initial upright deflection. These two criteria are required for a rhythm to be considered a "normal sinus rhythm." The common arrhythmias are reviewed in Chapter 49.

Axis

The QRS axis in the frontal plane is simply the direction of the mean QRS vector. Determination of the axis requires a knowledge of the vectors of each normal lead, as depicted in Figure 47.5. At younger ages, the axis may be nearly vertical (near $+90°$), but as people age, the axis moves gradually leftward and becomes more horizontal. Mild disagreement exists among authors as to the normal ranges for the QRS axis. The axis can be considered normal if it falls between $-30°$ and $+100°$. An axis between $-30°$ to $-90°$ is considered left axis deviation (Fig. 48.4). The pathologic process causing left axis deviation is usually block of the left anterior division(s) of the left bundle branch. An axis from $+100°$ to $180°$ is termed right axis deviation. Tables 48.2 and 48.3 list the most common etiologies of right and left axis deviation. Axes falling between $-90°$ and $180°$ may result from extreme left or right axis deviation and are quite uncommon.

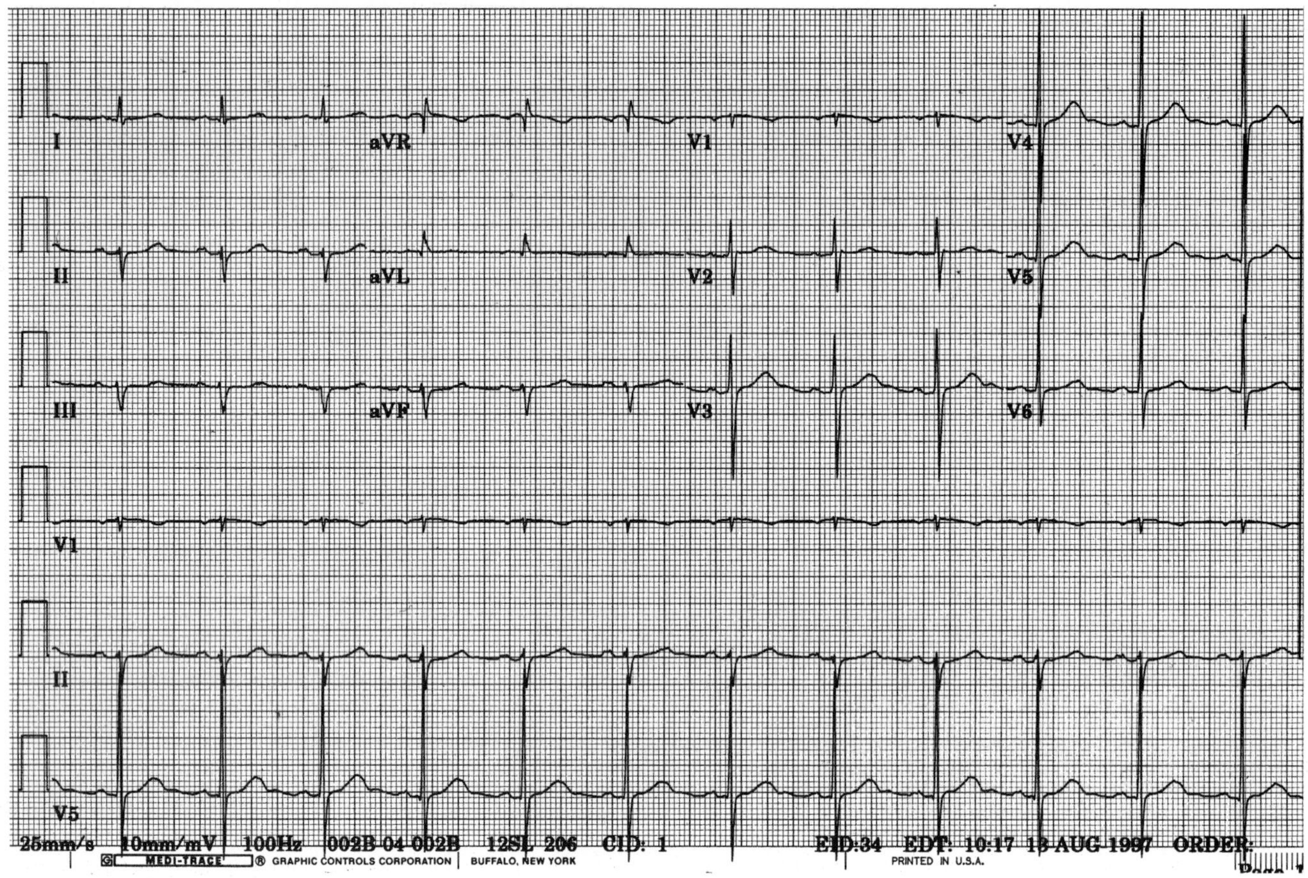

Figure 48.4. The QRS axis can be considered normal if it falls between −30° and +100°.

Table 48.2. Abnormalities Associated with Left Axis Deviation

Left anterior fascicular block
Left ventricular enlargement
Inferior myocardial infarction
Hypertensive heart disease
Cardiomyopathy
Congenital heart disease
Wolffe-Parkinson-White syndrome

Modified from Marriott HL. Practical Electrocardiography, 8th ed, 1988.

Table 48.3. Abnormalities Associated with Right Axis Deviation

Right ventricular enlargement
Left posterior fascicular block
Congenital heart disease
Mechanical shifts (i.e., emphysema, pneumothorax)
Dextrocardia
Wolffe-Parkinson-White syndrome
Normal variant

Modified from Wagner GS. Marriott's Practical Electrocardiography. 9th ed. Baltimore: Williams & Wilkins, 1994.

Plotting the mean voltage of deflection for leads I, II, and III on a grid and drawing a line from the origin through the intersection of the three lines is an accurate method to determine the mean QRS axis. However, this method is time consuming. An alternative method can be used that will reliably and quickly approximate the mean axis. First, estimate the QRS axis by determining which of the four quadrants (created by the intersection of leads I and a VF) contains the maximum QRS positive voltage. This can be quickly accomplished by looking at the QRS complex in leads I and aVF. If the predominant deflection of the QRS is positive in both, the axis must lie between 0° and +90°. If the complex is mainly upright in lead I but downward in lead aVF, the axis falls between 0° and −90°. Axes between +90° and +180° produce a downward complex in lead I and an upright complex in aVF. Once you have determined the quadrant in which the axis lies, find the limb lead which most nearly approximates a complex that has equal upward and downward deflections. This is often referred to as the isoelectric lead. A perpendicular line from this lead into the quadrant previously determined approximates the mean QRS axis. In Figure 48.4, the QRS complex is predominantly upright in lead I and mainly downward in lead aVF. Lead aVR is the most isoelectric lead, placing the axis at $-60°$, consistent with left axis deviation.

Intervals

The next step in the assessment of the ECG is the measurement of intervals. Figure 48.2 depicts the intervals measured on the ECG. The PR interval extends from the beginning of the P wave to the initial QRS deflection. This may be a Q wave or an R wave, depending on the morphology of the complex. This interval represents the time for the impulse to travel from the sinus node to the ventricles. Prolongation may reflect conduction abnormalities in the atrium, AV node, or His-Purkinje system. A normal PR interval in adults ranges from 120 and 200 msec. Each small box represents 40 msec. The normal PR interval may vary depending on the relative contributions of the sympathetic and parasympathetic nervous systems and the effect of medications on conduction through the AV node. A PR interval greater than 200 msec is termed 1st degree AV block, whereas a PR interval less than 120 msec is labeled a short PR syndrome.

The QRS interval may be measured in any limb lead. The QRS interval begins at the initial deviation from the baseline, either a Q wave or an R wave, and terminates at the end of the QRS, which may be an R wave or an S wave. A normal QRS interval is less than 100 msec. Common causes of prolongation of this interval include conduction defects such as bundle branch block, myocardial disease, and metabolic, electrolyte, and drug effects on the ventricular myocardium.

The QT interval encompasses both depolarization and repolarization of the ventricular muscle. It is measured from the onset of the QRS complex to the end of the T wave (see Figure 2.2). The QT interval is usually corrected for the ventricular rate by Bazett's formula, which is shown below.

$$QTc = \frac{\text{measured QT interval}}{\text{square root of the R-R interval (msec)}}$$

A normal, corrected QT interval is less than 440 msec. This interval may be prolonged by certain medications such as antiarrhythmic agents (quinidine, procainamide, disopyramide, sotalol, amiodarone), tricyclic antidepressants, electrolyte disorders (hypokalemia, hypocalcemia), ischemia, or myocardial disease. Congenital QT prolongation is associated with an increased risk of sudden cardiac death, due to a type of polymorphic ventricular tachycardia known as torsades de pointes.

Wave Form Analysis

The wave forms must be critically assessed in terms of their orientation, amplitude, contour, and position. The initial wave to interpret is the P wave. Knowledge of the basic vectors allows one to recognize normal from abnormal. The initial vector is directed leftward, inferiorly and anteriorly, as the right atrium is depolarized, followed by a leftward, inferior, and posterior vector generated by left atrial depolarization. The mean P wave axis in the frontal plane is between 0° and 90°, meaning that the P wave must be upright in lead II if it originates from the sinus node. In addition to being upright in lead II, the P-wave is upright in leads I, aVL, V3-V6, and is biphasic (initially upright then downgoing) in lead V1. The other leads exhibit variable P wave morphology. The amplitude of a normal P wave is usually less than 3 mm in lead II.

Next, note the QRS complexes and scan for any pathological Q waves. Small, narrow (<30 msec) Q waves in leads I, aVL, II, III, and aVF reflect the normal vector loop and are not indicative of previous myocardial infarction. The progression of the height of the R wave should increase across the precordial leads, with the transition zone (the lead where the R wave becomes greater than the S wave) usually occurring at lead V4. The increase in height of the R wave from V1 to V6 reflects closer proximity to the left ventricle, which has greater mass than the right ventricle.

The ST segments should be evaluated in each lead. Typically, the ST segment should be isoelectric (on the baseline) at the level of the PR or TP segment. ST segment depression or elevation may be abnormal. Many entities may affect the ST segment such as conduction system abnormalities, ischemia, ventricular hypertrophy, medications such as digitalis, and electrolyte and metabolic disorders.

T wave evaluation primarily involves ascertaining the T wave vector. In general, the T wave is directed toward the QRS complex. Abnormally flattened or inverted T waves (due to alteration of the T wave vector) may be caused by ischemia, infarction, hypertrophy, electrolyte disorders, hyperventilation, medications and non-cardiac illness.

▶ SUMMARY

A summary of the objective findings should be presented as the interpretation. The final interpretation must integrate the features into a common theme which includes consideration of the history and diagnosis. As in any area, repetition is the key to proficiency. Many hundreds of ECGs must be evaluated to achieve comfort with the numerous abnormalities and normal variants. Reading tracings in an organized fashion will allow the most accurate and concise interpretation.

Suggested Readings

Braunwald E. Heart Disease: A textbook of cardiovascular medicine, 5th ed. Philadelphia: W.B. Saunder Company, 1997.

Wagner GS. Marriott's Practical Electrocardiography. 9th ed. Baltimore, Williams & Wilkins, 1994.

396 399, 401 409, 410

 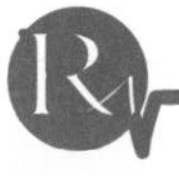 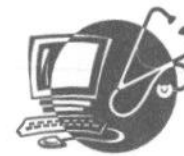

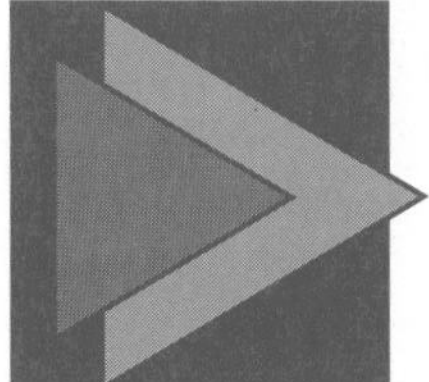

CHAPTER 49
Ischemia and Infarction

John A. Larry and Stephen F. Schaal

One of the most prevalent uses of electrocardiography is the identification of patients with myocardial infarction or myocardial ischemia. Monitoring the electrocardiogram (ECG) during exercise testing is a commonly used technique to assess whether myocardial ischemia is the etiology of chest discomfort.

MYOCARDIAL INFARCTION

Myocardial infarction results when blood flow to a region of heart muscle is interrupted by total occlusion of a coronary artery. ECG changes occur as a result of the impairment of flow to the myocardium. The initial manifestation is elevation of the ST segment and peaking of the T waves. The ST segment change is termed an injury current. The ST segments exhibit an upward convex shape as shown in Figure 49.1, an example of anterior myocardial injury. Within hours or days, the T waves invert and the ST segment gradually returns to baseline. Pathologic Q waves (or loss of R waves) may develop in the involved leads, depending on the location and extent of myocardial damage. These may develop soon after the occlusion or take several days to evolve. Q waves (or loss of R waves) occur due to the loss of electrical activity that normally results from the depolarization of that region of myocardium. Myocardial infarctions that do not develop Q waves are termed non-Q wave infarcts. Patients with a non-Q wave infarct have a better short term, but a worse long term prognosis compared to patients with Q wave infarcts.

The age of the infarct may be determined in relative terms. When ST elevation or hyperacute T waves are identified, acute injury is present. When Q waves are present, the ST segments have returned to baseline and the T waves remain inverted, the infarct is recent, between 2 weeks and 1 year old. These are often read as infarcts of indeterminate age. When the only manifestation is the presence of Q waves and no ST or T wave changes are present, the infarct is considered to be remote.

The ECG leads that exhibit changes permit determination of the region of myocardial infarction (Table 49.1). Figure 49.2 is an ECG from a patient with acute inferior wall injury. Note the ST segment elevation in leads II, III, and aVF. Inspection of Figure 49.3 shows loss of R wave in the precordial leads, consistent with an anterior wall myocardial infarction. The ST changes have resolved, but T wave inversions persist in leads V6, I, and aVL, suggesting this is a recent, but not acute infarction.

A common difficulty is differentiation of pathologic Q waves from those resulting from the normal depolarization sequence of the myocardium. The location, depth, and width of the Q waves may be useful in this determination. As previously stated, the normal vector loop of depolarization results in small Q waves in leads I, aVL, II, III, and aVF, V5, V6. These deflections are typically quite small in amplitude and narrow in width (less than 30 msec). Significant Q waves are typically greater than 30 msec, often at least one-third the height of the R wave, and occur in contiguous leads which reflect a particular region of the heart.

Myocardial infarction is not the only entity affecting ST segments. Causes of ST segment elevation other than myocardial injury are common. Pericardial inflammation present in **acute pericarditis** (Fig. 49.4) causes generalized ST segment elevation (all ECG leads), whereas acute injury due to an occluded coronary artery affects contiguous leads. In general, the ST segment typically has an upward concave appearance in pericarditis whereas the appearance is convex upward in the setting of myocardial injury.

Benign repolarization variants (also called early repolarization) are another common cause of ST segment elevation. These variants are most commonly seen in young African-American males but may be seen in other patients as well. Elevation of the J point from the baseline is present. The ST segments are elevated but exhibit a concave upward appearance; this helps in the differentiation from myocardial injury (Fig. 49.5).

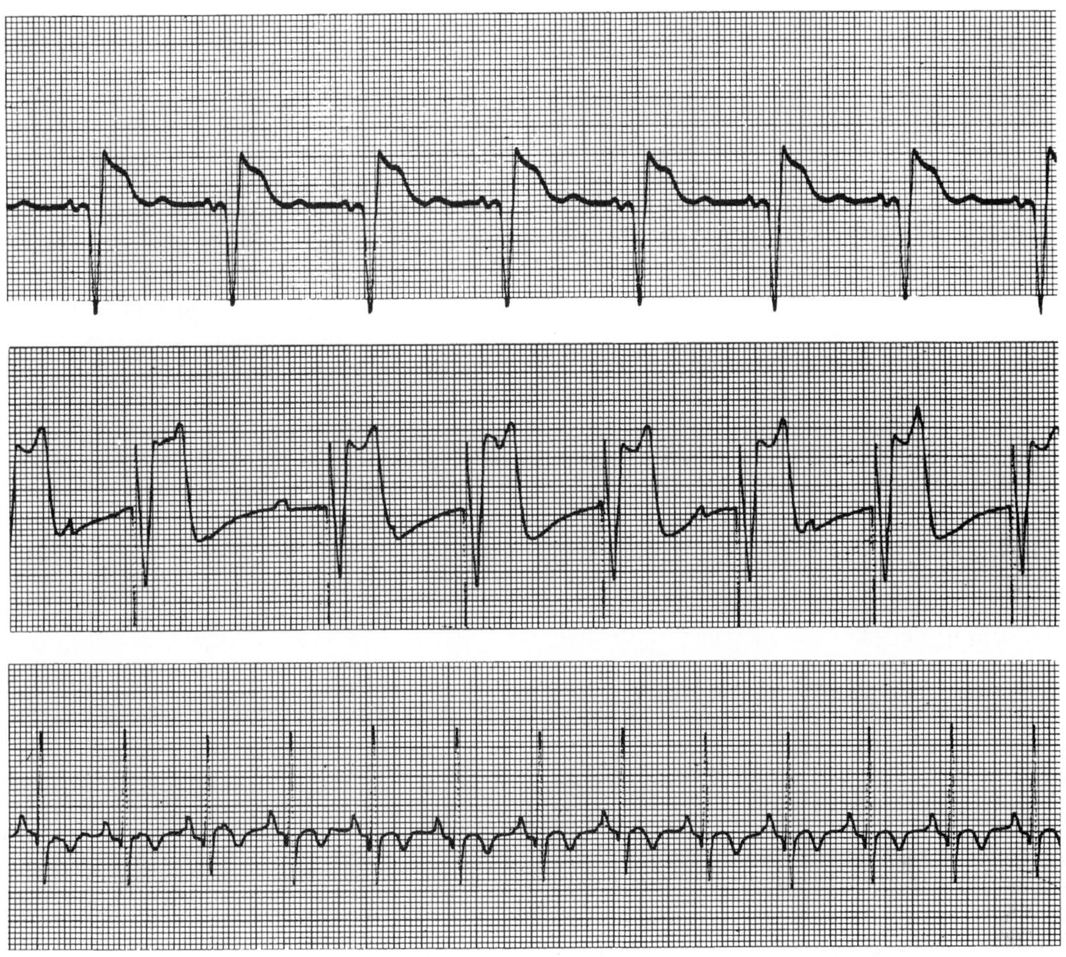

Figure 49.1. Anterior myocardial injury.

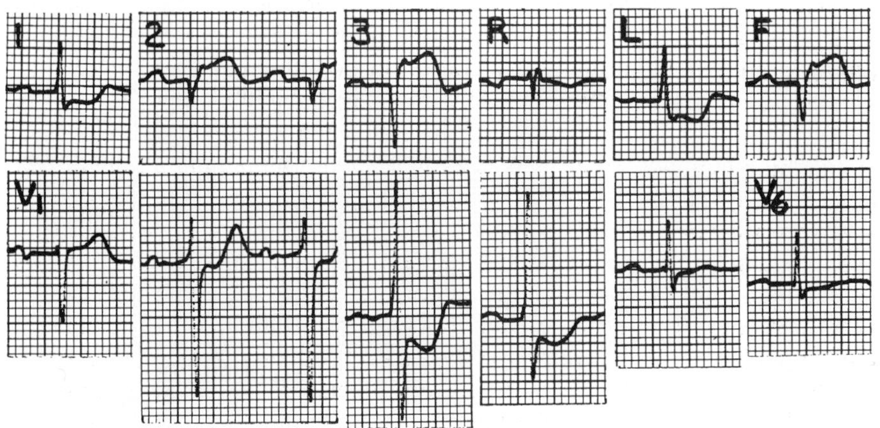

Figure 49.2. Acute Inferior wall injury.

Bundle branch blocks (see Figures 50.21 and 50.22) also exert influence on the ST segment. In the left bundle, the ST vector is directed away from the QRS vector resulting in elevated ST segments in the right precordial leads (Figure 50.22).

Table 49.1. Location of Myocardial Infarction/Ischemia

Location	Leads Affected
Anteroseptal	V1, V2
Anterior	V1–V4
Extensive anterior	V1–V6, I, aVL
Anterolateral	V3–V6, I, aVL
High lateral	I, aVL
Inferior	II, III, aVF
Posterior	V1, V2 (ST depression, tall R waves noted)

Persistent ST segment elevation after an infarction may be suggestive of **ventricular aneurysm** formation. This typically involves the anterior wall of the left ventricle and occurs after large infarcts. The presence of Q waves in the involved leads in a patient post myocardial infarction suggests this diagnosis.

MYOCARDIAL ISCHEMIA

When inadequate supply of blood flow exists to meet the demands of the myocardium, myocardial ischemia results. The patient often experiences chest pain with exertion. ECG changes include ST segment depression and/or inversion of the T waves (Fig. 49.6). Alteration in the ST segments and T waves is, in most cases, non-specific as numerous factors may contribute to similar appearing ST segment and T wave changes. Symmetrically inverted

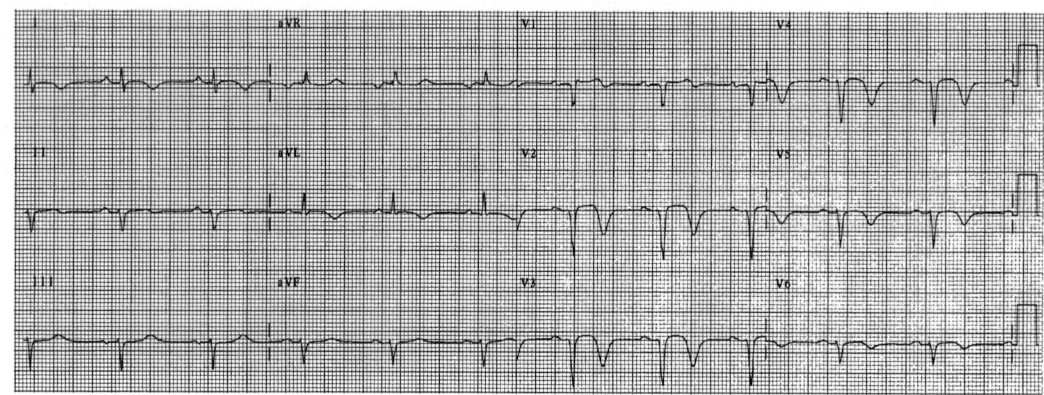

Figure 49.3. Anterior wall myocardial infarction.

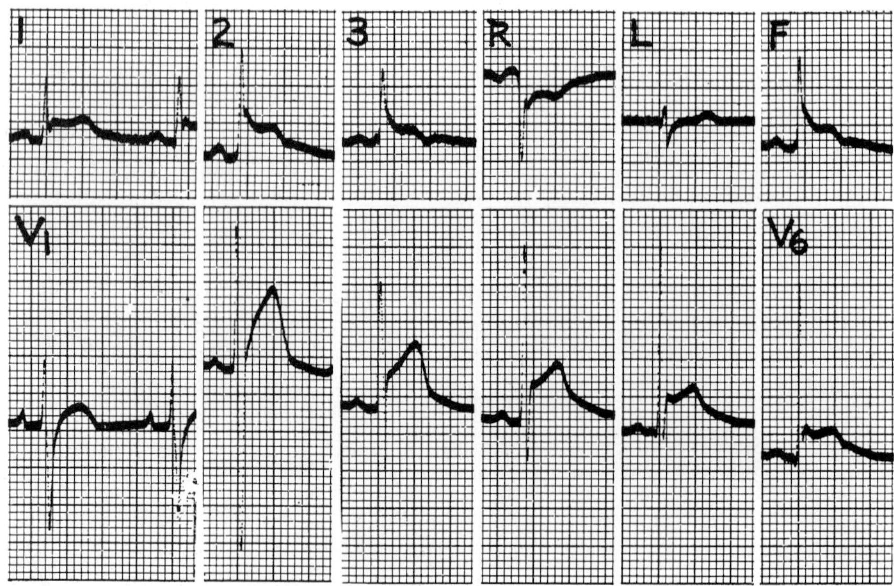

Figure 49.4. Acute pericarditis.

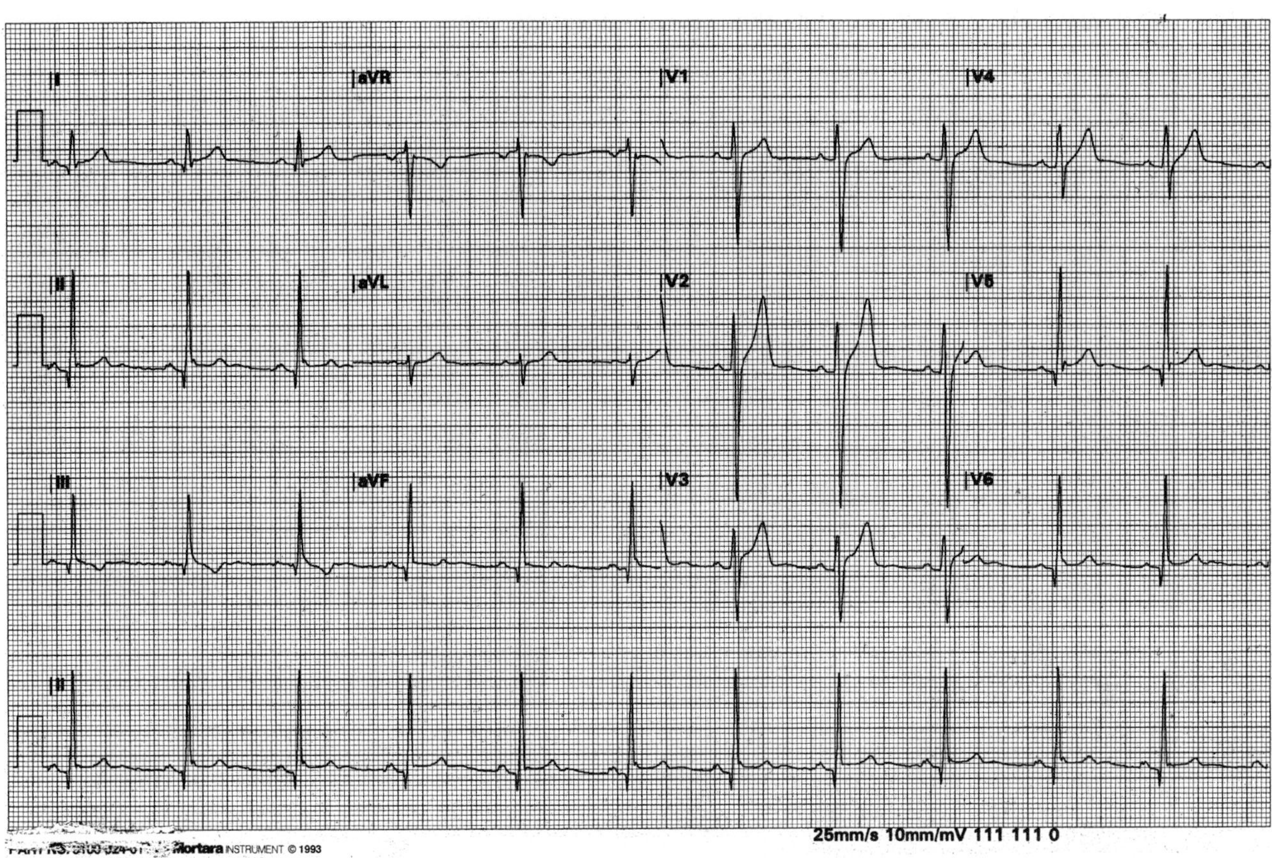

Figure 49.5. Repolarization variants.

T waves suggest ischemia, while other etiologies typically cause asymmetric inversion. Although many ECGs are interpreted as "non-specific ST and T wave changes," some of these changes may actually be the result of myocardial ischemia. The location of the ischemia may be determined by noting which leads exhibit the ST segment or T wave changes as seen in Table 49.1.

EXERCISE ECG TESTING

Monitoring the ECG during exercise testing affords the opportunity to detect **arrhythmias,** and to ascertain ischemic changes. Arrhythmias, discussed in Chapter 50, may be provoked during or after exercise. It is important for individuals performing exercise testing to be comfortable with the interpretation of these rhythm disorders and the, Advanced Cardiac Life Support (ACLS) protocols to treat them.

The lead placement for an exercise ECG deviates slightly from the standard 12-lead ECG. The leads typically placed on the right and left wrists are moved proximally to the upper chest near the shoulders. The lower extremity leads are moved to the lower abdomen. These recording sites reduce the motion artifact that occurs with movement of the extremities during exercise.

A history and examination are necessary to rule out contraindications to exercise testing. Continuous ECG monitoring is performed throughout the test and during the recovery. After exercise is initiated, a 12-lead ECG is recorded according to protocol and, additionally, during any symptoms or change in heart rhythm. Monitoring should continue for 4 to 6 minutes during recovery or until changes on the ECG have resolved. Ischemia may induce several changes on the ECG; the most common change is ST segment depression. When baseline ST abnormalities exist, the test becomes less specific. In addition to the magnitude of change, the character of the ST depression is important. Upsloping ST depression has less specificity for the presence of significant coronary disease than does horizontal or downsloping ST depression. Several clinical and electrocardiographic criteria exist for termination of the exercise study.

Because the subendocardial area of the left ventricular apex region is most often rendered ischemic during exercise, the ST segment shifts in V4, V5, and V6 are the most sensitive for detection of ischemia.

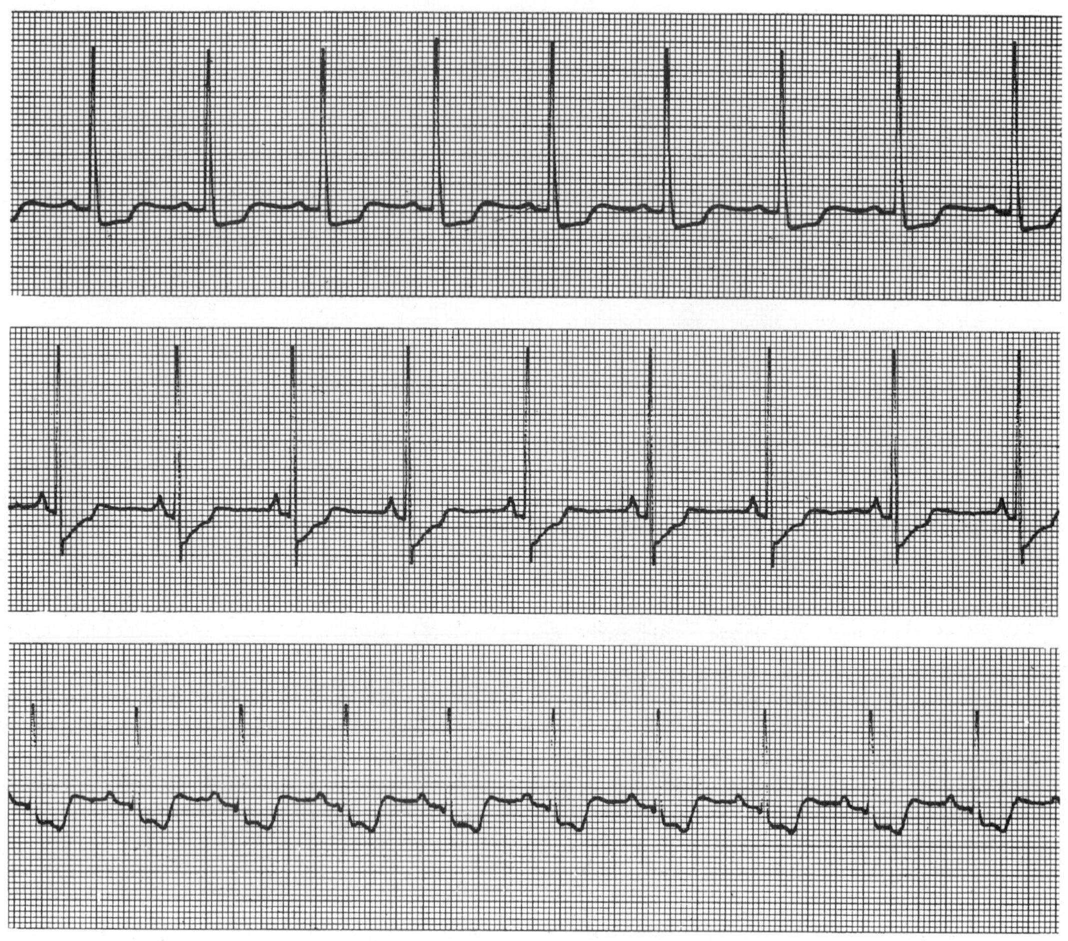

Figure 49.6. Myocardial ischemia.

▶ SUMMARY

Electrocardiography is useful in determining the presence of acute or remote infarctions and may detect resting ischemia. Combining exercise testing with ECG recording is a useful strategy to evaluate patients for the presence of exertional angina.

Suggested Readings

Braunwald. E. Heart Disease: A textbook of cardiovascular medicine, 5th ed Philadelphia: W.B. Saunder Company, 1997.

Wagner GS. Marriott's Practical Electrocardiography. 9th ed. Baltimore: Williams & Wilkins, 1994.

398 399, 403, 404, 405, 408

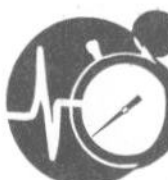

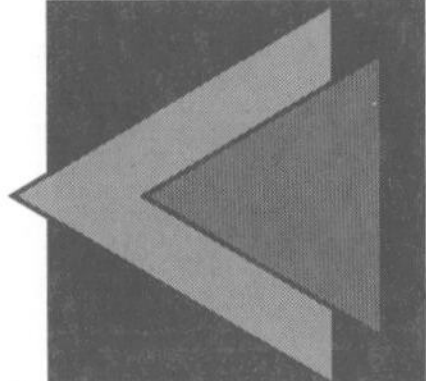

CHAPTER 50
DYSRHYTHMIAS

John A. Larry and Stephen F. Schaal

The sinus node is typically responsible for initiating depolarization of the myocardium. The impulse generated then travels through the atria, atrioventricular (AV) node, His-bundle branch-Purkinje system, and finally the ventricular myocardium. However, in patients with structural heart disease as well as those with normal hearts, deviations from the normal depolarization sequence occur. These abnormalities in heart rhythm are called arrhythmias (or dysrhythmias). Arrhythmias may be fast (tachyarrhythmias) or slow (bradyarrhythmias). This chapter examines the most common arrhythmias and the mechanisms responsible for their generation.

PREMATURE COMPLEXES

It is not uncommon for patients to exhibit either premature atrial complexes (PACs) or premature ventricular complexes (PVCs), especially during exercise testing when catecholamine levels are increased. PACs occur when a site in the atrium other than the sinus node depolarizes prematurely (Fig. 50.1). The resulting impulse traverses the AV node, bundle of His, bundle branches, and Purkinje system and in the absence of bundle branch block or myocardial disease, generates a narrow QRS complex.

Occasionally, the premature atrial complex occurs early enough that a portion of the conduction system may be refractory. If the impulse finds the AV node not recovered, the impulse will extinguish at that point and no QRS complex will result. These are referred to as "blocked PACs." The block at the AV node is physiological if the PAC occurs quite early. If the AV node conducts the impulse, but one of the bundle branches are refractory, the QRS complex will exhibit features of a bundle branch block (discussed later in this chapter), a phenomenon termed bundle branch aberration. If one of the fascicles of the left bundle is refractory when the premature beat arrives, the QRS complex may exhibit features of left anterior fascicular or left posterior fascicular block aberration. When a normal sinus beat alternates with a premature atrial contraction, this is called atrial bigeminy.

PVCs occur when a site in the ventricle fires before the next wave of depolarization from the sinus node reaches the ventricle (Fig. 50.2). These QRS complexes have bizarre, wide morphologies. Unlike PACs, these beats may not reset the periodicity of the sinus node, that is, the next sinus beat is often two cycle lengths from the beat prior to the PVC. A pattern of a sinus beat alternating with a PVC is termed ventricular bigeminy, and every third beat ventricular trigeminy. PACs and PVCs may occur in patients with normal hearts during rest or exercise, or they may be markers of underlying cardiac pathology.

MECHANISMS OF TACHYARRHYTHMIAS

Electrophysiologic mechanisms responsible for the generation of most cardiac arrhythmias have been identified as circus re-entry, enhanced automaticity, and triggered activity. The substrate for re-entry requires two pathways for current to travel. The first pathway depolarizes rapidly and recovers slowly, while the second depolarizes slowly but recovers rapidly (Fig. 50.3). Re-entry occurs when an area of altered conduction exists and unidirectional block occurs. If an impulse arrives prematurely at a time when the slow pathway has recovered but the fast pathway is refractory (not recovered from the previous depolarization), the impulse will conduct over the slow pathway. If conduction over the slow pathway reaches the fast pathway when recovered, the impulse may travel retrograde over the fast pathway. If the slow pathway has recovered, depolarization of the slow path will occur and a re-entrant loop is established.

Enhanced automaticity is another mechanism responsible for the generation of arrhythmias. In this situation, an increased rate of Phase 4 depolarization (see Figure 46.2) of a myocardial cell occurs, thereby reaching the

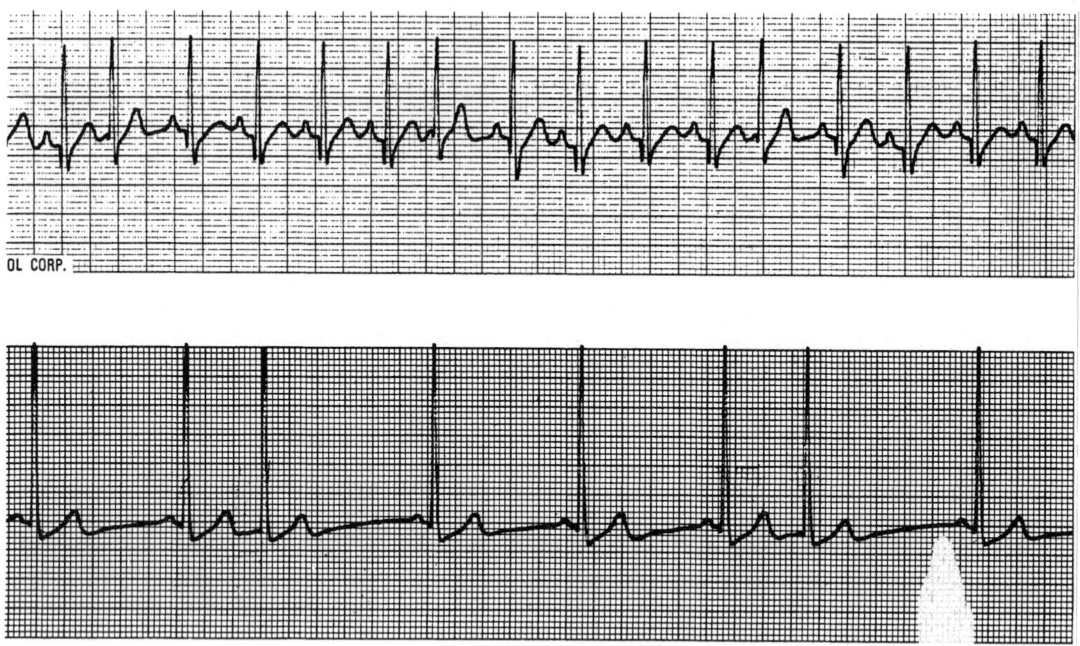

Figure 50.1. Normal sinus rhythm with premature atrial contractions. The third and seventh complexes represent PACs.

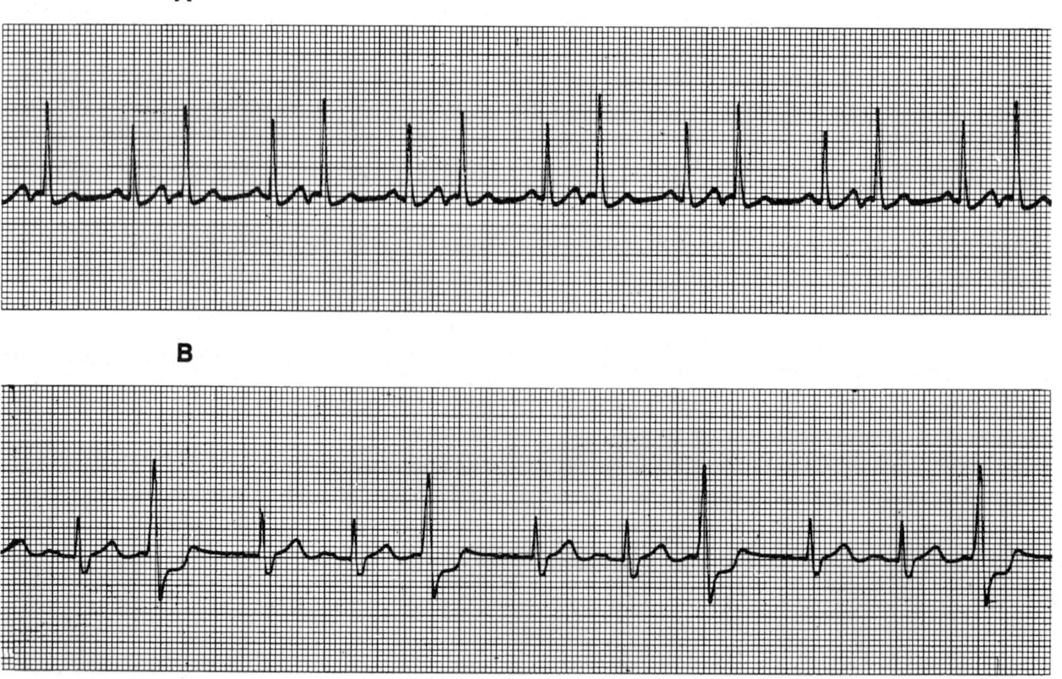

Figure 50.2. Normal sinus rhythm with PVCs in a bigeminal (**A**) or a trigeminal (**B**) pattern.

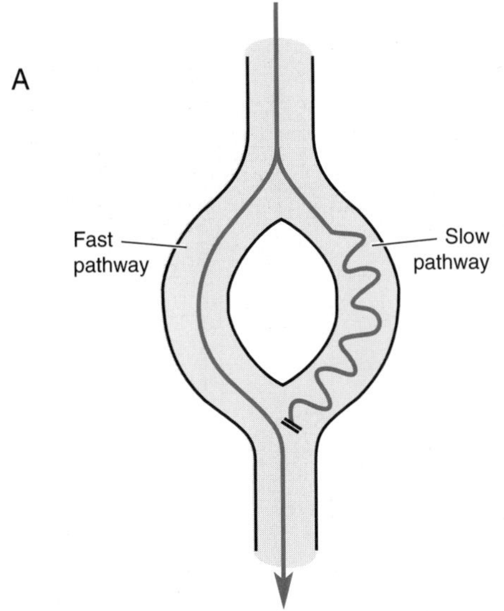

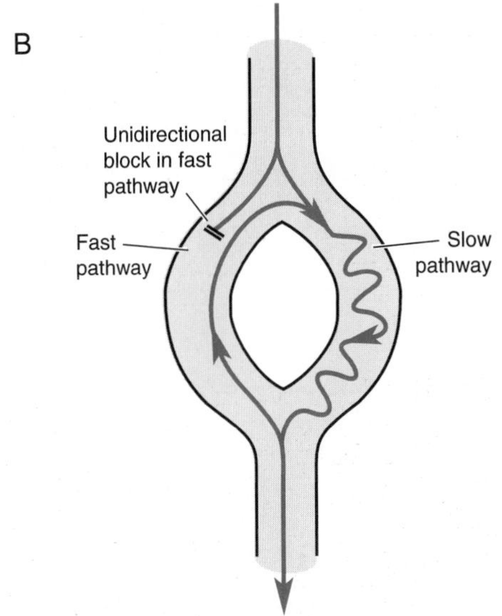

Figure 50.3. Schematic depicting substrate for reentrant arrthmias. **A,** Normal depolarization wave arrives finding both fast and slow patheways recovered from previous depolarization. Impulse travels via fast pathway to distal conducting tissue. **B,** A premature beat blocks in the fast pathway but is able to travel over the slow pathway which has a short refractory period. The impulse travels to the distal conducting tissue and also retrograde over the fast pathway, which by this time has recovered. If the slow pathway is recovered, a reentrant loop is generated, resulting in tachycardia.

threshold potential more rapidly than usual. Depolarization of the cell occurs and the impulse generated depolarizes the remainder of the myocardium.

A third mechanism of arrhythmias is called triggered activity, which exhibits features of both re-entry and automaticity. Myocardial cells may exhibit after-depolarization or increases in the membrane potential that occur during the repolarization phase of the action potential. These can be characterized as early after-depolarizations, which occur during Phase 3, and late after-depolarizations, which occur after Phase 3. If the magnitude of these after-depolarizations are great enough, depolarization may be triggered. Early after-depolarizations are related to conditions which prolong the action potential, such as antiarrhythmic agents (Type IA and III drugs), and electrolyte disorders such as hypokalemia and hypomagnesemia. Generally, the tachycardia develops after a pause. Delayed after-depolarizations occur in the setting of myocardial ischemia, digitalis toxicity, and congenital long QT syndromes. These after-depolarizations are tachycardia dependent and high catecholamine states contribute to the development of the tachycardia.

Circus re-entry, enhanced automaticity, and triggered activity may occur in any portion of the myocardium or specialized conducting tissue. The atrial myocardium, ventricular myocardium, SA node, AV node, and the His Purkinje system all may be susceptible to variations in conduction. The location of the abnormality and the underlying cardiac substrate governs the type of arrhythmia and its properties.

TYPES OF TACHYARRHYTHMIAS

Sinus Tachycardia

Sinus tachycardia (Fig. 50.4) is the result of enhancement of the rate of firing of the sinus node. The sinus node is under the control of the parasympathetic and sympathetic nervous systems and will therefore accelerate or decelerate depending on the physiological requirements. Sinus tachycardia results when increased activity of the sympathetic nervous system is present. These include situations such as fear, exercise, fever, hypovolemia, bleeding, thyrotoxicosis, hypoxia, or other acute illness. Decreased stroke volume in severe left ventricular dysfunction may also result in sinus tachycardia since the sympathetic nervous system is activated in an attempt to preserve adequate cardiac output.

Three key features of sinus tachycardia are important. First, patients typically exhibit a gradual increase in their heart rate (i.e., sudden acceleration from 80 beats per minute to 150 beats per minute does not occur). Second, although exceptions occur, the sinus rate typically does not exceed the maximum rate as calculated by the formula: **Maximum heart rate = 220 − the age.** Finally, the P wave vector must be normal.

Atrial Fibrillation

Atrial fibrillation (Fig. 50.5) is a relatively common arrhythmia which is the result of multiple re-entrant waves of electrical activity in the atria. These depolarization waves do not result in organized atrial contraction

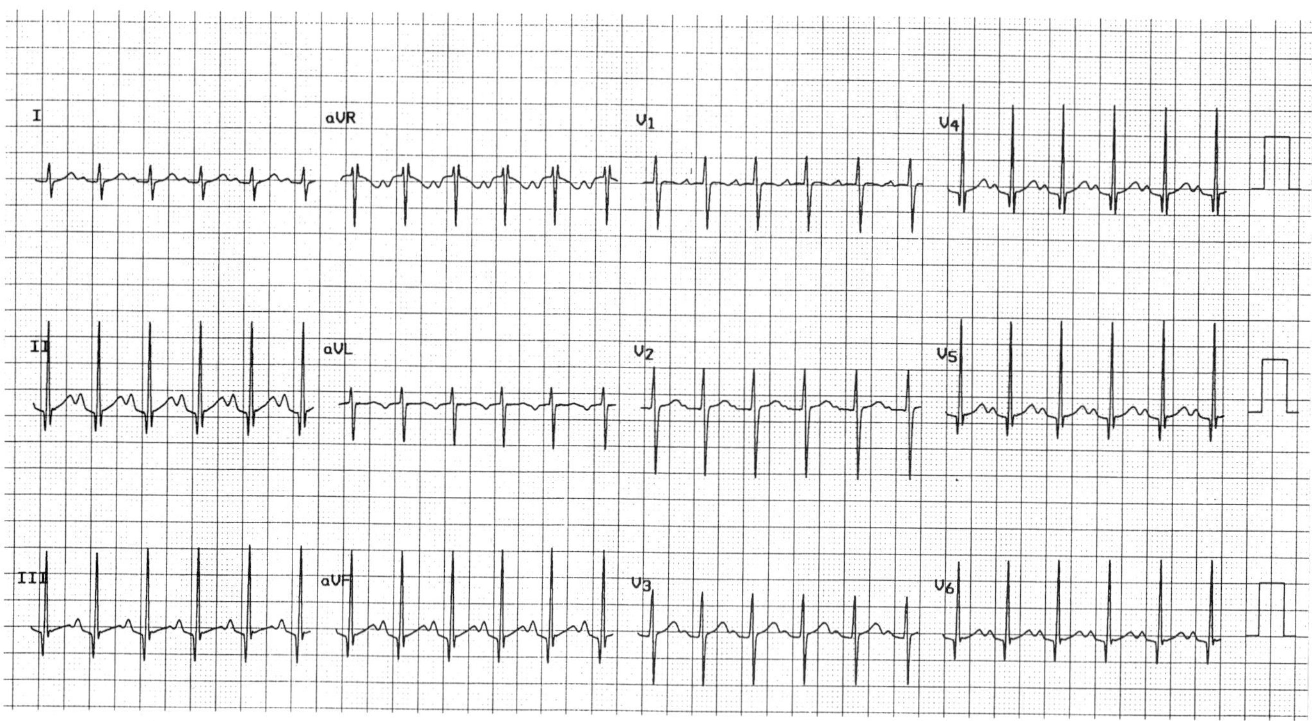

Figure 50.4. Sinus tachycardia.

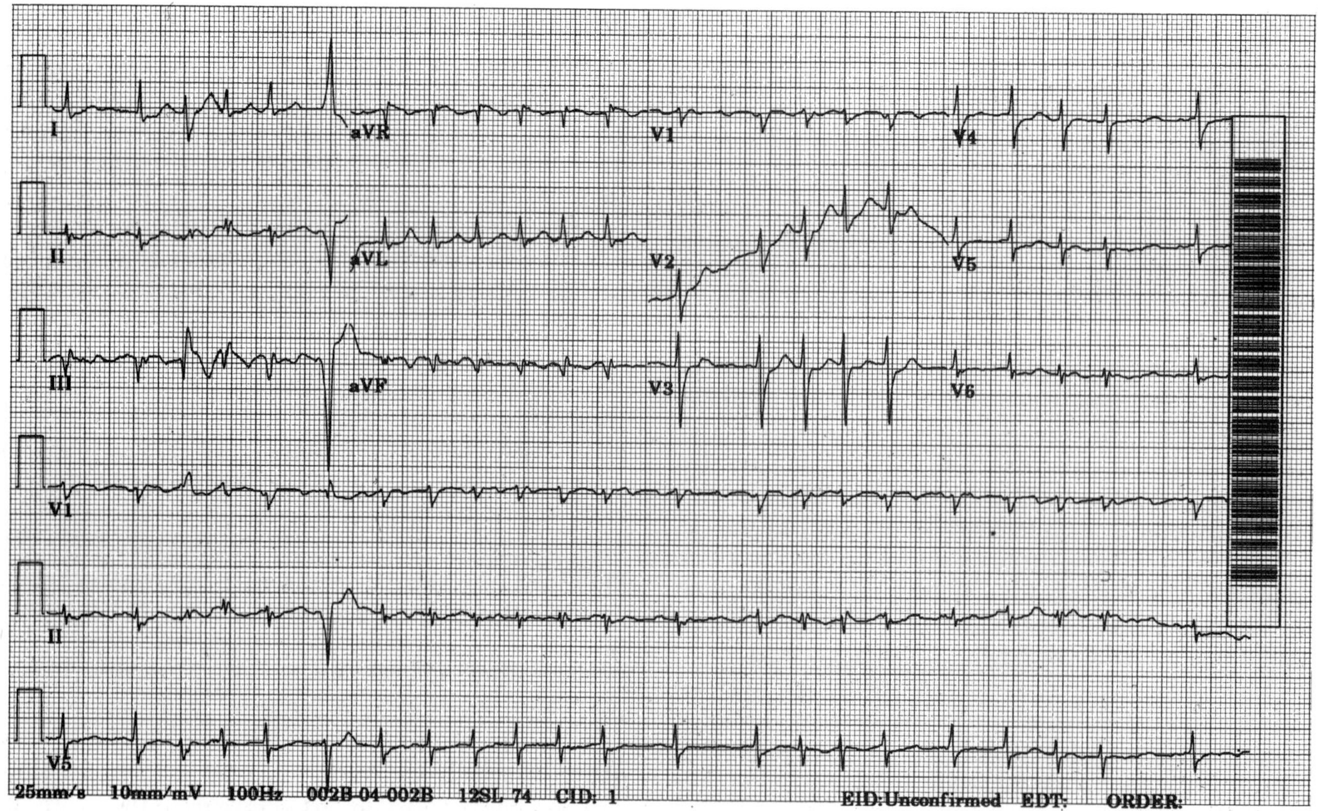

Figure 50.5. Atrial fibrillation with rapid ventricular response. The wide QRS complex likely represent aberrant ventricular conduction, although a PVC could not be excluded.

and the appearance of the atria has been described as a "bag of worms" when in fibrillation. The AV node is stimulated at frequent and irregular intervals by the very rapid atrial activity, resulting in an irregular heart rate (R-R response). The rate of the ventricular response is governed by the AV node refractory period. The hallmarks of atrial fibrillation are the absence of organized P wave activity and an irregular ventricular response. This rhythm has important consequences for the patient; the absence of a properly timed atrial contraction results in decline of the cardiac output (as much as 20% in those with relatively normal ventricles). In patients with cardiac disease, the cardiac output may decline by up to 40%. Atrial fibrillation may compromise ability to perform physical activities.

In addition, patients with atrial fibrillation are at increased risk of developing atrial thrombus that may embolize to the brain, kidneys, a peripheral artery, etc. The incidence of embolic stroke in patients with atrial fibrillation is five-fold the incidence of age-matched patients in normal sinus rhythm.

Treatment of atrial fibrillation is focused initially on decreasing the ventricular response with agents such as digitalis, calcium channel blockers (specifically diltiazem and verapamil), and beta-blockers which prolong the refractory period of the AV node. Anticoagulation is necessary prior to the restoration of normal sinus rhythm, which is usually attempted with Type IA, IC, or Type III antiarrythmic agents, namely quinidine, propafenone, sotalol, or amiodarone. Electrical cardioversion is required if the rhythm does not convert to normal sinus rhythm with the use of an antiarrhythmic drug.

Most patients with atrial fibrillation have underlying cardiac disease. A list of the common causes is presented in Table 50.1. Rarely, a patient may have lone atrial fibrillation, in which the arrhythmia exists in the absence of structural heart disease or other definable trigger. Because of the presence of underlying cardiac disease, even when successful restoration of sinus rhythm has been accomplished, almost 50% of patients have reverted to atrial fibrillation one year later.

Table 50.1. Cardiac and Non-cardiac Conditions Predisposing to Atrial Dysrhythmias

Hypertensive heart disease
Valvular heart disease
Ischemic heart disease
Cardiomyopathy
Congenital heart disease
Conduction system disease
Pericarditis
Thyrotoxicosis
Pulmonary embolus
Hypoxia
Holiday heart syndrome
Sepsis

Atrial Flutter

Atrial flutter (Figure 50.6) classically results from a macro-reentrant circuit in the atria, generating flutter waves at a rate of 250–350 atrial depolarizations per minute. The atrial waves are typically best seen in the inferior leads (II, III, aVF) and lead V1. As in atrial fibrillation, the ventricular rate depends on the refractory period of the AV node and the QRS complexes may be regular or irregular depending on whether a fixed or variable relationship exists between the atria and ventricles. The classic appearance of this rhythm is the sawtooth shape of the flutter waves noted in the inferior leads at a rates of 250–350 per minute. In the absence of medications or disease of the A-V node, 2:1 block exists such that one of every two atrial flutter waves are conducted to the ventricle. Consequently, whenever a ventricular rate near 150 beats per minute is detected, the tracing must be scrutinized for the presence of atrial flutter waves. The same underlying causes listed in Table 50.1 for atrial fibrillation apply to atrial flutter. In general, this rhythm may not persist for extended periods of time but often converts to sinus rhythm or, more commonly, degenerates into atrial fibrillation.

Patients with hypoxemia, hypokalemia, and other metabolic abnormalities as occasionally seen in chronic obstructive lung disease or congestive heart failure may exhibit a rhythm known as **multifocal atrial tachycardia** (Fig. 50.7). This rhythm, is likely due to multiple sites within the atrium functioning as the pacemaker of the heart, thereby generating multiple P wave morphologies. The AV node is stimulated at variable intervals by the atrial impulses, leading to irregular, narrow QRS complexes. Recognition of this rhythm depends on defining at least three different P wave morphologies in the same lead with irregular and, usually a rapid ventricular response.

Atrioventricular Nodal Reentrant Tachycardia

Atrioventricular nodal reentrant tachycardia (AVNRT) is a narrow complex tachycardia that occurs when a patient has two functional pathways in the AV node region. The pathways exhibit the classic characteristics that promote reentry: a fast pathway which depolarizes rapidly, but recovers slowly, and a slow pathway which depolarizes slowly but recovers quickly. The initiation of this rhythm is usually a premature atrial contraction timed such that it finds the fast pathway refractory and the slow pathway recovered. The PAC blocks in the fast pathway and conducts down the slow pathway. After the slow pathway depolarizes, the fast pathway has recovered, allowing the impulse to conduct in a retrograde fashion to the atria and again arrive at the slow pathway. This

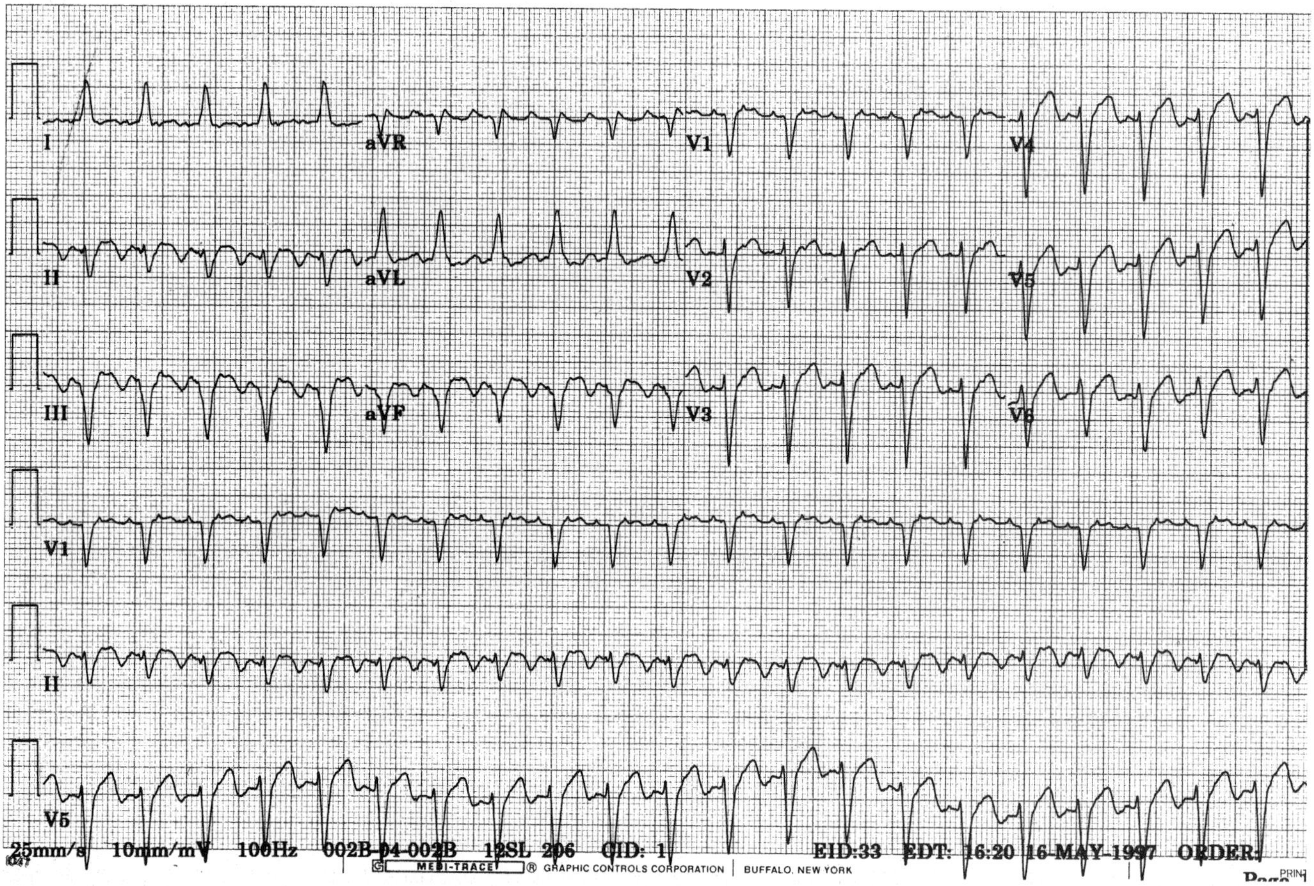

Figure 50.6. Atrial flutter with 2:1 AV conduction.

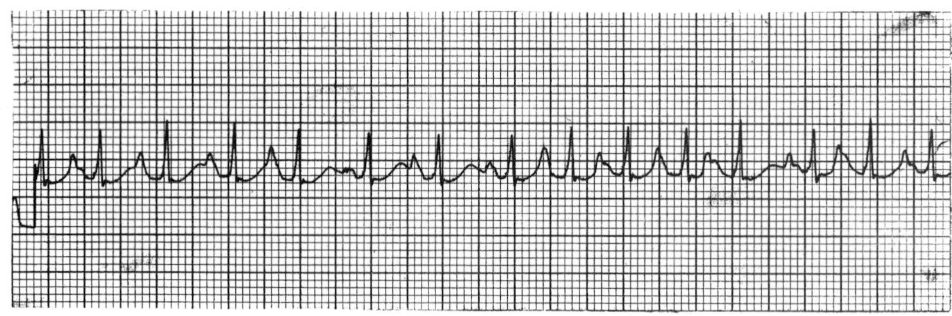

Figure 50.7. Multifocal atrial tachycardia.

results in a reentrant loop of depolarization traveling down the slow pathway and up the fast pathway. The atria and ventricles are depolarized nearly simultaneously. The P waves are typically inverted in the inferior leads (the atria are depolarized in a retrograde fashion from the AV node with the vector going superiorly) and may occur shortly after the QRS complex, or even simultaneously with the QRS complex such that the P wave cannot be visualized on the surface ECG (Fig. 50.8.).

Atrioventricular Reentrant Tachycardia

Atrioventricular reentrant tachycardia (AVRT) occurs in the setting of the substrate of an accessory pathway (AP). The AP is a muscle bridge of connection between the atria and ventricles. The onset of the tachycardia occurs when a PAC conducts over the AV node and returns to the atrium via retrograde conduction over the AP. Alternatively, depolarization from a PVC may travel retrograde over the accessory pathway stimulating the atrium and return antegrade down the AV node. The P waves are typically located at some interval after the QRS complex, usually greater than 100 msec (Fig. 50.9).

Atrial Tachycardia

Atrial tachycardia (Fig. 50.10) may be the result of rapid firing of an automatic or triggered atrial focus or reentry within the atrium. The ventricular rate depends on the atrial rate and the refractory period of the AV node. The P wave is of an altered morphology (exhibits a different vector from sinus rhythm) and the PR interval is often short.

Ventricular Tachycardia

Ventricular tachycardia (Figs. 50.11 and 50.12) is typically seen in patients with underlying heart disease, most commonly coronary artery disease with previous myocardial infarction or cardiomyopathy. Three or more

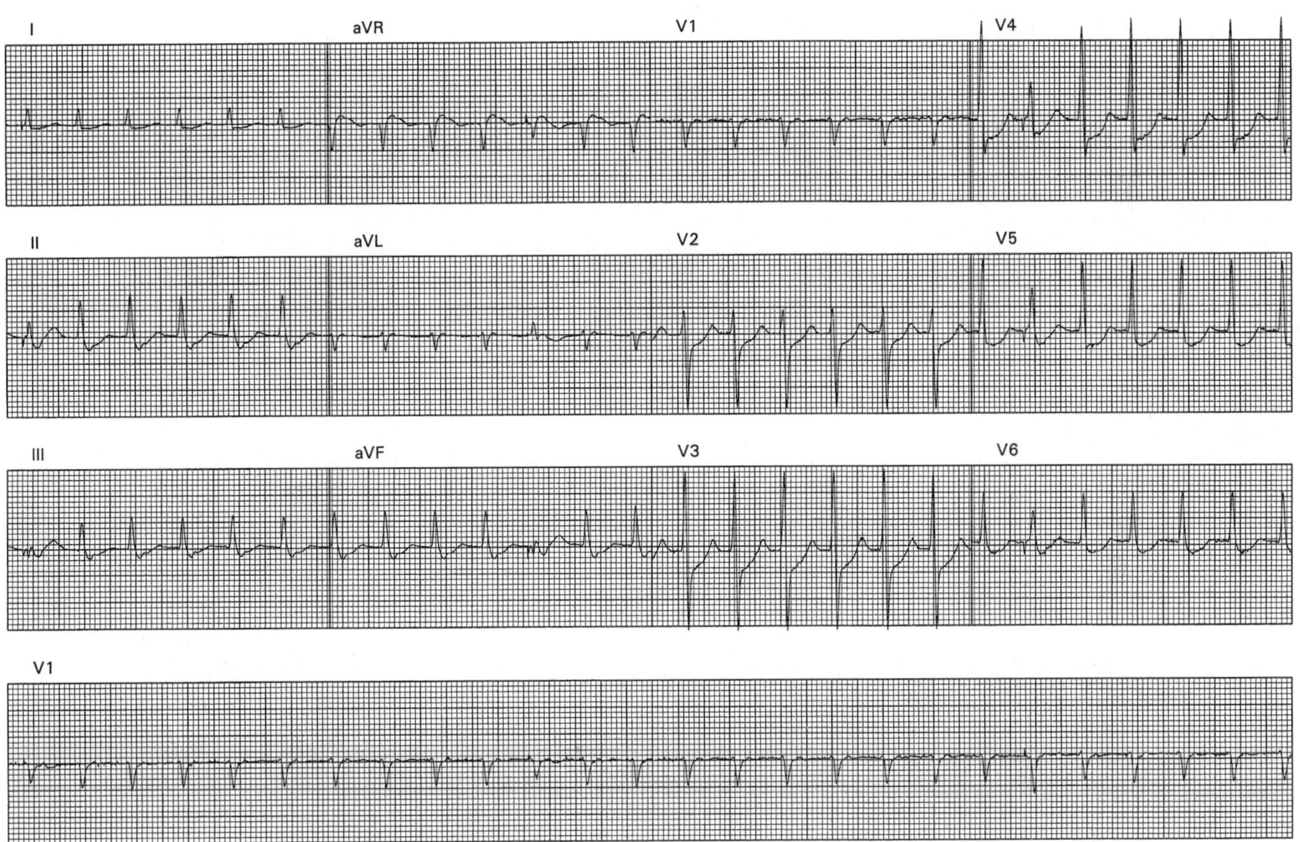

Figure 50.8. AV nodal re-entrant tachycardia. The P wave is "buried" in the QRS complex.

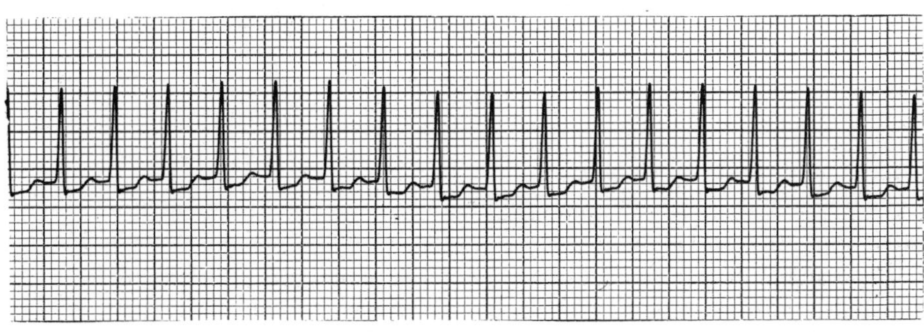

Figure 50.9. AV re-entrant tachycardia. Note the retrograde P waves present within the T wave.

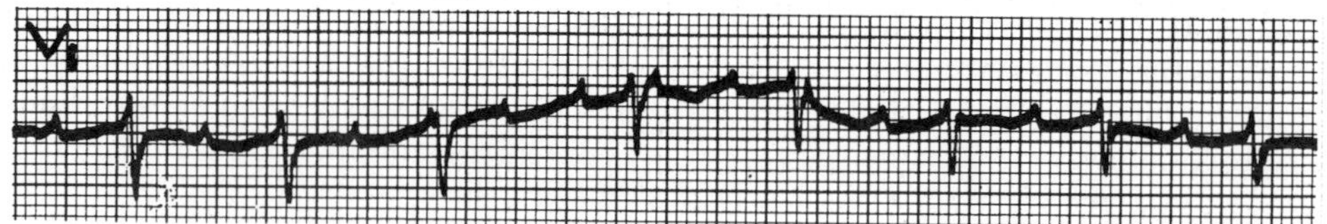

Figure 50.10. Atrial tachycardia with variable AV block. P waves label the atrial activity.

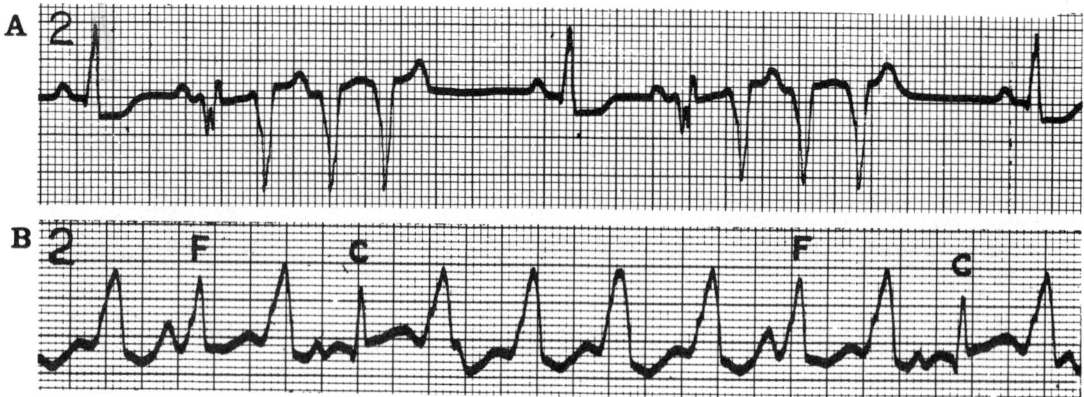

Figure 50.11. Normal sinus rhythm with a run of non-sustained ventricular tachycardia.

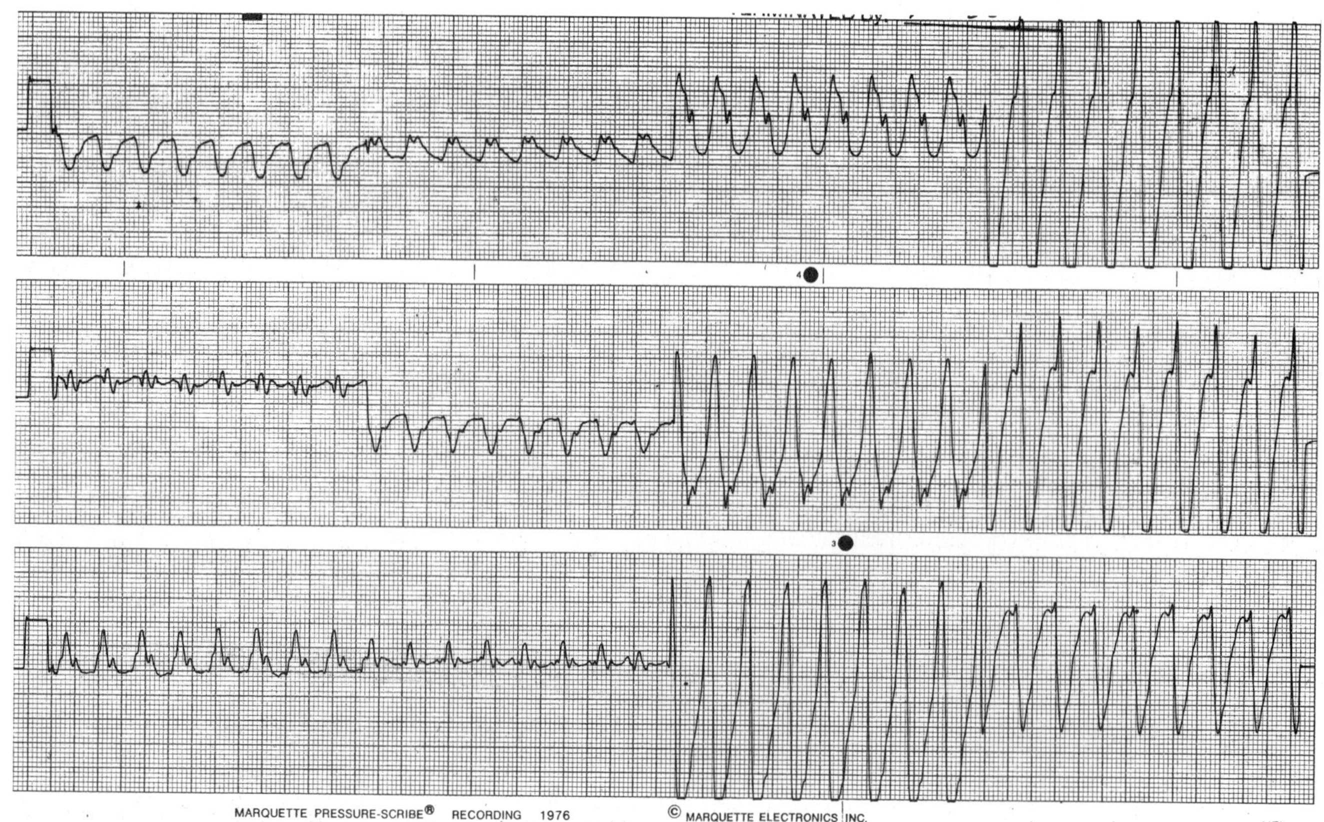

Figure 50.12. Sustained ventricular tachycardia (lasting longer than 30 seconds).

consecutive ventricular beats at a rate of 100 beats per minute defines ventricular tachycardia. Nonsustained ventricular tachycardia is a run of tachycardia lasting less than 30 seconds. Sustained ventricular tachycardia is defined as tachycardia lasting greater than 30 seconds or terminated because of hemodynamic consequences prior to 30 seconds. Ventricular tachycardia is usually recognized by the presence of a wide QRS complex (120 msec or greater), AV dissociation (the P waves and QRS complexes have no relationship) and a QRS complex that does not have the morphology of typical bundle branch block. Reentry is the most common mechanism of VT, however abnormal automaticity or triggered activity due to after-depolarizations may be responsible. Depending on the cardiac and hemodynamic status of the patient and the rate of the tachycardia, the patient may exhibit a normal blood pressure with minimal to no symptoms or be in cardiac arrest requiring immediate cardioversion.

Torsade de Pointes

Torsade de pointes is a type of ventricular tachycardia named because the morphology of the ventricular tachycardia appears exhibit a "twisting of the points." An example of this rhythm is shown in Figure 50.13.

Ventricualr Fibrillation

Ventricular fibrillation (Fig. 50.14) is a life threatening rhythm which is must be treated with immediate

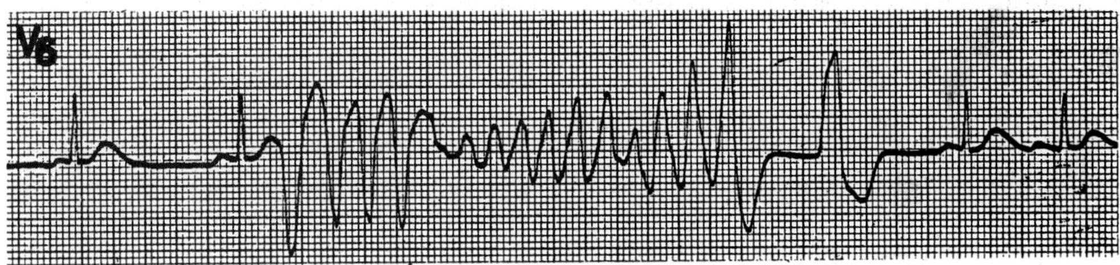

Figure 50.13. Torsade de pointes.

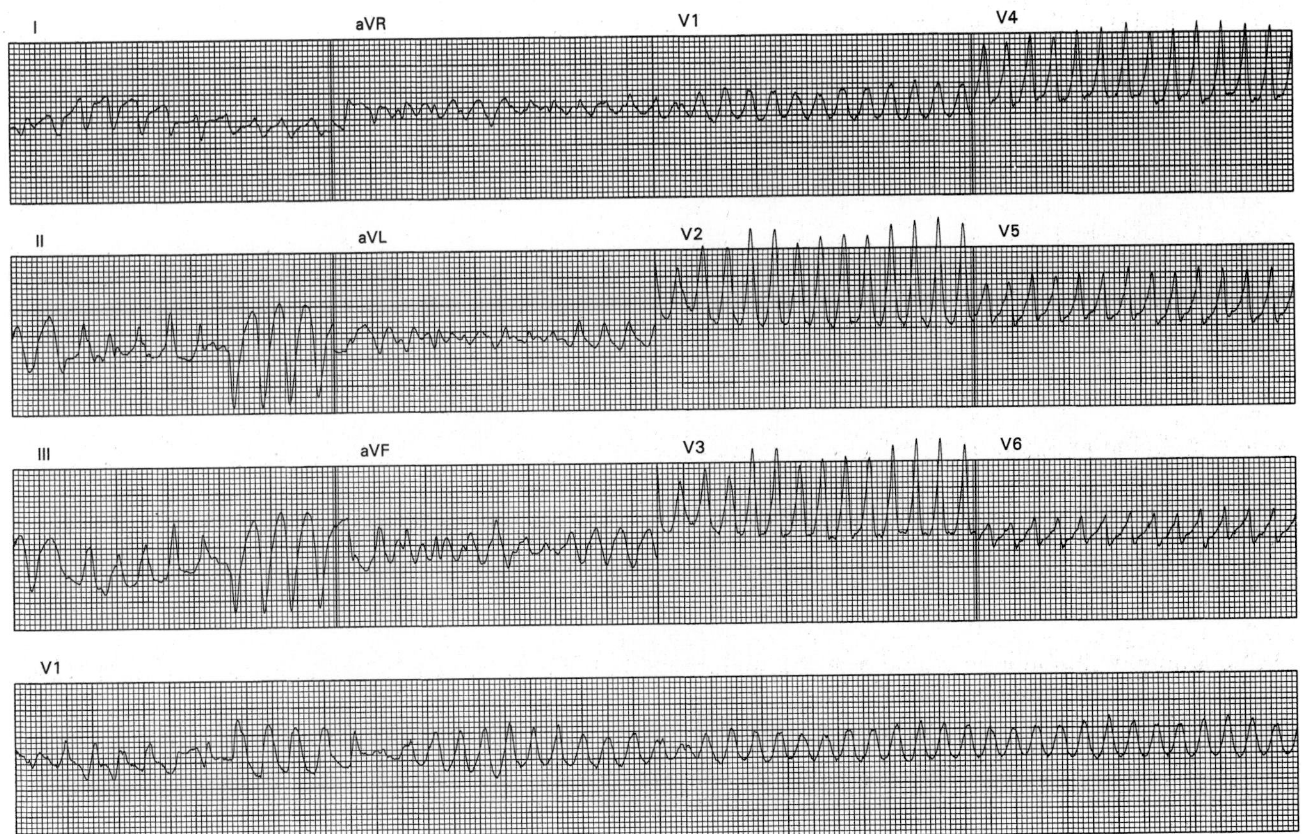

Figure 50.14. Ventricular fibrillation (coarse).

electrical defibrillation per Advanced Cardiac Life Support protocol.

BRADYARRHYTHMIAS AND DISORDERS OF THE CONDUCTION SYSTEM

Sinus Node Dysfunction

Sinus bradycardia (Fig. 50.15) occurs when the impulse originates from the sinus node at a rate less than 60 beats per minute. This may be seen in individuals who are well trained and exhibit high parasympathetic (vagal) tone, in patients who are receiving drugs that slow the heart rate (e.g., beta-blockers), or in individuals who have disease of the sinus node (sick sinus syndrome).

Sinus pauses may occur due to high vagal tone or disease of the sinus node. If the pause interval is a multiple of the intrinsic sinus rate, one may suspect **sinus exit block.** In this instance, the sinus node fires but the impulse does not conduct through the peri-sinus nodal tissue, such that the atrium is not depolarized. **Sinus arrhythmia,** a variation of the rate of firing of the sinus node, is commonly seen in younger persons, and does not reflect disease of the sinus node.

If the sinus node fails and none of the atrial cells take over the pacemaker role, the AV junction (His bundle region) may assume the role of pacemaker, resulting in a **junctional rhythm** (Fig. 50.16). This rhythm is typified by narrow QRS complexes which occur at regular intervals; the P waves often are generated by retrograde atrial conduction. P waves may occur during or after the transcription of the QRS complex. Typically, the AV junction has a much slower Phase 4 depolarization than the sinus node. Therefore, the normal junctional rate ranges between 40 and 60 beats per minute. Occasionally, the rate is more than 60 beats per minute; the rhythm is called **junctional tachycardia** or **accelerated junctional rhythm.**

Disorders of the AV node and His-Purkinje system

AV nodal disease may be due to a number of causes: infarction, ischemia, primary conduction system disease, and medication effect are the most common. The types of AV block are classified as follows:

1st degree AV block is simply prolongation of the P-R interval (see Fig. 48.3). This may be the result of intra-atrial or interatrial conduction delay, delayed

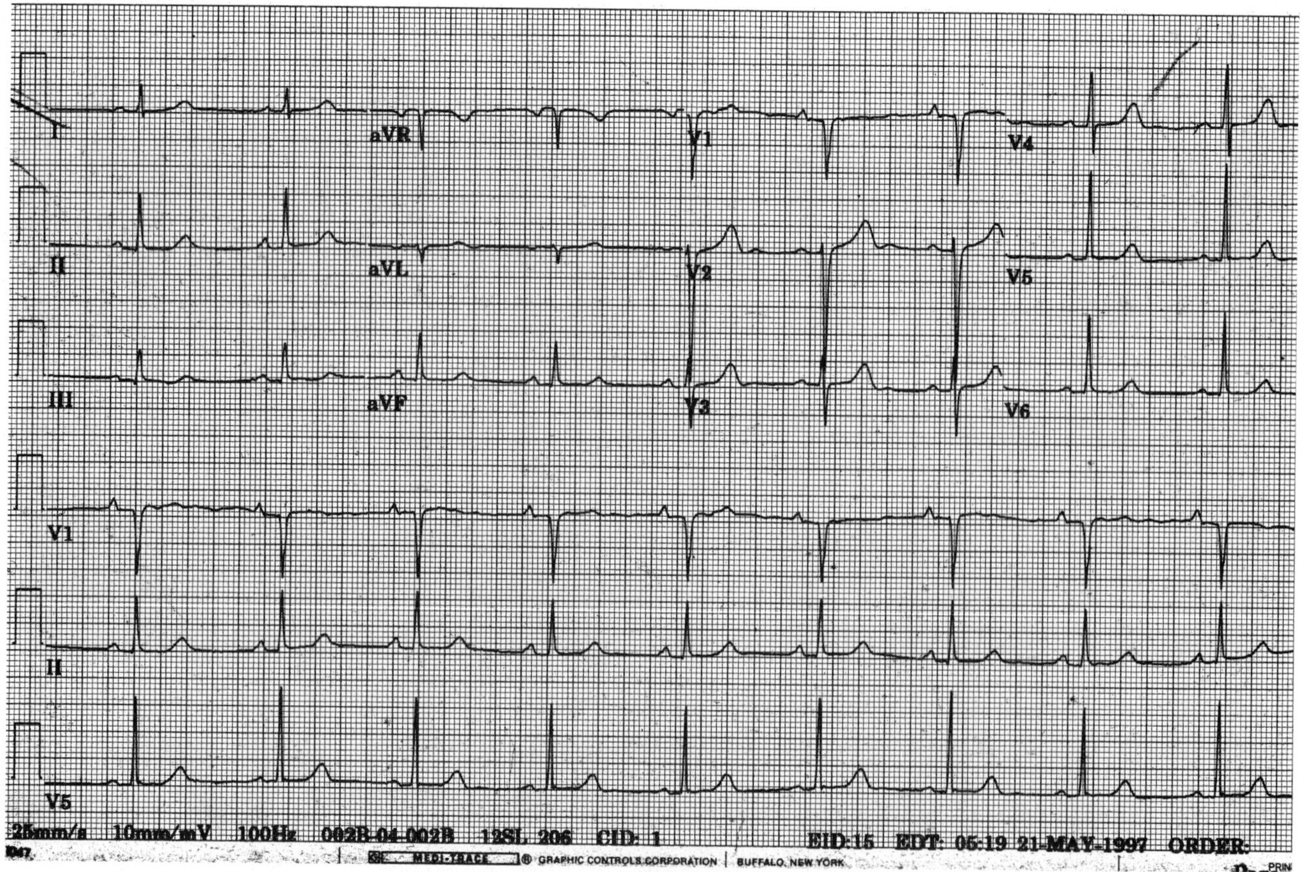

Figure 50.15. Sinus bradycardia.

conduction through the AV node, impaired conduction through the His-Purkinje system, or a combination of these.

2nd degree AV block may be divided into two types: *Mobitz Type I* and *Mobitz Type II*. In Type I (also known as Wenckebach) the disease process is usually present in the AV node. In Mobitz type I, the PR interval progressively lengthens with each beat until a P wave is not conducted to the ventricles (Fig. 50.17). In type II block, the disease usually is below the AV node in the His bundle-bundle branch region. The PR interval is fixed until a P wave is not conducted to the ventricles (Fig. 50.18). Type II block is often associated with a wide QRS complex. A rhythm disorder which may cause confusion is called *2:1 AV block* (Figure 50.19). The confusion arises with the semantics used to describe *arrhythmias*. Constant 2:1 AV block may represent 2nd degree type I or 2nd degree type II. Although the width of the QRS complex may be helpful, it is impossible to distinguish whether a progressively prolonging PR interval with a dropped beat or a fixed PR interval with every other beat dropped is present unless the onset or offset of 2:1 AV block is recorded. Further confusion results in the setting in which atrial flutter is present with 2:1 AV block. In this setting, no disease of the AV nodal-His bundle system exists; the refractory period of the normal AV node prevents the atrial impulses from reaching the ventricle in a one-

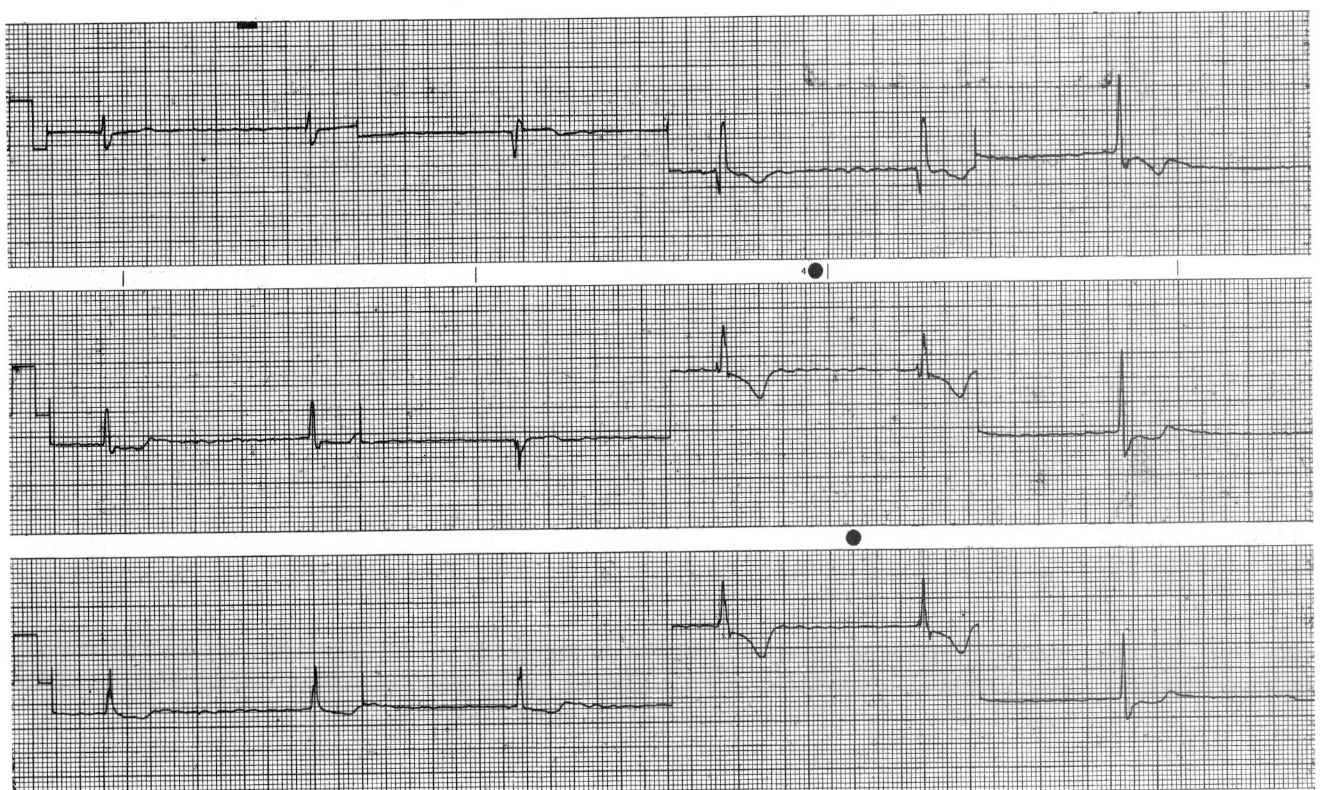

Figure 50.16. Junctional rhythm.

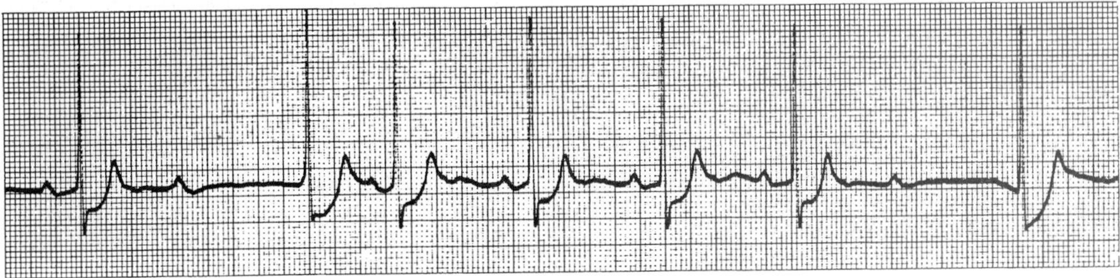

Figure 50.17. Second degree AV block, Type I.

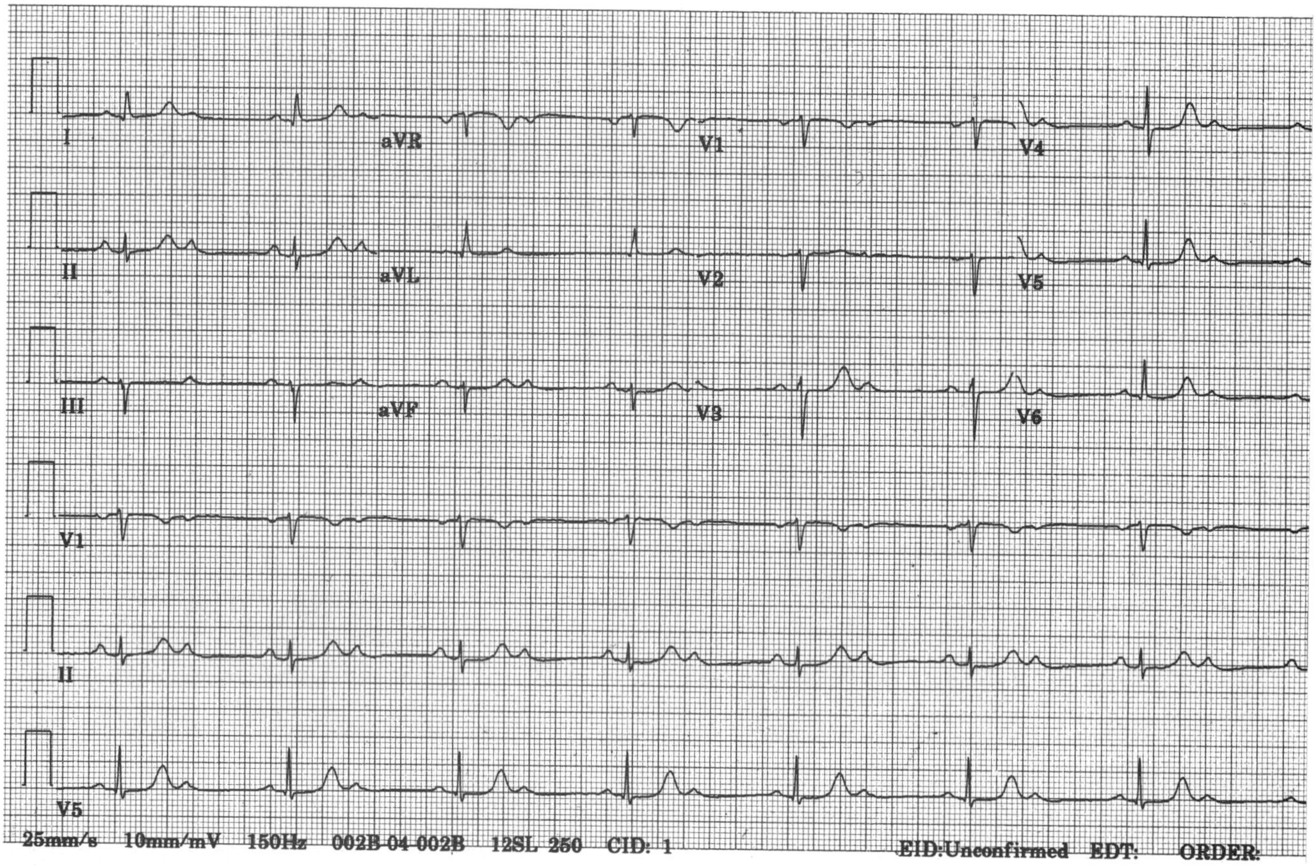

Figure 50.18. Second degree AV block, Type II.

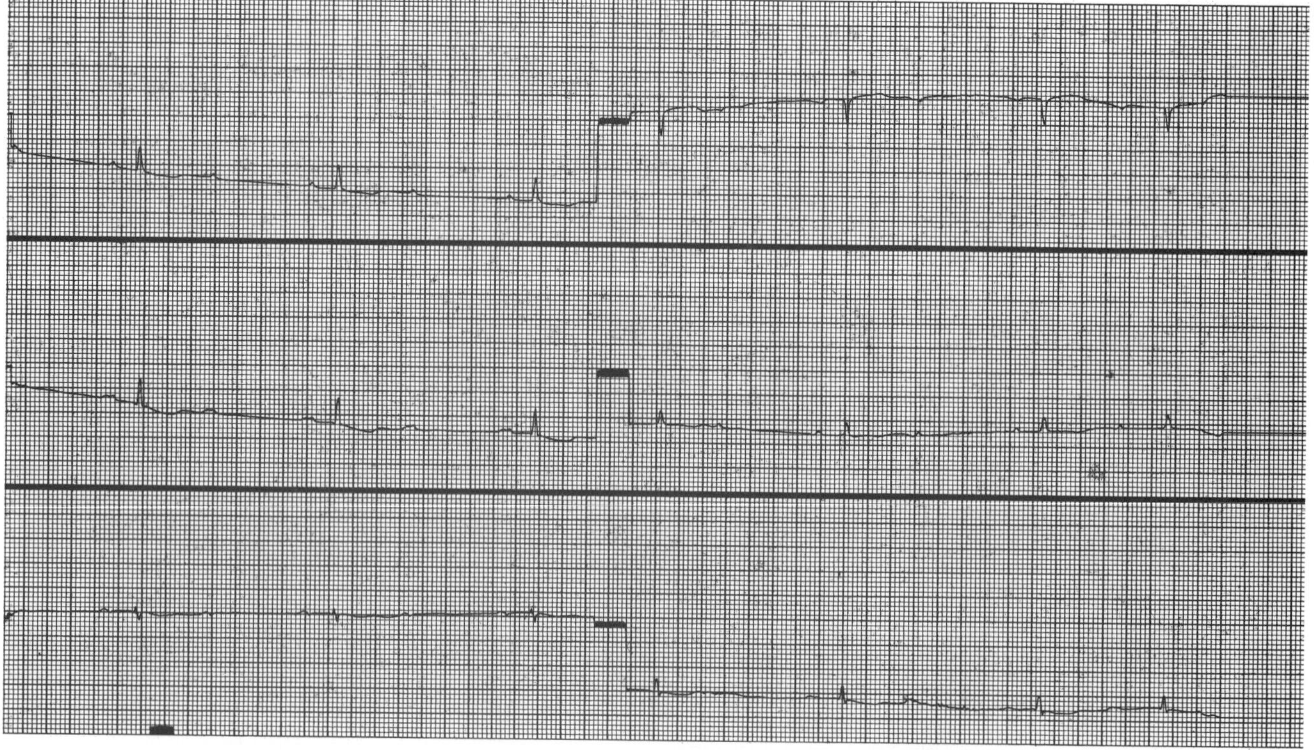

Figure 50.19. Normal sinus rhythm with 2:1 AV block–single lead.

to-one relationship. Therefore, depending on the clinical setting, 2:1 AV block may represent pathology below the AV node, pathology in the AV node, or no pathology.

Third degree (3rd) or complete heart block occurs when the atrial activity is unable to traverse the AV junction to generate a QRS complex (Fig. 50.20). The atrial rate is faster than the ventricular rate and the P waves have no influence on the QRS complexes. Depending on the site of origin of the QRS complexes, the QRS complexes may be narrow or wide.

DISORDERS OF THE BUNDLE BRANCHES AND FASICLES

Bundle Branch Blocks

When disease is present in one of the bundle branches, the QRS complex is wide (greater than 120

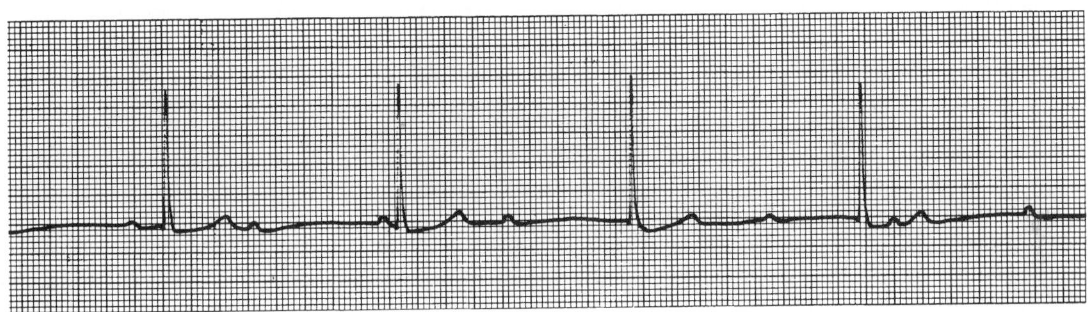

Figure 50.20. Complete heart block.

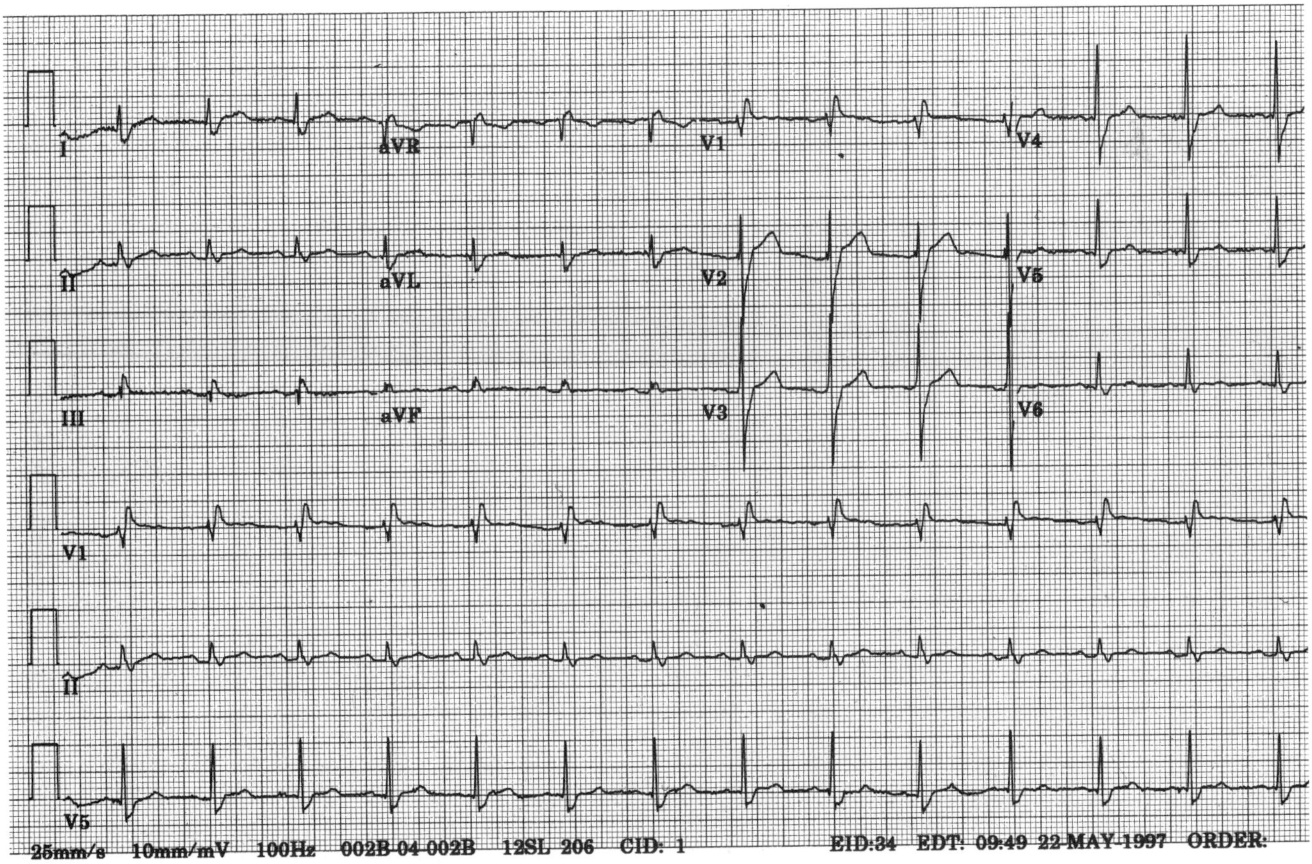

Figure 50.21. Normal sinus rhythm with right bundle branch block.

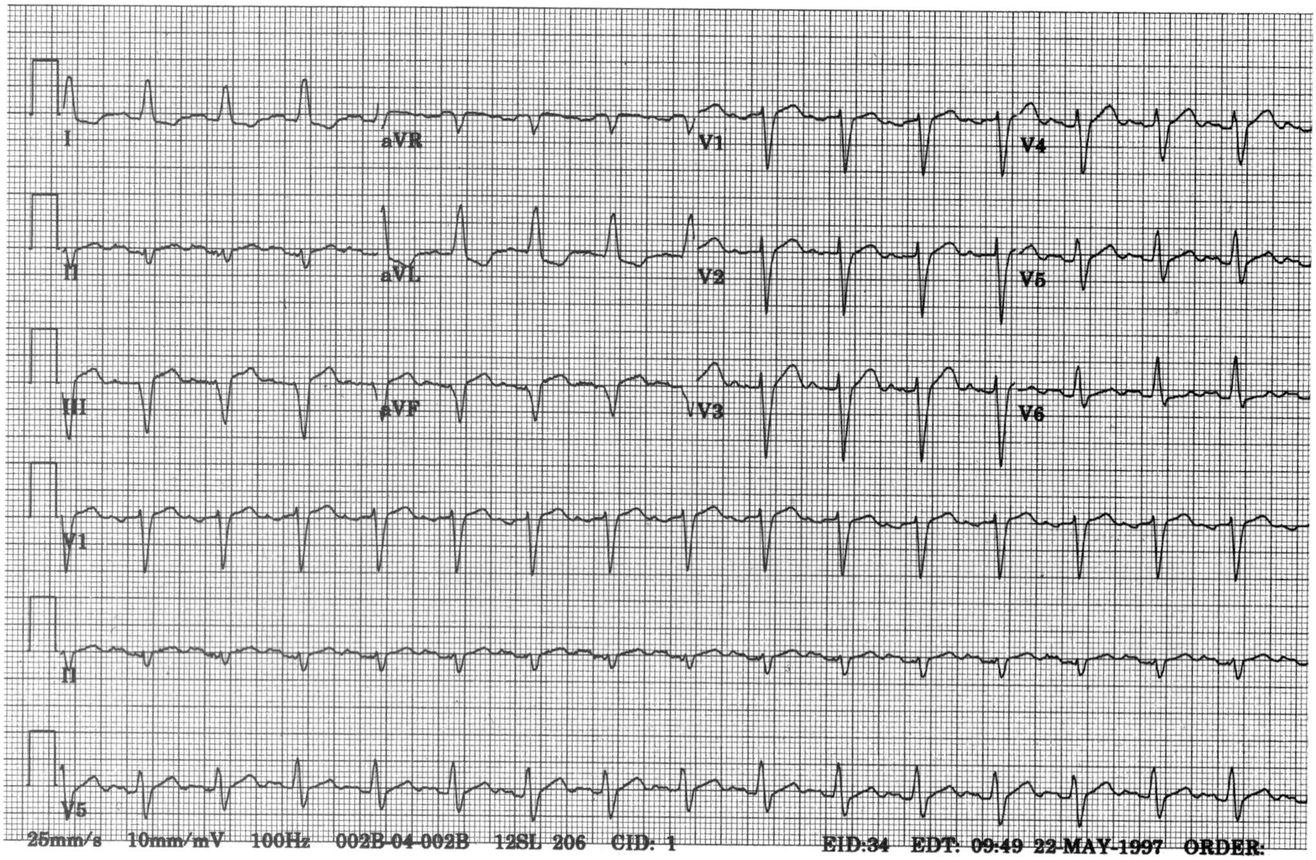

I aVR V1 V4

II aVL V2 V5

III aVF V3 V6

V1

II

V5

25mm/s 10mm/mV 100Hz 002B-04-002B 12SL 206 CID: 1 EID:34 EDT: 09:49 22-MAY-1997 ORDER:

Figure 50.22. Normal sinus rhythm with left bundle branch block.

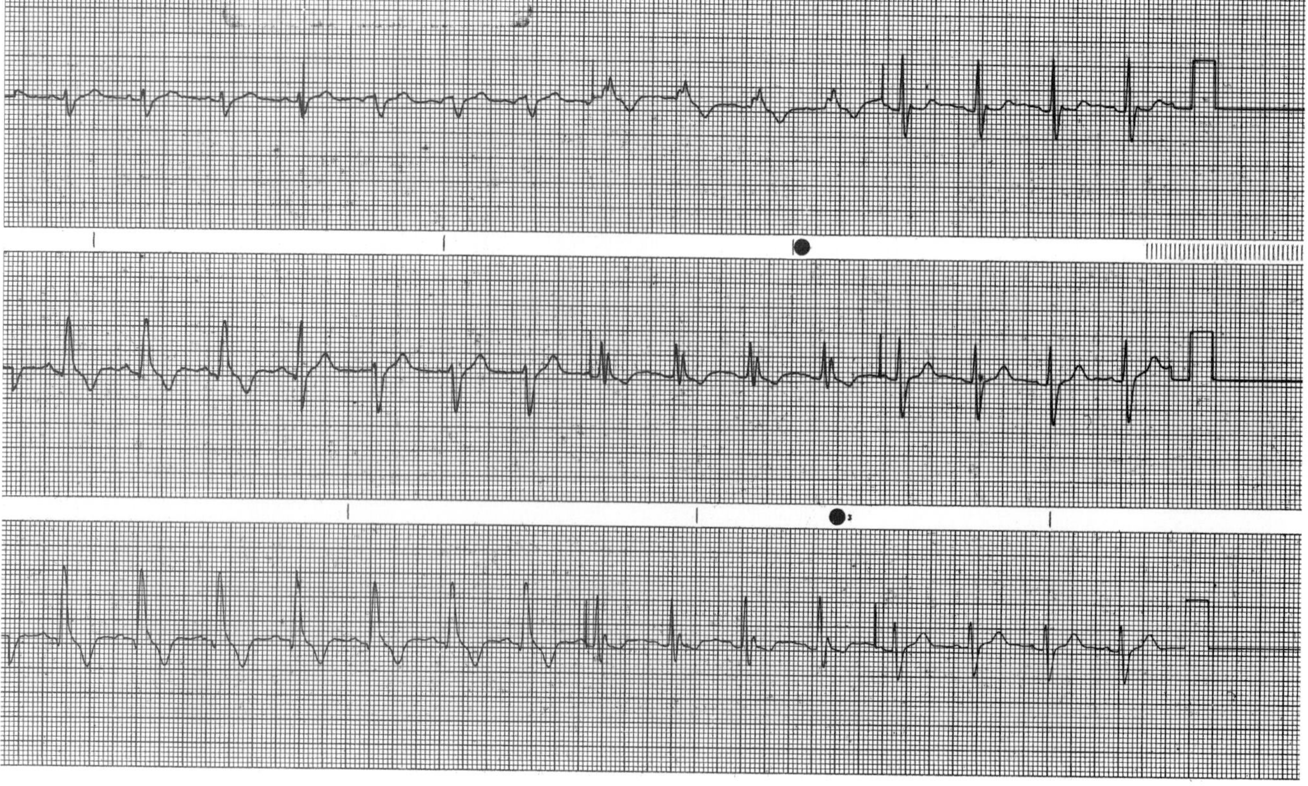

Figure 50.23. Normal sinus rhythm with right bundle branch block and left posterior fasicular block.

msec), wide QRS complexes may result from disease in the bundle branches, abnormalities of the ventricular myocardium, or the effects of drugs, electrolyte or metabolic disorders on the ventricular myocardium. Depending on the morphology of the QRS complex, these may be characterized as right bundle branch block, left bundle branch block, or nonspecific interventricular conduction defects.

In **right bundle branch block** (Fig. 50.21), activation of the left ventricle occurs prior to that of the right ventricle. The initial force due to left to right activation of the septum is normal. Consequently, the small Q waves seen in the inferior and lateral leads and the small R waves seen in leads V1 and V2 are unchanged. After the septum is depolarized, the impulse travels through the mass of the left ventricle, generating the initial portion of the QRS complex. After the left ventricle has been partially depolarized, the right ventricle depolarizes resulting in a terminal vector which is directed anteriorly and rightward. This results in a triphasic impulse in lead V1 often described as a "rabbit ears" configuration or an "RSR" complex. The abnormal depolarization results in abnormal repolarization with ST and T wave vectors directed away from the QRS complex in leads V1, V2, and sometimes V3. The presence of right bundle branch block does not prohibit electrocardiographic interpretation of ST changes in leads other than V1, V2, and V3 during an exercise test.

In **left bundle branch block** (Fig. 50.22), the initial force travels across the septum from right to left, thus altering the initial QRS deflection. This results in an initial negative deflection in lead V1 and an initial upright deflection in lead V6. As the remainder of the left ventricle is depolarized, the QRS vector continues to be toward V6. The depolarization of the right ventricle is mainly obscured by that of the left ventricle; therefore, little effect of right ventricle depolarization on the vector forces is noted. The repolarization pattern is altered in left bundle branch block, with the ST and T vector directed rightward and anteriorly. Consequently, the ECG may not be used to ascertain ischemic changes during an exercise study.

A QRS greater than 120 msec without the morphology of right or left bundle branch block is best termed a nonspecific intraventricular conduction delay.

Fascicular Blocks

Disease in the fasicles of the left bundle branch results in minimal prolongation of the QRS complex. Fascilicular block (hemiblocks) are recognized by their effects on the frontal plane axis. **Left anterior fascicular block** (see Figure 47.4) causes significant left axis deviation (greater than −30°), resulting in small Q waves in lead I and aVL, and small R waves in leads II, III, and aVF. **Left posterior fascicular block** (Fig. 50.23) produces right axis deviation, (usually 90–110°) with small Q waves in leads II, III, and aVF and small R waves in leads I and aVL. Unlike left bundle branch, these entities have no adverse effect on the ability to interpret ECG changes during an exercise test.

▶ SUMMARY

Many derangements in the normal depolarization sequence may occur. Three mechanisms for arrhythmia genesis have been described. By careful interpretation of the relationship between the P waves and QRS complexes, and the effect on other aspects of the ECG (i.e., axis, intervals, complex width and P wave and QRS vectors) one may readily ascertain the etiology of tachyarrhythmias, bradyarrhythmias, atrioventricular, and interventricular conduction defects.

Suggested Readings

Braunwald. E. Heart Disease: A textbook of cardiovascular medicine, 5th ed Philadelphia: W.B. Saunder Company, 1997.

Wagner GS. Marriott's Practical Electrocardiography. 9th ed. Baltimore: Williams & Wilkins, 1994.

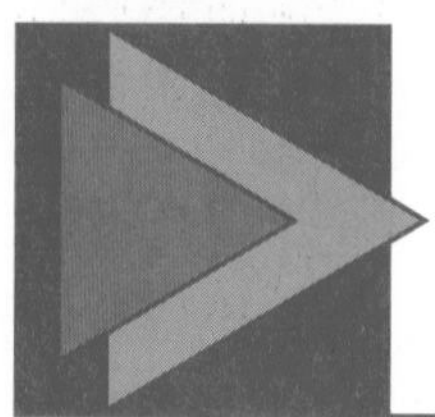

CHAPTER **51**

OTHER ABNORMAL ELECTROCARDIOGRAMS

John A. Larry and Stephen F. Schaal

There are other common pathologies of the heart that cause changes in the electrocardiogram (ECG). These include hypertrophic patterns, ECG changes mediated by pharmacologic agents or by electrolyte disorders, and conduction defects which often require pacemakers for correction and treatment. Some of the more common ECG patterns associated with them are discussed below.

VENTRICULAR HYPERTROPHY

While echocardiography remains the gold standard, chamber enlargement may be determined with a reasonable degree of accuracy by electrocardiography. Various criteria exist with different degrees of sensitivity and specificity. Below is a discussion of the most commonly used criteria that have reasonable sensitivity and specificity for determining vertricular hypertrophy.

Left Ventricular Hypertrophy

Left ventricular hypertrophy (LVH) or enlargement (Fig. 51.1), as detected electrocardiographically is associated with two mechanisms: hypertrophy of the walls or dilatation of the chamber. LVH is an important ECG finding, as it has been associated with increased morbidity and mortality. The terms enlargement and hypertrophy are often used interchangeably, although some experts do distinguish these entities. The most well known criteria for determining LVH are the **Estes criteria** (Table 51.1). This is a weighted scoring system in which points are assigned for certain characteristics. Increased voltage is the result of a greater mass of myocardium which must be depolarized. Repolarization changes develop with LVH which classically are described as a "strain pattern." The ST segments are depressed but exhibit an upward convexity and blend into a biphasic or inverted T wave. This pattern is most commonly seen in the inferior and lateral leads. Often, left atrial enlargement can be found in association with LVH. The QRS width may increase, and the time from the R wave to the S wave, the **intrinisicoid deflection,** also may increase. The tracing in Figure 51.1 would receive 11 points by the Estes scoring.

The **Scott criteria** (Table 51.2), another commonly used method for ECG analysis, are simpler to use. The voltage changes caused by the left ventricular enlargement are measured and used as an index for left ventricular enlargement. Consideration of the secondary changes in repolarization or in left atrial size are not used in the Scott criteria.

The presence of LVH on the baseline tracing may result in an indeterminate or false positive stress ECG. Because of this, evaluation for chest pain requires supplemental radionuclide imaging to confirm or exclude ischemia.

Right Ventricular Hypertrophy

Right ventricular hypertrophy (RVH) or enlargement (Fig. 51.2) is much less common than LVH. The major causes are pulmonary disease, valvular disease (particularly mitral and tricuspid), and congenital heart disease. A variety of electrocardiographic types of RVH have been described, but are beyond the scope of this chapter. Table 51.3 lists some of the electrocardiographic manifestations of RVH.

Left Atrial Enlargement

Left atrial enlargement (Fig. 51.1) may be inferred from changes in P wave morphology. The P wave changes of broadening and notching, when present, are usually best seen in lead II. A more sensitive finding is enlargement of the negative component of the P wave in lead V1. As previously noted, the negative deflection in lead V1 reflects left atrial depolarization, a posteriorly directed vector. In left atrial enlargement, the negative component in lead V1 is greater than one small box on the grid, that is, greater than 0.04 seconds in duration and 1 mm in amplitude.

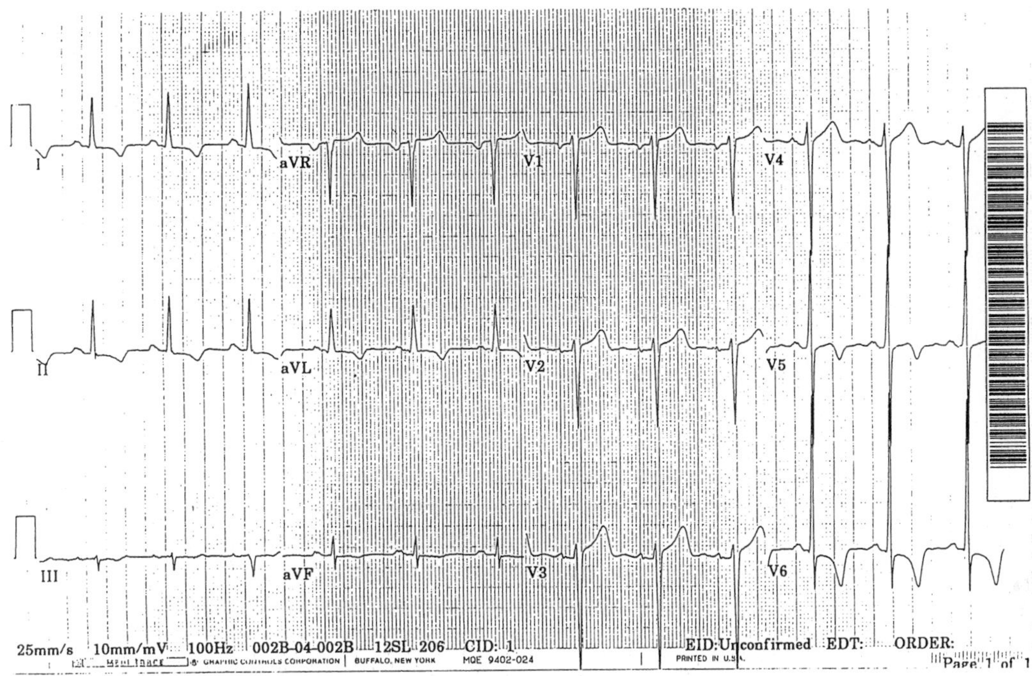

Figure 51.1. Left ventricular hypertrophy/left atrial enlargement.

Table 51.1. Estes ECG Criteria for the Determination of Left Ventricular Enlargement

	POINTS
1. Any of the following:	
R or S in limb lead ≥ 20 mm	
S wave in V1, V2, V3 ≥ 25 mm	
R wave in V4, V5, V6 ≥ 25 mm	3
2. Any ST shift:	3
Typical strain ST-T changes:	1
3. LAD > 15 degrees	2
4. QRS interval > 0.09 sec	1
5. Intrisicoid deflection > 0.04 sec	1
6. P-terminal force in V1 > 0.04	3
Total (LVH > 5 points, probable LVH > 4 points)	13

Modified from Wagner GS. Marriott's Practical Electrocardiography 9th ed. Baltimore: Williams & Wilkins, 1994.

Table 51.2. Scott ECG Criteria for the Determination of Left Ventricular Hypertrophy

Any one listed below:
1. S in V1 or V2 + R in V5 or V6 ≥ 35 mm
2. R in V5 or V6 ≥ 26 mm
3. R + S in any V lead ≥ 45 mm
4. R in I + S in III ≥ than 25 mm
5. R in aVL ≥ 7.5 mm
6. R in aVF ≥ 20 mm
7. S in aVR ≥ 14 mm

Modified from Wagner GS. Marriott's Practical Electrocardiography 9th ed. Baltimore: Williams & Wilkins, 1994.

Right Atrial Enlargement

Right atrial enlargement also produces changes in P wave morphology. Tall, peaked P waves (>3.0 mm) may be seen in lead II and the right sided chest leads. However, this criterion is less sensitive for right atrial enlargement than are the criteria for left atrial enlargement.

COMMONLY USED MEDICATIONS THAT AFFECT THE ELECTROCARDIOGRAM

Digitalis

Digitalis is an agent that is often used to treat patients with congestive heart failure or atrial arrhythmias. In addition to its effect of prolonging the refractory period of the AV node, digitalis effects the ST segment and T wave. Figure 51.3 demonstrates these changes. The ST segment appears scooped-out and depressed. These changes typically occur in the inferior and lateral leads. The presence of digitalis may yield false-positive stress ECG findings and additional imaging modalities may be required to increase the specificity of the study.

Quinidine

Quinidine is a commonly used anti-arrhythmic agent that is predominantly used to maintain sinus rhythm in patients with a history of atrial fibrillation. Historically, it has been used to treat ventricular arrhythmias, although recently it has been replaced with other agents and implantable defibrillators. Quinidine prolongs the QT interval on the ECG. Other agents in its class, **pro-**

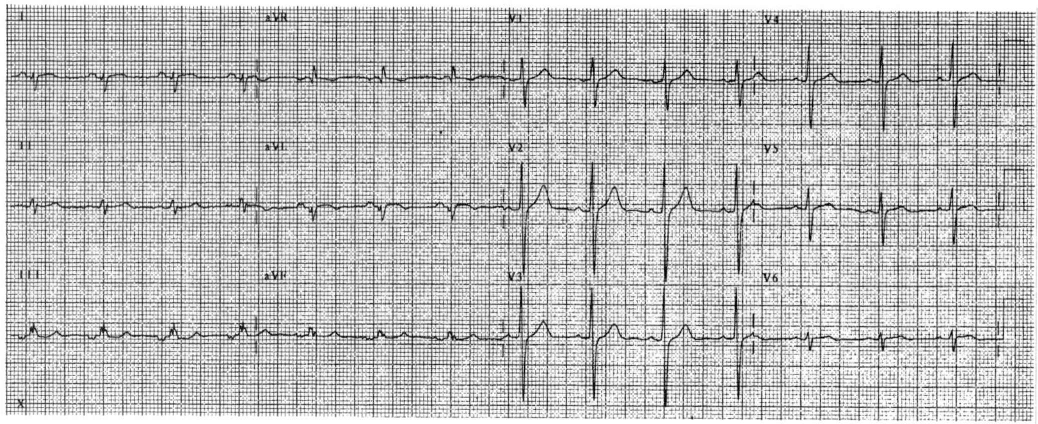

Figure 51.2. Right ventricular hypertrophy.

Table 51.3. Electrocardiographic Manifestations of Right Ventricular Hypertrophy

Right axis deviation
R wave in V1 than 7 mm
R in V1 + S in V5 or V6 10 mm
R:S ratio in V1 1.0
S:R in V6 1.0
Right intraventricular conduction defect
Right ventricular strain pattern in V1, V2, or II, III, and aVF

Modified from Wagner GS. Marriott's Practical Electrocardiography 9th ed. Baltimore: Williams & Wilkins, 1994.

cainamide and **disopyramide** have a similar effect. Some of the antidepressant agents, particularly the **tricyclic antidepressants,** may also prolong the QT interval. Significant prolongation of the QT interval predisposes the patient to Torsades de Pointes, which can be fatal.

ELECTROLYTE DISORDERS

Hyperkalemia is associated with a variety of ECG changes depending on the serum potassium. Initially the T waves become peaked (Fig. 51.4), followed by prolon-

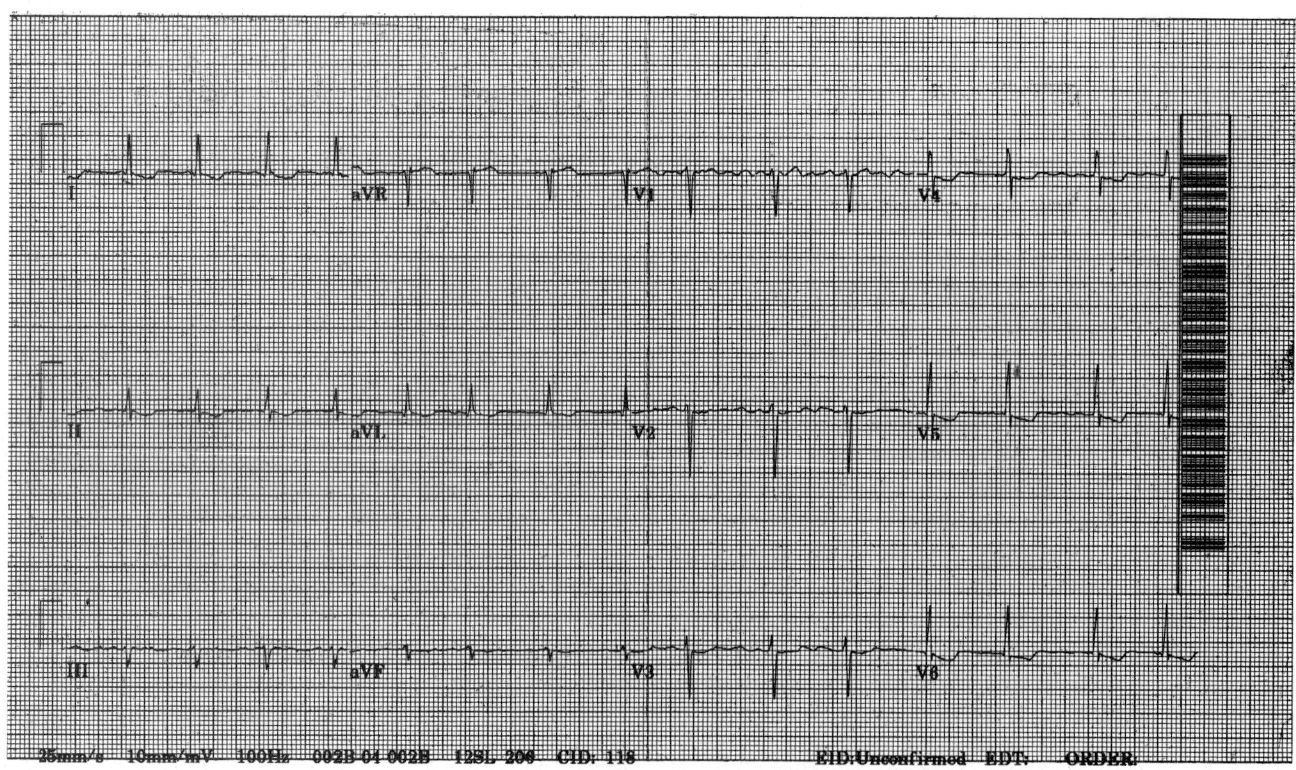

Figure 51.3. ST depression caused by digitalis.

Figure 51.4. Peaked T waves seen in hyperkalemia.

I
aVR
V1
V4
II
aVL
V2
V5
III
aVF
V3
V6
25mm/s 10mm/mV 100Hz 002B-04-002B 12SL 78 CID: 140
EID:Unconfirmed EDT: ORDER:

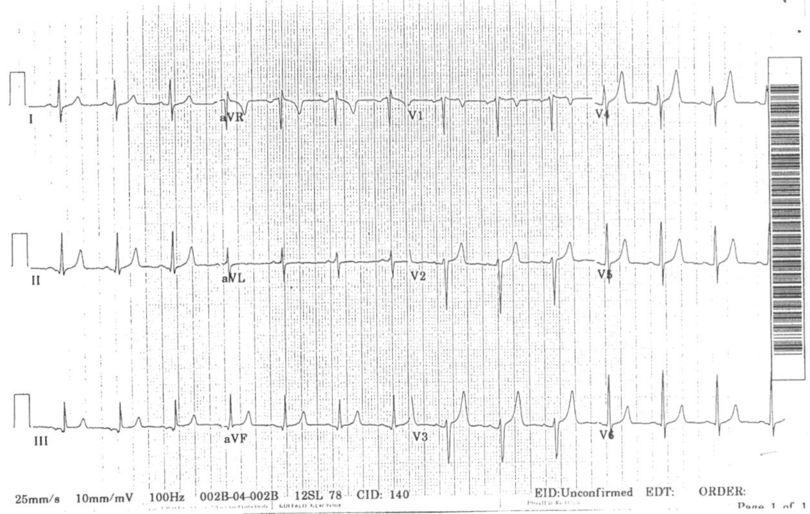

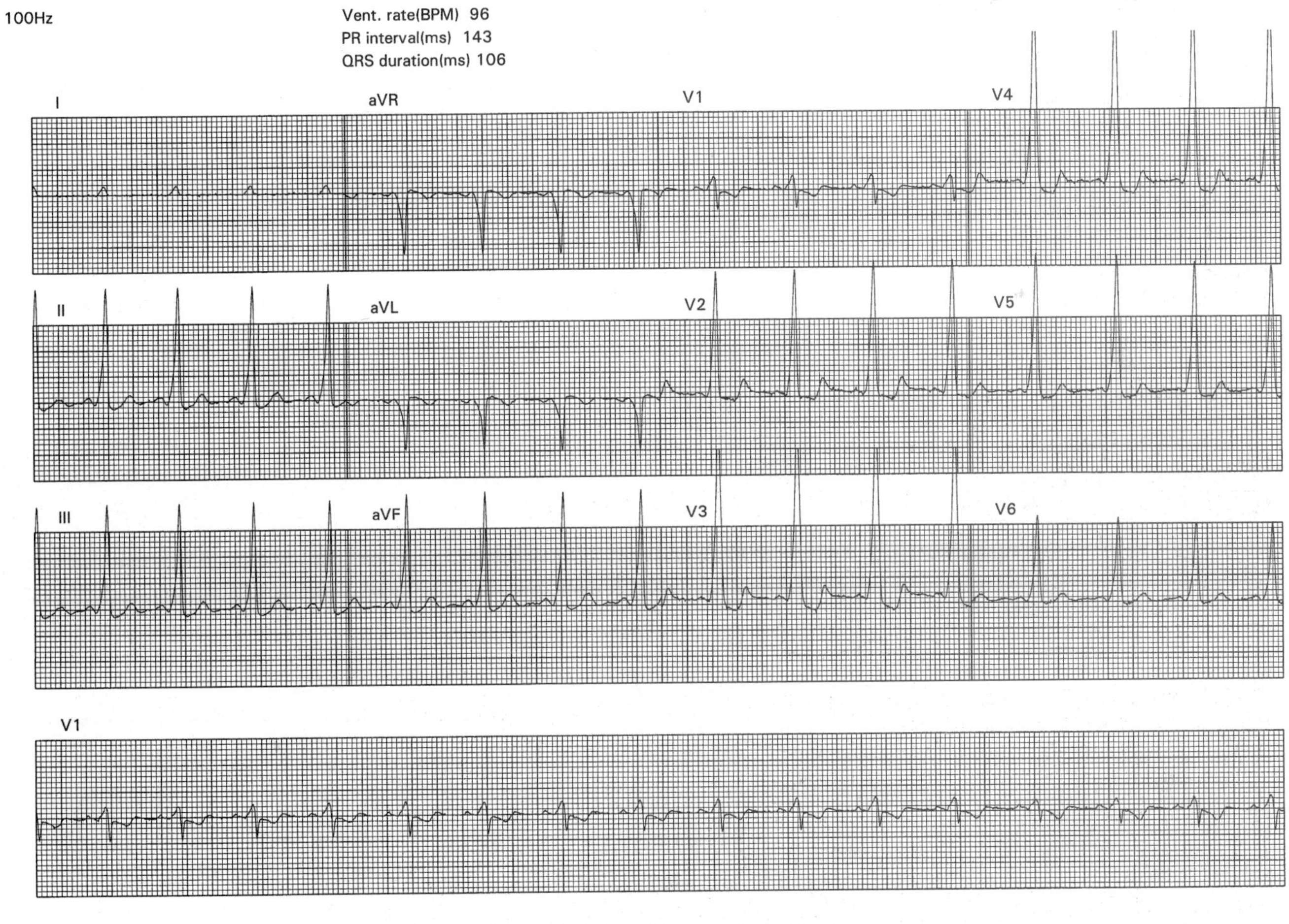

100Hz
Vent. rate(BPM) 96
PR interval(ms) 143
QRS duration(ms) 106
I
aVR
V1
V4
II
aVL
V2
V5
III
aVF
V3
V6
V1

Figure 51.5. Wolffe-Parkinson-White Syndrome.

gation of the QRS interval (not illustrated). Subsequently, the PR interval prolongs, and finally the P waves disappear. At extremely high levels of potassium the rhythm has the appearance of a sine wave.

Hypokalemia may cause diminution of the T wave voltage, prolongation of the QT interval, and rarely, ST segment depression. Prominent U waves may develop, although these can also be seen in the absence of potas-

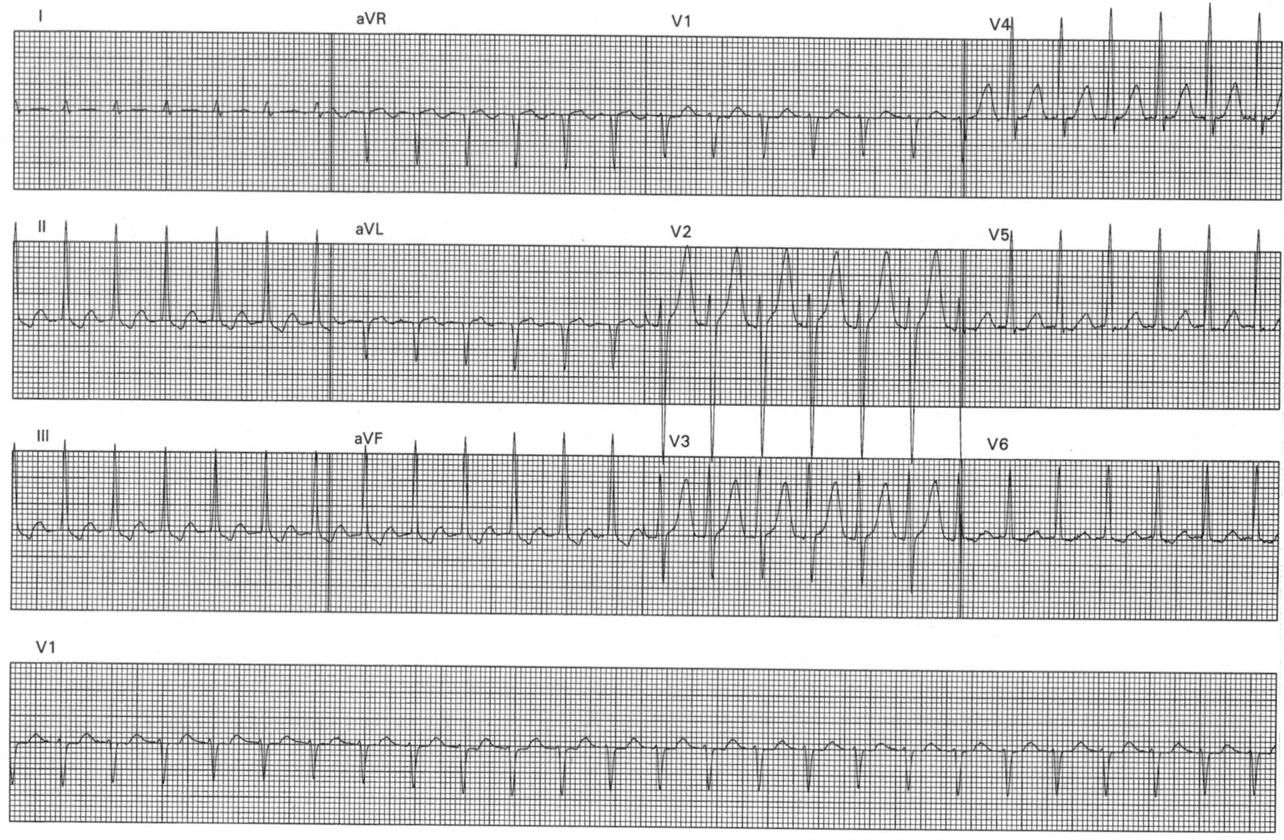

Figure 51.6. Orthodromic AV Reentrant Tachycardia.

sium abnormalities. **Hypercalcemia** results in shortening of the Q-T interval, while **hypocalcemia** prolongs the Q-T interval.

WOLFFE-PARKINSON-WHITE SYNDROME

Typically, the AV node is the only connection between the atria and the ventricles. In Wolffe-Parkinson-White syndrome there is an additional myocardial bridging connection between the atria and ventricles termed an accessory pathway. When the patient is in normal sinus rhythm, a short PR interval and a slurred QRS upstroke, termed a delta wave, are present (Figure 51.5). While patients with an accessory pathway may be asymptomatic, they are predisposed to three types of tachycardias: orthodromic AV reentrant tachycardia, antidromic AV reentrant tachycardia, and atrial fibrillation. When the reentrant loop travels antegrade over the AV node and retrograde over the accessory pathway, the tachycardia is referred to as **orthodromic** AV reentrant tachycardia (see Figure 51.6). This tachycardia has a narrow QRS complex. The alternative situation, when the impulse travels antegrade over the accessory pathway and retrograde through the AV node, results in a wide complex tachycardia, and is called **antidromic** AV reentrant tachycardia. Atrial fibrillation in patients with Wolffe-Parkinson-White syndrome may result in very rapid ventricular rates with hemodynamic instability. These arrhythmias can be provoked during exercise testing; therefore it is important to note the presence of the accessory pathway prior to testing and be alert for the development of a tachyarrhythmia.

Table 51.4. Standardized Pacemaker Code

1st letter: paced chamber
A = atria
V = ventricle
D = dual chamber
2nd letter: sensing chamber
A = atria
V = ventricle
D = dual chamber
3rd letter: mode of pacemaker
I = inhibit
T = trigger
D = both inhibit and trigger
4th letter: rate modulation present
R = rate responsive

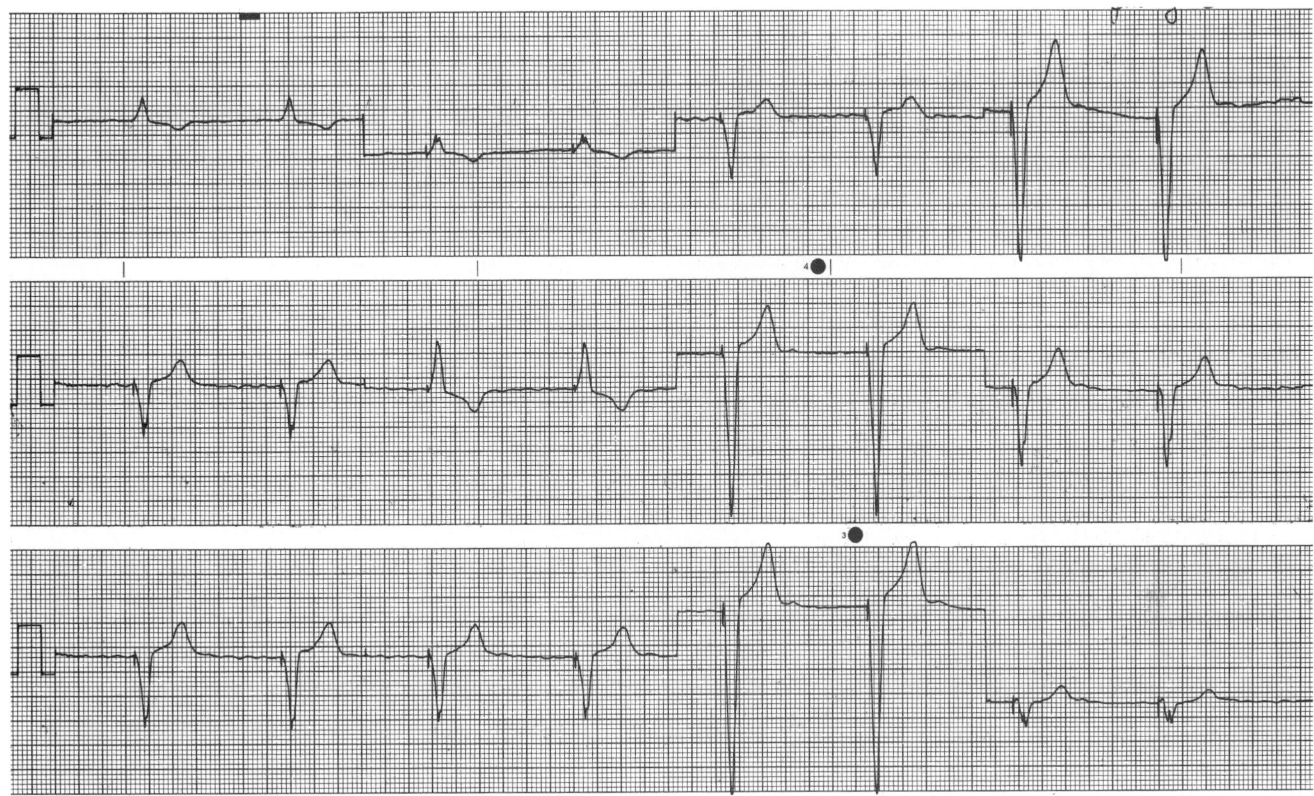

Figure 51.7. VVI pacemaker.

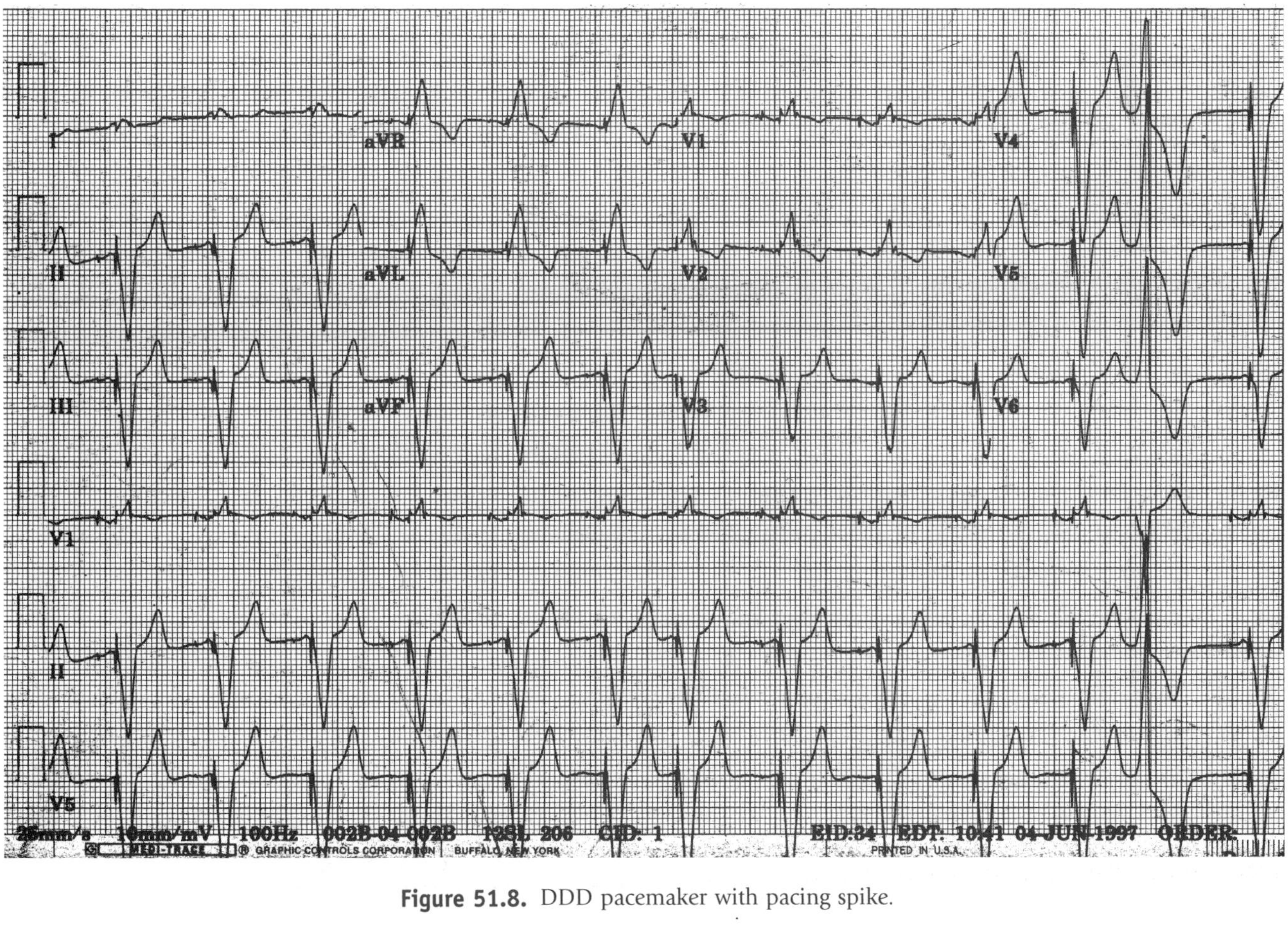

Figure 51.8. DDD pacemaker with pacing spike.

PACEMAKERS

A variety of pacemakers currently exist, and a comprehensive review is beyond the scope of this text. Nonetheless, many patients undergoing treadmill testing or entering cardiac rehabilitation programs have pacemakers. Pacemakers are inserted for patients with bradycardia due to disease of the conduction system. The most common reasons for pacing are sinus node dysfunction and atrioventricular block.

Pacemakers are described by a standardized code which has been adopted by both Europe and the United States. Table 51.4 shows the standard pacemaker code and describes the designation for each position in the code.

The simplest type of pacemaker is a VVI (Fig. 51.7). In this mode, there is a single pacing wire in the right ventricle which senses any impulses in the ventricle. If the rate is set at 60 beats per minute, the pacemaker senses for ventricular depolarization for the 1 second interval between depolarization of the SA node. If no impulses are detected during the pre-determined interval, the pacemaker delivers an impulse to the right ventricle resulting in ventricular depolarization. The timing interval is reset and the pacemaker begins to sense for ventricular impulses during the next interval. If an impulse is detected, the pacemaker is inhibited from firing, the timing interval is reset, and ventricular sensing restarted. Because the pacemaker is located in the right ventricle, the paced complexes have a wide morphology similar to left bundle branch block. Normally a pace artifact, or spike, is noted before the QRS complex. Due to the abnormal sequence of depolarization which exists in pacing, ST and T changes exist due to abnormal repolarization. This prevents interpretation of ST and T changes during an exercise study.

The most common pacemaker in use today is a DDD pacemaker (Fig. 51.8). This pacemaker has two leads, one in the right atrium and one in the right ventricle. This permits the maintenance of atrial and ventricular synchrony. Proper timing of atrial contraction to augment diastolic filling is more physiological. Depending on the underlying conduction disease and the programmed characteristics of the pacemaker, four scenarios may result on the ECG. These are depicted in Table 51.5.

Table 51.5. Complexes Seen in DDD Pacing

Native P wave	Native QRS
Paced P wave	Native QRS
Native P wave	Paced QRS
Paced P wave	Paced QRS

As many of the new pacemakers are rate responsive (DDDR), it is possible to see an increase in the paced atrial rate with exercise.

Rate responsive pacemakers use one of several strategies to detect the need for increased cardiac output. The most common sensor is a gyroscope located in the generator which senses movement of the upper body. Depending on the rate of vibrations sensed, the pacer will increase its rate based on a predetermined algorithm to the maximum programmed rate. A second sensor commonly used measures the respiratory rate and relative tidal volume to calculate minute ventilation. When the minute ventilation increases, so does the rate of the pacer.

▶ SUMMARY

Many cardiac and non-cardiac phenomenon can exert effects on the ECG. Some of the more common situations seen have been highlighted. Pacemakers are becoming more common as our population ages and one should not be surprised by the ECG findings in these patients. In order to be competent in ECG interpretation, repetition in reading tracings is essential. We hope to have provided a framework of understanding through which basic electrophysiologic principles govern the approach to electrocardiographic interpretation. The ECG remains an invaluable diagnostic tool; the better skilled the interpreter, the more information can be derived about the patients and their cardiac condition.

Suggested Readings

Braunwald. E. Heart Disease: A textbook of cardiovascular medicine, 5th ed Philadelphia: W.B. Saunder Company, 1997.

Wagner GS. Marriott's Practical Electrocardiography. 9th ed. Baltimore: Williams & Wilkins, 1994.

SECTION TEN

Exercise Programming

SECTION EDITOR: *Moira Kelsey, RN, MS*

29, 31, 148, 149, 150, 151, 152, 153, 154, 155, 156, 157, 168

178, 179, 180, 181, 187, 191, 193

CHAPTER 52

Cardiorespiratory Endurance

Robert G. Holly and James D. Shaffrath

Physical activity is defined as any bodily movement produced by skeletal muscles that results in energy expenditure. Exercise is defined as planned, structured, and repetitive bodily movement done to improve or maintain one or more components of physical fitness. The focus of this chapter is exercise planning or programming to increase cardiorespiratory (CR) fitness; however, some of the health benefits associated with less structured, but regular, moderate intensity physical activity will also be discussed (1, 2).

CR activities are those physical activities which cause an increase in the transport and uptake of oxygen by skeletal muscle. These activities, appropriately performed on a regular basis, increase CR fitness and lead to numerous health-related benefits (1, 2). However, CR exercise and activity performed inappropriately or by those for whom it is contraindicated may result in serious complications. Thus, it is important to understand both the general principles related to exercise programming and the actual approach to CR conditioning in order to safely meet the goals of the individual.

GENERAL PRINCIPLES

In this section the following topics are discussed:

- Principles of exercise adaptation
- Medical clearance and supervision
- Types of fitness
- Goal setting
- Components of an exercise session

Principles of Exercise Adaptation

A basic assumption in exercise programming is that something useful or beneficial occurs as a result of repeated bouts of exercise. This assumption is predicated on a number of physiological principles. The most central of these is the **principle of adaptation,** which states that, if a specific physiological capacity is taxed by a physical training stimulus within a certain range and on a regular basis, this physiological capacity will usually expand. Adaptation also depends upon two correlated physiological principles, **threshold** and **overload.** To elicit an adaptation, the physiological capacity must be challenged beyond a certain minimal level called the training threshold. If training stimulus exceeds this threshold level, it is a training **overload** and the process of physiological adaptation usually occurs. As the physiological capacities of the body expand, the initial training stimulus may be rendered sub-threshold, and the workload must be increased (**progression**) to maintain overload. The concept of progression also encompasses the practice of using very modest levels of work during the initial sessions of an exercise program. **Regression,** or deadaptation, refers to the transience of physiological enhancement from training that occurs when training ceases and the physiological capacities regress towards pretraining levels. **Retrogression,** on the other hand, refers to excessive taxing of physiological capacities, leading to their diminution. Retrogression can refer to either acute or chronic periods of excessive overload. That is, either a single bout or chronic bouts of excessive overload can cause retrogression. These principles are illustrated in Figure 52.1.

A final principle of central importance in exercise programming is the concept of **specificity.** Specific physiological capacities will expand only if they are stressed in the course of an exercise program. For example, it has been demonstrated that swimmers experience an 11% increase in swim ergometry performance over the course of a training season, but show no change in run time to exhaustion on a treadmill (3). Each of the above principles guides the design of an exercise program.

Medical Clearance and Supervision

Exercise training may not be appropriate for everyone. Patients whose adaptive reserves are severely limited by

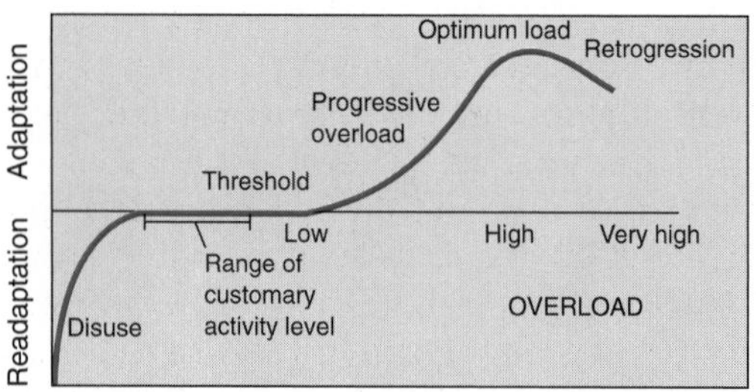

Figure 52.1. Illustration of the adaptive effects of decreased (disuse) and increased (overload) levels of physical activity relative to usual activity levels. See text for explanation of terms. (With permission from Adams WC. *Foundations of Physical Education, Exercise, and Sport Sciences.* Philadelphia: Lea & Febiger, 1991.)

pathologic processes may be unable to adapt to, or benefit from, exercise. In this small subpopulation of people with severe or unstable cardiac, respiratory, metabolic/systemic, or musculoskeletal disease, exercise programming may be fatal, injurious, or simply not beneficial, depending upon the clinical status and condition of the individual. The *ACSM Guidelines for Exercise Testing and Prescription* lists contraindications to both exercise training and testing (4). Medical clearance to exclude the presence of these conditions prior to beginning an exercise program is, thus, warranted for those with known disease or suggestive symptoms.

For individuals without known contraindications to exercise training, different levels of screening and supervision are appropriate relative to health and fitness status, goals, and personal preferences. These topics are covered in detail in the *ACSM Guidelines* and will only be discussed briefly here (4). The recommended level of screening prior to beginning or increasing an exercise program depends on the risk of the individual and the intensity of the planned physical activity (4). For individuals planning to engage in low to moderate intensity activities, the Physical Activities Readiness Questionnaire (PAR-Q) should be considered the minimal level of screening (5). A "yes" answer to any question indicates physician referral prior to beginning or increasing physical activity. The PAR-Q can be found in the *ACSM Guidelines* along with specific recommendations for screening.

Supervised exercise programs are recommended for those with low functional capacity (<8 METs) or poor health status. Beyond health and functional status, whether a person exercises under supervision depends primarily on goals and personal preference.

Types of Fitness

For the majority of individuals, the question is not whether, or in what setting will they benefit from exercise, but rather which of the benefits are desired outcomes. The principle of specificity implies that "fitness" is a diverse and varied group of related adaptations that may be differentially developed. Physical fitness has been defined as a set of attributes that people have or achieve that relates to the ability to perform physical activity (1). Those components of physical fitness that lead to increased vigor in daily life and help protect against degenerative diseases associated with physical inactivity are called the health-related aspects of fitness (4), namely, CR endurance, muscular strength and endurance, flexibility, and body composition.

CR or aerobic fitness is often refers to the constellation of improvements that enhance $\dot{V}O_2$max and/or aerobic work capacity. Clearly, CR conditioning is the primary focus of exercise programming for endurance athletes. CR conditioning is also a primary goal in cardiac rehabilitation programs since such training can enhance peripheral oxygen delivery, and, thus, help compensate for an impaired myocardium (6). Finally, this type of conditioning is also most strongly associated with health benefits in the general population (2, 4, 6–8).

Goal Setting

One of the first considerations in designing an exercise program is to prioritize the expected outcomes. Goal setting is, thus, an essential preliminary step in a successful program. The goals of an exercise program provide a focus for creating the detailed structure of the program. In general, goals should be set that realistically attempt to meet the medical, emotional, and functional needs of the exerciser within the context of limitations of time, interest and physical ability.

The first step in the goal setting process is to clarify stated goals or objectives. Occasionally, the stated goal reflects incomplete knowledge or unrealistic expectations about the effects of exercise training ("*I want to get off kidney dialysis using exercise*" or "*I want to lose 50 pounds without restricting my eating habits*"). In such cases, further education about the effects of training combined with clarification of priorities and values should result in more practical goal. There may be conflicts between the emotional and medical or functional needs ("*I want to run a 400 meter dash to show that I'm over my heart attack*"). Although the actual activities proposed may be unattainable or contraindicated, the exercise professional must recognize, respect, and attempt to address the emotional realities of the situation. Once the objectives have been clarified, the next step is to inventory resources for meeting these goals. If medical or physical limitations exist, these may define the scope of activities in the exercise program. Exploring past successes or failures with physical activity is often useful for identifying specific modes of exercise that may be enjoyable. Personal preferences for group or individual exercise should be considered. The location and cost of facilities or equipment needed for various modes of exercise should also be evaluated for convenience and affordability. Finally, a realistic appraisal of the time available for an exercise program can be made through examination of a personal calendar or date book.

Before a new exercise program is implemented, a means of evaluating effectiveness in meeting established goals should be considered. If the primary goal is "to feel better," evaluation may be as simple as assessing perception of well-being after 1 to 2 months of regular exercise. In many cases, especially where more concrete performance or physiological goals are stated, goal specific assessment is valuable. For most exercise programs, subjective evaluations or simple pre/post physiological evaluation of the goals is sufficient.

Record keeping is a powerful tool for meeting exercise goals and should be used in the implementation of a new exercise program. Most programs for health maintenance or recreation do not require this degree of vigilance for success; however, record keeping may be invaluable in programs for patients with major medical problems that may cause restriction of activity, individuals who are restarting exercise after many years of inactivity, exercisers for whom weight management is a major goal of their program, and performance oriented athletes.

To be useful, a record of physical activity should include day, date, time of day, type of exercise, an estimate of the external work or work rate (e.g., miles, watts, METs, etc.) and the physiological response (heart rate or rate of perceived exertion [RPE]). Symptoms or problems, such as specific, physical complaints ("left knee sore again"), or generalized symptoms ("couldn't catch breath for first 10 min") should be recorded. A carefully kept exercise record can provide early warning of impending overuse injuries and overtraining as well as powerful feedback about improvement or patterns of avoidance. In addition, the vagaries of human impulse and appetite are such that any person attempting to include dietary portion control or caloric restriction as a goal is likely to benefit from keeping a record, by kilocalories, weight, or volume, of all food consumed.

In summary, exercise programming is a purposeful activity. Identifying the goals of each participant clarifies and directs the development of a specific activity plan that addresses these goals while acknowledging the limitations of the exerciser. Evaluation of the effects and outcomes is part of this process. Certain groups may benefit further from keeping a record of their exercise (and dietary) activities.

Components of an Exercise Session

There are three basic components to any exercise conditioning session: warm-up, conditioning stimulus, and cool-down. An appropriate warm-up can improve sports performance and decrease risk of ischemic and dysrhythmic events (9, 10). Cool-down has these benefits as well as helping to clear metabolic waste from skeletal muscle. Warm-up and cool-down represent periods of metabolic and CR adjustment from rest to exercise and exercise to rest, respectively. Thus, the most appropriate types of warm-up and cool-down are activities similar to the conditioning stimulus activities, performed at approximately 50% of the stimulus intensity (9). Older individuals and those with or at increased risk of ischemic heart disease benefit from longer periods of warm-up and cool-down that may further decrease their risk of ischemic or dysrhythmic events (10). Warm-up and cool-down may take between 5–15 minutes depending upon the age and risk of the individual and time allotted for flexibility exercises. Stretching activities to increase flexibility are appropriate at these times, but should not substitute for those that alter metabolism. The conditioning stimulus may contain a period of aerobic conditioning, muscle conditioning or both. It may be as short as 20 minutes or in excess of 1 hour, depending upon the exercises selected (4, 7).

CARDIORESPIRATORY CONDITIONING

In this section the following topics are discussed:

- Benefits of CR activities and fitness
- Conditioning for health vs. fitness
- FITTE factors for increasing fitness
- Prescribing and determining exercise intensity
- Progression and maintenance
- Modifications for sport and activity-specific conditioning

Benefits of CR Activities and Fitness

The benefits of physical activity and fitness relative to health have been exhaustively reviewed and are summarized in Table 52.1 (2 ,4, 6, 11). Both CR conditioning and enhanced physical fitness decrease fatigue in daily activities, improve sports performance, and are associated with decreased all-cause, cardiovascular, and cancer mortality (12–15).

Conditioning for Health vs. Fitness

While there are unresolved issues concerning the appropriate dose of CR exercise necessary to achieve a specific response, in recent years it has become apparent that the level of physical activity necessary to achieve the majority of health benefits is less than that needed to attain a high level of CR fitness (Figure 52.2) (2, 8, 12–14, 16). For example, Blair and colleagues recently demonstrated that activity sufficient to cause only a small improvement in CR fitness may still have significant health benefits (14). Such research combined with the low physical activity level of the US population, has stimulated recommendations for levels of activity less

Table 52.1. Benefits of Increasing Cardiorespiratory Activities and/or Improved Cardiorespiratory Fitness

Decreased fatigue in daily activities
Improved work, recreational, and sports performance
Decreased risk of
Mortality from all causes
Coronary artery disease
Cancer (colon, breast)
Hypertension
Noninsulin dependent diabetes mellitus
Osteoporosis
Anxiety
Depression
Improved blood lipid profile
Improved immune function
Improved glucose tolerance and insulin sensitivity
Improved body composition
Enhanced sense of well-being
Decreased rate-pressure-product at a fixed workrate

N.B.: Many of the health benefits accrue due to physical activities which may have relatively little effect on increasing CR fitness (2).

than previously suggested for the general public (2, 8, 16). A recent joint statement from the Centers for Disease Control and Prevention (CDC) and the ACSM concludes that "every US adult should accumulate 30 minutes or more of moderate-intensity physical activity on most, preferably all, days of the week" (2). This recommendation differs from previous exercise recommendations by acknowledging the health benefits of more moderate intensity activities, by recognizing that benefits accrue from intermittent regular activity as well as regular continuous exercise, and by stressing the efficacy and safety of higher frequency activities when intensity is moderate and activities are non-impact. An example of activity meeting the CDC/ACSM criteria would be brisk walking over uneven ground at a 3–4 mph pace (3–6 METs), 3 times per day for 10–15 min each session, 5–7 days of the week. Using stairs instead of elevators is an additional means of engaging in intermittent moderate intensity exercise.

Reports of specific health benefits elicited by higher intensity exercise do not contradict the above recommendation (15). Thus, the CDC/ACSM recommendation complements, but does not replace previous recommendations which are based on the scientific evidence supporting the type of exercise needed to improve CR fitness (7). As suggested in Figure 52.2, the health benefits of physical activity/exercise exist along a continuum of intensity. Higher levels of exertion are likely to have specific health benefits (16).

FITTE Factors for Increasing CR Fitness

Exercise programming for fitness emphasizes focused training periods of at least 20–30 minutes duration, higher levels of exercise intensity, and, for those pursuing goals in specific activities or sports, a commitment to the principle of specificity. As such, the previous ACSM Position Stand remains a useful and accurate document for those goals that are focused on achieving a higher level of CR fitness (7).

The total training stimulus provided by an exercise program can be quantified by frequency (usually days per week), intensity, time (duration), and type of exercise. Coupled with the non-quantitative but crucial adherence factor of enjoyment, these factors form the acronym, FITTE. The minimum levels of the FITTE factors recommended by ACSM to achieve an increase in CR fitness are (4, 7):

- Frequency: 3–5 days/week
- Intensity: 50–85% of maximal oxygen consumption (VO_2max) (or 60–90% of maximal heart rate)
- Time: 20–60+ minutes/session, continuous activity
- Type: Aerobic (run, brisk walk, bike, swim, cross-country ski, dance)
- Enjoyment: Enjoyable aerobic activities

A major part of the art of exercise programming is to create a program that "fits" the unique needs of the individual and the performance demands of the specific sport or activity. A major part of this individualization is accomplished through differential emphasis of the interrelated FITTE factors. Different programs seeking to improve CR fitness begin at the lower end of the ranges listed above for each of the quantifiable FITTE factors and diverge as they focus more precisely on goals and functional demands of the selected activities. For example, an exercise program for health benefits is focused on frequent and enjoyable activity with broad latitude in the levels of exercise intensity, duration, and type (F i t t E).

Generally, there is an inverse relationship between the intensity and duration in a single session; that is, as intensity increases duration decreases or vice versa. It is for this reason that larger caloric expenditures can be prac-

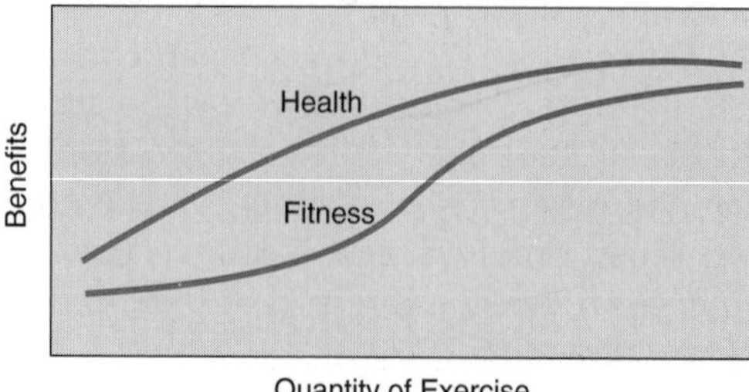

Figure 52.2. Theoretical representation of the relationship between the quantity of exercise and expected health and fitness benefits. Note that a level of exercise that has little effect on increasing fitness, may yield substantial health benefits. (With permission from William L. Haskell.)

tically achieved in exercise sessions of low to moderate intensity and longer duration. The total volume of work is described by frequency, intensity and time and may be expressed in kilocalories per week. Thus, for weight management programs, frequent enjoyable exercise periods of low to moderate intensity and longer duration ("F i T t E") will result in the largest weekly caloric expenditures. Finally, the athlete in competition seeks to perform an event at the highest possible intensity. Thus, for the athlete, it is intensity and type of activity which are most emphasized ("f I t T e"). The remainder of this chapter further details how the FITTE factors are tailored to the individual needs of those involved in specific activities.

Prescribing and Determining Exercise Intensity

Health benefits and caloric expenditure accrue even at low levels of intensity, therefore precise specification of intensity may not be necessary for an effective exercise program. If the goal is simply recreation or health, an adequate description of intensity might be "hard enough to increase breathing, but not hard enough to make you breathless or exhausted." The limitations of being rigidly quantitative with a cookbook approach to the prescription of intensity can be a recipe for disaster. Without proper application of knowledge of the principles of training and careful personal observation, no specific prescription of intensity is likely to result in optimal training.

The groups most likely to benefit from a precise determination of exercise intensity are, paradoxically, patients and athletes (17). Cardiac, pulmonary, or other patients with chronic disease who develop signs of exertional intolerance such as ischemia or hypoxemia at specific physiological workloads need a reasonably exact determination of intensity. This topic is discussed in the *ACSM Guidelines* (4). Endurance athletes, however, attempt to maintain a maximal overload stimulus without crossing over into retrogression. Answering two questions can help determine the optimal range of training intensity for the development of CR fitness:

1. What is the optimal range of training intensities for a particular individual?
2. How can this range of intensities best be determined in the course of training?

The threshold level for training intensity to initiate an adaptation in CR fitness is approximately 50% of $\dot{V}O_2max$, or 60% of maximal heart rate (7). Lower fit individuals may achieve significant training effects at intensities as low as 40% of $\dot{V}O_2max$, while those at higher levels of aerobic fitness may require intensities greater than 60% of $\dot{V}O_2max$. Training intensities above 50% of $\dot{V}O_2max$ generally facilitate greater improvement in aerobic capacity; whereas, training above the onset of blood lactate accumulation (OBLA) results in smaller gains, as well as increased risk of cardiovascular events, orthopedic injury, and lower compliance (7). For this reason, ACSM recommends programs emphasizing low to moderate intensity for most adults, with an upper limit of 85% of $\dot{V}O_2max$ (4, 7). Competitive athletes may require intensities above these levels to attain performance goals.

Therefore, the ideal intensity for an individual may range from 40% to 85% of $\dot{V}O_2max$. This range may even be applied in a single training session in some cases. For example, sports such as soccer and lacrosse feature a pattern of continuous, moderate aerobic activity punctuated by frequent surges of intensity up to and beyond $\dot{V}O_2max$. For these athletes, the optimal range of training intensities should include the range and pattern of intensity demands encountered in competition.

Intensity during training can be determined in a number of distinct and complementary ways. The goal is to guide efforts so that work occurs within the range most conducive to developing CR endurance (50–85% of $\dot{V}O_2max$). Quantitative laboratory measurements such as $\dot{V}O_2max$ or serum lactate level can precisely describe certain levels of intensity, but usually are connected to more readily available field measures of intensity, such as heart rate or RPE. The quantification of external work rate (such as speed of running or watts in cycle ergometry) complements the more usual measurements of the physiological response such as heart rate, lactate level or RPE. Comparing such markers of internal and external work intensity can provide unique and valuable information and both should be included in a system for monitoring progress. A decline in physiological response (e.g., heart rate) to a fixed rate of external work (160 watts of cycle ergometry) suggests a classic training effect. If, however, physiological responses become elevated at a fixed external work rate, this suggests retrogression (overtraining), incipient illness, environmental stress, or some other diversion of the physiological resources (18–21).

While laboratory methods may be used to precisely identify $\dot{V}O_2max$ or the OBLA, these are not necessary for successful intensity prescription and ultimately must be referenced back to techniques which can be employed by athletes during training. The most common means of determining exercise intensity in the field are based on either training heart rate range or non-heart rate methods of assessing intensity. Non-heart rate methods are most appropriate for the recreational exerciser, those working at low intensity to accumulate calories, exercisers without major medical problems, or the experienced exerciser with a well developed internal sense of work intensity. One such method is to estimate intensity of physical activity by using metabolic calculations or tables listing the metabolic cost of various activities at different levels of intensity (4, 22). A second method quantifies internal perception of intensity using a scale such as the Borg RPE scale (23). Activities eliciting perceived work intensities of 12–16, corresponding approximately to perceptions of light through hard, correlate well with intensities of 50–80% of $\dot{V}O_2max$. Perceptions of work as light (RPE of 11–12) are appropriate as initial exercise intensities for unconditioned subjects.

A final non-heart rate method of estimating work intensity is the "so-called" talk test. Exercising at or above OBLA and ventilatory threshold generally does not allow complete conversational sentences without pausing for breath. Thus, inability to complete simple sentences is a semi-quantitative test of ceiling intensity used by many apparently healthy adults in recreational programs. The use of these methods is further enhanced by combining them with determinations of intensity based on heart rate.

Heart rate is a useful means of prescribing exercise intensity since it increases linearly with oxygen consumption and intensity, is easily assessed, and can be cross-referenced with other objective and subjective indices of intensity. Heart rate methods are particularly useful for beginning exercisers, those with intensity-related medical problems such as angina, and competitive athletes. There are two basic techniques used to establish a training heart rate range. The first is to connect a specific heart rate with some other intensity-related marker, such as a measured oxygen consumption at 75% $\dot{V}O_2max$, an RPE of 12, or the onset of clinical events. In cardiac patients, it is common to identify the heart rate at which signs or symptoms of exertional intolerance (such as angina or ST depression) occur and use a training heart rate that is at least 10 beats per minute lower, depending on the setting in which the patient exercises and the severity of work intolerance. A second technique is to assign a range of training heart rates based on a percentage of the maximal heart rate. These methods are described in detail in the *ACSM Guidelines* (4).

In general, the recommended range for training intensity of 50–85% of $\dot{V}O_2max$ corresponds to 60–90% of the maximal heart rate (HR_{max}). It is important to note that HR_{max} estimated from equations such as 220–Age has a standard deviation of ±10–12 beats per minute (4). Therefore a predicted HR_{max} of 180 beats per minute, may actually be between 168 and 192 beats per minute. This emphasizes the importance of actually measuring HR_{max} (if safe and appropriate) whenever a precise estimate of intensity is required. HR_{max} can also be measured (in young, healthy individuals) by determining the pulse immediately after field tests such as 12 minute or 1.5 mile runs, if these are performed with true maximum effort.

During exercise, heart rate is usually quantified by counting a radial or carotid pulse. Assessing the carotid pulse requires gentle pressure at or below the level of the laryngeal cartilage to avoid disturbing carotid baroreceptors and potential atherosclerotic lesions which frequently occur at the carotid bifurcation beneath the angle of the mandible. Simultaneous palpation of carotid arteries bilaterally should be avoided. During cardiac emergencies, assessment of the pulse at the carotid is preferable to peripheral pulses because of concerns regarding cerebral perfusion.

Counting a Pulse Rate

To obtain a pulse rate, the following can be done:

1. Locate a pulse with the index and long fingers of one hand.
2. Count the number of pulsations in a given period of time.
3. For the highest precision, if timing is initiated simultaneously with a pulsation, this first pulsation is counted as "zero." If a second person is keeping time, or if there is lag between the initiation of timing and the first pulsation that is felt, the first pulse is counted as "one."
4. To determine the pulse rate multiply the number of pulse beats by the number of counting intervals in 1 minute.

   10 seconds = 6 intervals (multiply number of pulse beats by 6)
   15 seconds = 4 intervals
   20 seconds = 3 intervals
   30 seconds = 2 intervals

   [Note that the margin of error may be one pulse count within the counting interval which can lead to substantial errors in heart rate (in beats per minute) when short counting intervals are used. Longer pulse counts afford greater accuracy and provide more time for detection of some dysrhythmias.]

Locally telemetered heart rate monitors (heart watches) are commonly available and can be a useful aid in training, particularly for athletes or others desiring frequent, immediate feedback regarding exercise heart rate. It is important to note that the only advantages such monitors have over manual pulse counts are the ability to assess heart rate without interrupting exercise and the capacity for data storage. These devices do not perform any of the functions of a medical electrocardiographic monitor. Manual pulse counts have the advantages of detecting some forms of dysrhythmia and being constantly available to any person who carries a timepiece. Thus, it may be preferable to continue to use manual pulse counts in clinical or older populations.

It is important to recognize that the prescription of exercise intensity via heart rate is not rigidly quantitative. Exercise heart rate may be influenced by a number of factors other than work intensity and the presence of such factors may uncouple the connection between a given intensity-related event (such as the OBLA or a 5-minute/mile pace) and a specific heart rate. These factors include environmental conditions that influence heat dissipation (such as temperature, airflow, and humidity), the degree of rest or overtraining of the athlete, altitude, illness, and the timing and amount of specific cardiovascular medications. It is especially important to note environmental effects which impair the dissipation of heat. At the same absolute level of work intensity, heart rates may be 10–20 beats per minute higher during exercise in hot environments or in the absence of airflow (18–21).

Considering the above, it is apparent that cookbook approaches to prescribing exercise intensity are inappropriate. In three 40 year old individuals, using the equation 220 − Age to predict HR_{max} and a 75% training HR level, will result in a training heart rate of 135 beats per minute which may be detrimental to an individual with coronary disease, too low for a fit individual who is an experience exerciser or too high for an individual on medication which may inhibit increases in heart rate. A flexible and thoughtful approach to assessing and assigning exercise intensity will provide the most likely recipe for success.

Selecting Appropriate Modes of Exercise

It is also important that the mode of exercise be appropriate to individual goals and limitations. The apparently healthy adult seeking recreation or health benefits from exercise may engage in a wide range of physical activities, their choices guided by personal preferences which may change. For the athlete or competitive recreational exerciser, the mode of training will usually be tightly connected to the performance activity.

An important distinction among modes of training for those who are obese or have musculoskeletal problems is the distinction between high and low impact activities. Activities such as cycling, swimming, water aerobics, rowing, and low impact aerobics avoid the impact of body mass against the ground and may be better tolerated by those who are overweight or have orthopedic limitations. Some activities, which are technically low impact, such as cross country skiing or rollerblading, have a high fall potential and, thus, may not be appropriate for those with orthopedic problems. They may, however, be useful for younger athletes recovering from impact-related overuse injuries. It is particularly important among the FITTE factors that the type(s) of exercise selected be suitable and enjoyable to the participant.

Progression and Maintenance

The FITTE factors require change over the course of an exercise program to match progress. Just as an exercise session progresses through a warm-up stage to the conditioning stimulus, over a broader scale of weeks and months, a training program progresses through several discrete stages. Most training programs will feature three stages: initiation, improvement, and maintenance.

Initiation Stage

The initial stage of training allows time to begin the adaptive process. Typically, this is accomplished with lower intensity and shorter duration work and careful attention to signs of intolerance (particularly musculoskeletal or cardiopulmonary). The initial stage is the time to develop the habituation. A relatively high frequency of exercise (from 3 alternate days per week, up to 5–6 sessions/week) may assist this process, as long as other FITTE factors are maintained at low levels.

Suitable initial intensities may be from 40% of $\dot{V}O_2max$ (RPE of 11–12) to over 50% of $\dot{V}O_2max$ for individuals with higher aerobic capacities or experienced exercisers returning from time off from regular exercise. Appropriate initial levels of duration range from 12–15 to 40 minutes per session. Older, obese, or profoundly sedentary individuals may start with as little as 12–15 minutes (or less) of continuous exercise. In such situations, especially if the factor limiting duration is stable angina or claudication, intermittent exercise or multiple daily sessions may be helpful. If intensity is kept at a low to moderate level, sedentary, but otherwise healthy adults may be able to start with sessions of 20 minutes and experienced exercisers or high fitness athletes may begin with 30–40 minutes.

The exercise session, itself, may be modified during the initial stage of training by expanding the warm up period, using it to inventory potential signs of failure to adapt ("Let's stretch out our quadriceps now; is anyone sore here?"), providing information, and answering questions. The initial stage of training generally lasts 3–6 weeks, but may be expanded for those requiring additional time to adapt. The ability to conduct an exercise session independently and as prescribed at the upper levels of frequency (5–6 sessions/week) and duration (30–40 minutes) for 2 weeks without signs of excess fatigue or musculoskeletal overuse indicates that an individual is ready to progress.

Improvement Stage

In the improvement stage, expanding physiological capacities are further challenged. This stage is typified by the phrase "progressive overload." Small increments in the FITTE factors, particularly intensity and duration, may occur nearly every week. In fact, the challenge of the improvement stage is to appropriately increment training at a rate that continues to stimulate further advancement without causing overtraining and retrogression.

Several benchmarks of progression are discussed below, but self-observation of subjective and objective responses to training may be the most important. Failure to complete an exercise session, lack of normal interest in training, increased levels of heart rate or RPE at the same rate of external work, and an increase in minor aches and pains are all signs that progression may be too rapid (20). In an appropriately incremented improvement stage, interest and appetite for exercise will normally increase in tandem with the subjective and objective impressions that progress is being made. In general, frequency, intensity, and duration should not be incremented together in any single week, nor should total weekly training volume be advanced by more than 10% (17). Increasing duration by 5–10 minutes per session on a weekly basis is usually well tolerated, while incrementing intensity gradually through the range of 60–85% of aerobic capacity over a period of months is also tolerated. In a single session, progression of both intensity and duration not recommended; a single session of shorter-than-usual duration with higher levels of intensity may be well-tolerated.

In this stage, adjusting the training program is commonly accomplished by increasing one FITTE factor over another in a saltatory approach toward individual goals. Competitive athletes who train intensely and those encountering musculoskeletal or other physical obstacles impeding progress may benefit from the early incorporation of techniques such as cross training, which are more typical of the maintenance stage.

The adaptive potential of physiological function is finite and large increments in fitness, typical in the improvement stage, always taper at some point. Aerobic capacity can be expected to expand by approximately 5–30% in the course of a program following ACSM guidelines, while improvements of >30% rarely occur unless accompanied by a large reduction in body weight and fat (4). If training is discontinued, gains in fitness will regress by approximately 50% within 4–12 weeks (7). In general, after approximately 6 months of training, almost everyone will make the transition from improvement to maintenance.

The Maintenance Stage

The maintenance stage is typified by diversification of the training program and purposeful attempts to rotate and reduce the stresses of continued training. Diversification may take the form of using several modes of exercise to maintain enjoyment and explore new capabilities. This may be particularly important to life long programs with goals such as weight management or general health. For those with a goal of general health, frequency and duration may be reduced (up to a 50% combined reduction) without loss of functional gains if intensity is maintained (7). However, if other physical activity is not substituted, many of the health benefits of exercise which depend upon regular repetition may be lost (2). Therefore, reduced training frequency should be complemented by the addition of a variety of physical activities.

For those using the maintenance phase as a sustained period of performance or competition, diversification may be used as a means of reducing the potential for overuse injuries, particularly in programs with high training volumes or for participants with musculoskeletal limitations. Cross training, as this approach is often called, refers to using a variety of modes of CR endurance exercise (such as swimming, running, and biking) to maintain a high level of training stimulus for central aerobic adaptations such as enhanced stroke volume and expanded blood volume. This approach allows rotation of local fatigue and musculoskeletal stresses across a range of different muscle groups.

Cognitively, the maintenance stage is a time for enjoyment, surveillance, and reappraisal. It is a time for enjoying the fruits of labor by competing, engaging in new activities, or reducing the demands of weekly training. Surveillance for overuse injury must continue during the maintenance phase. Equipment and footwear should be re-evaluated. Finally, the goals of the program may be re-examined, physiological or performance testing repeated and new goals established. To advance performance and CR endurance further often requires special techniques such as periodization and isolation of performance demands.

Modifications for Sport and Activity-Specific Conditioning

Devising specific exercise programs for athletes to reach peak personal performance comprises the profession of coaching which exceeds the scope of this chapter. Some general principles will be discussed, however, with emphasis on modifying the components of a single training session to the demands of a particular sport or activity.

The three components of a CR conditioning session are the warm-up, the aerobic stimulus, and the cool down. In exercise programs specifically tailored to the goals and limitations of the individual, each component of the exercise session can be modified depending on the activity.

The warm-up should attempt to provide a transition from resting state to the exercise stimulus. Specifically, it is an opportunity to identify signs or symptoms of overuse, prepare specific muscle groups, and allow the CR system to adjust and prepare for higher intensity work. The most basic way in which the warm-up can be modified for specific activities is to use the specific muscle groups that are involved in the activity. The musculoskeletal segments should be moved through a similar range of motion as is used in the stimulus activity both to prepare the muscles and joints for exercise and to detect any residual soreness or other signs of injury or overuse. The intensity of the warm-up should gradually be increased over a 5 to 15 minute duration to about 50% of the intensity of the aerobic activity to follow. Before simple, repetitive activities such as running or cycling, the warm-up uses the same activity as the training stimulus, but at a lower rate. In this type of training session, stretching may be deferred until cool down. Before competitive events, warm-up should be expanded to include static stretching of muscle groups about to be used (after some light activity), followed by performance of the activity (at moderate intensity) prior to the start of the event.

Most sporting activities require sudden changes in intensity and rapid, powerful movements of multiple muscle groups and limbs over a wide range of motion, thus warm-up is especially important. In most cases, after some light activity, muscles that are used in the performance should be gently stretched before progressing to more intense simulations of the sport.

For racquet sports such as tennis, squash or racquetball, an adequate pre-competition warm-up takes about 15–30 minutes and includes range of motion and transitional metabolic activity for both the arms and the legs. Warm-up generally starts with gentle jogging around the court for at least 2 minutes, followed by several minutes of gentle, progressive static stretching of the major muscles of the arm and back (triceps, deltoid, pectorals, and latissimus dorsi) as well as each of the major muscles of the leg (with special attention to the gluteals and adductors which can be easily strained when stretching for a pass or volley). After stretching, shadow tennis, performed by moving through ground and overhead strokes without a ball, is followed by noncompetitive rallying. Hitting generally progress from soft ground strokes from the service line back to the base line, and then to overheads, lobs, and volleys.

Warming up for soccer may take a similar time period, but is more focused on preparing legs for ball handling and repetitive sprints. A typical pre-game warm-up starts with several minutes of light jogging around the field. Once warm and loose, gentle static stretching of all the major muscle groups of the legs with special attention to the quadriceps, hamstrings and adductors of the thigh is appropriate. Next, light work such as ball juggling, gentle dribbling in the center circle, or passing with a teammate may be followed by several wind sprints (with or without the ball) of 20 to 40 yards, increasing in speed and intensity.

It is the aerobic stimulus component of the exercise session that is most dramatically altered to match the patterns demanded by the sport or the limitations of the participant. Even in an individual sport such as running, the aerobic stimulus phase may range from a 3 hour continuous run at 55–60% $\dot{V}O_2$max for long distance runners, to a series of six 800 m intervals at >95% of $\dot{V}O_2$max completed in <25 minutes for a 3 kilometer runner.

In general, there are three basic patterns of aerobic stimulus activities: continuous, interval and circuit (24). Continuous exercise is probably the most common form of aerobic stimulus. It is best suited for those who perform a sustained, nearly single load work during the course of a sporting activity. Walking, hiking, distance running, and cycling are all activities where most exercise sessions are devoted to a continuous training stimulus. Some sustained sporting activities, such as cross country running, feature changes in work rate due to terrain or competitive tactics. Continuous training for these sports is sometimes modified to include such fluxes in intensity. Fartlek (from Swedish for "speed play"), where segments of a continuous run are completed at different speeds, is one example.

In interval training, intense bouts of short duration exercise are alternated with relief periods. Interval training is classically used by intermediate and middle distance runners as a means of providing a training stimulus to both the aerobic and anaerobic energy systems. It can also be used less formally by longer distance athletes wishing to improve a sustainable pace. For example, if a recreational half marathon runner desired to increase pace from 9:00 minute/mile to 8:45 minute/mile, one-half mile intervals at a 4:20 pace, with a half mile of jogging for recovery, repeated for 3–4 total miles may be an appropriate training session. After several weeks of this interval training once or twice a week, an 8:45 pace may be sustainable for a continuous run.

Circuit training refers to a similar pattern of intense work bouts alternated with relief periods; however, the work bout features a variety of work tasks. Circuit training is particularly appropriate for surge and recover sports that feature an array of physical qualities, such as soccer or basketball. An example of a circuit program might be a six station circuit, where each station is performed for 2:00 minutes interspersed with a 45 second recovery phase to move to the next station. A sample circuit session for basketball may involve six stations:

1. A set of short (<15 yard) line drills
2. As many jump shots as 2 minutes allows from a 16 foot perimeter
3. A series of plyometric rebounding tasks
4. A recovery station of free throws
5. A series of full court runs
6. Repetitive leaping to touch the backboard or rim

Circuit training is particularly appropriate for physically active occupations, such as fire fighting, where the job is often a linked series of specific, intense tasks (25). The degree of improvement in aerobic capacity using circuit training alone is modest (~8%), although work capacity in the specific activities may be increased to a greater degree. Therefore, in highly aerobic pursuits or programs intended to raise $\dot{V}O_2$max, circuit training is not recommended as the sole training stimulus (7).

The cool down need not be so specific as the warm-up or stimulus activity. The more intense and exhausting the event or conditioning session, the greater the requirement for gradual tapering of activity to avoid signs or symptoms upon transition to rest. After routine training, deep sustained stretching may be easier and more effective during the cool down. However, after injury or a maximal competitive event, rest, rehydration, and treatment of an injury usually takes precedence over deep stretching. Delayed onset muscle soreness appears to be related to muscle and connective tissue damage associated with eccentric contractions and does not seem to be prevented by stretching after the event (26).

Beyond modification of the components of a single exercise session, there are two additional important concepts in exercise programming for sports and activity. These are the concepts of isolation of specific physiological demands and periodization. Both techniques, like cross training, may be used to advance training beyond the maintenance phase into continued progression. Each however, has a different primary focus and range of application.

Isolation of specific physiological stress is done automatically by many experienced coaches. It is most appropriate in complex activities, such as sports that demand multiple physiological functions and involves "dissecting" the primary functional elements of the sport and providing more intense and focused training on each element in separate practice sessions. This isolation of distinct physiological stresses allows greater levels of overload for each element and also allows a rotation of specific stresses which may forestall overtraining and overuse injuries.

Periodization is an advanced training technique that divides the season or annual calendar into cycles or phases (27). These phases focus adaptive development so that peak performance is approached at the most advantageous time in the competitive schedule, while varying exercise mode, intensity and volume in order to diminish the possibility of overtraining (Figure 52.3).

Exercise programming for sport and specific activities is clearly based on the concept of fitting the details of training to the specific performance demands of the sport or activity. As such, it serves as a fitting closing example of a primary theme in this chapter: People become fit through programs that fit them. Designing CR training programs tailored to the goals, needs and limitations of each exerciser is a central skill of the exercise professional.

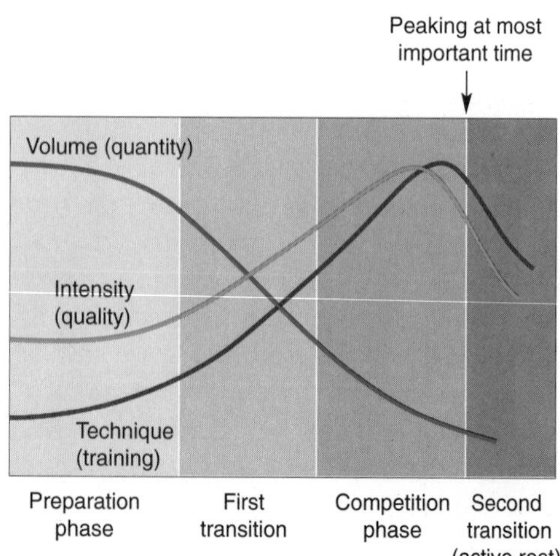

Figure 52.3. Interrelationships of volume intensity and technique for periodicity training.

References

1. Casperson CJ, Powell KE, Christenson GM. Physical activity, exercise and physical fitness: definitions and distinctions for health-related research. *Public Health Rep* 1985;100:126.
2. Pate RR, Pratt M, Blair SN, et al. Physical activity and public health. A recommendation from the Centers for Disease Control and Prevention and the American College of Sports Medicine. *JAMA* 1995;273:402.
3. Magel JR, Foglia GF, McArdle WD, et al. Specificity of swim training on maximum oxygen uptake. *J Appl Physiol* 1975;38:151.
4. American College of Sports Medicine. *ACSM Guidelines for Exercise Testing and Prescription for Exercise Testing and Prescription.* Baltimore: Williams & Wilkins, 1995.
5. Thomas S, Reading J, Shepard RJ. Revision of the Physical Activity Readiness Questionnaire (PAR-Q). *Can J Sport Sci* 1992;17:338.
6. Fletcher GF, Blair SN, Blumenthal J, et al. Statement on exercise: benefits and recommendations for physical activity programs for all Americans. A statement for health professionals by the committee on exercise and cardiac rehabilitation of the council on clinical cardiology, American Heart Association. *Circulation* 1992;86:340.
7. American College of Sports Medicine. The recommended quantity and quality of exercise for developing and maintaining CR and muscular fitness in healthy adults. *Med Sci Sports Exerc* 1990;22:265.
8. Harris SS, Caspersen CJ, DeFriese GH, et al. Physical activity counseling for healthy adults as a primary preventive intervention in the clinical setting. Report for the US Preventive Services Task Force. *JAMA* 1989;261:3590.
9. McArdle WD, Katch FI, Katch VL. *Exercise Physiology.* Philadelphia: Lea & Febiger, 1995.
10. MacAlpin RH, Kattus AA. Adaptation to exercise in angina pectoris. The electrocardiogram during treadmill walking and coronary angiographic findings. *Circulation* 1966;33:183.
11. Bouchard C, Shepard RJ, Stephens T, eds. *Physical Activity, Fitness, and Health.* Champaign, IL: Human Kinetics, 1994.
12. Powell KE, Thompson PD, Caspersen CJ, et al. Physical activity and the incidence of coronary heart disease. *Ann Rev Public Health* 1987;8:253.
13. Blair SN, Kohl HW, Paffenbarger RS, et al.: Physical fitness and all-cause mortality. A prospective study of healthy men and women. *JAMA* 1989;262:2395.
14. Blair SN, Kohl HW, Barlow CE, et al. Changes in physical fitness and all-cause mortality. A prospective study of healthy and unhealthy men. *JAMA* 1995;273:1093.
15. Lee IM, Hsieh CC, Paffenbarger, Jr. RS. Exercise intensity and longevity in men. The Harvard alumni study. *JAMA* 1995; 273:1179.
16. Haskell WH. Dose-response issues from a biological perspective. In: Bouchard C, Shepard RJ, Stephens T, eds. *Physical Activity, Fitness, and Health.* Champaign, IL: Human Kinetics, 1994.

17. Skinner JS. General principles of exercise prescription. In: Skinner JS, ed. *Exercise Testing and Exercise Prescription.* Philadelphia: Lea & Febiger, 1993.
18. Shaffrath JD, Adams WC. Effects of airflow and work load on cardiovascular drift and skin blood flow. *J Appl Physiol* 1984;56:1411.
19. Nadel ER, Cafarelli E, Roberts MF. Circulatory regulation during exercise in different ambient temperatures. *J Appl Physiol* 1979;46:430.
20. Lehmann M, Foster C, Keul J. Overtraining in endurance athletes: a brief review. *Med Sci Sports Exerc* 1993;25:854.
21. Rowell LB. *Human Circulation Regulation During Physical Stress.* New York: Oxford University Press, 1986.
22. Ainsworth BE, Haskell WL, Leon AS, et al. Compendium of physical activities. *Med Sci Sports Exerc* 1993;25:71.
23. Borg GA. Psychophysical bases of perceived exertion. *Med Sci Sports Exerc* 1982;14:377.
24. Fox E, Bowers R, Foss M. *The Physiological Basis for Exercise and Sport.* Madison: WC Brown & Benchmark, 1993.
25. Davis PO, Dotson CO, Santa Maria DL. Relationship between simulated fire fighting tasks and physical performance measures. *Med Sci Sport Exerc* 1982;14:65.
26. High DM, Howley ET. The effects of static stretching and warm-up on prevention of delayed-onset muscle soreness. *Res Q* 1989;60:357.
27. Roundtable. Periodization. *NSCA J* 1987;9:18.

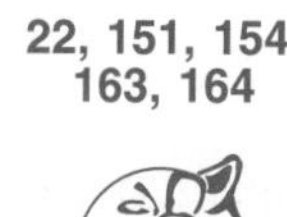
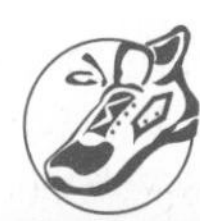
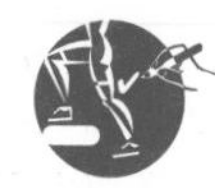

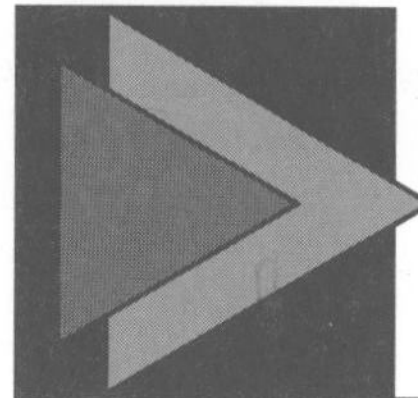

22, 151, 154, 163, 164 | 37, 39, 47, 48, 179, 184, 188 | 431, 432

CHAPTER 53
MUSCULAR STRENGTH AND ENDURANCE

Cedric X. Bryant, James A. Peterson, and James E. Graves

Strength (resistance) training has become more popular over the past 15 years. Until recently, resistance training was primarily performed by selected groups of athletes and by individuals desiring to enhance physique. Resistance training has become an integral component of the exercise program for an array of individuals including those interested in fitness, competitive athletes, children, older adults, and cardiac rehabilitation patients (1–8, 12, 25, 26).

Much of the increased popularity of resistance training can be attributed to successful education efforts regarding the number of positive benefits associated with resistance training. Commonly cited reasons to engage in resistance training include:

- Prevent and/or rehabilitate an injury
- Control body weight
- Prevent and/or treat osteoporosis
- Enhance athletic performance
- Manage stress

Given the increasing body of knowledge concerning the benefits of resistance training, it is not surprising that several professional organizations and numerous members of both the exercise science and medical communities recommend that individuals of all ages and both genders participate in medically sound resistance training programs. This chapter addresses the basic principles and guidelines needed to develop safe and effective resistance training programs for healthy adults and certain special populations.

RESISTANCE TRAINING PROGRAM CONSIDERATIONS

Resistance training is considered an important component of a comprehensive fitness program. A proper resistance training program should be based on several factors, including health and fitness status, goals of the participant, proper application of the basic principles of training, and the training environment.

Health and Fitness Status

Prior to initiating resistance training, participants should take certain precautions. Minimally, a health/medical questionnaire should be completed. One of the most widely used health/medical questionnaires is the Physical Activity Readiness Questionnaire (PAR-Q) (25). The PAR-Q is a relatively simple, yet valid query form used for screening individuals prior to beginning an exercise program.

A muscular fitness evaluation should be considered prior to initiating resistance training. Such information may serve several purposes. For example, initial level of muscular fitness can effect the magnitude and rate of improvement from resistance training (9). Generally, muscularly fit individuals do not improve as much or as quickly as untrained individuals, which can be important when establishing goals or in evaluating the effectiveness of resistance training. It is important to note, however, that some may not be capable of tolerating muscular fitness testing.

Goals

Once pre-exercise screening and assessment is complete, it is important to develop realistic goals and objectives for the resistance training program. Unrealistic expectations can lead to adverse outcomes, including discouragement, poor adherence, and injury. To enhance the likelihood that resistance training is based on appropriate expectations, an understanding of the physiological adaptations is important. Table 53.1 summarizes the effects of resistance training on morphological, biochemical, neural, anthropometric, and performance factors, (10). In addition, an extensive discussion of the chronic adaptations to resistance training can be found in Chapter 19.

Basic Training Principles

Overload and specificity are fundamental precepts of resistance training. Both relate to the ability to adapt to

Table 53.1. The Effects of Resistance Training on Morphological, Biochemical, Neural, Body Compositional, and Performance Factors

	Effect		
	Increase	Decrease	No Change
Morphological Factors			
• size of Type II (fast-twitch) muscle fibers	X		
• number of muscle fibers			X
• relative amount of muscle fibers			X
• number and size of myofibrils			X
• amount of contractile proteins	X		
• size and strength of connective tissue elements (e.g., tendons, ligaments, fascia, etc.)	X		
• bone mass and bone density	X		
Biochemical Factors			
• CP and ATP concentration	X		
• mitochondrial density		X	
• myokinase activity	X		
Neural Factors			
• discharge frequency of motoneurons	X		
• motor unit recruitment	X		
• synchrony of recruitment	X		
• neural inhibitions		X	
• motor skill performance	X		
Body Compositional Factors			
• total body weight			X
• lean body weight	X		
• fat weight		X	
• percent body fat		X	
Performance Factors			
• speed, power, balance, agility, and flexibility	X		

stress. Adherence to these principles elicits both structural and functional adaptations and resistance training that does not incorporate them cannot provide consistent improvement in muscular fitness.

Overload is accomplished when a greater than normal physical demand is placed on muscles or muscle groups. The amount of overload required is dependent upon the current level of muscular fitness. For example, a football player requires a different level of overload than a sedentary person. To produce strength and endurance gains, the muscular system must be progressively overloaded. In the context of resistance training, overload can be achieved by:

- Increasing the resistance or weight
- Increasing the repetitions
- Increasing the sets
- Decreasing the rest period between sets or exercises

By definition, overloading is dynamic (changing). In other words, as a muscle or muscle group adapts, a progressive overload is required to continue improvement.

A training intensity of approximately 40–60% of one repetition maximum (1 RM) appears to be sufficient for the development of muscular strength in most normally active individuals. Intensities of 80–100%, however, have been shown to produce the most rapid gain in muscular strength (11). However, due to the possibility of overtraining or injury, caution must be used when overloading a muscle or muscle group.

Specificity relates to the nature of changes (structural and functional, systemic and local) that occur in an individual as a result of training. These adaptations are specific, and occur only in the overloaded muscle groups or muscles.

The concept of specificity has other applications when applied to resistance training. Sports require specific movement patterns, which a properly designed program should consider. Although a sound, resistance training program should include exercises for all of the major muscle groups, it can be modified to address the unique demands of a particular sport or activity (12, 13). The resistance training program for a pitcher, for example, should emphasize the rotator cuff, the shoulder girdle, and the upper extremities more than resistance training for a soccer player, which focuses on the lower extremities and includes exercises to develop strength and endurance for the gluteals, quadriceps, hamstrings, abductors, adductors, and gastrocnemius.

One of the most controversial issues regarding specificity has been the debate over how to develop muscular strength versus muscular endurance. Based on the available literature, different programs should be employed for development of muscular strength versus muscular endurance (10–12). Muscular strength is the ability to generate force at a given speed (velocity) of movement, while muscular endurance is the ability to persist in physical activity or resist muscular fatigue (4, 12). Generally, strength is developed with more resistance and fewer repetitions, while muscular endurance requires low-to-moderate resistance and more repetitions (10–12). Adaptations occur at both the cellular level (metabolic adaptation) and at the fiber level (selective hypertrophy and motor unit recruitment patterns). It is important to note that both strength and endurance are developed, to some extent, regardless of the resistance training prescription because both fitness components exist on a continuum. However, one component may be emphasized, depending upon the specific resistance program prescription.

Strength gains also are dependent on the mode of resistance training (static, dynamic, isokinetic), the type of contraction (concentric, eccentric), the speed of contraction, and the joint position (11, 12). The extent to which and how these factors should be incorporated into the design of a resistance training program remains an ongoing topic of discussion.

The Training Environment

A wide variety of training methods and equipment exists for improving muscular fitness. Methods of resistance training are typically classified according to the type of muscular contraction (static, dynamic, or isokinetic).

Types of Muscular Contractions

During static (isometric) contractions, the muscle or muscle group involved maintains a constant length as resistance is applied and no change in joint position occurs. Research has demonstrated that static training produces improvements in muscular strength. The strength gains, however, are limited to the specific joint angles at which the static contractions are performed (12, 14–16). As a result, static training may have limited value in enhancing functional strength. Static training has also been associated with acute elevations in blood pressure, perhaps due to increased intrathoracic pressure during the performance of static contractions. Despite the limitations, static training appears to play a positive role in physical rehabilitation. For example, it is effective at maintenance of muscular strength and prevention of atrophy associated with the immobilization of a limb (e.g., application of a cast, splint, brace, etc.) (11, 12, 15).

Dynamic (isotonic) resistance training is another common method. If movement of the joint occurs during contraction, it is dynamic. If force is sufficient to overcome resistance and shortening of the muscle occurs (e.g., the lifting phase of a biceps curl), the contraction is concentric. When resistance is greater than force and the muscle lengthens during contraction, it is eccentric (e.g., the lowering phase of the biceps curl).

Most dynamic resistance training includes both concentric and eccentric action. Significantly heavier loads can be moved eccentrically; in fact, in non-fatigued muscle, the ratio of eccentric to concentric strength can be as high as 1.4:1.0 (11, 12). Further, at the onset of fatigue, the relative level of eccentric strength and eccentric:concentric ratio increases even more. Individuals who are eccentrically trained experience levels of delayed-onset muscular soreness (17, 18). Eccentric training can, however, play an important role in preventing and/or rehabilitating certain musculoskeletal injuries. For example, eccentric training, because it can affect deceleration capacity, has been demonstrated to be efficacious for treating hamstring strains, tennis elbow, and patellofemoral pain syndrome (19, 20).

Dynamic exercise can be further categorized into constant resistance and variable resistance. During constant resistance exercise, resistance applied does not change throughout the range of motion. Since force-production can vary significantly at different points in the range of motion, the potential gains are limited by inherent weak points on the strength curve of working muscle. On the other hand, during variable resistance exercise leverage advantages and disadvantages are changed over the range of motion, resulting in potential gains that are, theoretically, not restricted by variations in the strength curve of a muscle.

The other major type of resistance training, isokinetic exercise, involves constant speed muscular contraction against accommodating resistance. The speed of movement is controlled and the amount of resistance is proportional to the amount of force produced throughout the full range of motion. The theoretical advantage of isokinetic exercise is the development of maximal muscle tension throughout the range of motion. Research documents the effectiveness of isokinetic training (12, 15). Strength gains achieved during high-speed of training (i.e., contraction velocities of 180 degrees per second or faster) appear to carry over to all speeds less than that specific speed (21, 22). Improvement in strength at slow speeds of movement, however, has not been shown to carry over to faster speeds.

Types of Resistance Training Equipment

A variety of equipment is available to accommodate different types of training and different resistance training goals. Almost any type of resistance equipment enables individuals to meet training goals provided it allows an overload and that appropriate exercise guidelines are followed. Individuals should select equipment that is accessible and is consistent with personal needs and interests. Table 53.2 compares three common types of equipment on selected criteria. More detailed discussions of resistance equipment can be found in Chapter 77, and elsewhere (2, 13).

GUIDELINES FOR DEVELOPING MUSCULAR FITNESS

Specific guidelines for achieving muscular fitness are not as universally accepted as those for aerobic fitness.

Table 53.2. Comparative Overview of Various Types of Resistance Training Equipment

	Free Weights (Barbells/ Dumbbells)	Multi-station Machines	Selectorized Machines
Cost	*Low*	*Somewhat high*	*High*
Functionality	Excellent	Limited	Limited
Learning curve	Limited	Excellent	Excellent
Muscle isolation	Variable	Excellent	Excellent
Rehabilitation	Excellent	Excellent	Excellent
Safety	Relatively safe	Very safe	Very safe
Space efficiency	Variable	Excellent	Variable
Time efficiency	Variable	Excellent	Excellent
Variety	Excellent	Limited	Limited
Versatility	Excellent	Limited	Limited

There is considerable controversy regarding the most appropriate prescription for developing muscular fitness. However, there is growing awareness that moderate intensity resistance training should be an integral part of a comprehensive fitness program.

As with any exercise prescription, instructions regarding intensity, duration, and frequency, as well as guidelines for rate of progression and precautions are important. This information should be based on health and fitness status and personal goals and interests.

Muscular fitness can be developed through either static (isometric) or dynamic (isotonic and isokinetic) exercises. Dynamic resistance is recommended for most adults who wish to engage in basic resistance training. Further, because the primary objective of resistance training should be to develop total body muscular fitness in a safe and time-efficient manner, individuals should be encouraged to perform 8–10 different exercises to condition major muscle groups.

Appropriate resistance training for healthy adults should be based on the following guidelines and principles:

- Use a brief warm-up prior to performing resistance exercise.
- Adhere to proper techniques for performing each exercise.
- Perform at least one set of 8–12 repetitions of each exercise to the point of volitional fatigue. No "magic formula" exists regarding the number of sets and repetitions that provide optimal gains in muscular fitness for all individuals.
- Increase the resistance when a predetermined number of repetitions (typically 8–12) can be completed using proper form. Increases in resistance should be made gradually (e.g., increments of approximately 5%).
- Exercise at least 2 days per week. Recovery time (i.e., rest) is an important component of muscular growth and strength development and most individuals require approximately 48 hours to recover from a typical resistance training session. When training at very low loads (i.e., in certain therapeutic settings), more frequent training sessions may be tolerated.
- Perform both the lifting (concentric phase) and lowering (eccentric phase) portions in a controlled manner. Performing ballistic-type movements during resistance training can compromise safety and effectiveness.
- Perform each exercise through a functional range of motion. This helps ensure that joint mobility is maintained and, in some instances, enhanced.
- Maintain a normal breathing pattern; breath-holding may induce excessive elevations in blood pressure due to performance of a Valsalva maneuver.
- When possible, exercise with a training partner who provides feedback, assistance, and encouragement.

An understanding of resistance training equipment and the most commonly used methods for developing strength (as well as advantages and limitations) is basic to effective modification of the prescription for resistance training for specific conditioning needs and interests. Such modification is necessary to maximize the benefits from resistance training and to avoid injury. Many standard resistance training programs are described and well-illustrated in other publications (2, 13).

RESISTANCE TRAINING FOR SPECIAL POPULATIONS

Resistance training is useful for many special populations. For example, though modification is necessary, children can safely resistance train and benefit from the positive effects (3). Resistance training has also been demonstrated to be beneficial for various age-related medical conditions or in certain types of cardiovascular disease (4, 11). Not surprisingly, no age or gender restrictions exist for resistance training. Research documents that women experience similar benefits from resistance training as men and, under normal circumstances, do not develop large musculature (13). Furthermore, resistance training can be safely incorporated into an exercise regimen for pregnant women. In fact, the improved level of muscular fitness attendant to sound resistance training may serve to decrease the severity and/or incidence of orthopedic discomfort (4, 13).

Children

Until recently, the prevailing attitude among much of the medical community was that children (i.e., pre-adolescents) should not engage in resistance training because of concerns related to a lack of physical maturity. Collectively, these concerns appear to have focused on three issues:

1. Whether resistance training places excess stress on the musculoskeletal systems of adolescents.
2. Whether resistance training provides demonstrable benefits for children.
3. How resistance training programs for children should be designed to maximize benefits and minimize risks.

At least three major organizations have developed position papers making formal recommendations regarding children and resistance training (1, 2, 23). Research has demonstrated that resistance training for children, when properly performed, can be productive and beneficial (i.e., benefits outweigh risks) (1–3, 23). Unfortunately, despite the benefits, resistance training for children is not without some risk. Of concern is the potential that inappropriate resistance training may damage a developing skeletal system and the supportive tissues (2, 3). Lifting excessively heavy weights may significantly increase risk of growth cartilage injury. However, growth cartilage injuries associated with properly designed and supervised resistance training are rare. The risk of injury in resistance training in children is quite low, provided a proper lifting technique is used and appropriate demands are placed on the child.

There are no minimum age standards for resistance training in children. Several factors should be considered before beginning resistance training in children including:

- Ability to accept and follow instructions
- Desire to participate
- Basic motor skills and ability to safely perform exercises

Resistance training may be more appropriate for some children than others, depending on the aforementioned factors. Once the decision has been made, however, all resistance training programs for children must adhere to certain basic guidelines and principles, including:

- All children have developing musculoskeletal systems
- Proper training technique for all resistance training exercises is required.
- All exercises should be performed in a controlled manner and fast, jerky ballistic movement must be avoided.
- Resistance must be matched to the needs and structural limitations. Excess resistance can damage developing skeletal and joint structures. Each set of an exercise should consist of 8–12 repetitions. Adolescents should not exercise to the point of volitional muscular fatigue.
- Overload initially by increasing the number of repetitions, subsequently by increasing the resistance.
- The array of exercises selected should include at least one for each major muscle group (e.g., gluteals, quadriceps, hamstrings, pectorals, latissimus dorsi, deltoids, erector spinae, and abdominals). Perform one or two sets of 8–10 different exercises.
- Perform two resistance training sessions per week, with at least one rest day between sessions. Lower training volume reduces stress and allows other forms of physical activity.
- Perform full range, multi-joint exercises (e.g., leg press, lat pulldown, etc.), as opposed to single-joint exercises (e.g., leg extension, biceps curl, etc.), because such exercises facilitate development of functional strength.
- Achieve muscular balance in each session by alternating pairs of muscle groups (i.e., perform a pull exercise for each push exercise; see Table 53.3).

Appropriately trained personnel capable of providing proper strength training instruction must closely supervise all resistance training.

Table 53.3. Example of Suggested Exercise Order

	PUSH	PULL
Legs	Leg press	Leg curl
Chest & back	Bench press	Seated row
Shoulder & back	Military press	Lat pulldown
Arms	Triceps extension	Biceps curl
Trunk	Back extension	Abdominal curl

Seniors

Impaired muscular function has been linked to impaired functional ability in older adults. Ability to rise from a seated position, mobility (e.g., ambulatory ability), and balance are common functional disabilities in older adults. The long-range implication of lack of strength is limited independence. Appropriate resistance training may enhance overall function and well-being in older adults.

Resistance training may assist in effective management of osteoarthritis (24). Shared stress, around affected joints, by surrounding muscles and unaffected joints, can improve functional ability. Stronger muscles absorb more of the attendant stress on a joint, thereby reducing stress placed on affected joint surfaces.

Evidence indicates that resistance training slows bone loss and can increase bone density (12, 25). Osteoporosis is characterized by decreased bone mineral content (decreased density) and may be improved by resistance training. Further, training-induced improvements in muscular strength and balance may help prevent falls that cause many fractures among elderly osteoporotic women.

Resistance preserves muscle tissue during aging and may contribute to effective weight control through maintaining increased metabolic rate. In addition, most daily activities require some muscular fitness. With appropriate resistance training, older adults are more likely to maintain appropriate levels of muscular fitness and improved daily function.

Regardless of which specific resistance training protocol is adopted, several common sense guidelines for resistance training in older adults should be followed:

- Design a resistance training program to develop sufficient muscular fitness to enhance ability to live a physically independent lifestyle.
- Closely supervise and monitor initial sessions with trained personnel who are sensitive to the special needs and capabilities of older adults.
- Use minimum levels of resistance during the first 8 weeks to allow for adaptation of connective tissue elements.
- Instruct and use proper technique for performing all exercises.

- Instruct all older participants to maintain normal breathing patterns while exercising. Avoid Valsalva maneuvers.
- Overload initially by increasing number of repetitions and, subsequently, by increasing resistance.
- Use a resistance that can be comfortably lifted for at least six repetitions per set. Heavy resistance is potentially dangerous and damaging to skeletal and joint structure.
- Weights should be lifted and lowered in a slow, controlled manner. No ballistic movements should be allowed (to prevent orthopedic trauma to joint structures).
- Perform all exercises in a pain free range of motion (i.e., the maximum range of motion that does not elicit pain or discomfort). As positive adaptations occur, individuals may be able to gradually increase range of motion to improve flexibility.
- Perform multi-joint exercises (as opposed to single-joint exercises) that tend to assist in development of functional muscular fitness.
- The use of machines offers several advantages including:

    1. They require less skill to use
    2. They generally provide more support for the back by stabilizing body position
    3. They enable participants to start with lower levels of resistance (depending on the specific type of equipment)
    4. They typically enable increased resistance level through smaller increments (not true for all resistance training machines)
    5. They allow greater control of the exercise range of motion
    6. They generally provide a more time-efficient workout

- Don't overtrain. Two resistance training sessions per week is the minimum number required to produce positive physiological adaptation. While more frequent training may elicit larger strength gains, additional improvement is relatively small.
- Resistance training must be avoided during periods of active pain or inflammation in older adults with arthritis; exercise during these periods may exacerbate the inflammation.

The resistance training program should be performed on a regular basis throughout the year. Research demonstrates that cessation of resistance training results in rapid, significant loss of strength (12). When re-starting after a layoff, resume training with resistance levels equivalent to, or less than 50%, of the intensity prior to discontinuing. As adaptation occurs, slowly and progressively increase resistance.

Cardiac Patients

Historically, cardiac rehabilitation programs have focused almost exclusively on improving cardiorespiratory fitness, despite muscular fitness requirements for all activities of daily living, especially occupational tasks. The reluctance to include resistance training has been due, in part, to a belief that heavy resistance exercise places a strain on, rather than provides a training stimulus for, the cardiovascular system. However, appropriately prescribed and supervised, regular progressive resistance exercise training may favorably affect muscle strength, cardiorespiratory endurance, hypertension, hyperlipidemia, glucose tolerance, insulin sensitivity, and psychosocial well-being (4, 6–8). Both the American College of Sports Medicine (ACSM) and the American Association of Cardiovascular and Pulmonary Rehabilitation (AACVPR) recommend resistance training as an integral part of a comprehensive exercise program for cardiac patients, particularly the following types of individuals:

- Individuals whose occupations require extensive arm work (e.g., laborers, construction workers, auto mechanics, etc.). Improving strength and endurance of specific muscle groups involved in occupational activities allows such patients to be more capable of safely performing work-related duties, while concurrently diminishing the likelihood that other bodily systems might be overtaxed.
- Individuals with a desire to participate in leisure or recreational activities that involve extensive use of the upper extremities (e.g., racquet sports, gardening, etc.).
- Individuals with a desire to engage in resistance training, either to offset the atrophy that results from a sedentary lifestyle or to enhance physical appearance by favorably altering body composition. Such changes can positively affect level of self-esteem and psychological well-being.

Implementing a strength-training program for a cardiac patient should be based on needs, interests, and medical/health status. After specific needs and interests have been clearly identified, medical and health history should be carefully reviewed by a physician. The ACSM and AACVPR have guidelines to be used that assist in identification of coronary-prone individuals, for whom resistance training is safe and appropriate (25, 26). The ACSM and the AACVPR recommend the following inclusion criteria:

- 4 to 6 weeks post-myocardial infarction or coronary artery bypass grafting (CABG)
- 1 to 2 weeks following PTCA or other revascularization procedure, except CABG, without myocardial infarction

- Following 4 to 6 weeks in a supervised cardiovascular endurance program or completion of Phase II
- Resting diastolic blood pressure < 105 mm Hg
- Peak exercise capacity of > 5 METs
- Not compromised by coronary heart failure, unstable symptoms, or arrhythmias

Safety is the most important issue attendant to resistance training for cardiac patients. Specific guidelines for the safe and effective application of resistance training in cardiac patients have been developed by the AACVPR including (7, 25):

- Limit resistance training to patients who are asymptomatic or only mildly symptomatic.
- Initiate resistance training after a minimum of 12 weeks of aerobic training.
- Select an initial resistance allowing 10–12 repetitions of an exercise, comfortably to prevent soreness and injury. This level of resistance generally corresponds to approximately 60% of 1 repetition maximum. Training at this intensity can produce significant improvements in functional muscle strength.
- Use single-limb exercises (instead of double-limb) in patients who experience an exaggerated rise in blood pressure (BP) and/or rate pressure product (systolic BP × heart rate) during resistance training.
- Two to three sets of each exercise are recommended.
- Ratings of perceived exertion (6–20 RPE scale) should not exceed fairly light (11) to somewhat hard (13) during resistance training. Patients should not "strain."
- Avoid breath-holding. Breathe normally at all times.
- Increase resistance by 2.5–5 lbs when 10–12 repetitions can be comfortably accomplished; for high-risk adults and cardiac patients, the resistance should be increased only after at least 12–15 repetitions can be easily managed.
- Exercise muscles, generally, in a large-muscle to small-muscle order, 2–3 times per week. Include exercises for both the upper and lower extremities.
- Avoid excessive static contraction, handgripping (e.g., free weight bars, dumbbells, machine handles, etc.) if possible; high level, static contraction may evoke excessive blood pressure response.
- Discontinue exercise in the event of any contraindicative warning signs or symptoms, especially dizziness, abnormal heart rhythm, unusual shortness of breath, and/or chest pain.
- Rest periods should be relatively short (i.e., ≈ 1 minute), between both individual exercises and sets of exercises, to maximize muscular endurance and aerobic training benefits.
- Require patients to monitor and record heart rate response, RPE, and symptoms following each exercise, or set of exercises.

Pregnant Women

Many women are hesitant to continue resistance training during pregnancy because of the seemingly inconsistent and diverse opinions on the subject. Recently, however, specific advice for pregnant women interested in resistance training has been published (4, 13). Based on limited data, appropriate resistance training poses little risk to either the mother or the fetus, and may be beneficial. For example, proper resistance training provides a pregnant woman with an enhanced level of muscular fitness which may help compensate for the postural adjustments that typically occur during pregnancy and are often associated with low back pain. The activities of daily living may be performed with greater relative ease with an enhanced level of muscular fitness.

Experts, however, are relatively quick note that resistance training is not advisable for all pregnant women. The following recommendations regarding resistance training and pregnancy are appropriate:

- Women with any of the American College of Obstetrics and Gynecology (ACOG) contraindications for aerobic exercise during pregnancy should not participate in resistance training (Table 53.4) (4, 25).
- Women who have never participated in resistance training should not initiate one during pregnancy.
- Ballistic exercises should be strictly avoided, since pregnancy is associated with joint and connective tissue laxity which may increase susceptibility to injury.
- Women should be encouraged to breathe normally during resistance training, because oxygen delivery to the placenta may be reduced during breath-holding (i.e., a Valsalva maneuver).
- Heavy resistance should be avoided since it may expose the joints, connective tissue, and skeletal structures of an expectant woman to excessive forces. An exercise set consisting of at least 12–15 repetitions, without undue fatigue, generally ensures that the resistance is appropriate.
- As training occurs, overload initially by increasing number of repetitions and, subsequently, by increasing resistance.
- Resistance training on machines is usually preferred over free weights because machines require less skill and can be more easily controlled.

Table 53.4. Contraindications for Exercising During Pregnancy

1. Pregnancy induced hypertension
2. Preterm rupture of membrane
3. Preterm labor during the prior or current pregnancy
4. Incompetent cervix
5. Persistent second to third trimester bleeding
6. Intrauterine growth retardation

- If a specific exercise causes pain or discomfort, it should be discontinued and an alternative exercise used. The following warning signs or complications require physician consultation:

1. Vaginal bleeding
2. Abdominal pain or cramping
3. Ruptured membranes
4. Elevated blood pressure or heart rate
5. Lack of fetal movement

Limited research demonstrates that resistance training can be an integral part of a balanced exercise prescription during pregnancy. It appears that resistance training may assist in effective management of many of the rigors of pregnancy. Research also suggests that resistance training may not be appropriate for all pregnant women. Until more data are available, medical advice and physician recommendations should be obtained prior to resistance training during pregnancy. In addition, exercise prescription for resistance training during pregnancy should be individualized. As a general rule, exercise professionals designing resistance training programs for pregnant women should be conservative in the approach to manipulating resistance training variables.

▶ SUMMARY

Resistance training programs should be an integral part of a comprehensive fitness program. Health and fitness status, individual goals and basic principles of training should be considered when designing resistance training programs. Resistance training is generally safe for many special populations including children, older adults, and cardiac patients as long as appropriate precautions are observed. Exercise professionals should be aware of both the health status and the contraindications to exercise in all clients for whom resistance training is recommended.

References

1. Cahill B, ed. Proceedings of the Conference on Strength Training and the Prepubescent. Chicago: American Orthopaedic Society for Sports Medicine, 1988.
2. Kraemer WJ, Fleck SJ. *Strength Training for Young Athletes.* Champaign, IL: Human Kinetics, 1993.
3. Tanner SM. Weighing the risks: Strength training for children and adolescents. *Phys Sportsmed* 1993;21(6):105.
4. Peterson JA, Bryant CX. *The StairMaster Fitness Handbook.* Champaign, IL: Sagamore Publishing Co., 1995.
5. Munnings F. Strength training: Not only for the young. *Phys Sportsmed* 1993;21(4):133.
6. Bryant CX, Peterson JA. Strength training for the heart? *Fitness Manage* 1994;2:32.
7. Franklin BA, Bonzheim K, Gordon S, et al. Resistance training in cardiac rehabilitation. *J Cardiopulm Rehab* 1991;11:99.
8. McKelvie RS, McCartney N. Weightlifting training in cardiac patients: considerations. *Sports Med* 1990;10(6):355.
9. Hakkinen K. Factors influencing trainability of muscular strength during short term and prolonged training. *Natl Strength Cond Assoc J* 1985;7:32.
10. Kraemer WJ, Deschenes MR, Fleck SJ. Physiological adaptations to resistance exercise: Implications for athletic conditioning. Sports Med 1988;6:246.
11. DiNubile NA. Strength training. *Clin Sports Med* 1991;10(1):33.
12. Fleck SJ, Kraemer WJ. *Designing Resistance Training Programs.* 2nd ed. Champaign, IL: Human Kinetics, 1997.
13. Peterson JA, Bryant CX, Peterson SL. *Strength Training for Women.* Champaign, IL: Human Kinetics, 1995.
14. Graves JE, Pollock ML, Jones AE, et al. Specificity of limited range of motion of variable resistance training. *Med Sci Sports Exerc* 1989;21:84.
15. Knapik JJ, Mawdsley RH, Ramos NU. Angular specificity and test mode specificity of isometric and isokinetic strength training. *J Orthop Sports Phys Ther* 1983;5:58.
16. Gardner G. Specificity of strength changes of the exercised and nonexercised limb following isometric training. *Res Q* 1963;34:98.
17. Byrnes W. Muscle soreness following resistance exercise with and without eccentric contractions. *Res Q* 1985;56:283.
18. Talag TS. Residual muscular soreness influenced by concentric, eccentric, and static contractions. *Res Q* 1973;44:458.
19. Stanish WD, Rubinovich RM, Curwin S. Eccentric exercise in chronic tendinitis. *Clin Orthop* 1986;208:65.
20. Fleck SJ, Falkel JE. Value of resistance training for the reduction of sports injuries. *Sports Med* 1986;3:61.
21. Coyle E, et al. Specificity of power improvements through slow and fast isokinetic training. *J Appl Physiol* 1981;51:1437.
22. Lesme G, Costill D, Coyle E, et al. Muscle strength and power changes during maximal isokinetic training. *Med Sci Sports Exerc* 1978;10:266.
23. National Strength and Conditioning Association. Position statement on prepubescent strength training. *Nat Strength Condit Assoc J* 1985;7:27.
24. Ettinger WH, Burns R, Messier SP, et al. A randomized trial comparing aerobic exercise and resistance exercise with a health education program in older adults with knee osteoarthritis: The Fitness Arthritis and Seniors Trial (FAST). *JAMA* 1997;277(1):25–31.
25. Kenney WL, Humphrey RH, Bryant CX, eds. *ACSM's Guidelines for Exercise Testing and Prescription.* 5th ed. Baltimore: Williams & Wilkins, 1995.
26. American Association of Cardiovascular and Pulmonary Rehabilitation. *Guidelines for Cardiac Rehabilitation Programs.* 2nd ed. Champaign, IL: Human Kinetics, 1995.

1, 22, 161 37, 185, 186, 191

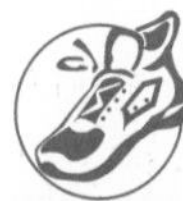

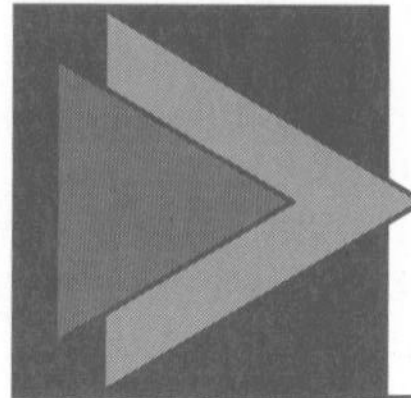

CHAPTER 54

Exercise Recommendations for Flexibility and Range of Motion

Denise M. Fredette

Flexibility is characterized by a ready capability to adapt to new and different or changing requirements and is applied, more specifically, to the range of motion (ROM) which occurs at a single joint or the total range of movement within a series of joints (1, 2). The adaptability that flexibility provides allows movement with fluidity, greater ease, coordination, and responsiveness (Table 54.1).

PHYSIOLOGY OF FLEXIBILITY

Neuromuscular Factors

Four proprioceptive sensory organ systems respond to a stretch stimulus (3, 4):

- The Golgi tendon organ (GTO)
- The intrafusal muscle fibers of the muscle spindle
- The pacinian corpuscle
- The Ruffini end organs in deep connective tissue and joint capsules.

These receptors are active during strong contraction or stretch. They inhibit or facilitate contraction, with a coordinated effect, to protect muscle from overcontraction or overstretch (4).

GTOs are located in muscle tendon and, when activated, reflexively inhibit contraction. GTOs signal a muscle that is being stretched to "relax." Muscle spindles are a sensory organ scattered throughout muscle tissue that reflexively activate muscle and concurrently inhibit the opposing, or antagonist, muscle. This response is known as the "stretch reflex" (4). If the stretch impulse is too great, muscle spindle input causes a protective contraction. The pacinian corpuscles and Ruffini end organs are stimulated by pressure from surrounding structures when joints are moved. Extreme pressure results in pain perception and withdrawal from a noxious stretch stimulus (3, 4).

Mechanical properties of connective tissue, the superstructure of muscles, tendons, and joint capsules, are also important. Within ground substance of connective tissue are fibroblasts that have an important role in connective tissue repair. Fibroblasts respond to injury by stimulating proliferation and fibrogenesis. They are involved in healing of defects in connective tissue, cartilage, tendon and adjacent connective tissue-like muscle (5). Gradual deformation of connective tissue is the goal of stretching a muscle. Microtrauma occurs in connective tissue in response to stretching, followed by recovery and repair. Repair leads to new fiber organization, thus greater extensibility in that tissue (4, 6). Connective tissue in muscle is composed of 80% plastin fibers and 20% elastin fibers giving myofascial tissue a great potential for extensibility (5, 7, 8). Hooke's law states that the amount of stretch (deformation) is proportional to the applied force (9). Current research on the response of connective tissue to an applied stressor indicates that a slow sustained stretch of 30–90 seconds is necessary to effectively get beyond elastic recoil properties of skeletal muscle and produce mild deformation that stimulates the fiber re-organization (7, 8). The stress strain relationship of tissues under stretch is demonstrated in Fig. 54.1.

WHO SHOULD AND SHOULD NOT STRETCH?

Everyone can learn to stretch regardless of age or initial flexibility. Emphasizing methods that are easy and gentle, and adapting the program to individual needs is important regardless of age. Children benefit from stretching as much as adults and high levels of fitness are not required to begin a stretching program.

Some individuals have naturally loose ligaments and connective tissue, thus joint capsules, ligaments and surface relationships may allow for excessive ROM. These hypermobile individuals should not be allowed to stretch into the extremes of ROM because as much joint stability should be maintained as possible.

During pregnancy the ligaments and connective tissue, especially of the pelvis, are softened by a hormone

Table 54.1. The Benefits of Increased Flexibility

- Reduced muscle tension and increased relaxation
- Maintain ease of movement
- Improved coordination by allowing for greater ease of movement
- Increased range of motion (ROM)
- Injury prevention
- Improvement and development of body awareness
- Improved capability for circulation and air exchange
- Decreased muscle viscosity, causing contractions to be easier and smoother
- Decreased soreness associated with other exercise activities

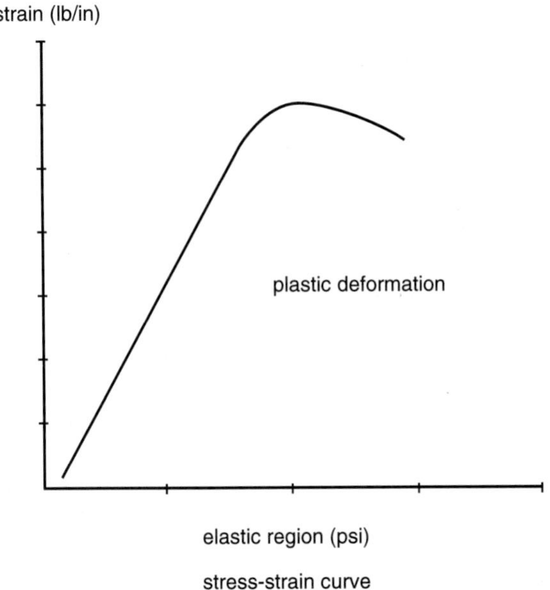

Figure 54.1. The Stress-Strain curve with the upward slope representing the Elastic Recoil Zone. The curve with the downward slope portrays the Plastic Deformation Zone.

called "relaxant." Excessive stretching during pregnancy is not recommended. It can lead to low back, sacroiliac and other hypermobility problems during and after pregnancy. The benefits of flexibility training are listed in Table 54.1. The contraindications and precautions for stretching and flexibility training are shown in Tables 54.2 and 54.3, respectively (10–12).

WHEN TO STRETCH

Individual preference determines appropriate time of day for flexibility exercise. Spontaneous stretching done properly at work, in the car, while watching television, or in the park is effective and desirable. Stretching before and after physical activity should be part of warm-up and cool-down. Warm-up with light activity, such as walking, before stretching is recommended. Warm muscle tissue accepts stretch easier than cold. Stretching is indicated after sitting or standing for long periods, especially during or after a long drive. Stretching can help prevent discomfort from periods of immobility.

FREQUENCY AND DURATION OF TRAINING

There is wide variation of opinion about the most effective frequency and duration for flexibility training. Beaulieu states that a stretch may be held for 10–15 seconds initially and gradually increased to 45–60 seconds over a 4–5 week period (13). Anderson suggests beginning with an easy stretch for 10–30 seconds followed by a "developmental" stretch for an additional 10–30 seconds (10). Moffatt recommends maintaining stretching posture for about 8–12 seconds (14). In contrast, Feldenkrais suggests taking 3–4 exercises and repeating those exercises slowly 3–4 times for a total of 30 minutes of exercise (15). Yoga practitioners dedicate 30–45

Table 54.2. Contraindications For Flexibility Training

- Motion limited by bony block at a joint interface
- Recent unhealed fracture
- Infection and acute inflammation, affecting the joint or surrounding tissues
- Sharp pain associated with stretch or uncontrolled muscle cramping that occurs when attempting to stretch
- Local hematoma as a result of an overstretch injury
- If contracture (desired functional shortening) occurs requiring stability to a joint capsule or ligament
- If contracture is intentional to improve function particularly in clients with paralysis or severe muscle weakness (e.g., tenodesis of finger flexors to allow grasp in an individual with quadriplegia)

Table 54.3. Precautions for Flexibility Training

- Stretch a joint through limits of normal ROM only
- Do not stretch at healed fracture sites for ~8–12 weeks post-fracture; after which, gentle stretching may be initiated
- In individuals with known or suspected osteoporosis, stretch with particular caution (e.g., men older than 80 years old and women over 65 years old, older spinal cord injured individuals).
- Avoid aggressive stretching of tissues that have been immobilized (e.g., casted). Tissues become dehydrated and lose tensile strength during immobilization.
- Mild soreness should take no longer than 24 hours to resolve after stretching. If more recovery time is necessary, then the stretching force was excessive.
- Use active comfortable ROM to stretch edematous joints or soft tissue.
- Do *not* over-stretch weak muscles. Shortening in these muscles may contribute to joint support that muscles can no longer actively provide. Combine strengthen and stretching exercise so that gains in mobility coincide with gains in strength and stability.
- Be aware that physical performance may vary from day to day.
- Set individual goals.

minutes each day to stretching (16, 17). The American College of Sports Medicine proposes that a stretch should last for 10–30 seconds (18).

Connective tissue deformation and neuroinhibitory effects require 30–90 seconds to effect tissue change and a relaxation response (4, 7, 8). Beaulieu states stretching should be done 10–20 minutes, 2–3 times per week (13). deVries found that stretching 30 minutes, two times per week results in improved flexibility within 5 weeks (19, 20). Feldenkrais and yoga practitioners recommend daily stretching exercise because of the relaxation benefits (15, 16).

HOW TO STRETCH

The guidelines shown in Table 54.4 are synthesized recommendations from Anderson (10, 21), Krusen, Kottke, Elwood (22), Kuland (23), Morris (2), Hittleman (17), Bersin, Bersin and Reese (15). It is helpful to have an exercise professional observe patients during the initiation of a stretch to assure proper alignment. Incorrect stretching can be ineffective and may be damaging. Proper alignment is defined as good biomechanical relationship of each joint to the joints adjacent to it.

TECHNIQUES USED TO GAIN FLEXIBILITY

Static Stretching

A static stretch is slow and sustained to increase motion at a particular joint when one segment is manipulated relative to another (2, 22). The advantages of static stretching include the following (19, 23–26):

- Decreased possibility of exceeding normal range of motion
- Lower energy requirements
- Less muscle soreness
- The types of static stretching include passive, active-assistive, active, and proprioceptive neuromuscular facilitation (PNF).

Table 54.4. Guidelines for Proper Stretching Technique

1. Determine posture or position to be used. Ensure proper position and alignment prior to the stretch.
2. Emphasize proper breathing. Inhale through the nose and exhale during the stretch through pursed lips, with the eyes closed to increase concentration and awareness.
3. Hold end points progressively for 30–90 seconds and take another deep breath.
4. Exhale and feel the muscle being stretched, relaxed, and softened so that further ROM is achieved.
5. Discomfort may increase slightly, but continue to focus on breathing.
6. Repeat the inhale-exhale-stretch cycle until the end of the available range for the day.
7. Do *not* bounce or spring while stretching.
8. Do *not* force a stretch while holding the breath.
9. Increase stretching range during exhalation encourages full body relaxation.
10. Slowly reposition from the stretch posture and allow muscles to recover at natural resting length.

Passive Stretching

Passive stretch requires assistance from another person or a device. Optimal passive stretch requires relaxation of all voluntary and reflex muscular resistance, which is often hard to achieve. A trust that the stretching partner will not go too far or too fast is essential (18). Types of passive stretching include (27):

- Manual stretching
- Prolonged mechanical stretching
- Cyclic mechanical stretching
- Self stretching.

Active Assistive Stretching

In active assistive stretching the muscle or joint being stretched may require assistance moving through the ROM because of weakness. The stretch requires the assistance of a partner and has the same limitations as passive stretching (18).

Active Stretching

During active stretching a muscle or joint is actively moved through the ROM. This technique requires greater energy than passive or static stretching and may elicit a stretch reflex and, thereby, cause the stretch to be improperly performed (18).

Proprioceptive Neuromuscular Facilitation

Types of PNF techniques for stretching include the contract-relax (hold-relax) stretch and the contract-relax-contract (hold-relax-contract) stretch (28). For contract-relax PNF, a muscle is contracted, relaxed, then further stretched into the available ROM during this brief relaxation phase. For contract-relax-contract, the same procedure is used, but subsequent contraction of the antagonist gains additional ROM. The disadvantage is the difficulty in teaching proper technique to patients and it is best accomplished with a partner. The end result is similar limitations to those with passive and active-assistive stretching (18). Hutton compared static, contract-relax and contract-relax-contract in effecting increased hamstring length and demonstrated contract-relax-contract to be most effective, but difficult to teach and more uncomfortable to perform (29). Etnyre compared static stretch to contract-relax PNF and contract-relax-antagonist contract PNF stretching and found the two PNF techniques to be more effective in both men and women for increasing hip and shoulder extension ROM (30).

Dynamic-Phasic-Ballistic Stretching

Dynamic, phasic, or ballistic activities refer to rapid movements requiring jerking and, often, bouncing movements (2). The disadvantages of this type of stretching outweigh the advantages. Ballistic movements predispose to muscle strain injury. A rapidly stretched muscle stimulates intrafusal muscle contraction (14). Ballistic movements are used to simulate sports-specific, pre-activity warm-up. Static stretching and plyometrics are recommended as safer options for warm-up flexibility. Studies conclude that static stretching is safer, requires less energy and may reduce muscle soreness associated with other exercise (19, 20, 29, 31, 32).

FLEXIBILITY EXERCISES

Specific examples of positions and postures for flexibility exercises are shown in Figures 54.2 to 54.7. These specific exercises attempt to address positions for almost

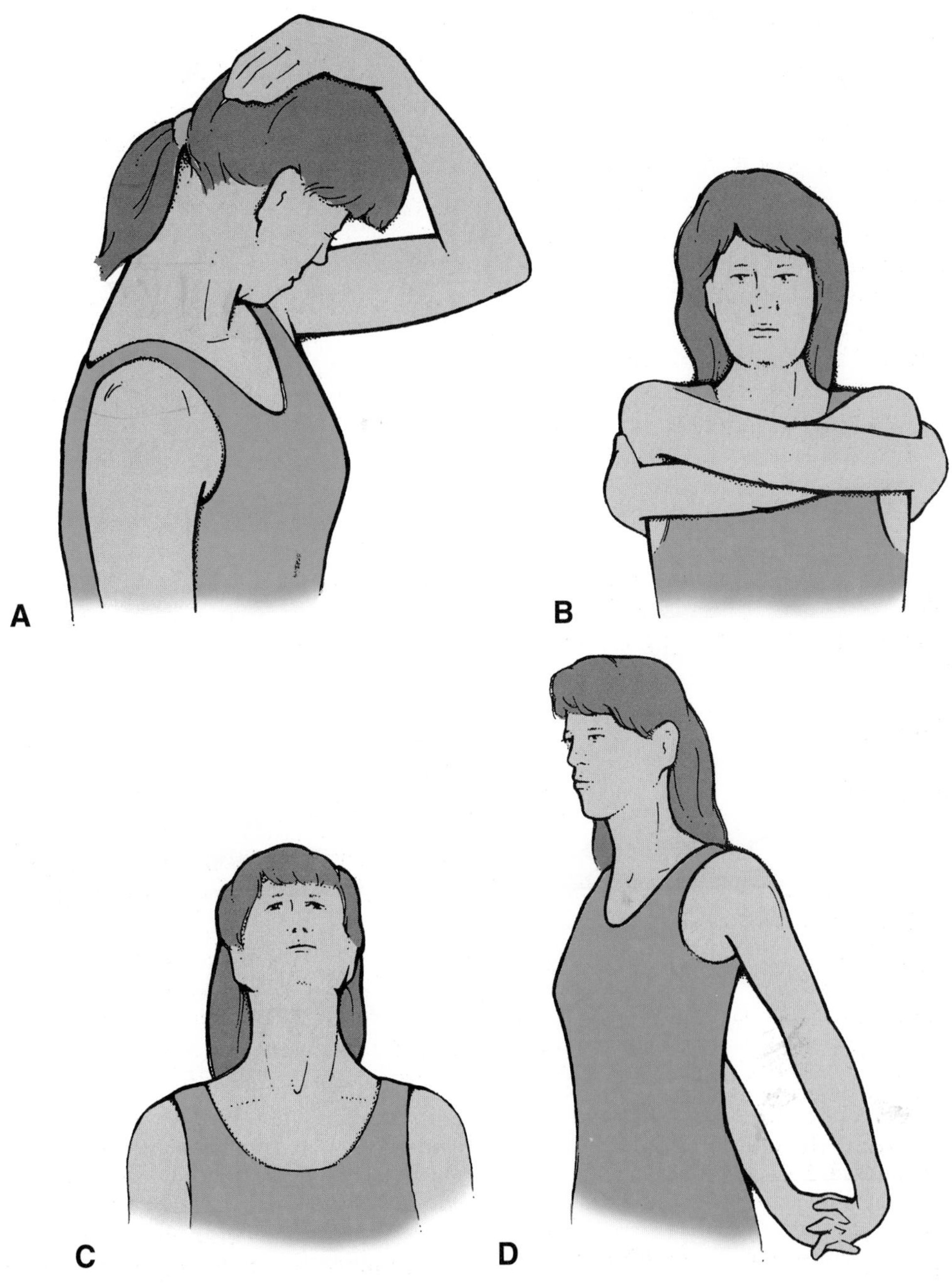

Figure 54.2. **A,** Neck Flexion (with gentle pressure): This technique can be used with side bending and a combination of side bending, flexion, and rotation. (Use caution with complaints of dizziness, avoid extension and rotation postures of the neck). **B,** Hugging/Shoulder Protraction Stretch: Reach across the body with both arms and grasp the shoulders. Inhale deeply, focusing the sensation of stretch between the scapulae. **C,** Neck Extension Stretch: Neck extension with jaw thrust to increase stretch on the anterior neck and jaw musculature. (Precaution: avoid complaints of dizziness). **D,** Anterior Chest Stretch: Shoulder extension, internal rotation and scapular retraction with full elbow extension and hands interlocked.

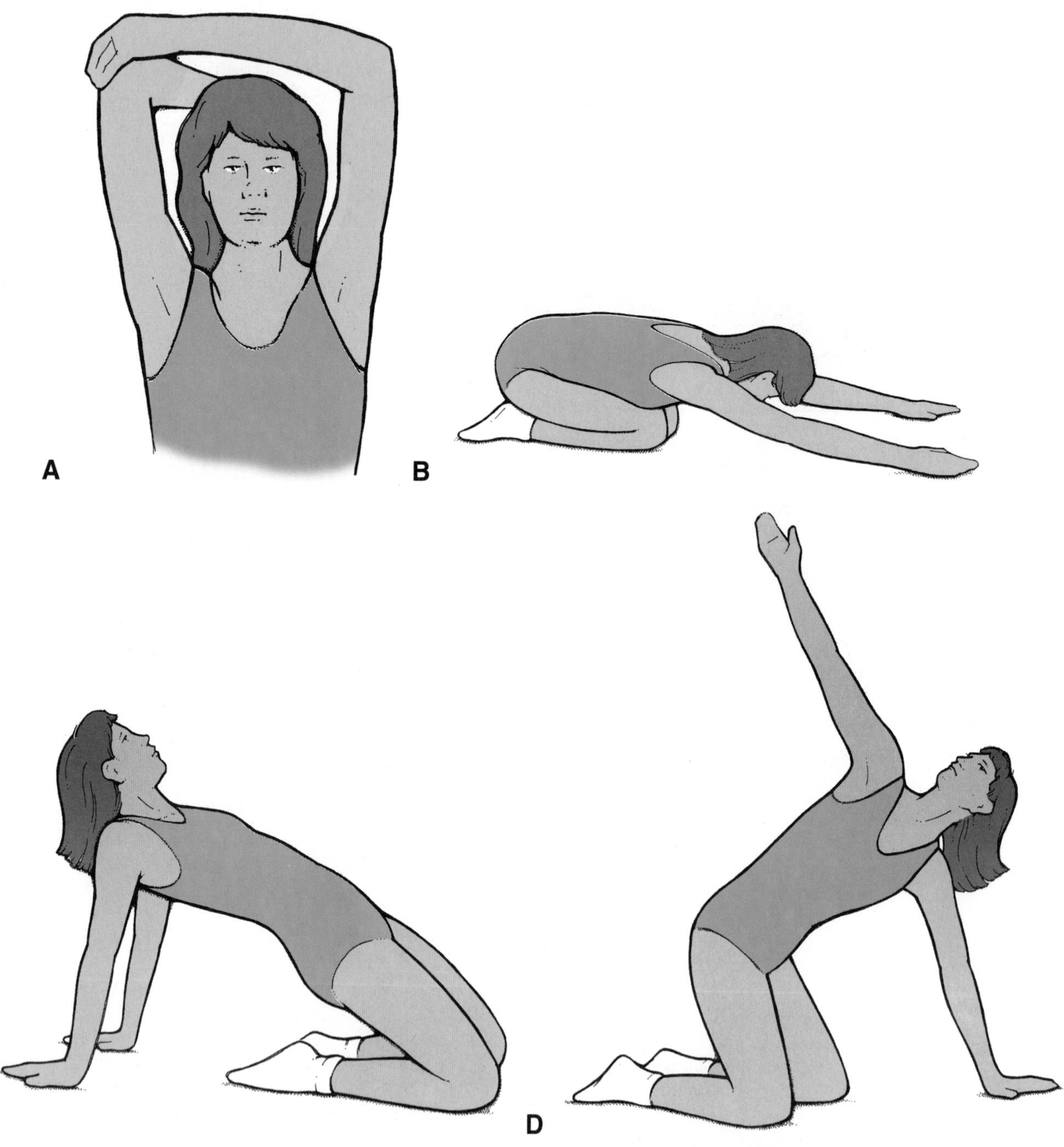

Figure 54.3. **A,** Triceps and Inferior Capsule Stretch: Full shoulder abduction—elbow is fully flexed and gentle overpressure is applied pulling toward the midline. (Precaution: Avoid overstressing the neck anteriorly in this posture). **B,** Latissimus Dorsi Stretch: Begin on hands and knees. The hands stay firmly planted and the person rocks backward on hips resting buttocks on calves. Proper position localizes stretch to low back and shoulder girdle. **C,** Thigh, Abdomen and Chest Stretch: Begin kneeling and reach posteriorly extending both arms and spine, bearing weight fully on hands. Press abdomen and hips anteriorly to localize stretch to chest, abdomen and thighs. **D,** Anterior Chest-Torso, Mild Rotation Stretch: Begin on hands and knees. Reach upward with one arm in extension and abduction. Allow the torso and head to rotate upward looking at the outstretched hand.

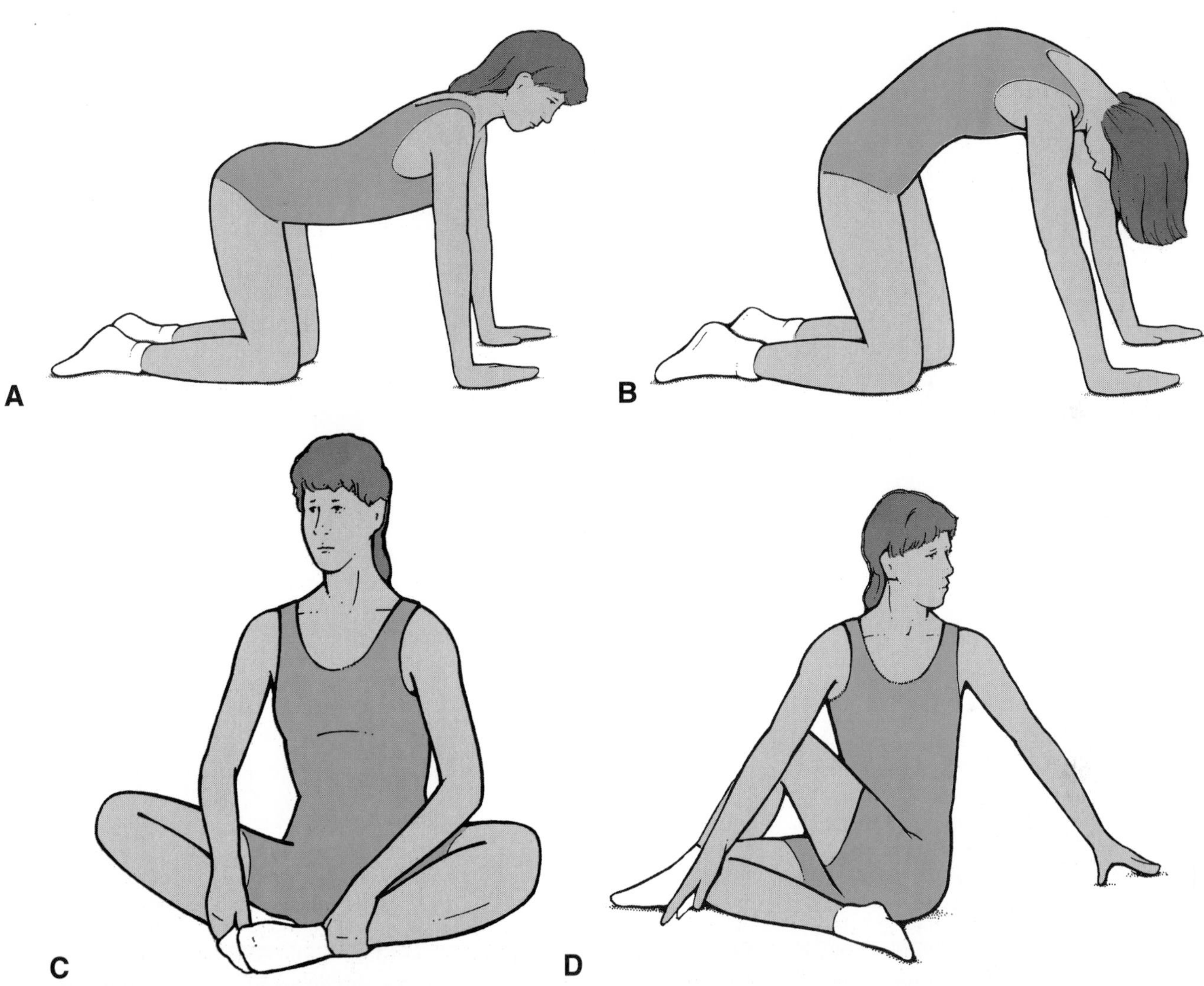

Figure 54.4. **A,** Full Spinal Segmental Extension Stretch: Begin on the hands and knees. Initiate extension of the sacrum, arching the back (extend) segment by segment, completing full extension from the lumbar to the cervical spine. **B,** Full Spinal Segmental Flexion Stretch: Begin on hands and knees. Initiate flexion of the sacrum, then lumbar, thoracic and cervical spine. Flexion of the thoracic spine is increased further by protracting both scapulae. **C,** Seated Adductor Stretch: Start in seated posture with an erect spine. Touch soles of feet together and bend knees, sliding the feet toward the midline. Allow knees to drop for increased hip abduction. With a straight back, lean forward to increase stretch in adductors. **D,** Combined Spinal Rotation, Hip Extension and Rotator Stretch: Begin seated with an erect spine. Both knees are flexed. Cross left leg over right leg. Right arm reaches for left knee and using the knee to assist the torso into left rotation. Inhale, on an exhalation attempt further spinal rotation. Reverse the stretch for right rotation.

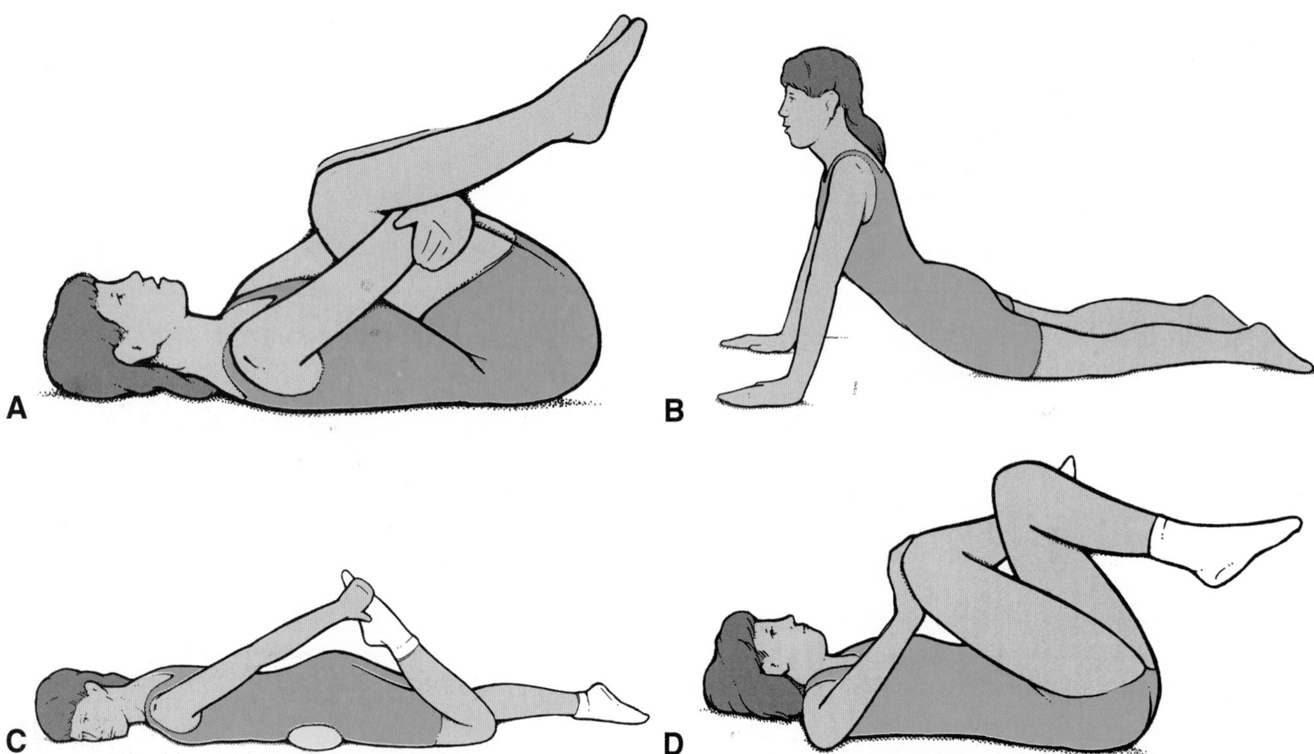

Figure 54.5. **A,** Bilateral Knee to Chest Stretch: Begin in the supine position. Pull both thighs to chest by supporting the back of the thigh with the hands. **B,** Full Spinal Extension Press Up Stretch: Begin in prone position. Place hands on the mat just below shoulder level and press upwards slowly. Maintain contact with the mat with front of thighs and pelvis. Evenly distribute spinal extension effort throughout the entire spine. (Precaution: Tightness in the thoracic spine restricts thoracic extension. This is a vulnerable area in the presence of osteoporosis. Propped on elbows is preferable for those with osteoporosis.) **C,** Quadriceps Stretch: Begin in prone position. To relieve stress on the low back, use a towel roll under the hips. Bend one knee toward the buttocks and hold the foot with one hand. A towel or rope can be used to assist reaching the lower leg. **D,** Hip Rotator Stretch: Begin in supine position. Cross one leg over forming a "figure 4" and flex both hips to or past 90°. The stretch is felt in the buttocks of the figure 4 leg.

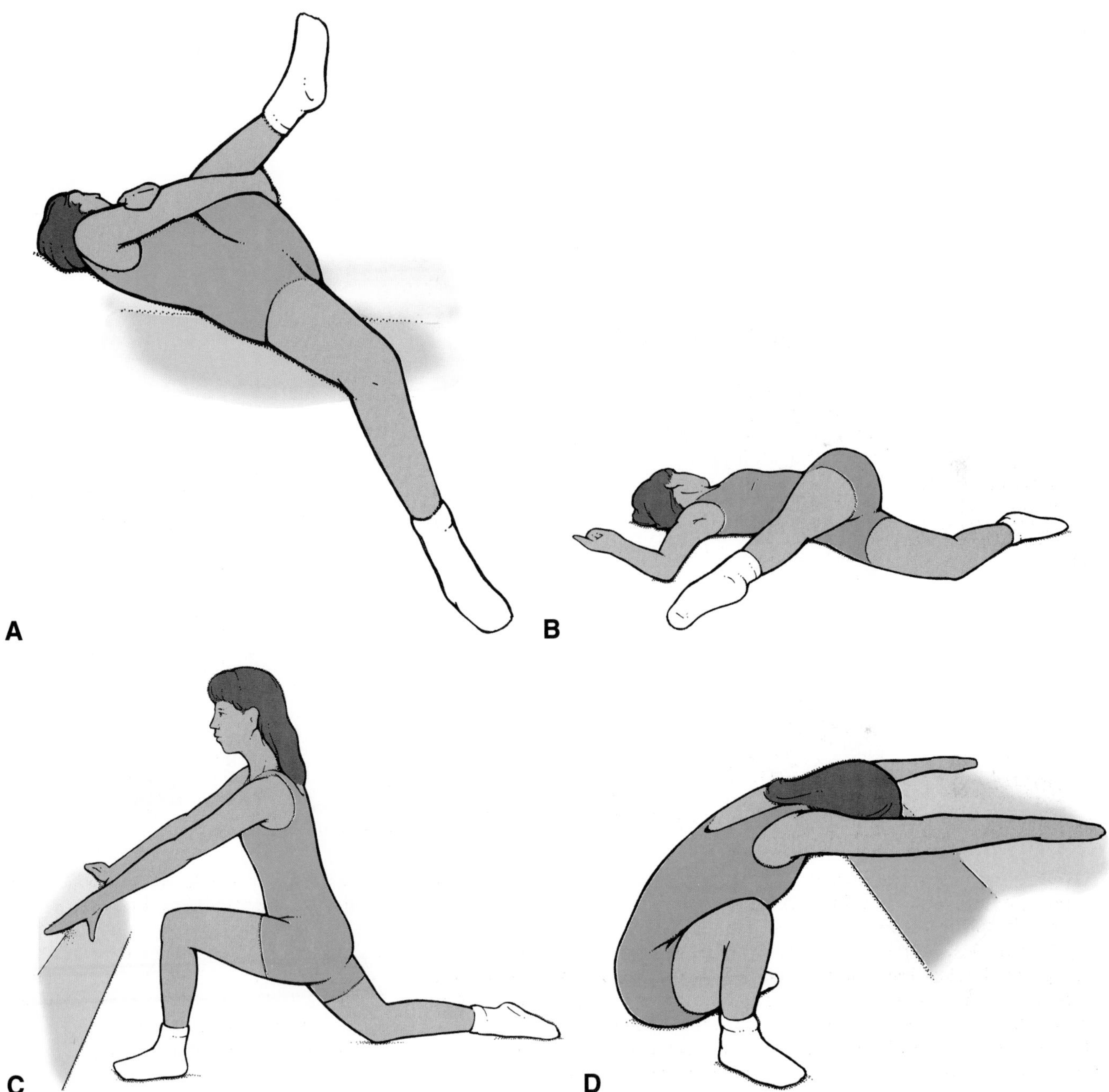

Figure 54.6. **A,** Hip Flexion Stretch: Begin in supine position. With one leg over the side of the exercise bench, flex the opposite leg as close to the chest as possible. The stretch is felt anteriorly in the hip and thigh of the hanging leg. **B,** Hip Internal Rotation, Adduction and Knee Extension Stretch: Begin in supine position. The stretch is horizontal adduction and internal rotation of the hip with fully extended knees. Rotate head in the opposite direction to aide keeping the shoulders flat against the mat. (Allowing knee flexion is a simpler technique). **C,** Forward Lunge Stretch: Begin in the standing position. Step forward with one leg, leaving the trailing leg in contact with the floor. The trailing leg stretches the anterior hip and thigh region. The forward leg is flexed at 90° at the knee and the hip causing a proximal hamstring stretch. **D,** Full Squat Stretch: Begin in standing position while holding a chair or table. Allow full adduction, external rotation and flexion at the hips. Careful attention to hip, knee and ankle alignment is important. Try to maintain both heels in contact with the floor.

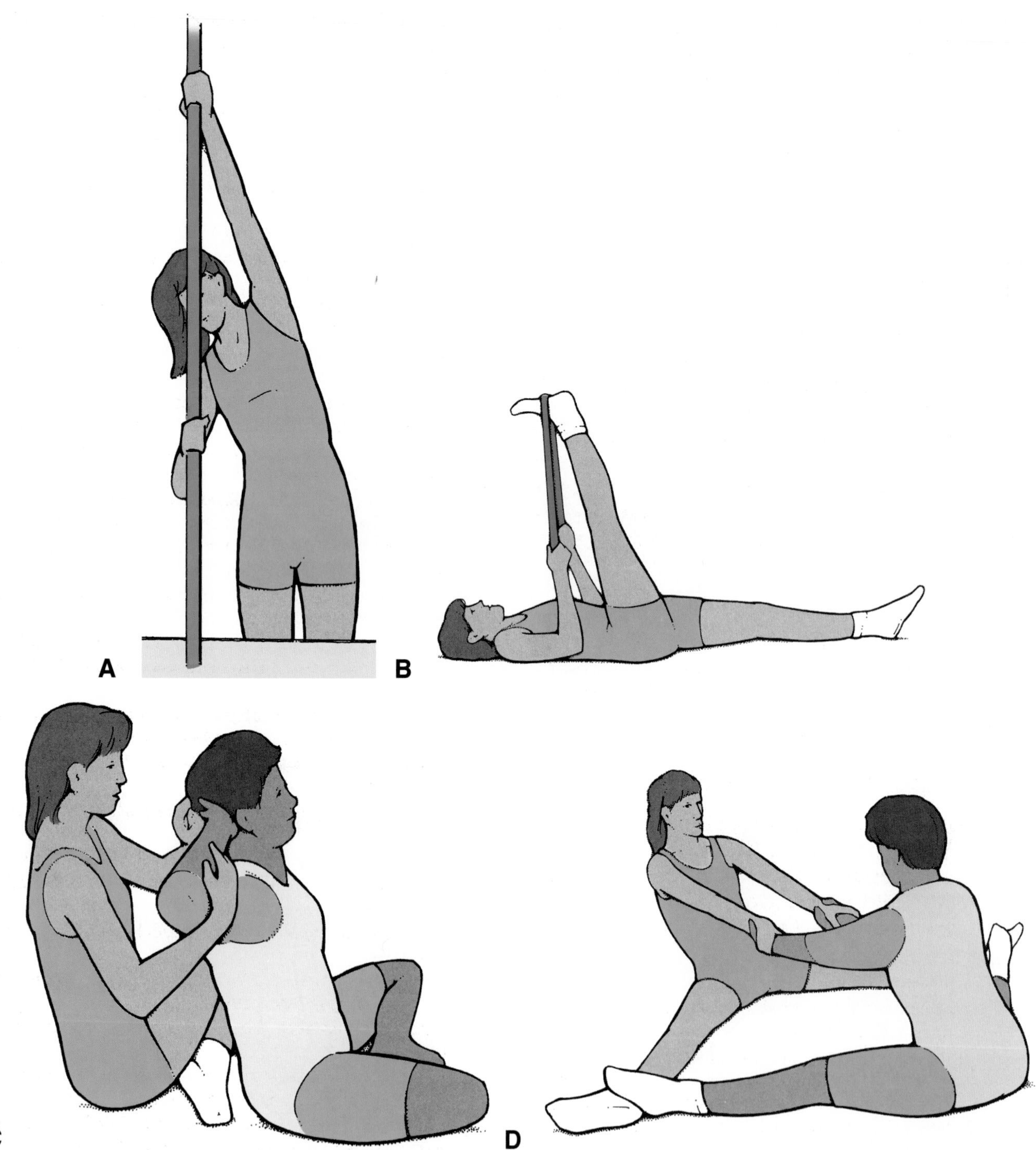

Figure 54.7. **A,** Long Dowel Rod Prop Stretch–Arm and Torso Stretch: Begin in the standing position. Place the pole on an exercise bench and slide the arm up the pole lengthening the shoulder girdle, spine, torso, and ribs. Use deep breathing to increase stretch between the ribs. **B,** Assisted Hamstring Stretch (using a long piece of rope): Begin in the supine position. Straight leg raise with the rope hooked around the sole of the foot and pull the leg into increasing hip flexion. (Simpler technique requires the rope be placed on the back of the calf.) **C,** Partner-Assisted Pectoralis Major Stretch: Begin with one partner sitting one behind the other. The partner receiving the stretch interlocks hands behind head. The partner assisting with the stretch places the knees against the "stretcher's" back and pulls gently on the arms creating an extension stretch for chest and upper back. (Precaution: This may be contraindicated in patients with osteoporosis.) **D,** Partner-Assisted Stretch of the Hip Adductors: Begin in a seated position facing a partner in full knee extension, full hip abduction, bracing the feet against feet. One partner gently and slowly pulls forward to increase the inner thigh stretch. Alternate stretching between partners asking for and giving feedback to assure safety.

every joint. Stretching techniques using props and partners are included for variety in relation to individual needs. Refer to Table 54.4 and follow illustrated and written directions for safe execution of these exercises. Also note that individual exercises or some combination of these exercises may be contraindicated in a variety of populations.

PLYOMETRICS

For optimum physical performance, an athlete trains for speed, strength, power, coordination, endurance, and flexibility. Plyometrics conditions through dynamic resistance exercise. Plyometrics were first applied to lower extremities by performing jumping-type exercises. Plyometrics has now been adapted for upper extremity and torso exercise using a weighted object, such as a medicine ball. Use of a medicine ball for resistance allows the individual to experience movement throughout the sport specific ROM. Chu describes plyometric exercises as beginning with rapid stretching (eccentric contraction) followed by shortening of the same muscle (concentric contraction) (12). This is known as the stretch/shortening cycle. The success of plyometrics is based on utilization of serial elastic properties and stretch properties of muscle. Under these loading conditions increased ROM and greater force with maximum metabolic efficiency is affected.

▶ SUMMARY

Physiological changes in connective and muscle tissue accompany flexibility training. Close attention to the proper technique, as well as precautions and contraindications to stretching is important in prescribing and teaching a safe, effective flexibility program.

Acknowledgments

A special thanks to Dr. Elizabeth Protas, Assistant Dean, School of Physical Therapy, Texas Woman's University, Houston, Texas. She was instrumental in advising and editing this chapter. A special thanks to Elizabeth Boswell Jones, MEd., for her help as a model and exercise consultant. Ms. Jones owns and directs the Physical Conditioning Center, a Pilates-based exercise studio in Houston, Texas.

References

1. Webster's Ninth New Collegiate Dictionary. Merriam-Webster, 1991.
2. Morris HF. *Sports Medicine Handbook.* 1st ed: Dubuque IA, William C. Brown Publishers, 1984;45–51.
3. McNaught M, Callender L. *Illustrated Physiology.* 3rd ed. New York: Churchill Livingston, 1975:241–245.
4. Per-Olof A, Rodahl K. *Textbook of Work Physiology.* 2nd ed. St Louis: McGraw Hill, Inc., 1977:72–79.
5. Bloom W, Fawcett DW. *A Textbook of Histology.* 10th ed. Philadelphia: W.B. Saunders, 1975.
6. Chamberlain G. Cyriax's friction massage: a review. *JOPST* 1982;14(1):16–22.
7. Garfin SR, Tipton CM, MuBarak SJ, et al. Role of fascia in maintenance of muscle tension and pressure. *J Appl Physiol* 1981;51:317–319.
8. Mozam K, Lawrence J, Keagy R. Muscle relationships in functional fascia. *Clin Orthop* 1978;150:403–409.
9. Bueche F. *Principles of Physics.* 2nd ed. St Louis: McGraw Hill Book Co., 1972:194–195.
10. Anderson B. *Stretching.* Bolinas, CA: Shelter Publication, 1980:10–110.
11. Altrig Z, Hoffman J, Martin J. *Clinical Exercise Testing Prescription and Rehabilitation.* 5th ed. Philidelphia: Lea & Febiger, 1992:123–126.
12. Chu D. *Plyometrics.* Livermore, CA: Bittersweet Publishing Co, 1989;8–15, 78–79.
13. Beaulieu JE. *Stretching for All Sports.* Pasadena, CA: The Athletic Press, 1980;5–50.
14. Moffatt RJ. Strength and flexibility considerations for exercise prescription. In: Blair SN, Painter P, Pate R, et al, eds. *Resource Manual for ACSM Guidelines for Exercise Testing and Prescription.* Philadelphia: Lea & Febiger, 1988.
15. Bersin D, Bersin K, Reese M. *Relaxercise Based on Feldenkrais Theory.* New York: Harper & Row Publishers, 1990:3-97.
16. Satchidananda YS. *Integral Yoga-Hatha.* Holt, Rinehart and Winston, 1970;11–65.
17. Hittleman A. *Hittleman's Yoga 28 Day Exercise Plan.* New York: Workman Publishing, 1969.
18. American College of Sports Medicine. *ACSM's Guidelines for Exercise Testing.* 4th ed. Philadelphia: Lea & Febiger, 1991.
19. deVries H. Evaluation of static stretching procedures for flexibility. *Res Q Exerc Sport* 1962;33:222–229.
20. deVries H. Physiology of Exercise. Flexibility 1981. *J Phys Ed Recreat Dance* 1980;52:41.
21. Anderson B. 8 Minute Stretch. *Women Sports Fitness* 1989; Nov-Dec:46–52.
22. Krusen, Kottke, Elwood. *Handbook of Physical Medicine and Rehabilitation.* 2nd ed. Philadelphia: WB Saunders, 1971;386–401.
23. Kuland D. *The Injured Athlete.* Philadelphia: JB Lippincott, 1982:165–176.
24. Karpovich PV, Hale C. Effects of warming up upon physical performance. *JAMA* 1956;162:1117–1119.
25. Jensen C. Pertinent facts about warm up. *Athletic J* 1975;56:72–75.
26. Martin BJ. Effects of warm up on metabolic responses to strenuous exercise. *Med Sci Sports Exerc* 1975;7:146–149.
27. Kisner C, Colby LA. *Therapeutic Exercise Foundations & Techniques.* 2nd ed. Philadelphia: FA Davis Co., 1990.
28. Knott M, Voss D. *Proprioceptive Neuromuscular Facilitation.* 2nd ed. New York: Harper & Row, 1968.
29. Hutton A. Three Techniques comparing stretching of the Hamstrings. University of California, 1979. (Abstract reported).
30. Etnyre BR, Lee EJ. Chronic and acute flexibility of men and women using three different stretching techniques. *Res Q Exerc Sport* 1988;59(5):222–228.
31. Agre JC. Static Stretching for Athletes. *Arch Phys Med* 1978;59:561.
32. Logan H, Egstrom GH. The effects of slow and fast stretching on sacrofemoral angle. *J Assoc Phys Mental Rehabil* 1988;15:85.

195, 196, 197, 198,
202, 206, 207, 209, 211

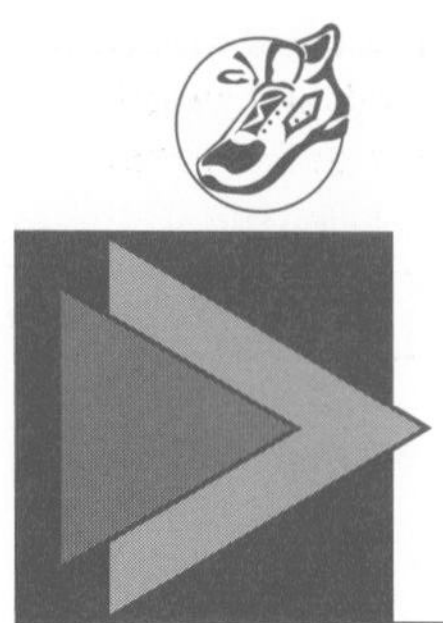

CHAPTER 55
NUTRITION AND WEIGHT MANAGEMENT

Rosemary Riley

Approximately one third of American adults are overweight (1). Obesity is associated with several chronic diseases, such as diabetes mellitus, hypertension, hypercholesterolemia, hyperinsulinemia, and hypertriglyceridemia, all of which increase the risk for cardiovascular disease (2). Severe obesity may limit the ability to exercise due to a low tolerance for activity or, perhaps, musculoskeletal problems. For individuals with severe obesity, exercise complements caloric restriction and promotes a more rapid weight loss. It can also facilitate an improvement in blood lipid profiles (3). However, complications of severe obesity may require a more aggressive clinical approach before a significant amount of physical activity can be initiated.

Exercise professionals who work with individuals involved in nutrition and weight management programs should understand the concepts of healthy nutrition and provide support for the behavioral changes necessary for successful weight management. A vital role for the exercise professional is to assist in the evaluation of programs to determine which are most likely to help the individual meet the weight management goals. The exercise professional should consult the state dietetic association to determine current regulations regarding nutrition counseling and the practice of dietetics.

SETTING A WEIGHT GOAL

Setting a weight loss goal is a complicated task, which requires negotiation and cooperation between the patient and the professional. Patients are often less concerned or motivated by health than by personal appearance. Goals should be realistic and achievable or the individual may be set up for failure.

There is little scientific consensus on the best method of setting a healthy weight goal. Body mass index (BMI) is often used to evaluate body weight. BMI is calculated from weight and height, but is not a measure of body composition. However, BMI correlates well with body fat in many populations. Since it is relatively easy to measure, it can provide a quick assessment of body composition. The National Institutes for Health has suggested that a BMI above 27 indicates obesity and a BMI above 30 indicates morbid obesity. The BMI is not as useful in defining underweight as it is in defining obesity. Nomograms are available for converting height and weight to BMI (see Chapter 70).

Epidemiological research indicates that a BMI of 21 to 22 is associated with the lowest risk for cardiovascular disease (3). Individuals with diabetes mellitus, hypertension, osteoarthritis, breast cancer, or endometrial cancer, or at risk for any of these conditions may benefit from maintaining a BMI of less than 27 (5–8). Research also indicates that significant health benefits can be achieved by losing only 10% to 20% of body weight, even if the ideal body weight is not reached (4, 9).

The Expert Panel on Healthy Weight recommends that adults maintain a BMI of less than 25.0 (10). Persons with BMI above 25.0 should develop a healthier weight goal, equivalent to a loss of approximately two BMI units (approximately 10 pounds) and maintain that weight loss 6 months before further weight loss. Obese individuals with a chronic disease or who are at risk for a chronic disease should consult a health care professional for weight reduction recommendations. These recommendations are suggested as an initial point for achieving goal weight. Intermediate goals for those with more ambitious objectives may help prevent discouragement and failure in reaching the goal weight.

ENERGY BALANCE

Weight loss generally occurs when energy expenditure exceeds energy intake, that is, when a negative energy balance is achieved. It is generally accepted that weight loss of 1 pound per week requires a negative energy balance of 3,500 calories per week, or 500 calories per day. This can be accomplished by

- Reducing daily caloric intake by 500 calories
- Reducing daily caloric intake by 250 calories and increasing daily energy expenditure by 250 calories, or some other combination of decreased intake/increased expenditure equal to a loss of 500 calories a day
- Increasing caloric expenditure (physical activity) by 500 calories per day.

The last option may be the most difficult for most obese individuals, who may not be able to tolerate the frequency, duration, or intensity of exercise needed to achieve this level of energy expenditure. A combination of moderate caloric restriction and moderate exercise is probably most likely to help the individual achieve the best result.

To improve compliance, the caloric restriction should be moderate, avoiding hunger and deprivation of favorite foods. The exercise component helps reduce stress, anxiety, and depression, which may trigger overeating. Exercise and activity can literally "get you out of the kitchen" or any location that contributes to unstructured eating. Individuals who exercise and conform to moderate caloric restriction achieve greater loss of fat mass and preserve lean body mass (11).

Exercise also establishes the types of behaviors required for weight maintenance. Research has shown that the best predictor of weight maintenance is continued regular exercise (12). Individuals can lose weight successfully without exercise, but successful weight maintenance without regular exercise is difficult.

Table 55.1. Estimation of Daily Energy Allowances at Various Levels of Physical Activity for Men and Women Aged 19–50

Level of Activity (kcal/kg per day)	Energy Expenditure
Very Light	
Men	31
Women	30
Light	
Men	38
Women	33
Moderate	
Men	40
Women	47
Heavy	
Men	50
Women	44

- *Very light activity* is defined as mostly seated and standing activities such as driving, typing, ironing, cooking, or playing cards.
- *Light activity* is defined as walking on level surfact at 2.5 to 3.0 mph such as housecleaning, child care, golf, restaurant trades.
- *Moderate activity* is defined as walking 3.5 to 4 mph, weeding and hoeing, cycling, skiing, and dancing.
- *Heavy* is defined as walking with a load or uphill, heavy manual labor, basketball, climbing, football, or soccer.

With permission from Food and Nutrition Board. Recommended Dietary Allowances, 10th ed. Washington, D.C.: National Academy Press, 1989.

DETERMINING CALORIC NEEDS

Current energy intake requirements can be determined in a number of ways, including dietary intake records, formulas that estimate daily caloric expenditure requirements for activity level and gender, or the arbitrary assignment of caloric restriction diets. See Chapter 46 for a detailed discussion of nutritional assessment.

Table 55.1 contains a list of factors that can be helpful in determining the daily energy requirements for a patient (14). The daily energy balance can be determined by simply estimating the daily energy requirement, increasing caloric expenditure (i.e., increasing physical activity) and/or reducing caloric intake proportionately.

The arbitrary assignment of caloric restriction is a third technique for meeting caloric requirements during weight reduction (13). Caloric ranges of 1,200 to 1,500 calories for women and 1,800 to 2,000 calories for men are common recommendations. Adjustments are generally made after a period of weeks, depending on compliance and results.

Caloric restriction plans of 1,200 calories or above are considered **moderate calorie-restricted programs,** or balanced calorie-deficit diets. A 1,200-calorie diet is believed to be the minimum level at which the recommended amounts of essential vitamins and minerals can be obtained without supplementation. Greater caloric restriction requires vitamin and mineral supplementation. Diet plans that provide 800 to 1,200 calories are considered low-calorie diets; plans that provide less than 800 calories are considered **very-low-calorie diets,** and should not be undertaken without medical supervision (19).

A 1,200-calorie diet, though considered moderate for many individuals, represents a very-low-calorie diet for morbidly obese individuals. For someone currently consuming 3,500 calories per day, the 1,200-calorie plan represents a 2,300-calorie deficit. This individual would be expected to demonstrate metabolic responses (i.e., decreased thyroid hormone activity, increased diuresis, and decreased blood pressure) similar to a nonobese individual on a very-low-calorie diet. The resulting rate of weight loss would be rapid, and requires medical supervision. A weight loss of 1 to 2 pounds per week, after the first 2 weeks, is considered safe. A faster rate of weight loss should be monitored by a health care professional, even when the caloric intake level is considered "safe."

FOOD PLANS

The foundation of any meal plan should be the *Dietary Guidelines for Americans,* 4th edition (1996) which includes the Food Guide Pyramid. The Dietary Guidelines encourage variety in intake, as well as moderation in fat, sugar, and alcohol consumption. The Food Guide Pyramid recommends a variety of foods, with a particular emphasis on grains, fruits, and vegetables. To incorporate these guidelines into a weight loss program, special attention must be paid to serving size and choosing mainly from food groups appearing in the lower half of the Food Pyramid (see Chapter 3.).

American Heart Association Recommendations

The American Heart Association (AHA) and the National Cholesterol Education Program (NCEP) have made more specific recommendations for a heart-healthy diet, including limiting total fat intake to provide less than 30% of total caloric intake; limiting saturated fat to provide less than 10% of total caloric intake, with polyunsaturated fat providing no more than 10% of total calories and the remainder of the fat intake provided by monounsaturated fat (15, 16). The AHA also recommends limiting cholesterol to less than 300 mg per day.

These recommendations are for healthy individuals over the age of 4 and do not limit total caloric intake. However, they are easily incorporated into a weight loss plan by specifying a number of grams of fat for dietary intake. Decreased fat is usually compensated for by increased intake of carbohydrates. Tables 55.2 and 55.3 illustrate details of the NCEP recommendations and contain a sample meal plan (16). The categories of naturally low-fat foods, such as grain products, fruits, and vegetables, allow more latitude with serving sizes, depending on the individual's caloric needs.

American Diabetes Association Recommendations

The American Diabetes Association (ADA) has also made dietary recommendations that can be used for weight loss (17). Although they were initially designed for individuals with diabetes mellitus, they represent a healthy eating plan for all individuals. This eating plan, commonly known as the **exchange system,** is also the basis of many commercial weight-loss plans. Food is divided into six groups (starches, milk, meat, fat, fruits, and vegetables) based on their carbohydrate, protein, and fat content. Within each group, a serving size for each food that yields similar calories and macronutrients is determined. These "exchanges" can be changed with other foods in another food group. As a result, these foods can be used interchangeably in creating a meal plan. The number of servings from each group is based on the individual's caloric needs for weight loss. The exchange system encourages a wide selection of food from different food groups and offers the advantage of providing an easy way to substitute one food for another while remaining within a caloric limit.

Table 55.2. National Cholesterol Education Program Diet Therapy Recommendations

	Recommended Intake (% total calories)	
Nutrient	Step I Diet	Step II Diet
Total Fat	30% of total calories	
Saturated Fatty Acids	8%–10%	7%
Polyunsaturated FA	Up to 10% of total calories	
Monounsaturated FA	Up to 15% of total calories	
Carbohydrates	≥ 55% of total calories	
Protein	Approximately 15% of total calories	
Cholesterol	< 300 mg/day	< 200 mg/day
Total calorie	To achieve and maintain desirable weight	

Table 55.3. NCEP General Recommendations for Food Choices

1. Six or more servings per day of breads, cereals, pasta, potatoes, rice, dried peas and beans.
2. Two or three servings per day of low-fat dairy products.
3. Up to 5 or 6 oz per day of lean meats, poultry, and fish.
4. No more than 6 to 8 teaspoons per day of fats and oils including fats and oils used in food preparation.
5. Five or more servings per day of fruits and vegetables.
6. No more than 4 egg yolks per week on Step I and no more than 2 per week on Step II.

Counting Fat Grams

Counting fat grams has become an accepted method for weight loss. The basis is restriction of fat intake, which also helps limit total caloric intake. Fruits and vegetables are not limited, but foods higher in fats (meats, cheeses, snack foods, etc.) are limited by a daily fat-gram allowance. Although the literature supports reduced fat intake without additional caloric restriction, epidemiological data demonstrates that Americans continue to get fatter even as the percentage of total calories provided by fat decreases (18). Total caloric intake remains the most important aspect of a weight loss plan.

Counting Calories

Calorie-counting may re-emerge as an acceptable method for weight loss, since individuals continue to gain weight as fat intake is lowered. A detailed calorie book and attention to the new food labels may allow individuals to count total calories. This may result in lower fat intake as it becomes clear to the individual that foods high in fat are also high in calories. This method allows the individual to consume favorite foods as long as the intake of other calories is reduced proportionately. The disadvantage of the calorie-counting plan is that the nutritional quality of the diet may be inadequate if the individual fails to select from a variety of food groups.

High-Protein Diets

High-protein diets with reduced fats and carbohydrates are usually associated with a low-calorie or very-low-calorie diet. They are based on the premise that a high protein intake preserves lean body mass during rapid weight loss. Examples of commercial variations of the high-protein diet include Medifast, Optifast, New Direction, and Health Management Resources (HMR).

The nutrient profiles of high-protein diets differ by the amount of carbohydrate and fat they contain. Some are very low in carbohydrates; the high protein/low carbohydrate profile results in mild ketosis. This type of diet, referred to as **ketogenic,** should contain 1.0 g to 1.5 g of protein per kilogram (kg) ideal body weight to preserve lean body mass, and should be supervised by a physician (20).

High-protein diets provide safe, rapid weight loss with dramatic improvements in many cardiovascular risk factors. However, for the weight loss to be maintained, the programs must provide intensive behavioral counseling, exercise guidelines and nutrition education. High-protein diet plans that limit carbohydrates until the evening meal are controversial and contradictory, and should be used with great caution.

General Recommendations

Health professionals should assist patients in choosing a safe and realistic weight loss plan that fits into the lifestyle of the patient. Healthy nutrition management is more than an eating plan and requires changes in other behaviors, as well. Most successful weight management programs include behavioral management in addition to a healthy eating plan. A program without record keeping, exercise, and social support should not be considered.

WEIGHT LOSS PROGRAM GUIDELINES

Selecting an appropriate weight loss program is difficult for the average consumer, given the myriad of diet/lifestyle books that promise great recipes, easy instructions and fast results. Furthermore, there are no regulations regarding weight loss programs, although the Food and Nutrition Board recently issued guidelines to help health professionals and consumers evaluate them (20). A primary goal of the document is to shift the concern from simply weight loss to weight management and improved health. The suggested means of accomplishing this attitudinal change is by emphasizing significant improvements in health and the reduction of risk factors that result from modest weight loss, especially if the loss is maintained. Three categories of weight management programs were presented:

- Do-it-yourself programs
- Non-clinical programs
- Clinical programs

Do-It-Yourself Programs

This category includes individual or group efforts to lose weight. They include Overeaters Anonymous, Take Off Pounds Sensibly (TOPS), and the use of Richard Simmons' Deal-A-Meal Plan, among others. Books, tapes, and worksite programs are included in this category. The distinguishing feature of these programs is a lack of individualization of the program by a professional.

Nonclinical Programs

This category represents many commercial programs. The program, calorie levels, and educational materials are established by a parent company and are consistent at all company locations. Examples of nonclinical programs include Weight Watchers, Jenny Craig, Diet Centers, and Nutri-System. Educational materials and program guidelines are often written by health care professionals, but the personnel delivering the program are usually lay leaders trained by the program. Often, successful program participants are used as group leaders or counselors.

Clinical Programs

Clinical programs and services are provided by a licensed professional who may or may not have special training in the treatment of obesity. They may be offered by a single health care professional or by a multidisciplinary team who coordinate the care of the individual. This team may include a physician, an exercise physiologist, a registered/licensed dietitian, a nurse, and a behavioral counselor. They may use a moderately reduced-calorie diet, a very–low-calorie diet, exercise, psychological counseling, drugs, surgery, or combinations of these modalities to help achieve weight loss and weight maintenance.

EVALUATION OF PROGRAMS

A framework for evaluating weight management programs, based both on the program and the consumer, has been developed (20).

Criterion I—Chosing the Appropriate Program

The purpose of the first criterion is to assure that consumers choose weight management programs appropriate for their needs and that the program provides resources appropriate to meet those needs. For example, a worksite program is generally not prepared to provide the medical supervision that someone with a chronic disease requires. Individuals with special needs require a program with health professionals available to provide medical supervision. Worksite programs can, however, provide social support, which is a critical factor in weight management.

Criterion II—Safety and Foundation of the Program

The safety and foundation of the program is considered in this criterion. Do-it-yourself and nonclinical programs should provide the following:

- Assessment of physical health and psychological status
- Nutrition information
- Physical activity
- Program safety

The minimum recommendation is that a self-administered health assessment be encouraged; optimally, the prospective participant should consult a health care professional prior to initiating a program. All programs should address both diet and physical activity. Weight loss programs without such changes cannot be successful in the long term.

Self-administered programs and nonclinical programs should be accompanied by minimal risk since there is little or no monitoring of health status during the program. Clinical programs should be especially safe considering the population served. The presence of health care professionals to monitor participants makes more aggressive diet and exercise strategies likely. Programs should provide information about staff qualifications and training. Credentials, qualifications, and experiences in nutritional management should be clearly indicated.

Criterion III—Long-term Results

The third criterion addresses outcomes. The four components of a successful weight management program are:

1. Long term weight loss.
2. Improvement in obesity-related comorbidities.
3. Improved health practices.
4. Monitoring the program for any adverse effects.

It is recommended that weight loss programs be judged on these components and that consumers should expect to receive information about each component when inquiring about the program.

While it is unlikely that do-it-yourself programs will evaluate outcomes, they can alert the consumer to the four issues delineated in Criterion III. The staff in nonclinical and clinical programs have personal contact with each participant, and should monitor weight loss and changes in participant health behaviors. Weight-loss programs should also educate patients with comorbidities about the potential need to adjust medications during weight loss. Furthermore, all programs should inform patients regarding the risks of weight loss, as well as the benefits.

Since long-term maintenance of a large amount of weight loss remains elusive for many people, additional weight-control program evaluation criteria have been established. These programs should be designed to ensure the following:

- Small weight losses are maintained
- Participants are successfully motivated to develop healthful eating habits
- Increased physical activity for participants
- Obesity-related comorbidities are reduced
- Quality of life improves
- Positive health-related knowledge and attitudes are developed.

Evaluation of the success of a program should not be based solely on participant weight loss, but on a variety of health-related outcomes.

▶ SUMMARY

A variety of methods are available to help obese individuals establish realistic and achievable weight goals, to provide food plans and to evaluate weight loss programs. The fitness professional has an important role in guiding the patient to the program most appropriate for the individual's needs and then to provide support through exercise recommendations and by reinforcing the behavioral strategies necessary for weight loss and weight maintenance.

References

1. Kuczmarski R, Flegal K, Campbell S, et al. Increasing prevalence of overweight among US adults. *JAMA* 1994;272:205.
2. Pi-Sunyer FX. Health implications of obesity. *Am J Clin Nutr* 1991;53:1595S.
3. Katzel L, Bleecker E, Colman E, et al. Effects of weight loss vs aerobic exercise training on risk factors for coronary heart disease in healthy, obese, middle-aged and older men. *JAMA* 1995;274:1915.
4. Kannel W, D'Agostino R, Cobb J. Effect of weight on cardiovascular disease. *Am J Clin Nutr* 1996;63S:419S.
5. Pi-Sunyer FX. Weight and non-insulin-dependent diabetes mellitus. *Am J Clin Nutr* 1996;63:426S.
6. McCarron D, Reusser R. Body weight and blood pressure regulation. *Am J Clin Nutr* 1996;63:423S.
7. Felson, D. Weight and osteoarthritis. *Am J Clin Nutr* 1996;63:430S.

8. Ballard-Barbush R, Swanson C. Body weight: estimation of risk for breast and endometrial cancers. *Am J Clin Nutr* 1996;63:437S.
9. Kanders B, et al. Long-term health effects associated with significant weight loss: a study of dose-response effect. In: Blackburn G, Kanders B, eds. *Obesity: Pathophysiology, Psychology and Treatment.* New York, NY: Chapman & Hall, 1994.
10. Meisler J, St. Jeor S. Summary and recommendations from the American Health Foundation's Expert Panel on Healthy Weight. *Am J Clin Nutr* 1996;63:474S.
11. Svendson O, et al. Effect of an energy restrictive diet, with and without exercise, on lean tissue mass, resting metabolic rate, cardiovascular risk factors, and bone in overweight postmenopausal women. *Am J Med* 1993;95:131.
12. Kayman S, Bruvold W, Stern J. Maintenance and relapse after weight loss in women: behavioral aspects. *Am J Clin Nutr* 1990;52:800.
13. Lichtman S, Pisarka K, Berman E, et al. Discrepancy between self-reported and actual caloric intake and exercise in obese subjects. *N Engl J Med* 1993;327(27):1893–1898.
14. Food and Nutrition Board. *Recommended Dietary Allowances.* 10th ed. Washington, DC: National Academy Press, 1989.
15. Chait, A et al. Rationale for the Diet-Heart Statement of the American Heart Association. Report of the Nutrition Committee. *Circulation* 1993;88:3008.
16. National Cholesterol Education Program. Second report of the Expert Panel on Detection, Evaluation, and Treatment of High Blood Cholesterol in Adults. (Adult Treatment Panel II). *Circulation* 1994;89:1329.
17. *Maximizing the Role of Nutrition in Diabetes Management.* Arlington, VA: American Diabetes Association, 1994.
18. Allred J. Too much of a good thing? An overemphasis on eating low fat foods may be contributing to the alarming increase in overweight among US adults. *J Am Diet Assoc* 1995;95:417.
19. National Task Force on the Prevention and Treatment of Obesity. Very low calorie diets. *JAMA* 1993;270:967.
20. Weighing the options: criteria for evaluating weight management programs. Washington, DC: National Academy Press, 1994. [Summary available in *J Am Diet Assoc* 1996;95:96.]

151 39 299 313

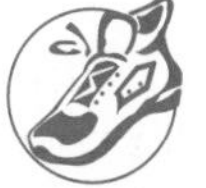   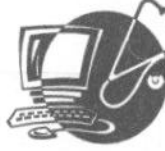

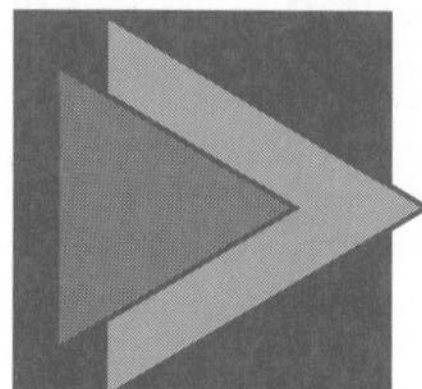

CHAPTER **56**

SPECIFICITY OF EXERCISE TRAINING AND TESTING

J. Larry Durstine and Paul G. Davis

Most athletes use training techniques that mimic movements used in competition in an attempt to train the same muscle groups required in the competitive event. For example, a soccer player spends more time in lower body training, while a kayak competitor requires more upper body training. In addition, athletes attempt to enhance specific energy systems used in competition.

Although the concept of specificity remains a basic premise of exercise training, cross-training has become particularly popular. Cross-training is the use of more than one mode of exercise (e.g., swimming and running) and/or training for more than one aspect of fitness (e.g., endurance, flexibility, and/or strength). Cross-training is often used to prevent injury, to maintain fitness while recovering from injury, or to supplement more specific training. Unfortunately, although some scientific evidence exists, much of the support for cross-training relies on testimony and could be coincidental.

Specificity also applies to exercise testing. Testing protocols that assess muscular strength do not accurately assess cardiorespiratory fitness. To test specific aspects of fitness, an activity-specific testing mode yields the most accurate results. Specificity is, therefore, an important consideration in testing or training for athletic competition, physical fitness, or rehabilitation after disease or injury. This chapter discusses specificity in terms of energy systems and movement. The applicability of combining different modes of exercise is also discussed.

ENERGY SYSTEMS AND FIBER TYPE

Adenosine triphosphate (ATP) must be generated for movement to occur. The speed and duration of movement determine how ATP is supplied for muscle contraction: Activities requiring sudden, high-intensity work, such as throwing, primarily use "stored" ATP (i.e., ATP that is already present in muscle cells); in short, high-speed events, such as the 100-meter run, most of the ATP is derived from the phosphocreatine system; in more sustained sprint events, such as the 400-meter run, energy is derived mainly through anaerobic glycolysis; and endurance activities (e.g., cross-country skiing or a marathon) rely primarily on oxidative (aerobic) metabolism for energy. Specific training is required to enhance the energy system that is predominant in energy production for a given event or sport. Likewise, an accurate assessment of the physiological characteristics required for an event requires an exercise test protocol that is specific for that event.

Endurance Training

In his early work, Holloszy examined the effects of a 3-month treadmill program on the skeletal muscle characteristics of rats and postulated the concept of specificity of training (1). Rats exercising 120 minutes per day, 5 days per week were able to run at submaximal speeds 6 times longer than rats exercising only 10 minutes per day 5 days per week. Endurance training was accompanied by a twofold increase in Krebs cycle and electron transport activity. Gollnick and King subsequently demonstrated an increase in both the number and size of mitochondria in endurance-trained skeletal muscle (2). An increase in mitochondrial activity promotes the use of fat as an energy substrate, thus delaying glycogen depletion and enhancing performance.

Endurance training is also accompanied by enhanced oxygen and substrate transport and increased capillary density. An increase in capillary density decreases the diffusion distance for oxygen and metabolic substrates (e.g., glucose and fatty acids) from blood to muscle. The concentration of myoglobin, which transports and stores oxygen within muscle, also increases during endurance training.

Substrate availability and use increases by other means during endurance training as well. Glycogen stores may increase, Type II (fast-twitch) muscle fibers may develop characteristics of Type I (slow-twitch) fibers, specifically, an increased number of mitochondria, and Type IIB (fast-glycolytic) fibers may convert completely to Type IIA (fast-oxidative) fibers (3). However, little occurs biochemically during endurance training to improve muscle strength or anaerobic power. Increased hexokinase activity, which facilitates glucose use, may be the most significant biochemical change accompanying endurance training that may affect anerobic power. Small increases in glycogen phosphorylase and phosphofructokinase (PFK) activity and ATP and phosphocreatine levels have also been reported following endurance training, but not in creatine kinase activity.

Strength Training

The primary change in skeletal muscle resulting from prolonged resistance training is increased muscle size (hypertrophy) due to an increased number of myofibrils (actin and myosin) and increased amounts of connective tissue. These changes occur in all major fiber types. During the first few weeks of training; however, these changes occur disproportionately to the gain in strength (4). Improved motor unit recruitment and efficiency rather than an increased amount of tissue seem to be responsible for initial gains in muscle strength (4).

As with endurance training, evidence of muscle fiber plasticity exists for strength training. The percentage of Type IIB fibers (fast-twitch, glycolytic fibers) usually decreases during strength training, perhaps because Type IIB fibers are either not recruited or are the last to be recruited (e.g., during a maximal contraction). As fiber recruitment increases, the histochemical properties of Type IIB fibers may change, so that they resemble the properties of Type IIA (fast-twitch, oxidative) fibers (4). The percentage of Type I fibers usually does not change.

Because a marked increase in oxidative enzyme activity occurs during endurance training, strength training may also be expected to be accompanied by increased anaerobic enzyme activity. In contrast, resistance training is associated with little change in glycolytic (PFK or lactate dehydrogenase) or nonglycolytic (creatine kinase or myokinase) enzyme activity. Additionally, muscle ATP and phosphocreatine levels do not increase.

Oxidative enzyme activity does not increase during strength training; in fact, the number of mitochondria per unit of muscle weight decreases with muscle hypertrophy (5). Myoglobin concentration may also decrease with muscle hypertrophy. On the other hand, some resistance training programs have been accompanied by an increase in capillary density (4).

Endurance and Strength Training

Endurance athletes often supplement training with resistance exercise. Athletes participating in events requiring strength often add endurance exercise to their training regimen.

Effects of Endurance Training on Strength

Endurance athletes have a lower-than-normal vertical jump. In fact, vertical jump decreases with endurance training and increases with cessation of endurance training (6). Conversely, previously inactive subjects undergoing simultaneous endurance and resistance training of the legs demonstrate improvement in leg strength and maximal oxygen consumption ($\dot{V}O_2max$) (7, 8). However, these training protocols have failed to elicit strength improvements similar to improvements identified when identical resistance training programs were administered without endurance training.

The above investigations used intense interval training (3–5 repetitions of 5 minutes each near $\dot{V}O_2max$) to improve $\dot{V}O_2max$. Under research conditions, less intense interval and continuous endurance training protocols have demonstrated that combined endurance and resistance training elicits improvement in strength comparable to that seen with strength training alone (9, 10). In addition, continuous endurance training was accompanied by an increase in $\dot{V}O_2max$ similar to that seen with intense interval training (i.e., approximately +18%) (8).

Effects of Strength Training on Endurance

Some studies have demonstrated that $\dot{V}O_2max$ increases during leg strength training, even in the absence of endurance-specific training (10, 11). However, this finding is inconsistent (Table 56.1) (12). Strength training alone and the addition of strength training in endurance-trained subjects were accompanied by increased cycling and running times to exhaustion at work rates representing 100% $\dot{V}O_2max$ without a concomitant increase in $\dot{V}O_2max$ (11, 13). Sale et al. demonstrated increased citrate synthase (a Krebs cycle enzyme) activity and an increased percentage of slow-twitch fibers in strength-trained vastus lateralis muscle (9). Increased capillary density in skeletal muscle may also contribute to the enhanced endurance demonstrated in these studies (4).

Some endurance athletes, therefore, may benefit from the addition of resistance training; middle distance athletes may benefit most, considering the increase in $\dot{V}O_2max$ and short-term endurance. Although power athletes do not gain strength from endurance training, low-to-moderate endurance training may provide benefits such as delayed fatigue, without compromising strength. Endurance training also helps maintain a desirable body composition. Individuals exercising for health and fitness should not be discouraged from including moderate levels of both endurance and strength exercise in an exercise program.

SPECIFICITY OF MUSCLE GROUP

Endurance Training

Athletes often use a variety of activities to improve performance. An improved performance may occur through cardiovascular, muscular, and neural changes. This section discusses how training these systems may cross-over to different activities.

Table 56.1. Effect of Strength Training on Endurance Variables[a]

Study (Ref #)	Training Duration		Cycle Ergometer $\dot{V}O_{2max}$ (L/min)	Treadmill $\dot{V}O_{2max}$ (mL/kg/min)	[b]Cycle Endurance (min)	[b]Treadmill Endurance (min)	[c]Lower Body One-Repetition Maximum (% change)	Fat-Free Mass (kg)
Hickson *et al.*, 1980 (11)	10 weeks	Pre-training:	3.40 ± 0.22	47.8 ± 1.5	278 ± 27	291 ± 14		[d]66.0
		Post-training:	3.54 ± 0.22*	48.8 ± 2.0	407 ± 32*	325 ± 12*		68.6
		Change:	4%	2%	47%	12%	40%*	4%
Hurley *et al.*, 1984 (12)	16 weeks	Pre-training:		36.1 ± 1.4				66.9 ± 2.6
		Post-training:		37.8 ± 1.3				68.8 ± 2.7*
		Change:		5%			33%*	3%
McCarthy *et al.*, 1995 (10)	10 weeks	Pre-training:	3.16 ± 0.12					65.9 ± 2.1
		Post-training:	3.49 ± 0.14*					68.1 ± 2.6*
		Change:	10%				23%	3%

[a] All values are listed as mean ± standard error.
[b] Endurance was measured as time to exhaustion at 100% pre-training $\dot{V}O_{2max}$.
[c] One-repetition maximum was analyzed as the average of the squat and leg extension (11), the average of the leg press, leg extension, and leg curl (12), and the squat (10).
[d] Fat free mass was not listed in (11), but was calculated from the listed body mass and percent body fat values.
* $p < 0.05$.

In addition to the metabolic changes that accompany endurance training, cardiovascular or "central" changes also occur. Central adaptation is reflected by increased maximum cardiac output ($\dot{Q}_{max}$), and peripheral adaptation is reflected by changed maximum arterial-venous oxygen difference (a-$\dot{v}DO_2$max). An increased $\dot{Q}_{max}$ results primarily from increased stroke volume; an increased a-vDO2max results from increased metabolic activity and, thus, increased intracellular use of oxygen.

Cross-training benefits are probably derived through central adaptations. This is suggested by comparisons between arm and leg performances where transfer of biochemical and neural factors is unlikely. Using arm ergometry as a training modality, Magel et al. demonstrated a 16% increase in $\dot{V}O_2$max measured on an arm ergometer compared to a 1% increase in $\dot{V}O_2$max when measured on a treadmill (14). The increased $\dot{V}O_2$max was attributed to an increased a-vO_2 diffmax, since $\dot{Q}_{max}$ and stroke volume did not change. In another study, arm ergometer training following cessation of leg ergometer training failed to preserve a leg training-associated increase in $\dot{V}O_2$max (15). In yet another study, 5 weeks of arm ergometer training in women was accompanied by an increase in a-$\dot{v}DO_2$max, $\dot{Q}_{max}$, stroke volume, and arm and leg $\dot{V}O_2$max, though $\dot{V}O_2$max assessed with arm exercises increased more than with leg exercises (16). Two different 10-week swim-training studies demonstrate increased swimming $\dot{V}O_2$max, but failed to demonstrate a change in running $\dot{V}O_2$max (17, 18). The different findings may be due to differences in the pre-training $\dot{V}O_2$max and/or differences in the training protocols (19).

Single-limb training has been used to investigate the transfer of training (Fig. 56.1). Saltin endurance-trained one leg for 4 weeks (20). The $\dot{V}O_2$max increased in both the endurance-trained and inactive legs, but the increase in the trained leg was significantly greater (23% vs. 7%). In addition, heart rate and blood lactate at a given submaximal work load decreased significantly when measured in the trained leg, only. On the other hand, succinate dehydrogenase (a Krebs cycle enzyme) increased in the trained leg, only. Results from both combined arm and leg training and single limb training studies suggest that transfer of training does result, but not to the same extent as in a more specific training mode.

In endurance training studies using the same limbs but comparing different modes of exercise (e.g., cycling vs. running), improvements in endurance were measured across modalities. Improvement may be detected better by testing subjects with the same exercise mode used in training. For example, 8 weeks of treadmill training increased both treadmill and cycle ergometer $\dot{V}O_2$max, but

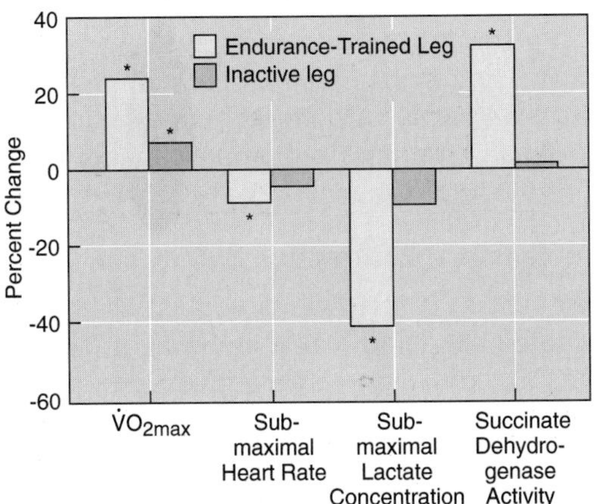

Figure 56.1. Effects of single leg endurance training on maximal oxygen consumption ($\dot{V}O_2max$), heart rate and blood lactate concentration at a given submaximal work rate (100 watts), and succinate dehydrogenase activity in vastus lateralis biopsies. In all cases, the endurance-trained leg demonstrated significantly greater change ($p < 0.05$) than did the untrained leg. An asterisk (*) indicates that significant change occurred due to endurance training. (Adapted from Saltin B, Nazar K, Costill DL, et al. The nature of the training response: peripheral and central adaptations to one-legged exercise. *Act Physiol Scand* 1976;96:289–305.)

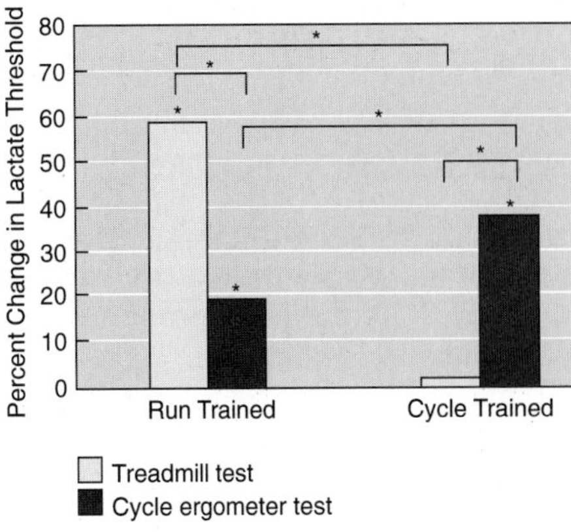

Figure 56.2. Change in oxygen consumption at lactate threshold following run-training or cycle-training when tested on either a treadmill or cycle ergometer. A large asterisk (*) above a bar indicates that oxygen consumption at lactate threshold changed significantly ($p < .05$) due to training. Small asterisks (*) between bars indicate different effects of training modes and testing modes. (Adapted from Pierce EF, Weltman A, Seip RL, et al. Effects of training specificity on the lactate threshold and $\dot{V}O_2$peak. *Intl J Sports Med* 1990;11:267–272.)

cycle ergometer training increased cycle ergometer $\dot{V}O_2max$ more than treadmill $\dot{V}O_2max$ (21). Increased function appears to be more accurately assessed using a testing modality similar to the training modality.

Pierce et al. trained groups with running or cycling at equal intensities (90% $\dot{V}O_2max$) and demonstrated similar increases in running and cycling $\dot{V}O_2max$ (22). Figure 56.2 illustrates that both modes of training result in higher $\dot{V}O_2$ at lactate threshold ($\dot{V}O_2LT$) during cycle ergometry (cycle > running), but only run training resulted in a higher $\dot{V}O_2LT$ during the treadmill exercise. This change is significantly greater than the change in $\dot{V}O_2LT$ demonstrated when cycle ergometer testing is used after run training. While some transfer of improved performance seems apparent, this study suggests that peripheral adaptation is more specific. Although the same muscles are used, cycling recruits fewer motor units than running. Therefore, biochemical changes that occur may not carry over to an activity using more muscle mass.

The above studies support both specificity and transfer of training. Although several studies indicate that central benefits gained from one mode of exercise training transfer to another mode, the extent of improvement in the training mode is usually greater. Improved $\dot{V}O_2max$ may be more likely to transfer from a large-muscle exercise (e.g., running) to a small-muscle exercise (e.g., cycling,) than vice versa. Many studies do not investigate changes in muscle metabolism; those that do, show little transfer of training (20, 22).

Although cardiovascular changes are primarily responsible for increasing $\dot{V}O_2max$, endurance may be enhanced more through changes in oxidative enzymes and glycogen storage. Finally, while transfer of training between different activities has been demonstrated, most studies of training transfer were conducted on previously inactive subjects. Therefore, the question of whether or not cross-training (i.e., the supplementation of training with an alternative activity) enhances performance is unresolved.

Strength Training

Since cardiovascular improvement does not occur as a result of resistance training, it is logical to expect strength training to be specific, with little or no transfer among motor units. However, neural adaptations occurring early during strength training are not entirely specific.

Single-limb resistance training is accompanied by strength gains in contralateral inactive muscle groups. Moritani and deVries found increased strength (35%) in trained as well as untrained (24%) elbow flexors (23). Ploutz et al. demonstrated increased strength in trained (14%) and untrained (7%) knee extensors, along with limited hypertrophy in trained muscle groups and no hypertrophy in untrained muscle groups (24). Integrated electromyography and magnetic resonance imaging indicates that fewer motor units are recruited per unit of force applied in both trained and untrained muscle groups (23, 24). These results suggest that the transfer of strength to contralateral, untrained muscle groups is due to neural adaptation. No evidence suggests that strength gain transfers to additional, untrained muscle groups (e.g., legs to arms or quadriceps to gastrocnemius).

SPECIFICITY OF MOVEMENT PATTERN

Specificity applies not only to energy systems and muscle groups, but also to movement patterns. Motor units used during training demonstrate the majority of physiological alterations; therefore, movement patterns are also specifically trained. The following factors affect motor unit recruitment:

- Body position and movement pattern
- Static or dynamic contraction
- Concentric or eccentric contraction
- Intensity, frequency, and duration of contraction

Body Position and Movement Pattern

Strength gain is specific to the angle of the joint at which training occurs. Thorstensson et al. trained subjects for 8 weeks, with free weights (squat training) and also with the vertical jump and standing long jump (Fig. 56.3) (25). Following training, a significant increase in squat strength was demonstrated, while leg press strength improved only about half as much. Interestingly, leg extension strength (measured statically) did not improve.

Body position may also affect the response to endurance exercise. In the supine position, stroke volume is near maximum. Therefore, at a given submaximal work rate in this position, the "passive" increase in stroke volume results in a lower heart rate and lower myocardial oxygen demand. These changes may permit some cardiac patients to exercise safely in a recumbent position (at higher work loads), perhaps facilitating enhanced improvement of functional capacity.

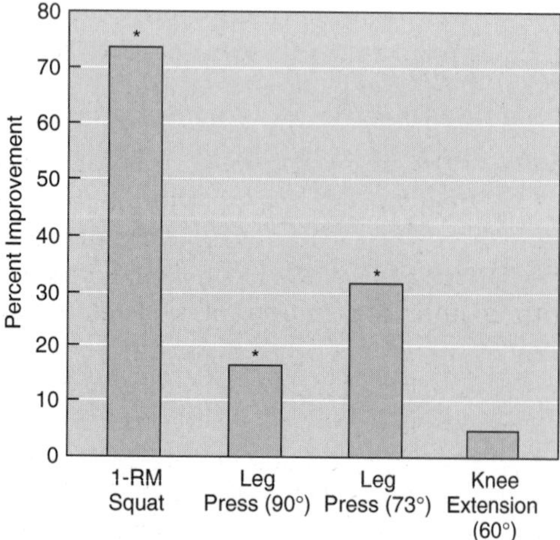

Figure 56.3. Effects of dynamic squat training on one-repetition maximum (1-RM) in squat and static strength in the leg press with the knee at 90°, the leg press with the knee at 73°, and the knee extension with the knee at 60°. An asterisk (*) indicates a significant improvement versus pre-training value ($p < .05$). (Adapted from Thorstensson A, Karlsson J, Viitasalo JH, et al. Effect of strength training on EMG of human skeletal muscle. *Acta Physiol Scand* 1976;98:232–236.)

Static Versus Dynamic Contractions

A static (isometric) contraction is applied against an immovable object and no joint movement occurs; whereas a dynamic contraction is accompanied by movement because the force overcomes the resistance or vica versa. Overload training using either type of contraction increases strength. However, the manner in which strength increases may be different. Static training increases strength at joint angles similar to those used in training. Therefore, static training is of little use for activities requiring dynamic movement. Duchateau and Hainaut demonstrated greater increase in static strength of the adductor pollicis following static training than following dynamic resistance training (26). On the other hand, a greater increase in the speed of contraction was seen following dynamic training than following static training.

In addition, static exercise accompanied by a Valsalva maneuver is contraindicated for most high-risk populations because it can produce a marked increased in blood pressure. The prolonged contraction increases total peripheral resistance and inhibits blood flow through muscle, and the Valsalva maneuver increases intrathoracic pressure, which can reduce venous return and stroke volume. These changes increase myocardial oxygen demand when cardiac output is reduced.

Concentric Versus Eccentric Contractions

There are two types of dynamic contraction: concentric (force is greater than the resistance and the muscle shortens) and eccentric (force is less than the resistance and the muscle lengthens). Lowering of a weight during a biceps curl is one example of eccentric contraction.

Although neither concentric nor eccentric contractions appear better suited for improving strength, eccentric contractions may enhance other types of adaptation. For example, both body-builders and ultramarathoners have large amounts of connective tissue within skeletal muscle, which may be a protective adaptation to cope with the high levels of force that must be exerted in these events (27). One disadvantage of having excess connective tissue may be that it inhibits motion in the antagonistic muscle. Excessive eccentric exercise also predisposes the athlete to overuse syndromes and muscle soreness (27).

Intensity, Frequency, and Duration of Contractions

In strength training, resistance moved and the number of repetitions and sets performed affects physiological adaptation. Competitive body builders, who typically use less resistance and more repetitions and sets than competitive weight lifters, often experience greater gains in muscle girth. This may, in part, be due to an increased amount of connective tissue (27). Additionally, although elite weight lifters may not continuously experience hypertrophy, strength may still increase substantially, perhaps due to an ability to recruit more motor units (4).

Fox et al. studied 8-week interval training programs of high power (19 repetitions of 30 seconds each) and low power (7 repetitions of 120 seconds each) (28). Figure 56.4 illustrates that both groups experienced similar increases in $\dot{V}O_2max$ and, although both groups had lower blood lactate concentrations after a 2-minute post-training run near $\dot{V}O_2max$, the lactate concentration in the low-power group was significantly lower than in the high-power group. Subsequently, it was demonstrated that long-duration training at a low intensity was accompanied by decreased anaerobic enzyme activity in both slow-twitch and fast-twitch muscle fibers and increased aerobic enzyme activity in Type I and Type IIA muscle fibers (29). Training at a higher intensity for a shorter duration increases anaerobic capacity in Type IIA muscle and Type IIB muscle and aerobic metabolism in Type IIB muscle. These data indicate that intense interval training is more beneficial for middle-distance events that rely on a blend of aerobic and anaerobic metabolism than for endurance performers who benefit more from longer, less intense training intervals and long-distance training.

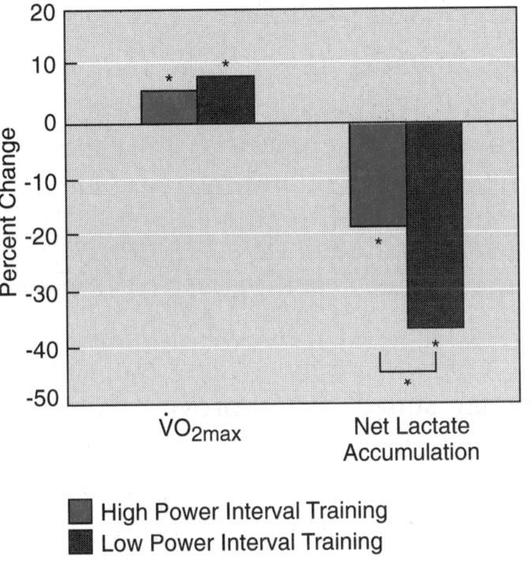

Figure 56.4. Effects of high power (19 repetitions of 30 seconds each) and low power (7 repetitions of 120 seconds each) treadmill interval training on maximal oxygen consumption ($\dot{V}O_2max$) and net blood lactate accumulation (increased lactate concentration following a single exercise session). Similar increases occurred in $\dot{V}O_2max$, but net lactate accumulation decreased more as a result of low power training than as a result of high power training ($p < 0.05$). (Adapted from Fox EL, Bartels RL, Klinzing J, et al. Metabolic responses to interval training programs of high and low power output. Med Sci Sports 1977;9:191–196)

In reality, serious competitors generally apply both types of training, but the ratio depends on the event.

SPECIFICITY AND OTHER COMPONENTS OF FITNESS

There are five major categories of health-related physical fitness:

1. Cardiorespiratory endurance.
2. Muscular strength.
3. Muscular endurance.
4. Flexibility.
5. Body composition.

This section discusses application of specificity to each component.

Cardiorespiratory Endurance

Specificity and endurance training were discussed previously in this chapter. Limited crossover of training effects exists between one mode of endurance activity and another. The most effective way to train for a particular activity is to practice that activity regularly. In addition, strength training of the same muscle group may increase endurance, but no evidence suggests that endurance training increases strength.

Specific testing protocols for assessing endurance were also discussed. A protocol inducing fatigue within 8 to 12 minutes assesses $\dot{V}O_2max$ most accurately. Uphill running on a treadmill can be used to assess $\dot{V}O_2max$ accurately, whereas a walking protocol is usually most appropriate for middle-aged and elderly subjects, if balance is not a problem. Additionally, body position and specific speed and resistance of contraction should be replicated as much as possible during training.

Muscular Endurance

Muscular endurance is the ability of a muscle or muscle group to repeat dynamic movements or to sustain static force over time. There is no clear distinction between cardiorespiratory and muscular endurance activities; both require contraction of skeletal muscle over extended time. However, cardiovascular endurance activities (e.g., distance running) are affected by cardiorespiratory limitations, and muscular endurance activities may be less affected. Muscular endurance activities (e.g., push-ups) generally require the athlete to overcome greater resistance and usually cannot be maintained as long as cardiorespiratory endurance activities. Muscular endurance activities also generally require greater anaerobic metabolic activity (anaerobic glycolysis) than aerobic metabolic activity for energy.

Training for muscular endurance can improve the efficiency of movement and acid–base buffering capacity. Trained athletes, therefore, often tolerate higher blood lactate concentrations than untrained persons.

Literature concerning the specificity of muscular endurance is scarce. Although some transfer from strength training is likely, optimal improvement in muscular endurance probably requires specific training. Therefore, training and testing should be activity-specific. Position, movement pattern, type of contraction (i.e., static versus dynamic, or concentric versus eccentric), and rate and resistance of contractions should be replicated during training.

Muscular Strength

Muscular strength is the amount of static or dynamic force that can be produced. Specificity of muscular strength was discussed earlier in this chapter. Strong evidence supports the importance of specific strength testing with respect to body position, movement pattern (including number of repetitions), and type of contraction. Single-repetition maximum testing is an excellent way of measuring strength; however, a 10-repetition maximum test may be a better indicator of muscular endurance.

Flexibility

Flexibility is the range of motion about a given joint or group of joints. Range of motion is limited primarily by the amount of soft tissue (including muscle and the joint capsule) surrounding the joint (30). Therefore, strength training resulting in hypertrophy and increased connective tissue mass may reduce the flexibility of joints involved in training. Flexibility can be increased or maintained through a regular stretching program and strength training exercises that move a particular joint through its full range of motion.

Body Composition

The two basic components of the body (fat and lean mass) respond differently to exercise training. Following several weeks of exercise training, the body composition may change slightly. The change is secondary to fat loss during endurance training, but may also be due to increased lean mass due to muscle hypertrophy in resistance training. Methods of assessing body composition (e.g., skinfold measurements), may be sensitive to certain components of body composition and, hence, may estimate exercise-related changes in body composition inaccurately.

For a significant amount of fat loss to occur, more energy must be expended than consumed. This is best achieved by reducing caloric intake and increasing physical activity. Endurance activity can be performed longer than resistance activity and is generally more useful for increasing caloric expenditure and fat loss. However, resistance training is more likely to preserve fat-free mass during weight loss and may help reduce fat (31). Therefore, weight loss programs should include both endurance and resistance training as part of the exercise program. Exercise should be prescribed to maximize total energy expenditure without undue fatigue. The optimal exercise prescription for weight control using resistance exercise remains unclear. More detailed information concerning weight control can be found elsewhere in this book.

▶ SUMMARY

A certain amount of training may be transferred between exercise training regimens. However, the need for specificity during training and performance testing is clear. In particular, the energy systems, the specific muscle groups, and the movements applied are important considerations.

Strength training may increase endurance, especially short-term endurance at high work loads. Endurance training does not increase strength, however, and may be detrimental to improvement in strength. However, moderate endurance training may not impede the development of strength and should be included in exercise programs designed to improve physical fitness.

A certain amount of training adaptations can be transferred from one training mode to another. This is primarily due to cardiovascular adaptation in endurance training and neural adaptation in strength training.

Position, movement pattern, type of contraction (static versus dynamic, concentric versus eccentric), and intensity, frequency, and duration of muscle contraction are all important factors in the specificity of muscular performance. Altering these factors during exercise training may significantly alter training results.

As specific as these points regarding the effects of training and training transfer may appear to be, it is important to note that most investigations supporting these conclusions were conducted with previously inactive subjects. The benefits of adding alternative modes of exercise to an established training regimen remain unclear.

The concept of specificity emphasizes a well-rounded program of exercise training. However, specificity applies to testing, as well. Task–specific testing is recommended for the assessment of both performance and performance improvement.

References

1. Holloszy JO. Biochemical adaptations in muscle. Effects of exercise on mitochondrial oxygen uptake and respiratory enzyme activity in skeletal muscle. *J Biol Chem* 1967;242:2278–2282.
2. Gollnick PD, King DW. Effect of exercise and training on mitochondria of rat skeletal muscle. *Am J Physiol* 1969;216:1502–1509.
3. Jansson E, Kaijser L. Muscle adaptation to extreme endurance training in man. *Acta Physiol Scand* 1977;100:315–324.
4. Kraemer WJ, Fleck SJ, Evans WJ. Strength and power training: physiological mechanisms of adaptation. *Exerc Sport Sci Rev* 1996;24:363–397.

5. MacDougall JD, Sale DG, Moroz JR, et al. Mitochondrial volume density in human skeletal muscle following heavy resistance training. *Med Sci Sports* 1979;11:164–166.
6. Dudley GA, Fleck SJ. Strength and endurance training: are they mutually exclusive? *Sports Med* 1987;4:79–85.
7. Hickson RC. Interface of strength development by simultaneously training for strength and endurance. *Eur J Appl Physiol* 1980;45:255–263.
8. Dudley GA, Djamil R. Incompatibility of endurance- and strength-training mode of exercise. *J Appl Physiol* 1985;59: 1446–1451.
9. Sale DG, MacDougall JD, Jacobs I, Garner S. Interaction between concurrent strength and endurance training. *J Appl Physiol* 1990;68:260–270.
10. McCarthy JP, Agre JC, Graf BK, et al. Compatibility of adaptive responses with combining strength and endurance training. *Med Sci Sports Exerc* 1995;27:429–436.
11. Hickson RC, Rosenkoetter MA, Brown MM. Strength training effects on aerobic power and short-term endurance. *Med Sci Sports Exerc* 1980;12:336–339.
12. Hurley BF, Seals DR, Ehsani AA, et al. Effects of high-intensity strength training on cardiovascular function. *Med Sci Sports Exerc* 1984;16:483–488.
13. Hickson RC, Dvorak BA, Gorostiaga EM, et al. Potential for strength and endurance training to amplify endurance performance. *J Appl Physiol* 1988;65:2285–2290.
14. Magel JR, McArdle WD, Toner M, et al. Metabolic and cardiovascular adjustment to arm training. *J Appl Physiol* 1978;45:75–79.
15. Pate RR, Hughes RD, Chandler JF, et al. Effects of arm training on retention of training effects derived from leg training. *Med Sci Sports Exerc* 1978;10:71–77.
16. Loftin M, Boileau RA, Massey BH, et al. Effect of arm training on central and peripheral circulatory function. *Med Sci Sports Exerc* 1988;20:136–141.
17. Gergley TJ, McArdle WD, DeJesus P, et al. Specificity of arm training on aerobic power during swimming and running. *Med Sci Sports Exerc* 1984;16:349–354.
18. Magel JR, Foglia GF, McArdle WD, et al. Specificity of swim training on maximum oxygen uptake. *J Appl Physiol* 1975;38:151–155.
19. Franklin BA. Aerobic exercise training programs for the upper body. *Med Sci Sports Exerc* 1989;21:S141–S48.
20. Saltin B, Nazar K, Costill DL, et al. The nature of the training response: peripheral and central adaptations to bonelegged exercise. *Acta Physiol Scand* 1976;96:289–305.
21. Pechar GS, McARdle WD, Katch FI, et al. Specificity of cardiorespiratory adaptation to bicycle and treadmill training. *J Appl Physiol* 1974;36:753–756.
22. Pierce EF, Weltman A, Seip RL, et al. Effects of training specificity on the lactate threshold and VO_2peak. *Intl J Sports Med* 1990;11:267–272.
23. Moritani T, DeVries HA. Neural factors versus hypertrophy in the time course of muscle strength gain. *Am J Phys Med* 1979;58:115–130.
24. Ploutz LL, Tesch PA, Biro RL, et al. Effect of resistance training on muscle use during exercise. *J Appl Physiol* 1994;6: 1675–1681.
25. Thorstensson A, Karlsson J, Viitasalo JH, et al. Effect of strength training on EMG of human skeletal muscle. *Acta Physiol Scand* 1976;98:232–236.
26. Duchateau J, Hainaut K. Isometric or dynamic training: differential effects on mechanical properties of a human muscle. *J Appl Physiol* 1984;56:296–301.
27. Stauber WT. Eccentric action of muscles: physiology, injury, and adaptation. *Exerc Sport Sci Rev* 1989;17:157–185.
28. Fox EL, Bartels RL, Klinzing J, et al. Metabolic responses to interval training programs of high and low power output. *Med Sci Sports Exerc* 1977;9:191–196.
29. Gillespie AC, Fox EL, Merola AJ. Enzyme adaptations in rat skeletal muscle after two intensities of treadmill training. *Med Sci Sports Exerc* 1982;14:461–466.
30. Johns RJ, Wright V. Relative importance of various tissues in joint stiffness. *J Appl Physiol* 1962;17:824–828.
31. Walberg JL. Aerobic exercise and resistance weight-training during weight reduction: implications for obese persons and athletes. *Sports Med* 1989;47:343–346.

31, 75, 77, 132, 133 140, 141

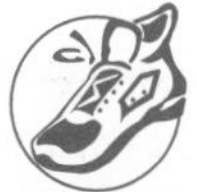

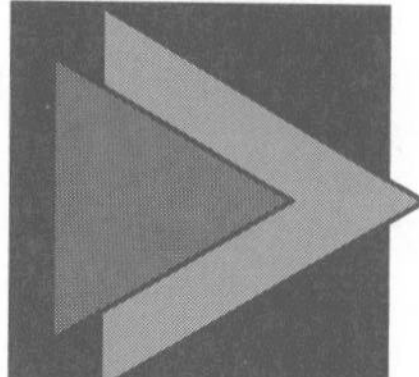

CHAPTER 57

Musculoskeletal Injuries: Risks, Prevention, and Care

John E. Kovaleski, Larry R. Gurchiek, and Daniel H. Spriggs

Most types of physical activities are considered beneficial because moderate exercise is an important element for general well being. The potential risk for musculoskeletal injury increases for all levels of participant with increasing physical activity, intensity, and duration of training. The incidence and severity of exercise-related musculoskeletal injuries can be reduced by understanding the associated risks, preventive measures, and care of the injury. This chapter identifies and describes the incidence and severity of some exercise injuries. Several etiological risk factors and mechanisms operative in injury recurrence and recommendations concerning injury prevention treatment are discussed.

INJURY INCIDENCE AND RISK FACTORS

The injuries most frequently associated with fitness-related activities are **overuse syndromes.** Running, for example, is associated with a high rate of musculoskeletal injury. Thirty-five to sixty percent of runners report injuries that resulted in reduced weekly running or required medical intervention (1, 2). The patellofemoral articulation and the foot are the most common sites of injury in runners. High-impact aerobics and dance also are associated with a high incidence of injury (3). The incidence of injury in aerobic dance is reported to be approximately 45% of students and 75% of instructors (4–6). Eighty percent of these injuries involved the lower leg and were related to high frequency (>3 times per week), improper footwear, and/or exercise on a hard, nonresilient surface (7).

With the increased interest in resistance and aerobic training, there has been an increase in the frequency and severity of musculoskeletal injuries, both from acute and overuse trauma. Despite the knowledge that sprains, strains, stress fractures, and soft tissue inflammation occur frequently during training, little is known about risk factors for such injuries.

Musculoskeletal injuries are attributed to the complex interaction of several risk factors that predispose physically active individuals to specific types of injury (8–10). Poor biomechanics is a common cause of microtrauma and is associated with overuse and fatigue. Past physical activity, current physical fitness, and present level of training also affect incidence of injury. Risk factors can be identified as intrinsic (Table 57.1) or extrinsic (Table 57.2).

Knowledge of risk factors is essential for reducing most injury rates. The sports medicine and exercise professional and participant must have an increased understanding of the short and long term risks of exercise. Improved understanding and identification of modifiable risk factors may lead to strategies and intervention to alter risk factors which may help prevent injury. The following discussion focuses on several fitness activities and those risk factors that can be encountered within the exercise setting.

Running

The overuse injury related to running is one of the most common injury conditions (11–13). Repetitive bouts of microtrauma leading to overt tissue injury cause overuse injuries. The etiologic factors related to musculoskeletal running injuries are factors related to the runner, running, and the running environment (2). Most investigations of running-related injuries involved cross-sections of runners at different levels of training (14, 15). Musculoskeletal injury increases exponentially with increased frequency and total volume of training (2, 7, 16, 17). Pollock et al. found that, with beginning jogger/runners who trained 30 minutes a day for 1, 3, or 5 days per week, 1 day of rest between exercise days may help prevent running-related injury (17). As functional capacity improves, frequency can be increased or the jogging alternated with lower impact modes of exercise.

Another common extrinsic risk factor related to overuse involves training errors. Training errors are reported in 60–80% of injuries to runners and are commonly caused by exceeding limits of duration or intensity, high rates of progression, and excessive hill running (18).

Table 57.1. Intrinsic Risk Factors Associated with Musculoskeletal Injury

- Bony alignment abnormalities
- Leg-length discrepancy
- Muscle weakness and imbalance
- Restricted ROM/inflexibility
- Joint laxity
- Body composition
- Previous injury
- Previous physical activity
- Gender
- Predisposing musculoskeletal disease
- Performing warming-up exercises
- Performing stretching exercises

Table 57.2. Extrinsic Risk Factors Associated with Musculoskeletal Injury in Sport

Excessive load on the body
- Type of movement
- Speed of movement
- Number of repetitions
- Footwear
- Surface

Training errors
- Excessive distances
- Fast progression
- High intensity
- Running on hills
- Poor technique
- Monotonous or asymmetric training
- Fatigue

Adverse environmental conditions
- Darkness
- Heat/cold
- Humidity
- Altitude
- Wind

Faulty equipment

Table modified from Strauss RH, ed. Sports Medicine. Philadelphia: WB Saunders, 1992.

Flexibility

Flexibility (range of motion) is influenced by bony and soft tissue structures surrounding the joint. Decreased flexibility is an intrinsic risk factor for musculoskeletal injury (8). Stretching exercises, performed as part of an exercise-specific training program to increase flexibility, are an important aspect of a training program. They should be performed before and after an exercise session. Increased flexibility decreases the incidence of musculoskeletal injury, minimizes or alleviates muscle soreness, and contributes to improved performance (19, 20).

Stretch refers to elongation or linear deformation of muscle and soft tissue. Stretching is important because it lengthens muscle tissue, thus increasing flexibility (and range of motion). People with decreased flexibility are at greater risk for muscle strain and musculoskeletal injury (4, 21). Jones et al. examined injuries associated with physical training among young men and observed that the most flexible and least flexible individuals are at higher risk of lower body injury than moderately flexible individuals (22).

Warm-up and Cool-down

The cardiovascular, respiratory, and neuromuscular systems can be put in a state of readiness for vigorous activity through warm-up exercises. Warm-up exercises gradually increase in intensity until myocardial blood flow and deep muscle temperature are suitable for exercise. Muscle that is not properly warmed is susceptible to injury (23). Increased muscle temperature improves elasticity of intramuscular connective tissue, increases metabolism, and increases potential magnitude and speed of contraction. Increased temperature and connective tissue elasticity may explain why warmed-up muscles can stretch to a greater length and require application of a greater force prior to being injured. Warm-up, therefore, reduces risk of muscle injury. Despite the theoretical support for warm-up, studies of warm-up do not demonstrate a clear advantage (8).

Walter et al. report that runners who "never warm up" compared to those who "always," "usually," or "sometimes warm up" have significantly reduced risk of running injury (24). This study also indicated that regular use of cool-down exercises was not associated with incidence of injury. There are some indications that training programs using stretching and warm-up can decrease incidence of injury. However, these programs have used several confounding variables and the effect of single factors has not been determined. At present, it appears that warm-up may be more important in performance than injury prevention.

Van Mechelen et al. conducted a 16-week study aimed at changing behavior with regard to warm-up, cool-down, and stretching exercise to evaluate the effect of health education on running injuries (25). The subjects were matched for age, weekly running distance, and general knowledge regarding injury prevention. The treatment was not effective in reducing running injuries. However, specific knowledge of warm-up and cool-down techniques improved in the treatment group. This finding suggests it is more effective to focus health education intervention strategies on behavior that is not conducted "naturally," such as warm-up, cool-down, and stretching. The study did indicate that modification of behavior with regard to early detection of symptoms of overuse injuries, full rehabilitation after injury, and distribution of training load are important predictors of running injury (24, 26, 27).

Other Risk Factors

Age is not associated with risk of exercise-related injury and, although several studies conclude that there are no differences in rate of injury between men and women gender, however, is a risk factor for women, participating in endurance training (1, 2, 27–29). For both men and women, contact sports cause more injuries than non-contact sports, with sprains and strains as the most common injuries (30). Whether injury rates are sport or exercise specific, rather than gender specific, is not clear. Nevertheless, structural differences (lower leg alignment, patellofemoral disorders, and foot problems) between women and men may play a role in injury incidence and type (11).

Diseases and disorders of the musculoskeletal system may directly increase risk for acute or chronic injury by interrupting normal structure and function of bone, joint, and soft tissue. The most common musculoskeletal conditions that present as risk factors include osteoarthritis, osteoporosis, chondromalacia, age-related musculotendineal degeneration, and malalignments (8).

Past exercise injury and poor physical fitness are associated with risk of musculoskeletal injury. Excessive weight has been found to predispose individuals to acute and overuse injuries as well as osteoarthritic changes in full weight-bearing, recreational activities. Physiological variables, such as low body fat and certain characteristics of body stature, may be risk factors for exercise and running-related injuries (e.g., stress fractures in females), although Jackson et al. observed no relationship between anthropometric data, physical fitness characteristics and sports injuries (16, 28, 31, 32). Definitive conclusions about the relationship between anthropometries and injury remain unclear.

Musculoskeletal injury is associated with exercise caused by a complex interaction of risk factors. In order to effectively reduce incidence and severity of injury, it is important to affect predisposing risk factors through education and clinical efforts on injury prevention.

INJURY PREVENTION

Attempts to improve or maintain fitness require awareness of injury prevention. Expanded participation in exercise results in greater potential for injury as number of participants and intensity and duration of training increase. Increased injuries has prompted development and promotion of several methods for prevention.

Pre-participation Screening

Exercise professionals should be encouraged to use health/fitness screening prior to initiating exercise programs for patients. Most pre-exercise screening is used to detect cardiopulmonary and metabolic contraindications to exercise. The American Academy of Family Physicians guidelines and objectives for pre-participation examination were developed for young athletes participating in high school and college sports programs (33). It may be appropriate to consider these or similar tools that emphasize obtaining a history of previous musculoskeletal injury.

Prevention of musculoskeletal injury can begin with pre-participation screening (Table 57.3). Identification of conditions, symptoms, and risk factors for injury along with more complete evaluation and musculoskeletal testing by a sports medicine professional should be part of pre-participation screening.

Basic Physical Fitness and Training

A well-rounded exercise program involves warm-up and cool-down, muscular strength and endurance exercise, flexibility training, and aerobic conditioning. Proper training techniques require attention to basic principles of specificity of exercise, overload, progressive resistance, and progression. Each program must be based on mode of activity, intensity, duration, and frequency. In addition, proper equipment (clothing and shoes) plays an important role in safe participation.

Warm-up and Cool-down

Each exercise session should be preceded by warm-up and followed by cool-down. These periods generally require 5–10 minutes. Prior to participation and prior to undertaking any exercise regimen, **general** and **specific** warm-up are essential. **General warm-up** increases internal temperature through active movement. General warm-up includes light activity such as jogging, stationary cycling, or calisthenics and is followed by slow stretching to enhance flexibility. **Specific warm-up** increases body and muscle temperature with activities involving movements similar to those involved in the activity. Cool-down includes light, general exercise such as walking or calisthenics, followed by stretching to maintain joint range of motion in muscle groups involved in the activity.

Flexibility Training

Flexibility training is a planned, regular exercise routine used to increase range of motion of a joint or system

Table 57.3. Objectives of the Musculoskeletal Pre-participation Screening

Primary Objectives	Secondary Objectives
Detect conditions that may limit participation	Determine general health
Detect conditions that may predispose to injury	Counsel on health-related issues
Meet legal and insurance requirements	Assess physical maturity
	Assess fitness level and performance

of joints. Flexibility warm-up is a deliberate and regular exercise performed immediately before activity to improve performance or reduce risk of injury (19, 34, 35). Although it is difficult to determine the ideal level of flexibility, a moderate level that permits efficient movement and reduces the likelihood of musculoskeletal injury is recommended (35, 36).

Cureton and Leighton discussed the benefits of flexibility in preventing injuries (37, 38). It is commonly held that a "short" muscle is more likely to be overstretched especially in ballistic activity and, therefore, is more susceptible to injury. Since the work of these early researchers, the value of flexibility exercises for prevention of musculotendinous injuries has been widely accepted, even though it is not well-substantiated (19).

Resistance Training

Resistance training supplements health-fitness programs to enhance muscle conditioning (8, 39). Muscles and other soft tissues subjected to exercise, including resistance training, exhibit increased ability to absorb mechanical load generated during activity. Evaluation is important to identify strength, muscle imbalance and flexibility deficits that occur and that appear to predispose injury. The first step when prescribing resistance exercise is to understand the components of the resistance exercise prescription. The order, resistance or load, number of sets, repetitions, and length of rest between sets should all be considered. Proper technique should be reinforced or improper technique corrected to avoid poor habits which may increase potential for injury and decrease effectiveness. Periodic review of the resistance training routine can prevent overtraining as well as enhance effectiveness by ensuring appropriate progression.

INJURY RECOGNITION

The exercise professional is often asked for advice or clinical opinion about an injury or need for referral. It is important to understand the role of non-licensed individuals in recognition or evaluation of injury. Because each situation is unique, only general guidelines are provided regarding the injury recognition process (40). See Tables 57.4 and 57.5 for a summary of common injuries, signs and symptoms, and associated causes and mechanisms of injury.

Management of musculoskeletal injuries follows a logical sequence as outlined in Table 57.6 The use of HOPS (History-Observation-Palpation-Special Tests) is especially important in obtaining information about the injury. A history of the injury, observation of the body part and limitation of movement, along with palpation of the injury provide invaluable information if obtained systematically. Performing special tests is generally beyond the knowledge and clinical skill base of exercise professionals and should be performed by a physician or health care professional specifically trained in injury examination (41).

Table 57.4. General Injury Classifications

Muscle Injuries	Major Signs and Symptoms
Acute	
Contusions	Soft tissue hemorrhage, hematoma, ecchymosis, movement restriction.
Strains	Hemorrhage, local tenderness, loss of strength/range of motion.
Tendon Injuries	Loss of strength & ROM; palpable defect.
Muscle cramps/spasms	Involuntary muscle contraction; muscle pain.
Acute-onset muscle soreness	Muscle pain, fatigue; resolves when exercise has ceased.
Delayed-onset muscle soreness	Muscle stiffness 24 to 48 hours after exercise; tenderness and pain.
Chronic	
Myositis/Fasciitis	Local swelling and tenderness.
Tendinitis	Gradual onset, diffuse or localized tenderness and swelling, pain.
Tenosynovitis	Crepitus, diffuse swelling, pain.
Bursitis	Swelling, pain, some loss of function.
Joint Injuries	
Acute	
Sprains	Swelling, pain, joint instability, loss of function.
Acute joint synovitis	Pain during motion, swelling, pain.
Subluxation/Dislocation	Loss of limb function, deformity, swelling, point tenderness.
Chronic	
Osteochondrosis	Joint locking, swelling, pain, disability.
Osteoarthritis	Pain, articular crepitus, stiffness, reduced ROM.
Capsulitis/Synovitis	Joint edema, reduced ROM, joint crepitus.
Bone Injuries	
Periostitis	Pain over bone, especially under pressure.
Acute fracture	Deformity, bone point tenderness, swelling and ecchymosis
Stress fracture	Vague pain that persists when attempting activity; local tenderness.

Injury Care

Injury management requires planning. Each acute or chronic injury should be evaluated and managed on an individual basis. This may involve immediate first aid and physician referral or simply advice about treatment and modifications of the exercise program. Regardless, the exercise professional must possess basic knowledge to deal with musculoskeletal injury.

Table 57.5. Common Acute and Chronic Exercise/Sport Injuries and Causes

Site	Condition	Injury Mechanism
Upper Extremity		
Shoulder region	Rotator cuff strain	Throwing; swimming freestyle
	Rotator cuff impingement	Use of the arm above the horizontal
	Acromio-clavicular joint sprain	Direct blow to the tip of the shoulder
	Anterior gleno-humeral dislocation	Forced-abduction, external rotation
Upper-arm	Bicipital tenosynovitis	Repeated forceful internal rotation of the upper arm
Elbow	Lateral epicondylitis	Repeated forceful extension of the wrist
	Medial epicondylitis	Repeated forceful flexion of the wrist
Wrist and hand	Carpal tunnel syndrome	Activities that require repeated wrist
	Strains and sprains	Falling on the hyperextended wrist
	Fractures	Falling on the outstretched hand
Lower Extremity		
Foot	Heel bruise	Contusion; sudden stop/go movements in running
	Plantar fasciitis	Leg length inequality; inflexibility of the longitudinal arch Tightness of the gastrocnemius-soleus muscle unit
	Retrocalcaneal bursitis	Pressure and rubbing by the upper edge of the sports shoe
	Metatarsalgia	Excessive pressure under the forefoot; fallen metatarsal arch
	Metatarsal stress fracture	Abusive training or overload; leg-length discrepancy; hyperpronation of the foot
Ankle/Lower leg	Inversion ankle sprain	Foot forced into inversion-plantar flexion
	Achilles tendon strain	Sudden excessive dorsiflexion of the ankle
	Achilles tendinitis	Training errors; tightness of the gastrocnemius-soleus unit
	Anterior/posterior tibial tendinitis	Faulty posture alignment; falling arches; overuse stress; training errors
	Stress fracture of the tibia/fibula	Overuse stress; biomechanical foot problems
Knee	Joint sprain	Direct straight-line or rotary forces
	Meniscal lesions	Excessive pressure (squatting) or shear forces
	Patellar subluxation/dislocation	Alignment abnormalities; quadriceps weakness
	Chondromalacia patella	Abnormal patellar tracking; anatomical variations
	Degenerative arthritis	Overuse stress
	Patellar or quadriceps tendinitis	Sudden or repetitive forceful extensions of the knee
	Ilio-tibial band friction syndrome	Overuse stress associated with running and cycling
Upper Leg	Quadriceps muscle strain	Weak muscles; sudden contraction as during jumping
	Hamstring muscle strain	Strength imbalance; tightness; explosive movements
Hip	Trochanteric bursitis	Increased Q-angle; leg-length discrepancy
Trunk		
Abdomen	Muscle strain	Sudden twisting of the trunk; reaching overhead
Spine	Lumbar strain and sprain	Faulty posture; lumbar lordosis; sudden abrupt extension contraction, sometimes combined with trunk rotation

Physiology of Injured Tissue

Most activity-related injuries result from macrotrauma (tension, shear, or compression) and microtrauma (**overuse** or **cyclic loading**). When forces exceed limits of the tissues, injury results and the response to injury is a systematic process of resolution. This process is similar for all types of soft tissue injuries and is also similar in bone with some modifications for bone formation through soft and hard callus formation and, finally, bone remodeling.

At the time of injury, mechanical trauma produces damage to cells. Because damaged cells cannot transport or process oxygen, nutrients, waste, and metabolites, they become necrotic. Capillaries or larger blood vessels may also be damaged causing hemorrhage. The immediate response to hemorrhaging is to activate coagulation and decrease blood flow to the area. Damage to tissues and cells from direct trauma is referred to as the primary injury. Treatment procedures have little effect on extent or severity of primary injury, with the exception of controlling hemorrhage. Swelling and additional tissue damage may continue, even after control of bleeding. Secondary hypoxic injury is likely to occur without proper treatment.

Secondary hypoxic injury results from reduction of blood and oxygen to undamaged cells and tissues as hemorrhage is physiologically controlled. In addition, internal and external pressure changes in undamaged cells may lead to further necrosis of tissue not directly affected by the primary injury. Fluid and blood plasma escaping from damaged cells produces edema. This increases in volume during secondary injury and the in-

Table 57.6. The Injury Recognition Process

1. Check vital signs and perform immediate first aid, if necessary.
2. Stabilize the individual and/or injury.
3. Identify injury:
   - **History** Subjective statements by the individual that include major complaints and a history of the injury, including description and mechanism, functional impairments, pain, and previous injury; also training level and changes, equipment used, and prior rehabilitation, etc.
   - **Observation** Inspect or look at the individual and the injured part. Note variation in size, swelling or skin discoloration, posture, gait, limping, joint range of motion, instability or deformity, and atrophy. Compare the injured part with the non-injured part, etc.
   - **Palpation** Using the fingers, carefully and gently feel the affected part, including soft and bony tissue structures. Examine for edema, skin temperature variations, deformity, point tenderness, etc
   - **Special Tests** Used to detect specific pathologies such as ligament stability, muscle strength and imbalances, circulation, etc.
4. Decide your course of action.
   - RICES
   - Referral to physician.
   - Return to activity.
5. Administrative procedures.
   - Record injury/incident in file.
   - Inform immediate supervisor.

flammatory phase. Proper treatment to control extent and amount of tissue damage and edema includes Rest, Ice, Compression, Elevation, and Stabilization (RICES).

The Healing Process

There are three phases of soft-tissue healing: inflammation, repair, and remodeling (40, 42). Each phase consists of a sequence of events that progress systematically. The optimal end result allows resolution of the injury allowing return to pre-injury level of activity. However, the end-result and length of time for complete healing is not only dependent on the severity of the injury, but also type and quality of treatment during each phase of the healing process.

Inflammatory Phase of Healing

The physiological reaction to tissue injury is inflammation. Signs and symptoms of inflammation include redness, local heat, swelling, pain, and loss of function. The purpose of inflammation is to localize injury, protect tissues from further damage, rid tissue of injurious agents and dead cells, and to prepare for the repair phase. White blood cells are attracted by chemotactic factors. Other cells that migrate to the area form new capillaries and connective tissue. Though inflammation is a necessary part of healing, chronic inflammation results when the cause of the injury is not eliminated (42, 43).

Repair Phase of Healing

The repair process begins within the initial hours after injury and is dependent upon resolution of the inflammatory phase. During this phase, proliferative and regenerative activity leading to scar formation and repair of injured tissue occurs. Most soft tissues (muscle, tendon, connective tissue) do not have the ability to regenerate the exact, specific tissue that was damaged, so healing occurs with formation of scar tissue. Initially, collagen fibers forming scar tissue are laid down randomly and are relatively fragile, but highly vascularized. Eventually, fibrous connective tissue than comprises scar tissue becomes stronger and less vascular. The following differences between scar tissue and normal tissue are significant because scar tissue is an inadequate early substitute for original tissue. In most cases:

1. Scar tissue is not as structurally strong as original tissue.
2. Scar tissue is not as elastic as original tissue.
3. Scar tissue is not supplied with as many blood vessels as original tissue.

Remodeling Phase of Healing

The remodeling phase overlaps with the repair phase because while some scar tissue is being formed, other scar tissue is being remodeled. The remodeling process involves realignment of collagen fibers so that scar tissue becomes stronger according to the tensile forces to which it is subjected. Strength of scar tissue continues to increase for 3 months to 1 year following injury. It is not uncommon for ligaments to take a year or longer to become completely remodeled. If excessive strain is placed on scar tissue during remodeling, the duration of the healing may be extended. If, however, an optimal level of stress is placed on remodeling fibers, stronger and more viable scar tissue is the result. Recommendations from a sports medicine specialist or physician for the appropriate time to begin exercise and the type and intensity of exercise following injury may be helpful for full resolution.

Treatment for Exercise-Related Injuries

Standard treatment procedures are divided into initial treatment (first aid) and follow-up treatment. Initial treatment for acute musculo-skeletal injuries is designated by the acronym RICES (42–44). Initial treatment should be administered for the first 24–72 hours depending on severity of the injury. The purpose of this procedure is to limit the amount of secondary hypoxic injury, control edema, and aid physiology of the inflammatory response.

Rest

Rest allows time to control the effects of trauma and to avoid additional tissue damage. Rest is a continuum ranging from complete rest to restricted activity (relative rest). The approximate rest time is relative to severity of the injury. Rest can be accomplished by immobilization, or with assistive devices such as a cane or crutches. Premature movement may increase hemorrhage and extent of injury, thus prolonging recovery time. Generally, pain should serve as a guide and movements causing pain should be avoided.

Ice

Application of ice is the first step in initial treatment. Ice, or some form of cold application, lowers the temperature of tissue reducing the metabolism of healthy cells. This lowers metabolic demands and controls edema, allowing healthy surrounding tissue to survive diminished blood flow and supply of oxygen. This, in turn, decreases secondary hypoxic injury (43). Cold applications are beneficial for reducing pain and muscle spasm that accompany musculoskeletal injury.

Ice is usually applied in a plastic bag, but commercial ice bags, chemical cold packs, and reusable ice packs are appropriate. An ice bag should be applied for 20 to 30 minutes approximately every 2 hours during the day. This procedure should be followed for the first 24–72 hours.

Compression

Compression controls edema and prevents fluid from accumulating in the injured area by increasing pressure outside of the vasculature. This promotes reabsorption of fluid. In addition, the support offered by a wrap decreases unnecessary and unwanted movement and may help relieve pain. Compression is accomplished with an elastic wrap or bandage.

Elevation

Elevation of an the injured area above the level of the heart (when possible) limits swelling and increases venous return by lowering capillary hydrostatic pressure and decreasing capillary filtration pressure. Controlling edema associated with injury also decreases tissue damage resulting in a smaller area of damaged tissue to be repaired.

Stabilization

Muscular spasm (termed "muscle guarding") and pain, both undesirable responses to injury, often occur in an attempt to protect the injured area. However, muscle spasm causes increased pressure on nerve endings resulting in increased pain resulting in more spasm, hence more pain. This vicious cycle of pain and spasm is commonly referred to as the pain-spasm cycle. Stabilization serves to support the injured area so surrounding muscles can relax. Early stabilization through use of braces and splints allows the muscle to relax, thus decreasing the pain-spasm-cycle.

Follow-up Procedures

Procedures that follow initial treatment are designed to allow return to the highest level of functional activity in the shortest time. Application of heat and cold are often prescribed after initial treatment is completed. Heat should not be applied during the acute inflammatory phase or when additional hemorrhage or swelling are likely to occur. The purpose of heat is to increase circulation and to reduce pain. Reduced pain allows movement of the injured part to begin more quickly with greater pain-free range of motion (42, 44).

While both heat and cold application are beneficial, exercise is the most important follow-up treatment procedure (43). Exercise is the most effective method to increase blood flow to an injured area, therefore, ice and heat should always be combined with exercise. Follow-up treatment should be directed by a sports medicine professional or a physician.

Medications

There are several medications available for treatment of inflammation and pain caused by direct trauma or overuse injury. Three non-narcotic drugs most often used are aspirin, Ibuprofen, and acetaminophen. Aspirin and ibuprofen are non-steroidal anti-inflammatory agents (NSAIDS) containing analgesic, antipyretic, and anti-inflammatory properties. They are non-prescription, over-the-counter (OTC) drugs (44).

Aspirin, a salicylate drug, and ibuprofen reduce pain, fever, and inflammation. Aspirin has been associated with a variety of adverse reactions including nausea, gastric discomfort, and decreased platelet aggregation. Although ibuprofen is tolerated by most individuals, gastric discomfort and stomach pain are indicative of poor tolerance. Acetaminophen has both analgesic and antipyretic effects, but does not have significant antiinflammatory capabilities. Aspirin-sensitive individuals should consult a physician before taking OTC pain relievers because cross-reactions may occur in individuals with known allergic reactions to aspirin.

OTC medications fulfill legitimate needs to relieve minor pain and discomfort. However, if dosage instructions are not followed, these products can be harmful. OTC and prescription medications should be discussed with a physician or pharmacist. Individuals with persistent pain or injuries that do not heal should consult a physician.

▶ SUMMARY

Musculoskeletal injury often results from the interaction of several identifiable risk factors. Since both intrinsic and extrinsic factors are involved, prevention must be practiced to reduce the incidence and severity of exercise injuries. When injury does occur, the exercise professional contributes by participating in education, care, referral, and physical conditioning of the individual. Only through educational efforts and clinical interaction between exercise professionals and sports injury specialists can prevention and reduction of exercise-related injuries occur.

References

1. Koplan JP, Powell KE, Sikes RK, et al. An epidemiologic study of the benefits and risks of running. *JAMA* 1982;248: 3118–3121.
2. Powell KE, Kohl HW, Caspersen CJ, et al. An epidemiologic perspective on the causes of running injuries. *Phys Sports Med* 1986;14:100–114.
3. Garrick JG, Gillien DM, Whiteside P. The Epidemic of Aerobic Dance Injuries. *Am J Sports Med* 1986;14:67–72.
4. Garrick JG, Requa RK. Aerobic dance: a review. *Sports Med* 6:169–179. 1988.
5. Mutoh Y, Sawai S, Takanashi Y, et al. Aerobic dance injuries among instructors and students. *Phys Sports Med* 1988;16:81–88.
6. Rothenberger LA, Chang JI, Cable TA. Prevalence and types of injuries in aerobic dancers. *Am J Sports Med* 1988;16: 403–407.
7. Richie DH, Kelso SF, Bellucci PA. Aerobic dance injuries: a retrospective study of instructors and participants. *Phys Sports Med* 1985;13:130–140.
8. Renstrom P, ed. *The Encyclopedia of Sports Medicine: Sports Injuries.* Oxford: Blackwell Scientific Publications, 1993.
9. Renstrom P, Kannus P. Prevention of Sports Injuries In: Strauss RH, ed. *Sports Medicine.* Philadelphia: WB Saunders, 1992.
10. Shephard RJ, Astrand PO, eds. *The Encyclopedia of Sports Medicine: Endurance in Sport.* Oxford: Blackwell Scientific Publications, 1992.
11. Arendt EA. Common musculoskeletal injuries in women. *Phys Sports Med* 1996;7(24):39–48.
12. Eggold JF. Orthotics in the prevention of runners' overuse injuries. *Phys Sports Med* 1981;9(3):125–131.
13. Mirking G. The prevention and treatment of running injuries. *J Am Podiatr Med Assoc* 1976;66:880–884.
14. Andrews JR. Overuse syndromes of the lower extremity. *Clin Sports Med* 1983;2:137–148.
15. Nieman DC. *Fitness and Sports Medicine: An Introduction.* Palo Alto, CA: Bull Publishing Company, 1990.
16. Blair SN, Kohl HW, Goodyear NN. Rates and risks for running and exercise injuries: studies in three populations. *Res Q Sport Exerc* 1987;58:221–228.
17. Pollock ML, Gettman LR, Milesis CA, et al. Effects of frequency and duration of training on attrition and incidence of injury. *Med Sci Sports Exerc* 1977;9:31–36.
18. James SL, BT Bates, LR Osternig. Injuries to runners. *Am J Sports Med* 1978;6:40–50.
19. Corbin CB, Nobel L. Flexibility: A major component of physical fitness. *J Phys Educ Rec* 1980;51(6):23–24.
20. Worrell TW, Perrin DH, Gansneder B, et al. Comparison of isokinetic strength and flexibility measures between hamstring injured and non-injured. *J Orthop Sports Phys Ther* 1991;13:118–125.
21. Liemohn W. Factors related to hamstring strains. *J Sports Med* 1978;18:71–76.
22. Jones BH, Cowan DN, Tomlinson JP, et al. Epidemiology of injuries associated with physical training among young men in the army. *Med Sci Sports Exerc* 1993;2(25):197–203.
23. Zarins B, Ciullo J. Acute muscle and tendon injuries in athletes. *Clin Sports Med* 1983;2(1):167–182.
24. Walter SD, Hart LE, McIntosh JM. The Ontario Cohort Study of running-related injuries. *Arch Intern Med* 1989;149:2561–2564.
25. van Mechelen W, Hlobil H, Kemper H, et al. Prevention of running injuries by warm-up, cool-down, and stretching exercises. *Am J Sports Med* 1993;21(5):711–719.
26. Macera CA, Pate RR, Powell K. Predicting lower-extremity injuries among habitual runners. *Arch Intern Med* 1989;149:2565–2568.
27. Marti B, Vader JP, Minder CE. On the epidemiology of running injuries. The 1984 Bern Grand-Prix study. *Am J Sports Med* 1988;16:285–294.
28. Macera CA, Jackson KL, Hagenmaier GW, et al. Age, physical activity, physical fitness, body composition, and incidence of orthopedic problems. *Res Q Sport Exerc* 1989;60: 225–233.
29. Kowal DM. Nature and causes of injuries in women resulting from an endurance training program. *Am J Sports Med* 1980;8:265–269.
30. DeHaven KE, Lintner DM. Athletic injuries: comparison by age, sport, and gender. *Am J Sport Med* 1986;14(3):218–224.
31. Jones BH, Bovee MW, Harris JM, et al. Intrinsic risk factors for exercise-related injuries among male and female army trainees. *Am J Sports Med* 1993;(21)5:705–710.
32. Jackson D, Jarrett H, Bailey D. Injury prediction in the young athlete: a preliminary report. *Am J Sports Med* 1978;6(1):6–11.
33. American Academy of Family Physicians. *Preparticipation Physical Evaluation.* Chicago: American Academy of Family Physicians, 1992.
34. Alter MJ. *The Science of Stretching.* Champaign, IL: Human Kinetics, 1988.
35. Aten DW, Knight KL. Therapeutic exercise in athletic training: principles and overview. *Athl Train* 1978;13:123–126.
36. Surburg PR. Flexibility exercise re-examined. *Athl Train* 1983;18:37–40.
37. Cureton TK. Flexibility as an aspect of physical fitness. *Res Q Sport Exerc* 1941;12:381–394.
38. Leighton JR. A simple objective and reliable measure of flexibility. *Res Q Sport Exerc* 1942;13:205–216.
39. Soukup JT, Maynard TS, Kovaleski JE. Resistance training guidelines for individuals with diabetes mellitus. *Diabetes Educ* 1994;20(2):129–137.
40. Arnheim DD, Prentice WE. *Principles of Athletic Training.* 9th ed. Madison, WI: Brown and Benchmark, 1997.
41. American Academy of Orthopaedic Surgeons. *Athletic Training and Sports Medicine.* 2nd ed. Park Ridge, IL: American Academy of Orthopaedic Surgeons, 1991.
42. Prentice WE. *Therapeutic Modalities in Sports Medicine.* 3rd ed. St. Louis: Mosby Year Book, 1994.
43. Knight KL. *Cryotherapy in Sport Injury Management.* Champaign, IL: Human Kinetics, 1995.
44. Prentice WE. *Rehabilitation Techniques in Sports Medicine.* 2nd ed. St. Louis: Mosby Year Book, 1994.

132, 133 114, 140 414

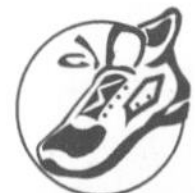
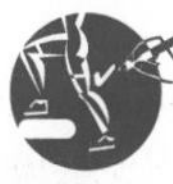
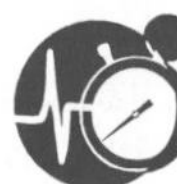

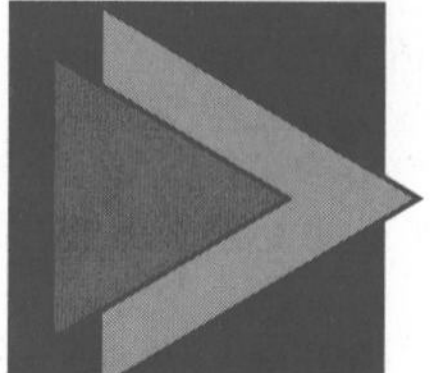

CHAPTER 58
Medical Complications of Exercise

Ben Levine, Julie Zuckerman, and Chris Cole

The potential medical complications of exercise are numerous (Table 58.1) (1). Fortunately, serious complications are rare and common complications are minor. Musculoskeletal and traumatic injuries are the most frequent hazards of exercise and are usually self-limited with only 10% to 20% requiring medical attention (2, 3). However, serious and even fatal events do occur during increased levels of activity, particularly in individuals who are not habitually active. This chapter focuses on these complications.

CARDIOVASCULAR COMPLICATIONS OF EXERCISE

Cardiovascular complications are cause for the most concern. Almost all such complications occur in individuals with underlying, acquired heart disease or congenital abnormalities. Individuals without heart disease have a low risk of a cardiac event during exercise. These complications can be divided into two general groups based on age. Cardiac problems in those older than 35 tend to be due to coronary heart disease (CHD) while those that occur in persons younger than 35 are usually secondary to cardiovascular structural abnormalities (4–6) (Fig. 58.1 and Table 58.2).

Complications in Those with Coronary Heart Disease

CHD is the leading cause of serious morbidity and mortality during high activity levels in those over 35 years of age. In a healthy population, a cardiac event during exercise is uncommon, but in those with underlying CHD, exercise may trigger an acute myocardial infarction (MI) and/or sudden cardiac death (4, 7–9). This risk was identified by Thompson in a paper reviewing all jogging-related deaths in Rhode Island over 5 years. Only one death per year per 7,620 joggers occurred, a relatively rare event. However, significant CHD was identified at autopsy in 92%, higher than would be expected based on a random population sample (4). In another review of 21 cases of sudden death during vigorous activity, CHD was present in 86% indicating that deaths during physical activity in those over 35 are usually due to CHD (7).

In the presence of CHD, competitive activity places the older athlete at a particularly increased risk of sudden death (4, 5, 10). Competition is defined as any event where external pressures, such as motivation to win and/or team participation, impair the athlete from appropriately ceasing exercise in spite of warning symptoms (e.g., chest pain or lightheadedness) (11). This problem was demonstrated in a review of sudden deaths among older athletes where over three-quarters of the fatalities occurred during competition (7). In addition, competitive activity was a factor in one-third of the jogging-related deaths in the Rhode Island study and in a series by Noakes, 20 of 28 marathon runners who died suddenly had reported symptoms of nausea, abdominal discomfort, dizziness, severe fatigue and even angina before death, but continued running (4, 12). It is, therefore, essential that all exercising adults be informed of the symptoms of cardiac ischemia and avoid continued exertion in the face of pain.

Recommendations for participation in competitive activities for athletes with coronary heart disease are found in the 26th Bethesda Conference report (11). This report suggests that athletes with CHD can be stratified into mildly and substantially increased risk groups based on the following:

- Left ventricular systolic function
- Exercise tolerance
- Presence of exercise-induced ischemia or complex ventricular arrhythmias
- Presence of hemodynamically significant coronary artery stenosis

Those athletes in the mildly increased risk group may participate in low dynamic and low or moderate static

Table 58.1. Potential Medical Complications of Exercise

Cardiovascular Complications
- Cardiac arrest
- Ischemia
  - Angina
  - Myocardial infarction
- Arrhythmias
  - Superventricular tachycardia
  - Atrial fibrillation
  - Ventricular tachycardia
  - Ventricular fibrillation
  - Bradyarrhythmias
  - Bundle branch blocks
  - AV nodal blocks
- Congestive heart failure
- Hypertension
- Hypotension
- Aneurysm rupture
- Underlying medical conditions predisposing to increased complications
  - Hypertrophic cardiomyopathy
  - Coronary artery anomalies
  - Idiopathic left ventricular hypertrophy
  - Marfan syndrome
  - Aortic stenosis
  - Right ventricular dysplasia
  - Congenital heart defects
  - Myocarditis
  - Pericarditis
  - Amyloidosis
  - Sarcoidosis
  - Long QT syndrome
  - Sickle-Cell trait

Metabolic Complications
- Volume depletion
- Dehydration
- Rhabdomyolysis
  - Renal failure
- Electrolyte disturbances

Thermal Complications
- Hyperthermia
  - Heat rash
  - Heat cramps
  - Heat syncope
  - Heat exhaustion
  - Heat stroke
- Hypothermia
- Frostbite

Pulmonary Complications
- Exercise induced asthma
- Bronchospasm
- Pulmonary embolism
- Pulmonary edema
- Pneumothorax
- Exercise-induced anaphylaxsis
- Exacerbation of underlying pulmonary disease

Gastrointestinal Complications
- Vomiting
- Cramps
- Diarrhea

Endocrine Complications
- Amenorrhea
- Complications in diabetics
  - Hypoglycemia
  - Hyperglycemia
  - Retinal hemorrhage
- Osteoporosis

Neurologic Complications
- Dizziness
- Syncope (fainting)
- Cerebral vascular accident (stroke)
- Insomnia

Musculoskeletal Complications
- Mechanical injuries
- Back injuries
- Stress fractures
- Carpal tunnel syndrome
- Joint pain/injury
- Muscle cramps/spasms
- Tendonitis
- Exacerbation of musculoskeletal diseases

Overuse Complications
- Overuse syndromes
- Over-training
- Over-exercising
- Shin splints
- Plantar fasciitis

Traumatic Injuries
- Bruises
- Strains and sprains
- Muscle and tendon tears and ruptures
- Fractures
- Contusions and lacerations
- Bleeding
- Crush injuries
- Blunt trauma
- Internal organ injury
  - Splenic rupture
  - Myocardial contusion
- Drowning
- Head injuries
- Eye injuries
- Death

competitive activity, but generally should not participate in intensely competitive activities. However, it was acknowledged that specific individuals with preserved left ventricular function, high exercise capacity and no evidence of inducible ischemia could be cleared for higher intensity competition. Those in the substantially increased risk group should restrict activities to low intensity, competitive sports. The Bethesda report offers a complete discussion of this topic including criteria for risk stratification (11).

Although more frequently seen in those over 35 years, coronary artery disease is occasionally identified as the cause of death in young athletes. For example, Maron identified three individuals ages 14, 19 and 28 years who died of premature atherosclerotic coronary artery disease (6). Eliciting a family history of premature atherosclerotic disease or unexplained death at an early age is crucial in screening. In addition, cholesterol screening can help identify those at risk.

The presence of documented CHD does not imply that all exercise must be curtailed. In fact, the risk of an adverse cardiovascular event is reduced by regular physical activity (8, 13, 14). This was demonstrated by Siscovick who retrospectively examined 133 deaths due to cardiac arrest and classified them according to activity level at time of cardiac arrest and by the amount of habitual vigorous activity. He documented that the overall risk of sudden cardiac death in habitually vigorous men was 40% less than in sedentary men (13). A similar reduction has been identified for the risk of acute MI. Mittleman interviewed 1,228 patients following MI and classified them according to frequency of heavy physical exertion per week. Those who were the most active had an almost 100 fold lower risk of onset of MI during heavy physical exertion, demonstrating the benefits of exercise in persons with CHD (8). Finally, regular exercise has clearly been shown to be an important factor in reducing the risk of CHD mortality and is to be encouraged in virtually all able individuals (14).

Complications in Those with Cardiac Structural Defects

While CHD is the leading cause of death during exercise in older individuals, anatomic structural defects are the foremost cause of sudden death in young athletes. All of these congenital abnormalities are rare, but the most common abnormalities are hypertrophic cardiomyopathy, coronary artery anomalies, and Marfan syndrome.

These three defects account for almost three-quarters of 158 deaths in young competitive athletes examined by Maron between 1985 and 1995 (Fig. 58.1) (6).

Hypertrophic Cardiomyopathy

Hypertrophic cardiomyopathy (HCM) and the closely related idiopathic concentric left ventricular hypertro-

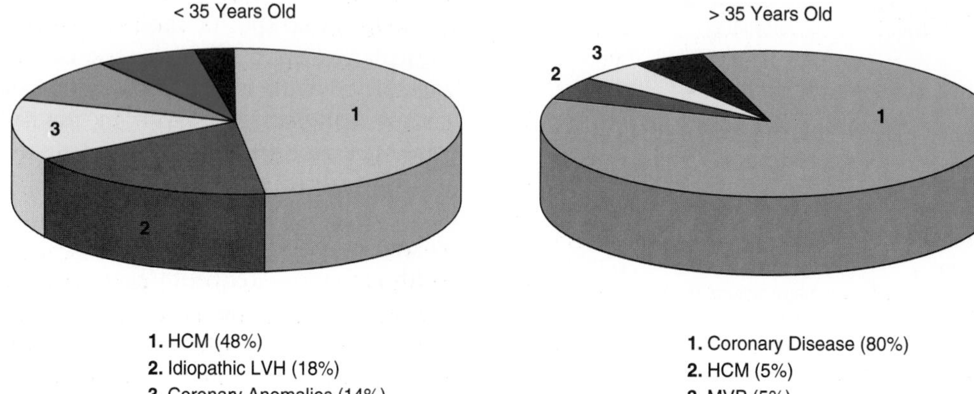

Figure 58.1. Causes of sudden death in athletes divided by age. (With permission from Maron BJ, et al. Causes of sudden death in competitive athletes. *J Am Coll Cardiol* 1996;7(1):204–214.)

phy, is the single most common abnormality found on autopsy in young athletes who die suddenly (5, 6). HCM is a genetic condition resulting in asymmetric thickening of the left ventricle, particularly the septum; it occurs in about 0.1% of the general population (15). Diastolic filling is impaired and, in about 25% of cases, is accompanied by left ventricular outflow tract obstruction. Symptoms may or may not be present and include dyspnea, angina, lightheadedness and syncope during exertion. Even when symptoms are absent, HCM may often be detected by physical examination. Physical findings include right-sided fourth heart sound, systolic ejection murmur along the left sternal border and systolic murmur at the apex increasing with amyl nitrate inhalation, assuming upright posture, or Valsalva maneuver.

HCM has a variable clinical course due to the wide spectrum of disease severity. Many individuals are asymptomatic and unaware of its presence. There is however a definite increased risk of death with HCM and the annual mortality rate reaches 1% (15). This risk is increased by heavy physical exertion. The mechanism whereby activity leads to sudden death is complex; arrhythmias (ventricular tachycardia/ventricular fibrillation) resulting from myofibrillar disarray as well as hypotension precipitated by exercise-related tachycardia both play a role. Arrhythmias occur as frequently in those with or without left ventricular outflow tract obstruction, with or without symptoms, even after surgical correction. Because of the high risk of a cardiac event during strenuous exercise, patients with HCM should not participate in most competitive sports except for those of low intensity. For additional information, review the Bethesda guidelines for high risk subsets (11).

Anomalous Coronary Artery

The second largest group of structural defects in young athletes who die suddenly are anomalous coronary arteries (Fig. 58.2). These arteries arise from and/or course through atypical locations and occasionally, due to anatomic position, an interruption of blood flow occurs resulting in sudden death. The risk of occlusion (blockage) is particularly high during or immediately after exercise.

All coronary artery anomalies are rare, but most common are the following:

- Left coronary artery arising from the anterior sinus of Valsalva (right cusp of the aortic valve) and coursing between the aorta and pulmonary trunk (Fig. 58.3) (16)
- Mural left anterior descending artery (LAD), which involves a tunneled segment of the LAD into the ventricular wall (17)

Less common coronary anomalies resulting in sudden death include the following:

- Single coronary artery
- Hypoplastic coronary arteries (small size or shortened course)
- Intussusception (inward convulsion) of a coronary artery
- Aneurysm of the coronary artery
- Acute-angled takeoff of the left main coronary artery (18, 19)

Marfan Syndrome

Marfan syndrome is an inherited connective tissue disease that predisposes affected individuals to develop aortic aneurysm. This condition is suspected in tall thin individuals (such as basketball or volleyball players) with physical characteristics consistent with Marfan's and a family history of sudden death. Possible physical find-

Table 58.2. Cardiovascular Abnormalities in 134 Young Competitive Athletes With Sudden Death

Primary Cardiovascular Lesion	No. (%) of Athletes	Median Age (Range)
Hypertrophy cardiomyopathy	48 (36.0)	17.0 (13–28)
Unexplained increase in cardiac mass[a]	14 (10.0)	17.0 (14–24)
Aberrant coronary arteries[b]	17 (13)	15.0 (12–23)
Other coronary anomalies	8 (6.0)	17.5 (14–40)
Ruptured aortic aneurysms[c]	6 (5.0)	17.0 (16–31)
Tunneled left anterior descending coronary artery	6 (5.0)	17.5 (14–20)
Aortic valve stenosis	5 (4.0)	14.0 (14–17)
Lesion consistant with myocarditis	4 (3.0)	15.5 (13–16)
Idiopathic dilated cardiomyopathy	4 (3.0)	18.0 (18–21)
Arrhythmogenic right ventricular dysplasia	4 (3.0)	16.0 (15–17)
Idiopathic myocardial scarring	4 (3.0)	20.0 (14–27)
Mitral valve prolapse[c]	3 (2.0)	16.0 (15–23)
Atherosclerotic coronary artery disease	3 (2.0)	19.0 (14–28)
Other congenital heart disease[d]	2 (1.5)	13.5 (12–15)
Long QT syndrome[e]	1 (0.5)	
Sarcoidosis	1 (0.5)	
Sickle cell trait[f]	1 (0.5)	
"Normal" heart[g]	3 (2.0)	18 (16–21)

[a] Includes 1 athlete with grossly normal heart but distinctly abnormal histologic architecture with marked disorganization of cardiac muscle cells and bundles, also, 2 of the 13 athletes with mildly increased mass had associated tunneled left anterior descending artery.
[b] Anomalous origin of the left main coronary artery from the right sinus of Valsalva in 13 (1 of these also showed acute-angled takeoff of the right coronary artery and 1 had a tunneled segment of LAD), anomalous origin of the right coronary artery from the left sinus of Valsalva in 2, anomalous origin of the left margin coronary artery (from between the left and posterior cusps) with acute-angled takeoff in 1, and origin of the LAD coronary artery from the pulmonary trunk in 1.
[c] Marfan syndrome was also present in 3 athletes with ruptured aortic aneurysm and in 1 with mitral valve prolapse.
[d] One athlete with secundum atrial septal defect and 1 with coarctation of the aorta.
[e] Also had anomalous origin of the right coronary artery from the left sinus of Valsalva.
[f] Judged to be the probable cause of death in the absence of any identifiable structural coardivascular abnormality.
[g] Absence of structural heart disease on standard autopsy examination.
With permission from Maron BJ, *et al.* Sudden death in young competitive athletes. JAMA 276:199–204, 1996.

ing include an outflow murmur and the presence of a pulsatile mass in the abdomen. If suspected, aneurysms can be screened with ultrasound. If undetected, these aneurysms may rupture during vigorous activity and cause death (20).

Diagnosis

Most underlying congenital conditions are difficult to detect. Of 134 athletes who died suddenly only 4 (3%) were suspected of having cardiovascular disease on routine prescreening physical exam and the cardiovascular abnormality responsible for death was correctly identified in only 1 (0.9%) prior to death (6). HCM may be suspected on finding an outflow murmur during physical exam or from a family history of sudden death at a young age and can be confirmed with echocardiography. However, routine screening of athletes with echocardiography is not cost-effective (21). Coronary artery anomalies, in contrast, are very difficult to identify prospectively. However, there may be prior episodes of syncope, exertional angina, or resting electrocardiographic (ECG) abnormalities (16). Some types of anomalous arteries may be excluded by echocardiography, but may be clearly visualized with magnetic resonance imaging. Those who are identified, particularly with the left coronary artery arising from the right cusp of the aorta, should not participate in competitive sports unless they have undergone surgical correction (11).

COMPLICATIONS OF EXERCISE TESTING

An exercise test is heavy physical exertion performed by an individual in a controlled setting. As such, the same complications seen in the general population during increased activity may occur. Most of these are, as in the general population, rare and range from minor to serious. To measure the level of risk, Atterhog prospectively studied 50,000 exercise tests in an unselected, clinical population (22). Documented complications were as follows: 2 deaths (0.4 per 10,000 tests); 2 cardiac arrests (0.4 per 10,000 tests) one of which died; 7 MIs (1.4 per 10,000) including one death; 2 cases of pulmonary edema (0.4 per 10,000 tests); and 2 cerebral vascular events (0.4 per 10,000 tests) (22). These rates were higher than those of a large retrospective study of 1,741,106 exercise tests done in the general population where 0.11 MIs and 0.02 fatal MIs occurred per 10,000 tests (23). Of those patients with complications almost 90% had suspected or proved heart disease reinforcing that those with CHD are at increased risk for cardiac events during exercise (22,23).

In those without known heart disease, exercise testing is a very low risk procedure. For example, no complications occurred in 380,000 exercise tests done in young individuals presumed to be free of heart disease (23). In addition, of 71,914 exercise tests performed at a single institution as part of a preventive medicine program only one cardiac complication occurred among persons without known CHD (24).

Arrhythmic Complications

Arrhythmias can be precipitated by exercise and may be encountered during exercise testing and cardiac rehabilitation. Two of the most serious arrhythmias are ventricular fibrillation (VFIB) and ventricular tachycardia (VTACH). Most cases of VFIB during exercise in the general population are fatal because they are not identified

Causes of Sudden Death in High School/College Athletes (1983-93)

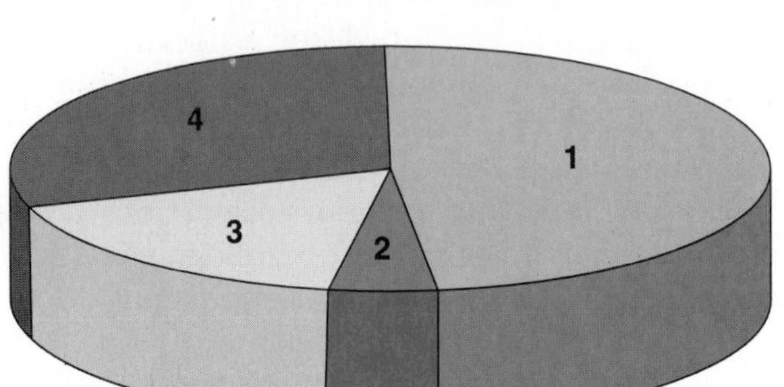

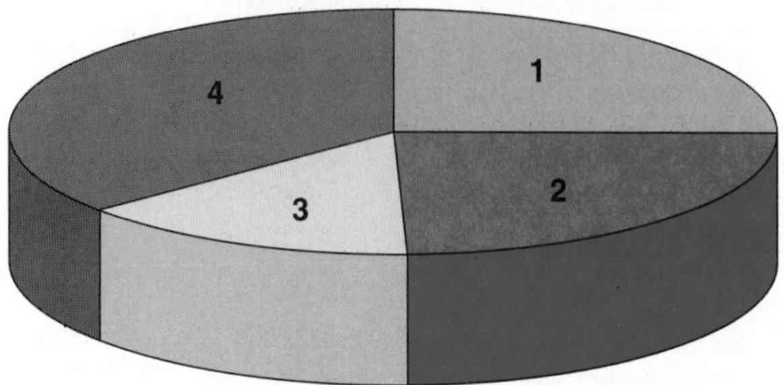

1. Hypertrophic Cardiomyopathy (48%)
2. Probable Hypertrophic Cardiomyopathy (5%)
3. Coronary Artery anomaly (14%)
4. Other (33%)

1. Intramural LAD (25%)
2. Anomalous Origin of LCA from R Sinus of Valsalva (24%)
3. Anomalous Origin of LCA from PA (13%)
4. Other (38%)

*22% of all deaths due to noncardiovascular causes

Figure 58.2. Causes of sudden death in high school/college athletes (1983–93). (With permission from Van Camp SP, et al. Nontraumatic sports deaths in high school and college athletes. *Med Sci Sports Exerc* 1995;27:641–647.)

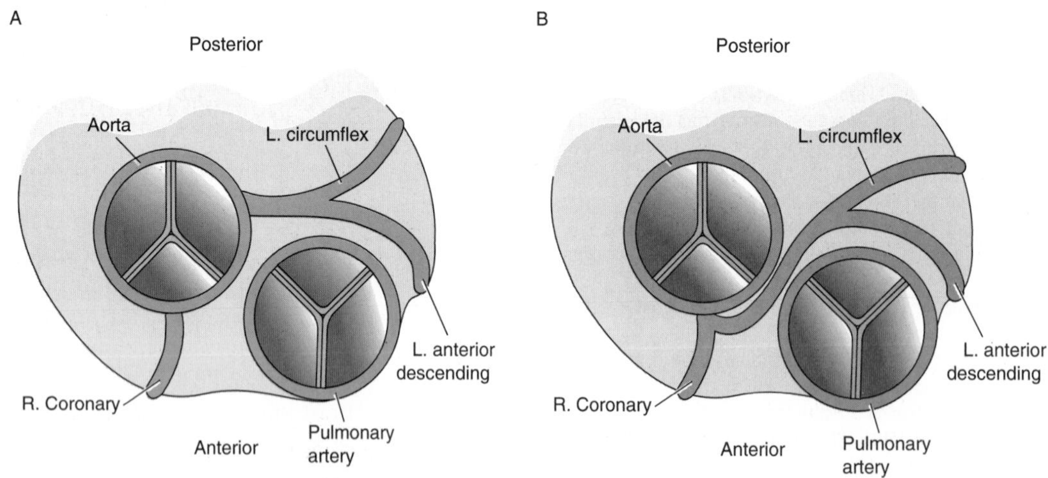

Figure 58.3 **A** and **B**. Anomalous coronary arteries.

and treated. During exercise testing and cardiac rehabilitation, however, participants are closely monitored and VFIB may be identified and its prevalence determined.

VTACH is a rapid arrhythmia of the ventricles that can degenerate to VFIB and usually suggests the presence of myocardial scar, rather than myocardial ischemia. It is slightly more common than VFIB and was found to arise 29 times in 50,000 exercise tests (5.8/10,000 tests) (22). Both VTACH and VFIB require immediate treatment with direct current cardioversion with a defibrillator.

Other arrhythmias that may occur during exercise testing are the following: atrial tachycardia (2/10,000 tests), sinus bradycardia (0.8/10,000 tests), atrial fibrillation (0.8/10,000 tests), atrioventricular (AV) nodal tachycardia (0.4/10,000), atrial flutter, second degree AV block and left bundle branch block (0.2/10,000 tests) (22). Arrhythmias are more likely to occur in those with a history of arrhythmia. Of 263 patients with a prior arrhythmia 24 (9.1%) had a subsequent arrhythmia during maximal exercise testing. In 3,444 patients with no history of conduction disturbance only 4 (0.1%) had sustained tachyrhythmia or bradycardia during testing (26). Therefore, for maximum safety persons trained in recognition and treatment of arrhythmias should be present during exercise testing and rehabilitation of high risk individuals.

Hemodynamic Complications

Besides monitoring electrical activity of the heart, monitoring of blood pressure should also be conducted during exercise testing. During dynamic upright exercise on a treadmill, systolic blood pressure (SBP) normally rises and diastolic blood pressure (DBP) remains the same or decreases slightly. Monitoring may reveal either a hypertensive (high blood pressure) or hypotensive (low blood pressure) response. A hypertensive response to exercise may occur in individuals with underlying hypertension. Relative indications to terminate exercise testing are a SBP > 260 or a DBP > 115 (27). Hypotension during exercise is a more ominous finding. A drop in SBP of greater than 20 mm Hg or a drop below resting standing blood pressure is strongly suggestive of extensive myocardial ischemia and is an absolute indication to stop the test (28).

Contraindications to Exercise Testing

Because exercise testing is a potentially dangerous procedure, it is crucial to identify those individuals at increased risk for complications and exclude them when necessary. All personnel involved in performing exercise testing should be familiar with contraindications categorized as absolute and relative. There are published guidelines for contraindications to exercise testing (27, 29).

In general, absolute contraindications are those conditions that could be aggravated by exercise or that may affect exercise performance. For example, exercise testing in an individual with unstable angina could precipitate MI or fatal arrhythmia. Severe aortic stenosis, dissecting aneurysm, and myocarditis increase the risk of a fatal complication. These contraindications are empirical, rather than based on clinical studies.

The experience level of the personnel conducting the test, access to emergency medical equipment and services, and the benefit of testing should be considered in the decision as to whether a safe exercise test can be performed with relative contraindications. In some cases, a decision to defer testing until the individual is treated and more stable is appropriate. Changes in the mode and protocol for exercise and/or endpoints for stopping the test can contribute to the safety of the test in some cases. The ability to monitor changes in the ECG and blood pressure is critical and the presence of a health care professional with extensive experience in exercise testing and a low threshold for stopping the test are crucial when the decision is made to proceed with testing.

Absolute and Relative Indications to Stop an Exercise Test

Indications to stop an exercise test are categorized as relative and absolute (27, 29, 31). Terminating a test is dependent upon the expertise and judgment of those supervising the exercise test. As with the contraindications, the setting and indications for the test may influence test termination. Increasing angina, hypotension, signs and symptoms of myocardial ischemia and serious arrhythmias are serious problems that may precipitate test termination. Other reasons, such as the technical inability to monitor the ECG and patient request are self-evident.

Relative indications for termination of an exercise test are findings that increase the level of concern and vigilance in those administering the test. Relative indications for termination rely heavily on the judgment of the personnel supervising the test and the decision to continue with the test should be made by an experienced health care professional, preferably with a physician in attendance or accessible during the test. In general, high risk patients should be treated more cautiously with a tendency to stop the test sooner, rather than later. In contrast, for low risk patients, interpretation of the relative contraindications may be more liberal.

Follow-Up After Terminating an Exercise Test

If an exercise test is terminated, the health care personnel supervising the test must carry out the appropriate course of action. Appropriate follow-up may include any or all of the following:

1. Notification of and attendance by a physician if one was not present during the exercise test.
2. Careful observation of ECG, blood pressure, and other signs and symptoms until the condition subsides or stabilizes.
3. Treatment (i.e., arrhythmias or angina) when qualified medical personnel are in attendance.
4. Phone contact with primary and/or referring physicians.
5. Transport to an emergency room or physician office.
6. Access to the emergency medical system.

Regardless of the course of action, documentation including ECG tracings, blood pressure recordings, and all test results should be provided to the physician.

COMPLICATIONS OF CARDIAC REHABILITATION

As previously discussed, habitual exercise decreases the risk of a cardiac event in those with CHD (8, 9). This important principle forms the basis for cardiac rehabilitation. Cardiac rehabilitation is an important aspect of post-ischemic care (patients who have unstable angina, have experienced MI or have undergone coronary artery bypass grafting) because it not only restores lost functional capacity, but also has beneficial effects on mortality. Because all of these individuals have CHD, the risk of complications is higher than the general population but is still, in general, low (30).

At one cardiac rehabilitation program, there were 5 episodes of exercise-induced VFIB during 75,000 person hours of supervised exercise (25). This would translate to one episode of VFIB a year for a program with 100 participants that met three times a week for an hour. All of these individuals had underlying CHD; in healthy participants, VFIB would be much less common.

Table 58.3 lists studies that have examined the risks exercise in apparently healthy individuals as well as of participants in cardiac rehabilitation programs (29). Two of the larger studies rely on data collected from surveys of cardiac rehabilitation centers. One survey done in 1978 found 1 non-fatal cardiac event for every 34,673 person-hours of cardiac rehabilitation activity and one death for every 116,402 hours of activity (31). The risk has since decreased. In a recent survey, the rates of non-fatal and fatal cardiac complications were 1 event per every 90,458 hours of activity and 1 event per every 783,972 hours of activity respectively; a further indication of the low risk of rehabilitation-induced complications (32). These events generally occurred when heart rate guidelines were exceeded, giving support to the importance of supervised, monitored exercise in high risk patients.

NONCARDIOVASCULAR COMPLICATIONS OF EXERCISE

Temperature-Related Complications

Temperature-related complications of exercise are a leading cause of noncardiovascular deaths in young athletes (5). Heat injury is a function of environment, degree of exposure, intensity of exercise, prior conditioning and the presence of pre-existing physical illnesses. Athletes are more prone to develop heat illness when they are not acclimatized to hot weather, are wearing heavy clothing (such as full football gear), are dehydrated, have sickle cell trait and/or are in a hot and humid climate (33).

Under these conditions a wide range of complications occur, ranging from minor to potentially fatal. The illnesses that may be precipitated by exercise in warm climates are heat rash, heat cramps, heat syncope, heat exhaustion and exertional heat stroke. Most of these problems are benign and self-limited, but heat exhaustion and exertional heat stroke are more serious conditions and may be fatal if not properly treated.

Table 58.3. Risk of Sudden Cardiac Arrest During Exercise Training

Study	Status	Activity	Monitoring	Supervision	Sudden cardiac arrests, events per hour
In the general population					
Vuori *et al.*	normal	cross-country skiing	none	none	1/600,000
Gibbons *et al.*	normal	jogging swimming tennis	none	none	1/375,000
Thompson *et al.*	normal	jogging	none	none	1/396,000
Vander	normal	jogging court games	none	none	1/888,000
Average for general population					1/565,000
Individuals with known heart disease					
Fletcher and Cantwell	cardiac	jogging	intermittent	present	1/6000
Leach *et al.*	cardiac	jogging	intermittent		1/12,000
Mead *et al.*	cardiac	jogging	intermittent	present	1/6000
Hartley	cardiac	jogging	intermittent	present	1/6000
Hossack and Hartwig	cardiac	jogging	none	present	1/65,185
Haskell	cardiac	mixed	intermittent	present	1/22,028
Van Camp and Peterson	cardiac	mixed	continuous	present	1/117,333
Hartley	cardiac	bicycling walking	intermittent	none	1/70,000
Fletcher	cardiac	mixed	intermittent	present	0/70,200
Average all cardiac					1/59,142

With permission from Fletcher GF, *et al.* Exercise Standards: A statement for healthcare professionals from the American Heart Association. Circulation 91(2):580–615, 1995.

Heat exhaustion is characterized by symptoms of intense thirst, goose-flesh, dizziness, fatigue, rapid pulse, muscle cramps, nausea and vomiting, syncope and, in advanced stages, circulatory failure. Heavy sweating usually persists throughout the course of illness. Core temperature remains < 40°C (104°F) and there is an absence of tissue injury. Heat exhaustion may progress to heat stroke.

Heat stroke is differentiated from heat exhaustion in that core temperature rises above 41°C (105.8°F) resulting in significant tissue injury. The skin may feel cool and the athlete often shivers, making it important to obtain core temperature for the diagnosis. Sweating may cease in heat stroke in contrast with heat exhaustion. When this occurs, body temperature regulation is lost and a true medical emergency arises. There may be associated mental status changes which may progress to convulsions and/or coma. Rhabdomyolysis, acute renal failure, hemolysis, myocardial infarction, hyperkalemia, hepatic necrosis can also develop and, if untreated, death often follows (34).

To treat heat exhaustion and exertional heat stroke, the victim should be moved to a cooler environment and the body cooled with fans, ice and wet cloths. Excessive clothing must be removed and the feet elevated. Intake of oral fluids should be encouraged. Heat stroke requires additional more intensive treatment (chilled intravenous saline and possibly hospitalization), but the above actions may be performed until trained medical personnel are present.

Heat illness may be prevented by avoiding the extremes of weather or by gradual adaptation to activity in hot climates. It is recommended that athletes curtail activities when the wet bulb-globe temperature, a measure of temperature, humidity and radiation index, is greater than 28°C (82°F) (35). In addition, maintaining adequate hydration is an important aspect of prevention.

Hydration-Related Complications

To maintain body temperature in a physiological range during exercise, sweating is necessary to promote heat loss. Water and electrolytes, mainly sodium and chloride, are lost in sweat. During prolonged exercise, this loss leads to dehydration (a loss of more water than sodium with a resulting rise in serum sodium) which impairs exercise performance. The amount lost is determined by the rate of sweating (dependent upon intensity of exertion), ambient temperature and humidity, amount of clothing and acclimation level of the athlete, as well as individual variation. Depending on these factors sweat rates can range from 0.5 to 3.7 l/hr. Children have lower sweat rates than adults.

Fluid ingestion during prolonged exercise is recommended to prevent significant dehydration (35). The ideal fluid is an isotonic carbohydrate-electrolyte solution which fulfills dual purposes of replacing sweat loss and providing carbohydrate fuel, such as glucose, to supplement tissue stores. Fluid replacement is generally not necessary for exercise lasting less than 30 minutes, but becomes more important with prolonged activity (36).

The exact amount of fluid that should be ingested during exercise is not established. The American College of Sports Medicine Position Paper on the Prevention of Thermal Injuries During Distance Running recommends that participants in foot races be encouraged to drink 100–200 ml of water every 2–3 km of the race (35). This is only a guideline and may be too much or too little fluid depending on the environment and the pace and sweat rate of the athlete. Over consumption of water can lead to hyponatremia (low serum sodium), a rare condition which may cause medical problems (37). Thus, a balance of fluid intake, neither too much nor too little, is key to optimize performance and avoid medical complications. Suggested guidelines to help achieve this balance are presented in Table 58.4.

COMPLICATIONS IN SPECIAL POPULATIONS

Exercise considerations in special populations such as those with chronic disease and pulmonary complications (asthma, exercise induced bronchospasm) are addressed elsewhere in this book. Complications in special populations, diabetes for example (see Chapter 31) are specific to the population and the disease state. Basic first aid for these and other common complications are listed in Table 58.5.

Table 58.4. Suggested Guidelines for Fluid Replacement During Prolonged Exercise

1. Immediately prior to exercise or during warm-up, ingest up to 300 ml of cool (~10° C) flavored water.
2. For the initial 60–75 minutes of exercise, ingest 100–150 ml of a cool, dilute (5.0 g/100 ml) glucose polymer solution at regular (10–15 minute) intervals. It seems unwarranted to consume carbohydrate (CHO) in amounts much greater than 30 g during this period, since only 20 g of ingested CHO are oxidized in the first hour of moderate-intensity exercise, irrespective of the type of CHO consumed or the drinking regimen.
3. After 75–90 minutes of exercise, the concentration of the ingested glucose polymer solution should be increased to 10–12 g/100 ml, to which 20 mEq/L of sodium should be added. Higher sodium concentrations, although possibly promoting rapid intestinal fluid absorption, are not palatable to most athletes. Potassium, which may facilitate rehydration of the intracellular fluid compartment, may be included in the replacement beverage in small amounts (2–4 mEq/L). For the remainder of the race, consume 100–150 ml of this solution at regular (10–15 minute) intervals. Such a drinking regimen will ensure optimal rates of both fluid and energy delivery, thereby limiting any dehydration-induced decreases in plasma volume, and maintaining the rate on ingested CHO oxidation at ~1g/min late in exercise.

With permission from Nokes TD *et al.*: Fluid and energy replacement during prolonged exercise. *Curr Ther Sport Med* 517–520, 1995.

Table 58.5. Possible Medical Emergencies and Suggested First Aid

PROBLEM	FIRST AID PROCEDURE
Heat cramps	Replace lost fluids. Increase sodium and potassium lost through excessive sweating.
Heat exhaustion and heat stroke	Move victim to shaded area; have victim lie down with feet elevated above the level of the heart. Remove excess clothing. Cool victim with sips of cool fluid; sprinkle water on him or her and on the facial area; rub ice pack over major vessels in armpits, groin, and neck areas. Victim should seek immediate medical attention and be given intravenous fluids as soon as possible.
Fainting (Syncope)	Leave the victim lying down. Turn on his or her side if vomiting occurs. Maintain an open airway. Loosen any tight clothing. Take blood pressure and pulse if possible. Seek medical attention because it is a potentially life-threatening situation and the cause of fainting must be determined.
Hypoglycemia (symptoms include diaphoresis, pallor, tremor, tachycardia, palpitations, visual disturbances, mental confusion, weakness, lightheadedness, fatigue, headache, memory loss, seizure, or coma)	May become life-threatening. Seek medical attention to treat cause. Give oral glucose solutions such as Kool-aid with sugar, non-diet softdrinks, juice, or milk. If patient is able to ingest solids, gelatin sweetened with sugar, mild chocolate or fruit may be given.
Hyperglycemia (symptoms include dehydration, hypotension, and reflex tachycardia, osmotic diuresis, impaired consciousness, nausea, vomiting, abdominal pain, hyperventilation, odor of acetone on breath)	May be life-threatening if it leads to diabetic ketoacidosis. Seek immediate medical attention. Rehydrate with intravenous normal saline. Correct electrolyte loss (K^+). Insulin.
Sprains/Strains	No weight bearing on affected extremity. Loosen shoes, apply a pillow or blanket type splint around extremity. Elevate the extremity. Apply bag of crushed ice to the affected area. Seek medical attention if pain or swelling persist.
Simple or compound fractures	Immobilize the extremity. Splint the extremity to prevent further injury to the bone or soft tissue. Use anything at hand as a splint. Do not attempt to reduce any dislocation in the field unless there is danger of losing life or limb. Seek immediate medical attention. Protect the victim from further injury.
Bronchospasm	Maintain open airway. Give bronchodilators via nebulizer if prescribed for patient. Give oxygen by nasal cannula if available.
Hypotension/Shock	Lie the victim down with feet elevated. Maintain open airway. Monitor vital signs (pulse, blood pressure). Call for immediate advanced life support measures because this is a life threatening emergency that requires intensive monitoring of vital signs, administration of intravenous fluids and drugs to maintain adequate tissue perfusion while evaluation is done as to the cause (i.e., hypovolemia, cardiogenic, sepsis, etc.).
Bleeding Lacerations Incisions Puncture wounds Abrasions Contusions	Apply direct pressure over the site to stop the bleeding. Protect the wound from contamination and infection. May need to seek medical attention; victim may need stitches, tetanus shot. If bleeding is severe, in addition to direct pressure, elevate the injured part of the body, and if an artery is severed, apply direct pressure over the main artery to the affected limb and seek immediate medical attention.

With permission from Strauss WE, *et al.* Emergency plans and procedures for an exercise facility. *ACSM Resource Manual for Guidelines for Exercise Testing and Prescription.* 2nd ed. Philadelphia: Lea & Febiger, 1993:373.

Besides knowledge of basic first aid, it is imperative that all persons involved in exercise testing and rehabilitation are trained in cardiopulmonary resuscitation (CPR). Certification may be obtained through the American Heart Association or the American Red Cross and classes are available in most cities.

Some individuals from these special populations will require medical evaluation before beginning a physical activity program. All persons at high risk of complication during exercise should be screened before making significant changes in activity level. The *ACSM Guidelines* gives further criteria for risk stratification and pre-test evaluation (27).

▶ SUMMARY

Despite the many potential complications of exercise, the risk for most individuals is low. Those individuals who are at increased risk for complications should be carefully screened and appropriately treated. For the remainder of the population, the benefits that may be gained from increased activity, such as improved cardiovascular, respiratory and musculoskeletal fitness, weight loss, reduced blood pressure and increased sense of well-being, far outweigh the potential risks.

References

1. Levine BD, Stray-Gundersen J. The medical care of competitive athletes: the role of the individual and the individual assumption of risk. *Med Sci Sports Exerc* 1994;26: 1190–1192.
2. Kraus JF, Conroy C. Mortality and morbidity from injuries in sports and recreation. *Ann Rev Pub Health* 1984;5:163–192.
3. Koplan JP, Siscovick DS, Goldbaum GM. The risks of exercise: A public health view of injuries and hazards. *Pub Health Rep* 1985;100(2):189–195.
4. Thompson PD, Funck EJ, Carleton RA, et al. Incidence of death during jogging in Rhode Island from 1975 through 1980. *JAMA* 1982;247(18):2535–2538.
5. Van Camp SP, Bloor CM, Mueller FU, et al. Nontraumatic sports deaths in high school and college athletes. *Med Sci Sports Exerc* 1995;27:641–647.
6. Maron BJ, Shirani J, Poliac LC, et al. Sudden death in young competitive athletes. *JAMA* 1996;276:199–204.
7. Opie LH. Sudden death and sport. *Lancet* 1975;1:263–266.
8. Mittleman MA, MaClure M, Tofler GH, et al. Triggering of acute myocardial infarction by heavy physical exertion. *N Engl J Med* 1993;329(23):1677–1683.
9. Willich SN, Lewis M, Lowel H, et al. Physical exertion as a trigger of acute myocardial infarction. *N Engl J Med* 1993;329(23):1684–1690.
10. Thompson PD, Klocke FJ, Levine BD, et al. 26th Bethesda Conference. Recommendations for determining eligibility for competition in athletes with cardiovascular abnormalities. Task Force 5: Coronary artery disease. *J Am Coll Cardiol* 1994;4(24):845–899.
11. Maron BJ, Mitchell JH. 26th Bethesda Conference. Recommendations for determining eligibility for competition in athletes with cardiovascular abnormalities. Revised recommendations for competitive athletes with cardiovascular abnormalities. *J Am Coll Cardiol* 1994;24(4):845–899.
12. Noakes TD. Heart disease in marathon runners: a review. *Med Sci Sports Exerc* 1987;19(3):187–194.
13. Siscovick DS, Weiss NS, Fletcher RH, et al. The incidence of primary cardiac arrest during vigorous exercise. *N Engl J Med* 1984;311:874–877.
14. Blair SN, Kampert JB, Kuhl HW, et al. Influences of cardiorespiratory fitness and other precursors on cardiovascular disease and all-cause mortality in men and women. *JAMA* 1996;276:205–210.
15. Wigle ED, Rakowski H, Kimball BP, et al. Hypertrophic cardiomyopathy, clinical spectrum and treatment. *Circulation* 1995;92:1680–1692.
16. Barth CW, Roberts WC. Left main coronary artery originating from the right sinus of valsalva and coursing between the aorta and pulmonary trunk. *J Am Coll Cardiol* 1986;7:366–373.
17. Morales AR, Romanelli R, Bovcek RJ. The mural left anterior descending coronary artery, strenuous exercise and sudden death. *Circulation* 1980;62:230–237.
18. Roberts WC, Glick BN. Congenital hypoplasia of both right and left circumflex coronary arteries. *Am J Cardiol* 1992;70:121–123.
19. Roberts WC, Silver MA, Sapala JC. Intussusception of a coronary artery associated with sudden death in a college football player. *Am J Cardiol* 1986;57:179–180.
20. Tahernia AC. Cardiovascular anomalies in Marfan's syndrome: The role of echocardiography and beta-blockers. *South Med J* 1993;86(3):305–310.
21. Maron BJ, Bodison SA, Wesley YE, et al. Results of screening a large group of intercollegiate competitive athletes for cardiovascular disease. *J Am Coll Cardiol* 1987;10(6):1214–1221.
22. Atterhog JH, Bjorn J, Samuelsson R. Exercise testing: A prospective study of complication rates. *Am Heart J* 1979;98(5):572–579.
23. Wendt TH, Scherer D, Kaltenbach M. Life-threatening complications in 1,741,106 ergometries. *Dtsch Med Wochenschr* 1984;109:123–127.
24. Gibbons L, Blair SN, Kohl HW, et al. The safety of maximal exercise testing. *Circulation* 1989;80:846–852.
25. Fletcher GF, Cantwell JD. Ventricular fibrillation in a medically supervised cardiac exercise program. *JAMA* 1977;238:2627–2629.
26. Young DZ, Lampert S, Graboys TB, et al. Safety of maximal exercise testing in patients at high risk for ventricular arrhythmias. *Circulation* 1984;70(2):184–191.
27. Kenney WL, Humphrey RH, Bryant CX, eds. *ACSM's Guidelines for Exercise Testing and Prescription.* Baltimore: Williams & Wilkins, 1995.
28. Dubach P, Froelicher VF, Klein J, et al. Exercise-Induced hypotension in a male population. *Circulation* 1988;78: 1380–1387.
29. Fletcher GF, Balady G, Froelicher VF, et al. Exercise standards: A statement for healthcare professionals from the

American Heart Association. *Circulation* 1995;91(2):580–615.
30. Haskell WL. The efficacy and safety of exercise programs in cardiac rehabilitation. *Med Sci Sports Exerc* 1994;26(7):815–823.
31. Haskell WL. Cardiovascular complications during exercise training of cardiac patients. *Circulation* 1978;57:920–924.
32. VanCamp SP, Peterson RA. Cardiovascular complications of outpatient cardiac rehabilitation programs. *JAMA* 1986;256(9):1160–1163.
33. Kark JA, Posey DM, Schumacher HR, et al. Sickle-cell trait as a risk factor for sudden death in physical training. *N Engl J Med* 1987;317(13):781–787.
34. Knochel JP. Pathophysiology of heat stroke. In: Hopkins, Ellis, eds. Hyperthermia and Hypermetabolic Disorders. Cambridge: Cambridge University Press, 1996;42–62.
35. American College of Sports Medicine. Position statement on the prevention of thermal injuries during distance running. *Med Sci Sports Exerc* 1987;19:529–533.
36. Noakes TD. Dehydration during exercise, what are the real dangers. *J Clin Sport Med* 1995;5:123–128.
37. Frizell RT, Lang GH, Lowance DC, et al. Hyponatremia and ultramarathon running. *JAMA* 1986;255:772–774.

SECTION ELEVEN

Human Development

SECTION EDITOR: *Douglas R. Southard, PhD*

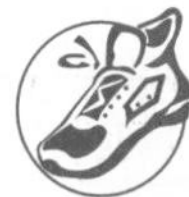

CHAPTER 59

Human Development and Aging

Mark A. Williams

Changes in human physiology over a life span are often categorized into time periods based upon calendar age to assist physicians, exercise professionals, and other health care practitioners in the evaluation of growth, changes in function with aging, and interventions that may impact physiologic function (Table 59.1). Although these distinctions can provide guidance, as a result of variations in growth and development, environment, aging, and disease, individuals often exhibit wide discrepancies between calendar and biologic age (1, 2).

THE IMPACT OF AGING

The aging categorizations in Table 59.1 facilitate the following review of physiological changes associated with aging. This chapter provides an overview of the impact of aging on selected physiological parameters important to exercise testing and prescription.

The Heart

The major limitation in attempting to describe structural changes in the heart associated with aging is that most investigations include individuals with cardiovascular disease. Thus, it is possible that changes associated with aging may be related in part to cardiovascular pathology in those studies. Nevertheless, in studies of normal men and women, aging-related increased left ventricular hypertrophy has been demonstrated between the second and seventh decades (3, 4). Increased afterload (the pressure overcome for left ventricular ejection to occur) resulting from increased peripheral resistance appears to be the primary mechanism for ventricular hypertrophy. With aging, elasticity of major blood vessels declines and often leads to increased systolic and mean blood pressure at rest and during exercise. Systolic blood pressure is as much as 40 mm Hg higher at rest and during submaximal exercise compared to younger adults (5, 6). However, the degree of left ventricular hypertrophy seen with advancing age is mild compared to pathologic conditions (4).

Several studies over the past 25 years show that resting cardiac output and stroke volume decrease with age. Results suggest that cardiac output decreases about one percent per year, from a mean of 6.5 liters per minute in the third decade to a mean of 3.9 liters per minute in the ninth decade (7). From 25 to 85 years, resting stroke volume decreases 30 percent, from 85 ml to 60 ml (6, 7). However, in subjects who have been carefully screened for coronary artery disease, investigators demonstrate that overall left ventricular function, using resting ejection fraction as an index, does not decline between 25 and 80 years (8). Estimates of volume, using echocardiography and gaited radionuclide scintigraphy, demonstrate that resting stroke volume does not decline with age. Since resting heart rate is also not age-related, these data suggest that resting cardiac output does not decline with increasing age in healthy individuals. Other work assessing intrinsic cardiac muscle function also indicates that resting myocardial performance is not affected by aging (3).

At any given level of work, cardiac output is somewhat lower in children than in adults (9, 10). However, during modest submaximal exercise, increases in stroke volume do not seem be related to aging. As one grows older, however, smaller increases in stroke volume and ejection fraction and greater left ventricular end-diastolic pressure are observed with increasing workloads. Maximal cardiac output in a 65-year-old person is 20-30% less than that in a young adult (11). A decrease in both maximal heart rate and maximal stroke volume contributes to decreased maximal cardiac output. By contrast, in the post-exercise period after high intensity exercise, heart rate recovery, return of oxygen uptake to baseline, and muscle power recovery occur faster in children than in young adults and adults (12–14).

Early left ventricular diastolic function is significantly reduced with increased age compared to systolic function (3, 15). This impairment of left ventricular filling may be related, at least in part, to the previously mentioned

Table 59.1. Stages of Aging

Neonatal	birth to 3 weeks
Infancy	3 weeks to 1 year
Childhood	
Early	1–6 years
Middle	7–10 years
Later	prebutertal: females 9–15 years males 12–16 years
Adolescence	6 years following puberty
Adulthood	
Early	20–29 years
Middle	30–44 years
Later	45–64 years
Senescence	
Elderly	65–74 years
Older Elderly	75–84 years
Very Old	85 years and above

age-related left ventricular hypertrophy which diminishes ventricular diastolic compliance. Doppler echocardiography confirms an age-related slowing of early diastolic mitral inflow (16).

Because peripheral vasculature provides the delivery system through which blood circulates, age-related changes in these blood vessels may limit cardiac performance and maximum perfusion of body tissues. Hemodynamic changes in the heart due to age-related increased aortic stiffness require greater left ventricular stroke volume, resulting in increased wall tension and myocardial oxygen consumption during systole. Substantial evidence suggests that resistance to ventricular emptying increases with age, which may partially explain the age-related increase in left ventricular hypertrophy previously described (17). Structural changes in the aorta and other large arteries are partially reflected clinically by a rise in systolic blood pressure and widening of pulse pressure with age. In addition, pulse wave velocity is consistently found to increase with age, indicating decreased arterial compliance (18).

Heart Rate

In children, heart rate is often elevated at rest (80–100 bpm), apparently as a result of reduced stroke volume relative to body size (1). This reduced stroke volume generally disappears with growth and increased levels of chronic physical activity. In combination with an increase in the capacity of blood to carry oxygen (hemoglobin increases through the late teens), resting heart rate decreases (to approximately 65–75 bpm).

A decline in maximal exercise heart rate with aging has been suggested (predicted maximum heart rate = 220 − age [± 10 beats]) although there is considerable variability (1). A decrease in myocardial sensitivity to catecholamines and the effect of prolonged diastolic filling occurring with aging appear to be responsible for this decline in heart rate. Decreased maximal heart rate with aging results in a 30–50% reduction in maximal exercise cardiac output from 25 to 85 years (19). Children, endurance-trained athletes, and active older adults are among those who frequently evidence variations from predicted maximum heart rate response. Maximum heart rates of 210–215 bpm have been observed in children, even though motivating children for a sustained effort to accurately determine maximal heart rate is difficult. In endurance athletes, values 5–10 bpm lower than predicted have been observed (20). Finally, many healthy older persons who maintain a lifelong commitment to physical activity can achieve heart rates higher than those predicted (21).

Maximal Oxygen Uptake

Aerobic capacity, assessed by maximal oxygen uptake ($\dot{V}O_2max$) appears to remain constant through childhood. There is, however, controversy concerning an apparent loss of $\dot{V}O_2max$ beginning about 12 years of age, perhaps related to decreased level of chronic physical activity (22). At adulthood, a steady, age-related decline in $\dot{V}O_2max$, averaging about one percent per year between 25 and 75 years (~5 $mlO_2/kg/min$ with each decade of aging), has been observed (23, 24). However, the degree to which this decline occurs is significantly affected by level of chronic physical activity. The decline parallels reduced maximal work capacity and is attributed to decreased maximal cardiac output and reduced maximal arterial-venous oxygen ($a\text{-}vO_2$) difference, as well as a loss of skeletal muscle mass (25, 26). Microstructural changes, including myofilament disorganization and changes in mitochondrial structure and distribution resulting in reduced oxidative capacity, may explain a reduced maximal $a\text{-}vO_2$ difference (27). Additionally, physical limitations resulting from a sedentary lifestyle, loss of coordination, lack of familiarity with required skills, and disabling diseases such as arthritis may also play a role in limiting $\dot{V}O_2max$ (28, 29). Conversely, individuals who are habitually active throughout life do not seem to demonstrate a similarly reduced $\dot{V}O_2max$ as sedentary individuals.

Pulmonary System

Lung compliance increases with age, while ability to expand the chest cavity becomes more limited (30). Residual volume increases by 30–50% and vital capacity decreases by 40–50% by age 70 (31). With exertion, increased ventilation becomes more dependent upon increased respiratory frequency rather than depth of respiration. The overall net effect is a 20 percent increase in the work of respiratory muscles (5). Despite these changes, respiratory function does not limit exercise capacity or the ability to benefit from exercise training unless lung function is severely impaired.

Skeletal Muscle and Strength

The relative proportion of fast and slow twitch fibers is largely determined at birth (1). The total number of muscle fibers is fixed at an early age, although considerable enlargement of muscle remains possible by fiber splitting and hypertrophy of existing fibers. Both boys and girls are capable of increased ability to generate muscular force, although children exhibit disproportionately less ability to generate upper body muscular force than adults. At adolescence, males exhibit rapid hypertrophy of muscle, disproportionately greater than observed in females at puberty. Thus, although ability to generate muscular force in active male children is similar to that of female children, postadolescent males are approximately 40% stronger than females. Both genders reach maximum levels of strength in the early 20s, followed by a plateau maintained into the mid-40s. Subsequently, there is accelerated loss of lean tissue associated with decrements in static and dynamic force generation as well as contractile speed. Thus, by 65 years, changes in the musculoskeletal system are demonstrated with great frequency, both in terms of skeletal muscle mass as well as decreased levels of physical activity (28, 32). Muscle function decreases approximately 25% by age 65 and by as much as 40% over a life span (33–36). Loss of muscle function appears to be due to decreased total fibers, decreased muscle fiber size, impaired excitation-contraction coupling mechanism, or decreased high-threshold motor units. Additionally, there may selective loss or atrophy (particularly after 70 years) of fast twitch (type II) fibers, although this is controversial and the cause unclear (37). At all ages, females appear to be more vulnerable to loss of lean tissue than males. As a result, the elderly must use a high proportion of available muscle mass for exercise, which may result in overuse and strain. Clinically, decreased strength and early onset of fatigue are observed.

It remains uncertain how much age-related loss of muscle function is an inevitable consequence of aging and how much it reflects decline in physical activity (37). Some data suggest that lean tissue mass can be sustained well into the seventh decade with an active lifestyle; others note than lean tissue can be maintained and function restored even into the ninth (38, 39). Evidence also suggests significant improvement in strength and, to a lesser degree, in muscle mass as the elderly participate in programs for strength improvement (39–46). Nonetheless, muscle function decline is directly the result of progressive decrease in the number of muscle fibers and cross-sectional area and decline in neuromuscular function resulting from disuse or loss of motoneurons (37).

Anaerobic power develops in parallel with changes in muscle mass through childhood into young adulthood, deteriorating in middle age corresponding to loss of muscle mass (1). Decreases of 45–60% from 25 to 65 years are observed in both genders although, as noted previously, such losses may be from physical inactivity, decreased neuromuscular coordination, decreased efficiency of movement, and decreased motivation.

Anaerobic capacity as described by peak blood lactate levels also develops through young adulthood. After exhaustive exercise, lactate concentrations in blood and muscle are greater in adults than in children, the latter having reduced levels of glycolytic enzymes and a smaller ratio of muscle mass to blood volume (47). Decreased motivation or neuromuscular coordination probably also contributes to reduced anaerobic capacity in children. Both sexes maintain a plateau of anaerobic capacity through about age 35, at which time there is increased loss of function. By age 65, anaerobic capacity declines to essentially the level of childhood even when subjects are highly motivated for testing.

Bone

Bone growth during childhood presents two primary problems because the epiphysis is not united with the bone shaft. First, overuse can result in epiphysitis during this growth period. Second, fracture may pass through the epiphyseal plate, leading to potential disruption of normal growth (1). Beginning at age 30 in females and age 40 in males, calcium content progressively decreases, leading to progressive bone loss with aging, although less rapidly in males. In women, loss occurs at a rate of approximately 1% per year after age age 35 and is particularly rapid during the five years after menopause. Men lose 10–15% by age 70 and 20% by age 80 (48–49). In women, the loss is greater, amounting to about 20% by age 65 and 30% by age 80. In both genders, by age 65, bone loss has generally progressed to a point where the elderly are predisposed to fractures. Bone fracture is a significant cause of morbidity and mortality in the elderly. Decreasing dietary calcium intake, diabetes mellitus, renal impairment, and lack of physical activity may accelerate bone loss. It appears that adequate mineral intake and progressive weight-bearing activity can stabilize calcium loss. In addition, hormone replacement therapy in women appears effective in limiting bone mass loss.

Degeneration or damage to articular cartilage results in a significant increase in incidence of osteoarthritis with aging (1). By age 60, as much as 80% of the population shows such evidence, although only about 15% present with symptoms. The contributions of overuse or trauma to this problem remain unclear.

Joints and Flexibility

A progressive loss of flexibility begins during young adulthood, resulting from a number of factors including disuse, deterioration of joint structures, and progressive degeneration of collagen fibers (1). Increased incidence of knee and back problems from osteoarthritis have been observed beginning with middle age and progressing through old age. Degeneration of joints, especially the spine, is often found in elderly persons (29). Weight-bearing activity may accelerate this onset. More judicious practice coupled with exercise training to promote strength may decelerate it (28, 29). Along with loss of strength described previously, loss of flexibility also plays a significant role in increased risk of falls and other injuries. The rate of deterioration accelerates beyond age 65, but less specific data are available for this age group.

Aging is also associated with changes in connective tissue (50). Connective tissue, including fascia, ligaments, and tendons, becomes less extensible. Range of motion, both active and passive, declines with advancing years. It is not clear whether this decreased flexibility occurs as a consequence of biological aging, degenerative disease, inactivity, or some combination of these factors.

Body Composition and Metabolism

In young children, the proportion of body fat ranges from 10% to 15%, with girls carrying slightly more body fat than boys of similar age (1). In addition, body surface area-to-mass ratio is greater in children than adults (9). In both adolescent males and females and into young adulthood, body fat percentage generally increases to 15–20% in males and 20–25% in females. In the moderately obese person, body fat that accumulates beyond normal is generally a result of imbalance of caloric intake and energy expenditure, the latter often decreasing with aging. Contributing to the decline of energy expenditure are several metabolic changes. The basal metabolic rate gradually decreases with aging as lean body mass decreases, while relative body fat increases (27, 51). In addition, glucose tolerance diminishes with age and is accompanied by increasing likelihood of developing non-insulin dependent diabetes mellitus (32). Thus, by middle age, body fat percentage may continue to increase beyond 20–25% in males and 25–30% in females. These values may continue to increase as one ages.

Renal Function, Fluid Regulation, and Thermoregulation

Renal function declines approximately 30–50% between the ages of 30 and 70 years (1). Along with this decline decreased acid-base control, glucose tolerance, and drug clearance occur. A general reduction in total cellular water occurs with aging, with a decline of 10–50% in total body water.

The primary maturational characteristics related to exercise in heat occur at late puberty or early adulthood. Prior to that time, children have a consistently lower sweat rate characterized by both lower absolute and relative amounts as well as increased core temperature required to start sweating. Differences are also noted in composition of sweat, particularly increased chloride (52, 53). Additionally, children tend to rely more on radiation and convection for heat dissipation than adults (9). The impact of aging predisposes older individuals to more rapid dehydration that may become particularly important during exercise through evaporative water loss and perspiration. In addition, many older adults take a variety of medications that may further confound limitations of thermoregulation.

Children have a greater surface area-to-mass ratio than adults, which enhances convective and radiative heat transfer between skin and the environment, making adaptation to cold environments more difficult (54). However, it has been suggested that other factors that mature with aging, such as thermogenic and vasoconstrictive responses, may also limit thermoregulation to cold in children. Beyond childhood, it has been demonstrated that core temperature regulation is detrimentally affected by aging (55–58).

Nervous System

Changes in the central and peripheral nervous systems include slowed conduction velocities and reaction times, which drop 15% by age 70 (59). Both incidence of sensory deficits, particularly hearing and vision, and threshold of perception for many stimuli increase. Changes such as these may be related to a 35–40% increase in falls by persons over age 60 (11, 27).

Immune System Function

It is widely agreed that immune system function declines with age (60–62). From peak immune system activity, around puberty, an overall decline of 5–30% over a normal life span is expected, with some functional indices dropping to 5–10% of young adult function. The end result is reduced resistance to pathogens and increased incidence of both tumors and auto-immune disorders.

Exercise Prescription and Exercise Training Response

The interplay of frequency, intensity, and duration of exercise training is responsible for the effectiveness of exercise training, but it is apparent that the age of the subject will also affect the relationship of these variables (1). Young children have difficulty sustaining the duration of effort, so frequency and intensity of training should be emphasized. There is no clear evidence that prepubescent children do not respond to aerobic training, nor is there any apparent physiological basis for suggesting that children are less suitable than adults to prolonged bouts of exercise, apart from some potential limitations described in Table 59.2 (63). The limitations related to sustained activity are probably related to preference for short-term intermittent activity, which are more "fun" than those which tend to be prolonged (and monotonous).

Table 59.2. Potential Limitations to Prolonged Exercise in Children

mechanical inefficiencies in movement
general limitations in the cardiovascular response to exercise
reduced sweating capacity
general limitations in ability to acclimatize
limitations with exercising in climatic extremes including:
heat intolerance as a result of high metabolic rate leading to excessive body heat
intolerance to cold

As one ages, higher intensities of effort are required to maintain or increase one's conditioning level. Such increasing intensity is not realistic for most of the population, primarily because of decreased motivation and increased risk of injury associated with high intensity exercise in an aging, often sedentary population. Thus, increased duration and frequency of exercise training take precedence, emphasizing caloric expenditure, particularly when health as opposed to fitness is the primary consideration (64, 65).

▶ SUMMARY

The impact of human growth and development has a clear impact upon the ability to participate in acute and chronic exercise. An understanding of expected changes in physiology as a result of these processes allows evaluation of both normal and abnormal responses to physical activity through the life continuum. The impact of aging may be a direct result of the aging process or may be a consequence of other aspects that become superimposed on the aging process. With aging, there is often a decline in habitual physical activity, poor nutrition, cumulative effects of long-term smoking, and increased chronic disease and depression, all of which adversely affect quantity and quality of life (60, 66). The contribution of appropriate health practices to offsetting the rapidity and degree of aging remains unclear.

References

1. Shephard RJ. Physiologic changes over the years. In: *ACSM's Resource Manual for Guidelines for Exercise Testing and Prescription.* 2nd ed. Philadelphia, PA: Lea & Febiger, 1993.
2. Timiras PS. Introduction: Aging as a stage in the life cycle. In: Timiras PS, ed. *Physiological Basis of Aging and Geriatrics.* 2nd Ed. Boca Raton, FL: CRC Press, 1994.
3. Gerstenblith G, Frederiksen J, Yin FCP. Echocardiography assessment of a normal adult aging population. *Circulation* 1977;56:273–278.
4. Sjogren AL. Left ventricular wall thickness in patients with circulatory overload of the left ventricle. *Clin Res* 1972;4: 310–318.
5. deVries HA, Adams GM. Comparison of exercise responses in old and young men. *J Gerontol* 1972;27:344–348.
6. Lakatta EG. Alterations in the cardiovascular system that occur in advanced age. *Fed Proc* 1979;38:163–167.
7. Brandfonbrener M, Landowne M, Shock NW. Changes in cardiac output with age. *Circulation* 1955;12:557–566.
8. Rodeheffer RJ, Gerstenblith G, Becker LC, et al. Exercise cardiac output is maintained with advancing age in healthy human subjects: cardiac dilatation and increased stroke volume compensate for a diminished heart rate. *Circulation* 1984;69:203–213.
9. Falk B, Bar-Or O, MacDougall JD. Thermoregulatory responses of pre-, mid-, and late-pubertal boys to exercise in dry heat. *Med Sci Sport Exerc* 1992;24:688–694.
10. Erikson BO, Grimby G, Saltin B. Cardiac output and arterial blood gases during exercise in pubertal boys. *J Appl Physiol* 1971:348–352.
11. Shephard RJ. *Physical Activity and Aging.* 2nd Ed. Rockville, Maryland: Aspen Publishers, 1987.
12. Hebestreet H, Mimura K-I, Bar-Or O. Recovery of muscle power after high-intensity short-term exercise: comparing boys and men. *J Appl Physiol* 1993;74:2875–2880.
13. Baraldi E, Cooper DM, Zanconato S, et al. Heart rate recovery from 1 minute of exercise in children and adults. *Pediatr Res* 1991;29:575–579.
14. Zamconato S, Cooper DM, Armon Y. Oxygen cost and oxygen uptske dynamics and recovery with 1 minutes of exercise in children and adults. *J Appl Physiol* 1991;71:993–998.
15. Gardin JM, Henry WL, Savage DD, et al. Echocardiographic measurements in normal subjects: evaluation of an adult population without clinically apparent heart disease. *J Clin Ultrasound* 1979;7:349–447.
16. Miyatake K, Okamoto J, Kimoshita N, et al. Augmentation of atrial contribution to left ventricular flow with aging as assessed by intra-cardiac doppler flowmetry. *Am J Cardiol* 1984;53:587–589.
17. Fleg JL, Gerstenblith G, Lakatta EG. Pathophysiology of the aging heart and circulation. In: Messeril FH, ed. *Cardiovascular Disease in the Elderly.* Boston: Martinus Nijhoff Publishing, 1988.
18. Avolio AP, Deng FQ, Li WQ, et al. Effects of aging on arterial distensibility in populations with high and low prevalence of hypertension, comparison between urban and rural communities. *Circulation* 1985;71:202–210.
19. Bruce RA, Fisher LD, Cooper NM, et al. Separation of effects of cardiovascular disease and age on ventricular function with maximal exercise. *Am J Cardiol* 1974;34:757–763.
20. Dal Monte A, Faina M, Menchinelli C. Sport-specific equipment. In: Shephard RJ, Astrand PO, eds. *Sports and Human Endurance.* Oxford: Blackwell Scientific Publications, 1992.
21. Sidney KH, Shephard RJ. Maximum and submaximum exercise tests in men and women in seventh, eighth, and ninth decades of life. *J Appl Physiol* 1977;43:280–287.
22. Shephard RJ. Maximal oxygen intake. In: Shephard RJ, Astrand PO, eds. *Sports and Human Endurance.* Oxford: Blackwell Scientific Publications, 1992.
23. Shephard RJ. Exercise and aging: extending independence in older adults. *Geriatrics* 1993;48:61–64.

24. Shvartz E, Reibold RC. Aerobic fitness norms for males and females aged 6–75 years: a review. *Aviat Space Environ Med* 1990;61:3–11.
25. Granath A, Jonsson B, Strandell T. Circulation in healthy old men studied by right heart catheterization at rest and during exercise in a supine and sitting position. *Acta Med Scand* 1964;176:425–446.
26. Julius S, Amery A, Whitlock LS, et al. Influence of age on a hemodynamic response to exercise. *Circulation* 1967;36: 222–230.
27. Shock NW. Physiological aspects of aging in man. *Ann Rev Physiol* 1961;23:97–122.
28. Fitzgerald PL. Exercise for the elderly. *Med Clin North Am* 1985;69:189–196.
29. Ike RW, Lampman RM, Castor CW. Arthritis and aerobic exercise. *Phys Sportsmed* 1989;17:128–139.
30. Mitman C, Edelman NH, Norris AH, et al. Relationship between chest wall and pulmonary compliance and age. *J Appl Physiol* 1965;70:1211–1216.
31. Smith EL, Serfass RC. *Exercise and Aging: The Scientific Basis.* Hillside, NJ: Enslow Publishers, 1981.
32. Rosenthal M, Doberne L, Greenfield M, et al. Effect of age on glucose tolerance, insulin secretion, and in vivo insulin action. *J Am Geriatr Soc* 1982;30:562–567.
33. Shephard RJ. *Body Composition in Biological Anthropology.* London: Cambridge University Press, 1991.
34. Aoyagi Y, Shephard RJ. Aging and muscle function. *Sports Med* 1992;14:376–396.
35. Shephard RJ, Montelpare W, Plyley M, et al. Handgrip dynamometry, Cybex measurements and lean mass as markers of the ageing of muscle. *Br J Sports Med* 1991;25:204–208.
36. Kasch FW, Boyer JL, VanCamp SP, et al. The effect of physical activity and inactivity in aerobic power in older men. *Phys Sportsmed* 1990;18(4):73–83.
37. Aoyagi Y, Shephard RJ. Aging and muscle function. *Sports Med* 1992;14:376–396.
38. Kavanagh T, Shephard RJ. Can regular sports participation slow the aging process? Data on masters athletes. *Phys Sportsmed* 1990;18(6):94–104.
39. Fiatarone MA, Marks EC, Ryan ND, et al. High-intensity strength training in nonagenarians. Effects on skeletal muscle. *JAMA* 1990; 263:3029–3034.
40. Butler RM, Beierwaltes WH, Rodgers FJ. The cardiovascular response to circuit weight training in patients with coronary disease. *J Cardiopulm Rehab* 1987;7:402–409.
41. Ghilarducci LE, Holly RG, Amsterdam EA. Effects of high resistance training in coronary artery disease. *Am J Cardiol* 1989;64:866–870.
42. Aniansson A, Gustafsson E. Physical training in elderly men with special reference to quadriceps, muscle, strength, and morphology. *Clin Physiol* 1981;1:87–98.
43. Kauffman TL. Strength training effect in young and aged women. *Arch Phys Med Rehabil* 1985;65:223–226.
44. Liemohn WP. Strength in aging: an exploratory study. *Int J Aging Hum Dev* 1975;6:347–357.
45. Moritani T, deVries HA. Potential for gross muscle hypertrophy in older men. *J Gerontol* 1980;35:672–682.
46. Perkins LC, Kaiser HL. Results of short-term isotonic and isometric exercise programs in persons over 60. *Phys Ther Rev* 1961;41:633–635.
47. Falk B, Bar-Or O, MacDougall JD, et al. Sweat lactate in exercising children and adolescents of varying physical maturity. *J Appl Physiol* 1991;71:1735–1740.
48. Aloia JF, Cohn SH, Ostuni JD, et al. Prevention of involutional bone loss by exercise. *Ann Intern Med* 1978;89: 356–358.
49. Smith DM, Khairi MR, Norton J. Age and activity effects on rate of bone mineral loss. *J Clin Invest* 1976;58:716–721.
50. Ippolito E, Natali PG, Postacchini F, et al. Morphological, immunochemical, and biochemical study of rabbit achilles tendon at various ages. *J Bone Joint Surg* 1980;62A:583–598.
51. Novak LP. Aging, total body potassium, fat free mass, and cell mass in males and females between ages 18 and 85 years. *J Gerontol* 1972;27:438–443.
52. Meyer F, Bar-Or O, MacDougall D, et al. Drink composition and the electrolyte balance of children exercising in the heat. *Med Sci Sport Exerc* 1995;27:882–887.
53. Falk B, Bar-Or O, MacDougall JD. Aldosterone and prolactin resonse to exercise in the heat in circumpubertal boys. *J Appl Physiol* 1991;71:1741–1745.
54. Smolander J, Bar-Or O, Korhonen O, et al. Thermoregulation during rest and exercise in the cold in pre- and early pubescent boys and in young men. *J Appl Physiol* 1992;72: 1589–1594.
55. Falk B, Bar-Or O, Smolander J, et al. Response to rest and exercise in the cold: effects of age and aerobic fitness. *J Appl Physiol* 1994;76:72–78.
56. Budd GM, Brotherhood JR, Hendrie AL, et al. Effects of fitness, fatness, and age on men's responses to whole body cooling in air. *J Appl Physiol* 1991;71:2387–2393.
57. Tankersley CG, Smolander J, Kenney WL, et al. Sweating and skin blood flow during exercise: effects of age and maximal oxygen uptake. *J Appl Physiol* 1991;71:236–242.
58. Young A. Effects of aging on human cold tolerance. *Exp Aging Res* 1991;17:205–213.
59. Elia EA. Exercise and the elderly. *Clin Sports Med* 1991;10: 141–155.
60. Shephard RJ, Shek PN. Exercise, aging and immune function. *Int J Sports Med* 1995;16:1–6.
61. Makinodan T, Bloom ET, James SJ, et al. Immunity and aging. In: Pathy MSJ, ed. *Principles and Practices of Geriatric Medicine.* Chichester: Wiley, 1994.
62. Miller RA. Aging and immune function. *Int Rev Cytol* 1991;124:187–215.
63. Shephard RJ. Effectiveness of training programmes for prepubescent children. *Sports Med* 1992;13:194–213.
64. Fletcher GF, Balady G, Froelicher VF, et al. Exercise standards: a statement for health care professionals from the American Heart Association. *Circulation* 1995;91:580–615.
65. US Centers for Disease Control and Prevention, American College of Sports Medicine. Physical activity and public health. *Sports Med Bull* 1993;28:7.
66. Hallfrisch J, Muller D, Drinkwater D, et al. Continuing diet trends in men: The Baltimore Longitudinal Study of Aging (1961-1987). *J Gerontol* 1990;45:M186–M191.

59, 60, 62 64, 65 68 314, 315, 317 391

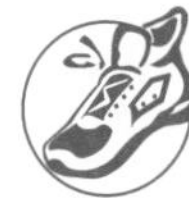

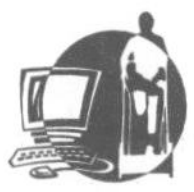
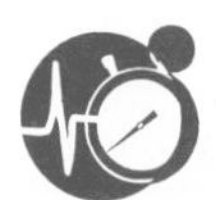

CHAPTER **60**

Exercise Testing and Prescription Considerations Throughout Childhood

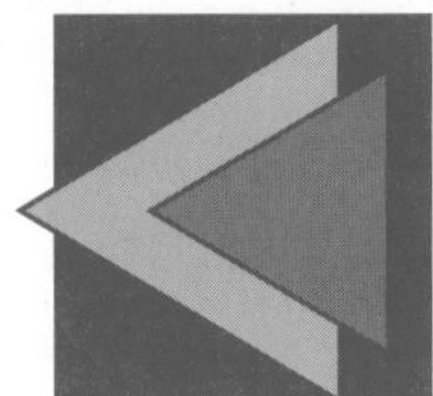

Linda D. Zwiren and Tina M. Manos

Unless otherwise indicated, this chapter refers to childhood as that period which ends with adulthood, and which is inclusive of preadolescence and adolescence. "Adolescence" is defined as ages 11 to 21 years, in accordance with the recent International Consensus Conference on Physical Activity Guidelines for Adolescence (1). Data on preadolescents are limited by experimental procedures that are not appropriate for use with children. The advent of non-invasive methods such as phosphorus magnetic resonance imaging (MRI) to study subcellular responses and muscle metabolism may lead to significant increases in that knowledge (2). It should be noted that there is substantial variability in growth status and maturity level for any given chronological age, making the distinction between preadolescence and adolescence imprecise. This chapter focuses on preadolescence; however, exercise prescription guidelines for adolescence have been added from the International Consensus Conference (3).

DEFINITIONS

While the terms **physical activity, physical fitness,** and **sports** are considered interchangeable, each term has a unique meaning and refers to a different concept. **Physical activity** is any bodily movement which increases energy expenditure. Therefore, an increase in physical activity can be a result of many different activities, including walking, gardening, vacuuming, climbing stairs, etc. Physical activity can be performed at various intensity levels. To increase physical activity levels of children means to decrease the time children are lying down or sitting and to increase the time they are moving.

Physical fitness refers to a set of individual physical attributes which can be improved by engaging in appropriate exercise programs. To improve health-related fitness includes increasing cardiovascular (endurance) fitness by engaging in large muscle group activities that significantly increase cardiac output and blood flow. Activities like jogging, running, swimming, or rollerblading must be performed at a given intensity, duration, and frequency (4). Increasing physical fitness may also include using resistance training or calisthenics to increase muscular strength, muscular endurance, and flexibility. Attaining and maintaining a reasonable and healthy body weight is also a component of health-related physical fitness.

Sports activities require specific skilled movements performed during organized game situations. To participate in sports, a certain level of motor fitness and the ability to perform skilled movements is required.

PHYSIOLOGICAL ASPECTS

Major differences in physiological responses to exercise exist between preadolescents and adults. The physiological characteristics of exercising children are presented in Table 60.1. Apart from low economy of locomotion and limitations of exercising in climatic extremes, no apparent underlying **physiological** factors have been identified that make preadolescents less suitable than adults for prolonged, continuous activities (5).

Although preadolescents can perform exercise over a wide variety of intensities and durations, they spontaneously prefer short-term intermittent activities with a high recreational component and variety rather than monotonous, prolonged activities. Physiologically, preadolescents may use oxygen more efficiently than adults, while they are less able to facilitate anaerobic pathways. Therefore, preadolescent children have greater aerobic ATP generation and higher cellular pH during exercise. In accordance with physiological profile and from a psychological viewpoint, children seem best suited to repeated activities of varying intensities lasting a few seconds, interspersed with short rest periods. This pattern, characterized by short bursts of activity, may optimize the anabolic effect of exercise in the growing child (2). The least suitable forms of exercise for preadolescent children, from a physiological viewpoint, are high intensity activities lasting 10 to 90 seconds (6).

Table 60.1. Physiologic Characteristics of the Exercising Child

FUNCTION	COMPARISON TO ADULTS	IMPLICATIONS FOR EXERCISE
Prescription Metabolic		
Aerobic		
$\dot{V}O_{2peak}$ (L/min)	Lower body mass	
$\dot{V}O_{2peak}$ (ml/kg/min)	Similar	Can perform endurance tasks reasonably well
Submaximal oxygen demand (economy)	Cycling: similar (18–30% mechanical efficiency); Walking and running: higher metabolic cost	Greater fatiguability in prolonged high-intensity tasks (running and walking); greater heat production in children at a given speed of walking or running
$\dot{V}CO_2$	Time required to increase $\dot{V}CO_2$ at onset of activity and to return to base line is significantly faster in preadolescents.	
Anaerobic		
Glycogen stores	Lower concentration and rate of utilization of muscle glycogen. Similar to adult levels by about age 16.	
Phosphofructokinase (PFK concentration)	Glycolysis limited because of low level of PFK. In children aged 11–14 years a variety of glycolytic enzymes are same as adults at maximal exercise.	Ability of preadolescent children to perform *intense* anaerobic tasks that last 10–90 seconds is distinctly lower than adults; same ability metabolically in brief, intense exercise.
Phosphagen stores	Stores and breakdown of ATP and CP are the same.	Same ability metabolically with very brief intense exercise.
Oxygen transient	Reaching steady state faster than adults. Shorter half-time of oxygen increase in children.	Preadolescent children reach metabolic steady-state faster; children contract a lower oxygen deficit; faster recovery; children therefore are well suited to intermittent activities.
LA_{peak}	Lower blood lactate levels at $\dot{V}O_{2peak}$	Individual variability is wide.
LA_{submax}	Lower at a given percent of $\dot{V}O_{2peak}$	Children perceive a given workload as easier.
HR at lactate threshold	Higher	Children are able to exercise closer to peak exercise levels than adults before LT is reached.
Cardiovascular		
Maximal cardiac output (Q_{max})	Lower due to size difference	Children are limited in ability to transport core heat to surface for dissipation during intense exercise in heat
Q at a given $\dot{V}O_2$	Somewhat lower	
Maximal stroke volume (SV_{max})	Lower due to size and heart volume difference	
SV at given $\dot{V}O_2$	Lower	
Maximal heart rate (HR_{max})	Higher	Up to maturity HR_{max} is between 195–215 beats/min
HR at submax work	At given power output and at relative metabolic load, child has higher HR	Higher HR compensates for lower SV
Oxygen carrying capacity	Blood volume, hemoglobin concentration, and total hemoglobin are lower in children.	
O_2 content in arterial and venous blood (C_aO_2-C_vO_2)	Somewhat higher	Potential deficiency of peripheral blood supply during maximal exertion in hot climates
Blood flow to active muscle	Higher	
Systolic and diastolic pressures	Lower maximal and submaximal	No known beneficial or detrimental effects on working capacity of child
Pulmonary		
Maximal minute ventilation V_{Emax} (L/min)	Lower	Early fatiguability in tasks requiring large minute volume
V_{Emax} (ml/kg/min)	Same as adolescents and young adults	
$V_{Esubmax}$	V_E at any given $\dot{V}O_2$ is higher in children	Less efficient ventilation, therefore greater oxygen cost of ventilation; may explain relatively higher metabolic cost of submaximal exercise.
Respiratory frequency and tidal volume	Marked by higher rate-(tachypnea) and shallow breathing	Physiological dead space is smaller than adults, therefore, alveolar ventilation is adequate for gas exchange.
Ventilatory threshold (VT)	VT occurs at a higher percentage of $\dot{V}O_{2max}$ in children	Children may rely more on aerobic metabolism to meet energy demands.
R_{max} ($\dot{V}CO_2/\dot{V}O_2$)	Lower in children	

Table 60.1. *(contintued)*

FUNCTION	COMPARISON TO ADULTS	IMPLICATIONS FOR EXERCISE
Perception		
RPE (rating of perceived exertion)	Exercising at a given physiologic strain is perceived as easier by children	Implications for initial phase of heat acclimatization
Thermo-Regulatory		
Surface area (SA)	Per unit mass, approx. 36% greater in children (percentage is variable; dependent on size of child, i.e., SA per mass may be higher in younger children and lower in older)	Greater rate of heat exchange between skin and environment. In climatic extremes, children are at increased risk of stress.
Sweating rate	Lower absolute amount per unit of SA. Greater increase in core temperature required to start sweating.	Greater risk of heat-related illness on hot, humid days due to reduced capacity to evaporate sweat; lower tolerance time in extreme heat.
Acclimatization to heat	Slower physiologically; faster subjectively	Longer and more gradual program of acclimatization required; special attention during early stages of acclimatization.
Body cooling in water	Faster cooling due to higher SA per heat-producing unit mass; lower thickness of subcutaneous fat	Potential hypothermia
Body core heating during dehydration	Greater	Prolonged activity; hydrate well before and force fluid intake during activity

Adapted from Zwiren LD. Exercise prescription for children. In: *ACSM Resource Manual for Guidelines for Testing and Prescription.* 2nd ed. Lea & Febiger: Philadelphia, 1993.

Since adolescent children (ages 11 to 21 years) can be pre-pubescent, pubescent, or post-pubescent, it is difficult to identify specific physiological responses of "adolescents." Pre-pubescent children have a physiological profile similar to that of a preadolescent. Physiologically, the post-pubescent adolescent responds to exercise as an adult. The precise physiological response of children going through puberty, therefore, depends on somatic growth and biological maturation.

SOMATIC GROWTH AND BIOLOGICAL MATURATION

It is important to keep children "naturally active." Activity level has a negative impact on somatic growth only if activity level falls below a biological threshold (2). There is no evidence that increasing levels of physical activity above this biological threshold will speed up the attainment of peak height velocity, skeletal maturation, or sexual maturation (7). At the other extreme, however, there is evidence that excessive training may have adverse effects and may result in a reduction of growth potential (8).

Bone Mass

While there is minimal research support (due to lack of longitudinal studies with appropriate research design) regarding physical activity and gaining bone mass genetic potential, adolescence is a critical time for bone density maximization. The International Consensus on Physical Activity Guidelines for Adolescents supports physical activity and exercise (especially weight bearing), including short bouts of intense daily activity and resistance training. It states that these are necessary for attainment of maximal genetic bone density (9). The positive effect of mechanical loading is attainable, however, only with adequate nutrition (sufficient calories and calcium) and appropriate hormonal status.

It is important to monitor the menstrual status of post-menarcheal females, since amenorrhea can have severe consequences on bone mass density. The American Academy of Pediatrics recommends intervention after onset of amenorrhea in physically active females to preserve normal bone development and to prevent skeletal demineralization (10).

The current recommendation is that females should be encouraged to engage in activities of all intensities. However, since disordered eating (inadequate calories for energy expended) coupled with intense exercise can lead to amenorrhea (which has consequences for loss of bone mass and osteoporosis), it is imperative that sufficient caloric intake of nutrient dense foods is promoted in active adolescents (11). (See Table 60.2 for signs associated with eating disorders.)

PRECAUTIONS FOR EXERCISING IN CLIMATIC EXTREMES

Preadolescent children have higher energy expenditure at any given submaximal walking or running speed, therefore they produce excessive body heat. This higher metabolic load (children have higher oxygen consumption [$\dot{V}O_2$] per unit of body mass), in addition to a poor sweating capacity, large surface-to-mass ratio, and immature cardiovascular system (see Table 60.1), causes

Table 60.2. **Danger Signals**

ANOREXIA NERVOSA	BULIMIA NERVOSA
• has lost a great deal of weight in a relatively short period	• develops eating rituals and eats small amounts of food (e.g., cuts food into tiny pieces or measures everything before eating extremely small amounts)
• continues to diet although already thin	• prefers to eat alone
• reaches weight goal and immediately sets another goal for further weight loss	• becomes obsessive about exercising
• remains dissatisfied with appearance, claims to feel fat	• appears unhappy much of the time
• loses menstrual periods	• exercises often but retains or regains weight
• binges regularly (eats large amounts of food, empties refrigerator; food disappears)	• disappears into the bathroom for long periods of time
• purges regularly (uses diet pills, caffeine, water pills, diuretics)	• appears depressed much of the time

With permission from Casper RC. Fear of fatness and anorexia nervosa in children. In: Cheung LWY, Richmond JB, eds. Child Health, Nutrition, and Physical Activity. Champaign, IL: Human Kinetics, 1995.

children to have less tolerance for exercising in heat and greater susceptibility to heat stress (6). The American Academy of Pediatrics (AAP) recommends light weight clothing, limited to one layer of absorbent material, to expose skin, and facilitate evaporation of sweat. Wet clothes should be replaced by dry and rubberized suits should not be used (12).

Children have low tolerance to extreme heat or cold. However, when exercising in neutral or moderately warm climates they thermoregulate as effectively as adults, and, depending on the degree of maturation of sweat glands, cardiorespiratory organs, mechanical efficiency, physical fitness, and body composition, they exhibit exercise-heat tolerance similar to adults (13, 14). The AAP emphasizes "that heat related disorders are particularly pronounced in races that exceed 30 minutes in duration" (5). Activities lasting 30 minutes or longer should be reduced whenever relative humidity and air temperature are above critical levels (Table 60.3).

While preadolescent children do have characteristics that increase the risk of heat illness, it is not dangerous for children to exercise in hot and humid environments. Preadolescent children are more likely to suffer from heat exhaustion than other heat illnesses. Adolescents are more likely to be victims of heat stroke when competing in stressful thermal environments (14).

Acclimatization

Preadolescent children tend to lag behind adults in the **rate** of physiologic acclimatization and, therefore, should have a longer, more gradual program. The AAP recommends that intensity and duration should be initially lower and gradually increased over 10–14 days (12). Children can acclimate to some extent when they exercise in neutral environments and when they rest in hot climates; however, they acclimatize subjectively faster than adults. Therefore, especially during early stages of acclimatization, children may feel capable of performing exercise in the heat, despite marked physiologic heat stress.

Table 60.3. **Weather Guide for Prevention of Heat Illness**

AIR TEMPERATURE (°F)	DANGER ZONE (% RELATIVE HUMIDITY)	CRITICAL ZONE (% RELATIVE HUMIDITY)
70	80	100
75	70	100
80	50	80
85	40	68
90	30	55
95	20	40
100	10	30

With permission from Haymes EM, Wells CL. *Environment and Human Performance.* Champaign, IL: Human Kinetics, 1986.

FLUID REPLACEMENT

During continuous activity of more than 30 minutes, fluid should be replaced at a rate of 100–150 ml every 15–30 minutes, even if the child is not thirsty (12, 13). Bar-Or recommends that replacement fluids for children not exceed 5 mEq/L Na^+ (0.3 g/L NaCl), 4 mEq/LK K^+ (0.28 g/L KCl), and 25 g/L sugar (13). Haymes and Welles suggest that children weighing 40 kg should ingest 150 ml of cold water every 30 minutes during activity (15). There does not seem to be any benefit from ingesting carbohydrate drinks (i.e., sport drinks) over water in preadolescent children who are well-hydrated (16).

OVERUSE INJURY

There has been an increase in children experiencing overuse injuries (17). Overuse injuries are caused by repetitive microtrauma to the musculoskeletal system (18). Risk factors for overuse injury include:

- Significant change in intensity, duration, frequency, or type of training
- Musculotendinous tautness (inflexibility) in early adolescence
- Imbalance of strength and flexibility
- Anatomic malalignment of lower extremities
- Incorrect biomechanics
- Improper footwear
- Training on hard surfaces
- Excessive loading of the back during growth spurts (17–19)

It is estimated that one-half of overuse injuries in children are preventable (19). Prevention involves improvement in musculoskeletal fitness and sports-specific skills and monitoring of growth rate to identify periods of accelerated growth when vulnerability may be greatest. Therefore, training should be modified by gradual progression with less than a 10% increase in training time, distance, or number of repetitions (19). The AAP recommends that pediatricians consider the risks of distance running when advising parents and children. However, at the present time, data do not support precluding children from distance running (5).

EXERCISE PRESCRIPTION

Large Muscular Activity

The recommendation for adults to lower risk for all-cause and coronary heart disease mortality is an energy expenditure of approximately 11–13 kJ/kg/d (3 to 4 kcal/kg of body weight/day), equivalent to approximately 30 minutes of brisk walking (20). To increase health-related fitness the exercise prescription guidelines are to engage in repetitive large muscle activity for 30–60 minutes at an intensity of 50–85% maximal oxygen uptake 3 to 5 times a week. In addition, health-related fitness includes resistance training for muscle strength and endurance and flexibility exercise (4).

For preadolescent children, the recommendation is 30–60 minutes of accumulated activity per day (6–8 kcal/kg body weight/day) to ensure that when children reach adulthood, they will meet the adult standard (11). Younger children generally do not like prolonged exercise without rest periods; therefore, exercise prescription for sustained large muscle activity for a minimum of 20 minutes may be discouraging and interfere with enjoyment (21). Increased energy expenditure coupled with appropriate eating habits is a major component of multidisciplinary programs for both prevention and management of obese children (22).

For preadolescent children, the primary goal is to maintain activity, to enjoy movement, and to develop lifelong activity habits. To accomplish these goals preadolescent children should be:

- Allowed to be naturally active
- Allowed to control the intensity and duration of the activity (21)
- Enjoying the activity
- Encouraged to play outside away from the television and computer (23)
- Involved with organized activities where emphasis is placed on gaining basic motor and sport skill competency since the motorically competent adult (who can play a variety of sports or who can participate in dance) will be more likely to participate in activity throughout life (7)
- Provided active role models by parents/guardians and family members

Multidisciplinary intervention programs should be implemented for children who are sedentary, obese, or disabled. Girls may require additional support to be physically active (23).

For adolescent children, motor and sport skill acquisition should be emphasized. The specific recommendation for activity and exercise to improve health-related fitness from the International Consensus Conference on Physical Activity Guidelines for Adolescents is found below (3).

Guideline 1: All adolescents should be physically active daily, or nearly every day, as part of play, games, sports, work, transportation, recreation, physical education, or planned exercise, in the context of family, school, and community activities. Adolescents should do a variety of physical activities as part of their daily lifestyles. These activities should be enjoyable, involve a variety of muscle groups and include some weight bearing activities. The intensity or duration of the activity is probably less important than the fact that energy is expended and a habit of daily activity is established. Adolescents are encouraged to incorporate physical activity into their lifestyles by doing such things as walking up stairs, walking or riding a bicycle for errands, having conversation while walking with friends, parking at the far end of parking lots, and doing household chores.

Guideline 2: Adolescents should engage in three or more sessions per week of activities that last 20 minutes or more at a time and that require moderate to vigorous levels of exertion. Moderate to vigorous activities are those that require at least as much effort as brisk or fast walking. A diversity of activities that use large muscle groups are recommended as part of sports, recreation, chores, transportation, work, school, physical education, or planned exercise. Examples include brisk walking, jogging, stair climbing, basketball, racquet sports, soccer, dance, swimming laps, skating, strength (resistance) training, lawn mowing, strenuous housework, cross-country skiing, and cycling.

The promotion of active lifestyles and lowering obesity rates is dependent on community support, availability of safe and accessible facilities, media exposure and advertising and socioeconomic and political factors. It is imperative to look at the broader picture for promotion of activity, especially for minorities, individuals with disabilities, and individuals in lower socioeconomic levels where safe facilities and other cost-related factors may prohibit activity. Children with an illness or disability may require specific or modified exercise prescription (4, 13, 24, 25). Specific prescriptions may also be recommended for hypokinetic children or for those with two or more risk factors for coronary artery disease.

STRENGTH TRAINING

Strength is the maximal force or torque developed by a muscle, or muscle group, during a maximal voluntary contraction. **Muscle endurance** is the ability of a muscle, or muscle group, to exert force continuously (without producing movement) or repetitively (while producing or resisting movement). **Power** is the rate at which work is performed. **Strength training** uses a variety of methods to increase ability to exert or resist force (11, 26). Strength training usually involves a series of repetitions against a resistance. Greater repetitions and lower resistance effects muscle endurance, whereas fewer repetitions with greater resistance produces strength gains (27). **Weight lifting and power lifting** are competitive sports in which maximal weight is lifted in a single attempt (28). **Body building** is a competitive sport in which the participants use various methods to develop muscle size, symmetry, and definition (29).

Consideration of the potential benefits of training (e.g., strength gains, injury protection, improved sports performance, psychological benefits, and learning of proper techniques) should be weighed against potential risks (e.g., low back injury, growth plate injury in adolescents, as well as other acute and chronic musculoskeletal injuries, "weight lifter's blackout," and hypertension) (30). It is generally agreed that the benefits of participation for a child with the emotional maturity to follow directions outweigh the risks with supervision by a well-trained adult (28–30).

Strength testing and training equipment should be adaptable to body size (28). Field and laboratory tests for muscular strength and endurance are described in the literature (26). Recommendations for strength training in children are numerous and fairly consistent across multiple sources (4, 24, 28, 30, 31). Strength training programs for children should be characterized by:

- Close, continuous, trained supervision
- Adequate warm-up
- High repetitions per set (no less than 6 to 8 repetitions per set)
- Adequate recovery between sessions (frequency of no more than 2 to 3 days a week)
- Emphasis on proper form
- Inclusion of flexibility exercises (especially during adolescent growth spurts)

In the early stages of a program, children can use body weight as resistance, and specific lifts should be introduced using little or no load with emphasis on technique. Overload is initially achieved by increasing repetitions, followed by increased resistance. It is recommended that children avoid weight lifting, power lifting, and body building as well as the use of high resistance in strength training programs until Tanner stage 5 of developmental maturity (29). It is generally agreed that strength training should be one component of the exercise program for increasing fitness or performance, but should not be the sole component.

It is clear that strength gains can be realized with minimal risk of injury in prepubescent and pubescent children (28). Preadolescents make similar but smaller absolute strength gains compared with adolescents and young adults in response to similar resistance training programs. As in adults, the gains are dependent on training load. Training-induced strength gains are lost during detraining (30).

GRADED EXERCISE TESTS

Rationale for Exercise Testing

Some reasons for using exercise testing in pediatric populations are listed in Table 60.4. Application of graded exercise testing (GXT) to specific diseases or problems is beyond the scope of this chapter. More detailed information is available (32, 33). In many cases, the GXT is best used as an affirmation that exercise can be performed safely. For research purposes, the legality and ethics of involving children should be carefully considered and informed consent of both parent and child should be obtained (34).

Ergometers

The same types of ergometers can be used with children and adults, although treadmill testing is preferable for children (especially under age 7 years). Premature, local muscle fatigue and inability to maintain required or accurate cadence may prevent children from reaching maximal values on a cycle ergometer. Most children must be taught correct use of ergometers. Cardiorespiratory measurements should be directly assessed, since estimation of maximal values from submaximal $\dot{V}O_2$ is

Table 60.4. Rationale for Exercise Testing in Pediatric Diagnosis

Measure physical working capacity
1. Assess daily function—establish whether daily activities are within physiological functioning level
2. Identify deficiency in specific fitness component—muscular endurance and strength may limit daily performance rather than aerobic capacity (e.g., muscular dystrophy)
3. Establish a baseline before onset of an intervention program
4. Assess effectiveness of an exercise prescription
5. Chart the course of a progressive disease (e.g., cystic fibrosis, Duchenne muscular dystrophy)
Exercise as a provocation test
1. Amplify pathophysiologic changes
2. Trigger changes otherwise not seen in the resting child
Exercise as an adjunct diagnostic test
1. Non-invasive exercise test can be used for screening to determine the need for an invasive test
2. Assessing the severity of dysrhythmias
3. Assessing functional success of surgical correction
4. Assessing adequacy of drug regimens at varying exercise intensities
Assessment and differentiation of symptoms
1. Chest pains (asthma from myocardial infarction)
2. Breathlessness (bronchioconstriction from low physical capacity)
3. Coughing
4. Easy fatiguability
Instill confidence in child and parent
Motivation or compliance in intervention program

Adapted from Bar-Or O. Exercise in pediatric assessment and diagnosis. *Scand J Sport Sci* 1985;7:35–39.

not reliable because efficiency of gait is variable (13). Handrails and the support system for gas-analysis equipment should be modified (35).

When using an ergometer, an electronically braked cycle ergometer is preferred because power output is not dependent on pedal rate. Pedaling rates of 50–60 rpm are recommended for mechanically braked ergometers (13). Special pediatric ergometers or existing ergometers modified in children ages under 9 years. The handlebars, seat height (angle of the knee joint in the extended position is 150°) and pedal crank length (13 cm for age 6 years; 15 cm for age 8 to 10 years) should all be adjusted (13, 33). In addition, smaller resistance increments may be required, therefore resistance indicators on the cycle ergometer should be in 5-watt gradations. Some special population children may require an arm ergometer for testing. Some test procedures (e.g., radionuclide imaging and echocardiography) are more easily accomplished on a cycle ergometer (33).

Protocol

A variety of protocols are appropriate for children (13, 32, 33, 36). Some are similar to those used in adults, but in some instances, modification of initial power output and subsequent incremental increases are necessary. The specific protocol selected depends on:

- The goals and objectives of the test
- The measurements to be obtained
- Whether submaximal and/or maximal data are required
- The abilities and limitations of the patient

A GXT is not required prior to initiating an exercise program for asymptomatic children.

Supervisory Personnel

A physician with training in exercise testing, along with training in the performance of exercise tests in children with disorders of varying severity, should assume responsibility for directing diagnostic exercise testing although actual conduct of the test may be delegated to qualified personnel (33). A physician should be actively involved in testing for the following conditions (13, 33):

- Serious rhythm disorders
- Aortic stenosis with gradients >50 mm Hg
- Myocardial disease
- Cyanotic heart disease
- Advanced pulmonary vascular disease
- Ventricular dysrhythmia with heart disease
- Coronary artery disease
- ACSM certified individuals can perform/supervise maximal exercise testing in normal children for research purposes (33).

Contraindications to Exercise Testing in Children

In addition to the contraindications listed in the *ACSM Guidelines*, the following are also contraindications to exercise testing of pediatric patients. Children who have (4, 13, 33):

1. Dyspnea at rest or whose 1-sec forced expiratory volume (FEV_1) or peak expiratory flow is less than 60% of predicted value.
2. Acute renal disease or hepatitis.
3. Insulin-dependent diabetes and did not take insulin as prescribed or who are ketoacidotic.
4. Acute rheumatic fever with carditis.
5. Severe pulmonary vascular disease.
6. Poorly compensated heart failure.
7. Severe aortic or mitral stenosis.
8. Hypotrophic cardiomyopathy with syncope.

Criteria for Test Termination

Criteria for stopping an exercise are similar to those for adults included in the Guidelines (4). Attainment of peak $\dot{V}O_2$ and/or maximal heart rate are termination criteria for exercise testing in children.

Maximal Oxygen Uptake ($\dot{V}O_2max$)

Evidence for a plateau in children is less common than in adults, therefore, $\dot{V}O_2$ peak values are the norm (36). Data on intraindividual variation in $\dot{V}O_2max$ indicate, however, that acceptable data can be obtained even if criteria for identifying a plateau in $\dot{V}O_2max$ are not always satisfied (13, 36).

Maximal Heart Rate

Children with weakened or atrophied (e.g., muscular dystrophy or cerebral palsy) peripheral musculature, congenital heart block (and a number of other congenital heart defects), anorexia, and those receiving beta-blocker therapy may have reduced maximal heart rate (HR) (4, 13). Younger children attain a higher HR_{max} than adults (see Table 60.1). Maximal heart rate usually does not change until after puberty when there is a decrease of 0.7 or 0.8 beats per minute per year. Treadmill exercise results in a slightly higher HR_{max} than does cycle ergometry (33).

▶ SUMMARY

Exercise, exercise testing, and exercise training are safe in children. Children may respond differently to exercise and exercise training and may have different needs, requirements, and desire for activity than adults. They should be encouraged to be spontaneously active, but planned exercise with skill development is also important. Caution during exercise in climatic extremes is important. Exercise testing is not contraindicated in children, but additional precautions exist.

References

1. Sallis JF, Patrick K, Long BJ. Overview of the international consensus conference on physical activity guidelines for adolescents. *Ped Exerc Sci* 1994;6(4):299–301.
2. Cooper DM. New horizons in pediatric exercise research. In: Cameron CJR, Bar-Or O, eds. *New Horizons in Pediatric Exercise Science.* Champaign, IL: Human Kinetics, 1995;1–24.
3. Sallis JF, Patrick K. Physical activity guidelines for adolescents: Consensus statement. *Ped Exerc Sci* 1994;6(4):302–314.
4. American College of Sports Medicine. *ACSM's Guidelines for Exercise Testing and Prescription.* 5th ed. Baltimore: Williams & Wilkins, 1995.
5. American Academy of Pediatrics Committee on Sports Medicine. Risks in running for children. *Pediatrics* 1990;86(5):656–657.
6. Bar-Or O. Exercise in childhood. In: Walsh RP, Shephard RJ, eds. *Current Therapy in Sport Medicine, 1985–1986.* Toronto: C.V. Mosby, 1985.
7. Bar-Or O, Malina RM. Activity, fitness, and health of children and adolescents. In: Cheung LWY, Richmond JB, eds. *Child Health, Nutrition, and Physical Activity.* Champaign, IL: Human Kinetics, 1995;79–124.
8. Zwiren LD. Exercise in children and youth. In: Shepard RJ, Miller H, eds. *Exercise and the Heart in Health and Cardiac Disease.* New York: Marcel Dekker, 1992.
9. Bailey DA, Martin AD. Physical activity and skeletal health in adolescents. *Ped Exerc Sci* 1994;6(4):424–433.
10. American Academy of Pediatrics (AAP). AAP Committee on Sports Medicine. Amenorrhea in adolescent athletes. *Pediatrics* 1989;84:394–395.
11. Rowland TW. *Exercise and Children's Health.* Champaign, IL: Human Kinetics, 1990.
12. American Academy of Pediatrics. Climatic heat stress and the exercising child. *Phys Sport Med* 1983;11:155–159.
13. Bar-Or O. *Pediatric Sports Medicine for the Practitioner: from Physiologic Principles to Clinical Applications.* New York: Springer, 1983.
14. Armstrong LE, Maresh CM. Exercise-heat tolerance of children and adolescents. *Ped Exerc Sci* 1995;7(3):239–252.
15. Haymes EM, Wells CL. *Environment and Human Performance.* Champaign, IL: Human Kinetics, 1986.
16. Meyer F, Bar-Or O, MacDougall D, et al. Drink composition and the electrolyte balance of children exercising in the heat. *Med Sci Sport Exerc* 1995; 27(6):882–887.
17. Macera CA, Wooten W. Epidemiology of sports and recreation injuries among adolescents. *Ped Exerc Sci* 1994;6(4):424–433.
18. American Academy of Pediatrics, Committee on Sports Medicine and Fitness (1991). *Sports Medicine: Health Care for Young Athletes.* Elk Grove Village, IL: American Academy of Pediatrics, 1991.
19. American College of Sports Medicine. The prevention of sport injuries of children and adolescents. *Med Sci Sport Exerc* 1993;25(8):1.
20. Blair SN, Clark DG, Cureton KJ, et al. Exercise and fitness in childhood: implications for a lifetime of health. In: Gisolfi CV, Lamb DR, eds. *Perspectives in Exercise Science and Sports Medicine.* Indianapolis: Benchmark, 1989;401–422.
21. Pangrazi RF, Corbin CB, Welk GJ. Physical activity for children and youth. *JOPERD* 1996;67(4):38–43.
22. Pate RR. Physical activity in children and youth: Relationship to obesity. *Contemp Nutr* 1993;18(2).
23. Klesges RC, Malott JM, Boschee PF, et al. The effects of parental influences on children's food intake, physical activity, and relative weight. *Intl J Eating Disord* 1986;5:335–346.
24. Goldberg B, ed. *Sports and Exercise for Children with Chronic Health Conditions.* Champaign, IL: Human Kinetics, 1995.
25. Small E, Bar-Or O. The young athlete with chronic disease. *Clin Sport Med* 1995;14(3):709–726.
26. Gaul CA. Muscular strength and endurance. In: Docherty D, ed. *Measurement in Pediatric Exercise Science.* Champaign, IL: Human Kinetics, 1996;225–258.
27. Wathen D. Load assignment. In: Baechle TR, ed. *Essentials of Strength Training and Conditioning.* Champaign, IL: Human Kinetics, 1994.
28. National Strength and Conditioning Association (NSCA). Position paper on prepubescent strength training. *Natl Strength Cond Assoc J* 1985;7(4):27–31.
29. American Academy of Pediatrics (AAP), Committee on sports medicine. Strength, training, weight and power lift-

ing, and body building by children and adolescents. *Pediatrics* 1990;86:801.
30. Blimkie CJR. Resistance training during preadolescence. Issues and controversies. *Sports Med* 1993;15(6):389–407.
31. Freedson PS, Ward A, Rippe JM. Resistance training for youth. In: Grana WA, Lombardo JA, Sharkey BJ, eds. *Advances in Sports Medicine and Fitness* (Vol. 3). Chicago: Year Book Medical Publishers, 1990;57–65.
32. Rowland TW. Aerobic exercise testing protocols. In: Roland TW, ed. *Pediatric Laboratory Exercise Testing: Clinical Guidelines.* Champaign, IL: Human Kinetics, 1993;19–41.
33. American Heart Association (AHA). Guidelines for exercise testing in the pediatric age group. *Circulation* 1994;90(4): 2166-2179.
34. Armstrong N, Welsman JR. Assessment and interpretation of aerobic fitness in children and adolescents. *Exerc Sport Sci Rev* 1994;22:435–476.
35. Docherty D, ed. Introduction. In: *Measurement in Pediatric Exercise Science.* Windsor, ON (Canada): Human Kinetics, 1996;1-13.
36. Léger L. Aerobic performance. In: Docherty D, ed. *Measurement in Pediatric Exercise Science.* Windsor, ON (Canada): Human Kinetics, 1996;183–224.

61, 62 64, 65, 66 67, 68 314, 315, 316, 317

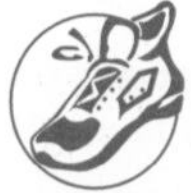  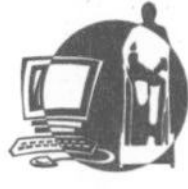 

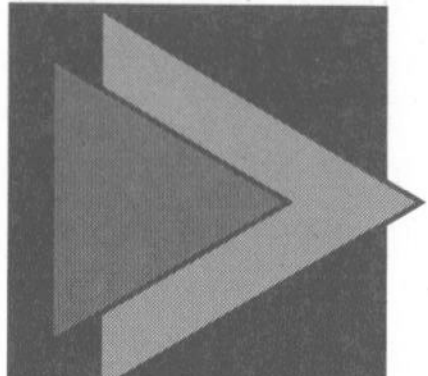

CHAPTER 61
EXERCISE PROGRAMMING FOR OLDER ADULTS

Gregory W. Heath

Older adults (≥ 65 years) who engage in regular physical activity have increased physical working capacity, decreased body fat, increased lean body tissue, increased bone density, and lower rates of coronary artery disease (CAD), hypertension, and cancer (1–6). Increased physical activity is also associated with longevity (7). The benefits of regular physical activity and exercise can enhance the quality of life for older individuals, improving their capacity for work and recreation, and altering the rate of decline in functional status (8). In the design and prescription of exercise for older adults, a number of physiological, anatomical, and behavioral characteristics should be considered to ensure a safe, effective, and enjoyable experience.

PHYSICAL ACTIVITY IN OLDER ADULTS

Maximum oxygen uptake ($\dot{V}O_2max$) declines steadily with age; however, the level of activity influences this change (1). The prevalence of physical inactivity during leisure time among older adults is approximately 33% (11). In contrast, 25% of older adults report engaging in moderate levels of physical activity regularly. Participating in moderate exercise five or more times per week is important because of the potential health benefits that can be accrued in this age group with this level of physical activity (12, 13). Clearly, the majority of older adults are not sufficiently active.

In consideration of the effect of aging and inactivity on $\dot{V}O_2max$, many older adults just beginning a regular program of physical activity have low levels of cardiorespiratory fitness. The age-associated decline in fitness may also be exacerbated by the presence of pathology. Therefore, the initial exercise prescription requires that it be tailored to this population.

Overcoming Pre-existing Pathology

In spite of the increased likelihood of chronic pre-existing conditions, older individuals can obtain benefits from regular endurance exercise training that are similar to those observed in younger adults (15). For example, $\dot{V}O_2max$ can increase significantly in sedentary older adults persons when they engage in regular endurance activity. Lower heart rate, blood pressure, and blood lactate levels can be demonstrated with regular submaximal endurance exercise (15, 16).

Coronary artery disease (CAD) is the most prevalent chronic disease in the elderly (15). Often cardiovascular limitations associated with aging result from CAD or complications of the disease. There are a number of contraindications for exercise in older adults with pre-existing CAD and other forms of heart disease. However, the exercise prescription can usually be adapted for the less severe contraindications.

Respiratory function does not limit exercise capacity unless pulmonary function is significantly impaired, as in cases of chronic obstructive pulmonary disease (e.g., emphysema or chronic bronchitis). The ventilatory changes associated with aging do not interfere with the ability to manifest significant improvements in $\dot{V}O_2max$ after training (17).

BENEFITS OF REGULAR EXERCISE IN OLDER ADULTS

A lifetime of regular physical activity appears to delay the slowing of reaction times associated with aging; however, the results of studies of exercising in previously sedentary older individuals are inconclusive (18). Although few researchers have documented the positive or negative effects of regular physical activity on psychological function, some investigators report decreased levels of anxiety and an increased sense of well-being in older adults who exercise (19, 20).

Increased strength, with mild to moderate muscle hypertrophy, has been demonstrated with regular strength training in older adults (21, 22). Regular weight-bearing exercise can cause increased bone density in middle-aged and older women, and men who exercise regularly have higher bone densities than sedentary men (23). Flexibility programs for older adults significantly improve range of motion in the neck, shoulder, wrist, back, hip, knee, ankle, and other joints (16). Regular physical activity increases lean body mass and decreases body fat among older participants (3). Alterations in glucose and lipid metabolism have also been demonstrated in older individuals engaging in regular endurance activity and there have been reports of improved glycemic control in diabetics (24).

The pharmacologic status of older adults is important to consider when developing an individualized exercise program. Vigorous exercise may affect the activity of some medications (e.g., decreased insulin requirement or increased sensitivity to dehydration), and some medications (e.g., beta blockers) can affect the patient's response to exercise.

Specific personality, attitudinal, and behavioral characteristics have been identified in older adults which predict improved adherence to regular physical activity. These include greater self-efficacy, intention, and perceived control (25–27). Regular physical activity can be effective in maintaining functional independence, enhancing the sense of well being, and reducing anxiety in the older adult (28, 29).

MEDICAL HISTORY AND SCREENING FOR EXERCISE PROGRAMMING

Exercise programming for older adults is usually offered in three different ways (30–32):

- Program-based, consisting primarily of supervised exercise training.
- Exercise counseling and exercise prescription followed by self-monitored exercise.
- Community-based, which is self-directed and self-monitored.

Supervised Exercise Programs

In supervised exercise programs and programs offering exercise counseling and prescription, participants should complete a brief medical history and risk factor questionnaire (33). In this way, important information regarding potential limitations and restrictions for the activity program may be obtained. Guidelines require physician approval for older participants prior to beginning a program of moderate or vigorous exercise. Furthermore, participants should be encouraged to consult a physician with any questions regarding medical status.

After the medical history is obtained, participants should undergo a preprogram evaluation to document baseline measurements in flexibility, aerobic endurance capacity, and strength. These baseline measures are crucial not only for prescribing the appropriate level of physical activity, but also in monitoring progress through repeat assessments. The assessment need not be sophisticated, but measurements should be standardized.

By observing gait and movement from a seated to standing position, the health care professional may be able to identify sensory impairment, impaired equilibrium, or orthostatic hypotension. Strength testing may take the form of a simple grip strength test combined with a modified push-up and sit-up. Cardiorespiratory endurance capacity can be assessed by appropriate field tests, such as a 12-minute walk/run or step test, or a submaximal bicycle test to assess heart rate and blood pressure (34). These tests are intended to evaluate submaximal functioning. In appropriately screened individuals, they are relatively safe and effective, and provide data needed to develop an exercise prescription and physical activity education program. Potential participants with documented CAD, diabetes mellitus, or risk factors for these diseases should be referred for diagnostic exercise tolerance testing as well as functional assessment.

Community-based Exercise Programs

In community-based, self-monitored programs, medical clearance is usually the decision of the participant. The physical activity promotion campaign attempts to educate the older population regarding precautions and recommendations for moderate and vigorous physical activity (1). The message should provide steps for older adults to begin a regular program of physical activity. These steps should include:

- Awareness of pre-existing medical problems (e.g., CAD, arthritis, osteoporosis, or diabetes mellitus)
- Consultation with a physician or other appropriate health professional before starting a program
- Information on different types of activity and instructions on selecting an activity appropriate for the individual
- Principles for intensity, duration, and frequency of activity
- Principles for initiation and progression of activity
- Principles for monitoring symptoms of excessive fatigue
- Recommendations for making exercise fun and enjoyable

GENERAL EXERCISE PRESCRIPTION GUIDELINES

Mode of Activity

Many older individuals who participate in regular exercise programs or want to do so have significant limitations. Exercise programs for persons with degenerative joint disease (including osteoarthritis), which is common in this age group, must be appropriately modified.

An emphasis on minimal or nonweight-bearing, low-impact activities, such as cycling, swimming, chair, and floor exercises, may be most appropriate. Activity may be contraindicated initially for individuals with restricted mobility in the knees and hips, or with restricted movement to and from the floor. Most older adults are able to engage in moderate walking activities. Individualization of the mode of activity, including variation of activity and adjustments for participant bias and preference, is important. Caution should be exercised when persons with degenerative joint disease participate in calisthenics. However, modified stretching and strengthening may be used. Recommendations for modification of activities for patients with selected chronic conditions are listed in Table 61.1.

Frequency

Emphasis is placed on increased frequency of exercise in older adults (5 to 7 days per week), as it may enhance or promote the maintenance of endurance capacity as well as flexibility. In addition, increased frequency enhances compliance and leads to a greater probability of assimilation of physical activity into a daily routine (36).

Duration

Twenty to forty minutes of endurance activity per session is an appropriate goal for most older adults. However, pathophysiological limitations may indicate a need for a shorter duration (10–15 minutes) repeated 2 to 3 times a day. In contrast, some age-related limitations may require that the intensity of exercise be decreased and, thus, the duration increased (up to 60 minutes, if possible).

Intensity

Intensity is critical due to general medical and physiological limitations that often exist in older individuals (36). For participants with CAD or at high risk for CAD, the exercise prescription should be based on the results of a recent diagnostic exercise test. An appropriate exercise prescription based on target heart rate or metabolic equivalent (MET) level and adjusted for symptoms and/or electrocardiographic changes can be formulated. The young-old (aged ≤75 years) may have a peak work capacities greater than 7 METs; whereas the old-old (aged >75 years) frequently have peak work capacities of less than 4 METs. Medical and physical activity status may vary significantly, and generalization of workload can be difficult. The use of MET levels to establish intensity after assessment of work capacity is useful. Rate of perceived exertion (RPE) is effective in regulating intensity in older individuals (37).

Progression of Activity

A gradual increase in physical activity is most appropriate after initiation of exercise; 4–6 weeks is usually adequate for most older participants to progress from moderate to vigorous conditioning. Another 4–6 weeks may be necessary to achieve maintenance level. Individual variability in fitness and adaptation to exercise usually dictates the rate of progression.

Table 61.1. Modification of the Exercise Prescription: Selected Aging-Related Conditions

Condition	Recommended Modification
Degenerative joint disease	Non-weight bearing activities such as stationary cycling, water exercises, and chair exercises. Emphasis placed on interval activity. Low resistance—low repetition strength training.
Coronary artery disease (CAD)	Physician oversight. Symptom-limited activities. Moderate level endurance activities preferred (i.e., walking, slow cycling), although at physician's discretion more vigorous activities can be prescribed. Low resistance, higher repetition strength training. (see Chapter 16)
Diabetes mellitus	Daily, moderate endurance activities. Low resistance, higher repetition strength training. Flexibility exercises. Monitoring of symptoms and caloric intake. In the presence of obesity, non-weight bearing exercises may be indicated.
Dizziness, ataxia	Chair exercises may be preferred. Low resistance, low repetition strength training. Moderate flexibility activities with minimal movement from supine or prone to standing positions.
Back syndrome	Moderate endurance activities (i.e., walking, cycling, chair exercises). Modified flexibility exercises; low resistance, low repetition strength training; modified abdominal strengthening activities; water activities.
Osteoporosis	Weight-bearing activities with intermittent bouts of activity spaced throughout the day. Low resistance, low repetition strength training, chair level flexibility activities.
Chronic obstructive lung disease	Moderate level endurance using an interval or intermittent approach to exercise bouts. Low resistance, low repetition strength training; modified flexibility and stretching exercises.
Orthostatic hypotension	Minimize movements from standing to supine and supine to standing. Sustained moderate endurance activities with short rest intervals. Emphasize activities that minimize the changing of body positions.
Hypertension	Emphasize dynamic large-muscle endurance activities; minimize isometric work and focus on low resistance, low repetition isotonic strength training.

LEADING AN EXERCISE PROGRAM FOR OLDER PARTICIPANTS

Planning

Community-based exercise programs require an assessment of resources and participant preferences prior to implementation. The use of focus groups is an appro-

sical activity needs. This
nation about local facili-
social barriers to exercise,
nned exercise program.
ouraged to provide input
es to be provided. Com-
with local and regional
de valuable planning in-
gencies can provide dem-
older adults and lists for
ontacts. The promotion of
be focused, often with dif-
et groups. This allows the
lequate subset of the older
gramming.
for older adults should be
neory. Physical activity is a
ng should establish behav-
or participation. Programs
of physical, environmental,
of activity are more likely
participant adherence. The
nysical activity behavior ap-
n to increasing participation
lly with older adults (38).

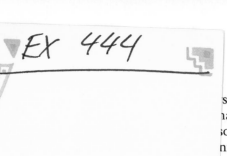

The exercise facility should have adequate lighting and ventilation. Because of the prevalence of hearing impairment in older adults, background noise in exercise facilities should be limited so that the participants can hear instructions clearly. A resilient surface is more accommodating and less likely to result in injury. For the same reason, well-cushioned mats are recommended for floor exercises.

EXERCISE LEADERSHIP

Programming

Programs should offer a variety of activities designed not only for conditioning, but also for fun and enjoyment. A staff that is well trained, amiable, and ACSM-certified is preferred. Many programs succeed without the best facility or equipment because staff members are empathetic, knowledgeable, and fun. Knowledge of the community and its resources is important, since the sites selected for exercise programming should be convenient and accessible.

Emergency Skills

Staff involved in supervised programming should be certified in Basic Life Support cardiopulmonary resuscitation (BLS-CPR) and knowledgeable about basic first aid. Familiarity with major medical disorders of older adults (e.g., CAD, diabetes, arthritis and hypoglycemia) assures a safer environment for exercise. An emergency plan is required in supervised programs. Information about emergency contacts and the primary physician should be available for each participant. Participants in a supervised program or for whom exercise counseling and prescription is provided should know their medical and pharmaceutical regimens and how they influence exercise. A pattern of referral for medical consultation should be available if participants do not have a primary physician.

SUMMARY

As the aging population grows and the effects of physical inactivity predominate in this population, exercise programs for older adults are of increasing importance. Regular physical exercise has many physiological and psychological benefits in both apparently healthy and chronically ill older adults. Although programming may require different planning processes than for younger individuals and exercise prescription often requires adaptation, the importance of community programs and resources for older adult exercise programs cannot be underestimated.

References

1. Bortz WM. Disuse and aging. *JAMA* 1982;248:1203–1208.
2. Sidney KH, Shephard RJ, Harrison JE. Endurance training and body composition of the elderly. *Am J Clin Nutr* 1977;30:326–333.
3. Smith DM, Khairi MR, Norton J, et al. Age and activity effects on rate of bone mineral loss. *J Clin Invest* 58:716–721, 1976.
4. Paffenbarger RS, Hyde RT, Wing AL. Physical activity as an index of heart attack risk in college alumni. *Am J Epidemiol* 1978;108:161–175.
5. Tipton CH. Exercise, training, and hypertension: an update. *Exerc Sport Sci Rev* 1991;19:447–505.
6. Lee IM, Paffenbarger RS, Hsieh CC. Physical activity and risk of developing colorectal cancer among college alumni. *J Natl Cancer Inst* 1991;83:1324–1329.
7. Paffenbarger RS Jr, Hyde RT, Wing AL, et al. Physical activity, all-cause mortality, and longevity of college alumni. *N Engl J Med* 1986;314:605–613.
8. Shephard RJ. Exercise and aging: extending independence in older adults. *Geriatrics* 1993;48:61–64.
9. Lakatta EG. Cardiovascular reserve capacity in healthy older humans. *Aging* 1994;6:213–223.
10. Heath GW. Physical fitness and aging: effects of deconditioning. *Sci Sports* 1994;9:197–200.
11. Siegel PZ, Frazier EL, Mariolis P, et al. Behavioral risk factor surveillance, 1991: monitoring progress toward the nation's year 2000 health objectives. *MMWR* 1993;42(SS-4):4–6.
12. Crespo CJ, Keteyian SJ, Heath GW, et al. Leisure-time physical activity among US adults. *Arch Intern Med* 1996;156:93–98.
13. Pate RR, Pratt M, Blair SN, et al. Physical activity and public health—a recommendation from the Centers for Dis-

ease Control and Prevention and the American College of Sports Medicine. *JAMA* 1995;273:402–407.

14. National Center for Health Statistics. *Healthy People 2000 Review, 1993*. Hyattsville, MD: Public Health Service, 1994: 7–13.
15. Van Camp SP, Boyer JL. Cardiovascular aspects of aging. *Phys Sports Med* 1989;17:121–130.
16. Brown M, Holloszy JO. Effects of walking, jogging and cycling on strength, flexibility, speed and balance in 60–72-year-olds. *Aging* 1993;5:427–434.
17. Smith EL. Special considerations in developing exercise programs for the older adult. In: Matarazzo JD, Weiss SM, Herd JA, et al., eds. *Behavioral Health: A Handbook of Health Enhancement and Disease Prevention*. New York: John Wiley & Sons, 1984.
18. Spirduso WW. Reaction and movement time as a function of age and physical activity. *J Gerontol* 1975;30:435–440.
19. Barry AJ, Page JF, Steinmetz JR, et al. Effects of physical conditioning on older individuals: motor performance and cognitive function. *J Gerontol* 1966;21:192–199.
20. Sidney KH, Shephard RJ. Attitudes towards health and physical activity in the elderly: effects of a physical training program. *Med Sci Sports Exerc* 1977;8:246–252.
21. Frontera WR, Meredith CN, O'Reilly KP, et al. Strength conditioning in older men: skeletal muscle hypertrophy and improved function. *J Appl Physiol* 1988;64:1038–1044.
22. Rogers MA, Evans WJ. Changes in skeletal muscle with aging: effects of exercise training. *Exerc Sport Sci Rev* 1993;21: 365–379.
23. Chow R, Harrison JE, Notarius C. Effects of two randomized exercise programmes on bone mass of healthy postmenopausal women. *Br Med J* 1987;295:1441–1444.
24. Seals DR, Hagberg JM, Hurley BF, et al. Effects of endurance training on glucose tolerance and plasma lipid levels in older men and women. *JAMA* 1984;252:645–649.
25. McAuley E. Self-efficacy and the maintenance of exercise participation in older adults. *J Behavior Med* 1993;16:103–113.
26. Courneya KS. Understanding readiness for regular physical activity in older individuals: an application of the theory of planned behavior. *Health Psych* 1995;14:80–87.
27. Emery CF, Hauck ER, Blumenthal JA. Exercise adherence or maintenance among older adults: 1-year follow-up study. *Psych Aging* 1992;7:466–470.
28. Emery CF, Pinder SL, Blumenthal JA. Psychological effects of exercise among elderly cardiac patients. *J Cardiopulm Rehab* 1989;9:46–53.
29. Stewart AL, King AC, Haskell WL. Endurance exercise and health-related quality of life in 50- to 65-year-old adults. *Gerontologist* 1993;33:782–789.
30. Brown M, Holloszy JO. Effects of low intensity exercise program on selected physical performance characteristics of 60- to 71-year olds. *Aging* 1991;3:129–131.
31. Barry HC, Eathorne SW. Exercise and aging: issues for the practitioner. *Med Clin North Am* 1994;78:357–376.
32. King AC, Haskell WL, Taylor CB, et al. Group- vs home-based exercise training in healthy older men and women. A community-based clinical trial. *JAMA* 1991;266:1535–1542.
33. Smith EL, Gilligan C. Physical activity prescription for the older adult. *Phys Sports Med* 1983;11:91–101.
34. Hagberg JM. Exercise assessment of arthritic and elderly individuals. *Baillieres Clin Rheum* 1994;8:29–52.
35. King AC, Haskell WL, Young DR, et al. Long-term effects of varying intensities and formats of physical activity on participation rates, fitness, and lipoproteins in men and women aged 50 to 65 years. *Circulation* 1995;91:2596–2604.
36. King AC, Taylor CB, Haskell WL. Effects of differing intensities and formats of 12 months of exercise training on psychological outcomes in older adults. *Health Psych* 1993;12:292–300.
37. Hassemen P, Ceci R, Backman L. Exercise for older women: a training method and its influence on physical and cognitive performance. *Eur J Appl Physiol Occup Physiol* 1992;64:460–466.
38. Marcus BH, Simkin LR. The stages of exercise behavior. *J Sports Med Phys Fitness* 1993;33:83–88.

SECTION TWELVE

MODIFICATIONS OF HEALTH BEHAVIOR

SECTION EDITOR: *Douglas R. Southard, PhD*

92 96 319 322 327

CHAPTER 62
HEALTH COUNSELING SKILLS

Douglas R. Southard and Barbara H. Southard

Chapters in this section on psychology and behavior modification provide resource material useful to counselors in health and fitness settings. This initial chapter presents an overview and addresses interpersonal communication issues common to all health counseling environments. Chapter 63 examines the concept of adaptive vs. maladaptive mechanisms of coping with life stressors. This is followed by a chapter describing common forms of psychopathology often associated with an inability to cope in an adaptive manner. Basic principles of modifying behavior, along with elements of stress management and social support, critical components in all lifestyle interventions, are presented in Chapters 65–67. Finally, the remaining chapters cover counseling issues specific to exercise promotion, dietary intervention, and smoking cessation.

HEALTH COUNSELING SKILLS

Counselors in health promotion settings serve four significant functions. The first is to **develop rapport and convey a sense of empathy** for the challenges participants confront in making and maintaining lifestyle changes. The second function is to **assess health-related behaviors** in terms of their impact on optimum functioning and risk for disease, which includes understanding the perspective of the participant on how these behaviors contribute to health and quality of life. This second function also includes assessing the current state of readiness for change. The third function is to **facilitate change** through discussion of potential benefits and problems associated with implementing a lifestyle change. This function allows participants to make informed decisions consistent with personal values. Finally, the counselor is in a key position to assist the participant in **managing transient life crises** which may include allowing the participant to ventilate feelings while skillfully expressing empathy. The counselor must also be sufficiently knowledgeable regarding psychopathology to identify participants needing referral for further evaluation and possible treatment.

Function 1: Developing Rapport and Conveying Empathy

Acceptance

The counselor should set a tone of openness and acceptance during initial conversations with the participant. It is particularly important to refrain from appearing judgmental regarding lifestyle or health history. Such a perception on the part of the participant could affect the type of information the participant is willing to disclose, or the accuracy of the information. To act in a nonjudgmental manner is not easy, particularly if values conflict, as is often the case in the area of health behaviors. Therefore, it is important for the counselor to separate personal values and beliefs from that of the participant. Only then can the counselor begin to respond in an objective as well as empathetic manner, both verbally and nonverbally.

Expressing Empathy Through Active Listening

Empathy has been defined as the ability to understand people from their frame of reference rather than your own (1). Empathy can be conveyed by expressing a desire to comprehend through the use of active listening responses. This involves identifying what the participant is experiencing and then paraphrasing it back. Such paraphrasing serves to ensure that the counselor has made an accurate interpretation and also conveys that the counselor is truly attempting to listen and understand what is being said. For example, a counselor might respond to a participant's complaints by saying "You seem frustrated with not being able to jog as fast as you would like." This response is particularly effective as it identifies and reflects the emotional component of the experience. Such statements facilitate the development of rapport and self-disclosure.

In contrast, expressing sympathy conveys an attempt to actually experience another's feelings (e.g., "I've had the same thing happen to me") or to imply pity for the experienced (e.g., "I'm sorry that you are having a problem"). Although such responses are useful in some limited situations, in general, the counselor should be careful not to convey that personal experiences are exactly the same as the participant or that an expression of sympathy is only given because it is socially appropriate. However an empathetic response, as noted above, is almost always helpful.

Active listening can also be conveyed through the use of questions designed to clarify a statement or probing for additional information. For example, if a participant said, "I've tried to stop smoking, but every time I do I gain a ton of weight and go right back to smoking again anyway. The only thing I change is my weight, and that's not a good change either." A clarifying response would be, "When you say a ton of weight, just how much do you really mean?" A more probing response would be, "Can you tell me how you tried to stop smoking? Did you take a class, use a transdermal patch, or go cold turkey?"

At times, the counselor may wish to summarize the report with the intention of identifying a general theme or rephrasing a story in a succinct way. Using the above example, a summarizing response might be: "So you've tried unsuccessfully to stop smoking, and as a result you weigh more than before you tried to quit." An interpretative response is different from summarizing in that it goes a step further and offers some insight regarding the problem that goes beyond what has been stated. For example, an interpretative response to the same example could be: "You've tried to quit smoking, just ended up gaining weight, and now maybe you're just a little afraid that if you try again, you'll end up gaining even more weight." Interpretations are a little riskier than summarizing statements and generally are used after establishing good rapport and a comfortable counseling relationship.

Non-verbal Communication

Communication between counselor and participant includes both verbal and non-verbal components. Although the verbal portion of a message is often easiest to describe, the non-verbal component is also an extremely important mode of conveying information (1). Non-verbal communication, such as maintaining good eye contact, is essential to the development of rapport and expression of empathy. Humans respond to non-verbal communication, even if they are not specifically aware of what they are sensing and responding to. Experienced counselors, however, are particularly alert to seeing and hearing non-verbal communication. For example, when asked about his diet, a participant may report "I kept up with it fairly well." Based upon the verbal report, one might suspect the participant is doing well. However, poor eye contact and inflections in the tone of voice and hesitant, low-energy speech might suggest that compliance with the prescribed diet may not have been "fairly well." Such incongruence between verbal and non-verbal components should prompt the counselor to consider a gentle, inquisitive confrontation regarding the issue (e.g., "You say you are keeping up with your diet but you seem hesitant when talking about it. I'm wondering if you could share with me any problems you might be having?").

Non-verbal communication can be divided into three main categories. **Kinesics** refers to body movements which convey information, such as eye contact, hand gestures, winking, body position, and facial expressions. Poor eye contact, extremely low levels of body movement, or a flat or sad facial expression are particularly important cues for the counselor to observe and monitor. Characteristics of speech, such as voice inflections and changes in volume are collectively referred to as **paralinguistics.** These characteristics often modify the meaning of the verbal content. The example at the beginning of this section in which the voice inflection conflicts with verbal statements regarding dietary compliance provides an example of how important it is to be aware of paralinguistics in sorting out the true meaning of the words.

Finally, characteristics of interpersonal space, such as seating arrangements and interpersonal distance, are included in the non-verbal component of **proxemics.** Awareness of proxemics is vital to achieving an atmosphere conducive to successful counseling. For example, a participant is more likely to feel comfortable during individual counseling if the counselor uses a small, private room, where there are minimal barriers (e.g., having only the corner of a desk rather than a large desk between counselor and participant) and where the chairs, temperature, noise level, etc., are comfortable and appropriate. On the other hand, in a group counseling session, the room should be larger in order to comfortably accommodate more people. In addition, a room that is noisy or lacking in privacy might hinder open sharing and communication. Finally, arranging chairs in a circle so that all participants can make eye contact with each other can facilitate open discussion in group sessions.

Function 2: Assessing Health Related Behaviors

Behavioral Assessment

The importance of obtaining a comprehensive history of health-related behaviors cannot be over-emphasized. In addition to self-report, a particularly useful strategy for gathering data during the assessment phase is to have the participant track or self-monitor health behaviors, preferably in a graphic format over a prescribed period of time. It may also be helpful to involve family members and significant others in the interview process. Frequently, people close to the participant have valuable insight into health behaviors and can provide information that the participant may not aware of or is not able, willing, or ready to disclose. Thus, these important sources often supply the "missing links" or "holes" in what a counselor has been able to glean. In addition, they can also provide the counselor with a better understanding of the social environment in which the participant will attempt to make lifestyle changes.

Motivational Assessment

Health-related behaviors must be placed in the context of the values and overall lifestyle of the participant. Whereas one cannot "motivate" individuals directly, one can appeal to what motivates them. Motivations for health-related behavior change, however, may not be the same for the participant and the health professional. The challenge is to find common ground where health-enhancing recommendations also meet a valued participant need. For instance, the counselor may suggest a regimen of regular aerobic exercise to increase the cardiopulmonary endurance. The initial response may be a lack of perception of a significant need to engage in such activity, since the participant is currently very functional. Careful questioning, however, may reveal that the participant discontinued hunting several years ago due to lack of strength and endurance. In this case, the task would be to connect the need for cardiopulmonary endurance with the desire to once again participate in a valued recreational activity. Once this match is realized and appreciated, the task is to help the participant develop clear, well operationalized goals to be achieved within a specific time frame.

Function 3: Facilitating Change

Counselor's Role

The task of the counselor is to serve as a facilitator of change more than as simply a prescriber of change. Thus, the counselor and participant should work together to discuss, develop, and agree on a plan for change. In doing so, the counselor should be wary of the tendency to overwhelm the participant with a barrage of verbal commands and written materials designed to promote compliance. Simplicity is often a key to success.

During this partnership the counselor should always keep in mind that the ultimate goal for the participant is to accept and maintain responsibility for personal behavior. Dependency on the counselor is a real threat to long-term maintenance, one that is not readily apparent to those new to the counselor role. Therefore, it is critical that the counselor encourage independence. For example, the counselor may facilitate social support and link rewards for success to family and friends, rather than solely from the counselor. In addition, the participant must be encouraged to accept personal responsibility for making the change and solving related problems which arise on a day-to-day basis.

In preparing for behavior change, it is often helpful to assist the participant in identifying all of the benefits as well as the costs of the behavior change. Consider having the participant list the benefits on one side and costs on the other side of a piece of paper. Then ask the individual to compare and to determine whether the benefits truly outweigh the costs. The role of the counselor during this process is to help the participant explore all the possibilities in terms of costs and benefits, including those that may not have been considered. Once identified, discussion can be focused on methods to decrease the costs and accentuate the benefits. Unfortunately, this exercise is often bypassed in the haste to "get on with" the behavior change. Such a seemingly "intellectual" exercise puts the behavior change into perspective and provides a frame of reference that can be used to advantage during difficult times in the behavior change process. For instance, the written list can be saved for use during relapse when the patient may have "lost" perspective and to bring back the original frame of reference in terms of the cost/benefit ratio.

Participants often have mixed feelings regarding the adoption of a new behavior (e.g., exercise) or cessation of a valued behavior (e.g., smoking, high fat diet, etc.). It is therefore not uncommon to hear a participant say, "I want to lose weight," only later to admit that he/she doesn't want to change eating habits. When the counselor suspects a conflict, gentle confrontation may be a very useful technique. This entails restating the two conflicting points and probing for clarification. For example, "Mary, I need you to help me. You've said that you really want to exercise more often and that 5:30 p.m is the best time for you. Still, you rarely are able to make it. What are you saying to yourself when you are making the decision not to exercise?" Although an extremely useful technique, confrontation, if not carefully worded, can be uncomfortable for both participant and counselor. Hence, gentle confrontation is generally employed once rapport has been established. Chapter 64 provides an overview of additional techniques relevant to modifying health related behaviors.

Working in Groups

Group counseling is an alternative or supplement to individual counseling. Groups can be designed specifically for the efficient conveyance of information or for a combination of information and social support. Some groups address a variety of related issues (e.g., ongoing cardiac rehabilitation support group) while others are more time limited and focused on a specific topic (e.g., weight loss, anger control, etc.). Small group formats offer several advantages over individual counseling. First and foremost is social support. Participants can sometimes "hear" information and advice better from other participants than from professional counselors. They may also "see" themselves in other participants and begin to better understand some of their own problems. Participants can also offer important feedback to other participants in a way that counselors cannot. Additionally, a small group allows participants to "give" support, encouragement, feedback, etc., in an altruistic manner, a gesture which has been shown to be of significant psychological benefit (2).

Powerful as these small groups can be, it is important that the counselor be prepared to deal with potential problems that may arise. This requires informing the group from the beginning regarding the rules of confidentiality, instructing them to speak about their own challenges using "I" statements, and cautioning them against giving extensive "advice" to others on how to solve their problems.

Function 4: Managing Transient Life Crises

Types of Crises

Counselors in health and fitness settings routinely encounter participants experiencing one or more life crises. Some of the more common types include: interpersonal stress involving marital, family, and significant others; financial stress involving changes in job status or outstanding medical bills; crises due to loss of health or function, and crises involving legal problems (see Chapter 63 and 64). Crisis management can be conceptualized as a series of five basic steps.

1. Listen actively and express empathy. Do not take responsibility for or try to solve problems quickly unless related to a safety issue under your control.
2. Assess for imminent danger (harm to self or others). Notify appropriate authorities or refer to other health care providers as necessary.
3. Assist the client in clarifying problems and identifying options.
4. Facilitate the development of a plan of action. This may use individual, family, community, and professional resources.
5. Follow-up with the participant in person or by phone to determine the effectiveness of your counseling and/or referral.

Managing Crises in Small Groups

While groups offer an excellent environment for facilitating behavior change, they may be uncomfortable for both practitioner and participants if significant emotional distress is present. Episodes of crying, anger outbursts, and interpersonal conflict are particularly uncomfortable. "Knee-jerk" reactions to either ignore the event or take immediate action to restore a peaceful environment may not be the most effective. Rather, it may be more appropriate to use active listening skills that focus on the process (e.g., "John, this seems to make you angry," or "Helen, you seem upset when talking about this issue.") and to acknowledge that such feelings are reasonable and/or acceptable (e.g., "It's OK to cry, these are difficult issues to deal with"). Tissues should be available and offered to those who cry. Interpersonal conflict within the group can also be openly acknowledged; however, it is essential to minimize escalation through the use of facilitator input (e.g., "Bob, can you describe what it is about Henry's behavior that bothers you without verbally attacking him?").

▶ SUMMARY

Health counselors can enhance the development of rapport and facilitate behavior change through using active listening responses and by paying careful attention to non-verbal, as well as verbal forms of communication. Assessment of health related behaviors should include self-monitoring data and reports from significant others when possible. It is also important to identify and appeal to aspects of the behavior change that the participant finds inherently motivating. Counselors can facilitate change by gently confronting participants when they present with conflicting thoughts or feelings regarding behavior. Long-term success is increased when counselors promote self-reliance and emphasize the development of problem solving skills. Counselors also have an important role in assisting individuals as they attempt to make behavior changes while coping with common life crises. The therapeutic success can be enhanced through the use of small group work as a supplement or alternative to individual counseling.

References

1. Cormier WH, Cormier LS. *Interviewing Strategies for Helpers: Fundamental Skills and Cognitive Behavioral Interventions.* Pacific Grove, CA: Brooks/Cole Publishing Co, 1993.
2. Yalom ID. *The Theory and Practice of Group Psychotherapy.* 3rd ed. New York: Basic Books, Inc., 1985.

Suggested Readings

Purtilo R. *Health Professional and Patient Interaction.* 4th ed. Philadelphia: W.B. Saunders Company, 1990.

Sotile WM. *Psychosocial Interventions for Cardiopulmonary Patients: A Guide for Health Professionals.* Champaign, IL: Human Kinetics, 1996.

98 318, 319, 320 322 329

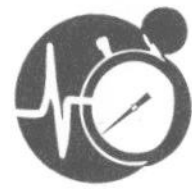

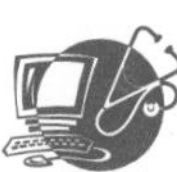

CHAPTER 63
STRESS AND COPING

Wesley E. Sime and Kathryn Hellweg

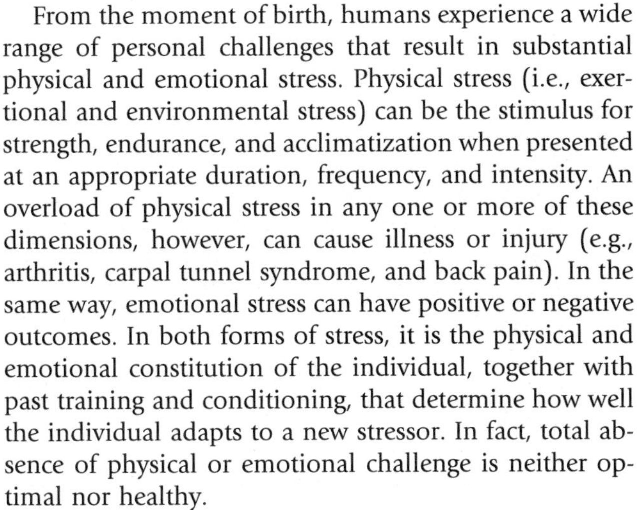

From the moment of birth, humans experience a wide range of personal challenges that result in substantial physical and emotional stress. Physical stress (i.e., exertional and environmental stress) can be the stimulus for strength, endurance, and acclimatization when presented at an appropriate duration, frequency, and intensity. An overload of physical stress in any one or more of these dimensions, however, can cause illness or injury (e.g., arthritis, carpal tunnel syndrome, and back pain). In the same way, emotional stress can have positive or negative outcomes. In both forms of stress, it is the physical and emotional constitution of the individual, together with past training and conditioning, that determine how well the individual adapts to a new stressor. In fact, total absence of physical or emotional challenge is neither optimal nor healthy.

Healthy, vibrant working adults who become ill suddenly and unexpectedly (e.g., cardiac patients) are likely to be highly stressed. The change in lifestyle (diet, exercise, etc.), temporary limitations in work capability and threat to the identity (e.g., loss of a sense of physical prowess) induced by the sudden change in health status are substantive stressors. For men in particular, the ego-threatening compromise in physical ability can be devastating and depressing. Many patients become self-conscious about the medical attention required and resist acknowledging the disease state. Family members who sincerely express concern and put forth reminders to help the patient follow medical orders or maintain limits or restrictions on eating and working may become the target of angry, defensive reactions.

Family members are likely to experience a variety of emotional responses, ranging from fear of losing a close relative to irritability over failure to follow prescribed behavioral changes. Special efforts are recommended to provide emotional support for spouses and to elicit their cooperation in both understanding the patient and in reinforcing positive behavioral changes as needed. Social support from family and friends has a buffering effect on cardiovascular response (e.g., reduced blood pressure and heart rate) to stressful challenges (1, 2).

Throughout this chapter, many healthy and appropriate stress coping principles are described, including the accurate appraisal of an undesirable event (e.g, a heart attack) as a means of developing physical and emotional hardiness, and participation in a well-designed rehabilitation program. Some of these principles are based on pioneering work on the psychophysiological effects of stress and the stress-reducing effects of exercise (3–6).

STRESS AS A CHALLENGE FOR POSITIVE OR NEGATIVE OUTCOMES

Considerable empirical experience shows that a program of progressively increasing emotional or cognitive challenge is both healthy and invigorating. Individuals who are confronted with reasonable task demands and who meet such demands usually feel personally satisfied as well as better able to cope with new challenges. The ability to adapt to new circumstances and to cope with apparent threats is most important for emotional as well as physical health, especially cardiovascular health. "The coping process has been described as one of constant change in cognitive and behavioral reactions to manage external or internal demands that the individual appraises as taxing to existing resources" (8).

Coping with stress can be either positive or negative as illustrated in Figure 63.1. Using a work stress model, this figure shows how a healthy, capable employee who is beset by overwhelming burdens, challenges, or demands can emerge from the travail successfully with increased confidence, higher self-esteem, and a sense of hardiness gained from having faced a difficult challenge and being committed to having a positive outcome. The figure also shows how the person who views the task as burdensome, who gains little satisfaction from the work, who worries and frets, and gets little substantive relaxation (i.e., recreation), and who may also be sleep-de-

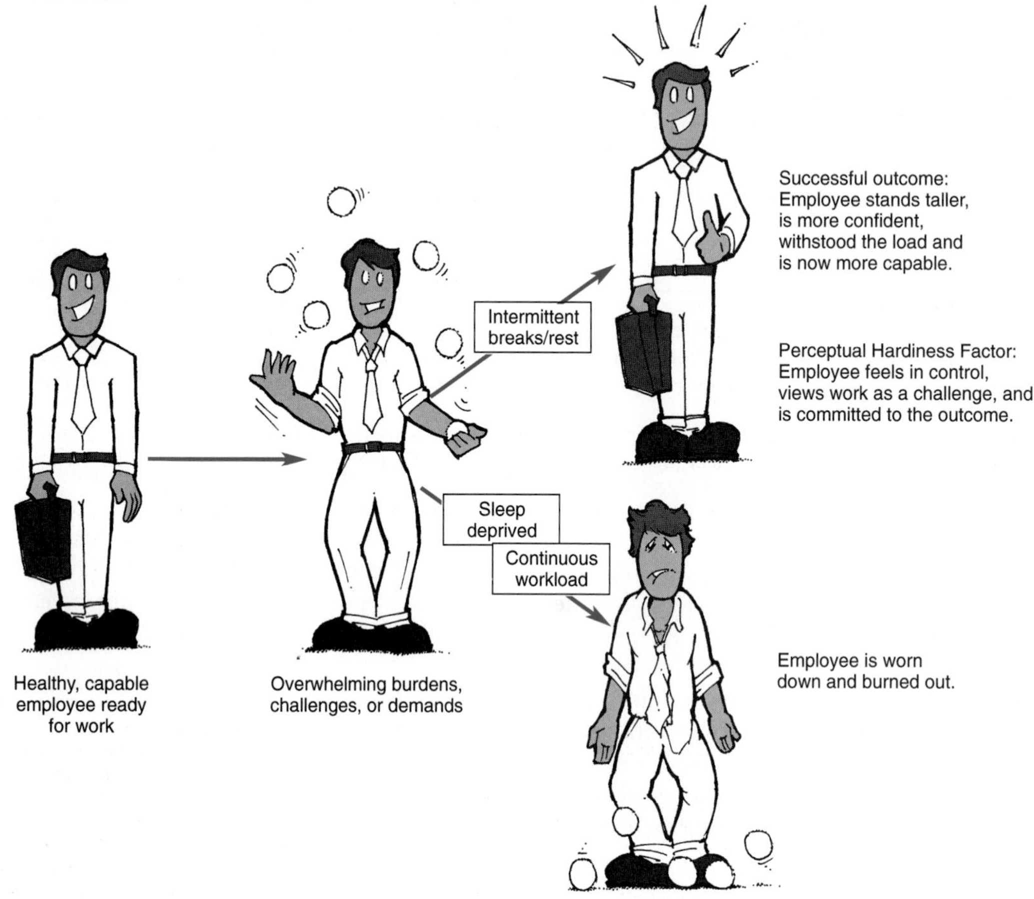
Successful outcome:
Employee stands taller,
is more confident,
withstood the load and
is now more capable.
Intermittent
breaks/rest
Perceptual Hardiness Factor:
Employee feels in control,
views work as a challenge, and
is committed to the outcome.
Sleep
deprived
Continuous
workload
Employee is worn
down and burned out.
Healthy, capable
employee ready
for work
Overwhelming burdens,
challenges, or demands

Figure 63.1. Illustration of positive and negative outcomes in reaction to stressful situations.

prived is more likely to burn out. While the model presented in this illustration is oversimplified, it provides patients with a clear picture of the effects of overwork coupled with little personal satisfaction.

The concept of emotional stress or distress is controversial, partly because the stimulus "load" of the stressful event or circumstance is difficult to describe objectively. In exertional and environmental stress, the units of "load" are clear and generally universal (e.g., foot/pounds, kilocalories, and atmospheric pressure); in humans, however, emotional load is determined in part by personal interpretation, which is influenced greatly by personality factors and past experience. Personality variables can be assessed objectively and will be discussed in detail throughout this chapter. However, past experiences are more difficult to assess objectively and vary widely with the degree of traumatization and accumulation over time. For example, some individuals exhibit remarkable tolerance for prior traumas, while others are extremely sensitive to the occurrence of even a single distressing event (e.g., events causing embarrassment, terror, anger, or hopelessness), allowing it to cause substantial distress.

Individual variation in coping styles may account for variations in sensitivity to stressful events. The response to stress may be unique. Ordinarily, a stressful circumstance may be thought of as an immediate threat or acute challenge. For a cardiac patient, the stress is initially acute, due to a fear of death. The initial period is followed by the long-term uncertainty of other potential compromises (e.g., inability to work) and complications. A heart attack is perhaps most worrisome to patients because a quick and fatal incident is always a serious possibility. The irony is that when patients worry about future ills and when they are prone to emotional outbursts, their risk for coronary disease increases (9). As a result, it is extremely important to make patients aware of the risks associated with acute and chronic stress exposure and help them develop coping skills.

COPING WITH STRESS

A number of situational and personality factors influence the appraisal of stress. A description of factors associated with job stress is provided in Tables 63.1 and 63.2. These items are presented as a concept (e.g., nov-

Table 63.1. Situational Factors That Influence Appraisal of Stress Using Job Stress Examples

SITUATIONAL FACTORS	DESCRIPTION	EXAMPLE
Novelty (with negative history)	Facing a new situation with a history of harm, danger, or loss in similar past experiences	New job assignment while having experienced embarrassment or failure in previous assignments
Predictability (consequence, no control)	Recognizing warning signals of impending threat without option to prevent it	Seeing indications that a bad outcome might result from a new job assignment
Imminent threat with time to worry	Knowing that harm, danger, or loss will likely occur, but not knowing when it will occur	Receive notice that job layoffs are expected sometime in the near future
Incubation period and length of exposure	Time period prior to stressful event as well as duration of exposure	Job layoffs will occur in 30 days and could last 3–6 months or longer
Anticipation of a time limited event	Not knowing when an event is going to occur but knowing that it won't last very long	Rumors that a layoff is inevitable in the near future, but layoffs never last more than a week or two
Acute versus chronic exposure	Immediate short-term exposure contrasted with regular intermittent threats of extended losses	Taking a cut in pay to obtain a stable, secure job versus keeping a lucrative job risking frequent layoffs
Situational ambiguity	Lack of clarity or insufficient information to make an appraisal of degree of threat	Rumors threaten job security, but no one knows which areas will be affected

Adapted from R. Lazarus and S. Folkman. Stress, Appraisal and Coping. Spring Publishing Co., New York, 1984, pp. 55–115.

Table 63.2. Personality Factors that Influence Appraisal of Stress Using Job Stress Examples

PERSONALITY FACTORS	DESCRIPTION	EXAMPLE
Personal uncertainty	Confusion in one's mind about the meaning of the warning signals or the degree of threat	Received notice of promotion or transfer, but not able to evaluate the risks versus the benefits
Commitment and risk-taking	Level of drive, determination, motivation, investment, persistence, planning, e.g., will to live	Making the choice to continue battling against adversity despite being vulnerable to embarrassment or disappointment
Belief system	Perceptual lens through which the events or circumstances are viewed and interpreted	Interpreting new opportunities in light of past experiences, personal values, etc.
Cognitive appraisal	The evaluation process of taking inventory; assessing loss or gain and options for future risk	Lost my job, but what advantages, disadvantages, result, e.g., more time to look for better job or to start a new business or profession
Stress coping	Individuals differ widely in sensitivity and vulnerability to various exposures to stressful circumstances	Anger, depression, anxiety, denial, guilt, challenge, vengeful, persistence, helplessness

Adapted from R. Lazarus and S. Folkman. Stress, Appraisal and Coping. Spring Publishing Co., New York, 1984, pp. 55–115.

elty) followed by a description (e.g., a new situation complicated by negative experiences in similar situations) and an example of how each factor influences the ability to cope with stress in a job setting. The situational factors include novelty, predictability, imminent threat (with time available to worry), incubation, exposures, anticipation of time-limited events, acute versus chronic exposure, and ambiguity.

The personality factors that influence the degree of stress reaction include:

- Personal uncertainty (confusion)
- Commitment and risk-taking
- Personal belief system (perception)
- Cognitive appraisal (taking inventory of advantages, disadvantages and options when facing a crisis)
- Inherent stress coping strategies (denial vs. feeling guilty; challenged vs. feeling helpless).

People can have situational ambiguity, but know exactly what decision to make when the stressor occurs; that is, an individual can have situational ambiguity without personal uncertainty. The greater the situational ambiguity, the more strongly personality factors influence the effect of stressful situations. Careful examination of the job examples (Table 63.1) reveals a wide variety of unique individual outcomes that emanate from the peculiar threat of each situational and personality variable as it relates to job security. Many cardiac patients have a history of high job stress preceding the onset of disease and can expect to experience some difficulty returning to the same level of job performance after treatment (10).

The relationship of stress to illness includes a critical role for cognitive appraisal. As described by Lazarus, it is the foundation of the Specificity of Illness Model, which suggests that any personal-environmental stressor is first mediated by individual appraisal which then determines the extent to which physiological disturbance and possibly illness occur (11). Emotions vary with the way an individual constructs and evaluates events or relationships in light of personal goals and expectations. Conflicts and adverse events affect the individual to the degree that cognitive interpretation of the event allows. This theory serves as the basis for several stress management techniques presented in Chapter 66 (2).

INHERENT STRESS COPING REACTIONS

Several additional inherent stress coping reactions distinguish stress coping from coping techniques specifically used to change attitudes or behaviors to manage stress. The limited discussion in this chapter will focus on denial, emotion-focused coping, problem-focused coping, and social-focused coping.

Denial

Interestingly, denial is sometimes a healthy response to stress. While denial appears to be negative and nonproductive (i.e., a closed-minded effort to minimize the problem), it has a few benefits. For example, if no constructive solution to an immediate problem is possible, denial can temporarily alleviate distress. In the instance of an anticipated job lay-off, for example, worry becomes needless if no immediate action can be taken. Denial can also be viewed as a strange mode of positive thinking (it will never happen to me), as long as it does not interfere with the ability to perform necessary job functions. On the other hand, denial is risky for cardiac patients when it precludes an early diagnosis and proper treatment. Regardless, the concept of denial can be beneficial as long as necessary therapy and medications are not neglected.

Emotion-Focused Coping

Emotion-focused coping is one of several natural reactions to an overwhelmingly stressful experience. Classic examples of emotion-focused coping include anger (toward self or others), avoidance, rationalization, rejection, and distancing. These are nonphysical, passive responses to stress; however, it is possible that an active response, such as exercise, may facilitate emotional coping. For example, exercise allows patients to distance themselves from stressful issues and allows them to work through their thoughts while working off physical tension. If anger is the predominant emotion, then some form of ballistic, vigorous exercise (e.g., punching a bag or stomping on a stair climber) can help dissipate the tension associated with emotion. Ironically, some individuals seem to need to embellish an angry response before the stressor can be overcome and recovery ensues. Relief comes only after a period of self-blame or self-punishment that allows the individual to fully experience the distress.

Problem-Focused Coping

Problem-focused coping is a far more appropriate means of responding to a crisis or any seriously distressing situation when a solution is available. The process includes both external and internal analysis. The **external analysis** includes the following steps:

1. Defining the problem.
2. Generating alternative solutions.
3. Weighing the alternatives.
4. Choosing the best alternative.

The **internal analysis,** which is designed for introspection of inherent self-defeating attitudes and behaviors) involves the following steps:

1. Changing goals to eliminate the problem.
2. Reducing ego involvement in the outcome.
3. Learning new skills to overcome the problem.
4. Developing new behaviors and new reinforcers to maintain those behaviors.

These are essential steps in crisis management, and should be offered as a part of the rehabilitation process.

Social-Focused Coping

Social-focused coping includes other people in the coping process. It also requires a minimum level of social skills. Individuals must be able to express their needs effectively and behave somewhat appropriately in order to elicit the cooperation and support that is required. This method of coping also tends to generate more problem-solving options and facilitates the use of group activity to negotiate potential solutions. One critical issue is to determine whether a personality problem exists that tends to bring on unnecessary challenges. If so, a referral to a psychologist or family counselor may be appropriate.

Interpretation, personality, and past experience cloud the ability to objectively measure emotional workloads or the demands of a particular task or experience. Therefore, the combination of physical, behavioral, cognitive, and emotional responses by the individual to a realistic stressor becomes the only measurable factor in the stress-illness equation, with physical and behavioral responses being the most objective and reliable factors.

OBJECTIVE INDICATORS OF FAILURE TO COPE

Physical responses indicating "failure to cope" include measures common in cardiac rehabilitation (e.g., increased heart rate, blood pressure, rate pressure product, etc.) and other less familiar parameters of heart health (e. g., peripheral resistance, peripheral blood flow, electrodermal response and electromyography). Other common physical signs and symptoms of stress are listed in Chapter 5 (12).

The most common and observable behavioral indicators of inadequate stress coping skills include irritability, fear, anger, anxiety, and depression. To some extent, these phenomena are observable and as such, can be recorded and documented in event-provoked circumstances such as a structured interview for Type A behavior patterns. Similarly, depression can be measured objectively through observation during an interview or by using a psychological screening instrument, such as the Beck Depression Inventory (13). Staff who suspect depression should refer the patient to a psychologist for testing and possible counseling, since depression is an important predictor of survival (14). For a comprehensive assessment, the entire array of behavioral and cognitive/emotional elements of stress can be determined through self assessment using a battery of questionnaires, such as the state/trait measures of anxiety, anger, hostility, self-deception, Type A personality, and hardiness (Table 63.3).

Self-reports of stress-coping are often influenced by situational factors and are subject to personal openness, honesty, and perceptual awareness. More specifically, some individuals fail to report behaviors that appear to be socially undesirable or reflect badly upon their character. Others are candidly honest, but inaccurate in their reporting, failing to report certain moods (e.g., depression) and behaviors (e.g., hostility) that are obvious to others, but not to themselves. Thus, it is important to interview the spouse and perhaps other family members to obtain more detailed information about the true coping ability of the individual in stress to determine the role of personality in the disease process.

STRESS HARDINESS AND COPING

Hardiness is defined as an internal resource facilitating resistance to stress. This personality construct applies to individuals who have a sense of commitment and a feeling of control, which allows them to view problems as mere challenges. Recent evidence suggests that hardiness is a valid indicator of long-term psychosocial adjustment in patients with coronary heart disease (15).

Several discrete personality subtypes (hardy, distressed, inhibited, repressed) have also been useful in predicting future risk of coronary heart disease (16). Hardy individuals tend to use active coping techniques; they are self-assured and resilient, which helps them to adjust easily to stressful difficulties. A higher risk for heart disease is found in individuals who are distressed (dissatisfied with self and others), inhibited (insecure and low in self-expression), or repressed (avoid confrontation and deny emotions). Overall, the difference between hardy individuals and others seems to lie in their appraisal of adverse events. In hardy individuals, events

Table 63.3. Measures of Stress and Coping Appropriate for Cardiac Rehabilitation Patients

State/Trait Anxiety (23)	State anxiety is the acute experience of distress at the moment, while trait anxiety is the tendency to feel anxious in general for no apparent reason.
Depression (13)	Feeling dejected with loss of interest and possible change in weight, appetite, increased fatigue, agitation, fatigue guilt, shame, low self-esteem, and self destructive tendencies.
State/Trait Anger (23)	The short-term immediate reaction to a provocation eliciting an emotional response is state anger. By contrast, the tendency to hold back the outward expression of severe disgruntlement and to turn the expression of angry inward is the trait anger measure.
Hostility Measures (25)	The experience of severe annoyance and anger compounded by profound verbal display or cynical portrayed with resentment, unpleasantness, and discourteousness.
Shapiro Control Inventory (17)	Patients who feel in control or having the ability to gain control as needed versus those who fear losing control have no control emotions, ability, power, etc.
Jenkins Activity Survey-Questionnaire (26)	Assessment of type A behavior pattern featuring three essential components: 1) speed and impatience; 2) hard driving and aggressive; and 3) high job involvement.
The Stress Profile (21)	The Stress Profile is a comprehensive measurement instrument that features elements of personal vulnerability to stress as well as strengths in coping by emotion-focused and problem-focused methods. It includes an appraisal of the patients work stress situation.
Kobasa's Hardiness Scale (27)	The concept of "hardiness" is defined as an internal resource facilitating stress resistance. This personality construct describes individuals who have three important personality qualities: 1) a sense of commitment; 2) a feeling of control; and 3) the ability to view problems as mere challenges.

appraised as less threatening and more controllable elicit less stress reactivity (9). Likewise, hardy individuals tend to have a strong sense of coherence, such that life circumstances are more comprehensible, manageable, and meaningful for them (17).

FACILITATING RESILIENCE AND STRESS COPING CONTROL

The amount of stress induced by a heart attack or a recent diagnosis of cardiac disease may vary with several personality factors. For some individuals, the fear of dying may compound the reaction to ordinary treatment and therapy; for others, a heart attack or surgery may be an acceptable reason to avoid a noxious job situation or strong justification for needing help with a marginally unbearable workload. As such, the convalescence period may produce some unintentionally rewarding experiences known commonly as "secondary gain." Initially, a patient may experience emotional shock due to a crisis that occurs without warning. From a psychological standpoint, the patient may feel helpless, panicky, and confused, then tend to go through withdrawal and denial. Hopefully, during the recovery phase, there will be an opportunity for reality testing, wherein the best and the worst of the situation is recognized so that a healthy recovery can be pursued.

In general, coping is described as the continuous process of adjusting thoughts and behaviors to avoid, manage, or ignore some form of threat or challenge (Fig. 63.1). Unfortunately, there are numerous inherent constraints that can compromise effectiveness of coping, including fear of public embarrassment, fear of failure, fear of success, feeling helpless, guilty or distrustful, and not wanting to appear "needy." In the worst cases, some individuals are so personally conscientious that they never seek assistance because they would feel obliged to return the assistance, and that sense of personal indebtedness is simply intolerable.

Issues of control, or lack thereof, also tend to compromise the effectiveness of various coping instincts. Some individuals have a greater need for control than others, especially when coping with stress. Some interesting manifestations of control must be considered in light of "coping" among patients.

1. Primary control is an attempt to change the environment.
2. Secondary control is an effort to fit in better.
3. Predictive control involves guessing about future risks to avoid distress.
4. Illusory control involves aligning with the most likely outcome to share in the success for stress relief.
5. Interpretive control involves developing a logical rationale, so that understanding why bad things happen provides some stress relief.
6. Vicarious control involves becoming associated with other powerful influences to share in their success.

Efforts have been made to assess several dimensions of control related to cardiovascular risk (18). Some individuals have either a sense of being in control or having the ability to gain control as needed. At the other extreme are individuals who have either a fear of losing control or a sense of having no control over such things as emotions, ability, power, etc. The Shapiro Control Inventory describes four specific dimensions of controlling behavior:

- Positive assertive (decisive leader)
- Negative assertive (manipulative or over-controlling)
- Negative yielding (timid, indecisive)
- Positive yielding (trusting, accepting)

Unfortunately, no single homogeneous control profile in cardiovascular disease has been clarified; rather, several combinations of these profiles are associated with increased risk (18).

Patients often feel out of control following a heart attack or bypass surgery. However, those who view a problem as a challenge, who also feel commitment to family and a sense of control over their destiny are more likely to survive and thrive (19). Fortunately, it is possible to assess these and other psychosocial coping behaviors using a comprehensive stress profile in rehabilitation (20).

The Stress Profile is a comprehensive instrument that can elicit candid patient responses to personal and professional areas of concern for stress and coping (Fig. 63.2) (21). It is designed to screen elements of personality that are vulnerability to stress as well as coping strengths, while assessing work stress concerns. Results of the assessment are provided in graphic illustrations by category (psychosocial, work environment, family relationships, major life events, hassles versus satisfactions, self-perception, coherence, coping skills, stress reactions, and burnout). Each patient is encouraged to review the results with a staff member to confirm the accuracy of the assessment and to make a plan of action that reduces the causes of stress and enhances coping skills.

Several other complicating factors must be dealt with in order to strengthen coping behaviors. Many patients are emotionally challenged by exercise tolerance testing used for diagnosis and for exercise prescription. Even an exercise training program can be viewed as a stage for performance and evaluation. By comparison, these experiences are similar to having test anxiety. Fortunately,

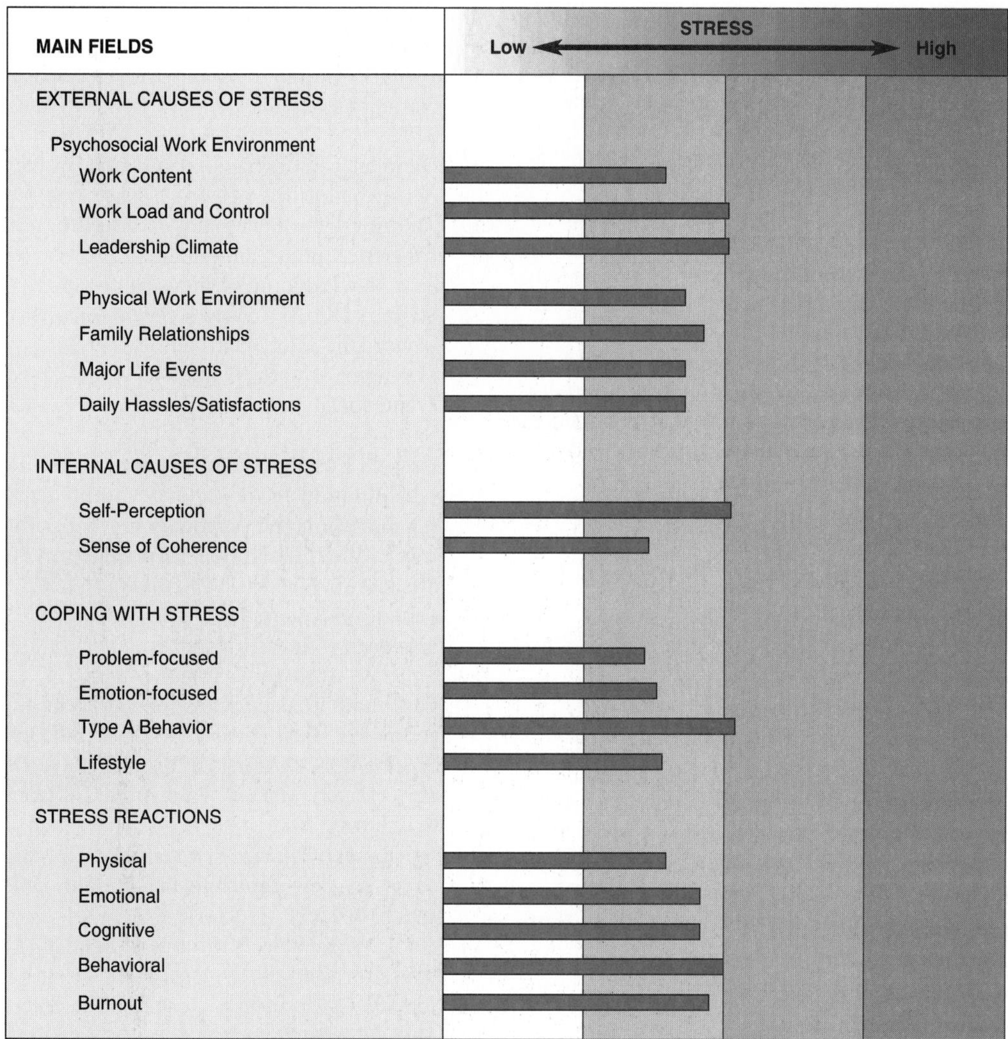

Figure 63.2. Main Field Output from the Stress Profile.

it has been possible to reduce test anxiety and improve performance (22).

Getting patients to communicate well and socialize among themselves may be one of the most important ways of reducing situational anxiety in the clinical testing and training environment. Finally, it should be noted that many patients have a legitimate fear of dying. While death is inevitable, it is often hard to recognize and accept the fact that cardiovascular function is compromised and that risk of death, in a number of months or years, is high.

▶ SUMMARY

The above is an attempt to provide a realistic and meaningful discourse on the most relevant issues related to coping with stress. That stress is a challenge which can be met in widely diverging ways is clearly evident from the illustration in Figure 63.1. A variety of situational and personality variables are presented (Tables 63.1 and 63.2) that influence perception and appraisal of the degree to which a stressful event provokes a distressful outcome. There are several inherent coping reactions (denial, emotion, social and problem-focused coping) that interact within each person, making them more, or less, vulnerable (or hardy) in the face of difficult circumstances. Recognizing the need for control (with positive and negative implications for assertiveness or manipulative behavior) among cardiac patients is critical to long-term survival. Lastly, the use of an interactive interview and a plan of action for coping with real-world stressors is strongly recommended.

References

1. Gerin W, Pickering T. Social support as moderator of cardiovascular reactivity: a test of the direct effects and buffering hypothesis. Proceedings of the Society of Behavioral Medicine Meeting. Boston MA, April 1994.
2. Sotile W. Stress management. Resource manual for guidelines for exercise testing and prescription. In Roitman J, ed. *Resource Manual for Guidelines for Exercise Testing and Prescription* 3rd ed. Philadelphia, PA: Lea & Febiger, 1998.
3. Sime W, McKinney M. Stress management applications in the prevention and rehabilitation of Coronary Heart Disease. In Blair S, Painter P, Pate R, et al., eds. *Resource Manual for Guidelines for Exercise Testing and Prescription.* 1st ed. Philadelphia, PA: Lea & Febiger, 1988.
4. Sime W, McGahan M, Eliot R. Stress management and Coronary Heart Disease: Risk assessment and intervention. In: Durstine JL, King A, Painter P, et al, eds. *Resource Manual for Guidelines for Exercise Testing and Prescription.* 2nd ed. Philadelphia, PA: Lea & Febiger, 1993.
5. Sime W. Psychophysiological (emotional) stress testing for assessing coronary risk. *J Cardiovasc Pulm Tech* 1980;8:27.
6. Sime W. Psychological benefits of exercise. *Adv Inst Health* 1984;1(4):15–29.
7. Reference deleted.
8. Lazarus R. Progress on a cognitive-motivational-relational theory of emotion. *Am J Psychol* 1991;46(8):819–834.
9. Eliot RS. *From Stress to Strength: How to Lighten Your Load and Save Your Life.* New York, NY: Bantam Press, 1994:24–42.
10. Maschewsky W. Psychosocial working conditions in industry and coronary heart disease. Proceedings of the First International Symposium on Work Environment and Cardiovascular Disease. Copenhagen, Denmark, June 1995.
11. Lazarus R, Folkman S. *Stress, Appraisal and Coping.* New York, NY: Springer Publishing Co, 1984:55–115.
12. Sime W, Eliot RS, Solberg EE. Stress and coronary heart disease: epidemiology and risk assessment. In: Roitman JL, et al, eds. *Resource Manual for Guidelines for Exercise Testing and Prescription.* 3rd ed. Baltimore: Williams & Wilkins, 1998.
13. Beck AT. *Depression. Causes and Treatment.* Philadelphia, PA: University of Pennsylvania Press, 1972.
14. Frazure-Smith N, Lesperance F, Talajic M. Depression following myocardial infarction. *JAMA* 1993;270:1819–1825.
15. Drory Y, Florian Y. Long-term psychosocial adjustment to coronary artery disease. *Arch Phys Med Rehab* 1991;72:326–331.
16. Denollet J. Biobehavioral research on coronary heart disease: where is the person? *J Behav Med* 1993;16:115–141.
17. Antonovsky A. Personality and health: testing the sense of coherence model. In: Friedman HS, ed. *Personality and Disease.* New York, NY: Wiley, 1990:155–177.
18. Shapiro DH. *The Shapiro Control Inventory.* New York: Behaviordyne Inc, 1994.
19. Rosengren A, Orth-Gomor K, Wedel H, et al. Stressful life event, social support and mortality in men born in 1933. *Br Med J* 1993;307:1102–1110.
20. Lisspers J, Hallgren D, Hallgren I, Setterlund S. Changes in rehabilitation factors after a comprehensive program for rehabilitation and secondary prevention of CHD. Proceedings of the International Conference on Stress and Health. Stockholm, Sweden, September, 1996.
21. Setterlund S, Larsson G. The stress profile: a psychological approach to measuring stress. *Stress Med* 1995;2:85–92.
22. Sime W, Ansorge C, Olson J, Parker C, Lukin M. Coping with math anxiety: stress management and academic performance. *J Coll Student Pers* 1987;28(5):421–437.
23. Spielberger CD, Gorsuch RL, Lushene R. *The State-trait Anxiety Inventory Manual.* Palo Alto, CA: Consulting Psychologist Press, 1970.
24. Spielberger C, Grier K, Greenfield G. Major dimension of stress in law enforcement. *Fl Frat Order Pol J* Spring 1982;10–12.
25. Cook W, Medley D. Proposed hostility and phasic-virtue scales for the MMPI. *J Appl Psych* 1954;38:414–418.
26. Jenkins C, Zyzanski S, Rosenman R. *Jenkins Activity Survey Manual.* New York, NY: The Psychological Corp, 1979.
27. Kahn S. *Fact Sheet for Third Generation Hardiness Test.* Arlington Heights, IL: The Hardiness Institute, 1986.

97 319 321, 322, 323, 326 327, 328, 329

CHAPTER 64
PSYCHOPATHOLOGY

C. Barr Taylor and Nancy Houston Miller

Exercise professionals encounter a variety of psychological issues and problems in leading and conducting exercise programs. Many of these problems not only affect participation, but also other aspects of the participant. This chapter provides an overview of some more important issues and problems, as well as discusses how to cope with them. Instructors should be able to identify major psychopathological problems and provide referral as needed.

CRISIS

Perhaps the most general psychological event affecting participants in exercise programs is personal crisis. A crisis can be defined as a usually brief period when demands from an event exceed ability and resources to cope, leading to distress (1). People in crisis may feel hopeless, anxious and/or tense. Other common feelings are fear, anger, guilt, embarrassment, and shame. A high level of anxiety often impedes thinking and impairs coping. A crisis is necessarily a very stressful period in one's life and stress coping techniques, as described in Chapter 63, are often useful.

The most common crises are situations such as physical illness, status and role change, rape, physical abuse, divorce, or loss of a loved one. People in crises should not be considered mentally ill, yet their distress should be taken seriously. Frasure-Smith et al. telephoned myocardial infarction patients on a regular basis following the event (2). During each phone call, patients were assessed with a brief psychological tool to determine level of distress. Those exhibiting extreme distress were given home visits and assistance for coping with what was most commonly a crisis. This relatively simple intervention had a significant impact on survival.

Determining whether a person is in crisis is usually not difficult, since most people who are distressed appear distressed. People may cope with a crisis by avoiding customary habits (like attending an exercise program). Thus, unplanned absence may be caused by a crisis.

Crisis Management

There are four general steps to crisis management. The exercise professional should become familiar with these steps and assist patients in crisis in coping. The steps in crisis management include:

- Psychosocial assessment
- Development of a plan
- Implementation of the plan
- Follow-up

Psychosocial Assessment

The purpose of assessment is to determine the origin of the problem and to try get a sense of the cause and how well the patient is coping. Individuals require adequate resources (financial, social, etc.) to resolve a crisis. Attempts should be made to determine whether an individual is suicidal or might harm someone else. The key risk factors for suicide are found in Table 64.1 (3). Prediction of suicide is difficult, but the possibility should be entertained when any of the features listed in Table 64.1 are exhibited.

If the exercise professional suspects depression or suicidal tendencies, the participant should be asked directly whether there is contemplation of suicide. One might say, "You seem pretty down, have you had any recent thoughts of hurting yourself or even killing yourself?" Participants with physical illness who feel helpless and hopeless are at particularly high risk for suicide. Any suggestion that suicide is a possibility should be followed up to determine seriousness of intent. A common belief is that asking about suicide may plant the idea; this is not true.

An open discussion about suicidal feelings is helpful in and of itself and can set the stage for referral. Participants who are suicidal or dangerous and unable care for

Table 64.1. Risk Factors for Suicide

1. Previous suicide attempt
2. Overt or indirect suicide talk or threats
3. Current plan for how to kill him/herself
4. The means to kill him/herself
5. Depressed mood
6. Significant recent loss, e.g., spouse, job
7. Unexpected change in behavior or attitude
8. Elderly, male, isolated with chronic illness
9. Sense of hopelessness, helplessness, loneliness, exhaustion, "unbearable" psychological pain
10. Alcohol, drug abuse or intoxication
11. Failing health, particularly if previously independent

themselves should be referred for immediate professional treatment. Suicide crisis centers and community mental health centers can provide advice and recommendations about referral. Participants may also be taken to hospital emergency rooms. One should ensure that there is an **immediate** place to go and transportation. Suicidal individuals should not transport themselves for treatment, but rather should be accompanied.

Occasionally the exercise professional may encounter a potentially violent patient or client. Some groups are at increased risk for violence, such as young males, urban, violent cultural subgroups, alcohol or drug users or abusers. Individual predictors include past history of violence, active use of alcohol, physical abuse as a child, or history of brain injury. All threats of violence should be taken seriously. The exercise professional must be willing to seek assistance from police as necessary for reasons of security and safety.

Most crises, however, are not accompanied by emergency situations. Further assessment includes answering questions such as:

1. To what extent has crisis disrupted normal life patterns?
2. Is the individual able to hold a job?
3. Can the person handle responsibility of daily living?
4. Has crisis disrupted the lives of others?
5. Has crisis distorted perception of reality?
6. Is the usual support system present, absent, or exhausted?
7. What are the available resources?

Development of a Plan

Crisis management involves the development and assistance in management of the plan. For exercise professionals the focus is usually on referral and follow-up, as well as assisting in prevention from discontinuing an exercise program.

Implementation of the Plan

The third step in crisis management involves drawing on the personal, social, and material resources to assist in overcoming a crisis. This role is usually left to the mental health professional, and the role of the exercise professional is assistance with referral.

Follow-up

Continued support and reinforcement of the plan and support of positive actions are the final, critical stage of the plan. Support in the environment of the patient is important to maintaining the plan and to resolution.

DEATH AND DYING

Most exercise programs have participants who lose or have lost a loved one. Grieving individuals are at increased risk for relapse to old habits, dropping out of exercise programs, illness, injury, and even mortality. Support from an exercise professional can help prevent or minimize these outcomes. The exercise professional should be aware of the basic processes affecting a grieving individual.

While the nature and course of grief is complex, individual and strongly affected by background, psychology, culture, beliefs and experience, many aspects of grieving are universal (4). Immediately upon loss of a loved one, grieving individuals appear emotionally numb, seemingly disbelieving the loss. This period is followed by pangs of grief—periods of crying and yearning—which are interspersed with longer periods of anxiety, despair, and unreality. The grieving person may experience anger, self-reproach, bewilderment, and many other emotions in the struggle to make sense of the loss. Sometimes anxiety escalates to full-blown panic attacks or hyperventilation, and despair to serious depression. The grieving person may have transitory hallucinations of the lost one being near at hand or even speaking to them. As time passes the intensity and frequency of the grief diminish and there are longer periods of apathy and despair. Appetite is decreased. The grieving person avoids the future and may remain disengaged. The death of a loved one forces most people to reevaluate many of their assumptions and habits and new roles must be adopted. The transition to this new role is often resisted. Eventually, normally within 4–6 months, reorganization, recovery and, perhaps, new insight and meaning take place for the grieving person.

The exercise professional should be aware of changing moods and the course of bereavement. Some studies suggest that those who repress grief are more likely to remain depressed and disabled than those who express grief. The exercise professional should be supportive and communicative, allowing the expression of grief, yet being respectful of privacy.

While there is no single "normal" grieving process, some symptoms or behaviors may indicate problems. These include:

- Not exhibiting a sense of loss (at least in the first month or so after loss of the loved one)
- Acquisition of symptoms of illness like those experienced by the deceased
- Increase of psychosomatic illnesses
- Excessive withdrawal
- Excessive hostility or fury
- Intense depression

In fact, grieving individuals are at increased risk for depression; grief is a significant risk factor for suicide. Exercise professionals may monitor the grieving participant particularly with respect to the final two domains. Participants who are having extreme trouble with grieving or exhibit depression or suicidal tendencies should be referred to mental health counselors.

Exercise programs may also have participants who are dying or who die during the course of participation in the program. This is especially true when programs operate in a community over a long periods of time or deal with medically ill populations. When deaths occur, the exercise professional should inform the group and, perhaps, acknowledge the contributions the participant may have brought. Support for those close to the participant is particularly important. Writing to family members is encouraged.

PSYCHOSOCIAL ASSESSMENT

A general psychosocial assessment may be helpful in routine evaluation of participants. Some simple screening tools can help identify major problems. These tools can be followed with more sophisticated instruments or assessments as required. Although there are a variety of important problems, the general domains for assessment include:

- Depression
- Anxiety
- Drug and alcohol abuse
- Eating disorders
- Stress/coping/type A
- Family/social support

One approach is the use of a simple screening tool that may help identify individuals requiring assistance. Table 64.2 provides an overview of a psychosocial screening tool used in the Stanford Cardiac Rehabilitation Program (5). A score of 5 or greater on the first four items indicates a potential problem requiring follow-up. Questions 7–10 are the "CAGE" questionnaire, an instrument widely used to screen for alcohol abuse (6). Two or more positive answers suggest alcohol abuse or dependence and indicate the need for follow-up. Follow-up clinical questions should be guided by criteria described below.

Questions 14 and 15 are used to determine degree of social isolation; however, there is no simple instrument that adequately assesses social isolation. Social isolation is often defined as the absence of social support. Social support includes emotional, physical, monetary, and instrumental (e.g., availability of transportation) support. Each of these domains needs to be assessed in potentially isolated individuals.

The American Association of Cardiovascular and Pulmonary Rehabilitation has published outcome measures for cardiac and pulmonary rehabilitation programs (7). Many of those described can be used to provide more information about depression, anxiety, and other psychological factors.

DEPRESSION

Depression affects 5–10% of adults during their lifetime (8, 9). In addition to feeling "down," depression is often accompanied by somatic symptoms (Table 64.3). Depression following myocardial infarction (MI) has been associated with poor prognosis post-MI, including increased mortality and morbidity (10–12). Depressed patients may exhibit psychomotor retardation, easy crying, and a sad face. They often feel helpless and hopeless and exhibit self-reproach. Especially relevant to assessment is that depression is frequently accompanied by suicidal feelings. Suicidal feelings in depressed patients should be assessed directly and patients should be referred for care, following the aforementioned guidelines for emergency crises.

Hospitalization for psychiatric care is sometimes necessary, but more often depressed patients recover with outpatient professional treatment, medication, and passage of time. The symptomatology of depression makes exercising difficult, but exercise appears to be beneficial (13).

Patients hospitalized for MI often feel depressed. This feeling usually resolves after return home. Moderate or worsening depression persisting 2–3 weeks after returning home and resuming usual activities requires further evaluation. Such patients should be considered for referral to local mental health professionals or the primary care physician.

ANXIETY DISORDERS

Anxiety affects everyone at some time in life (14). Severe anxiety, however, can lead to avoidance and restriction of activities and may be associated with severe de-

Table 64.2. Psychosocial Questionnaire

Name ______________________ **Date** ______________

For the first four questions, please circle a number on the scale following each item to show how much you are troubled now by each emotion.

1. Feeling miserable or depressed

1	2	3	4	5	6	7	8	9
Hardly		Slightly		Moderately		Markedly		Very Severely

2. Feeling irritable or angry

1	2	3	4	5	6	7	8	9
Hardly		Slightly		Moderately		Markedly		Very Severely

3. Feeling tense, anxious, or panicky

1	2	3	4	5	6	7	8	9
Hardly		Slightly		Moderately		Markedly		Very Severely

4. Feeling under stress or pressure at work or at home

1	2	3	4	5	6	7	8	9
Hardly		Slightly		Moderately		Markedly		Very Severely

5. Would you like help with any of these areas?

   Depression: No _____ Yes _____ Anxiety: No _____ Yes _____

   Anger: No _____ Yes _____ Stress: No _____ Yes _____

6. Do you ever drink alcohol?

   _____ No (go to #13) _____ Yes

	No	Yes
7. Have you ever felt you ought to cut down on your drinking?	_____	_____
8. Have people ever annoyed you by criticizing your drinking?	_____	_____
9. Have you ever felt bad or guilty about your drinking?	_____	_____
10. Have you ever had a drink first thing in the morning ("eye opener") to steady your nerves or get rid of a hangover?	_____	_____

11. About how often do you drink alcohol?

1 Daily or almost every day	4 Once or twice per month
2 3 or 4 times per week	5 Less often than once per month
3 Once or twice per week	6 Never

(Table 64.2 Continued)

12. How many of these alcoholic beverages do you drink during an average **WEEK**?

_____ # of 12-oz bottles or cans of beer, ale, etc.
_____ # of 4-oz glasses of wine, sherry, port, etc.
_____ # of shots (one shot = 1.5 oz) of vodka, rum, scotch, whiskey, burbon, tequila, or gin (including mixed drinks and cocktails)
_____ # of after-dinner drinks or liqueurs

13. Do you ever use illegal drugs?
_____ No _____ Yes

14. Do you live alone?
_____ No _____ Yes

15. Do you have enough help at home?_____

Thank you for your responses to these questions. This information will remain confidential.

Table 64.3. Symptoms of Depression

Emotional features
depressed mood, feeling blue
irritability, anxiety
loss of interest
withdrawal from others
preoccupation with death
Cognitive features
feeling worthless or guilty
hopeless, in despair
poor concentration
indecisive
suicide feelings
Vegetative features
fatigue, lack of energy
trouble sleeping
loss of appetite
weight loss or gain
lack of interest in sex
looks depressed

pression and panic attacks. Acute anxiety can often be resolved with reassurance or brief periods of psychotherapy. Chronic anxiety is sometimes secondary to depression, but may represent a primary anxiety disorder. The three most common clinical anxiety disorders are:

- Generalized anxiety disorder
- Panic disorder (with and without agoraphobia)
- Social phobia

Generalized anxiety disorder is characterized by excessive worry and signs of motor tension (e.g., trembling, muscle tension, restlessness), autonomic hyperactivity (e.g., sweating, dry mouth, and frequent urination), vigilance, and scanning (e.g., feeling keyed up or on edge all the time).

Panic disorder is characterized by recurrent panic attacks, which are discrete periods of apprehension or fear accompanied by symptoms such as dyspnea, palpitations, choking, chest pain or discomfort, sweating, dizziness, fear of going crazy, and/or being out of control. The initial panic attack usually occurs in the early 20s and may occur spontaneously. Many patients with panic disorder develop severe phobic avoidance (agoraphobia). Such patients are not likely be able to participate in an exercise program, but participation is beneficial.

Social phobia is characterized by a fear of social situations. Participants who appear shy or unnecessarily embarrassed in public may require special encouragement to participate in exercise programs. Chronic anxiety can occur secondary to psychiatric problems other than depression, such as alcoholism, drug abuse, and schizophrenia. It can also be caused by medical problems, such as hyperthyroidism, hypoglycemia, and temporal lobe epilepsy. Some patients with anxiety report unpleasant symptoms with exercise. Use of diagnostic treadmill testing can reassure anxious patients of safety and can assist the exercise professional in identification of contraindications to exercise (15). Furthermore, exercise may help reduce symptoms in patients with severe anxiety disorders (13).

ALCOHOL AND DRUG ABUSE

Alcohol or drug abuse is indicated by a maladaptive pattern of use, leading to clinically significant impairment or distress manifested by:

1. Tolerance (a need to increase amounts of the substance to achieve intoxication or desired effect or markedly diminished effect with continued use of the same amount of the substance).
2. Withdrawal.

3. Use in larger amounts or over a longer period than intended.
4. Persistent desire or unsuccessful efforts to cut down or control use.
5. Extensive time and effort spent to obtain the substance.
6. Impairment of social, occupational, or recreation activities because of use.
7. Continued use despite knowledge of having a persistent or recurrent problem related to use.

Confrontation may be necessary if the exercise professional suspects abuse (e.g., the patient smells of alcohol, reports black-out periods, or seems preoccupied with alcohol). This involves directing attention to something that the client may not be aware of or is reluctant to admit. Confrontation should only address observable facts and not infer motives or emotional state. For example, a post-MI participant who is intoxicated at the time of an exercise session and is disruptive may require confrontation. An example of an overly aggressive confrontation follows:

- **Exercise professional:** You have been drinking. You had better not drink before you come here.

A more appropriate confrontation might be:

- **Exercise professional:** You seem to be acting funny today. Have you been drinking?
- **Participant:** Nah.
- **Exercise professional:** I can smell alcohol on your breath. When did you last have something to drink?
- **Participant:** Oh, a couple of beers about an hour ago.
- **Exercise professional:** I can't allow people to exercise here if they have been drinking. Will you make sure you have not been drinking before you come next time?

Most of us are uncomfortable with direct confrontation, but it may be necessary as well as useful. However, choosing the appropriate time and circumstance is important, particularly if a participant may become violent; generally the time to confront is not when a participant is intoxicated.

Table 64.4. Clinical Picture of Anorexia Nervosa

Loss of more than 25% premorbid body weight
Distorted body image
Fears of weight gain or of loss of eating control
Adolescent and young adult women primarily affected
Perfectionist behavior
Refusal to maintain normal body weight
No known physical illness on account for weight loss

Patients who appear to be or admitt to abusing alcohol may benefit from referral. The Yellow Pages under "Alcoholism Information" or "Drug Abuse and Addiction Information" is an excellent place to look for treatment resources. The Council on Alcoholism or Council on Alcohol and Drug Abuse are good resources. Alcoholics Anonymous (AA) or Narcotics Anonymous (NA) may also be helpful. The National Clearinghouse for Alcohol and Drug Information (1-800-729-6686) can also provide local or state treatment resources.

DISORDERED EATING

Bulimia Nervosa

Bulimia nervosa is characterized by the following (16):

1. Recurrent episodes of binge eating (rapid consumption of large amounts of food over short periods of time).
2. Feeling of a lack of control over eating during binges.
3. Self-induced vomiting, use of laxatives or diuretics.
4. Strict dieting, fasting, or vigorous exercise in order to prevent weight gain.
5. Persistent overconcern with body shape and weight.

Food consumed during a binge is usually high in calories, sweet and easy to swallow. Binges usually occur secretly and food is eaten quite rapidly with little chewing. A binge ends because of abdominal discomfort, sleep, social interruption, extreme guilt, or induced vomiting. Bulimia is more common among exercisers than nonexercisers. Bulimic patients often feel guilty about the disorder and are likely to suffer from some depression. Frequent vomiting can lead to dental erosion. Electrolyte imbalance and dehydration can occur and may lead to serious physical complications (17). Cognitive/behavioral psychological interventions are effective in assisting bulimic patients reduce symptoms and treatment should be encouraged (16). The National Association of Anorexia Nervosa and Associated Disorders (708-831-3438) is a good resource.

Anorexia Nervosa

Anorexia nervosa is a rare, life-threatening eating disorder. Table 64.4 provides a clinical description of anorexia nervosa (16, 18). Most anorectic patients exercise to excess. If anorexia is suspected, a weight and dietary history should be obtained, and, if possible, the percentage of body fat should be measured.

Anorectic patients are effectively treated by professionals specializing in eating disorders, but an exercise professional can play an important role through confrontation about the seriousness of the disorder and by insisting that the person seek treatment. Once therapy has begun, the exercise professional can assist in designing a program for normal eating and activity emphasizing health and proper nutrition, not weight, and by providing psychological support.

ORGANIC BRAIN DISEASE

Organic brain disease is rarely encountered in most exercise programs, but the exercise professional should be aware of the signs of organic brain disease including:

- Sudden, unexplained change in personality or behavior (including a significant change in personal appearance)
- Difficulty remembering information, particularly newly presented information
- Confusion
- Difficulty in finding words
- Impairment in planning and organizing

Sudden onset of such symptoms may indicate an acute, serious, medical condition. If organic brain disease is suspected, it is important to enlist social support to facilitate referral for the participant.

HOW TO MAKE A REFERRAL

Referrals from the exercise professional may be more effective under the following circumstances:

- The participant feels that the exercise professional cares and has an understanding of the problem.
- The participant accepts need for referral and the referral is likely to lead to improvement.
- The exercise professional is familiar with the mental health professional to whom referral is being made.
- Follow-up is obtained.

Empathy, listening carefully about concerns, and being supportive are important parts of the referral process. Participants may be more likely to accept recommendations under these circumstances and success in obtaining referral and treatment may be more successful. Most depressed and anxious patients suffer and may be happy to seek treatment. The alcoholic or drug abuser who may deny or minimize the problem is more difficult to refer. Such patients may require confrontation in a clear, directive fashion. Finally, follow-up to determine whether the referral occurred and treatment has ensued is important.

▶ SUMMARY

The role of the exercise professional in psychopathology is both evaluative and supportive. Evaluation and assessment requires fundamental knowledge of basic situations and problems which might arise as well as the ability to propose and guide participants to referral. Support requires empathy, reinforcement of positive behavior and ongoing rapport necessary to gain trust and confidence of all participants.

References

1. Hoff LA. *People in Crisis.* 2nd ed. Menlo Park, CA: Addison-Wesley, 1984.
2. Frasure-Smith N, Prince R. Long-term follow-up of the ischemic heart disease life stress monitoring program. *Psych Med* 51:485, 1989.
3. Ghosh TB, Victor BS. Suicide. In: Hales RE, Yudofsky SC, eds. *Synopsis of Psychiatry.* Washington, DC: American Psychiatric Press, 1994.
4. Parke CM. Bereavement. In: Doyle D, Hanks GW, Macdonald N, eds. *The Oxford Textbook of Palliative Medicine.* Oxford: Oxford University Press, 1994.
5. Miller NH, Taylor CB. *Lifestyle Management in Patients with Coronary Heart Disease.* Champaign, IL: Human Kinetics Publishers, 1995.
6. Ewing JA. Detecting alcoholism: The CAGE Questionnaire. *JAMA* 252:1905, 1984.
7. AACVPR Outcomes Committee, et al. Outcome measurement in cardiac and pulmonary rehabilitation. *J Cardiopulm Rehab* 15:394–405, 1995.
8. American Psychiatric Association. *Diagnostic and Statistical Manual of Mental Disorders,* 4th ed. Washington, D.C.: American Psychiatric Association, 1994.
9. AHCPR. Depression Primary Care, Volumes 1 and 2. Rockville, MD: USDHHS, AHCRP Publication No. 93–0551, 1993.
10. Carney RM, Rich MW, Freedland KE, et al. Major depressive disorder predicts cardiac events in patients with coronary artery disease. *Psychosomatic Med* 50:627, 1988.
11. Levine JB, Covino NA, Slack WV, et al. Psychological predictors of subsequent medical care among patients hospitalized with cardiac disease. *J Cardiopulm Rehab* 16:109, 1996.
12. Allison TG, Williams DE, Miller TD, et al. Medical and economic costs of psychologic distress in patients with coronary artery disease. *Mayo Clin Proc* 70:734–742, 1995.
13. Benight CC, Taylor CB. The effects of exercise on improving anxiety, depression, emotional well-being and elements of Type A behavior. In: Elliot DL, Goldberg L, eds. *Exercise as Medical Therapy.* Philadelphia: FA Davis, 1994: 319–332.
14. Taylor CB, Arnow B. *The Nature and Treatment of Anxiety Disorders.* New York: The Free Press, 1988.
15. Taylor CB, King R, Ehlers A, et al. Treadmill exercise testing and ambulatory heart rate measures in patients with panic attacks. *Am J Cardiol* 60:48J, 1987.
16. Agras WS. *Eating Disorders: Management of Obesity, Bulimia, and Anorexia Nervosa.* New York: Pergamon, 1987.
17. Harris RT. Bulimarexia and related serious eating disorders with medical complications. *Ann Intern Med* 99:800, 1983.
18. Garfinkel PE, Garner DM. *Anorexia Nervosa: A Multidimensional Perspective.* New York: Brunner/Mazel, 1982.

Suggested Readings

Colgrove M, Bloomfield HH, McWilliams P. *How to Survive the Loss of a Love.* Los Angeles: Prelude Press, 1991.

Gonda TA, Ruark JE. *Dying Dignified.* Menlo Park, CA: Addison-Wesley Press, 1984.

91, 92 95, 97 101, 102

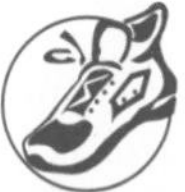  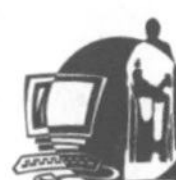

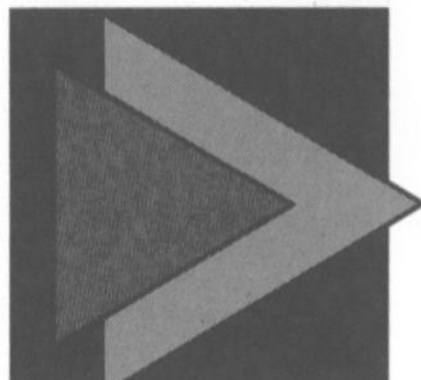

CHAPTER 65
PRINCIPLES OF HEALTH BEHAVIOR CHANGE

C. Barr Taylor and Nancy Houston Miller

Assisting people to begin and maintain health behavior change is a challenge for even the most experienced counselor. Nevertheless, behavioral scientists have identified some strategies that, if systematically applied, are useful in initiation and maintenance of health behavior change.

One model for health behavior is derived from social learning theory, a comprehensive analysis of human functioning in which human behavior is assumed to be developed and maintained on the basis of three interacting systems: behavioral, cognitive, and environmental (1, 2). Social learning theory emphasizes the human capacity for self-directed behavior change. Willingness to change is related to self-efficacy (self-confidence), which is influenced by four main factors:

1. Persuasion from an authority
2. Observation of others
3. Successful performance of the behavior
4. Physiological feedback

Social learning theory is a useful model for understanding why people change; behavioral therapy provides methods and strategies for effecting and maintaining behavior change. Many excellent and detailed discussions of behavior change programs are available (3–6).

Other theoretical models have added useful ideas for conceptualizing behavior change. Fishbein and Ajzen emphasize the importance of expectations and attitudes as precursors to behavior (7). The Health Belief Model also places emphasis on the role of beliefs in determining health care behavior (8). In this model, the important variables influencing behavior include the readiness to change, perceived benefit of change, and cues to action and modifying factors, such as knowledge and socioeconomic background. Prochaska and DiClimente have described how behavior change occurs, beginning with precontemplation, which leads to contemplation, preparation for change, actual behavior change, and maintenance of change (9). The model has been refined and expanded over the past 15 years and extended to a number of problem behaviors (10). Also, cognitive and behavioral processes used in changing health behaviors have been examined, particularly in relationship to exercise (11). Finally, comprehensive models of behavior change involving systems and even community factors have been developed; these models may provide helpful ideas for designing more effective programs (12, 13).

In this chapter, the person helping another person make a health behavior change—a physician, nurse, exercise specialist, fitness professional, or health educator—is referred to as the **instructor;** the person making the changes is the **participant.**

HEALTH BEHAVIOR CHANGE MODEL

Health behavior change can be conceptualized as occurring in stages, arbitrarily divided into antecedent, adoption, and maintenance phases (Fig. 65.1). The antecedent stage includes precontemplation, contemplation, and preparation for change components of the Prochaska and DiClimente Stages of Change model (10). Antecedents refer to all conditions that exist that can assist, initiate, hinder, or support change. Observing the benefits a friend receives from exercising may serve as an antecedent or stimulus for motivation to begin an exercise program. Adoption refers to the early phases of a behavior change program. Maintenance applies to later phases when the participant is undergoing behavior change.

Antecedents

People sometimes decide to change for reasons that they do not understand or that are beyond control. A chance encounter with a friend who has made important changes and looks better, an illness, a caustic remark from a co-worker, and loose clothes that become tight

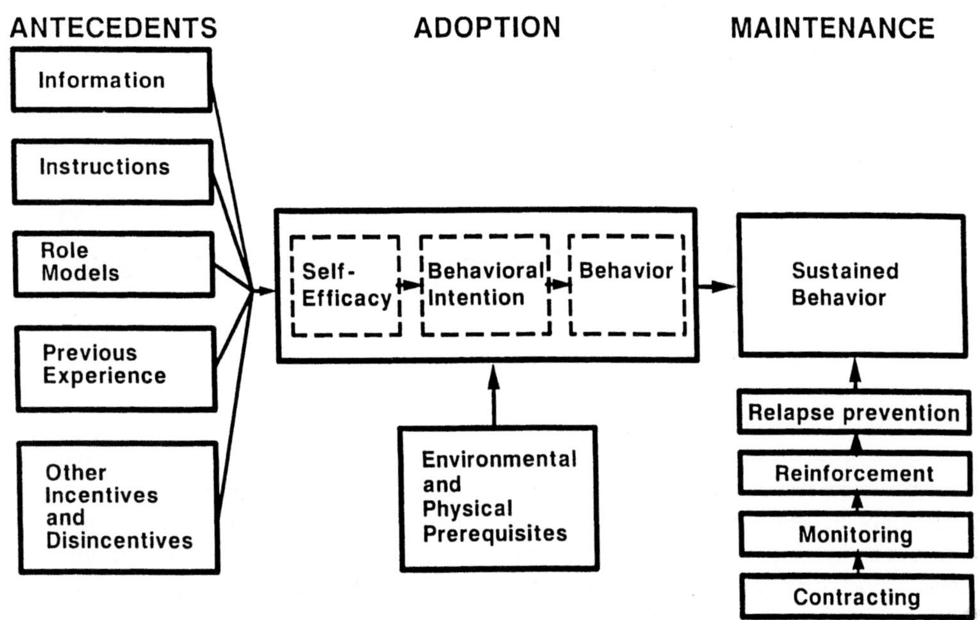

Figure 65.1. Health behavior change can be conceptualized as occurring in stages, arbitrarily divided into antecedent, adoption, and maintenance phases.

are all events that may initiate a health behavior change. Nevertheless, social learning theory predicts that certain antecedents to behavior change can be identified that are useful in increasing intention to change. The phrase **intention to change** is preferable. **Motivation,** the customary term describing willingness to change, implies dichotomy (the individual will or will not change), whereas intention implies a continuous psychological state. If you ask a person to rate their intention on a scale from 0 to 10 in which 0 indicates no intention to change and 10 indicates certainty, people with little intention are not likely to change, whereas those persons with higher scores of intention are more likely to change (14). Intentions frequently change and can be influenced by factors listed in Figure 65.1. For motivated individuals, environmental cues such as posters or notes on bulletin boards may stimulate a behavior change.

Information

Intention to change often begins with information. Information should be presented in simple and clear ways using language that is understandable. Thirty to forty percent of the public reads at a 7th grade level or lower. Information is most effective when combined with instructions about how to make changes. Although pamphlets, self-help books, and hand-outs are often used to communicate health information, most people read 10–15% of such material unless they are extremely interested or are held accountable. Some audiences who would seem to benefit most from information may ignore it. For instance, smokers ignore messages about the risks of smoking, nonexercisers know less about benefits of physical activity than exercisers, and less educated groups may not read lengthy or complicated materials. Knowledge critical to behavior change should be tested prior to initiating a program so myths and misperceptions can be corrected.

Instructions

Instructions to change a particular behavior (persuasion) from a person of authority is a powerful antecendent to behavior change. Health care professionals are considered the most credible source of information by the public. Persuasion from an authoritative figure should occur in a kind but firm manner. People reluctant to make health behavior change listen for ambivalence in the message. They are not, for example, likely to follow this message: "Smoking is bad for your health; you should think about stopping." They are more likely to be affected by: "You must stop smoking." Instructions should be clear, achievable, and accompanied by necessary information about how to change. In addition, instructions should be reinforced by reminders and feedback. Participants should be asked to repeat the critical information.

Models

Role models, whether family, friends, or other credible sources (e.g., health professionals), can facilitate change by allowing the participant to see how other individuals make change, react to change, generalize change to different types of situations (e.g., how people practice food changes at home, in restaurants, and in grocery stores), and cope with difficult situations to maintain healthy habits. People undergoing health behavior change can benefit from being asked to think of persons they know or admire who have made changes. Videotapes or films demonstrating how individuals make changes and the effect of change can be effective in increasing intention to change.

Previous Experience

Previous experience is a major factor in determining initiation of a new health behavior. People are more likely to repeat a behavior if it was helpful in the past. Previous experience may also lead to superstitious health traps. A cold that seemed to resolve more rapidly than usual may, for example, be associated with taking a vitamin whether or not it is helpful. The level of confidence to try a new behavior is largely determined by previous experience. Review of previous success or failure may assist with the change process. Examination of a previously unsuccessful attempt at exercise, for example, may assist in adopting the behavior in a future attempt. People often need to develop new skills to be more effective before change can occur. Developing new skills leads to increased confidence and intention to change.

Other Incentives and Disincentives

Other incentives and disincentives are important antecedents for health behavior change. Incentives should be built into a program and should outweigh the disincentives. Clients should be encouraged to answer the question, "How can I make sure that I benefit from this program?" Some of the benefits may be obvious, such as exercising to feel and look better, while other benefits may not be as obvious, such as exercising to prevent disease. Reducing disincentives when beginning a health program is equally important. A participant may begin exercise at an inconvenient time, in a place that does not appeal to them, or with an activity that is not enjoyable. Such disincentives almost ensure that a program will be short-lived.

Careful attention to antecedents can influence intention to adopt behavior change. With sufficient information, compelling instructions, appropriate models to change, positive physiological feedback, increased confidence to change, and maximized incentives and minimized disincentives, a health behavior change is more likely to be adopted.

An examination of the antecedents for change answers the questions:

- What does the participant need to know about reasons for and methods of bringing about change?
- What instructions (persuasion) have been given from significant people about the importance of making changes?
- What are existing and potential models for change?
- What has been the past success with making this or comparable changes?
- How confident is the participant that change can be accomplished this time?
- What can be done to increase confidence?
- What are the potential incentives and disincentives?

Adoption

When to intervene or encourage adoption of a new behavior should be guided by clinical experience and science and facilitated by carefully listening to participant needs and interests. Continued, gentle reminders may be useful, even for a chronic smoker who has refused to quit many times in the past. Simply asking a person to try a new behavior (e.g., increase activity or alter diet) may be sufficient to instigate change. Medical or personal crises may present an incentive, and often an opportunity, for change. However, at times it is important not to push the participant beyond current willingness to change. Questions like, "Are you ready to try (some behavior change)?" or "Do you want to consider (some behavior change)?" may assist the instructor whether to encourage further change.

Goal-setting is an important part of the adoption phase. Asking participants to list goals and to identify areas where assistance is needed may be effective. A number of studies have demonstrated that more flexible, individually tailored and achievable goals increase adherence to change. Goals should be specific, not global, and short-term, but linked to longer-term goals. A useful way to determine whether a goal is likely to be achieved is to determine level of confidence (using a scale from 0–100%, "no confidence" to "entirely certain") for attaining the goal in a given time frame. Participants reporting 70% or more are likely to be able to do so. In setting goals it is important to ensure that needs, goals and preferences are included in the goals setting process.

Once a person intends to make a behavior change and is confident of success, the adoption of change is often precipitated by **cues to action.** For instance, many people begin a health care program on the basis of symptoms or general state of being. Such physiological and emotional feedback cues people to change and is critical in influencing maintenance. Smoking relapse often occurs in the first few days after quitting because withdrawal symptoms may overwhelm intentions. Poorly conditioned people may stop exercising at the beginning of an exercise program because of unpleasant feelings, such as shortness of breath.

Certain environmental and physical prerequisites are often necessary for health behavior change and should be discussed with participants. Such prerequisites for exercising include:

- Clothing and equipment
- Access to facilities
- Necessary written materials
- A release from a physician, if appropriate.

The early stages of change are often the most difficult. Replacing one activity, even a self-destructive one, with another involves many subtle and important shifts in life. Cigarette smokers who quit often state they feel as though they have lost a good friend. Availability and support are particularly important at such times.

Maintenance

Once a behavior is adopted, other factors determine maintenance. Behavior that satisfies (reinforcing) or causes less discomfort is more likely to be maintained. Four strategies may prove useful in enhancing maintenance:

1. Monitoring and feedback of change (monitoring).
2. Making the activity as satisfying as possible (reinforcement).
3. Anticipating relapse or interruptions (relapse prevention).
4. Making a formalized commitment (a contract).

Monitoring

Self-report, diary, physiological, or other types of monitoring are useful for maintaining behavior change and assisting instructors in determining progress. Monitoring forms may be used by instructors for review and problem solving. In addition, monitoring through use of self-reports and diaries provides participants with important feedback that may increase likelihood of maintenance. Goals vary, but cognitive-behavioral and physiological goals should be developed as appropriate. Monitoring forms should be simple and convenient.

Reinforcement

Positive reinforcement is a powerful factor for sustaining change. Many environmental stimuli are natural reinforcers (e.g., food, water, sexual activity, and warmth). Other activities may be social or symbolic reinforcers, such as attention, praise, money, and awards. Recognition from peers or games and competition can help maintain a behavior. However, it is important to realize that reinforcers are idiosyncratic, that is, reinforcment to one participant may not reinforcment to another. Several excellent references about reinforcement are available (15, 16).

Relapse Prevention

Various techniques can assist participants with relapse or prepare for interruptions or other events that may cause discontinuation of a program. The relapse prevention model is derived from studies of alcoholics and smokers attempting to change. Marlatt observed that even one cigarette might lead to total relapse and that preparation for situations in which the cigarette urge is strongest (e.g., while drinking or experiencing stress) could help to prevent relapse (17). This model can be applied to other behaviors. For instance, the Stanford Cardiac Rehabilitation Program staff encourages people to monitor exercise to improve maintenance and identify clear signals for relapse, such as an actual or anticipated reduction in exercise frequency, and to develop strategies to deal with potential relapse.

Upon initiation of an exercise program, participants are encouraged to write what they will do when illness, injury, or changes in schedule interrupt exercise. Some examples may be:

- Asking a jogging partner for a reminder after return from vacation
- Leaving a money deposit with a friend that is refundable when re-starting exercise after an illness
- Asking an instructor to call periodically to inquire about exercise

Participants who stop exercising for an extended time may require additional effort to overcome the lapse, but the principles are similar. Note that relapse prevention focuses on decreasing rather than increasing behavior.

Contracts

Written contracts are also useful to maintain change and to help with maintenance. Instructors should not make contracts that are unrealistic or unlikely to be achieved. Behavior change is dynamic and goals should be assessed, updated, and revised as necessary. Problem-solving may be important for goals that are not achieved. In problem-solving, a participant identifies a list of possible solutions, develops a plan for implementing these solutions, tries them, evaluates results, and repeats the process if the initial solutions are not successful.

DEVELOPING A PROGRAM

A program consists of the antecedent, adoption, and maintenance phases of behavioral change, how the interventions associated with this phase are sequenced and integrated, and the interaction between the instructor and the client. An example of the components integrated into the Stanford exercise studies of moderate exercise is detailed in Table 65.1 (18).

Organization

Implementing behavior change requires time. Programs should ensure that such time is available for both

Table 65.1. Elements of Exercise Program Design

Antecedents and Adoption
Written description of benefits of exercise
Assessment of expectations;
Review of expectations to make them realistic
Assessment of confidence;
Skills training to enhance confidence
Videotape instruction on warm up and maintaining heart rate within guidelines
Physical examination, treadmill, weight, and skinfold assessment
Experimentation to identify most enjoyable locations
Maintenance
Monitoring
Weekly diaries of exercise duration and intensity
Heart rate monitor with auditory feedback
Reinforcement
Social: Biweekly phone calls from staff group meetings
Monetary: None built into program
Physical: Three and six-month treadmill test and weight assessment
Symbolic: T-shirts
Accomplishment: Monitoring confidence, psychological variables
Contracts: None built into program
Relapse prevention
Participant develops own plans for coping with interruptions of exercise

the instructor and the participant. A session immediately prior to exercise class devoted to education and behavior change may be helpful. This session can be used to present new information, review progress toward goals, share solutions for problems, etc. It is also to allow instructors time with peers and administrators to formally review behavioral aspects of the program. Such sessions can be spent evaluating educational material, reviewing progress of clients, problem-solving, and designing new aspects of intervention.

The components listed in Table 65.1 can be easily organized into a step-by-step approach to a behavior change program. The initial step is asking a participant to consider change. Often people intend to adopt one behavior, but recommending additional health behavior changes may be important, such as recommending that an exerciser also stop smoking. Suggesting such changes can be difficult, but few people resent a thoughtful attempt to assist in improving health.

The second and perhaps most important step is to provide information, instructions, and models for change. This includes reviewing past experiences, building confidence for change, reducing disincentives, and increasing incentives to change.

The third step is to request a commitment that is specific in time and place for when the new behavior will occur. The final step is to develop, with the participant, a way to monitor progress of the new behavior and to determine when and how progress will be reviewed. Early in the adoption phase, the participant should be trained in relapse prevention. Problem-solving should be used as necessary to help overcome difficulties. Such problem-solving can occur in the whole group, at the beginning or the end of a session, via telephone, or in a face-to-face counseling session.

Instructor Qualities

Different instructors achieve different outcomes, even within the same program. Instructors seem to be more effective when participants feel that the instructor is competent, likes them, understands them, and is interested. This relationship translates into a bond between instructor and participant that helps to make the program effective. Role-playing of typical participant situations with peers and receiving feedback is a particularly good way for instructors to develop interpersonal skills.

Overpersistence with an unwilling participant is a problem for some instructors. Instructors who assume too much responsibility for the actions of another person are particularly likely to be overpersistent. Unfortunately, overpersistent instructors often begin to resent inaction, feel chronic frustration, or devote too much time to that participant. To avoid these problems, instructors should have guidelines about when a program or request for change may be discontinued. In one YMCA program, participants meet with the coordinator to review reasons for noncompliance, to solve problems, and to set measurable compliance goals. A second meeting is scheduled if the participant continues to be noncompliant. If the participant fails to comply after a second meeting, a termination meeting is scheduled to discontinue the program. During the termination meeting, the coordinator explains that this program is not appropriate for the participant and that, in light of the hazard of noncompliance both to the participant and to persons who might be influenced by noncompliance (e.g., overexerting), the participant should not continue in the program.

▶ SUMMARY

Social learning theory is the basis for a model for understanding behavior change. Behavior therapy helps to develop many effective change procedures. Information, instructions, models, increasing confidence in performing exercise, as well as maximizing incentives and minimizing disincentives, can increase intention to change and may lead to actual adoption of the behavior. Once adopted, maintenance can be improved by monitoring and feedback, reinforcement, relapse prevention, and the use of contracts.

References

1. Bandura A. Self-efficacy: Toward a unifying theory of behavioral change. *Psychol Rev* 84:191,1977.
2. Bandura A. *Social Foundations of Thought and Action: A Social Cognitive Theory*. Englewood Cliffs, NJ: Prentice-Hall, 1986.

3. Agras WS, Kazdin AE, Wilson CT. *Behavior Therapy: Toward an Applied Clinical Science.* San Francisco: WH Freeman, 1979.
4. Miller NH, Taylor CB. *Lifestyle Management in Patients with Coronary Heart Disease.* Champaign, IL: Human Kinetics Publishers, 1995.
5. Watson DL, Tharp RC. *Self-directed Behavior Change.* Monterey: Brooks/Cole, 1981.
6. Blumenthal JA, McKee DC. *Applications in Behavioral Medicine and Health Psychology: A Clinician's Source Book.* Sarasota, Fl: Professional Resource Exchange, 1987.
7. Fishbein M, Ajzen I. *Belief, Attitudes, Intention and Behavior.* Reading, Mass: Addison-Wesley, 1975.
8. Becker MH, Maiman LA. Sociobehavioral determinants of compliance with health and medical care recommendations. *Med Care* 13:10, 1975.
9. Prochaska JO, DiClimente CC. Stage process of self-change of smoking: Toward an integrative model of change. *J Consult Clin Psychol* 51:390, 1983.
10. Prochaska JO, Velicer WF, Rossi JS, et al. Stages of change and decisional balance for 12 problem behaviors. *Health Psych* 13:39, 1994.
11. Marcus BH, Simkin LR. The transtheoretical model: Applications to exercise behavior. *Med Sci Sports Exerc* 26:1400, 1994.
12. Winett RA, King AC, Altman D. *Psychology and Public Health: An Integrative Approach.* New York: Pergamon Press, 1989.
13. Green LW, Kreuter MW. *Health Promotion and Planning: An Education and Environmental Approach.* Mountain View, CA: Mayfield Publishing Co., 1991.
14. Taylor CB, Houston-Miller N, Killen JD, et al. Smoking cessation after acute myocardial infarction: Effects of a nurse-managed intervention. *Ann Intern Med* 113:118, 1990.
15. Goldfried M, Davison CC. *Clinical Behavior Therapy.* New York: Holt, Rinehart & Winston, 1976.
16. Cautela JR, Kastenbaum RA. Reinforcement survey schedule for use in therapy, training, and research. *Psychol Rep* 29:115, 1967.
17. Marlatt GA, Gordon JR, eds. *Relapse Prevention: Maintenance Strategies in the Treatment of Addiction.* New York: Guildford Press, 1985.
18. Gossard D, et al. Effects of low and high intensity home exercise training on functional capacity in healthy middle-aged men. *Am J Cardiol* 57:446, 1986.

97, 99 321, 324 327, 329

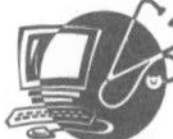

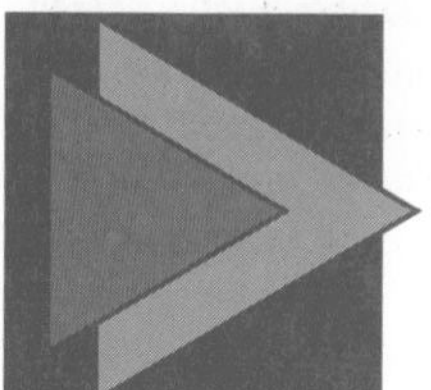

CHAPTER 66
STRESS MANAGEMENT

Wayne M. Sotile

The rubric and techniques of stress management training can be effectively used to address many goals and problems of rehabilitation and health-promotion. A plethora of interventions have been described in stress management literature and no single model is universally accepted. In an effort to systematize this disparate body of information into a set of practical guidelines for providing brief counseling in medical settings, Sotile proposed the Effective Emotional Management (EEM) model depicted in Figure 66.1 (1). This model integrates key components for promoting stress hardiness, both in healthy and rehabilitating populations. It is emphasized that this is only one of many ways of structuring stress management efforts.

THE EFFECTIVE EMOTIONAL MANAGEMENT MODEL

As illustrated in Figure 66.1, a comprehensive stress management program should emphasize education in five areas:

1. The physiological and psychological aspects of stress.
2. Relaxation methods.
3. Ways to manage personality-based coping patterns.
4. Relationship skills.
5. Cognitive control.

The EEM model proposes that stress management counseling be based upon the ability to cope with the demands of daily living, which is enhanced if the patient is helped in two broad ways. First, teach patients to disrupt problematic coping progressions by making more adaptive cognitive, behavioral, physiological, or interpersonal choices. Second, assist patients in creating supportive environments and social networks. Stress hardiness is enhanced when the "territory" in which an individual lives provides a reasonable "fit" between daily demands and inner needs, wants, and values. Living "territory" can be defined by three factors that fill life: situations, processes, and relationships.

Situations are where time is spent and include community, neighborhood, job setting, church, clubs, and health care facilities. Processes are the ways in which self-care is provided; physically, psychologically, emotionally, and spiritually. Therein lies typical stress management topics, such as exercise, attending to thinking patterns, managing nutritional choice, etc. Relationships refer not only to relations with intimate others and friends, but also to relationships with health care providers, colleagues, and acquaintances.

Through supportive interaction, psychoeducation, and coaching, stress management training should help patients create situations, processes and relationships that enhance their functioning. In this way, health care providers become part of the nurturing influence in patients' lives.

PRACTICAL APPLICATIONS

Stress management training is implemented in various treatment venues, ranging from brief, informal consultation delivered during administration of typical medical care to formal presentation of a systematically-delivered program. Depending on the treatment format, interventions might focus on some or all the factors discussed below.

Clarification of Emotional and Psychological Symptoms

"Being stressed" is typically equated with "being anxious." However, the stress response actually yields a variety of physical and emotional manifestations. Information from Table 66.1 illustrates various emotional concomitants that may accompany different stages of the stress response. Explaining this fact can highlight the need for stress management training.

Help Identify the Causes of Stress

Most patients perceive that major causes of stress lie outside of the realm of control. Effective emotional man-

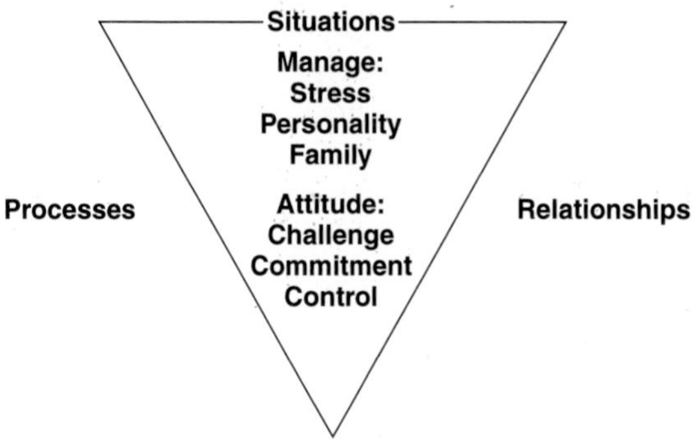

Figure 66.1. Effective Emotional Management. (With permission from Sotile W. *Psychosocial Interventions for Cardiopulmonary Patients: Guidelines for Health Professionals.* Champaign, IL: Human Kinetics, 1992.)

Table 66.1. Physical and Emotional Aspects of Stress

Physiological Aspects	Emotional Correlates
Fight or flight	Anxiety Alarm Anger
Conservation withdrawal	Numbness Vulnerability
General Adaptation Syndrome	Depression and problems in each of the following areas: physical emotional cognitive
Neurochemical depletion or "jamming"	Clinical depression or anxiety disorders

With permission from Sotile W. Psychosocial Interventions for Cardiopulmonary Patients: *A Guide for Health Professionals* by W. Sotile. Champaign, IL: Human Kinetics, 1996. Reprinted with permission.

agement hinges on learning to identify and manage those aspects of the coping process that are controllable, even when faced with uncontrollable external circumstances. Various standardized or clinician-developed inventories and exercises facilitate this aspect of stress management training.

For example, the numbers and types of transitions faced by the patient may be assessed with the Holmes-Rahe Social Readjustment Scale, or a thought diary can be used to track cognitive coping patterns (1, 2). A values inventory can assess behavioral choices that may (or may not) be made in daily life that are harmonious with inner needs and wants (3). Finally, video material can broaden the awareness of various stressors, provide vicarious learning about ways to cope, and normalize stress management as integral to healthy living.

Assist with Pinpointing Reactions to Stressors

Comprehensive stress management training incorporates education regarding the ways that cognitions and personality mediate stress responses.

Thinking Patterns

In addition to coaching ways to monitor and disrupt maladaptive thinking habits, stress management counseling should help patients and significant others, clarify attitudinal paradigms that shape world views and organize approaches to fitness or rehabilitation. The importance of optimism in promoting physical health should be emphasized and cognitive habits that perpetuate a state of optimism can be learned.

In addition, patients should be instructed in the importance of embracing the **three C's of stress hardiness** suggested by Kobasa and colleagues (5). Stress management capability is enhanced if coping with a given stressor is viewed as a **challenge**, if the individual is **committed** to facing that challenge, and if the individual learns what is necessary to gain a reasonable sense of **control** over the coping process. Patients should be asked to define stressors. For example, is the situation being faced a punishment, a relief, an opportunity, a beginning, an ending, a warning, or a tragedy?

Personality-based Coping Patterns

Comprehensive stress management training involves recognizing and aborting stress-generating, personality-based coping patterns. Discussion of this important topic need not be esoteric or extensive. Table 66.2 outlines a concise, common sense model for conceptualizing per-

Table 66.2. What Drives You? Coping Patterns and Pitfalls

Driver	Underlying Hope	Coping Pitfalls
Being strong	To be nurtured	Numbness, loneliness, anger
Being perfect	To feel good enough	Guilt, anxiety, obsessive preoccupation, aloofness
Trying hard	To feel deserving of rest and enjoyment	Exhaustion, stress, depression, joylessness
Pleasing others	To feel understood and appreciated	Exhaustion, withdrawal, guilt
Hurrying	To feel finished	Frazzled and chaotic feelings
Being careful	To feel safe	Free floating, fear, obsessive worrying

With permission from: Sotile W. Heart Illness and Intimacy: How Caring Relationships Aid Recovery. Baltimore, MD: Johns Hopkins University Press, 1992.

sonality-based coping patterns, the underlying hopes, and potential pitfalls of various modes of coping. Medical input should be delivered in language matching the personality-based coping style and its corresponding underlying hope. Extensive guidelines for incorporating this information into the delivery of medical care are available from Sotile (1, 6).

Type A Behavior Pattern

Type A behavior patterns (TYABP) amplify any coping tendency. This is not a unidimensional coping pattern, and no one evidences all of the characteristics of this syndrome; however, it is estimated that upwards of 70% of individuals evidence at least one pronounced Type A coping habit. It is prudent to integrate information regarding this syndrome into a stress management program. Comprehensive treatment programs for TYABP have been described (7, 8). Minimally, intervention should focus on education and coaching regarding the importance of managing hostility, a topic to be discussed below.

Relaxation Techniques and Use of the Relaxation Response

The term "relaxation training" is used in the health literature to refer to various interventions, including yoga, training in self-hypnosis, progressive muscular relaxation, breathing exercises, and biofeedback. There is no convincing evidence that one form of relaxation therapy is more effective than others (1). Relaxation can be quickly learned through instruction in identification of naturally occurring or previously learned relaxation strategies. For example, recalling sensations and/or techniques employed during Lamaze methods for childbirth, past classes in yoga or meditation, or prayer can help a person relax. All may be effective ways of "relaxing" that already exist in the coping repertoire, but are not typically identified as methods of relaxation. Instructing the patient to concentrate on a multisensory memory of such a time—elaborating the sights, smells, sounds, and bodily sensations of the experience—can produce an altered state of hypnotic-type relaxation (1).

Biofeedback is another method for learning control of voluntary and involuntary physiological functions using visual or auditory cues. Digital displays, auditory feedback, and/or graphic representations of the effects of emotional arousal on various physiological functions such as heart rate, blood pressure, skin temperature and palmar sweating are commonly used (9, 10). Through trial-and-error, patients learn cognitive strategies for controlling these functions. Biofeedback is typically offered in 2–5 sessions as an adjunct to stress management training.

In clinical practice, combinations of relaxation training strategies are most often used. For example, diaphragmatic breathing may be paired with progressive muscular relaxation and guided imagery. In guided imagery, a relaxed patient is encouraged to replace distressing images with images that enhance a sense of well-being. This may involve visualizing the healing or strengthening of certain body parts or systems. Comprehensive guidelines for such healing imagery are available (11).

The relaxation state is a fertile time for use of cognitive rehearsal that can bolster confidence in stress management skills. This method pairs the state of relaxation with imagery of upcoming events during which a relaxation response would enhance adaptive coping (1). Similarly, through imagery, the state of relaxation can be deepened with specific verbal, kinesthetic, or visual cues, which can then be used repeatedly (e.g., throughout the day) to trigger brief periods of relaxation. This is an effective method of pattern disruption in stress management training.

Use of Exercise as a Tool for Stress Management

Although it is controversial whether regular exercise in and of itself leads to lasting psychosocial benefits, the clinical experience strongly suggests that exercise is an effective way for stressed individuals to enhance their sense of self-control and coping self-efficacy (1, 12). Thus, regular exercise should be incorporated into stress management efforts. Aerobic exercise of moderate intensity and duration decreases muscle tension acutely and should therefore be recommended as a prelude to relaxation training (9).

Interpersonal Skill Training

No program of stress management is complete without psychoeducation and skill-building of interpersonal factors. Sensitizing individuals to the effects they have on others, teaching appropriate assertive behavior, and teaching anger management strategy should also be considered. Individuals locked into Type A coping habits may create especially taxing interpersonal environments (6, 13). Sotile pointed out that highly hostile patients are likely be motivated to learn new interpersonal skills if they are presented with facts that implicate hostility and anger as dangerous to health (1). Excellent summaries of this information are available (14–16).

In addition, it should be emphasized that the construct of "high hostility" actually contains three distinct components (15):

- Anger—an unpleasant emotion ranging from irritation to rage
- Aggression—overt behavior such as attacking, destructive, or hurtful actions
- Hostility—the emotion of anger that perpetuates a tendency to distrust others and to wish to inflict harm on them

The cognitive mediators of hostility can be treated with various cognitive retraining strategies. Aggressive behavior is best treated through training in the use of alternative, adaptive behaviors, such as methods of assertion and conflict resolution. Extensive guidelines for assertion training are available (17). In addition, through role playing or with the aid of audio- or videotaped interactions, patients can learn to attend to various aspects of communication style, such as what is said (i.e., words, nonverbal sounds) and how it is said (i.e., voice quality, tone, and volume), body movements, facial expressions, and gestures. Extensive models for structuring anger management interventions are available (1, 14, 16).

OUTCOMES

Sotile summarized the positive effects of various forms of stress management training documented in a broad-based research literature (1). Relaxation techniques have been shown to reduce anxiety, heart rate, respiratory rate, and muscle tension in normal populations. They are beneficial in treating medical disorders such as headache, insomnia, and hypertension. The benefits of providing brief relaxation training to patients anticipating surgery has also been documented. Sime et al. discussed the fact that training in relaxation can enhance response to exercise (9). For example, Benson et al. found that oxygen consumption at a fixed workload is significantly lower (4%) when subjects use relaxation during exercise on a bicycle ergometer (18).

Stress management interventions of various types have been shown to be effective in reducing systolic blood pressure and anxiety (19). Cognitive therapy is effective for reducing anger (16). Biofeedback, especially in conjunction with relaxation training, is effective in treating hypertension and for individuals who show exaggerated TYABP (20, 21).

The importance of regular aerobic exercise as a stress management tool is well documented. In nonmedical populations, regular exercise diminishes anxiety, muscular tension, and depression and increases stress management ability and general feelings of well-being and self-esteem. In addition, it has been shown to reduce the cardiovascular impact of emotional stressors (1).

The importance of supportive family relationships, especially spouse support, is apparent in promoting health behavior change such as smoking cessation, dietary modifications, and adherence with exercise (22). In addition, spouse support is a crucial component of effective management of various psychosocial issues for recovering medical patients (23, 24).

Combination approaches to stress management are especially effective, for both healthy and diseased (cardiopulmonary) populations (1). Stress management intervention emphasizing exercise reduces exaggerated cardiovascular reactivity and enhances control of arrhythmias and psychosocial functioning (25). Van Dixhoorn demonstrated the benefits of incorporating relaxation therapy, consisting of systematic breathing therapy, into formal cardiac rehabilitation through decreased failure rates (up to 50%) (26). Finally, marked positive changes in TYABP have been documented from extensive treatment programs combining group support and stress management in both healthy and cardiac populations (7, 8).

INTEGRATING STRESS MANAGEMENT TRAINING INTO A FORMAL REHABILITATION PROGRAM

Below is a curriculum for a model stress management training program that can be incorporated into the educational portion of a rehabilitation program. It is based upon clinical experiences and relevant literature (9, 27). This program involves four weekly lecture/discussion group sessions of 60 minutes each and a 20–30 minute relaxation training session conducted immediately following exercise held once per week. The relaxation training is tape recorded and patients should be encouraged to use the tape during a daily relaxation practice session of 10–20 minutes. Patients should also be encouraged to invite a significant other to attend all sessions, especially session three. Video and audio taped material can be used to stimulate discussion.

Week 1

Topics
- Overview of program
- The physiology and psychology of stress
- Self-directed exercises for pinpointing stressors

Audiovisuals
- Video regarding emotional reactions to illness.

Sample discussion questions
- What are your major stressors at this time?
- What changes have you faced in the past two years?
- What are your physical and emotional signs of stress?
- What do you typically do next when these stress symptoms occur?

Homework
- Listen to selected audiotape regarding stress management.
- Practice relaxation exercise daily for 20-to-30 minutes.
- Keep a thinking journal.

Week 2

Topics
- Brief overview of personality-based coping patterns
- Brief discussion of Type A behavior pattern
- Outline of anger and assertion training skills

Audiovisuals

Video regarding coping strategies and Type A behavior

Sample discussion questions:

What did you learn from your thinking log?

How does your personality compel you to cope when stressed?

How are you Type A? Your loved ones?

What are small changes that you can make to disrupt your typical stress-generating coping patterns?

Homework

Listen to audiotape regarding relationship issues.

Practice relaxation and monitor Type A coping styles.

Week 3

Topics

Discussion of the importance of social support

Description of families as teams

Operationalization of what support means

Audiovisuals

Videos regarding relationship issues and the importance of social support post-illness.

Sample discussion questions

In facing illness, what problems do patients and their spouses (or other significant partners) share?

What problems are unique to each group?

How are children or grandchildren affected?

Which family reactions are helpful to the patient?

Which are not helpful?

Where do each of you get your support?

Homework

Discuss with loved ones exactly *how* they can be supportive.

Listen to audiotape regarding guidelines for managing intimate relationships.

Week 4

Topics

Review of progress

Ways to use relaxation and cognitive strategies to cope

Pinpointing desired areas of change in relationships

Goal-setting regarding overall emotional management

Audiovisuals (None)

Sample discussion questions

How would your life need to be six months from now in order for you to feel satisfied that you truly have learned to better manage stress?

List two specific stress management goals that you will address in the upcoming weeks.

What are challenges that face you, individually and in your family, in the immediate future?

What resources do you have available to you to help face these challenges?

References

1. Sotile WM. *Psychosocial Interventions for Cardiopulmonary Patients: A Guide for Health Professionals.* Champaign, IL: Human Kinetics, 1996.
2. Holmes TH, Rahe RH. The social readjustment scale. *J Psychosomatic* Res 11:213,1967.
3. Sotile WM, Sotile MO. *The Medical Marriage: A Couple's Survival Guide.* New York: Birch Lane Press, 1996.
4. Seligman ME. *Learned Optimism.* New York: A. Knopf, 1991.
5. Kobasa SC, Maddi SR, Puccetti MC, et al. Effectiveness of hardiness, exercise and social support as resources against illness. *J Psychosomatic Res* 29:525,1985.
6. Sotile WM. *Heart Illness and Intimacy: How Caring Relationships Aid Recovery.* Baltimore, MD: Johns Hopkins University Press, 1992.
7. Friedman M, Ulmer D. *Treating Type A Behavior and Your Heart.* New York: A. Knopf, 1984.
8. Roskies E. *Stress Management for the Healthy Type A: Theory and Practice.* New York: Guilford Press, 1987.
9. Sime WE, McGahan M, Eliot RS. Stress management and coronary heart disease: Risk assessment and intervention. In: *ACSM's Resource Manual for Guidelines for Exercise Testing and Prescription.* Philadelphia: Lea & Febiger, 1993:489–506.
10. Schwartz MS. *Biofeedback: A Practitioner's Guide.* New York: Guilford Press, 1987.
11. Naparstek B. *Staying Well with Guided Imagery.* New York: Warner Books, 1994.
12. Emery CF, Pinder SL, Blumenthal JA. Psychological effects of exercise among elderly cardiac patients. *J Cardiopulm Rehab* 9:46,1989.
13. Smith TW, Anderson NB. Models of personality and disease: An interactional approach to Type A behavior and cardiovascular risk. *J Person Soc Psych* 50:1166,1986.
14. McKay M, Rogers P, McKay J. *When Anger Hurts.* San Francisco, CA: New Harbinger Publications, 1989.
15. Smith TW. Hostility and health: Current status of a psychosomatic hypothesis. *Health Psych* 11:139,1992.
16. Williams R, Williams V. *Anger Kills.* New York: Harper, 1993.
17. Alberti R, Emmons M. *A Guide to Assertive Living: Your Perfect Right.* San Luis Obispo, CA: Impact Publishers, 1982.
18. Benson H, Dryer T, Hartley H. Decreased VO_2 consumption during exercise with elicitation of the relaxation response. *J Hum Stress* 4:38,1978.
19. Bosley F, Allen TW. Stress management training for hypertensives: Cognitive and physiological effects. *J Behav Med* 12:77,1989.
20. Kaufman PG, Jacob RG, Ewart CK. Hypertension intervention pooling project. *Health Psych* 7:209,1988.
21. Stoney CM, Langer AW, Stutterer JR, et al. A comparison of biofeedback assisted cardiodeceleration in Type A and B men: Modification of stress-associated cardiopulmonary and hemodynamic adjustments. *J Psychosomatic Med* 49:79,1987.
22. Sotile WM, Sotile MO, Ewen GS, et al. Marriage and family factors relevant to effective cardiac rehabilitation: A review

of the risk factor literature. *Sport Med Train Rehab* 4: 115,1993.

23. Sotile WM, Sotile MO, Sotile LJ, et al. Marriage and family factors relevant to cardiac rehabilitation: An integrative review of the psychosocial literature. *Sport Med Train Rehab* 4:217,1993.
24. Sotile WM. The intimacy factor in cardiopulmonary illness: A practical model for structuring interventions. *J Cardiopulm Rehab* 13:237,1993.
25. Blumenthal JA, Emery CF, Walsh MA, et al. Exercise training in healthy Type A middle-aged men: Effects on behavioral and cardiovascular responses. *Psychosomatic Med* 50: 418,1988.
26. Van Dixhoorn J, Duivenvoorden HJ, Staal HA, et al. Physical training and relaxation therapy in cardiac rehabilitation assessed through a composite criterion for training. *Am Heart J* 118:545,1989.
27. Dracup K, Meleis A, Baker K, et al. Family focused cardiac rehabilitation: A role supplementation program for cardiac patients and spouses. *Nurs Clin North Am* 19:113,1984.

Suggested Readings

American Heart Association. Healthy Heart. Video series. American Heart Association HA, 7320 Greenville Ave., Dallas, Texas.

Levin R. Portrait of a Heartmate. Video series. Heartmates, Inc., Minneapolis, MN.

Naparstek, B. Health Journeys. Audiotape series. Time Warner AudioBooks, Los Angeles, CA.

Sotile WM. Controlling Yourself During Uncontrollable Times. Audiotape. Winston-Salem, NC.

Sotile WM. Coping With Heart Illness. Video series. Human Kinetics, Champaign, IL.

Sotile WM. High-Powered Lives Need High-Powered Relationships. Audiotape. Winston-Salem, NC.

Sotile WM. Thriving, Not Just Surviving. Audiotape. Winston-Salem, NC (1993c).

For an extensive list of audiovisual aids available for rehabilitation settings, contact the American Association of Cardiovascular and Pulmonary Rehabilitation, 7611 Elmwood Avenue, Suite 201, Middleton, WI 53562.

90, 91, 95 328

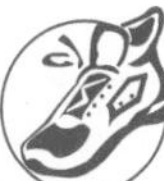

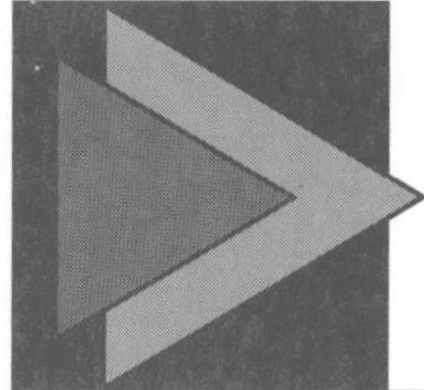

CHAPTER **67**

Enhancing Social Support and Group Dynamics

Paul M. Ribisl and Sally A. Shumaker

Measurement of social support and understanding its role in influencing physical activity outcomes in preventive and rehabilitative programs has not received the attention that it perhaps deserves. Yet, oddly enough, social support has the potential to be one of the most influential factors affecting the success of intervention strategies in preventive and rehabilitative programs because it can have a direct impact upon adherence. Well-designed programs with state-of-the-art facilities and equipment conducted by well-trained staff may be compromised, or even fail, if social support of participants or patients is inadequate.

DEFINITION

Social support has been defined as "the comfort, assistance, and/or information one receives through formal or informal contacts with individuals or groups" (1). It can also describe both the **structure** of the social environment and the **resources** or functions such environments provide. Structural support refers to the size, density, complexity, symmetry, and stability of family, friends, coworkers, health professionals, and community resources (i.e., the social network). Resources refers to the perception of the availability of support and of the resources provided (i.e., social support). Both dimensions are often combined in measures of social support.

IMPORTANCE OF SOCIAL SUPPORT

Social support has a significant role to play in both the etiology of and the recovery from illness and disease. There is a considerable literature linking social support to health outcomes (2–4). Two major theories have been proposed regarding the role of social support in disease etiology:

- The **direct hypothesis**
- The **buffering hypothesis**

The direct hypothesis infers creation of a positive effect, improved self-esteem, and a sense of stability and control. These lead to the development of healthful behaviors such as smoking cessation, improved diet, and increased physical activity. In the buffering hypothesis, people are protected from the pathogenic effects of stress by instilling coping behaviors and reducing reactivity to perceived stress (5).

In preventive and rehabilitative programming, the focus should be on understanding how social support interacts with the intervention strategies used in these programs to promote positive outcomes. Specific interventions typically include smoking cessation, dietary intervention/weight control, psychosocial stress management, physical activity, education, and adherence to prescribed medications. Unfortunately, the prevailing literature provides us with an incomplete understanding of how social support may influence outcomes associated with these intervention programs.

SOCIAL MILIEU IN HEALTH BEHAVIORS: AN OVERVIEW

Efforts to use social support in intervention programs must capitalize on the different forms that social support takes for individuals of different ages. Research on parental influence on physical activity patterns of children is inconsistent; however, several studies demonstrate that parental social influence is effective (6–8).

For **pre-school children,** parents appear to be most influential in the development of positive health behaviors, while siblings and playmates play a minor role. Parents prompting children to play outdoors instead of allowing them to play video games or watch television has been shown to be effective for increasing level of activity (9). Programs developed in pre-school may influence shaping these behaviors as well. Taylor et al. give examples of how social support can be used to increase physical activity in children including (6):

- Providing information on physical activity
- Viewing a child play or practice
- Discussing physical activity with the child
- Offering to exercise with the child
- Assisting the child in physical activity interests by providing transportation to practice and games

In **elementary school,** parents continue to be the most influential source of support, but classmates and school programs begin to play a greater role. The widespread loss of scheduled physical education classes in American public schools along with increased attraction of passive activity such as television and computer games has significantly diminished the opportunity for daily physical activity in this age group. While young children are fairly active, the levels of physical activity actually declines about 50% during the school years (10).

These same forces continue to operate in **secondary school,** however, peer influence from classmates and friends assumes a greater role than parents during adolescence. Nevertheless, Anderson and Wold have demonstrated that parental encouragement is closely correlated with physical activity level in adolescents (11). However, Sallis points out that if adolescents identify with a peer group that values and participates in activity, then the group creates a supportive environment; in contrast, the group becomes a deterrent if it devalues physical activity (12). For most adolescents, organized sports and school programs are the major opportunities available for regular physical activity and both coaches and team members provide a significant source of social support for continued participation.

In the young adult of **college age,** peers or classmates exert the primary influence and provide the major source of support for healthful behaviors. While alcohol, tobacco, and other drug use may be initiated in middle-school or high school, early adulthood is a critical time for maintenance of good health habits because peers can exert a powerful influence on these behaviors during a vulnerable time. This may also be the first time that individuals live away from home and make personal food choices without parental control or influence. While some colleges offer courses on healthful lifestyles, the exposure is brief and peer influence has a greater potential to affect behavior.

For most **middle-aged** adults, a spouse, friends, or co-workers are the major sources of support in the form of encouragement, participation in physical activities, and providing assistance, such as child care (12). Individuals in the workforce face different challenges than those who are at home raising families. Finding the time and setting to exercise during the workday is difficult for most, especially the blue-collar worker, while for mothers with children at home, there is the challenge of finding time to exercise in addition to the expense of child-care. These barriers are sufficient to cause a large proportion of the middle-aged to remain physically inactive. Social support in the form of co-workers to exercise with at work or, in the case of the mother at home, having friends or family to assist with child-care, may make the difference between being active and inactive. Also, Danielson and Wanzel indicate that women have better attendance in fitness classes when accompanied by a companion, while Wankel found that a buddy system positively influences adherence in exercise settings (13, 14).

The major sources of social support for the **older adult** are the spouse, friends, and community social systems. Physical activity benefits to older individuals are substantial and this group may need physical activity more than any other age group. Disability from chronic disease is most prevalent in this group and maintaining independence for Activities of Daily Living (ADLs) is closely linked with an active lifestyle. Yet Cousins points out that this group may encounter a number of factors that increase the difficulty of becoming active, such as disapproval from a spouse, lack of peer involvement, discouragement from the immediate family, and inadequate encouragement from physicians (15). There are other barriers to being physically active in the older adult. Shephard cites the following that must be recognized and overcome (16):

- The absences of a suitable companion
- Lack of transportation to the exercise site
- Limited sight or hearing
- Cognitive, emotional, or behavioral problems

GROUP DYNAMICS IN EXERCISE PROGRAMS

Various sources of social support exist within a formal exercise program, including exercise professionals and exercise participants. It is important to recognize that both have the potential to exert positive or negative influences.

Enhancing the Supportive Atmosphere

Exercise professionals are crucial to a supportive atmosphere and offer, perhaps, the dominant influence on compliance of participants. Individuals often, but not always, prefer to be among participants who are similar in age, gender, fitness level, and physique. Older adults do not want to feel "out of place" and, as Shephard points out, it is often better for the sake of role modeling to use an older person to lead an exercise class since research suggests that a very fit class leader may further weaken self-efficacy and motivation among the frail elderly (16, 17).

There are times when certain participants can have a negative social influence on the conduct of group exercise classes. The following discussion addresses some of the more common types of negative influence that may be encountered.

Chronic Complainers

Chronic complainers should be interviewed carefully to determine whether the cause of the complaint is physical. It is possible that there are legitimate physical ailments (arthritis, joint problems, back problems, etc.) that make exercise uncomfortable, and medical attention may be warranted. If the complaints are due to dissatisfaction with the program or leadership, then address them directly. Some individuals are general malcontents and are often tolerated; however, if the person is disruptive to the program, ask them to either modify the behavior or to leave the program (and find other program arrangements).

Disrupters/Comedians

These individuals must be dealt with at the first sign of disruption to minimize the effects on other participants. Usually, the need for attention can be channeled into productive activity by having them take a leadership role in the class. Allowing them to lead warm-up exercises or help in another way may satisfy attention-getting needs that otherwise lead to disruptive behavior. It should be noted that, depending on the class make-up, a "comedian" participant may in some way enhance the mood of the class. However, if the behavior poses a danger to other participants or detracts from program participation, then they should be dealt with directly regarding modifying the behavior.

Noncompliers

Noncompliers may either under-exert or over-exert during the activity portion of a program. Those who fail to comply by exercising under the prescribed threshold should be educated on the benefits of overload and encouraged to exercise at appropriate levels. However, since program dropout rates are higher from vigorous activity than from moderate intensity activity, there is a downside to pushing individuals beyond a certain point (18). In addition, for the sedentary person who has rarely exercised, a gradual period of adjustment is required in order to learn to tolerate increased levels of discomfort that are commonly accepted by a veteran exerciser. A discussion with a sympathetic exercise professional along with matching them with another participant who can share experiences may help such participants.

In contrast, those who over-exert pose a significant safety hazard to themselves by exercising above the recommended upper limit (19). The value of pacing should be emphasized. They may also be paired with another patient, preferably a former over-exerter who has modified exercise style. As Sotile has pointed out, the over-exerter's orientation to "hurry up" and "try harder than the next person" is counter-productive to the concept of a safe, individualized exercise threshold (20).

RESEARCH ON SOCIAL SUPPORT IN CARDIOPULMONARY REHABILITATION

Convincing evidence exists that social support is protective of cardiovascular health. Orth-Gomer cites both cross-sectional and longitudinal studies demonstrating that lack of social support and weak social integration are associated with elevated risk of myocardial infarction (21). In one study, the influence of stressful life events on all-cause mortality in middle aged men was examined (22). Only those men with adequate emotional support seemed to be protected. Further work substantiates that when standard CAD risk factors are controlled, two factors emerge as the strongest independent risk contributors to myocardial infarction in middle-age men—smoking and lack of social support (23).

The literature on social support in cardiac rehabilitation has been directed primarily at influences on adherence to physical activity. Much of this research focuses exclusively on spouse support rather than on a full network or the support available within a formal program (i.e., other participants and professional staff) (24–26). Most studies are retrospective, examining multiple factors, including social support, that influence compliance in the form of attendance or adherence to a healthful behavior. While the majority findings support the notion that social support is positively related to adherence to healthful behaviors, what is lacking is experimental research in which social support is manipulated to determine whether it is an independent variable and has significant influence on improving outcomes (adoption or maintenance of healthful behaviors).

Dracup states that the available evidence suggests that enhanced social support is a relatively powerful but relatively untested component of cardiac rehabilitation and that a major problem with the research is that it is difficult to differentiate the effects of social support on patient outcomes from the other interventions provided within a cardiopulmonary rehabilitation program (27). Patients receiving social support from family and friends are more likely to be compliant with modification of behaviors associated with risk factors and spousal support is a known predictor of program adherence in cardiac rehabilitation (28, 29). A recent pilot study demonstrated that even a brief session with family members instructing them on how to be supportive of exercise behavior can be effective in getting patients to be more physically active outside the formal program (30). Other supportive evidence comes from the Heart Smart Family Health Promotion program that focuses on the entire family system rather than individuals (31). The format minimizes lecture and maximizes awareness, skills development, problem-solving, and real-life application over a 12–16 week agenda. This program has demonstrated positive changes in cardiovascular risk factors and can be applied to both clinical and health-promotion settings.

OUTCOMES AND MEASUREMENT OF SOCIAL SUPPORT

In order to provide evidence that a specific intervention is effective, outcomes that reflect change in important parameters of social support should be defined and measured. Kaplan discusses the complex issues associated with the measurement of health outcomes in social support research and concludes that while social support is associated with a lower rate of mortality from cardiovascular disease, studies linking social support to health are problematic (4). This is partly due to problems associated with conceptualization and measurement, as well as a lack of a consensual definition of social support. While efforts continue in regard to the development of valid and acceptably reliable measures of social support in the cardiopulmonary rehabilitation literature, a consensus does exist that the phenomenon of social support is sufficiently robust and warrants inclusion as an important psychosocial parameter in cardiopulmonary rehabilitation.

Despite continuing debate regarding specific instruments, it makes sense to use the best of what is available until further research yields more definitive measures of social support and its influence on the course of patient treatment in cardiopulmonary rehabilitation. The following measures of social support may be considered appropriate.

The MOS Social Support Survey

This survey is a brief, multi-dimensional, self-administered social support survey that has been used in both healthy populations and in patients with chronic conditions (32). It identifies four functional support scales, including **tangible, affectionate, positive social interaction,** and **emotional/informational** support. The instrument has excellent psychometric properties and has been used extensively in clinical research. Brief descriptions of the four types of support are as follows:

- Tangible Support: Someone to help you if you were confined to bed, take you to a doctor if needed, prepare meals, or help with daily chores.
- Affection Support: Someone who shows you love and affection, hugs you, and makes you feel wanted.
- Positive Social Interaction: Someone to have a good time with, get together with for relaxation, and do something enjoyable with.
- Emotional Support: Someone to listen when you need to talk, give advice in a crisis, confide in and share private worries and fears, and who understands your problems.

This survey provides a total score as well as separate ratings of each of the four types of support that can identify those who lack sufficient social support.

The Health Support Index (HSI)

Evidence suggests that success rates of programs designed to change health-related behaviors (diet, exercise, and smoking habits) may be influenced by the availability of social support for these targeted changes (33, 34). In an effort to focus on how social network members provide support related to desired behavioral changes, the HSI is used to assess existing social support for planned changes in health-related behaviors. It measures two theoretically distinct aspects of social-environmental support for health-related behavior change: supportiveness and modeling. Each component is assessed by a subscale of the HSI. The validity and reliability of the HSI indicates that it may be a promising tool for evaluating social support for the modification of health-related behaviors (34).

The Social Provisions Scale (35)

This survey measures six separate provisions related to social support received from friends, family members, coworkers, etc. These are as follows:

- Attachment
- Social integration
- Reassurance of worth
- Guidance
- Opportunity for nurturance
- Reliable alliance.

This scale can also be modified to indicate support for specific health-related behaviors such as smoking, dietary intake, stress management, and physical activity.

RECOMMENDATIONS FOR PRACTICE

How we should use measures of social support to improve outcomes in cardiopulmonary rehabilitation requires speculation, because there is little published research for guidance. It is prudent to assess level of social support at entry using instruments such as the **MOS Scale** or the **Social Provisions Scale** to determine whether levels of social support present a threat to compliance. While it may not be possible to alter the social support and network involving family, friends, and coworkers, it may be feasible to look for ways to provide supplemental social support for those who have the greatest need. This could be in the form of increased attention during program participation, written materials for home use, periodic phone calls and/or home mailings to encourage compliance, and establishing support groups that meet outside of regular program hours. While the research on social support continues to provide more scientific evidence of its effectiveness, clinical experiences over the past two decades provide empirical evidence that social support, in many forms, is a powerful factor for promoting and sustaining health behavior change.

References

1. Wallston BS, Alagna SW, DeVellis BM, et al. Social support and physical health. *Health Psych* 2:367–391, 1983.
2. Cohen S, Syme SL, eds. *Social Support and Health.* New York: Academic Press, 1985.
3. Shumaker SA, Czajkowski SM, eds. *Social Support and Cardiovascular Disease.* New York: Plenum Press, 1994.
4. Kaplan RM. Measures of health outcome in social support research. In: Shumaker SA, Czajkowski SM, eds. *Social Support and Cardiovascular Disease.* New York: Plenum Press, 1994.
5. Cohen S, Kaplan JR, Manuck SB. Social support and coronary heart disease: Underlying psychological and biological mechanisms. In: Shumaker SA, Czajkowski SM, eds. *Social Support and Cardiovascular Disease.* New York: Plenum Press, 1994.
6. Taylor WC, Baranowski T, Sallis JF. Family determinants of childhood physical activity: a social-cognitive model. In: Dishman RK, ed. *Advances in Exercise Adherence.* Champaign, IL: Human Kinetics Publishers, 1994.
7. McKenzie TL, Sallis JF, Nader PR, et al. Beaches: An observational system for assessing children's eating and physical activity behaviors and associated events. *J Appl Behav Anal* 24:141–151, 1991.
8. Dennison BA, Straus JH, Mellits E, et al. Childhood physical fitness tests: Predictor of adult physical activity levels? *Pediatrics* 82:324–330, 1988.
9. Epstein LH, Smith JA, Vara LS, et al. Behavioral economic analysis of activity choice in obese children. *Health Psych* 10:311–316, 1991.
10. Sallis JF, Nader PR, Broyles SL, et al. Correlates of physical activity at home in Mexican-American and Anglo-American preschool children. *Health Psych* 12:390–398, 1983.
11. Anderssen N, Wold B. Parental and peer influences on leisure-time physical activity in young adolescents. *Res Q Exerc Sport* 63:341–348, 1992.
12. Sallis JF. Influences on physical activity of children, adolescents, and adults or determinants of active living. *Phys Activity Fitness Res Dig* 1(7):3, 1994.
13. Danielson R, Wanzel R. Exercise objectives of fitness program dropouts. In; Landers D, Christina R, eds. *Psychology of Motor Behavior and Sport.* Champaign, IL: Human Kinetics, 1977:310–320.
14. Wankel LM. Decision-making and social-support strategies for increasing exercise involvement. *J Cardiac Rehab* 4:124–135, 1984.
15. Cousins SO. The role of social support in later life physical activity. In: Quinney HA, Gauvin L, Wall AE, eds. *Toward Active Living.* Champaign, IL: Human Kinetics, 1994.
16. Shephard RJ. Determinants of exercise in people aged 65 years and older. In: Dishman RK, ed. *Advances in Exercise Adherence.* Champaign, IL: Human Kinetics Publishers, 1994.
17. Sidney KH, Shephard RJ. Attitudes towards health and physical activity in the elderly: Effects of a physical training programme. *Med Sci Sport* 8:246–252, 1977.
18. Dishman RK, Sallis JF. Determinants and interventions for physical activity and exercise. In: Bouchard C, Shephard RJ, Stephens T, eds. *Physical Activity, Fitness, and Health: International Proceedings and Consensus Statement.* Champaign, IL: Human Kinetics, 1984:214–238.
19. American College of Sports Medicine. *ACSM's Guidelines for Exercise Testing and Prescription.* 5th ed. Baltimore: Williams & Wilkins, 1995.
20. Sotile WM. *Psychosocial Interventions for Cardiopulmonary Patients.* Champaign, IL: Human Kinetics, 1996.
21. Orth-Gomer K. International epidemiological evidence for a relationship between social support and cardiovascular disease. In: Shumaker SA, Czajkowski SM, eds. *Social Support and Cardiovascular Disease.* New York: Plenum Press, 1994.
22. Rosengren A, Orth-Gomer K, Wedel H, et al. Stressful life events, social support, and mortality in men born in 1933. *Br Med J* 307:1102–1105, 1983.
23. Orth-Gomer K, Rosengren A, Wilhelmsen L. Lack of social support and incidence of coronary heart disease in middle-aged Swedish men. *Psychosomatic Med* 55:37–43, 1993.
24. Knapp D, Gutmann M, Foster C, et al. Exercise adherence among coronary artery bypass surgery (CABS) patients. *Med Sci Sport Exerc* 15:120, 1983.
25. Burkett PA. Practical issues for increasing exercise adherence. *J Cardiopulm Rehab* 12:18–19, 1992.
26. Oldridge N, Ragowski B, Gottlieb M. Use of outpatient cardiac rehabilitation services: factors associated with attendance. *J Cardiopulm Rehab* 12:25–31, 1992.
27. Dracup K. Cardiac rehabilitation. The role of social support in recovery and compliance. In: Shumaker SA, Czajkowski SM, eds. *Social Support and Cardiovascular Disease.* New York: Plenum Press, 1994.
28. Gianetti VJ, Reynolds J, Rign T. Factors which differentiate smokers from ex-smokers among cardiovascular patients: A discriminant analysis. *Soc Sci Med* 20:241–245, 1985.
29. Andrew GM, Oldridge NB, Parker JO, et al. Reasons for dropout from exercise programs in post-coronary patients. *Med Sci Sport Exerc* 11:376–378, 1979.
30. Dominick KL, Ribisl PM, Rejeski WJ, et al. Social support strategies improve physical activity outcomes in cardiac rehabilitation. *J Cardiopulm Rehab* 14:335, 1994.
31. Johnson CC, Nicklas TA. Health ahead—the Heart Smart Family approach to prevention of cardiovascular disease. Am J Med Sci 310(Suppl 1):S127–32, 1995.
32. Sherbourne CD, Stewart AL. The MOS social support survey. *Soc Sci Med* 32:705–714, 1991.
33. Robbins SR, Slavin LA. A measure of social support for health-related behavior change. *Health Education* 19(3):36–39, 1988.
34. Colletti G, Brownell KD. The physical and emotional benefits of social support: Applications to obesity, smoking, and alcoholism. In: Hersen M, Eisler RM, Miller PM, eds. *Progress in Behavior Modification.* New York: Academic Press, 1982:110–179.
35. Russell D, Cutrona CE. The provisions of social relationships and adaptation to stress. In: Jones WH, Perleman D, eds. *Advances in Personal Relationships.* Greenwich, CT: JAI Press, 1987.

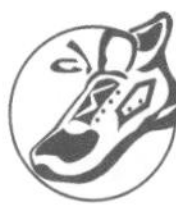

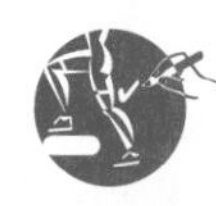

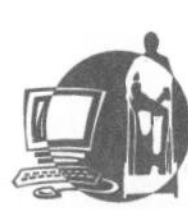

CHAPTER 68
PHYSICAL ACTIVITY PROMOTION: ANTECEDENTS

Abby C. King and Michaela Kiernan

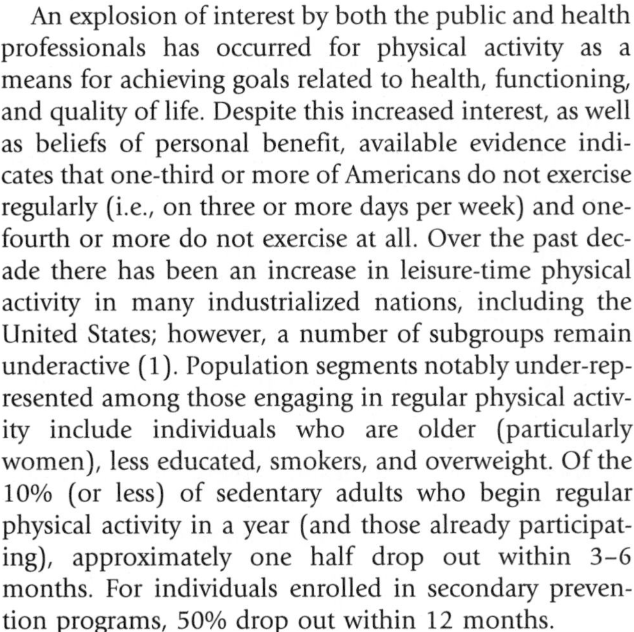

An explosion of interest by both the public and health professionals has occurred for physical activity as a means for achieving goals related to health, functioning, and quality of life. Despite this increased interest, as well as beliefs of personal benefit, available evidence indicates that one-third or more of Americans do not exercise regularly (i.e., on three or more days per week) and one-fourth or more do not exercise at all. Over the past decade there has been an increase in leisure-time physical activity in many industrialized nations, including the United States; however, a number of subgroups remain underactive (1). Population segments notably under-represented among those engaging in regular physical activity include individuals who are older (particularly women), less educated, smokers, and overweight. Of the 10% (or less) of sedentary adults who begin regular physical activity in a year (and those already participating), approximately one half drop out within 3–6 months. For individuals enrolled in secondary prevention programs, 50% drop out within 12 months.

Such statistics indicate that assisting individuals to stay regularly involved in physical activity is a challenge requiring creativity and patience. In addition, finding ways to encourage the extremely sedentary to adopt a more active lifestyle represents an increasingly important public health goal. Exercise professionals can take advantage of the current public enthusiasm for becoming more active, as well as the growing literature suggesting strategies that can be effective for enhancing participation in physical activity.

THE ADHERENCE PROBLEM

In some ways, physical activity may be a unique health behavior, governed by factors that differ somewhat from other health behaviors (2–4). Certainly the demand for regularity in performing physical activity to benefit throughout life calls for innovative methods of studying the process that makes regular exercise habitual. Additionally, factors influencing initial adoption and early participation in exercise may differ from those affecting subsequent maintenance. Stages of change models may better identify strategies that will work for individuals in different stages and levels of exercise participation, e.g., persons contemplating joining an exercise program, those in the early stage of exercise adoption, or those committed to maintaining a program across the long-term. Such models draw extensively from social cognitive theory and other theories of behavior change (5, 6). Although the understanding of this process is generally not extensive, a number of potentially important variables have been identified (6).

SOCIAL/COGNITIVE THEORY

Though no single theory allows full explanation why individuals become or stay active, efforts to understand such health behaviors by placing them in the context of a social learning/social cognitive model of health behavior change has helped. The social cognitive approach, broadly defined, views such behavior as being initiated and maintained through a complex interaction of personal, behavioral, and environmental factors and conditions. Past experiences with physical activity, views of physical activity in general and different forms of activity in particular, the extent of current activity-related knowledge, skills, and beliefs, and how the surrounding environment either helps or hinders efforts to increase physical activity all play a role in influencing how active the individual currently is and will remain.

The social learning/social cognitive theoretical approach emphasizes ability to regulate behavior through setting goals, monitoring progress towards these goals, and modifying the physical and social environment to support the goals. Observational learning and modeling by others is an important influence on behavior. Self-efficacy (i.e., belief in ability to successfully perform a specific behavior or activity) and outcome expectancies (i.e., belief that the behavior leads to a desired outcome) are identified to be the critical factors influencing which behaviors are attempted and with what level of effort before a person gives up.

In addition to social cognitive theory, other conceptual models or approaches that have been applied include the health belief model, the locus of control model, relapse prevention models, the theory of reasoned action, and expectancy-value decision theories (7). To date few have been as heuristic as the social cognitive perspective in helping to shape effective intervention.

Social cognitive and related approaches to understanding physical activity behavior have been supplemented in recent years with increased appreciation for the place of psychological readiness in changing physical activity patterns. Such psychological readiness interacts with and can be influenced by the types of personal, behavioral, program-related, and environmental factors described below.

Personal Factors

Among the demographic factors found to be associated with physical activity participation are the following:

- Gender—women participate less in vigorous activity, especially at younger ages
- Age—increasing age is associated with lower levels of physical activity
- Educational attainment—educational level is positively associated with leisure-time physical activity

Meanwhile, demographic factors such as occupation and race or ethnicity have less consistent relationships with leisure-time physical activity. Though few studies have specifically examined differences by race, some have demonstrated that African-American women are consistently less active than Caucasian women (7). There is some evidence that physical activity levels may, to some extent, "run in families;" however, reasons (i.e., genetic, behavioral, environmental, or some combination of these factors) are currently unclear.

Health factors have been shown to have consistent relationships with physical activity level. People with medical problems or disabilities are more likely to be inactive. Smoking status is related to lower levels of physical activity in some, although not all populations, as well as associated with higher drop-out rates from vigorous leisure-time exercise programs.

Overweight and obese individuals have been consistently found to be less active in a range of activities, including both leisure-time and routine activity such as walking and taking stairs. It is, however, unknown why overweight and obese individuals are less active. It is possible that engaging in physical activity is more aerobically challenging and physically difficult due to weight. However, it may also be that attending exercise classes or engaging in physical activity is stressful for some subgroups of overweight individuals who are dissatisfied with physical appearance. People may be more dissatisfied (about appearance) when in situations eliciting thoughts about appearance and may actively avoid situations that exacerbate feelings of dissatisfaction (8). Exercise, especially in a group with a focus on appearance and social comparison, may be one such situation. Cognitive strategies including correcting size and weight estimates-of-self relative to peers, norms, and objective standards, and behavioral strategies such as incremental exposure to a target situation have been demonstrated to improve body image for normal weight individuals (9, 10). Such approaches may also be helpful for overweight individuals that have extreme body dissatisfaction and indicate the desire to engage in increased physical activity.

In addition to demographic and health factors, variables influencing initial participation in regular physical activity include the following:

- Past experiences with physical activity
- Perceptions of health status as well as exercise ability and skills
- Self-efficacy beliefs, defined as the level of confidence in the ability to successfully perform a specific physical activity regimen
- Outcome efficacy beliefs (i.e., belief that physical activity has value for health, fitness, or related outcomes)
- Perceived exercise enjoyment and satisfaction
- Perceptions related to access to exercise facilities, lack of time, and exercise intensity;
- Understanding of how increased physical activity relates to personal benefits, both in the short term, as well as in the long term

In addition, rating of self-motivation may be related to continued participation in exercise. Importantly "self-motivation" may be learned when defined as an ability to find rewards for behavior independent of external rewards available for that behavior. This concept is preferable to definitions of motivation that place responsibility for nonadherence on internal processes related to "personality" or similar constructs. These latter definitions, aside from being unfair by ignoring extrapersonal influences on behavior (e.g., the environment), do not provide the exercise professional with a firm direction for intervention.

Though many of the abovementioned factors are associated with initial participation in physical activity, relatively few appear to substantially influence length of maintenance of an exercise regimen. Factors that may are smoking status, weight, self-efficacy, and perceived lack of time. Other factors likely have an effect on continued participation are ongoing enjoyment of the physical activity program, as well as the perception of barriers such as scheduling, illness, travel, and other factors that can impede physical activity participation.

Behavioral Factors

Behavioral factors include the skills to carry out physical activity to facilitate exercise-related benefits while minimizing injury and boredom. Such skills include knowledge and use of behavioral and psychological strategies that assist negotiation of barriers and pitfalls that inevitably interfere with regular activity.

A useful behavioral skill may be as simple as knowing how to plan ahead by identifying and preparing for periods when disruption to exercise is likely (e.g., during holidays). This type of strategy is known as relapse prevention (11). Studies applying relapse prevention strategies, either alone or in combination with other behavioral strategies, suggest their utility in promotion, adoption, and maintenance of physical activity (11–13). Another potentially effective strategy is implementation of a decision balance-sheet, whereby careful evaluation of expected or experienced benefits and costs of participating are compared. Other self-regulatory skills that appear to promote physical activity participation if used regularly are self-monitoring of progress, realistic short- and longer-term goal setting coupled with ongoing feedback related to success, and the use of self-rewards (7).

Environmental and Program Factors

A number of environmental and program-based factors can influence initial participation as well as longer-term adherence. These include the following:

- Family influences and support–individuals reporting spouses to be neutral or unsupportive of physical activity are more likely to drop out
- Proximity and access to facilities (for those persons preferring facility-based activities)
- Weather
- Regimen flexibility
- Convenience of activity (real or perceived)
- Immediate cues and prompts in the environment promoting physical activity (e.g., reminders to exercise)
- Immediate consequences of activity

The social environment can have major impact on both physical activity adoption and maintenance. Family participation and support as well as parental level of physical activity are associated with increased physical activity in some population groups. Social support from friends or coworkers may also have a positive effect. In addition, physicians and other health professionals can positively influence physical activity behavior. Although surveys suggest that physician advice is considered to be potentially important with respect to health behaviors, relatively few physicians discuss physical activity practices with patients. Barriers to physician counseling on physical activity include lack of confidence in ability to effectively advise patients (often stemming from lack of knowledge and/or training), lack of time, lack of knowledge related to the most appropriate referral sources in the community, and limited reimbursement for these services. As part of Project PACE, funded by the Centers for Disease Control and Prevention, a physician-based brief physical activity assessment and counseling protocol is available for use in the clinical setting (14).

The type of physical activity (e.g., swimming, brisk walking, aerobic dance), as well as intensity, duration, and frequency can influence subsequent participation levels. The format in which the activity is offered (e.g., class, home-based with or without partners) may also have an important effect on both initial participation and longer-term adherence. Although the majority of exercise programs are offered in a class or group format, evidence indicates that the public generally prefers programs offered outside a formal group. There are important benefits to long-term adherence with adequately structured home-based regimens (13). The mode, intensity, frequency, duration, and location of physical activity must meet the needs of differing groups of individuals. For example, women report stronger preference for videotaped exercise and aerobic dance than men. Similarly, the workplace has been shown to be preferred for physical activity in some groups (7).

Immediate consequences, including observance of physical activity-related benefits and enjoyability of activity, are other program-related factors likely to have strong impact on adherence. Conversely, sedentary people persist principally because it is immediately reinforcing and attempts to become physically active are likely to result in immediate aversive consequences. Thus, the task of the health professional is to ensure that initial attempts to exercise are painless, enjoyable, and reinforcing. Although time constraints are typically noted as major reasons for inactivity, regular exercisers complain as much as those persons who are not regularly active. Thus, perceived available time may reflect, in large part, priority on being active rather than actual time limitations.

In light of the substantial prevalence of inactivity, there is growing interest in physical and psychological health benefits of moderate intensity physical activity. Traditionally, research examining health benefits of exercise focus on the relationship between exercise training and physical fitness. It was assumed that health improved as a result of exercise only if requisite increases in physical fitness (i.e., mainly cardiorespiratory fitness) occurred. To achieve increased cardiorespiratory fitness, it is necessary to participate in exercise that is relatively vigorous, continuous, and aerobic. Recommendations for exercise involved the rhythmical and aerobic use of large muscle groups, 3–5 days/week, at 60–90% of maximum heart rate, for 20–60 minutes. These recommendations have been considered a **threshold** exercise prescription for health benefits.

However, a new conceptual paradigm based on epidemiological data broadens the focus to include health benefits from activity (15). It is now assumed that health benefits can be gained from diverse types of physical activity, such as walking, stair climbing, gardening, and household tasks rather than only from aerobic exercise. Additionally, the dose of physical activity includes moderate intensity (not just vigorous) activities as well as the utility of activity accumulated intermittently (rather than continuously). The current recommendations also acknowledge increased health benefits are likely to accrue with increased amounts and/or intensity of physical activity. However, a growing body of research demonstrates that moderate intensity physical activity, such as walking, is more appealing to many than more vigorous intensity programs (7).

The results from a recent two-year study of 269 healthy, initially sedentary middle-aged men and women who had been randomly assigned to one of three different physical activity programs suggested 6 different clinically meaningful subgroups of people who were at either low, moderate, or high risk of poor adherence by the second year of their physical activity program (16). For instance, persons who had been assigned initially to a community-based exercise class offered three times per week throughout the study period and who had a body mass index (i.e., body weight in kg/height in m^2) of 27 or greater were at particularly high risk for poor adherence throughout the two-year study period (i.e., only 7.7% of this subgroup achieved exercise adherence rates of at least 66% or greater by the second year). In contrast, individuals who had been initially assigned to a supervised home-based physical activity program and who reported low initial stress levels were at relatively lower risk for poor exercise adherence throughout the two-year study period (i.e., more than half of this subgroup achieved exercise adherence rates of at least 66% or greater across the two-year period). Continued research in this area using applications of such clinical decision-making approaches will help to further refine our understanding of those subgroups of people, defined through a combination of biologic, psychosocial, behavioral, and exercise program-specific factors, for whom tailored interventions are particularly indicated.

SIGNAL DETECTION

Signal detection methods were originally used by engineers to detect physical stimuli (e.g., auditory signals). They have been applied in medicine to develop diagnostic methods and tests. Signal detection can be used to define, through application of algorithms consisting of a series of simple "and/or" decision rules, distinct groups that are mutually exclusive and maximally discriminated from each other. More recently, applications of signal detection methods that define a "signal" as a behavioral outcome (e.g., presence or absence of smoking behavior or regular exercise participation) have been discussed (17). A strength of signal detection in behavioral research is that it allows for full use of all data available for each variable being evaluated, thereby eliminating problems related to missing data that accompany the use of multiple regression approaches (17).

▶ SUMMARY

The factors that most strongly influence initial adoption are probably different from those that affect maintenance (18). Currently noted variables clearly constitute part of the factors relevant in affecting activity levels, many of which have yet to be identified. Because of the complex interrelationships among these variables, many individuals may have difficulty explaining problems with starting or maintaining exercise without monitoring activity. Some factors, identified as predictive of inactivity (e.g., smoking status or being overweight) are present in those who may reap the most benefits from regular physical activity, those who are least likely to adopt or maintain an activity program. Finally, the variety of factors implicated indicates the importance of developing programs and strategies that fit the needs and preferences of different population groups. This "tailoring" can be contrasted with more typical methods of fitting individuals into existing programs. By tailoring physical activity to the population or individual, exercise professionals may positively influence initial drop-out rate (during the critical period i.e., the first 3–6 months) as well as during later periods. Systematic research evaluating specific methods of tailoring programs is increasingly indicated. In addition, applications knowledge of endurance exercise should be systematically applied to other dimensions of physical activity, including strength and flexibility training.

The use of linear regression methodologies to define factors associated with physical activity participation has limited understanding of the manner in which various personal, behavioral, program-specific, and environmental factors combine to identify subgroups at particular risk for poor physical activity adherence. Recent applications of clinical decision-making approaches, such as signal detection analysis, show promise in helping to define in a meaningful way subgroups of people at risk for poor exercise adherence, thus for whom tailored programs may be able especially effective (17).

Acknowledgments

This work was supported in part by PHS grant #AG-12358 from the National Institute on Aging awarded to Dr. King.

References

1. Stephens T, Caspersen CJ. The demography of physical activity. In: Bouchard C, Shephard RJ, Stephens T, eds. *Physical Activity, Fitness, and Health: International Proceedings and Consensus Statement.* Champaign, IL: Human Kinetics Publishers, 1994:239–256.
2. Dishman RK. Compliance/adherence in health-related exercise. *Health Psychol* 1:237–267, 1982.
3. Oldridge NB. Compliance with exercise rehabilitation. In: Dishman RK, ed. *Exercise and Public Health.* Champaign, IL: Human Kinetics Publishers, 1988:283–304.
4. Martin JE, Dubbert PM. Exercise adherence. *Exerc Sport Sci Rev* 13:137–167, 1985.
5. Bandura A. *Social Foundations of Thought and Action. A Social Cognitive Theory.* Englewood Cliffs, NJ: Prentice Hall, 1986.
6. Marcus BH, Takowski W, Rossi JS. Assessing motivational readiness and decision making for exercise. *Health Psych* 11:257–261, 1992.
7. King AC, Blair SN, Bild DE, et al. Determinants of physical activity and intervention in adults. *Med Sci Sports Exerc* 24: S221–S236, 1992.
8. Haimovitz D, Lansky LM, O'Reilly P. Fluctuations in body satisfaction across situations. *Intl J Eating Dis* 13:77–84, 1993.
9. Rosen JC, Saltzberg E, Srebnik D. Cognitive behavior therapy for negative body image. *Behav Ther* 20:393–404, 1989.
10. Butters JW, Cash TF. Cognitive-behavioral treatment of women's body image dissatisfaction. *J Consult Clin Psych* 55:889–897, 1987.
11. King AC, Frederiksen LW. Low-cost strategies for increasing exercise behavior: The effects of relapse preparation training and social support. *Behav Modification* 4:3–21, 1984.
12. Belisle M, Roskies E, Levesque JM. Improving adherence to physical activity. *Health Psychol* 6:159–172, 1987.
13. King AC, Haskell WL, Taylor CB, et al. Group- vs home-based exercise training in healthy older men and women: A community-based clinical trial. *JAMA* 266:1535–1542, 1991.
14. Calfas KJ, Long BJ, Sallis JF, et al. A controlled trial of physician counseling to promote the adoption of physical activity. *Prevent Med* in press.
15. Pate RR, Pratt M, Blair S, et al. Physical activity and public health: A recommendation from the Centers for Disease Control and Prevention and the American College of Sports Medicine. *JAMA* 273:402–407, 1995.
16. King AC. Using signal detection methods to predict exercise adherence in adults [abstract]. *Ann Behav Med* 17(Suppl):S041, 1995.
17. Kraemer HC. Assessment of 2 × 2 association: Generalization of signal detection methods. *Am Stat* 42:37–49, 1988.
18. Sallis JF, Haskell WL, Fortmann SP, et al. Predictors of adoption and maintenance of physical activity in a community sample. *Prev Med* 15:331–341, 1986.

91, 92, 94 95 101

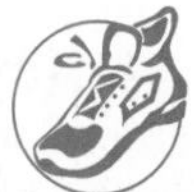

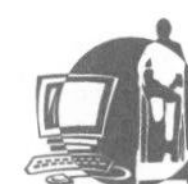

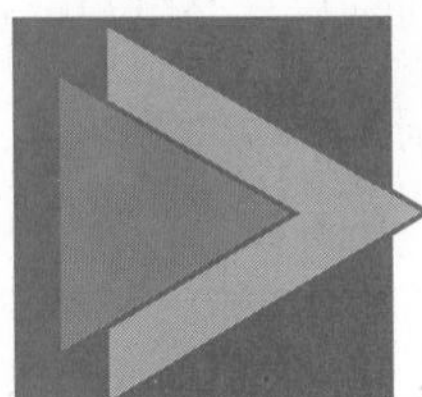

CHAPTER 69

Physical Activity Promotion: Adoption and Maintenance

Abby C. King and John E. Martin

A growing number of health behavior change theories and models have been applied physical activity behavior, with varying results (1). Among the most heuristic of these approaches is the application of social learning/social cognitive theories (2). These theories, previously described (see Chapter 68), focus on the dynamic relationship between personal attributes and resources, the behavior targeted for change, and influences of the physical and social environment in shaping adoption and maintenance of the targeted behavior. Along with similar conceptual approaches, they provide a framework for development of physical activity interventions.

In recent years such theories have been augmented with stage-based approaches, such as the transtheoretical model, in which different phases and processes potentially involved in the acquisition and maintenance of health behaviors are described (3). In combination with social learning/social cognitive theories and similar approaches, such stage-sensitive models may help identify groups of people at varying levels of psychological readiness for change, allowing more targeted intervention. However, it should be noted that social cognitive theory and similar approaches, as well as stage-based approaches to intervention, have not often been applied in a comprehensive fashion in physical activity intervention research. In addition, the majority of physical activity intervention studies focus on endurance exercise, often ignoring other forms of activity, such as strength and flexibility training, that are important components of fitness. While more systematic work is needed in this area, some promising strategies—drawn primarily from social learning/social cognitive approaches—for facilitating physical activity participation in early, as well as later, stages of physical activity acquisition have been clarified.

INCREASING ADOPTION AND EARLY ADHERENCE

Adoption of increased physical activity patterns can be enhanced through paying particular attention to factors in previously described personal, behavioral, environmental, and program-related spheres.

Personal and Behavioral Factors

With respect to personal factors, previous experience with physical activity should be explored, along with unreasonable beliefs and misconceptions about exercise (e.g., "no pain, no gain," older individuals should not be active because they need to "conserve their energy," etc.). For example, many potential exercisers believe that exercise is inherently painful and, therefore, aversive; these individuals must be told and shown that this statement is untrue. Sedentary individuals are often unaware of the utility of moderate activities (e.g., brisk walking) that may be more appealing than more structured, vigorous activity regimens. Behaviorally, many sedentary individuals benefit from specific instruction (accompanied by actual rehearsal and feedback) on appropriate ways of performing specific activities (e.g., jogging, striding, cycling, and warmup exercises) to obtain health-related benefits while avoiding injury.

In addition to activity-related attitudes, knowledge, and skills, a physical activity program should be personally relevant, both in terms of type of activity (or activities) and goals. For example, if stress reduction is a motivating factor, activities that can be helpful in reducing stress (i.e., not overly competitive, noisy, or demanding) should be targeted. Examples of such activities include brisk walking, jogging, or bicycling conducted outdoors in pleasant surroundings that allow time to "get away from it all."

Additional useful measures include structuring appropriate expectations concerning physical activity (what can and cannot be accomplished) as early as possible, stressing the many benefits of making change, as well as exploring perceived barriers to increasing physical activity (e.g., unreasonable expectations, fear of embarrassment, failure, boredom). A simple questionnaire regarding expectations can provide an exercise professional with early clues to such expectations.

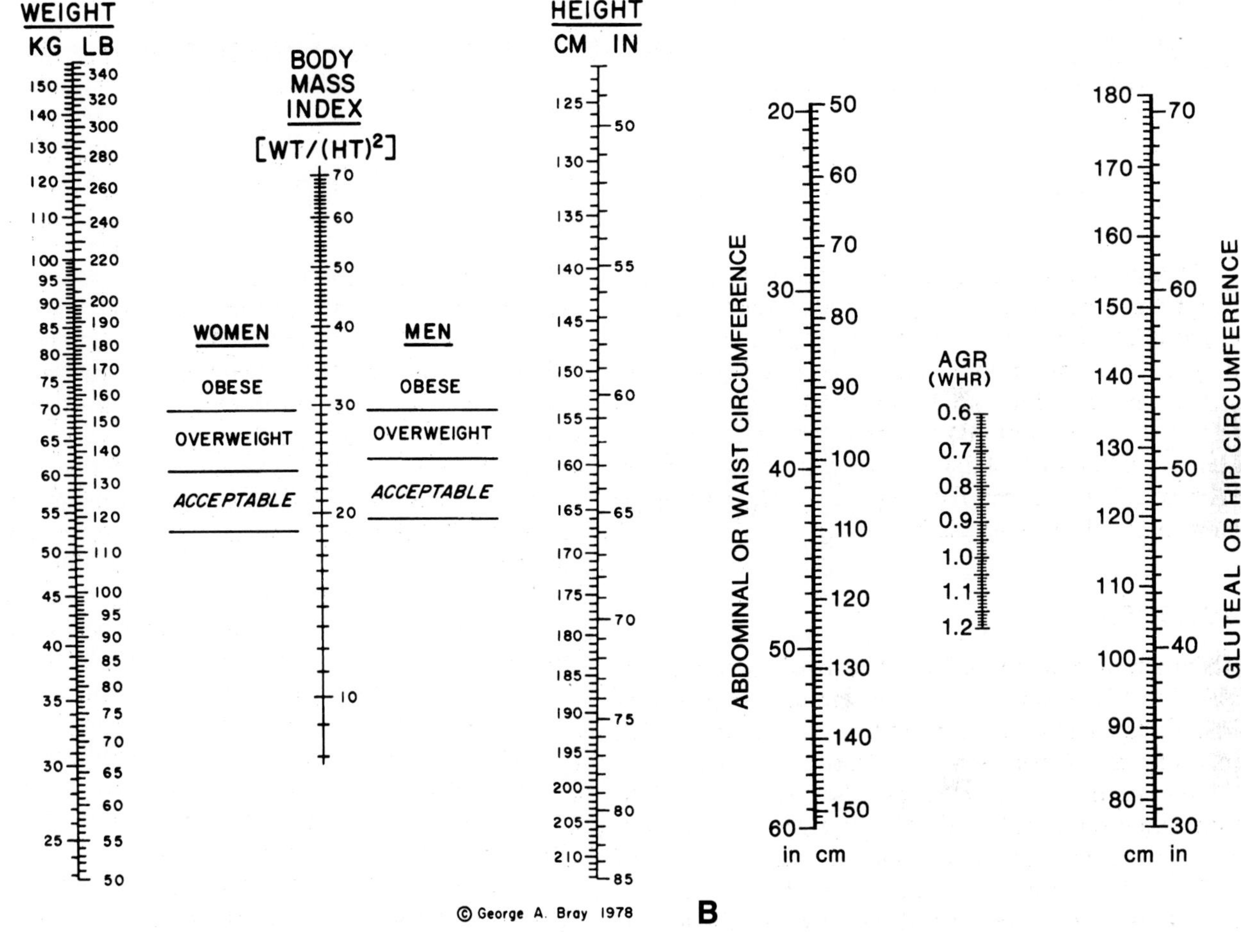

Adult Intervention Guidelines

BMI kg/m²		
19—34 years	>35 years	
< 25	< 27	Normal; refer to waist-to-hip ratio
25—27	—	Intervention indicated if there is a family history or presence of heart disease, type II diabetes, hypercholesterolemia, or hypertension.
> 27	> 27	Intervention indicated even in the absence of another risk factor

C

Figure 70.1. **A,** Nomograms for Body Mass Index (BMI) and Waist-to-Hip Ratio (WHR). **B,** Also shown are recommendations for adult interventions based on BMI and classification of health risk based on WHR. (BMI nomogram reprinted from Bray GA: Definitions, measurements, and classification of the syndrome of obesity. *Int J Obesity,* 1978; 2:99, WHR nomogram reprinted from Bray GA, Gray DS. Obesity: Part I—pathogenesis. *West J Med* 1988;149:429.)

logical aspects of obesity reveals few significant differences between overweight and average-weight persons. Even when psychological distress occurs in overweight persons, the distress may be either cause or consequence. Recent research has, however, identified two psychological factors that may be especially salient among overweight persons: body image dissatisfaction and binge eating problems.

Overweight persons tend to suffer more from negative body image and are more likely to have problems with binge eating than their average weight peers. The presence of binge eating is associated with increased risk for psychological problems.

Interest in physiological factors focus on the concept of a body weight "**set point.**" The set point theory proposes a "natural weight" for each individual, i.e., the weight the body seeks to protect against pressures to be too heavy or too thin. A set point above the ideal destines a "battle" against physiology in an attempt to lose weight. The concept of set point is appealing because it leads a search for factors that regulate body weight, but whether a set point exists is controversial. The practice of working with overweight individuals requires walking a fine line between acknowledging the importance of biology and painting a pessimistic physiological picture of weight change.

Recent research demonstrates that body weight is, in large part, controlled genetically. It is estimated that approximately 30–50% of the variance in body weight is explained by genetics. Moreover, the pattern of body fat distribution (e.g., upper or lower body) also appears to be genetically influenced. Studies also indicate that resting metabolic rate (RMR), which accounts for roughly 70% of daily expenditure, but varies considerably, is also influenced by genetics.

Genetic investigations of obesity, bolstered by recent technological advances, represent a particularly promising avenue that may soon contribute to a better understanding of overweight. A specific gene believed to contribute to obesity has recently been identified and cloned. In mice, this gene mutates and appears to produce extreme obesity and Type-II diabetes. Evidence also suggests that a specific secreted protein (leptin) may function as part of a signaling system that regulates the size of body fat deposits. Such research may someday lead to the development of pharmacological interventions for weight and fat regulation.

The findings that weight and fat distribution seem to be strongly influenced by biological and genetic factors, do not, however, suggest dieting is ineffective. They do suggest that individuals should adopt more **reasonable** goals and should avoid wholesale pursuit of aesthetic or even health "ideals." Overweight individuals **inherit only the tendency for obesity and the extent of its expression can be influenced by diet and exercise.**

IMPORTANCE OF EXERCISE IN WEIGHT CONTROL

Accumulated evidence demonstrates the importance of exercise in weight control. First, overweight persons are rarely physically active; however, inactivity may be either the cause or consequence of overweight. Second, people in weight loss programs who maintain the loss are most likely to exercise. Finally, the most convincing evidence comes from studies in which those attempting to lose weight are randomly assigned to groups that do or do not exercise with dietary change. Many, but not all, experimental controlled studies demonstrate that exercise in combination with diet produces greater weight loss than diet alone. The available controlled studies of exercise and diet that include post-treatment follow-up assessments are consistent—exercise facilitates long-term weight loss. Since successful weight loss maintenance, rather than short-lived weight loss, is universally viewed as the biggest challenge faced by obese persons, available data suggest that exercise should be included in weight control programs.

Exercise has been used as a component of weight control programs for years, but it is generally treated as a formality. Professionals were skeptical about compliance because the prospect of exercise to someone with the physical burden of excess weight is daunting. There are compelling reasons, however, to **emphasize physical activity.** Exercise professionals should be aware of the benefits of exercise and enthusiastic about the role of exercise in weight control. Describing the benefits to those attempting to lose weight can provide an added incentive to become more physically active.

Exercise Expends Energy

Exercise uses calories. It is a mistake to believe that caloric expenditure from low-level activity is adequate to permit increased food intake. The cumulative effects of exercise over long periods of time are substantial, so even modest levels of activity can be beneficial. The caloric expenditures of various physical activities are detailed elsewhere.

Exercise May Suppress Appetite

There is more animal than human evidence of this, but exercise may help to suppress appetite in some persons, while some individuals increase caloric intake to offset increased expenditure. The effects of exercise on appetite, therefore, may be either neutral or positive. It may be helpful to schedule exercise at times of day when overeating is common.

Exercise Counteracts the Ill Effects of Obesity

Exercise reduces morbidity and mortality via a number of possible mechanisms. Exercise has positive effects on blood pressure, serum cholesterol, body composition, and cardiorespiratory function, and obese persons are at increased risk for abnormalities in these areas. Some of the benefits of exercise are independent of weight loss. In fact, some research indicates that exercise may be necessary to achieve desired health outcomes of dietary interventions.

Exercise Improves Psychological Functioning

Changes in anxiety, depression, general mood, and self-concept are noted in those who maintain an exercise program, perhaps through increased sense of personal control. These psychological changes may enhance dietary compliance in someone attempting to lose weight.

Exercise Can Minimize Loss of Lean Body Mass

Up to 25% of weight lost through dieting alone is lean body mass (LBM). Overweight people typically have increased LBM as well as fat, but loss of LBM during dieting is potentially dangerous if protein reserves in essential areas of the body are depleted. LBM loss decreases when diet is combined with exercise. Aerobic exercise and resistance training have both been found to minimize the loss of LBM. Because endurance activities are commonly part of exercise programs, the potential for decelerating loss of LBM via resistance weight training is an important area for further research.

Exercise May Counteract the Metabolic Decline Produced by Dieting

Caloric restriction produces a rapid reduction of resting metabolic rate (RMR). The decline may be up to 20%, and because RMR accounts for 60–70% of total energy expenditure, it has substantial implications. This reduction in RMR may account, in part, for the "plateau" reached by many when weight loss slows or stops, even if caloric intake is stable. Exercise increases RMR, but the magnitude and duration of increase are unknown. How the type, frequency, intensity, and duration of exercise can be altered to offset the metabolic decline produced by dieting is not clear.

EXERCISE ADHERENCE

As is the case with dieting, compliance with exercise is a major challenge. In addition to providing education regarding the importance of exercise for weight control, the professional can enhance compliance in several ways.

Emphasize Psychological Benefits

The psychological benefits of exercise can be substantial. In addition to expending energy and improving health, exercise can enhance self-esteem, provide motivation, decrease anxiety, and buffer individuals against stress (a common trigger for overeating). The exercise professional can do much to enhance adherence by stressing that every time some form of physical activity is performed, it represents a positive step. Motivationally, it is important to keep track of such "success" (e.g., parking and walking to the mall), which may contribute to a feeling of greater **personal control.**

Be Sensitive to the Excess Weight

When sedentary people state what prevents them from exercising, it commonly involves being "too busy." This "barrier to exercise" can often be overcome by creative scheduling and by alerting people to the benefits of exercise. This reason, however, often masks other, more important barriers. One such barrier is excess weight itself. Becoming active can be difficult, tiring, and painful under the added workload of obesity. People should be assisted with setting reasonable exercise goals and expecting reasonable amounts of time to elapse before high levels of activity can be accomplished.

Negative self-image is another obstacle to exercise. It involves associations that plague many people, particularly those persons who have been overweight since childhood and/or are characterized by negative body image. They are likely to be self-conscious and embarrassed about their body and the mere prospect of exercise evokes negative feelings. Prescription of levels of activity consistent with abilities and fitness level, assisting individuals to select enjoyable activities, and sensitivity to body image concerns are all of importance.

Avoid an Exercise Threshold

A common question is, "How much should I do?" to which the response is the well-accepted, three-part equation involving **frequency** (3 times per week), **intensity** (70% maximum heart rate), and **duration** (15–30 minutes). Use of this prescription implies an exercise "threshold," that is, exercise must be done at a specific level to be beneficial. This threshold may be a useful incentive for some, but represents a deterrent to others.

Recent research has demonstrated that modest physical activity and modest weight loss both have significant health benefits. Relatively low levels of activity are associated with decreased mortality. Modest exercise also predicts weight loss. Moreover, surprisingly small weight losses can normalize blood pressure among some obese hypertensive subjects and improve control among obese Type II diabetics.

Exercise professionals should make a specific point about exercise and activity, **any exercise/activity is better than none.** Moreover, it should be underscored that such an effort represents a positive commitment. **Consistency may be more important than the type or amount of exercise.**

Select the "Right" Exercise

The selection of a realistic and appropriate exercise program is a key predictor of adherence. People are more likely to continue activities that are enjoyable. Two questions can be asked as a starting point: **Is it fun?** and **Will you do it regularly?** The exercise professional can assist in choosing activities that will match lifestyle and schedule. For obese individuals, the choice of low-impact activities is particularly important. For many, obese or lean, regular walking represents a potentially rewarding option.

Prevent Injury

Physical discomfort and injury represent frequent reasons for attrition from exercise. Exercise professionals should assist patients in establishing gradually progressive exercise programs that minimize discomfort and potential for injury, including attention to appropriate clothing and footwear. Care should be taken to prevent overheating and dehydration.

A COMPREHENSIVE APPROACH TO WEIGHT CONTROL

Overweight is not easily remedied by simple advice to "eat less and exercise more." Important elements of programs should have a broad base considering three factors: nutrition, exercise, and behavior change.

There is a wide range of options for weight control programs. Self-directed approaches, self-help groups, commercial programs, behavioral approaches, hospital-based programs (including very-low-calorie-diets), professional counseling, pharmacological treatments, and surgery are among the approaches that are successful. Although some treatments produce significant short-term weight loss, average weight losses are far from "optimal" and are difficult to maintain over time. Obesity is increasingly viewed as a chronic, ongoing problem that, for many people, requires lifestyle change, not simply short-term efforts.

Therefore, educated referrals are an important aspect of working with overweight persons. Unfortunately, clinical judgment must be relied upon for making such referrals, because research does not provide clear guidelines about matching patients to effective treatment. A **stepped-care** approach prescribes the least intensive interventions first (e.g., self-directed programs), especially for persons who are not significantly overweight, followed by more intensive treatment (e.g., hospital-based) for those who have been unable to succeed in other programs. Matching individuals to specific treatments is based on personal needs and program characteristics. For example, psychological counseling might be indicated in someone with significant distress or for binge eaters in addition to methods that address weight. Obese binge eaters are characterized by higher levels of psychological problems and greater body image distress than non-bingers and appear to derive fewer benefits from traditional weight-loss programs.

COMPONENTS OF EFFECTIVE TREATMENT

Nutrition, exercise, and behavior change represent three key elements of weight control programs. The integration of behavioral components into comprehensive weight control programs seems to produce improvements in general well-being and result in fewer negative psychological effects than dieting alone. Several references for weight control are cited in the reference section.

Behavior Change

Lifestyle and behavior change are cornerstones of effective treatment. Behavioral interventions are critical to ensure such changes and should focus on more than eating and exercise habits. They involve teaching individuals the relationship between **antecedents** (i.e., events, thoughts, and feelings leading up to eating), **behaviors** (i.e., eating, binging, etc), and **consequences** (i.e., events, thoughts, and feelings that follow eating and can determine subsequent problematic eating). In addition, individuals can be taught specific **coping skills** to change eating and exercise patterns and to overcome problems that interfere with change. Teaching coping skills to overcome difficult situations and prevent negative reactions is, perhaps, the most important treatment intervention.

Exercise

Exercise is a key component of weight control as stated above. Consistency, adherence, and enjoyment are the goals rather than intensity or mode of exercise. Exercise professionals should work with patients to set reasonable short-term physical activity goals that contribute to achieving intermediate-term goals of consistent lifestyle activity coupled with regular bouts of moderate exercise. Successful integration of both lifestyle and programmed exercise behaviors into long-term lifestyle change can be enhanced by consideration of the specific needs of overweight persons (see Exercise Adherence).

Nutrition

Adequate nutrition and decreased calorie intake relative to expenditure (negative energy balance) are general goals of dietary intervention. There are three primary methods for monitoring caloric intake. First, count calories. Instruction relative to specific servings and portion sizes from basic food groups with a defined total calorie intake are given. A second method involves the American Dietetic Association (and the American Diabetic Association) food exchange plan. Individuals are instructed concerning "exchanges" within food groups; each exchange represents a specific amount of food within group. Exchanges are equivalent in nutrition and calories. Finally, the Food Guide Pyramid, recently developed by the U.S. Department of Agriculture, encourages specific servings from various food groupings. Each approach may be acceptable in appropriate circumstances. Personal preference (of patient and professional) can be used to select one method. Reducing both overall caloric intake and fat intake appears to be more effective than fat-reduction alone.

Negative Energy Balance

Although numerous methods exist to arrive a recommendation for caloric intake, the following approach is recommended. Generally, 1500 kcal/day for males and 1200 kcal/day for females is used as a starting point. Modify caloric consumption depending on the individual and activity and a weekly goal of 1–2 lb weight loss. Calorie intakes below 1000 kcal/day should be medically monitored.

Determination of caloric intake necessary to produce a 1–2 lb weight loss per week can be difficult because various, complex factors can influence metabolic requirements. For example, reducing calorie intake by 500 per day (3500/week), is associated with a one pound (per week) weight loss only over large population groups, but there is considerable variability both individually and over time. Thus, a dietary record may aid in adjusting intake to help establish specific calorie goals.

Adequate Nutrition

Nutrition requirements should be carefully considered when selecting the approach to weight reduction. Inadequate nutrition during weight reduction can have serious medical consequences. Hypocaloric diets must be nutritionally adequate especially with respect to protein, vitamin, and mineral intake. Moreover, diet composition may influence various mechanisms relevant to weight control such as diuresis, appetite, and satiety.

Very-Low-Calorie-Diets

A particularly aggressive approach to weight loss involves very-low-calorie diets (VLCD). These involve fasting with either a powdered supplement or small amounts of lean meat, fish, or fowl. Calorie levels range from 400–800 kcal/day and programs vary considerably in the quality of behavioral and nutritional intervention. Recent research has indicated that there is little advantage to VLCDs with < 800 calories/day.

These diets are typically used in individuals 40% or more over ideal weight and should be medically supervised. They are appealing because weight loss is rapid (2–3 lbs/wk for women, 3–5 lbs/wk for men) and because food choice is not an issue. Long-term maintenance, however, can be a problem. The initial studies with one year follow-up demonstrated good maintenance of weight loss when VLCD is combined with a high-quality behavioral program. Results from three- and five-year follow-up, however, indicate nearly total recidivism. While it may be premature to abandon these diets, individuals should be cautioned about the probability of relapse. In the meantime, research examining methods for sustaining impressive losses produced by these diets is needed.

Cognitive Change

Thoughts and attitudes about self, nutrition, and exercise play key roles in weight maintenance. It is important to assist people to become **actively** aware of thoughts. Often "**automatic**" thoughts, or overlearned responses to particular situations, influence feelings and have a profound impact on dietary compliance. Examples are self-deprecating thoughts following dietary violations, adoption of unreasonable goals, and all-or-none thinking (e.g., foods are "legal" or "illegal" or being "on" or "off" a diet). Teaching awareness of these thoughts and ways to substitute more objective thoughts can be effective. The exercise professional can also help individuals **focus on progress** (not shortcomings) and look for **problems in behaviors and situations** (not characterologic defects).

Social Support

The social environment influences health behavior. Social support represents a potential positive resource for dietary change, however, some individuals benefit from social support, whereas others may not. Some individuals prefer privacy in weight loss programs, whereas others benefit from social support. It is helpful to examine this issue with individuals and to teach those who would profit from such reinforcement methods for eliciting and sustaining the support.

Relapse Prevention

Maintaining weight loss is the greatest challenge that those attempting to lose weight face. Many individuals "successfully" lose weight numerous times only to regain it. This problem of relapse has negative psychological and medical consequences. Recent research demonstrates that individuals whose body weight fluctuates repeatedly over time (e.g., cycles of weight loss and gain) may be at increased risk for coronary heart disease compared to individuals with stable weight.

We view relapse as a process, not an outcome. Those attempting to lose weight, regardless of their motivation, commitment, or level of success, inevitably experience temptations and, almost universally, have episodes of overeating. How a dieter **copes** with such situations may determine whether that isolated event (i.e., temptation or lapse) escalates into repeated overeating (relapse), leads to abandonment of the diet (collapse), or, ideally, leads to increased confidence and continued maintenance. Relapse prevention techniques have been developed to identify potential **high-risk** dieting situations and develop **coping skills** to overcome those situations.

In those cases in which lapses do occur, individuals must be taught to avoid negative reactions and to react instead with an attempt to learn from the lapse, solve problems for future events, and renew commitment to the program.

PHARMACOLOGICAL TREATMENTS

Recent advances in biology and genetics coupled with a shift towards viewing obesity as a chronic bio-behavioral disorder of energy regulation and metabolism have led to an explosion of interest in pharmacologic approaches to treatment. There are ten FDA-approved drugs for weight control which influence the adrenergic system (amphetamine-like compounds). Two previously FDA-approved drugs (dexfenfluramine and fenfluramine) which influence the serotonergic system, have been abruptly removed from the market and are no longer approved for treatment of obesity. One of these drugs (fenfluramine) was one part of the popular "fen-phen" combination with phentermine (a centrally acting adrenergic drug with low abuse potential that remains on the market). A series of recent studies identified two potential major health risks associated with these medications: primary pulmonary hypertension and heart valve abnormalities.

The adrenergic drugs are generally associated with about 1 kg/week weight loss that is regained soon after discontinuation. Such drugs are generally not recommended because of the potential for abuse. In the context of controlled research studies with obese patients, some serotonergic compounds have been shown to produce impressive short-term weight loss; however, weight is gradually regained following discontinuation. One recent study found that drug treatment combined with comprehensive dietary and behavioral treatments produced significantly greater weight loss than placebo in obsese patients. This study suggests the potential effectiveness of combining specific pharmacological and behavioral treatments for achieving and sustaining long-term weight control. Research is ongoing to determine the efficacy and safety of existing and new medications for obesity.

Medications represent only one part of a comprehensive weight control program. Advantages of drug treatments must be balanced against side-effects and risks. However, the risks of obesity also need to be considered and balanced against the risk of drug treatments. Severe obesity with coexisting medical complications due to the obesity might warrant consideration of the potential risks and benefits. The recent "phen-fen" problem has also demonstrated that obesity drugs should not be prescribed for non-obese persons. The FDA has recommended that approved obesity medications be used only in persons with BMI >30 (or >27 if medical co-morbidities are present). The National Institutes of Health National Task Force on the Prevention and Treatment of Obesity has taken a cautious stance on long-term use of pharmacotherapy for obesity and has called for further research before the drugs are used on a broad scale.

▶ SUMMARY

Obesity is a significant health problem. Complex physiological, genetic, cultural, and psychological factors contribute to the problem and it cannot be attributed solely to weak willpower or personal deficit. Exercise is an important predictor of success for weight reduction, therefore increased physical activity is a key goal for those who wish to lose weight. Compliance may be jeopardized, however, if special physical and psychological burdens of being overweight are not considered. Regardless of the level of intervention, a comprehensive program involving nutrition, behavior, cognitions, and social support, in addition to exercise, appears to hold the greatest promise for long-term results. The high frequency of relapse and potential psychological and medical consequences emphasize the need for aggressive work in relapse prevention.

Continued research to better understand the complex biological and psychological aspects of weight regulation is important and may lead to the identification of pharmacologic approaches to enhance the effectiveness of treatment components. Consistency and lifestyle change are key goals in all weight reduction programs.

Suggested Readings

Abenhaim L, Moride Y, Brenot F, et al. Appetite-suppressant drugs and the risk of primary pulmonary hypertension. *N Engl J Med* 1996;335:606–616.

Agras WS, Telch CF, Arnow B, et al. Weight loss, cognitive-behavioral, and desipramine treatments in binge eating disorder: An additive design. *Behav Ther* 1994;25:225.

Atkinson RL. Use of drugs in the treatment of obesity. *Ann Rev Nutr* (in press).

Ballor DL, Katch VI, Becque MD, et al. Resistance weight training during caloric restriction enhances lean body weight maintenance. *Am J Clin Nutr* 1988;47:19–25.

Brownell KD. *The LEARN Program for Weight Control.* 6th ed. Dallas: American Health Publishing Co., 1994.

Brownell KD, Fairburn CG, eds. *Eating Disorders and Obesity: A Comprehensive Handbook.* New York: Guilford Press, 1995.

Brownell KD, Rodin J. Medical, metabolic, and psychological effects of weight cycling. *Arch Intern Med* 1994;154:1325.

Brownell KD, Rodin J. The dieting maelstrom: Is it possible and advisable to lose weight? *Am Psychol* 1994;49:781.

Brownell KD, Wadden TA. Etiology and treatment of obesity: Towards understanding a serious, prevalent, and refractory disorder. *J Consult Clin Psychol* 1992;60:505.

Friedman MA, Brownell KD. Psychological correlates of obesity: Moving to the next research generation. *Psychol Bull* 1995;117:3.

Goldstein DJ, Potvin HJ. Long-term weight loss: the effect of pharmacologic agents. *Am J Clin Nutr* 1994;60:647–657.

Grilo CM. The role of physical activity in weight loss and weight loss management. *Med Exerc Nutr Health* 1995;4:60.

Grilo CM, Pogue-Geile M. The nature of environmental influences on obesity: A behavior genetic analysis. *Psychol Bull* 1991;110:520.

Guy-Grand B, Apfelbaum M, Crepaldi G, et al. International trial of long-term dexfenfluramine in obesity. *Lancet* 1989;2:1142.

Kurz X, van Ermen A. Valvular heart disease associated with fenfluramine-phentermine. *N Engl J Med* 1997;337;1772–1773.

Manson JE, Faich GA. Pharmacotherapy for obesity: do the benefits outweigh the risks? *N Engl J Med* 1996;335:659–660.

McArdle WD, Katch FI, Katch VL. *Exercise Physiology: Energy, Nutrition, and Human Performance.* 3rd ed. Philadelphia: Lea & Febiger, 1991.

Pavlou KN, Krey S, Steffee WP. Exercise as an adjunct to weight loss and maintenance in moderately obese subjects. *Am J Clin Nutr* 1989;49:1115–1123.

Rippe JM, Ward A, Porcari JP, et al. Walking for health and fitness. *JAMA* 1988;259:2720–2724.

Schlundt DG, Hill JO, Pope-Cordle I, et al. Randomized evaluation of a lowfat and libitum carbohydrate diet for weight reduction. *Intl J Obesity* 1993;17:623.

Vogler GP, Sorensen TIA, Stunkard AJ, et al. Influences of genes and shared family environment on adult body mass index assessed in an adoption study by a comprehensive path model. *Intl J Obesity* 1995;19:40.

Wadden TA, Foster GD, Letizia KA. Response of obese binge eaters to behavior therapy combined with very low calorie diet. *J Consult Clin Psychol* 1992;60:808.

Wadden TA, Van Itallie TB, Blackburn GL. Responsible and irresponsible use of very-low-calorie-diets in the treatment of obesity. *JAMA* 1990;263:83.

Weintraub M. Long-term weight control: The National Heart, Lung, and Blood Institute funded multimodal intervention study. *Clin Pharmacol Ther* 1992;51:581.

Wilfley DE, Grilo CM, Rodin J. Group psychotherapy for the treatment of bulimia nervosa and binge eating disorder: research and clinical methods. In: JL Spira, ed. *Group Therapy for the Medically Ill.* New York: Guilford Press, 1997;225–295.

Wilson GT: Behavioral treatment of obesity: Thirty years and counting. *Adv Behav Res Ther* 1994;16:31.

Wood PD, Stefanick ML, Williams PT, et al. The effects on plasma lipoproteins of a prudent weight-reducing diet, with or without exercise, in overweight men and women. *N Engl J Med* 1991;325:461-466.

Yanovski SZ. Binge eating disorder: Current knowledge and future directions. *Obesity Res* 1993;1:306.

Zhang Y, Proenca R, Maffei M, et al. Positional cloning of the mouse obese gene and its human homologue. *Nature* 1994;372:425.

91 277

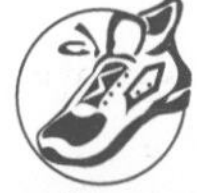

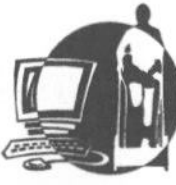

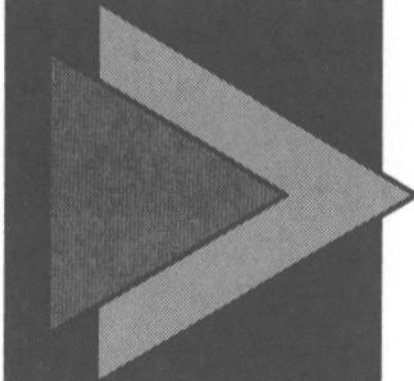

CHAPTER 71
SMOKING CESSATION

Andrew Gottlieb

HEALTH RISKS OF SMOKING

Cigarette smoking is the leading preventable cause of premature death from heart disease, lung disease, and cancer. Of the 46 million Americans who smoke regularly, approximately 420,000 die of premature illness each year. Worldwide, the negative impact of cigarette smoking on health is staggering. According to a recent survey conducted by the World Health Organization (WHO), 3 million people die each year from smoking related illnesses (1). By the year 2020, the death toll will rise to 10 million per year! Of the people alive today, roughly half a billion will die of tobacco related causes. American women are disproportionally affected. Though 5% of women live in the United States, 50% of women worldwide who die from smoking-related causes live in the United States.

Although most people are aware of the link between smoking and cancer, far fewer individuals understand the causal relationship between smoking and heart disease. The risk of heart disease is directly related to number of cigarettes smoked. Smoking one pack per day doubles the risk compared to nonsmoking; smoking more than one pack per day triples the risk. The main mechanisms affecting the development of heart disease are effects of carbon monoxide. Nicotine in tobacco smoke causes increases in heart rate and blood pressure, which increase the work of the heart. It also may increase platelet adhesiveness, changing blood viscosity. Carbon monoxide interferes with the ability of red blood cells to carry oxygen, thereby reducing oxygen delivered to heart muscle.

HEALTH BENEFITS OF QUITTING SMOKING

The health benefits of quitting smoking are immediate and substantial. They extend to young and old and to those with and without smoking related disease. Smoking cessation represents the single most important step that smokers can take to enhance length and quality of life (2).

Although risk from smoking is cumulative, increased risk of cancer and heart disease drops rapidly after stopping smoking, even if the person has smoked for many years (3, 4). After 2 1/2 years of nonsmoking, risk of lung cancer is reduced by 50%. Within 3–5 years of nonsmoking, risk of a heart attack is similar to a nonsmoker and within 5–10 years, risk of major health problems decreases to levels only slightly greater than those who have never smoked. Besides the obvious major health benefits, many other benefits result, including increased energy, improved sense of smell, ability to exercise more easily, and higher self esteem.

WHY PEOPLE SMOKE

To counsel smokers effectively, it is useful to understand that both physical and psychological components drive smoking behavior (5, 6). Physical dependence on nicotine is one major factor. Each cigarette puff delivers a "hit" of nicotine to the brain within 7 seconds, making smoking one of the most effective drug delivery systems known. The average smoker may self-administer 50,000 to 70,000 nicotine doses a year. Nicotine appears to have both stimulating and tranquilizing effects, depending on dosage. Evidence exists that nicotine may increase the production of brain hormones, such as beta-endorphins. This effect may explain why nicotine can reduce perception of pain and increase feelings of well-being. Smokers can "fine-tune" emotional response by varying puff rate and depth to control the amount of nicotine delivered to the brain. Thus, a smoker literally has fingertip control of emotional and physical responses, reducing the need for other coping techniques. Once a person becomes dependent on these effects of smoking to function normally, quitting becomes extremely difficult.

The other major component is conditioned psychological dependence. The thousands of nicotine doses received each year are linked to situations and emotional states. Each of these situations and emotional states becomes a cue to the smoker that it is time for a cigarette puff. Situational cues include such things as drinking coffee or an alcoholic beverage, talking on the phone, watching TV, finishing a meal, or driving. Other cues are negative emotions, such as anger, frustration, stress, or boredom. Further, dropping blood levels of nicotine trigger withdrawal symptoms that also bring on smoking.

CESSATION

The Quitting Process

The experience of quitting smoking varies considerably among smokers. Some smokers quit "easily" and report surprise at how much easier than expected it was; some report that quitting was the most difficult thing that they ever attempted, while others report some degree of difficulty between these two extremes. Some report that physical factors are the primary difficulty, some the psychological factors, and others report both.

Withdrawal from nicotine can produce a variety of effects, including craving for tobacco, increased anxiety, increased irritability, increased restlessness, difficulty concentrating, headache, drowsiness, and gastrointestinal disturbances. These symptoms are generally most intense for the first 2–3 days after cessation, then decrease, but increase again around day ten, and finally decrease gradually thereafter. The acute phase of nicotine withdrawal is generally over within 2–4 weeks, although some withdrawal symptoms such as the urge to smoke may continue for months or even years. The number and severity of withdrawal symptoms reported varies in number from none to many and in severity from mild to severe. (Nearly 90% of smokers experience at least one withdrawal symptom.)

Most smokers quit a number of times before achieving long term abstinence. The majority of smokers who relapse do so within the first 6 months after quitting; some relapse years after cessation, but this is the exception. As the duration of abstinence increases, relapse becomes less likely (2). Many smokers are able to quit for short periods, but maintaining smoking cessation is a major challenge.

Approaches to Smoking Cessation

Most people who have quit smoking report doing so on their own, without the help of a formal program or a health professional. Formal smoking cessation programs can be helpful to those smokers who cannot quit on their own, often those who smoke more heavily and are more addicted (7, 8).

In order to guide a smoker to appropriate assistance for smoking cessation, it is important to know the options available, the effectiveness, as well as potential barriers to participation (cost, location, time, and cultural biases) (7). The appropriateness of a group program vs. individual sessions with a health professional should be considered. When examining effectiveness, it is important to look at the long term quit rate of a strategy or program, since relapse is common. Some programs boast high initial quit rates but fail to report long term relapse rates. There is no "magic bullet" (at any cost) that can guarantee long-term quitting. However, there is help in a variety of forms to assist any smoker who would like to quit.

Smoking cessation techniques include the following:

- Pharmacological interventions
- Behavioral interventions
- Other strategies such as acupuncture and hypnosis.

Stop smoking programs are available in a variety of formats:

- Self-help materials (with or without minimal contact)
- Group meetings
- Individual sessions with a health professional.

Many studies have been conducted evaluating various behavioral and pharmacological smoking cessation approaches, allowing us to identify with some confidence the approaches that work.

PHARMACOLOGICAL INTERVENTIONS

Early Approaches

Early pharmacological interventions included Pronicotyl, a spice tablet, and silver acetate, which were supposed to make cigarettes taste foul when inhaled. They were generally ineffective, or only minimally effective. Lobeline, a nicotine analogue, sold as CigArrest, Bantron, and Nicoban, has no advantage over a placebo. More recently, some researchers have reported that clonidine hydrochloride reduced tobacco withdrawal symptoms and facilitated smoking cessation. Research findings, unfortunately, have been mixed regarding effectiveness of clonidine (9, 10).

Nicotine Replacement Medication

The most promising pharmacological interventions (currently in widespread use) are nicotine replacement via nicotine polacrilex (Nicorette) and transdermal nicotine patch (Habitrol, Nicoderm, Nicotrol, and Prostep). Both are available over-the-counter and are designed to provide a partial substitute for nicotine obtained from cigarettes to make the initial phase of tobacco withdrawal less unpleasant, allowing new ways of coping with the behavioral aspects of smoking cessation (unlinking smoking-related cues from actual cigarette smoking) to be learned. Nicotine nasal spray is available by prescription only.

Nicotine replacement treatment should be used for at least 10–12 weeks following quitting; many smokers require 6 months treatment, some will need treatment for 1–2 years before successfully tapering off nicotine medication.

Nicotine Gum

Nicorette (nicotine polacrilex) 2 mg and 4 mg, available since 1984 by prescription (and available over-the-counter since 1996), has nicotine bound to a resin base (nicotine gum). When the medication is chewed, nicotine is released and is absorbed through the oral mucosa. For maximum benefit, the patient chews 12 or more pieces of gum a day. The suggested dosing is as follows:

- Weeks 1 through 6: one piece every hour
- Weeks 7 through 10: tapering
- Week 12: discontinuing use

Patients should be instructed carefully in how to chew the gum, since optimal use is quite different than regular chewing gum. Current costs of Nicorette gum may exceed $400 for a 12 week treatment program. Buying the starter kits rather than the refill kits may decrease cost up to 30%.

Most researchers report impressive improvement in quit rate, but usually when combined with behavioral counseling or follow-up. The 4 mg gum is more effective than 2 mg gum for highly nicotine dependent smokers (smokers who smoke > 25 cigarettes a day), yielding 2-year quit rates of 34% (4 mg) vs. 6% (2 mg) (11).

Researchers continue to examine ways to increase effectiveness of nicotine polacrilex. Clear chewing instructions and a behavioral change component accompany a Nicorette prescription (12, 13). When advising a smoker, it is important to guide the individual to either a behavioral program in which nicotine polacrilex use is an integral part or to a physician who will provide good follow-up care along with this medication.

Studies show that the effectiveness of nicotine polacrilex 2 mg is influenced by the behavioral intervention component that accompanies it (5, 6). If there is no behavioral component and if a physician simply calls a prescription to a pharmacy, nicotine polacrilex is no more effective than placebo after 1 year of follow-up; however, if the behavioral intervention is even minimal, a significant effect can be expected. By adding nicotine polacrilex to physician advice, studies indicate that the one year quit rate increases from approximately 5% to 9%; adding physician advice and follow-up increases quit rates from 15% to 27%; and by adding comprehensive group counseling program increases quit rates from 16% to 38%. Studies where behavior modification is combined with nicotine polacrilex are associated with one year quit rates of over 40%. Now that nicotine polacrilex is available without prescription, it is more important that some type of behavioral support or follow-up be encouraged.

Nicotine Patch

The nicotine patch was approved in the United States in late 1991 and is currently available over-the-counter. Patches provide a much easier route for nicotine delivery than nicotine polacrilex, making both smokers and health professionals happy they are available. Nicotine patches are not the "magic bullet," however.

Patches come in three sizes, 30 cm^2, 20 cm^2, and 10 cm^2, delivering nicotine for 24 hours/day (Habitrol, Nicoderm and Prostep) or 16 hours/day (Nicotrol). The 24 hours/day patches deliver 21, 14 and 7 mg nicotine/day (30 cm^2, 20 cm^2, and 10 cm^2 respectively), while the 16 hours/day patches deliver 15, 10 and 5 mg nicotine/day. Nicotine patches are applied once a day. Most smokers use the 24 hour patches and begin with the 21 mg patch, subsequently tapering to 14 and 7 mg patches. Most smokers who use the 16-hour patches, start with the 15 mg patch and taper to the 10 and 5 mg patches.

Approximate costs are about $4 per day of treatment. Recommended treatment duration is 8 weeks for light smokers, and 10 weeks for heavy smokers, for a total cost of about $280-$400.

Whether to use a 24-hour patch or a 16-hour patch probably depends on how strong the craving for cigarettes is in the morning. Those with intense morning craving may do better on a 24-hour patch, but a 16-hour patch produces less sleep disruption and fewer nightmares. In a study of 935 participants, 6-month sustained abstinence rates for those receiving the nicotine patch were significantly higher than for those receiving placebo (26% vs. 12%, respectively). Good results have been demonstrated with nicotine patch therapy as long as there is regular contact with the patient. Nine group-counseling sessions over 12 weeks resulted in 26% non-smoking rates at 6 months (14). Seven regular physician visits over 18 weeks of patch therapy produced 34% cessation rates at 6 months (15). Even brief weekly telephone follow-ups during 6 weeks of patch therapy yielded a 21% quit rate at 6 months (16). As with nicotine polacrilex, more needs to be learned about increasing the effectiveness of the nicotine patch.

Combining the use of nicotine gum with nicotine patch may provide better relief of nicotine withdrawal symptoms than either drug alone (17). Although no smoking cessation studies have been performed that support this, a nicotine patch can provide a baseline level of nicotine, while gum adds nicotine in high risk situations. The overall dose of nicotine would still be less than that attained by smoking.

Nicotine Nasal Spray

Nicotine nasal spray is aqueous nicotine delivered into nasal pathways using a device similar to that used to deliver intranasal steroids. Nicotine nasal spray may be helpful for heavy smokers who do not get adequate relief using nicotine gum or patches. Available by prescription as Nicotrol NS, nicotine nasal spray delivers nicotine in a quickly absorbed form, resulting in blood nicotine levels that peak within 4–15 minutes, between 2–12 ng/ml. Some 20% of users achieve a blood nicotine level similar to that derived from smoking one cigarette. Dosing is 1 mg of nicotine per two sprays (one in each nostril). Maximum daily dose is 5 per hour, or 40 per day, with a treatment time of 3 months. However, according to the package insert, 32% of spray users reported feeling dependent, therefore the potential for addiction may be higher than with patch or gum (18).

Cost is approximately $40 per 10 mg, or about one hundred doses. At a recommended dosing of 1–2 doses per hour, cost for 10 weeks of treatment is between $450-$900. All of these nicotine medications seem to be safe. The most common side effects are local, such as skin irritation from patches or heartburn from nicotine gum and nasal irritation from nicotine spray. Contrary to press reports from July 1992, a nicotine patch does not cause heart attacks (19).

Cigarettes deliver nicotine more rapidly than any of the medications. Next is nicotine nasal spray, followed by nicotine polacrilex, and, slowest (but steadiest), a nicotine patch. Thus it may be that nicotine nasal spray best simulates the nicotine bolus effect of smoking cigarettes, but whether this will make it difficult to give up the spray remains to be seen (19).

Other Pharmacologic Approaches: Buspirone and Buproprion

Buspirone (Buspar) is a non-benzodiazepine anti-anxiety medication. One randomized, double blind, placebo-controlled trial demonstrated that participants using buspirone had 4-week abstinence rates of 47% compared to 16% for placebo (20). Buspirone may be useful, either alone, or in combination with nicotine gum or patches, especially for smokers who use cigarettes to cope with anxiety.

A series of interesting findings relate cigarette smoking and depression. Although the lifetime prevalence of major depression is 3.7–6.7 %, in the general smoking population it is 27%, and it is 46–61% in smokers who present for treatment. Of those with major depression, 74% smoke, in contrast to 26% of the general population. Further, the quit rate of those with major depression is about half that for smokers with no psychiatric diagnosis (21, 22).

Thus it appears that some smokers use smoking to control depression. For those smokers, concomitant treatment with an antidepressant may be helpful. The only published studies on antidepressants and smoking are on buproprion (Wellbutrin). One found 55% of patients treated with buproprion abstinent at 6 months as compared to 0% treated with placebo (23). Another study of 190 people showed 40% of buproprion-treated patient abstinent at 4 weeks compared with 24% of placebo treated subjects (24). Evaluation of smokers for depression using the Beck Depression Inventory (Center for Cognitive Therapy, Philadelphia) or other similar instrument and concomitant treatment for depression may significantly improve smoking cessation results.

BEHAVIORAL INTERVENTIONS

Behavioral interventions including components such as self-monitoring, contracts, and assertiveness skills training are often included in smoking cessation programs. As previously stated, these components may increase long-term effectiveness. One of the most effective techniques is rapid smoking. When properly administered, this approach has long-term abstinence rates of 64–70%. Rapid smoking is a multicomponent treatment that involves several different elements, including relapse prevention training (see subsequent discussion) and rapid smoking, in which the patient inhales smoke from his own cigarette every 6 seconds until he no longer wants to take another puff. The procedure creates an aversion to smoking that, when combined with skills training, leads to good cessation outcomes. This technique must not be attempted without support and guidance from a health professional. It is used more rarely now because it requires good medical support. In addition, other, non-aversive methods have become more widely available.

Relapse prevention is a useful behavioral approach to maintaining smoking cessation. Relapse prevention teaches anticipation of those situations where temptation to smoke may be present and development of new coping techniques for avoiding relapse in these situations (25). Simple questionnaires can be used to measure confidence in ability to resist smoking during exposure to high-risk situations (26). These questionnaires may be helpful in determining the types of coping skills on which to focus attention.

The relapse prevention approach is particularly valuable in smoking cessation. As Mark Twain said, "Quitting smoking is easy; I have done it many times." Staying quit is difficult.

OTHER TECHNIQUES

Smokers are often attracted to acupuncture or hypnosis as "the magic bullet" or as an easy way to achieve long term smoking cessation. Controlled studies fail to show any positive correlation between acupuncture and smoking cessation (27). Hypnosis can be provided individually or in groups for one or multiple sessions and is often combined with other behavioral techniques. Study methodology makes it impossible to evaluate the effectiveness of hypnosis as an aid to long term cessation.

STOP SMOKING PROGRAMS

Programs are available in a variety of formats. In a self-help or minimal intervention format, one attempts smoking cessation without the continued assistance of health professionals, trained leaders, or organizations; reliance on self is the primary method with a self-help book or guide to assist in devising ways to quit and stay off cigarettes. A study using the American Lung Association, Freedom From Smoking in 20 Days (one of the many manuals available), reports a 1-year quit rate of 5% (vs. 2% for controls). Generally, self-help programs report substantially lower quit rates than more formal programs, but are low cost and generally widely available. Efforts are underway to maximize effectiveness of self-help programs (28).

Programs in a group format provide a support group. The content, cost, and providers of these programs vary, but generally health organizations, as well as commercial groups, offer these programs. Few well designed studies have been completed to evaluate this type of program. When specific programs advertise high success rates, it is important to inquire about long term (ideally one year, but minimally six months) rates and the method for determining those rates.

Some smokers prefer working with a health professional on an individual basis. Under this format, it is important to inquire about approaches used and qualifications of the health professional. Typically the health professional is a physician, nurse, or counselor of some type. Research projects (at medical schools, universities or other medical facilities) can often provide another resource for smokers.

HOW TO HELP SOMEONE STOP SMOKING

Exercise professionals are often asked to help with smoking cessation in individual cases. The following guidelines may be useful as aids to promote successful quitting.

Advise the Smoker to Quit

Advice to quit from a health professional with good rapport may have substantial impact. For example, studies show that 60 seconds of definitive advice from a physician has substantial impact on long term (1 year) quit rate, increasing it 17-fold in one study (29). Advice should be clear, succinct and unequivocal regarding the dangers of smoking and the benefit of quitting. Timing the discussion to occur when a patient is experiencing symptoms caused by, attributed to, or exacerbated by smoking such as coughing, shortness of breath, or angina may be especially effective. Avoidance of moralism or punitive action is important. Emphasize the benefits experienced after quitting and advise the patient to completely eliminate tobacco products. There are NO healthy tobacco products and virtually no smokers can smoke in a limited way.

Help Develop a Specific Plan for Cessation

Help the smoker choose a specific quit date. A specific quit date helps prepare for nonsmoking. Review prior quit attempts to evaluate what was helpful and identify problems. Reframe past relapses in a positive light by emphasizing that past attempts can teach something useful. Say that most successful long term quitters have made more that one attempt to quit.

Inform the smoker about resources in the community such as self-help or minimal contact programs, group programs, and individual health professionals who work in smoking cessation. A list of programs with names and phone numbers for additional information is helpful, as well as information about the components, format, cost, and effectiveness of the intervention. Good sources of information concerning local programs include:

- Local universities
- Medical groups, hospitals
- Agencies such as American Cancer Society, American Lung Association and the American Heart Association
- Inform the patient about over-the-counter nicotine replacement options such as nicotine gum or patches.

Encourage Quitting Efforts and Provide Support During Difficult Times

Help motivate by asking about positive health benefits or other positive occurrences resulting from quitting, such as increased stamina, better breathing, less coughing, and improved sense of smell. Reassure that withdrawal symptoms are temporary and are signs that dependence on nicotine is diminishing. Since relapse is common after quitting, ask about difficult times and help identify ways to cope.

Some smokers may not be ready to quit immediately, but will express readiness at a later date. Those not ready to quit are sometimes concerned about the negative impact of quitting or ability to succeed; these factors should be addressed if they are clearly expressed. Gentle, but firm, reminders about the importance of quitting can influence motivation to make the attempt.

Respond to Concern about Weight Gain

Smokers may express concern about weight gain, either as a reason not to quit or after cessation. Approximately 80% of those who quit gain weight after cessation. The average weight gain is approximately five pounds. Increased food intake and/or decreased energy expenditure may be partially responsible for post-cessation weight gain. The health benefits of smoking cessation far exceed any risk from the average weight gain (2). It is useful to tell the patient that 100 pounds have to be gained before impact of gaining weight equals that of continued smoking. Suggestions such as increasing physical activity, eating low-fat sweets in response to an increased desire for sweet foods, having low calorie snacks available, etc. may be helpful. The best way to avoid excessive weight gain is to increase levels of physical activity and exercise.

▶ SUMMARY

Cigarette smoking is the leading preventable cause of death. Smoking cessation has major and immediate health benefits. Advice to quit smoking from a health professional with good rapport may have substantial impact. Millions of smokers have quit successfully; however, for some quitting is difficult. Both physical and psychological factors contribute to maintaining cigarette smoking behavior. There is no "magic bullet" but help is available. Most smokers quit without assistance and most successful long term quitters have made many short term quit attempts before achieving long term abstinence.

A variety of techniques in a variety of formats are available to help smokers who want to quit but are unable to do so without assistance. Programs that include nicotine replacement in combination with behavioral intervention seem to provide the best results. There are a number of options for nicotine replacement, and both nicotine gum and nicotine patches are now available without a prescription.

It is important to encourage smokers to quit, and to provide clear information and support to help increase chances of success. The good news is that even small interventions seem to have large effects, especially compared to no intervention. Thus with a little knowledge and persistence, a professional can have a powerful positive effect on the health of patients.

ACKNOWLEDGEMENTS

Thanks to David Sachs, M.D., who gave feedback and input into the original preparation of this chapter and whose research writings had a significant influence on the author's thoughts about smoking. Also thanks to Barbara Newman, who helped with a prior revision of this chapter.

References

1. University of California at Berkeley Wellness Letter, Vol. 12, Issue 5, Feb. 1996.
2. U.S. Department of Health and Human Services. The Health Benefits of Smoking Cessation. Public Health Service, Centers for Disease Control, Center for Chronic Disease Prevention and Health Promotion, Office on Smoking and Health. DHHS Publication No.(CDC) 90-8416, 1990.
3. Sachs DPL. Cigarette smoking: health effects and cessation strategies. *Clin Geriatr* Med 1986;2:337–362.
4. Schuman LM. The benefits of cessation of smoking. *Chest* 1971;59:421–427.
5. Sachs DPL, Leischow SJ. Pharmacologic approaches to smoking cessation. *Clin Chest Med* 1991;12(4):769–791.
6. Sachs DPL. Advances in smoking cessation treatment. *Curr Pulmon* 1991;12:139–198.
7. Fiore MC, Novotny TE, Pierce JP, et al. Methods used to quit smoking in the United States. Do cessation programs help? *JAMA* 1990;263:2760–2765.
8. Glynn TJ. Methods of smoking cessation—Finally some answers (editorial). *JAMA* 1990;263:2795–2796.
9. Glassman AH, Stetner F, Walsh BT, et al. Heavy smokers, smoking cessation, and clonidine: results of a double-blind, randomized trial. JAMA 1988;259:2863–2866.
10. Franks P, Harp J, Bell B. Randomized, controlled trial of clonidine for smoking cessation in a primary care setting. *JAMA* 1989;262:3011–3013.
11. Tonnesen P, Fryd V, Hansen M, et al. Effect of nicotine chewing gum in combination with group counseling on the cessation of smoking. *N Engl J Med* 1988;318:15–18.
12. Pomerleau OF, Pomerleau CS, eds. Nicotine Replacement-A Critical Evaluation. *Progress in Clinical and Biological Research* Vol 261. New York: Alan R. Liss, Inc., 1988.
13. Sachs DPL. Nicotine polacrilex: practical use requirements. *Curr Pulmon* 1989;10:141–158.
14. Transdermal Nicotine Study Group. Transdermal nicotine for smoking cessation. Six-month results from two multicenter controlled clinical trials. *JAMA* 1991;266:3133–3138.
15. Sachs DPL, Sawe U, Leischow SL. Effectiveness of a 16 hour transdermal nicotine patch in a medical practice setting, without intensive group counseling. *Arch Intern Med* 1993;153:1881–1890.
16. Westman E, Levin E, Rose J. The nicotine patch in smoking cessation: a randomized trial with telephone counseling. *Arch Intern Med* 1993;153:1917–1923.
17. Fagerstom KO, Schneider N, Lunelle E. Effectiveness of nicotine patch and nicotine gum as individual versus combined treatments for tobacco withdrawal symptoms. *Psychopharmacology* 1993;111:271–277.
18. Package insert, Nicotrol NS. Pharmacia AB, Sweden.
19. Sachs PL, Fagerstom KO. Medical management of tobacco dependence: Practical office considerations. *Curr Pulmon* 1995;16:239–249.
20. West R, Hajek P, McNeill A. Effect of buspirone on cigarette withdrawal symptoms and short term abstinence rates in a smokers clinic. *Psychopharmacology* (Berl) 1991;104: 91–96.
21. Hall SM, Munoz, RF, Reus VI, et al. Nicotine, negative affect, and depression. *J Consult Clin Psychol* 1993;61:761–767.
22. Glassman AH, Helzer JE, Covey LS, et al. Smoking, smoking cessation and major depression. *JAMA* 1990;264: 1546–1549.
23. Ferry LH, Robiins AS, Scariati PD, et al. Enhancement of smoking cessation using the antidepressant bupropion hychochloride. *Circulation* 1992;86:I-167.

24. Ferry LH, Burchette RJ. Evaluation of bupropion versus placebo for treatment of nicotine dependence. Oral paper presented at the 147th Meeting of the American Psychiatric Association, Philadelphia, May 26, 1994.
25. Marlatt GA, Gordon J. Relapse Prevention: *Maintenance Strategies in the Treatment of Addictive Behaviors.* New York: Guilford Press, 1985.
26. Condiotte MM, Lichtenstein E. Self-efficacy and relapse in smoking cessation programs. *J Consult Clin Psychol* 1981;49:648–658.
27. Ter Riet G, Kleijnen J, Knipschild P. A meta-analysis of studies into the effect of acupuncture on addiction. *Br J Gen Prac* 1990;40(338):379–382.
28. Glynn TJ, Boyd GM, Gruman JC. Essential elements of self-help/minimal intervention strategies for smoking cessation. *Health Educ Q* 1990;17(3):329–345.
29. Russell MAH, Wilson C, Taylor C, et al. Effect of general practitioners' advice against smoking. *Br Med J* 1979;2: 231–235.

SECTION THIRTEEN

Program Management

SECTION EDITOR: *Tracy York, MS*

177, 192, 221

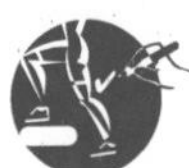

128, 225, 228, 233, 269, 273, 274
279, 280, 281, 282, 283, 284

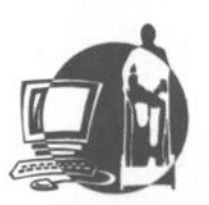

CHAPTER 72
HEALTH AND FITNESS PROGRAM DEVELOPMENT

Sandy Minor

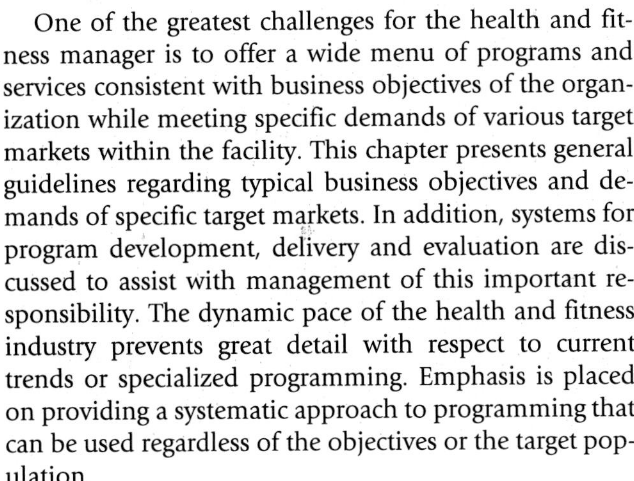

One of the greatest challenges for the health and fitness manager is to offer a wide menu of programs and services consistent with business objectives of the organization while meeting specific demands of various target markets within the facility. This chapter presents general guidelines regarding typical business objectives and demands of specific target markets. In addition, systems for program development, delivery and evaluation are discussed to assist with management of this important responsibility. The dynamic pace of the health and fitness industry prevents great detail with respect to current trends or specialized programming. Emphasis is placed on providing a systematic approach to programming that can be used regardless of the objectives or the target population.

PROGRAMMING BASED ON FACILITY OBJECTIVES

As the fitness industry has matured over the past decade, facilities have become more similar with respect to general design and types of equipment. It is likely, for example, that a prospective participant will find a similar range of cardiovascular equipment (treadmills, stair machines, bicycles, rowers, and skiers) available in both community-based centers and commercial settings. As a result, programming has become the primary product differentiating facilities in the marketplace. For this reason, it is important that a menu of programs be designed to closely align with the specific mission and business objectives of that particular fitness setting.

The following section outlines four general categories of business that exist within the health and fitness industry. A description of typical business objectives in each of these categories is discussed to provide the health and fitness manager with a reference point. In reality, regardless of the category of business, there are likely to be several objectives within the business plan of a given organization. It is the responsibility of the health and fitness manager to clearly identify objectives and to construct a menu of programs and services based on these objectives. The categories of business in the health and fitness industry include commercial, community, corporate, and clinical.

Commercial Settings

Commercial fitness facilities are usually operated to make a profit. Private athletic clubs, country clubs, and spas are examples of commercial fitness facilities. It is important to recognize that programming can contribute to profitability in several ways. Programs can generate revenue directly through assessment of additional fees for services. Personal fitness training is an example of a successful revenue generating program that is popular in commercial settings. In addition to fee-for-service programs, complimentary programs may also be consistent with the profit objective by providing assistance in selling and retaining members. Participants may make a decision to join based largely on types of programs and services offered. In addition, the decision to continue paying monthly dues is largely based on use of the facility and success in meeting individual goals. Programs that encourage regular participation and effective facility use can have a positive impact on member retention and, therefore, a positive effect on profitability.

Community Facilities

The objective of most community fitness facilities is service to as many members of a specific target market as possible. YMCAs, Jewish Community Centers, community recreation centers, and university recreation centers are examples of community settings. These are nonprofit organizations and generally, to cover expenses within the organization, they charge minimal fees. Depending on the popularity of a program, some programs may operate at a profit to support other programs that service the community.

Corporate Settings

Corporate fitness facilities are usually operated to reduce employee health care costs and increase employee productivity. Programs in this environment are funded, in part, by the company and directed at preventing unnecessary medical expenses. In addition, programs can be utilized to improve employee morale and assist in recruiting new employees. Corporate fitness programs may exist independent of a fitness facility. Many health and wellness programs are delivered at corporate worksites using conference room facilities for educational programs and health fairs, individualized health risk appraisals, and written health information in the form of articles and newsletters. Outdoor activities such as walking, running, and cycling clubs can also be offered without a fitness facility.

Clinical Setting

If a clinical facility operates as a for-profit entity, programs are conducted with similar objectives to those in a commercial setting. In the case of a non-profit facility, objectives similar to corporate or community fitness business are assumed. Based on the above commercial and community settings, it is increasingly difficult to define the menu of programs for a facility based solely on a general category. For example, for a hospital that insures subscribers on a capitated basis, a health and fitness facility may be developed with several objectives. The hospital may operate a "corporate" business for its employees in an attempt to control health care costs and to improve employee productivity and morale. The facility may also be available as a "community" business for its health insurance subscribers to maintain healthy lifestyle and lower the use of medical services. Finally, the hospital may also use the facility as a "commercial" business to position itself as a wellness-oriented health care provider, thus having a positive effect on health insurance sales to additional subscribers.

For this reason, it is important that the health and fitness manager design a menu of program offerings based not only on the type of facility, but more importantly on the specific mission and objectives of the facility and the specific needs of the participant.

PROGRAMMING BASED ON TARGET MARKET OBJECTIVES

Regardless of the category, the participant base (target market) has its own set of objectives (needs) related to health and fitness. Understanding and identifying the range of objectives is essential to the development of a menu of fitness programs and services. The following describes three typical individual objectives of those considering participation in a health and fitness program. Participant needs are rarely limited to a single category and often change over time. It is important to recognize the range of participant needs and to offer a variety of programs and services that meet as many of these needs as possible. Proper identification of participant needs not only contributes to successful programming, but also to long term participant retention. The more diverse the menu of services offered, the more likely participants will continue to use the facility as objectives change. Objectives related to health and fitness can be described in the categories of health, fitness, and performance.

Health Goals

People often consider participation in a health and fitness program to improve health or prevent onset of disease. Programming for this population involves education and behavior modification. Initial assessments, such as Health Risk Appraisals, provide individuals with important information related to health status, as well as a benchmark to measure improvements.

For exercise programming, regular physical activity should be emphasized. Program development should be divided into initial, improvement, and maintenance phases. The initial phase involves a gentle introduction to activity emphasizing regular participation and proper technique. The improvement phase involves a progressive increase in frequency, intensity, and duration of activity. The maintenance phase involves variations in program design to maintain level of fitness that has been achieved as well as adherence to the program. Participants who have health-related objectives may need to spend more time in the initial phase of exercise programming before proceeding to the improvement phase. Incentive programs are important in the maintenance phase of exercise programming.

Fitness Goals

Participants with these goals participate in a program to "get in shape" or "lose weight." While the goals can be very specific, they often center around looking and feeling better. Emphasis in programming for this population involves individualized exercise prescription based on participant goals emphasizing the improvement phase of exercise programming.

Performance Goals

These participants have specific fitness goals that center around performance improvement for a specific activity. Athletes, first time competitors, and participants undergoing rehabilitation are included in this category. Specific exercise prescription with frequent re-evaluation is necessary. Measuring outcomes is essential to assess effectiveness in meeting specific participant goals.

STRATEGIC PROGRAMMING AND PROGRAMMING SYSTEMS

The process of developing a menu of program offerings for a given facility is a four-step process that involves needs assessment, program planning, program implementation, and program evaluation (Fig. 72.1).

The Needs Assessment

The purpose of a needs assessment is to determine the specific needs and interests of the target market. This information, combined with industry trends and organizational objectives can assist in clearly defining a menu of programs and services. Options for conducting the needs assessment include the methods discussed below.

Target Market Surveys

The purpose of a target market survey is to determine level of interest for a prospective participant in specific health and fitness programs. Questions must be carefully constructed and sample groups selected by random process so that accurate and relevant information is obtained. In the case of a start-up operation, where initial programming decisions may have a significant financial impact on the design of the facility, consideration of a consultant for conducting a thorough market analysis is recommended. While it may be expensive, the relative cost of renovating a facility to accommodate different programming justifies the money invested in a market analysis prior to facility design and construction.

Focus Groups

Focus group interviews, though sometimes considered a second phase, can be conducted in an interactive way to obtain detailed information regarding prospective participant interests in specific programs. Focus groups can also be used to obtain more complete information regarding pricing, scheduling, and other details related to specific program plans. Outside consultants can conduct the interviews, allowing the business to observe potential participants from an observation room (out of view). The involvement of a third party in the interview process can make participants more comfortable and less intimidated in expressing views.

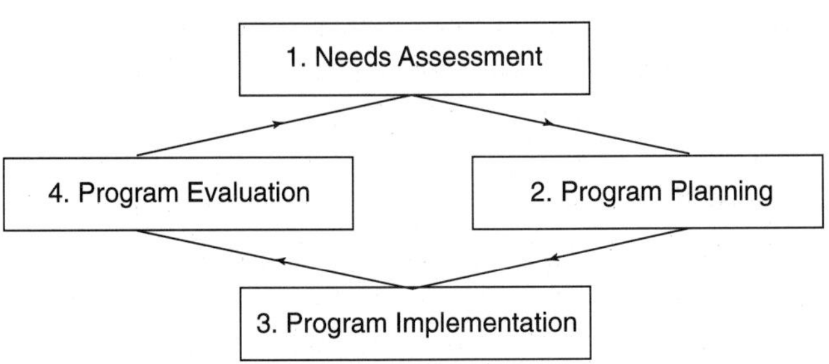

Figure 72.1. Outline for development of effective programs. (With permission from Patton B, et al. *Developing and Managing Health/Fitness Facilities.* Champaigne IL: Human Kinetics, 1989.)

Participant Surveys

If new programming is being considered in an existing facility, a survey of participants provides valuable insight, since future participants are likely to have similar needs and interests. These surveys can be distributed through billing statements, at specific programs, and as part of registration for other activities. Regardless of the method used, participation is likely to increase if there is an incentive to complete the survey.

Current Program Evaluations

As part of complete program delivery, evaluations should be conducted on a periodic basis for all programs offered within a facility (see next section for further details). These program evaluations provide valuable information regarding adaptations for existing programs, as well as identification of opportunities for new program development. This process should be ongoing and includes analysis of revenue, expenses, attendance records, participant satisfaction, and attainment of program goals and objectives.

Surveys of Staff, Management, and Advisory Committees

Input from staff, management, and other experts provides important insight, as well as an important base of support during the marketing phase. Staff directly in contact with participants often have valuable insight. Line staff are exposed to informal suggestions and complaints that help them formulate ideas regarding programming. Managers often have important input regarding operational issues and financial considerations related to the overall objectives. Finally, expert advisors from the community provide a perspective from outside the facility. Experience often helps to identify trends and new business opportunities, as well as assists in later stages of program planning. In addition, the involvement of line staff and management during early phases of needs assessment builds a strong base of support for marketing the program to prospective participants. Staff are more likely to feel ownership and to be more supportive and informed about the details of the program during the marketing phase.

Health Screening and Fitness Assessment Results

Identifying specific goals and objectives for programs is essential to evaluating success later. When programs are directed at specific changes in health or fitness status, pre-testing provides important information regarding programming priorities. For example, a corporate site may consider implementing a health and fitness program to lower the need for medical care and, in doing so, offer initial health risk appraisal on employees to obtain data regarding prevalent health risk behaviors. From this information, informed decisions can be made about cost-effective programs for reducing these risk factors.

Health Care Utilization Reports

Reports on health care utilization assist an organization in identifying programming opportunities based on the type of health care services used. A corporate worksite may be experiencing a large number of claims related to back pain and injury; programming decisions based on a goal of reducing back injuries through education, exercise and ergonomic workstation adjustments are then logical.

Community Agency Data

Organizations such as the American Heart Association, American Lung Association, American Red Cross, and U.S. Public Health Department provide a wealth of information regarding prevalence of disease and risk factors in the population. In addition, these agencies may also provide resources including well researched and developed "turn key" programs, referrals of independent contractors and marketing materials for risk factor intervention.

Program Planning

When the needs assessment is complete and there is sufficient interest to support development of a specific program, the planning process begins. All program planning should include a long-term vision so that short-term planning then becomes a means by which that long-term vision is achieved. Program planning includes those aspects discussed below.

Identifying Program Objectives

The first step in program planning is to define the general business and specific program objectives. Clearly defined objectives provide the basis upon which all program decisions are made. In addition, they allow for evaluation of success and assist in development of effective marketing materials. General business objectives must be consistent with objectives of the organization. Examples of general objectives include:

- Generating net revenue
- Improving participant retention
- Acquisition of new participants
- Community service

Objectives are usually program specific. Examples include:

- Improving performance or fitness
- Providing education (classes or materials) about a specific wellness topic
- Reducing risk factors, such as body fat, blood pressure, or cholesterol

Defining the Target Market

The next step in program development is to define the specific characteristics of people who are likely to participate. Determine whether the market size is adequate to meet the objective based on the initial needs assessment.

Organizational Staff Structure

Effective program planning begins with designation of specific responsibilities within the programming team (staff). Programs are most successful when there is broad input from both management and front line staff. If possible, planning should include those who will be responsible for delivery. A project leader should be designated and responsibilities divided among members of the team.

Program Content

This portion of planning involves specific decisions about content. Content planning includes development of lecture outlines, lesson plans, audiovisuals, handouts, and activity plans.

Delivery Model

The delivery model is largely dependent on the objectives, characteristics of the target market and projected number of participants. Decisions regarding the delivery model include:

1. Location: It must be accessible and convenient for the target market as well as meeting specific program needs.
2. Scheduling: The program must be convenient and not compete with other activities which aim at this target market.
3. Pre-activity screening and waivers: Required assessments and specific waivers of liability and informed consent forms should be clearly identified.
4. Staff-to-participant ratio: This should be defined in advance so that enrollment limits can be established and accurate budgeting is possible.
5. Follow-up: A plan for follow-up with participants at the conclusion of the program may include evaluation and assessment, rewards, reassessment, and opportunities to continue.

Marketing and Sales Plan

The marketing plan defines the message and the specific methods to be used to inform potential participants. Since most marketing activities have financial implications, it is especially important that marketing be carefully designed with a clear message and identification of a specific target market. Typical marketing activities include advertising, newsletter articles, brochures, flyers, bulletin board displays, posters, information sessions and demonstrations. A sales plan outlines direct action to be taken to secure sales. Sales training should be conducted with all involved staff. Communication techniques, use of scripts and rehearsal through role playing sessions can make staff more effective in communicating the benefits to prospective participants.

Budget Development and Program Pricing

Once program planning is complete, specific pricing and budgets can be established including expenses such as salaries, employee taxes and benefits, marketing expenses, sales commissions, program materials and equipment, and facility use charges. Pricing can then be established based on projected number of participants and desired net revenue; break even participation volume should be established. In order to conduct programs within established budgetary guidelines, revenues and expenses should be reviewed throughout all phases of program delivery.

Program Implementation

Program implementation involves carrying out the design created during the planning phase. Implementation involves hiring staff, carrying out marketing and sales, and delivering program components according to the plan. It is important to recognize that the implementation phase is a dynamic process that continually rolls back into small planning phases as new participant needs are identified. The most effective programs are created with enough flexibility to make immediate changes in the delivery model when needs are identified.

Program Evaluation

Program evaluation should be conducted throughout implementation and immediately at the conclusion of the program. Evaluation assesses effectiveness in meeting program objectives (outcomes), as well as success in carrying out specific components of plan (process). In addition, instructor performance and participant satisfaction should be evaluated.

Computers

Use of computers is essential for effective management of health and fitness programs. Desktop publishing allows cost-effective marketing, spreadsheet and data base programs assist in data collection, tracking and reporting, and specialized software programs are available which allow for detailed participant management. A fully integrated package allows input of personal data, health history, fitness assessment information, program participation and participant goals and interests. This data assists in planning through identification of specific needs. Program effectiveness can be evaluated through participation records, pre- and post-fitness assessment. Finally, group reports can be generated for purposes of communicating with corporations and HMOs regarding outcomes related to investments in wellness programs.

Outcome Evaluation

The first step in evaluating the outcome of a specific program is to refer to the originally stated general business and specific program objectives. These provide a reference point for measuring success. A cost-benefit analysis should be conducted to identify all expenses and assign a dollar value to all benefits so that the overall cost or savings of a program can be calculated. Table 72.1 illustrates examples of business objectives and specific program objectives as well as appropriate methods of evaluation.

Process Evaluation

Process evaluation is the assessment of success in carrying out specific components of a plan. Process evaluation is conducted throughout program delivery through direct supervision and participant suggestion. When possible, changes in delivery should be immediate. At the conclusion of the program, process evaluation can be conducted through a review of records and completion of participant questionnaires (Fig. 72.2).

Process evaluation should assess the following:

- Appropriateness of the facility
- Completion of screening procedures, waivers, and informed consents
- Appropriateness of the schedule
- Performance of the staff

Table 72.1. Program Evaluation

Evaluation of Business Objectives	
Generate net revenue	Complete financial analysis of revenue vs. expenses
Improve client retention	Tracking of length of stay in the facility for participants vs. non-participants
Acquisition of new clients	Track clients reasons for joining the facility
Provide community service	Measure number of participants
Evaluation of Specific Program Objectives	
Improving performance	pre/post measurements of specific tasks
Improving fitness level	pre/post fitness measures
Providing education	pre/post participant questionnaires assessing their knowledge on a specific topic
Lowering risk factors	pre/post fitness assessments, health risk appraisals, medical screenings

Other models exist which include the sale of food and nutritional supplements. These programs are popular in fitness facilities because of the revenue potential. It is important to fully investigate the products to ensure that accuracy of claims and product safety.

Group Exercise Classes

Group exercise classes can add an important dynamic to health and fitness programming. Such classes allow for a low cost option to provide instruction, motivation and guidance in specific exercise programs. Most facilities have expanded group program offerings to include resistance training, flexibility, body sculpting, sport specific conditioning, pre/postnatal, child, and active older adult exercise, martial arts, yoga, various types of dance, and a variety of aerobic activities that uses equipment such as steps, slides and spinning bikes.

Program types and time schedules vary depending on the resources available and the number of participants. For example, a small club may offer a limited number of the most popular group exercise classes during prime time use hours, whereas a larger facility with several studios may offer a wider variety of programs concurrently. The health and fitness manager must stay current on programming trends by attending conferences, reading journals, and using continuing education programs. In addition, it is important that participant needs are assessed on a regular basis to ensure that program offerings are appropriately scheduled.

▶ SUMMARY

Required skills for group exercise instructors are similar to those for other exercise professionals with emphasis on strong group leadership qualities. A good knowledge base in risk factor screening and exercise program design for apparently healthy and special populations is essential. Facilities should require that all group exercise instructors hold certifications from a nationally recognized organization such as the ACSM. As with the personal training staff, the health and fitness manager is responsible for being informed about various certifications and deciding which will be required (or accepted) by the organization.

Suggested Readings

American College of Sports Medicine. *ACSM's Guidelines for Exercise Testing and Prescription.* 5th ed. Baltimore: Williams & Wilkins, 1996.

Patton B, et al. *Developing and Managing Health/Fitness Facilities.* Champaigne IL: Human Kinetics, 1989.

129, 227, 234, 235, 236, 237, 238, 240, 242, 243, 244, 245, 275, 285

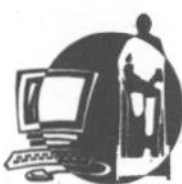

441, 443

CHAPTER 73
PERSONNEL ISSUES

Brent Darden

The greatest asset of a successful company is its people. The collective talents of a diverse group of individuals (the workforce) represent the defining characteristics of any organization. If employees know and understand their job responsibilities and how it relates to other areas of the business, better performance and better services can be provided by the employees (1). Although facilities and programs initially draw participants, staff can have an influence on continued customer use of the facility. How personnel issues are managed, in large part, determines effectiveness of the workforce (those responsible for meeting organizational objectives).

HIRING

Effective hiring is essential to success, particularly in a service-oriented business. A systematic, organized, and positive approach toward selection increases the chances of a mutually beneficial relationship between employer and employee. In addition to inconvenience of employee turnover, the negative impact on the customer and cost of recruiting, hiring and training a new employee is substantial. Time and preparation invested prior to hiring results in more satisfied employees and better-functioning organizations.

Developing Job Descriptions

Creating an effective job description begins with defining the responsibilities and expectations of the position. A properly constructed job description helps to ensure that the best person is hired; it also serves as a valuable reference throughout the term of employment. Key points for developing a job description include:

1. Fit the job title to the job.
2. Identify reporting relationships.
3. Include a summary statement of the job.
4. Describe each duty and responsibility.
5. State the qualifications required.
6. Indicate the status of the position.
7. State the physical requirements.
8. Specify hours, shifts and work schedule.
9. Emphasize the role of the position within the organization.
10. Assign responsibility for upholding mission statement/core values.

Recruitment

If the job description is complete, soliciting applicants is the next step in the hiring process. Locating health and fitness professionals who are technically qualified and who possess excellent "people skills" can be critical to the use of the facilities and programs. Although traditional methods of advertising open positions (e.g., local newspapers) may provide viable candidates, networking through fitness industry contacts and advertisements in professional trade journals usually produce better results. Posting the position with local colleges, professional associations, and placement services may also be effective.

Selection

A systematic comparison of applicant qualifications with the job description helps to narrow the pool of applicants to the 3-5 top candidates for interview. A thorough evaluation of educational background, certification, experience, and references is important.

Educational Background

In light of the rapid growth of the industry as well as the continued challenge to bring credibility to the profession, a minimum of a Bachelor's degree should be required for most positions. There are innumerable related degrees and, although the degree title is typically based on a specialization, the differences between them are often negligible and rarely should be a determining factor when processing applications. Health and fitness professionals usually have expertise in either health promotion or fitness leadership. Health promotion specialists are generally competent in needs assessment, program planning, implementation, and evaluation in a variety of health-related areas. Fitness leadership specialists may be more proficient in exercise testing and prescription, fitness training and exercise class leadership (2). Proficient exercise professionals may possess skills and/or experience in both areas.

Certification

Requirements for some type of certification has become standard. The benefits of certification obtained through a credible provider are obvious; however, there are many providers and quality of the certification must be considered. Acknowledgment of nationally recognized and widely accepted certification programs is prudent. Recommended standards for various positions can be found in ACSM's Health/Fitness Facility Standards and Guidelines (Table 73.1) (1).

Experience

Beyond the obvious advantages of previous employment in the health and fitness industry, look for related skills that may be beneficial. Customer service, sales, teaching, management, and supervisory experiences and many other such skills are transferable.

References

Most applicants carefully select only positive references. Still, it is important to check these references. The nature of the adjectives used to describe the candidate in a conversation may provide useful insight.

Interviewing

The interview is, perhaps, the most critical part of the hiring process. The paramount skill for effective interviewing is listening. The "85/15" rule is a good rule of thumb: the candidate should do 85% of the talking, the interviewer, 15%. At least 3 or 4 top candidates should be interviewed in a consistent manner by the one or more staff (the same for each interview). Prepare in advance, set aside uninterrupted time, and avoid rushed hiring decisions.

There are numerous interview methods, but a panel consisting of several current staff may to yield the best

Table 73.1. Organizations Offering Health/Fitness Professional Certifications

Organization	Certifications	Workshops/Examinations
American College of Sports Medicine Box 1440 Indianapolis, IN 46206-1440 (317)637-9200	*Rehabilitative Tract* Exercise test technologist Exercise specialist Program director *Health/Fitness Tract* Exercise leader Health fitness instructor Health fitness director	Workshops Written and practical examinations
American Council on Exercise P.O. Box 910449 San Diego, CA 92191-0449 (800)825-3636	Aerobics instructor Personal trainer	Workshops Written examinations
Aerobics and Fitness Association of America 15250 Ventura Blvd. #200 Sherman Oaks, CA 91403 (818)905-0040	Personal training Weight training Basic aerobics instructor Advanced step aerobics instructor	Workshops Written and practical examinations
Cooper Institute for Aerobics Research 12330 Preston Road Dallas, TX 75230 (800)635-7050	Health promotion director Physical fitness specialist Lifestyle coordinator Aquatic specialty Program director specialist Total well being-physicians Group exercise leader Biomechanics of strength training	Workshops Written and practical examinations
National Strength and Conditioning Association P.O. Box 38909 Colorado Springs, CO 80937-8909 (719)632-6722	Personal training Strength conditioning Resistance exercise programming	Written and practical examinations
YMCA of USA 101 North Wacker Drive Chicago, IL 60606 (312)977-0031	Physical fitness specialist	Written and practical examinations

results. A standardized interview report facilitates more objectivity. Structure the interview by asking all applicants the same questions in the same manner. Table 73.2 provides a sample of interview questions. Avoid the tendency to jump to conclusions based on first impressions. Ensure that the questions are legally permissible. Equal Employment Opportunity Commission (EEOC), Affirmative Action, the Americans with Disabilities Act (ADA) and other laws strictly prohibit discrimination (3). Each interview session should include:

1. Introduction: Establish a rapport.
2. Explain the interview process: Include the time length and format.
3. Interviewer questions: Ask open-ended questions.
4. Candidate questions: Opportunity for candidate to ask questions.
5. Closing remarks: Review job opportunities, let applicant know the next step.

Table 73.2. Interview Questions

1. What part of your work has given you the greatest feeling of achievement and satisfaction?
2. What part of your work have you found the most frustrating or unsatisfying?
3. Describe a work-related problem you had to face recently. What procedures did you use to deal with it?
4. What have you done to make your job easier or more rewarding?
5. How do you determine which activities should have top priorities in your time?
6. Under what kinds of conditions do you do your best work?
7. Describe the best or worst person for whom you have worked. Why did you have this reaction?
8. How do you keep informed about what's happening in your field?
9. In your mind, what is the greatest thing that distinguishes a superior employee from someone who gives typical good performance?
10. Why did you choose the career for which you are interviewing?
11. What do you consider to be your greatest strengths and weaknesses?
12. What motivates you to put forth your greatest effort?
13. What two or three accomplishments have given you the most satisfaction? Why?
14. Why did you decide to seek a position with this company?
15. How does this job fit into your career path?
16. What did you like and dislike most about your previous job?
17. How do you think your present (past) superior would describe you?
18. What traits or qualities do you most admire in someone who was your immediate superior?
19. What is most important to you in a job?
20. Why did you leave your prior job(s)? (Get full explanation)
21. How would you define customer service?
22. What qualities/characteristics do you believe are most important for this position?
23. What are some general tactics you might use when dealing with an upset customer?
24. What are your short- and long-term career goals? Why are you the best choice for this job?

Once the selection has been made, an offer letter should be drafted that includes the following:

- Job title
- Start date
- Rate of pay (expressed in dollars per hour or amount per pay period for salaried individuals)
- Acceptance deadline

Do not overstate the responsibilities or opportunities associated with the position. After a position has been filled, candidates who were not selected should be notified, thanked for their time and interest, and assured that their information will be placed on file for future consideration.

COMPENSATION

Payroll costs are usually the highest expense associated with operating a business. The traditional approach to determining appropriate compensation begins with establishing a wage-based scale. A sensible and fair salary should be commensurate with the job and the skills required. A comparison of salaries for similar positions outside the organization governs compensation decisions. Consider the following factors when making comparisons:

- Type of business (corporate, commercial, hospital, non-profit, university)
- Type of facility (multi-purpose, fitness, medical)
- Size of facility
- Location of facility (region of country—city, suburb or rural)
- Financial status (yearly revenue generated)

Incentive-based compensation management is a viable alternative in many settings. This method is based on the philosophy that employees are motivated to perform and financially rewarded for achieving specific or measurable goals. Some form of a commission structure may be applicable in many departments and at virtually all levels of staffing. Careful review of the incentive structure, with assistance from a financial expert if possible, should occur before implementation of such a system. Important points include the following:

1. Incentives should be based on factors over which the individual has control.
2. Use a relatively short interval for reward.
3. Use simple methods for calculating earned commissions/bonuses.
4. Level of incentive should mirror level of performance.
5. A reward system should encourage teamwork.

Sources of information regarding personnel issues include state employment commissions, local human resource associations, and health and fitness professional organizations.

EMPLOYEE BENEFITS

The significance of a benefits program can not be overstated. The quality of staffing is key in separating a program from the competitors, making it essential to attract the best employees possible. Most benefits are not required by law, but are critical in decision making for potential employees. Staff often perceives the benefits package as an indicator of care and concern by the organization for individuals. While fair compensation is certainly the primary concern, vacation/sick days, paid holidays, insurance, 401K plans, and support of continuing education are standard items in a benefit package. Some form of an employee wellness program should be a prerequisite for organizations in the health and fitness industry. A good benefits program helps attract and, perhaps retain, quality employees.

STAFF DEVELOPMENT

Productive employees are the most valuable asset and acting accordingly will foster a positive support system throughout the organization. It is imperative to the health and success of both the individual and the organization that staff development include training, supervision, and the potential for growth (2). The attention and energy required to adequately fulfill these three objectives may be underestimated and, in fact, diminished if not approached conscientiously.

Staff Training

The training process is essential for all employees and should be viewed as an ongoing process regardless of position or tenure. The groundwork for peak performance begins with new employee orientation. Introducing the mission statement, core values, philosophy of service, organizational structure, coworkers, responsibilities, and members are all requisite. Orientation should be an enjoyable experience that familiarizes the employee with daily operation, responsibilities, expectations, and their role in the team concept. Exposure to the different departments, services, equipment, facilities, and personnel helps establish a broader base of understanding. A checklist can provide direction to the orientation process and ensure that all areas are covered.

Supervision

Personnel management can be one of the most rewarding aspects of supervision. Open, effective communication is paramount during the initial phases of training and during the rest of the employees tenure. Improved communication is one of the most frequent answers given by employees asked for suggestions that would positively impact the workplace. Combining opportunities for exchange of information through staff meetings, group discussions, and memos with an "open-door" philosophy fosters a sense of support. Employees should be encouraged to "Always Seek Knowledge" (ASK) through industry periodicals, training videos, seminars, workshops/conferences and any other avenue possible. Staff training should incorporate visual, auditory and kinesthetic properties, whenever possible, to accommodate individual learning preferences. The health and fitness industry is constantly changing with new research findings, improved training techniques, and state-of-the-art equipment requiring that exercise professionals remain informed and up-to-date.

LEADERSHIP

Providing guidance to employees is a challenging role. There is no single best technique for managing people. References abound, including 1-minute management (Blanchard & Johnson, 1982), management by walking around (Peters & Austin, 1985; Peters & Waterman, 1982), humanistic management (Herzberg, 1966; Maslow, 1965, McGregor, 1967), total quality management (Deming, 1980), principle centered leadership (Covey, 1990), motivation (Nash, 1985; Tarkenton, 1986; Zigler, 1986), goal setting (Locke & Latham, 1984), and standard management practices such as management by objectives (Drucker, 1980) (4). All of these management philosophies have been demonstrated to be successful and have advantages and disadvantages. No single theory is best in every situation. Optimally, a manager should understand and incorporate the basic concepts of sound management principles into a strategy that fits personal leadership style. People generally respond well to leaders who have high expectations and genuine confidence in them. An effective leader provides direction, channels employee efforts toward a single desired outcome, and empowers staff. A basic five step plan for coaching people is as follows (5):

1. Tell employees what you want them to do.
2. Show what good performance looks like.
3. Let the employees do it.
4. Observe employee performance.
5. Praise progress and/or redirect efforts.

A common tenant of proactive management is to "catch" people doing something right and recognize their contribution. Companies that believe money is a sole motivation for work are destined to lose some good people. Praising accomplishments provides psychological rewards critical to satisfaction in any professional setting. The manager should strive to develop win-win agreements that are mutually beneficial. Creating an environment that is results-oriented and based on a standard of excellence requires attention to detail and constant awareness of opportunities for improvement. Treating staff with respect, valuing opinions, and following the golden rule will help insure a content and motivated staff. It is also interesting to note that "admirable" characteristics most often cited in a leader are based on attitude rather than aptitude. Traits such as a positive attitude, enthusiasm, determination, and confidence were seen as most desirable (4).

GROWTH

All employees are interested in opportunity for personal and professional growth. Promotion, increased pay, expanded responsibilities, continuing education, professional affiliation, attendance at industry conferences, public speaking, and committee service are all viable options. Growth typically mirrors experience and is a result of learning and change (2). Continual growth requires a cooperative effort by the employee and supervisor (employer).

TIME MANAGEMENT

Personal time management is a most useful skill. Part of success can be attributed to the ability to distinguish what is urgent from what is important. The ongoing challenge to use time wisely requires the ability to focus on goals, objectives, and priorities, both personal and organizational. There are many systems and philosophies for time management. The goal is to use an approach that matches personal management style and to evaluate success regularly. Make a conscious choice to handle telephone calls, meetings, paperwork, unannounced visitors, and other potential time wasters efficiently. By objectively analyzing how time is spent and recognizing that time-related problems can typically be controlled, steps can be taken to improve time management skills. A proactive source on time management is *First Things First* by Stephen R. Covey.

PERFORMANCE REVIEWS

A performance appraisal provides an opportunity for communication between the supervisor and the employee to discuss expectations (from each party) and how well those expectations are being met. Performance appraisals are not adversary proceedings, or opportunities for socialization. They are essential communication between people with a common purpose (3). Employees want to know their level of performance and cannot be expected to improve if unaware of level of performance. Preparation for performance review should focus on desired outcomes of the appraisal session. Feedback and appraisal should be based on what has been seen, heard, and measured about performance. The overall objective of a productive performance review is to bridge the gap between present and ideal performance (Table 73.3).

A meaningful performance review allows the opportunity to reinforce positive behavior and correct unsatisfactory performance. Appraisals should presented with thoughts of the future within the organization and should lay the groundwork for upcoming reviews. In an appraisal discussion, four fundamental areas should be covered (6):

1. Measurement of performance against goals and standards.
2. Recognition of the contributions.
3. Correction of new or ongoing performance problems.
4. Establishment of goals and/or standards for the next appraisal period.

MANAGING CONFLICT

Managing conflict is a learned skill that, with effort, can be refined. Conflicts always arise and dealing with them in a productive manner can promote harmony or diversification between individuals and/or an organization. Developing a management style based on mutual achievement and win-win agreements fosters an atmosphere of cooperation. Covey's philosophy of conflict resolution begins with a win-win performance agreement that clarifies expectations by making the following five elements explicit (7):

- Desired results
- Guidelines
- Resources

Table 73.3. Performance Review Tips

- If a review will be critical in nature, try not to schedule it on a Friday so the employee can start taking action right away
- Schedule mid-morning meetings when both parties are fresh
- Create a formal, but non-threatening environment
- Focus the discussion on the job not the person
- Ensure that the employee does the majority of the talking
- Use open-ended questions whenever possible
- Practice active listening
- Emphasize the importance of employee's contributions
- Clearly communicate expectations
- Balance positive and negative feedback
- Encourage the employee to give feedback and express expectations
- Provide a copy of the review to employee

- Accountability
- Consequences

By approaching conflicts with an open mind and exploring options, both parties can formulate a mutually desirable outcome. Taking a thoughtful stance with employees or customers by using questions rather than accusations helps avoid defensiveness and redirects anger into communication and understanding. Investing time and effort toward enhancing conflict resolution skills is beneficial.

TERMINATION

If repeated attempts to correct unfavorable behavior are not successful, termination may be the best option. The discharge of an employee should not come as a surprise to either party if performance evaluations have been handled conscientiously and a progressive system of discipline has been followed. A sequence of warnings and disciplinary actions designed to allow the employee to correct the offending behavior should be documented. Graduated steps include an oral warning, written warning, probation, and ultimately, termination. Termination is rarely a pleasant experience, but the effort should be to treat the employee fairly and with respect. In a confidential and formal atmosphere, the employee should be told directly that they are being discharged with a concise explanation of the reason(s). Although it is appropriate to actively listen to the response and carefully answer questions, avoid arguing and leave no doubt that the decision is final. Before concluding the meeting, explain any severance considerations including extended medical benefits. A human resource representative (if available) should be included in termination proceedings to assist with communicating details of the severance package and for support throughout the process. Careful review of the reason(s) for termination may help avoid legal action for wrongful termination by an employee.

ORGANIZATIONAL STRUCTURE

The organizational structure, such as the one depicted in Figure 73.1 identifies responsibilities, reporting relationships, and the framework for accomplishing organizational objectives. Depending on the size and setting of the program, the health and fitness director and program director may be a combined position. Most often, responsibilities are split with the program director assuming the lead role for programatic activities, such as educational efforts, wellness, recreation, and services for special groups (e.g., seniors, youth), and the health and fitness director overseeing exercise prescription, fitness

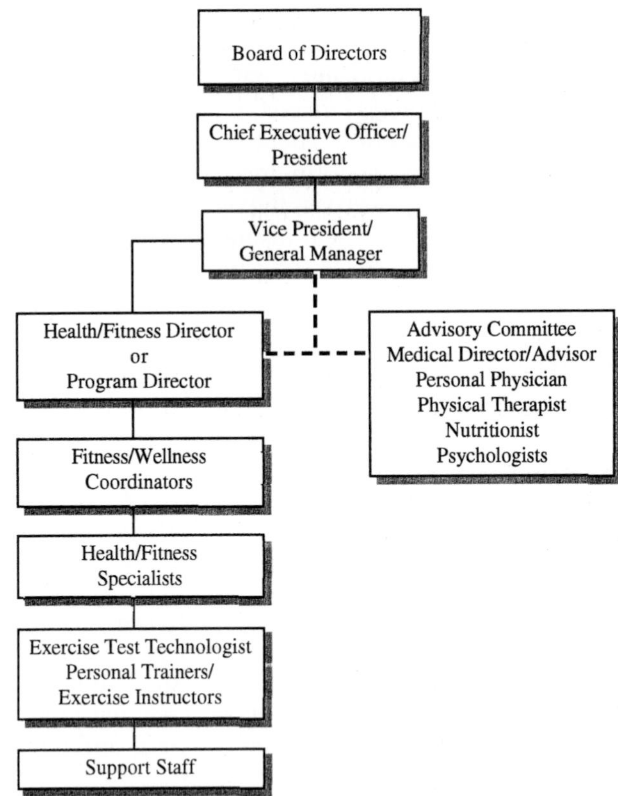

Figure 73.1. Sample organizational structure.

testing, exercise classes, personal training, and supervision of exercise activity areas.

Support staff include receptionists, service desk representatives, secretaries, clerical workers, custodians, and maintenance personnel. Medical support may be provided directly by an on-staff medical director (rarely found outside hospital-based programs), or indirectly by a medical advisor who offers guidance and evaluates policies and procedures or special cases as required. Establishing an advisory committee and/or developing a network including a combination of health-related professions such as a physical therapist, nutritionist, psychologist, and physician adds credibility and contributes expertise to a comprehensive program. The director of the program should work closely with the medical liaison or referring physician to ensure that appropriate protocols are followed, restrictions are adhered to, and follow-up including documentation is thorough.

The actual design of an organizational chart expresses the emphasis of programs and, as such, should be presented in a manner reflecting that. Variations of the traditional structure illustrated in Figure 73.1 may be circular to exemplify an interrelated structure or inverted to portray a participant driven philosophy. Commercial, non-profit, corporate, hospital, clinical, church, and university based programs, though similar in many regards, require different mixes of professional staff.

EXTERNAL SERVICES

It is often appropriate to seek outside services for assistance in delivering comprehensive programs. Consultants, subcontractors, interns, and volunteers often help provide these services in a cost-effective manner. In addition to avoiding the overhead cost of having permanent staff on the payroll, external sources offer specialized expertise and can supply trained personnel quickly. Outside services that are frequently used include:

- Medical/fitness testing
- Exercise class instruction
- Educational seminars
- Needs assessments
- Equipment maintenance
- Computer support
- Health intervention programs

Prior to engaging an outside service, it is important to define the scope of assistance required and, afterward, to monitor the quality of service provided. Follow up, including evaluation, guides future decisions for contract renewal. Assistance with special events, fitness programs, walks or runs, tournaments, and promotions is typically supplied by volunteers. Actively recruiting volunteers from program participants or other resources provides an influx of assistance along with diverse talents (an invaluable contribution to any program). It is very important to recognize volunteers for that contribution.

EMPLOYEE ASSISTANCE PROGRAMS (EAPs)

Perhaps the ultimate goal of health promotion/wellness programs is to increase awareness of health issues. A desire to educate and motivate the public to take personal responsibility for their health lies at the core of wellness strategy. Prevention and early detection of health-related problems is a common goal of health promotion services and EAPs. While wellness initiatives invariably emphasize care for physical health, a holistic approach must include the emotional and psychological health as well (the fundamental concern of EAPs). Speakers, counseling, and other services focusing on such topics as stress, parenting, relationships, managing change, dependency, and related subjects are frequently addressed in EAPs. Cross-promotion between these organizations is mutually beneficial, especially since many companies actively encourage employees to use EAP self referral services, which are always confidential.

▶ SUMMARY

Taking steps to ensure the highest quality staff requires a strategic approach and an ongoing commitment to develop individual talents. Hiring the best person for the job is paramount and should be given great consideration. Establishing a positive, comfortable work environment is the foundation of a successful organization. As employees are treated, so employees treat the customer.

References

1. Sol N, Foster C. *Organizational Structure and Professional Staffing. American College of Sports Medicine Health/Fitness Facility Standards and Guidelines.* Champaign, IL: Human Kinetics, 1992.
2. Patton RW, Grantham WC, Gerson RF, et al. Staff selection and development. In: Wilmoth S, Mount C, Gilly H, eds. *Developing and Managing Health/Fitness Facilities.* Champaign, IL: Human Kinetics Books, 1989.
3. Maddux RB. Are you ready for better appraisals? In: Crisp MG, ed. *Effective Performance Appraisals.* 3rd ed. Menlo Park, California: Crisp Publications, Inc., 1993.
4. O'Dooley P. Medical Certificates. *Flight Plan For Living–The Art of Self Encouragement.* New York: Master Media Ltd, 1992.
5. Shula D, Blanchard K. Overlearning. In: Cryderman L, ed. *Everyone's A Coach.* New York: Zondervan Publishing, 1995.
6. Maddux RB. How to prepare for more effective appraisals. In: Crisp MG, ed. *Effective Performance Appraisals.* 3rd ed. Menlo Park, California: Crisp Publications, Inc., 1993.
7. Covey SR, Merrill AR, Merrill RR. Empowerment from the inside out. In: Covey SR, ed. *First Things First.* New York: Simon & Schuster, 1994.

225, 246, 247, 248, 249, 250, 251, 252, 253, 254, 255, 256

216

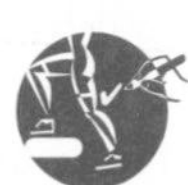

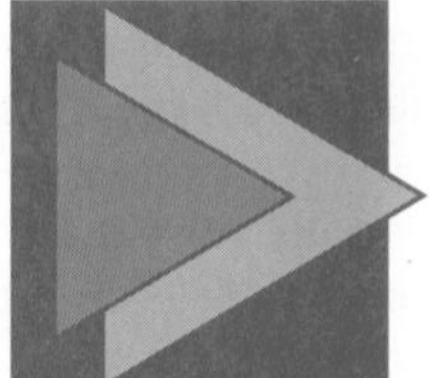

CHAPTER 74
FINANCIAL CONSIDERATIONS

Frank Ancharski

The financial considerations of any organization, whether for-profit or not-for-profit, in a university or community setting, corporate or private health club, is often the driving force behind major decisions. Fitness professionals too often view **the bottom line** as a necessary evil for which someone else is responsible. The exercise professional is preoccupied with the work of fitness and may have little understanding and appreciation for the impact of dues or programming fees on revenue. A corporate fitness director may favor public relations and staff morale rather than determining annual capital improvements. Certainly, the public perception of an organization and the satisfaction of employees in the work environment is vital to the success of an organization. However, the reality of financial considerations for any organization cannot be overlooked. This chapter concerns the need to embrace and understand basic financial issues rather than allowing accountants, business managers and corporate "higher-ups" be solely responsible.

BASIC TERMS AND PRINCIPLES

Financial management, in the health and fitness field, is basically not different from any major corporation. The most notable difference is the responsibility a corporation may have to stock holders if it is publicly held. Few companies in the health and fitness industry have such an obligation. Recently, however, firms such as Bally's Total Fitness and Sports Club Company of Los Angeles have offered Initial Public Offerings (IPO) with limited success (1). The industry is relatively young and other firms are likely to follow.

Typically, an ACSM-certified health and fitness director or program director is employed by a private or public entity with no publicly held stock. If the parent company trades on the market, the facility in which they work only remotely affects the performance of the company (in the stockholders' eyes). Some examples include corporate fitness facilities (e.g., Johnson & Johnson, Ford Motor Company). University recreation centers, not-for-profit hospital programs, or commercial health clubs are not usually concerned with stockholder obligations. In either case, the following basic terms of finance apply (2).

Real Assets

Tangible assets such as furniture, fixtures, and equipment (FF&E) and buildings. Intangible assets such as technical expertise, trademarks and patents are considered real assets.

Financial Assets

Sometimes referred to as securities, these assets are commonly either shares of stock, cash, accounts receivable, bonds, bank loans or lease obligations.

Value

Whether an organization is deciding to build a facility, finance capital improvements, or provide working capital, it should begin by valuing the investment. In other words, what is the return on investment (ROI). Unless the ROI is very near or better than what an investor can get in the market, obtaining private or bank investors becomes a difficult task. An investor will usually decide on a balance between risk and reward. A high ROI with limited risk and/or investment is generally a preferred scenario. The determination of ROI is done by averaging the expected cash flow over the life of the project divided by the average annual cash flow by the initial investment outlay. ROI is sometimes referred to as ROA (Return On Assets) (3).

For example, if the average annual cash flow (over 5 years = \$50k, 60k, 70k, 100k, 120k) is \$60k and the initial investment is \$400k, then the ROI = Average Annual Cash Flow ÷ Initial Investment. In this case, \$60k

÷ \$400k = 15%. An average ROI of less than 20% is considered excellent.

Net Profit (Loss)

Net profit (or loss, if this is the case) is calculated using information for costs (variable and fixed) and revenue as illustrated below.

- **Operating Profit** = Revenue − Variable Costs (costs which may change)
- **Net Profit** = Operating Profit − Fixed Costs (costs which remain the same); when revenues exceed variable costs and fixed costs
- **Net Loss:** when variable costs and fixed costs **exceed** revenues

Capital

Capital is money available for new equipment and facility improvements. When capital is invested in a lump sum, it is considered a fixed cost and is "debt" to an investor who may use an **ROI** valuation to determine if the return is worth the investment. A facility may decide to lease equipment if sufficient capital is unavailable or may consider borrowing. In either case, both a lease payment or a bank loan debt are usually reflected in fixed costs.

Working Capital

Working capital is defined as **current assets** minus **current liabilities.** Equity or Owner's Equity is not included when determining working capital. On a balance sheet, total assets must equal total liabilities (4). Current assets, including cash in the bank and accounts receivable make up a portion of total assets (Table 74.1). Accounts receivable are assets that have been earned for a performed service or delivered product, but have not been received. Current liabilities, such as accounts payable, taxes, salaries and wages, are considered a part of total liabilities. Accounts payable are liabilities payable to a party who has performed a service or has delivered a product to a recipient of those services or products.

Working capital is of primary concern early in a project because of the possibility of a net loss (variable costs and fixed costs exceed revenue). Working capital must be obtained through investors, donations, personal savings or bank loans to finance a net loss until revenues exceed variable and fixed expenses. Unlike capital, which is used for real assets such as FF&E, working capital can take the form of cash or accounts receivable and can be used to finance operating costs.

Break-even

In many settings such as a not-for-profit, hospital, corporate or university, a break-even point analysis is reserved for evaluating wellness (e.g., weight loss or smoking cessation) or usage incentive programs (e.g., "rowing the Colorado River" using a rowing machine or "climbing Mount Everest" using a stair climber). When valuing a facility, a break-even point analysis occurs when revenue is equal to expenses. As illustrated in Figure 74.1, the break-even point analysis for a program or facility occurs when revenue and expenses are equal or when revenue exceeds expenses. In Figure 74.1, break-even occurs in year two. This also coincides with the point at which working capital is no longer necessary and a net profit results. A net surplus is a synonym for net profit in not-for-profit facilities.

Table 74.1. Sample Balance Sheet

ASSETS	LIABILITIES
Short-term	Short-term
Cash	Accounts payable
Marketable securities	Short-term debt (notes payable)
Accounts receivable	Accruals (taxes due, salaries, wages)
Inventory	
Long-term	Long-term
FF & E, plant	Debt
Less: Depreciation	Preferred stock
Net: FF & E, plant	Equity (owner's equity)
	Stock
	Retained earnings
Total Assets	**Total Liabilities**

FF & E, furniture, fixtures, and equipment.

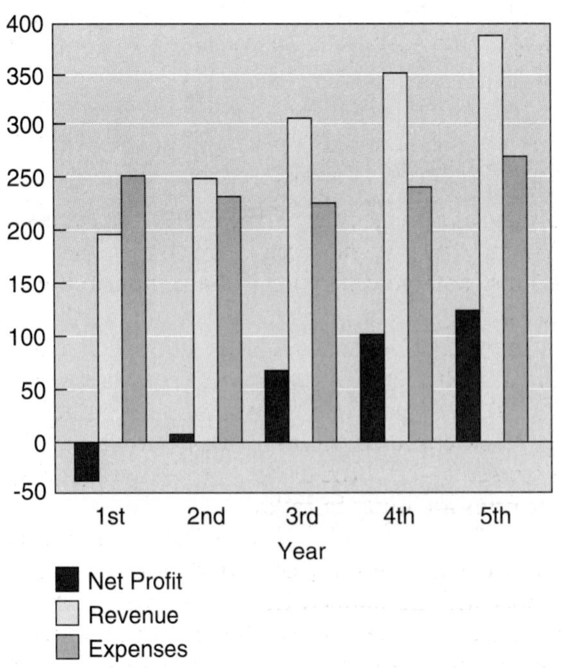

Figure 74.1. Sample break-even profitability graph.

Time and Opportunity

This principle is analogous to spending more than income allows in the short term. An opportunity may present and, although long-term benefit is evident, short term financing is unavailable. There are times, when convinced of such an opportunity, it pays long-term benefits to undertake expenses, even in the absence of sufficient revenue to cover them. A director must face the inevitable fact that windows of opportunity can be small and moving forward on a program or a project is important to the overall mission and goals of an institution.

People

The basic principles of finance include **people** because real assets and financial assets alone do not comprise a successful facility. Assets, though tangible, are not brought to life without cooperation, team work and support of people who must carry out the business. While there is a fiduciary responsibility to understand and manage the financial aspects of a business, the director must not lose sight of the dynamics of a business driven by people.

Business Organization

There are various types of business organization. The influence of taxes and personal risk weigh heavily in the process of deciding which organization type should be used. The main types are listed below.

Sole Proprietorship

The name defines this form of organization. Sole means a single individual owns the business. This is the simplest, least expensive form of business to start. Often, simply a license or registration is required to begin operation. Few government regulations apply and earnings are subject to personal income tax. A major disadvantage is the difficulty in obtaining significant capital to initiate or grow such a business. Additionally, the personal liability to creditors for a business debt is extensive.

Partnership

A partnership can be either an informal agreement or a formal written document filed with the state government. Partnerships have limited governmental constraints and are personally taxed proportionately to the percentage of ownership. This form of business is advantageous in that it can consolidate the skills and resources of each partner. Transfer of ownership or the death of a partner can cause problems in this type of business. Partnership does carry financial liability including exposure to personal assets if obligations cannot be met by other partners.

Corporation

This form of business is more formal and is heavily influenced by laws and stockholders, who are free from debt liabilities. The operations of a corporation are governed by the charter and bylaws. The risk for owners is limited and a wide variety of investors may be attracted to the business. Transferability is easier than either of the two previously mentioned forms of business. The corporation is completely separate from managers and owners. Changes in those positions do not affect operations.

S-Corporation

This form of business is a hybrid of a partnership and corporation formally known as Sub-Chapter S Corporation in the IRS tax code. At times, a small business with grand growth plans begins as an "S-corp." This entity combines the advantages of all of those above without the accompanying disadvantages. There is limited risk and exposure to personal assets and partners cannot be taxed twice on salary and business income. A partner is free to distribute dividends avoiding the complexities of a partnership.

BUDGET DEVELOPMENT AND FORECASTING

Budgets are necessary to forecast financial expectations and goals, to provide accountability, track progress of actual versus projected (budgeted) results, and allow for justification and scrutiny. Completing an accurate, reliable budget without a computer is virtually impossible in today's business world.

Capital Budget

The difference between a capital budget and an operational budget is in the purpose. A capital budget is developed to plan for FF&E and cosmetic improvements generally for 1 year, but at times multi-year projections may be made. Exercise equipment, renovating and/or expansion plans are addressed in this type of budget. Major changes planned for a facility are detailed in the capital budget and should be carefully monitored and implemented, costs should be tracked, time lines adhered to, and final audits and evaluation made. Competitive bids should be procured to obtain favorable price options.

The cost for capital expenditures are depreciated or amortized over the useful life of the equipment or by the amount permitted using Generally Accepted Accounting Principles (GAAP). The depreciation cost is often found under fixed expenses on the financial statements. The director should encourage owners or investors to regularly re-invest a portion of profits (often 1–5% of gross revenues) to maintain the facility.

Operating Budget

An operating budget is a plan detailing goals for expected revenues and expenses to operate a facility. Operating costs are the "costs of doing business." Ideally, in most if not all settings, revenues for participant use (e.g., membership fees and ancillary income, wellness

Table 74.2. Sample Budget

ACSM Fitness Center

	Existing Clients	Monthly	New	Average Fee	CXLS	Total	Total $
ENROLLMENT PROJECTIONS							
Jan	700	45	0	150	0	750	42,12
Feb	750	45	75	150	23	803	44,32
Mar	803	45	75	150	24	853	46,64
Apr	853	45	65	150	26	893	47,38
May	893	45	55	150	27	921	47,62
June	921	45	50	150	28	943	48,11
July	943	45	50	150	28	965	49,10
Aug	965	45	50	150	29	986	50,06
Sept	986	45	60	150	30	1,017	52,48
Oct	1,017	45	65	150	30	1,051	54,58
Nov	1,051	45	70	150	32	1,090	56,85
Dec	1,090	45	50	150	33	1,107	55,54
TOTAL MEMBER REVENUE:							594,84

OTHER REVENUE:	
Smoking Cessation	1200
Massage	16200
Guest Fees	35000
1-1 training	32400
Weight Management	12000
Pro-Shop	1200
Rest	3000
Wellness Programs	1200
Misc	10000
Total Other Revenue	112200
MEMBER REVENUE	594,848
OTHER REVENUE	112,200
TOTAL REVENUE	707,048

PAYROLL PROJECTIONS	
General Manager	35000
Sales 1	35000
Administrator	20000
Fitness Director	26000
FT Fitness 1	22000
FT Fitness 2	20000
PT Fitness	21840
Receptionist	25000
Aerobics	18000
Nutrition	9500
Cleaning	24000
Bonus	8000
TOTAL PAYROLL	264340
TAXES	34364
BENEFITS	18240
TOTAL SALARIES	316944

EXPENSE PROJECTIONS	
TOTAL OPERATING EXPENSES:	
SALARIES TAX & BENEFITS	316944
MARKETING	48000
MAINTENANCE/REPAIR	
HVAC	1500
Equipment	2400
Exterminating	1200
Other	500
TOTAL MAINTENANCE	5600
OPERATING SUPPLIES	
Cleaning Supplies	1200
Locker Room	3000
Other Supplies	1500
Towels	2000
TOTAL SUPPLIES	7700
OTHER EXPENSES	
Printing	3600
Postage	3000
Travel Seminars	2000
Uniforms	6000
Misc	1000
Programs	500
Office Supplies	600
Telephone	7200
TOTAL OTHER EXPENSES	10800
TOTAL FIXED EXPENSES:	
Cam	24000
Debt	10000
Insurance	18000
Leasing	8400
Management Fees	48000
Rent	70705
Utilities	
Elec	36000
Gas	4800
Water	2000
TOTAL UTILITIES	42800
TOTAL FIXED	264705
TOTAL EXPENSES	653749
NET PROFIT/(LOSS)	53,299

(With permission from McCarthy J. Fund Allocation has become critical. Club Business International. 1990.)

programs, pro shops, personal training, etc.) should exceed projected expenses. Start-up facilities and not-for-profit facilities may be the exception. Expenses are usually broken into two categories, operating and fixed. See Table 74.2 for a sample budget.

Assumptions for the Budget

When preparing the operating budget, one should be aware that expenses increase continually. A critical portion of the budget is development of "assumptions." In this attachment, a line-item by line-item explanation with supporting calculations is critical (e.g., enrollment fees, pay raise percentages, cost of uniforms, etc.). See Table 74.3 for an example of assumptions which correspond to line items on the budget.

Though perhaps initially tedious, the process is worth the effort. During budgetary approval, all parties privileged to the justification of the numbers make better decisions. This process is useful for preparing the budget, explanation of variances throughout the year and planning for next year.

Development, evaluation, revision and approval of a budget is usually a lengthy process and adequate time must be allotted. If the fiscal year matches the calendar year, September through November is an acceptable time table for the budget process, allowing for all levels of approval. Prior to each budget meeting, the director should gather general ledgers (line item explanation of paid invoices), current financial statements, and assumption pages for current year and projected year (5).

Including department supervisors, administrators, and key personnel in the budget development process helps employees "buy-into" the expectations established and informed employees contribute to success. Each supervisor who participated in the process should be given a final copy of the operating budget. On a monthly basis, financial statements, should be distributed to supervisors to compare actual numbers to budget. A monthly action plan is established to remain "on budget," make adjustments for the coming month, and adjust for any revenue shortfall or excess expense.

Table 74.3. Assumptions for Budget Preparation

LINE ITEM	ASSUMPTIONS
Revenue	
New Enrollment Fees	Each new member pays 50% of current months dues plus one full month and an average enrollment fee of $75 each
Guest Fees	Project 10 members/day paying $10/visit 7 days/week for 52 weeks
Expenses	
Payroll: Reception	4 part-time employees each working 20 hours for $6.00/hr for 52 wks. Each will receive a 5% raise in June
Uniforms	10 new full uniforms at $50/uniform (jacket, pants, shorts, shirt) three times/year. Staff pays via payroll deduction for "seconds"
Insurance	Increased $100/month compared to last year at $1,500/month

FINANCIAL INDUSTRY TRENDS

The fitness industry has many organizations that monitor and support financial performance. The International Health Racquet Sports Association (IHRSA) is well recognized by commercial, for-profit facilities. They perform and provide analysis of industry trends to clubs. Some of the more significant numerical trends noted in the year 1994–1995 are noted below (6):

- 8.1% of the population exercises in facilities
- The largest age group exercising in facilities is 35–45 years
- 4 million people became 50 years of age in 1996
- 34% of growth will be in the "senior" market
- 22% of business comes from corporate accounts
- The most profitable clubs have low attrition rates and high revenue generating participants
- Average attrition rate is 36%
- Payroll represents 40% of gross revenue
- Net growth in membership was 6.8%
- Revenue/participant is $445
- Indoor square feet/participant is 10
- Revenue/square foot is $63
- Net income (profit) is 9.3%
- Average annual fees are $693

Expense Model

In the 9-year period from 1980 to 1989, the industry expense model changed. The following model (Table 74.4) is determined by using line item expense as a percentage of total gross revenue (e.g., gross revenues = $100k, payroll = $40k, then payroll is 40% of gross revenues).

The former 60/40 operations-to-fixed expense model has been replaced by the 65/35 model. This model clearly represents the challenge to maintain conservative profit margins (10%). Profit is considered a fixed expense because the model is a "zero sum model." However, it is clear from Figure 74.1 (break-even chart) that net profit is not always fixed. The primary factor in the change to the expense model is usually payroll (wages and benefits). Because of the current litigious society in the United States, insurance has also contributed to the challenge of producing a profit.

Taxes

A noteworthy trend is the attention tax-exempt organizations are receiving from the IRS. Currently, fitness fa-

Table 74.4. **Expense Model**

	1980			1989	
	RANGE (%)	AVG. (%)		RANGE (%)	AVG. (%)
Operating Expenses					
Payroll	24–26	25		33–37	35
Utilities	7–9	8		7–9	8
Repairs & maint.	6–8	7		5–7	6
Marketing	4–6	5		4–8	6
Admin. equip. & supplies	2–4	3		2–3	2.5
Club equip. supply	2–4	3		2–3	2.5
Legal/Accounting	2–4	3		1–3	2
Cost of goods[a]	5–7	6	Insurance[a]	2–4	3
Total operating expense	51–69	60		56–74	65
Fixed expenses					
Debt service[b]	14–16	15		14–16	15
Depreciation[c]	8–10	9	Reserve/Replace[c]	4–6	5
Real estate taxes[b]	2–4	3		2–3	2.5
Insurance[b]	2–4	3		2–3	2.5
Profit/(Loss)	8–12	10		8–12	10
Total fixed expense	34–46%	40%		30–40%	35%

[a] Referred to pro shop, restaurant and massage, personal trainers, seminar & lessons performed by independent contractors. These items deleted in 1989 to compare equally.

[b] Occupancy cost is used in place of Debt service, Real Estate Taxes and Insurance for leasehold facilities.

[c] Reserve for replacement replaces depreciation as genuine fixed cash expense. (7)

With permission from McCarthy J. Fund allocation has become critical. Club Business International 1990.

cilities may be organized as either taxable or tax-exempt entities (7). The primary advantage a tax-exempt entity enjoys is simply in tax savings, which are often significant and carry a competitive advantage over commercial, for-profit settings. Certain restrictions, however, are placed on tax-exempt organizations including continuing proof of benefit to the community. In addition, they should provide services that cannot be found in for-profit settings within the community. Additionally, organizations labeled as 501 C (3) must restrict activity for ancillary income (8).

FINANCIAL STATEMENTS AND EXPENSE MANAGEMENT

Analysis of financial statements should be conducted monthly with written variance reports and action for the coming month. Assumption pages and general ledgers can be used to explain variances and to generate action points. Information should be shared with supervisors who help prepare budgets and are accountable for line items within specific departments. The financial statement should include a comparison of actual revenue/expenses vs. budgeted for both current year-to-date and previous year. Often statements will use the IHRSA 65/35 model track distribution of expenses and compare to industry norms (9).

Comparisons of actual financial performance to budget should be used as a guide for evaluating performance. Most directors do not carry forward excess profit or "earmark" net profit. Such discipline insures profits are not used for future expenses. Each month should be evaluated separately and profit reserved for times when profit may be minimal (e.g., summer months or year-end) when year-to-date profit may be depleted.

Financial statements usually reflect revenue problems, not expense problems. Over time, revenue shortfall becomes a serious problem of diminishing returns. Cutting expenses to maintain profit projections can confront this problem; however, there is usually a point when continual expense cutting affects service and, ultimately, revenue.

When faced with such a challenge, the sense of urgency to generate revenue cannot be overstated. Often, enrollment or membership revenue accounts for 80% or more of total income (10). This is an area where much of the manager's time and effort should be concentrated. If marketing efforts are not planned properly or the results tracked diligently, effectiveness cannot be determined. The critical precursor to membership revenue is marketing ("outflow"). Planning ahead for marketing (e.g., direct mailings, newspaper ads, health fairs) and enhancing sales skills are paramount to correcting revenue shortfall. Remaining revenue can be enhanced by creating profit centers, such as yoga or Tai Chi classes, ballroom or line dancing, spa services, scuba lessons or group trips such as sporting or theater events to fill revenue gaps (10).

Allocation of operating costs may be dictated by industry norms, historical information and management style. These variable costs usually rise each year. Control of such costs can be insured by using a "budget bank." Similar to home budgeting and check book balancing techniques, below is an example of a "budget bank":

Income – Recurring or Fixed Expenses

= Operating or Expense Variable

where:

Income: projected revenue from budget
Recurring Expenses: mortgage, utilities, depreciation, payroll
Operating Expenses: marketing, uniforms, seminars & training, printing, telephone, office, pool and laundry supplies, etc.

The amount left for operation should be treated as an expense. Each check is deducted from the previous balance. When the "budget bank" balance reaches zero, all ordering would be ceased until the next budget month. This process repeats monthly. The key benefit of using this type of process to manage expenses when incurred (at the point of ordering), not when invoices arrive or after financial statements are produced. This is a **prospective** tool, whereas financial statements are a **retrospective** tool. If used correctly and carefully, the budget bank should never "bounce."

There are many other ways to manage expenses, but a director must become very knowledgeable with the detail on financial statements. A thorough understanding of general ledgers, assumption pages and cost operational issues improves fiscal fitness. Some techniques used by industry professionals to diagnose problems and confront expense management are listed below (10–13).

Services

- Review plant, accountant, attorney, and equipment contracts bi-annually.
- Tabulate class attendance weekly. Cut low attendance classes.
- Track use of day care and courts.
- Keep inventory of exercise equipment, laundry and other equipment parts.
- Employee money savers: use staff to recruit interns from colleges, offer incentives to staff to recommend employees and recruit at job fairs.

Supplies

- Restrict use of copier or use coded keypad access.
- Lock storage areas for office supplies, pro shop and uniforms and limit key distribution.
- Use 1–3 vendors for major purchases or supplies.
- Stick to a "budget bank" and record when order is placed not when invoice is received.
- Use purchase order system with organized procedures and approval processes.
- Check unit costs regularly. Watch for abrupt increases with regular vendors.

Fixed Costs

- Confirm property taxes with local property assessment board.
- Ask local utility companies to audit use and recommend changes and improvements.
- Shop insurance costs yearly.

Advertising/Marketing

- Purchase graphic software and hire/train staff for in-house newsletter production and promotion.
- Co-market with restaurants, schools and community or national events (e.g., smoking cessation class that coincides with the Great American Smokeout).
- Use independent market feasibility analysis to determine site of facility. A poor location cannot overcome superior services, equipment, facilities and staff.
- Purchase demographic report on target market.

Hidden Expenses

- Block access to directory information and shop all long distance carriers. Look for carriers who bill on the lowest incremental time and audit number of phone lines in use.
- Check postal rates for options on pre-sort, zip code +4 and bar codes.
- Shop credit card fees.
- Recognize that bank charges are negotiable.
- Use brokers to shop for disability insurance.
- Contest unemployment claims. Not doing so shows precedent to existing staff and rate increase with each successful claim.
- Change job classification categories (laundry attendant to housekeeping personnel) and add as many as possible for facility to lower worker compensation insurance.

FACTORS AFFECTING DECISIONS

Not every decision can or should be made in a purely financial fashion, using only budgetary or financial data. Haste in decision making leads to some of the biggest mistakes. The day-to-day process of dealing with multiple situations, being consumed by multiple priorities, and days filled with endless interruptions lends credence to the "haste makes waste" axiom.

Lack of planning contributes to poor decisions. Disregard for planning is precipitated by giving little time dedicated to "thinking." With the tasks required of a director including budgeting, financial statement review, program evaluation, staff allocation, market analysis and community development (to name a few), planning cannot be successfully performed without "quiet" planning time.

Below are two examples of how this quiet time might be used to make important decisions concerning operations which contain financial consideration, but for which finances may not be the determining factor.

Decision 1: Staff positions can be examined for level of contribution and whether hiring or layoff is necessary. Examine performance reviews and scheduling grids to insure maximum staffing levels. Hire less people and expect more from them. Higher pay may be possible to help retain key personnel. "Brainstorming" such as this can generate ideas that may lead to solutions.

Decision 2: The marketing department may project from competitive market analysis that bicycle "spinning" classes would create a competitive advantage and attract additional members. If the amount of new enrollments due to spinning classes exceeds the cost of the bikes, instructors and other equipment within a short time, the decision is clear. The major variable is the confidence in enrollment projections. However, the capital budget may be reduced by 10% forcing greater scrutiny of the spinning over, for example, replacing a chlorinating system for the pool. Space may be premium, thus a program, though financially beneficial, may not be possible. Formal planned evaluations of programs are necessary to justify the time and money being used. Attendance, cost of materials and revenue generated should be considered during an evaluation of a program.

Another "kink" in this "spin scenario" is that current members may prefer another use for the space. If staff is not in tune with existing (and prospective) member needs, then the addition of such classes may be a mistake. Also, if retention improves because existing members needs are met or exceeded by adding space for stretching (or spinning classes), then additional revenue may be made available for other capital items.

The constant barrage of decisions for a facility is no small job. It can be an "adventure" to seek feedback of superiors, subordinates and members. Once all such input is digested, a director sometimes uses "instinct" to make the right decision.

Additionally, there is community obligation. Hospitals, universities and health clubs are giving back to the community and educating the public. If the fitness industry is to be a torch bearer for exercise and health, then proactive involvement with local charities or business chambers must occur.

▶ SUMMARY

The competition among and between profit and not-for-profit organizations, and hospitals, recreation and university fitness centers is increasing. Each entity is coming under scrutiny from constituents. Shareholders, taxpayers (in some cases), and investors in for-profit commercial settings all demand justification for dollars spent. The pressure to justify costs and enhance financial performance is shared by all directors despite location.

It is no longer sufficient to positively influence morale and productivity of an organization or to decrease absenteeism and health care costs of participants. The "bottom line" knows no bias when it comes to facilities and organizations. Success may depend on open mind, basic financial knowledge and "fear" that the bottom line may be exorcized. Financial considerations have become as important as influencing behavior to increase exercise habit. The more this is accepted, the better all facets of the organization can be coordinated and directed toward success.

References

1. Caro R, King D, Davis N. Developing an Exit Strategy. San Diego, CA. IRSHA National Convention, 1996.
2. Healy RA, Myers SC. *Principles of Corporate Finance.* New York: McGraw-Hill, 1988.
3. Weston JF, Copeland TE. *Managerial Finance.* New York: CBS College Publishing, 1986.
4. Lowery AJ. *How To Become Financially Successful By Owning Your Own Business. A Step-By-Step Guide To Independence and Profits.* New York: Simon & Schuster, 1981.
5. Krieger G. The Budget Process-"The Right Stuff." San Diego: IHRSA National Convention. 1996.
6. Profiles of Success. The IHRSA/Gallup Survey. Boston, 1995.
7. McCarthy J. Fund allocation has become critical. *Club Bus Intl* 1990.
8. Coopers & Lybrand. Tax Implications of Hospital Owned Fitness Facilities. Boston, 1996.
9. Profiles of Success. The IHRSA/Gallup Survey. Boston, 1995.
10. Handley A. Setting up new profit centers. *Club Indus* January 1995.
11. Sattler TP, Doniek CA. Trim the extra fat from your facility. *Fitness Manage* April 1996.
12. Morris BA. Cost Control Tactics For The 90's. *Club Indus* April 1995.
13. Caro R. Attacking hidden expenses. Parts I, II, III, IV. *Club Insider* June 1994, July 1994, October 1995.

104 116, 138, 139 147, 271

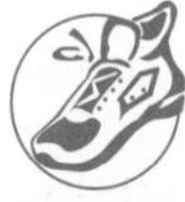

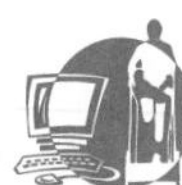

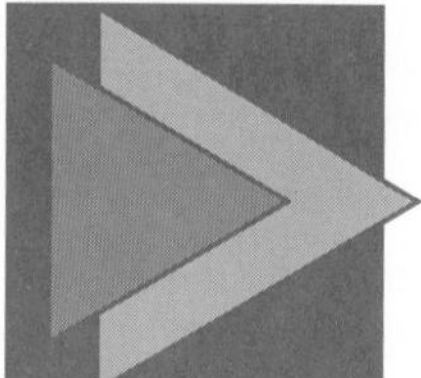

CHAPTER 75
LEGAL CONSIDERATIONS

David L. Herbert and William G. Herbert

Legal considerations represent an important dimension of service for those administering fitness evaluations and exercise tests, engaging in physical activity counseling and exercise prescription, or providing health-related fitness programs for adults. One area of paramount concern to exercise leaders, fitness instructors, rehabilitation specialists, and program administrators is the professional-client relationship and activities performed within the legal confines of that relationship. Other considerations with special legal significance include the physical setting and area within which program activities are conducted, the specific purpose for which exercise services are performed, the equipment used and the techniques employed with the exercise participant.

The law influences exercise personnel in each of these domains, as well as others. It also is important to note that legal expectations are substantially affected by the work environment (recreational, commercial, or clinical settings) and by the clientele served (whether engaged in vigorous sports activities, participating for health promotion purposes, and/or following rehabilitation protocols related to diagnosed disease). Regardless of the situation, it is fundamental to recognize that sensitivity to legal issues and application of risk management principles may enhance the quality of service and client satisfaction, and reduce the occurrence of service-related injuries, the likelihood of personal injury litigation, and the extent of damage to the provider in the event of legal claim and suit.

Laws affecting these matters vary considerably from state to state. Nonetheless, there are certain legal principles with broad application to exercise testing, prescription, and leadership. All exercise program personnel should be cognizant of these principles and endeavor to develop practices aimed at reducing risks of negligence-type litigation and, concomitantly, to maintain safe care of clientele.

In carefully screened and supervised adult populations, the risks of serious cardiovascular accidents in exercise programs is low. Even for those with some signs of disease who undergo clinical tests, the cardiovascular complication rate is ~ 2/10,000, and for selected cardiac patients following moderate intensity exercise the rate is < 1/35,000 (1, 2). Indeed, occurrences are uncommon and only a fraction of cases have resulted in legal claims against exercise professionals. Nonetheless, there is a growing trend of exercise-related claims being processed through the legal system, especially with regard to claims against physicians involving exercise testing (3–5). Even though tort reform proposals might help stem this trend, the future portends an ever-increasing risk of claim and suit for health-care professionals generally; exercise professionals are not likely to escape the problem.

TERMINOLOGY AND CONCEPTS

Almost invariably, legal claims against exercise professionals center on either alleged violations of contract or tort law. These two broad legal concepts, along with written and statutory laws, define and govern most legal relationships between individuals, including activities of exercise professionals with clients.

Contract Law

The law of contracts defines undertakings that may be specified among individuals. A legal contract is simply a promise or performance bargained for and given in exchange for another promise or performance, all of which is supported by adequate consideration (i.e., something of value).

In examining exercise testing and prescription activities, the law of contracts affects the relationship established between exercise professionals and clients. The client may receive physical fitness information and recommendations on exercise training. Likewise, the professional may perform exercise testing services in exchange for payment, reimbursement, or some other consideration of value. This contract relationship also encompasses any related activities that occur before and after exercise testing, such as health screening prior to testing and exercise prescription after testing and evaluation. If expectations during this relationship are not fulfilled, lawsuit for breach of contract may be instituted. Such potential suits allege non-fulfillment of certain promises or a breach of alleged warranties that the law sometimes imposes on many contractual relationships.

Apart from the professional-client relationships, contract law also has implications for inter-professional relations such as those with equipment companies, independent service contractors, and employees.

Informed Consent

Aside from breach of contract claims arising from a lack of promise fulfillment, claims against exercise professionals can be based upon a type of breach of contract for failure to obtain adequate informed consent from exercise participants. Although claims based on lack of informed consent, founded upon contract principles, are somewhat archaic, suits based upon such failures are still put forth in some jurisdictions. More frequently today, however, such claims are brought forth in connection with negligence actions rather than breach of contract suits. To subject another individual to a specific exercise procedure both properly and lawfully, the client must give informed consent to the procedure. Informed consent is intended to ensure that the client entered into the procedure with full knowledge of the material, relevant risks, any alternative procedures available that might satisfy certain of the objectives, and the benefits associated with that activity. This consent can be express (written) or implied by law simply as a function of how the two parties to the procedure conducted themselves. To give valid consent to a procedure, the individual must be of lawful age, not be mentally incapacitated, know and fully understand the importance and relevance of the material risks, and give consent voluntarily and not under any mistake of fact or duress (6). Written consent is certainly preferable to any oral or implied form of consent and expressly demonstrates the process should later questions arise as to whether that was the case.

In many states, programs are required to provide adequate information on the informed consent process to ensure that the participant knows and understands the risks and circumstances associated with the procedure. In such states, a so-called "subjective test" is used to determine whether that person understood and comprehended the risks and procedures associated with the matter at hand. Other states have adopted a less rigid rule and provide an objective test to determine the existence of a consent to a procedure or treatment. Under this test, the legal determination centers on whether the participant, as a reasonable and ordinary person, understood the facts and circumstances associated with the procedure in order to give voluntary consent. Even though some states do not require the use of informed consent for nonsurgical procedures or when a test is performed for healthcare-related purposes, adherence to the processes is a professionally desired approach. Examples of informed consent documents for exercise testing and training programs are available elsewhere (6–9).

Suits arising from the informed consent process frequently occur where an injured party claims that a professional was negligent in the explanation of the procedure, including the risks, and that the participant would not, but for the negligence of the professional, have undergone the procedure. These cases are often decided upon the testimony of expert witnesses who determine whether the professional engaged in substandard conduct in securing the informed consent. These informed-consent cases can involve claims related to contract law, warranties, negligence, and malpractice. Suits arising from alleged deficiencies in the informed consent process related to testing, exercise prescription, or physical activity have become more commonplace. The law is moving toward a requirement for ever broadening disclosure of risk to participants. Some courts have even gone so far as to require the disclosure of all possible risks, as opposed to those which are simply material (10). Such a requirement imposes unusual burdens on programs and raises substantial medico-legal concerns (11). These concerns require individual analysis and response.

One element of the informed consent process relates to confidentiality and disclosure of personal and sensitive information that may be gathered from the client in the course of evaluating health status or delivering health-exercise services. Provision should be made in the informed consent or other documentation to secure the written authorization to disclose specific test results, exercise progress reports, etc., to health-care professionals who have a "need to know," such as a primary-care physician. Written authorization might also be secured from clients in situations where there is an intent to use data in reporting group statistics for program evaluation or research purposes, even when such information is presented in ways not identifiable with the client. Many states, and the federal government, have promulgated privacy statutes which may affect the release of personally-identifiable material regarding a program participant. The application of these laws to a program and rights to release information will depend on a variety of factors that only a local counsel can properly address.

Tort Law

A tort law is simply a type of civil wrong. Most tort claims affecting exercise professionals are based on allegations of either negligence or malpractice, causing personal injury or death.

Negligence

Although negligence cannot be precisely defined (legally), it is regarded as failure to conform one's conduct to a generally accepted standard or duty. A legal cause of action based on claims of negligence may be established given proof of certain facts, specifically, that one person failed to provide **due care** to protect another to whom the former owed some duty or responsibility and that such failure proximately caused some injury to this latter person (6).

Thus, the legal validity of negligence claims is typically established through a specific process that examines certain facts and establishes whether:

- A defendant owed a particular duty or had specific responsibilities to some person who has issued a claim of negligence
- There were one or more failures (breaches) that occurred in the performance of that duty, as compared to a particular set of behaviors that were expected (due care, standard of care)
- The injury or damage in question was attributable to the established performance failure(s), that is, they were the **proximate cause** of the injury or damage.

When negligence claims arise, the matter of whether or not an exercise professional provided due care is an issue of critical importance. Once a duty is established, the nature and scope of expected performance is usually determined by reference to current published standards and guidelines from peer professional associations. Standards of care are discussed in a different section of this chapter. Ultimately, the most effective shield against claims of negligence may be the daily pattern of adhering to and documenting compliance with the most relevant published guidelines.

Malpractice

Malpractice is a specific type of negligence action involving claims against defined professionals. Malpractice actions generally involve claims against certain professionals who have **public authority to practice** (arising from specific state statutes) for alleged breaches of professional duties and responsibilities toward patients or other persons to whom they owed a particular standard of care or duty (6). Historically, malpractice claims have been confined actions against physicians and lawyers. By statute or case law, however, some states have expanded this group to include nurses, physical therapists, dentists, psychologists other health professionals. Very recently, Louisiana became the first state to pass legislation to license and regulate exercise practitioners who work under the authority of physicians with patients in cardiopulmonary rehabilitation treatment programs (12, 13). The Louisiana State Board of Medical Examiners is now developing policies and procedures for administering this new law. There are specific provisions in the Louisiana Act that will affect practitioners in a variety of ways. Some of these are not easily predicted, but the more obvious possibilities include level of autonomy in practice, changes in availability and provisions of liability insurance, costs of such insurance, and new exposure to claims of malpractice.

DEFENSES TO NEGLIGENCE OR MALPRACTICE ACTIONS

Properly given informed consents can sometimes be used as legal defense to claims based on either tort or contract principles. In such cases, defense counsel may seek to characterize a consent as **an assumption of risks of the plaintiff.** Assumption of risks of the procedure, however, is often difficult to establish without an explicit written statement or clear conduct that demonstrates such an assumption. In addition, an assumption of risks never relieves the exercise professional of the duty to perform in a competent and professional manner. Even where a valid informed consent/assumption of risks is obtained, a spouse, children, and/or heirs can sometimes independently file suits against the exercise professional for loss of consortium-type claims (even when the participant could not have asserted these claims because of his or her own assumption of risks) (14).

In some jurisdictions, it may be advisable or even necessary to obtain consent from a participant, a spouse, and perhaps, in limited number of states, to make it binding on any children or the executor, administrators, and heirs to an estate. Certainly such consents should be binding on estates if certain of these negligence/malpractice claims are to be successfully avoided from those quarters (15, 16).

Informed consents often are confused with so-called **releases.** Releases are statements sometimes written into consent-type documents that contain **exculpatory** language, that is, wording that professes to relieve the provider from any legal responsibility in the event of an injury or death due to any error or omission or even negligence. These releases also are sometimes referred to as **prospective waivers** of responsibility and, in some states, may be disfavored. Moreover, in a medical setting the use of such releases, with certain limited exceptions, has been declared invalid and against public policy. In non-medical settings, however, particularly with certain ultra-hazardous activities, such as with auto racing, sky diving, and with certain other exercise-related activities, the use of such releases may be valid in some jurisdictions and under certain circumstances, if properly drafted and utilized. In fact, when well-defined and properly written, such documents may be of substantial benefit to programs.

Several other defenses to claims of negligence or malpractice are also available. In some states, for example, proof of negligence by the participant, referred to in law as **contributory negligence,** can preclude any recovery of damages from a defendant. In many states, however, this rule has been modified by adoption of a so-called system of **comparative negligence.** Under this latter rule, negligence of the injured party is compared with negligence of all defendants in the case. Then, if the negligence of the injured party is found to be less than that of all defendants in the case or in some states in any case, the plaintiff is allowed to recover, although in an amount reduced by the sum of the negligence of the injured party (6).

Liability insurance is an effective mechanism to protect against financial loss, in the event of claim and suit. Such insurance policies provide an insurance-paid defense for any covered claims and suits, as well as **indemnification** from any judgment or settlement that is not excluded from the terms of coverage—up to the limits of said coverage.

STANDARDS OF PRACTICE

Standards of practice (or care) express how contemporary services should be delivered to give reasonable assurance that desired outcomes will be achieved in a safe manner. In most professions, such standards are developed and periodically revised by consensus among professionals or national associations of providers. Standards documents address what are considered to be benchmark methods, procedures, processes, etc., that are applied in almost all settings regardless of location, resources, and/or training of the provider.

In reality, the national standard of practice at any point in time typically is influenced by a variety of sources including published statements from professional associations, government policies, state and national government regulations, etc. In recent years, the promulgation of standards has increased dramatically in fitness and health-care fields. This circumstance mandates that professionals stay abreast of new pronouncements and regulations. Without knowledge of the most relevant and current standard-type documents and incorporation of those tenents into the operating protocols and records of service fulfillment, the individual practitioner becomes more vulnerable to damage and loss in the event of legal challenges arising from personal injury lawsuits.

The reason for this derives from the critical role that **standards of care** play in the legal arena. To clarify, consider that in law, proof of negligence consequent to injury of a client (plaintiff) is often dependent on whether it can be established that there was a clear causal connection between the injury to the client and what the professional did (commission) or failed to do (omission). To establish what should or shouldn't have been done in a given case, the court relies heavily upon interpretations from these standard-type documents. The use of these standards in certain cases dealing with exercise testing and exercise leadership has already occurred (4).

Several organizations have published documents that influence the legal standard of care in the health-fitness and exercise rehabilitation fields. Some of the more important are those of the American College of Sports Medicine (ACSM), the American Heart Association (AHA), American Association of Cardiovascular and Pulmonary Rehabilitation (AACVPR), the Agency for Health Care Policy and Research (AHCPR), the American College of Cardiology (ACC), the American Medical Association (AMA), the International Health, Racquet Sports Club Association (IHRSA), and the Aerobics and Fitness Association of America (AFAA) (7–9, 17–24). Documents from these organizations vary in scope and applicability. Professionals should carefully examine services, uses of technologies and procedures, and clientele, before deciding which standards and guidelines are most applicable.

Published guidelines may be incomplete or not entirely uniform. In the event of participant injury or death, such deficits may create confusion rather than provide a solution for the professional behavior expected in a specific exercise setting. In the area of exercise testing, standards of the ACSM, the AACVPR, and the AHA are somewhat inconsistent with regard to the need for significant involvement of a physician during graded exercise testing (7–9, 17, 18, 25).

On the matter of exercise prescription, one AHA publication explicitly identifies the nurse as an individual who may "assess physical activity habits, prescribe exercise, and monitor responses in healthy persons and cardiac patients" (17). Another contemporary AHA source acknowledges that cardiac patient exercise may be appropriately supervised by physicians, nurses, or exercise physiologists, as long as supervisors are trained and their respective duties are consistent with state statutes governing the practice of medicine and certain other allied health-care professions (18). If deficiencies or disparities in the published guidelines have implications for safety and legal exposure for a particular local exercise service situation, the development of "low risk" protocols and procedures may be a matter of critical importance that requires advice of local counsel.

Health-care professions are in the midst of a movement that will eventually see written standards and guidelines covering nearly every major dimension of care. Fitness and rehabilitation professionals are being similarly affected and must keep up to date with consensus publications that affect services. To reduce medicolegal risks, it is prudent to adopt the most stringent standards possible. Fulfillment is of equal importance. So practitioners should not only engage in updating program operating manuals to verify adoption of current standards, but also document day-to-day client records of service delivery to show "what was done and how it was done."

In fact, documentation is vital to many aspects of risk management, not just verification of adherence to standards. Documentation should include contemporaneous recording of critical response levels that arise in exercise testing or training (e.g., important symptoms, estimations of effort, and activity demand, along with signs suggestive of myocardial ischemia, or poor ventricular response) and annotations about how these are referred in a timely way to appropriate health care providers. It also encompasses notations on program incidents, especially care delivered in emergency situations (perhaps the most crucial of settings to demonstrate (after the fact) what and when essential steps were performed). Follow-up should always be performed and program records maintained to verify the outcome of the situation whenever emergent and non-emergent exercise program incidents occur.

In the case of emergency readiness, records should be maintained to provide evidence that regular and frequent emergency drills are performed. Dated logs listing staff duties and providing a place to check adequacy of performance/error corrections in emergency drills are helpful for this purpose. Formal drills prepare staff for rapid and effective response when a genuine emergency arises. If a legal challenge should arise, the documentation may be most helpful in establishing that a particular standard was adopted and followed on a routine basis within the program setting.

Forms also may be developed for staff to use routinely in assuring standardization in other areas where injury and/or legal risks are considered significant, e.g., for instructing new clients in exercise routines or explaining specific cautions for avoidance of injury, for staff use in routine inspection of equipment and facilities, etc. Effective forms demonstrate a link to a standard that has been adopted for critical areas of service. Routine annotation of client records by staff helps show a pattern of consistent fulfillment.

UNAUTHORIZED PRACTICE OF MEDICINE AND OTHER ALLIED HEALTH PROFESSIONAL STATUTES

In recent years, the growing prominence of exercise testing and other health-fitness services increasingly places exercise professionals in collaborative roles with licensed health-care providers. This evolution has stimulated a variety of initiatives to clarify roles and responsibilities, promote professionalism, and increase professional opportunities. Competency certifications of the ACSM (e.g., Health-Fitness Instructor℠ and Exercise Specialist℠), the AACVPR Core Competency position statement for Cardiac Rehabilitation Specialists and efforts to establish licensure are illustrations of initiatives that affect positioning of specialists and/or greater role delineation (13, 23).

Providing exercise services with some degree of independence in collaboration with licensed providers can create legally precarious circumstances for the exercise professional. A prime example of confusion in this area is reflected in questions that often arise about the competency and legal authority needed to provide emergency cardiac care in community or clinic based settings for exercising cardiac patients. The emergency response standard in this situation is clear and universal in calling for a defibrillator, crash cart with artificial airways, suction pump, emergency drugs, etc., and current competency of an on-site provider who is able to administer Advanced Cardiac Life Support skills of the AHA when needed (7, 9, 26). The provider of emergency services, however, must understand that she/he cannot assume such duties, unless the physician in charge has given written **standing orders** to that effect **and** the individual has legal authorization under state statutes to accept such standing orders. This is almost never the case for the nonlicensed exercise professional, with or without current successful training in an ACLS program of the AHA.

Compounding these problems is the emergence of the health care reform movement. A significant part of this evolution is aimed at reducing costs using paraprofessionals in ever-increasingly important treatment roles. In fact, various states have undertaken efforts to expand nursing practice and other medical practice laws beyond mere observation, reporting, and recording of patient signs/symptoms. Various physician assistant or similar paraprofessional laws allow more nonphysicians to have expanded treatment authority when dealing with patients.

Until this ongoing process (healthcare reform) is completed, however, some nonphysicians who engage in certain practice that might be characterized as engaging in the practice of medicine or some other statutorily-defined and controlled allied health profession. In such situations, the nonlicensed provider runs the risk of engaging in unauthorized practices that could lead to both criminal and civil sanctions. Many states have defined the practice of medicine broadly so that persons engaged in exercise testing and prescription activities could, under some circumstances, fall within the ambits of such statutes.

As previously indicated in this chapter, published standards are not always definitive in expressing roles and responsibilities for exercise professionals, particularly with regard to services for clients with documented diseases or even those with no outward signs of disease (e.g., silent myocardial ischemia). Thus, without the presence or assistance of a licensed physician or other allied health professional for certain aspects of these exercise services, claims as to the unauthorized practice of medicine could be put forth. Under some of these state statutes, such practices are often classified as crimes, usually misdemeanors, punishable by imprisonment for less than 1 year and/or a fine.

In addition, a person found to have engaged in the unauthorized practice of medicine or some other allied health profession faces (after the fact) the legal expectation to provide an elevated standard of care in the event of participant injury or death. Under this rule, the actions of an exercise professional is compared to an assumed standard of care of a physician or other allied health professional acting under the same or similar circumstances. In the event that the actions do not meet this standard (which the nonphysician or allied health professional cannot meet because of inadequacies of knowledge, skill, authorization and experience), liability may result.

SUMMARY

This discussion is a brief overview of the potential legal problems facing the exercise professional. As more and more participants are exposed to organized exercise programs the actual number of untoward events, avoidable or otherwise, will inevitably rise. Increased numbers of these occurrences will result in negligence-type claims that will ultimately find resolution in court. The probabilities of such traumatic actions are low, particularly for individuals and organizations that operate programs in a manner commensurate with accepted professional standards. Awareness of the areas of special legal vulnerability and adoption of legally sensitive practices, however, will keep the risks of litigation low and concurrently lead to safer and more efficacious programs. Professionals would be well advised to keep up to date and current as to developments in this ever-changing medico-legal field (6).

References

1. Rochmis P, Blackburn H. Exercise tests: a survey of procedures, safety and litigation experience in approximately 170,000 tests. *JAMA* 1971;217:1061.
2. Haskell WL. Cardiovascular complications of outpatient cardiac rehabilitation programs. *JAMA* 1978;57:920.
3. *DeRouen vs. Holiday Spa Health Clubs of California.* Superior Court of County of Los Angeles, Case No. C346987 (Dismissed upon settlement 1985).
4. *Tart vs. McGann.* U.S. District Court, Southern District of New York, Case No. 81-CIV-IL-3899 (ELP 1981). Cited in 697 F. 2d 75 (2d Cir. 1982).
5. Reference deleted.
6. Herbert DL, Herbert WG. *Legal Aspects of Preventive and Rehabilitative Exercise Programs.* 3rd ed. Canton, OH: Professional Reports Corporation, 1993.
7. American College of Sports Medicine. *Guidelines for Exercise Testing and Prescription.* 5th ed. Philadelphia: Lea & Febiger, 1995.
8. American College of Sports Medicine. *ACSM's Health/Fitness Facility Standards & Guidelines.* Champaign, IL: Human Kinetics, 1992.
9. American Association for Cardiovascular and Pulmonary Rehabilitation. *Guidelines for Cardiac Rehabilitation Programs.* 2nd ed. Champaign, IL: Human Kinetics, 1995.
10. *Hedgecorth v. United States.* 618 F. Supp.627 (E.D. Mo, 1985).
11. Herbert DL. Informed Consent Documents for Stress Testing to Comport With *Hedgecorth v. United States. Exerc Stand Malpract Rep* 1987;1:81.
12. Louisiana licenses clinical exercise physiologists! [editorial]. *Exerc Stand Malpract Rep* 1995;9:56. (Reproduction of the licensing act included.)
13. Herbert WG. Licensure of clinical exercise physiologists: Impressions concerning the new law in Louisiana. *Exerc Stand Malpract Rep* 1995;9:65.
14. Child Sues for "Loss of Consortium." *Lawyers Alert* 1984;3:249.
15. Herbert WG, Herbert DL. Exercise testing in adults: legal and procedural considerations for the physical educator and exercise professionals. *JOHPER* 1975;46:17.
16. Koeberle BE. *Legal Aspects of Personal Fitness Training.* Canton, OH: Professional Reports Corp, 1990:35–38.
17. American Heart Association. The AHA Medical/Scientific Statement on Exercise. *Circulation* 1992;86:340.
18. American Heart Association. The AHA medical/scientific statement on cardiac rehabilitation programs. *Circulation* 1994;90:1602.
19. American Association for Cardiovascular and Pulmonary Rehabilitation. *Guidelines for Pulmonary Rehabilitation Programs.* Champaign, IL: Human Kinetics, 1993.
20. Agency for Health Care Policy and Research. *Cardiac Rehabilitation.* Clinical Practice Guideline No. 17. Rockville, MD: US Department of Health and Human Services (Publication No. 96–0672), 1995.
21. American Physical Therapy Association, Cardiopulmonary Specialty Council. *Specialty Competencies in Physical Therapy: Cardiopulmonary.* Manhattan Beach, CA: Board for Certification of Advanced Clinical Competence, American Physical Therapy Association, 1983.
22. Cooper PG, ed. *Aerobics Therapy & Practice.* Sherman Oaks, CA: Aerobics and Fitness Association of America, 1985.
23. American Association for Cardiovascular and Pulmonary Rehabilitation. Core competencies for cardiac rehabilitation specialists. *J Cardiopulm Rehabil* 1994;14:87.
24. Herbert DL. Preparing to meet new industry standards for health and fitness facilities: Where do we go from here? *Exerc Stand Malpract Rep* 1993;7:40.
25. American Heart Association. The AHA medical/scientific statement on exercise standards. *Circulation* 1990;82:2286.
26. American Heart Association. Guidelines for cardiopulmonary resuscitation and emergency cardiac care. *JAMA* 1992;268:2171.

215, 222 224, 276

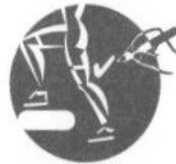
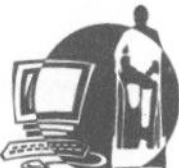

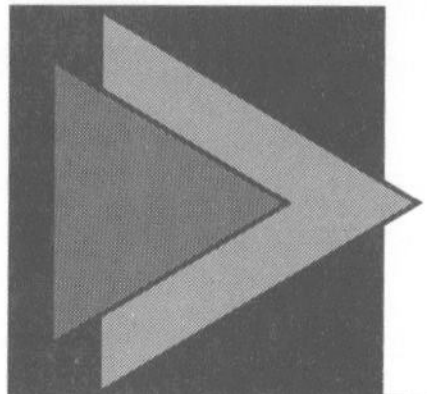

CHAPTER 76 OPERATIONS

Nestor Fernandez, II

Managing the operations of a health and fitness facility requires a thorough understanding of the facility, staffing, and customer concerns. A detailed operational plan that identifies key areas as well as potential problems is necessary in operating a well-managed facility. The following chapter outlines areas that require attention to maintain a well-managed facility.

PROCEDURES

Procedures help establish guidelines to address operational demands. Their main purpose is to establish guidelines for safety, cleanliness, member satisfaction and employee support. Procedures should be thorough, clearly written, easily performed and tracked, and communicated to employees at all levels and departments and must be regularly reviewed to evaluate effectiveness. Procedures that no longer work toward the goal of establishing guidelines for safety, cleanliness, member satisfaction, and employee support should be eliminated. Most procedures should be invisible to the customer, and rather than being obstacles to delivering outstanding service, work toward providing outstanding customer service.

There are several essential procedures that ensure successful facility and operations management. Baseline procedures that require special attention are the procedures for opening and closing the facility. These procedures typically belong to an individual employee without management supervision and/or support on the premises during the time they are performed.

Opening and Closing Procedures

Member/customer expectations require that businesses are accessible during scheduled hours of operation. The opening shift (usually staffed by the front desk) for many facilities requires minimal staffing, often only one or two employees. This in itself may cause problems should anything happen to the employee(s) entrusted with these duties. Procedures should be in place for such occurrences to minimize the negative effects.

An opening checklist prepares the facility for use prior to admitting members/customers into the facility. It identifies basic safety issues (lighting, equipment, alarms, etc.), as well as all pre-presentation preparation, including cash register count, restocking supplies, and cleanliness. A pre-presentation walkthrough of the entire facility is highly encouraged to ensure that the building, equipment, and common areas are visually presentable and ready for use. A checklist with space to report problems is required. The operations supervisor should be responsible for reviewing the checklist and addressing problems and concerns upon arrival.

In the event that problems keep the facility from opening, a backup plan should be in place. Employees responsible for opening the facility should have access to telephone and pager numbers of staff that can open in an emergency, and emergency staff should be on call and available by phone or pager.

Closing checklist procedures are similar to opening, except that special attention is placed on securing the facility (Fig. 76.1). All points of entry, including windows, elevators, and maintenance doors, should be secure. All electrical equipment, including computers, televisions, and stereos, should be off. If the employee is leaving the facility while other personnel (such as housekeeping or maintenance) remain, there should be a system in place to identify the last person in the building. That person has final responsibility for securing the facility, engaging alarms and locking the final exit door.

The opening employee should review the closing checklist from the prior evening for problems or areas of concern before opening. Once the facility is open for business and adequately staffed for operations, a supervisor or department head should review both the opening and closing checklist. Problem areas should be reviewed and corrected. All corrective actions should be communicated to the reporting employee(s).

__________ Announce the Club will be closing 1-hour before Club close and repeat every 15-minutes.

__________ Clean Sports Desk area.

__________ Stock supplies for the next day: In and Out Sheet, Guest Registration, office supplies, etc...

__________ Log-in remaining Lost & Found items.

__________ Check out all remaining members and guests.

__________ Count cash register, make "X" report, "Z" report and prepare drop bag.

__________ Turn off the computer.

__________ Lock main doors.

__________ Close handicap entrance doors.

__________ Lock women's locker room entrance. Turn off all lights in the women's locker room.

__________ Check aerobics studio doors and lights.

__________ Turn off basketball court, free weight and pool hallway lights.

__________ Lock pool door.

__________ Lock double doors in cardio room.

__________ Turn off all lights in men's locker room.

__________ Turn off all lights on third and second floors, making sure that marketing office door is locked.

__________ Put the safe drop bag in the safe and punch out.

__________ Turn off the lights in Sports Desk area, making sure that Child Care and Pro Shop doors are locked.

__________ Return Allen wrench to lock box, and lock the lock box.

__________ Set the alarm.

__________ Exit through main doors and push doors in securely at the bottom.

__________ Drive home safely.

ALL AREAS OF THE BUILDING MUST BE CHECKED FOR CLEANLINESS AND/OR MAINTENANCE ISSUES.
PLEASE INDICATE ANYTHING THAT NEEDS IMMEDIATE ATTENTION BELOW:

Figure 76.1. Sample closing checklist.

Facility Quality Control

Developing a safe, clean, easy to use, and visually appealing environment is the responsibility of every employee. Failures in these areas are common reasons for member dissatisfaction, and maintaining staff attention to this responsibility is important. Review of forms, control of the process, and problem solving facility quality is the ultimate responsibility of the general manager.

A facilities director, director of operations, or general manager (depending on distribution of responsibility and size of the facility) should perform a regularly scheduled facility inspection to evaluate every component of the facility. All areas of presentation and safety, both interior and exterior should be reviewed with a checklist. Regularly scheduled facility inspections help to ensure continuous maintenance of high use areas. Checklists include a variety of components, including:

- Wall repairs
- Paint condition
- Cleanliness of air vents
- Carpeting
- Lighting

The condition and cleanliness of fitness equipment should also be included. Inspections may be broken down into daily inspections (for general housekeeping and presentation) and monthly inspections (for larger projects such as patching and painting of walls, equipment replacement or lighting and ventilation) (Fig. 76.2). Regardless of frequency, the ultimate goal is to ensure that responsible staff are looking with a discriminating eye at all aspects of the facility, seeing potential problems, and observing each component of the facility from a customer's point of view.

Many facilities schedule annual club "shutdowns," when the facility is closed for business so deep cleaning can be performed. In addition, large projects that may be difficult to accomplish while members are present and facilities are in use can be completed. Projects commonly completed during these closures include:

- Court resurfacing
- Area remodeling
- Extensive painting
- Swimming pool resurfacing or cleaning
- HVAC and plumbing repairs

Because the facility is closed to normal operations, these projects can be completed without disturbing members/customers. In the long run this contributes to maintaining the quality of the facility.

Manager On Duty Procedures

The use of a "Manager On Duty" (MOD) system is a method whereby continuous evaluation of facility quality and staff performance may occur. The MOD system is composed of specific senior staff with proven leadership skills used to monitor, support, and execute service strategies and standards. The MOD must be visible and available for line staff and members at all times. This system is especially useful during high-use hours and when senior staff are less likely to be present (such as evenings and weekends). The MOD should be trained in all areas of operations so that any problem can be effectively resolved. This includes:

- Knowledge of all department operations
- Shift hours
- Emergency procedures
- Schedule of events and programs

MOD guidelines and reports should be established to insure that all areas of the operation are monitored and inspected regularly.

Emergency Procedures

Most states require that employees undergo job-specific safety training. Prudent safety training includes proper operation of equipment, as well as training in lifting and back health. Employers may be required to have a safety action plan, as well as ongoing training to meet state or local insurance requirements. Consult with local government offices and/or business insurance carriers to determine the requirements.

Detailed facility evacuation plans should also be developed and communicated to all staff. An evacuation plan covers all necessary steps to evacuate the facility, emphasizing safety of members and staff. All required information (phone numbers, contact names, etc.) should be maintained in a central location (usually the front desk) for easy, quick access. Regular review and update of the information and procedures, as well as ongoing staff training, provides assurance of a safe environment for members and staff.

SERVICE

Every business must determine the level of service that customers expect and exceed it. A business that delivers consistently good service outperforms the competition and maintains customer satisfaction. Facilities should evaluate customer expectations, as well as their ability to deliver those services, then organize operations to support delivery of services up to those standards. Standards, determined from customer feedback, are the blueprint for the training, implementation, and continuous revision of a service delivery system. A more detailed discussion of program planning and marketing can be found elsewhere in this book.

Identify Member Expectations

Customer expectations drive the facility, programs, planning and budget. An organization must seek and fa-

DATE:

		STATUS
CARDIO ROOM	Carpet	
	Ceiling Tiles	
	Air Vents	
	Mirrors	
	Mats	
	Baseboards	
	Walls - patching	
	Walls - paint	
	Trash Cans	
	Water Fountain	
	Equipment - cleanliness	
	Equipment - repair	
	Televisions	
	Newspaper Racks	
FITNESS TESTING OFFICE	Carpet	
	Ceiling Tiles	
	Air Vents	
	Baseboards	
	Walls - patching	
	Walls - paint	
	Trash Cans	
	Telephone	
	Office Furniture	
FITNESS OFFICE	Carpet	
	Ceiling Tiles	
	Air Vents	
	Baseboards	
	Walls - patching	
	Walls - paint	
	Trash Cans	
	Telephone	
	Office Furniture	
POOL HALLWAY	Carpet	
	Ceiling Tiles	
	Air Vents	
	Baseboards	
	Walls - patching	
	Walls - paint	
	Handicap Ramp	
	Pool Doors	
	Women's Locker Room Door	
	Men's Locker Room Door	
SWIMMING POOL	Perimeter Landscaping	
	Flower Pots	
	Pool Deck	
	Pool Deck Matting	
	Running Track	
	Pool Furniture - repair	
	Pool Furniture - cleanliness	
	Aquatics Equipment	
	Shower	
	Walls - patching	
	Walls - paint	
	Rear Gates	

Figure 76.2. Club walk through.

FREE WEIGHT ROOM	
Carpet	
Ceiling Tiles	
Air Vents	
Baseboards	
Walls - patching	
Walls - paint	
Mirrors	

RACQUETBALL COURTS	
Floors	
Walls	
Air Vents	
Lighting	

BASKETBALL COURTS	
Floors	
Walls	
Air Vents	
Lighting	
Score board	
Basketball nets, rims and backboard	
Emergency exit door	

CHILD CARE ROOM	
Carpet	
Ceiling Tiles	
Air Vents	
Linoleum floor	
Bathroom	
Baseboards	
Walls - patching	
Walls - paint	
Sink	
Equipment - cleanliness	

SPORTS DESK/LOBBY	
Floors	
Ceiling Tiles	
Air Vents	
Countertops	
Baseboards	
Walls - patching	
Walls - paint	
Telephones	
Lighting	
Stairs	
Handicap hallway	
Porter Room	

WOMEN'S LOCKER ROOM	
Carpet	
Ceiling Tiles	
Air Vents	
Mirrors	
Mats	
Baseboards	
Walls - patching	
Walls - paint	
Trash Cans	
Water Fountain	
Cardio equipment - cleanliness	
Cardio equipment - repair	
Television	
Restroom stalls	
Toilets	
Restroom dispensers	

Figure 76.2. *(continued).*

Lighting	
Vanity dispensers	
Telephones	
Bulletin boards	
Signage	
Tanning room - supplies	
Tanning room - equipment	
Tanning room - walls	
Tanning room - floors	
Jacuzzi	
Cold dip	
Showers - tile	
Showers - dispensers	
Showers - lighting	
Showers - air vents	
Showers - partitions	
Shower heads	

MEN'S LOCKER ROOM

Carpet	
Ceiling Tiles	
Air Vents	
Mirrors	
Mats	
Baseboards	
Walls - patching	
Walls - paint	
Trash Cans	
Water Fountain	
Cardio equipment - cleanliness	
Cardio equipment - repair	
Television	
Restroom stalls	
Toilets	
Restroom dispensers	
Lighting	
Vanity dispensers	
Telephones	
Bulletin boards	
Signage	
Tanning room - supplies	
Tanning room - equipment	
Tanning room - walls	
Tanning room - floors	
Jacuzzi	
Cold dip	
Showers - tile	
Showers - dispensers	
Showers - lighting	
Showers - air vents	
Showers - partitions	
Shower heads	

ACTION ITEMS:

Figure 76.2. *(continued).*

cilitate input from membership. Annual questionnaires and focus groups covering every component of the facility including cleanliness, staff responsiveness and customer service, program offerings, and facility improvements are methods for gathering information. Information gathered must be carefully reviewed to form an overall picture representing customer expectations. Reporting results back to the customers is important.

Focus groups can be organized around specific programs or areas of the facility. Focus groups can and should be composed of staff as well as customers. Once member expectations are identified, they must be integrated into training and communication of service standards (Table 76.1).

Customer Service

Customer service training is critical to delivering good service. Training programs orient new employees to the service standards and support continued improvement and development of all staff. The training should provide a blueprint for the "perfect" delivery of service. Regularly scheduled training programs to reinforce service standards are important across the facility and at all levels of the organization.

The service delivery system should be specific and detailed, yet flexible enough to allow employees to solve unexpected problems. Policies and procedures should guide employee actions. However, employees should be empowered to make decisions in keeping with the spirit of the service standards. In addition, senior staff must convey a sense of leadership that not only reviews and enforces service standards, but also models them through behavior and action.

PLANNING

Facilities should establish an annual operational plan to determine staffing requirements and scheduling for special programs and events. Staffing requirements address several factors, including:

- Seasonal staffing requirements
- Vacation scheduling
- Dates when all staff are expected to be available
- Annual facility closing for comprehensive maintenance and cleaning

Developing an annual programming calendar prepares for extraordinary demands on facility and staff and prevents scheduling conflicts.

Seasonal Usage

The annual operational plan complements the annual budget. Forecasting demands on human and facility resources creates a clear picture of the costs associated with each. Planning for seasonal help is important for clubs with summer programs, outdoor pools, catering operations and other specialty departments or programs.

Seasonal help must be hired and trained in advance. Advertising and recruiting staff with specific skills that are in demand during peak seasons should be anticipated prior to the beginning of the season. Although these staff may be "temporary," regular orientation (similar to permanent employees) is important. Performance standards should be similar to other employees to insure seamless service delivery.

Facilities that experience extraordinary use during peak seasons should prepare by developing a preventative maintenance checklist to address needs specific to that season. Repairs or maintenance required should be scheduled prior to the peak period so that service is not interrupted. Commonly replaced parts and components should be stocked in anticipation of repair or maintenance required due to high use.

Scheduling

An annual operations plan not only accounts for additional staff, but also scheduling to meet the needs of peak use. Careful tracking of traffic through the facility and anticipation of planned programs and events helps organize scheduling. Scheduling vacations and block-out times is important to efficient facility operation. An operations calendar outlines events and programs that may require full or additional staffing. This allows staff to request vacation time around block-out times.

COMMUNICATION

Continued maintenance of a well-managed facility requires ongoing communication of operational demands between all departments and staff. Management must facilitate information sharing from all sources as procedures are performed, member expectations are identified, and operational plans are executed. This information can

Table 76.1. Service Standard

We provide all that enter with a sense of "home." The Club is a place where people feel safe, secure, comfortable, and sheltered from the stresses of the outside world.

- Remember to be an amiable host at the Club and encourage the staff to do the same (smile, have eye contact, say hello, good morning, etc.).
- Stay agreeable, friendly and helpful even when being confronted.
- Coach the staff in maintaining a friendly, calm, helpful attitude.
- Encourage and coach the staff to treat the member as their personal guest at all times.
- Coach and assist the staff in solving member problems in a swift and friendly manner.
- Take the initiative and authority to do whatever you think is appropriate to satisfy member needs.
- Encourage and coach the staff to empathize with the members' plight or situation at all times.

I. Review of last week's meeting:

II. Program/Operational Concerns:

-
-
-
-
-
-
-
-
-

III. Current Week's "To Do List"

	TASK	COMPLETION DATE	STATUS	COMMENTS
1	____________	( )	( )	
2	____________	( )	( )	
3	____________	( )	( )	
4	____________	( )	( )	
5	____________	( )	( )	
6	____________	( )	( )	
7	____________	( )	( )	
8	____________	( )	( )	
9	____________	( )	( )	
10	____________	( )	( )	

IV. This weeks schedule: week beginning - ____________

MONDAY ____________

TUESDAY ____________

WEDNESDAY ____________

THURSDAY ____________

FRIDAY ____________

SATURDAY ____________

SUNDAY ____________

**MUST BE RECEIVED BY THE GENERAL MANAGER BY 10:00A.M.
EVERY MONDAY.**

Figure 76.3. Weekly objectives.

then be used to develop the best action plans for continued growth and development.

Daily communication focuses on issues and items in the day-to-day operation require attention. These are typically reported from opening and closing checklists, inspection reports, and/or MOD reports. The problems should be resolved quickly. Operational concerns should also be addressed during weekly manager meetings or regular department head (or supervisor) meetings. Each department head should have a clear understanding of the operational condition of their area and its impact on customer satisfaction (Fig. 76.3). Changes and improvements in operations can be communicated through regularly scheduled, club-wide staff meetings to insure that all staff receive important information. Continued, clear communication between all levels of the organization helps to maintain a high level of customer satisfaction and employee morale. Ultimately, this can positively effect the bottom line.

▶ SUMMARY

Operation of a facility includes all aspects important to daily and continuous management of the facility. Procedures and checklists for operating all aspects of the facility are critical to efficient and effective management. Customer service is crucial to the success of any facility and is part of the operational plan. Planning and communication for operations and management of a facility help assure ability to meet customer needs and thereby satisfy customer demands.

Suggested Readings

Patton RW, Corry JM, Gettman LR, et al. *Implementing Health and Fitness Programs.* Champaign, IL: Human Kinetics, 1986.

Patton RW, Grantham WC, Gerson RF, et al. Staff Selection and Development. In: Wilmoth S, Mount C, Gilly H, eds. Developing and Managing Health/Fitness Facilities. Champaign, IL: Human Kinetics, 1989.

Patton RW, Grantham WC, Gerson RF, et al. *Managing Health/Fitness Facilities.* Champaign, IL: Human Kinetics, 1989.

Sol N, Foster C. *Organizational Structure and Professional Staffing. American College of Sports Medicine Health/Fitness Facility Standards and Guidelines.* Champaign, IL: Human Kinetics, 1992.

Storlie J, Baun WB, Horton WL. *Guidelines for Employee Health Promotion Programs: Association for Fitness in Business, 1992.* Champaign, IL: Human Kinetics, 1992.

137, 142, 188 165, 166, 265, 267

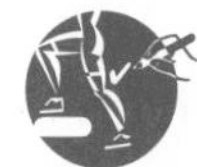

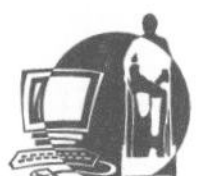

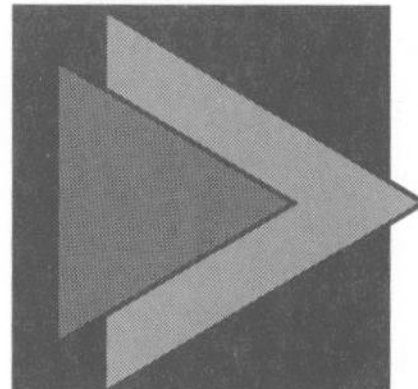

CHAPTER **77**

Equipment Selection, Purchase and Maintenance

Mike Caton

Selecting, purchasing, and maintaining exercise equipment can be a challenging process. The growing number of equipment options, advancements in technology, and monetary risks make purchasing equipment increasingly difficult. This chapter provides basic information about equipment selection, purchase and maintenance, whether stocking a new facility, replacing existing equipment, or considering a new product on the market.

EQUIPMENT SELECTION

New equipment may be requested for several reasons:

- Long waiting lines at existing equipment
- High repair costs of outdated equipment
- Member requests
- An intriguing piece seen in a trade journal

In any case, it is vital to make an informed decision without allowing emotions to lead to a costly mistake (Table 77.1).

Need

Before purchasing any equipment, the first step is to confirm the need. Ask the following questions:

- Is this equipment necessary?
- Is the product in question a legitimate option or a fad?
- Is the equipment suited for the demographics of membership?
- Is it affordable?

Space

The next step is to evaluate availability of space by examining dimensions of the equipment and the available space. For example, a treadmill may not be the best choice if the space is narrow or near a walkway. A climber, because of the small space requirements, may be more favorable. Equipment layout is another factor that must be considered, including the location of the appropriate electrical outlets. It is also important to allow for traffic flow and to avoid blocking emergency access to an exit.

Gathering Information

Gathering product information is the next step. Review and compare as many equipment choices as possible. Fitness trade magazines, trade shows, and equipment vendors are excellent resources for attaining this information. Trade magazines and journals provide reader service cards and often publish an annual guide listing names and numbers for all equipment manufacturers. In addition to advertisements featuring a variety of brand names, monthly issues also have an advertising index in each issue.

Trade shows make it easy to gather information. The differences between brands are more obvious and choices become clearer and narrow very quickly when direct comparison is possible.

CARDIOVASCULAR EQUIPMENT

Cardiovascular equipment is no longer solely limited to bikes, treadmills and rowers. The marketplace has an array of cardiovascular modalities from which to choose. Each modality has positive attributes, and there is no best choice for every environment or situation. This section reviews and discusses popular choices of cardiovascular exercise equipment and discusses their advantages and disadvantages.

Treadmills

Treadmills are consistently among the favorites in fitness settings. Treadmills have distinct advantages. Most people do not require time to learn the activity because walking and running are natural activities. The participant is supporting their body weight with their legs. Leg

Table 77.1. Equipment Selection Checklist

1. Determine needs, validity, and budget.
2. Evaluate facility for space, safety, and power requirements.
3. Gather product information from resources such as trade journals, trade shows, and distributors.
4. Evaluate products for safety in terms of design, biomechanics, and electrical circuitry.
5. Investigate reputation of manufacturers for quality, service history, financial stability.
6. Compare cost of products.
7. Evaluate products on basis of aesthetics.
8. Check references of current users. Lists can be obtained from manufacturers.
9. Compare warranties for length and comprehensiveness.
10. Determine service points provided by manufacturers in terms of availability of local service and parts.
11. Use product.
12. Compare products in terms of learning curves, familiarity of movements, and accessibility.
13. Determine most effective purchase plan.
14. Purchase equipment.

muscles are larger and require more energy while exercising, so heart rate can be raised and kept in the target range, leading to sustained training for an increased length of time without extensive local fatigue. Intensity of exercise can be changed easily by increasing speed or elevation. Treadmills also have some disadvantages. Weight-bearing exercise may be more difficult for those with weight problems or orthopedic injury. In these cases, non-weight-bearing exercise may be more appropriate. Also, treadmills are large, making them difficult to accommodate with respect to space.

Stationary Bikes

The stationary bicycle is popular and time-tested. Among the advantages are the following:

- Cycling is a motion that most people are comfortable performing
- Little time is required for habituation
- It is non-weight bearing and, therefore, no impact

For these reasons, the bike can be an ideal mode of exercise in rehabilitative settings. However, those using a bicycle ergometer may have difficulty raising their heart rate to target range, and maintaining it may be difficult due to local fatigue.

Recumbent Bikes

Recumbent and semi-recumbent bicycles are very popular and have become standard in many facilities. The seat is more comfortable than traditional bicycle seats. These bicycles may be beneficial for special populations due to back support. Safety is increased because of the wide base of support and the ease of mounting and dismounting.

The disadvantages are similar to other non-recumbent, stationary bicycles. Maintaining target heart rate may be more difficult than on upright bicycles due to the supine position. Local fatigue can also be a consistent problem on these bicycles.

Stairclimbers

Stairclimbers, or stairsteppers, are another popular cardiovascular exercise option. The advantages of stairclimbers include:

- The motion of stepping or climbing is familiar to most users, making it easy to learn.
- It is weight-bearing, thus allowing an easily sustained elevated heart rate.
- It is low-impact.
- Climbers occupy less space than many other types of equipment.

Rowers

Though a legitimate form of cardiovascular exercise, rowing machines have never enjoyed the popularity of most other modalities and have decreased in popularity recently. Rowing uses large muscles of the legs as well as the large, upper body muscles of the arms and back; raising and sustaining target heart rate is relatively easy. Rowing is a non-weight-bearing and no-impact exercise.

On the negative side, the rowing motion is unfamiliar to most users, making it difficult to learn. Additional emphasis on proper instruction is required. Also, rowers require significant floor space (especially in length) and may require specially shaped space.

Cross Country Skiers

Cross country ski machines have become commonplace in fitness centers. Skiers offer some advantages. Large muscle mass (upper and lower body muscle groups are used) is used during exercise, and therefore target heart rate range is easily reached and sustained. Though weight-bearing, cross-country skiing is non-impact.

Most people are unaccustomed to this activity and experience difficulty in learning the skill. Despite the disadvantage, ski machines enjoy a great deal of positive press as well as very effective marketing. Consequently, many exercisers try skiers more than once in an attempt to learn the skill.

Other Cardiovascular Equipment

The exercise equipment industry has produced several equipment innovations that have not had the opportunity to demonstrate longevity. Although the fate of these new products is yet to be determined, their current popularity warrants attention. The first and most popular new classification of cardiovascular exercise equipment is the fitness rider. This type of exercise uses a pushing motion with the legs in conjunction with a rowing motion of the arms. The disadvantage is that it uses unfamiliar motions and is non-weight-bearing; heart rate may be difficult to elevate and local fatigue may also be a problem. However, there is almost no learning curve. The immediate success of this product seems to depend on effective target marketing to a deconditioned population. The fact that the exercise is non-weight-bearing and no-impact is also an advantage.

The fitness walker has also become popular in the commercial fitness market. This activity is best described as a cross between walking and cross-country skiing. It is weight-bearing, non-impact, and uses muscles of the upper and lower body, allowing for a sustained elevated heart rate. It provides all the benefits of cross country skiing and has a very short learning curve.

RESISTANCE TRAINING EQUIPMENT

In recent years, resistance training has become one of the most popular forms of exercise. This growing popularity has compelled manufacturers to extend the market and types of equipment. Where there was once a single multi-station unit with one exercise option per muscle group, there are now multiple machines and free weights, offering several exercise options for each muscle group. Expanding demographics of the exercising population have caused manufacturers to change the appearance of equipment, creating broader market appeal.

Types of Equipment

Manufacturers of resistance training equipment offer three different types of resistance training machines; isotonic, variable resistance, and isokinetic. Isotonic resistance training is provided by free weights and machines in which the resistance remains constant throughout the range of motion. Variable resistance machines, by changing the radius of a cam, increase the resistance through part of the range of motion coinciding with the biomechanics of contraction. Isokinetic machines increase resistance at the point of maximum force while controlling the speed of contraction. This is accomplished through the use of systems including hydraulics or motors.

Resistance training machines come in a variety of styles and shapes. Although the majority are "selectorized" (using a weight stack), some manufacturers offer plate-loaded equipment with manually placed weight plates instead of weight stacks. In many cases this plate-loaded equipment looks and feels similar to the selectorized counterparts. This type of machine can be purchased at a much lower cost than selectorized machines.

The increased popularity of variable resistance machines has diminished the demand for free weight training. Barbells and dumbbells continue to offer a cost effective means of supplying resistance training equipment. Most recently, developers have added dual-axis machines, which offer resistance in multiple planes. This type of exercise is more consistent with natural movement patterns.

SAFETY CONSIDERATIONS

Safety is of primary importance when selecting fitness equipment. Health and fitness facilities are obligated to members to provide a safe exercise environment.

1. Ensure that all electrical plugs are secured and grounded.
2. Treadmills should have emergency cut-off switches that are easily accessible.
3. Safety instructions should be mounted on all equipment.
4. Ensure that equipment accommodates different body sizes and types. Adjustable seats, back pads, and leg pads should be available.
5. The machines must restrict joint movements beyond normal range of motion.
6. Back pads should never force loss of the natural curve of the spine.
7. Bench width should provide support without restricting the movement of the upper arm in supine exercises.
8. Free weight racks must be wide enough to accommodate the width of an Olympic bar, decreasing the risk of pinching a hand when re-racking a weight. The apparatus must be constructed properly to sustain adequate amounts of weight.

When considering the purchase of a piece of equipment, it should be "tried out." Purchasing equipment based on advertisements is not recommended. Direct experience to determine workmanship, comfort, and biomechanical appropriateness is imperative. An exercise session on the equipment provides a more accurate feel for the machine.

DECISION-MAKING FACTORS

Once needs are determined and product information has been gathered, the evaluation process begins. Factors in evaluation include cost, aesthetics, references, warranty, support and training, and maintenance.

Cost

The cost of a product is often the first question. If the product costs more than budget allows, buying the equipment is not feasible. However, though cost is a major factor, it should not be the only one, and purchasing a piece of equipment because it is the least expensive may be a mistake. Many factors determine cost, including quality of the materials used, manner of assembly, and sales volume.

Aesthetics

Appearance of equipment is rightfully part of the decision-making process. It is important that all equipment fit with the desired look of a facility. Beyond decor, some equipment may appeal more to certain demographics. For example, large, high profile pieces of weight lifting equipment might appeal to members interested and skilled in weight lifting, but may intimidate members of a wellness-oriented facility.

References

When considering any exercise equipment, request references of current owners from the manufacturer, including familiar companies if the product in question is unfamiliar or new to the facility. An equipment manufacturer may make quality treadmills, but inferior bicycle ergometers.

Warranty

Manufacturer's warranty is another important issue. The length of the warranty and exactly what is covered are considerations. Most manufacturer warranties on strength equipment place a different warranty period on moving parts and upholstery than on metal frames. One way to determine practical life of any piece of equipment prior to need for replacement, repair, or refurbishing is to determine the warranty period.

Support and Training

Many companies provide a representative to help set up equipment and train staff and members on proper usage. Amount, speed, and quality of support provided is also important. Some equipment may require minimal support after installation and training while other types (e.g., computer-based or automated equipment) may require continued support. For some types of equipment these may be critical factors in purchasing.

Maintenance

All equipment requires maintenance. Determining the level of local service is a concern. Most major companies train local technicians to service and stock parts. Review the local company and obtain references. Some fitness facilities take advantage of trial periods or demonstrations offered by equipment manufacturers. In these situations, facilities may allow members to assist in the decision, but some managers believe this may be a negative situation because members may become attached to a piece of equipment that is, ultimately, not purchased.

After potential suppliers are identified, request a bid and layout. At this point, with a narrowed field, a decision may be based on cost. Bids may be formal or informal and may involve some negotiating. A minimum of three bids should be obtained for all purchases.

EQUIPMENT PURCHASING OPTIONS

Before making a final decision, some purchasing options that should be considered: buying new, buying used, or leasing.

Buying New Equipment

The first option is buying new equipment outright. Although payment structures can be negotiated, most manufacturers require 50% down and the balance at the time of installation. It is important to know whether freight and installation will be an added cost. Some facilities prefer to withhold 10% of the cost for 30 days to insure satisfactory installation, training, and support.

Buying Used or Refurbished Equipment

A second option is buying used or refurbished equipment. There are many equipment dealers specializing in refurbished and used equipment. They resell at prices of up to 30–50% less than new equipment. This is a good option, especially for resistance equipment, since resistance equipment is well-made and sturdy; many used pieces are considered as good as new. The same is generally not true of cardiovascular equipment. The warranty on most cardiovascular equipment is usually 2 years, as opposed to 10 or more for resistance equipment. Most fitness facilities maintain resistance equipment at least as that long. Older equipment is considered outdated and is likely to have excessive "wear and tear."

Leasing

Leasing equipment may be a consideration if funds to obtain the equipment outright are not available. Some manufacturers work through leasing companies to make this possible. Leasing requires a smaller initial cash outlay, allowing the organization to acquire more equipment. Leasing to own often provides better selection, better warranty, and sometimes buy-back options. In addition, tax credits may be available for leased equipment. However, leasing is usually considered high risk and interest rates may be high.

EQUIPMENT MAINTENANCE

A maintenance program can extend the life of equipment. Some facilities have staff who are knowledgeable and experienced in repairing equipment or dedicated to maintenance. Other clubs use the services of an outside person or company to complete preventive maintenance as well as repair. The advantage of on-staff employees to service equipment is that response time is shorter. The disadvantage is that a staff maintenance worker, because of a lack of training on intricacies of equipment, may misdiagnose a problem and delay the repair. In addition, facilities rarely stock adequate parts and must order them, resulting in more delay. Regardless of the approach, exercise equipment must undergo regular preventive maintenance to extend its life and save more expensive repair costs in the future.

Internal Maintenance

While some maintenance is more suited for a trained professional, there are details that designated staff can perform regularly to reduce cost. This is internal maintenance. Much of internal maintenance is cleaning, which is the single most effective means of preventing premature breakdown. Some claim that the life of a piece of cardiovascular equipment can be doubled by cleaning. A preventive maintenance program can cut expenses as much as 50%, therefore, an effective internal maintenance program is critical. The checklist in Table 77.2 is an example of an effective maintenance schedule.

Upholstery

Upholstery on resistance training equipment is considered one of the most important parts of the equipment because it is the point of contact between people using the equipment. Regular disinfecting is required. Some forms of herpes skin virus have been shown to survive on a warm, moist surface for up to 6 hours. Regular cleaning also prevents drying and cracking caused by oils and salts from perspiration. The most common areas for cracking are the points at which the head and elbows are supported. Another cause of upholstery damage is the buckles of weight lifting belts. The use of belts on this equipment should be avoided. It is easy and cost effective to replace upholstery on high use areas. Other steps that can prolong the life of the equipment are listed in Table 77.3.

It is important to track repair performed on all equipment. See Table 77.4 for an example of a repair log for fitness equipment. These forms can be an important tool in communicating with a repair company. In addition, with good records, the upkeep cost on each piece of equipment can be determined. One commonly accepted rule of thumb can help determine when to replace equipment that requires constant and costly upkeep. If the cost of repair over 2 years is greater than the cost of new unit, or if a single repair costs 50% of the cost of a new unit, replace the unit.

After it is determined that a single piece or an entire line of equipment is too costly to maintain, there are two options: replace or refurbish. Refurbishing is a viable alternative to replacing equipment because of the cost savings, although it is not always the best decision. Re-

Table 77.3. Resistance Training Equipment Monthly Checklist

General
- Wax upholstery with a hard floor wax (monthly).
- Remove pads at first sign of cracking.
- Stock back-up pads.

Frames
- Inspect for cracks in welds (monthly).
- Apply factory touch-up paint to chipped areas to prevent spreading as needed.
- Inspect for loose nuts and bolts (monthly).
- Clean chrome parts with a chrome polish (monthly). Household cleaners will fade the finish.
- Apply car polish to painted surfaces (quarterly).
- Remove rust with fine steel wool and apply polish to surface as needed.
- Replace worn or missing warning decals.
- Replace worn hand grips and seatbelts.

Moving parts
- Inspect all parts and connections (monthly).
- Replace any worn, stretched or frayed cables, belts, or chains.
- Lubricate bearings and bushings with a Teflon type-lubricant when metallic dust or shavings or when squeaking or grinding sounds appear.
- Lubricate chains with chain lubricant (monthly).

Weight Stack
- Clean guide rods with an aerosol cleaner that leaves no residue (weekly).
- Apply a light coating of a Teflon lubricant to the guide rods (weekly).
- Clean chrome weight stacks with a chrome polish (weekly).

Table 77.2. Cardiovascular Equipment Maintenance Checklist

Treadmills
- Check tension and alignment of walking belt (monthly)
- Check speed calibration (monthly)
- Check grade calibration (monthly)
- Lube drive belt (monthly)
- Lube elevation gears (monthly)
- Wax walking deck (Bi-annually)

Bicycles
- Lube chain (Bi-annually)
- Check crank bearings (monthly)
- Check seat (monthly)
- Check tension and RPM sensor (monthly)
- Lube pedals (Bi-monthly)

Steppers
- Lube pivots (quarterly)
- Grease sprockets (quarterly)
- Lube chains (quarterly)
- Check chain tension (quarterly)
- Tighten drive belt (quarterly)

Rowers
- Oil chains (quarterly)
- Check RPM sensors (quarterly)
- Inspect seat bearings (quarterly)

Note: In addition, it is important that all pieces be cleaned throughout each day to remove perspiration, dust, dirt and other elements that may come into contact with equipment and people.

Table 77.4. Fitness Equipment Repair Chart

Fitness Equipment Repair Chart

Date	Equipment	Serial No.	Problem	Date Repaired	Order #	Cost

furbishing cardiovascular equipment may not be a good decision because life span is comparatively short. However, refurbishing resistance training equipment, especially free weight and plate-loaded equipment, is a good investment because of their long lifespans. Another consideration is the amount of structural damage sustained. If the frame has been exposed to large amounts of rust or heat (e.g., from a fire), refurbishing is not a good idea. High levels of rust or heat can weaken stress joints and make a unit unstable.

EXERCISE TESTING AREAS

An area should be set aside for exercise testing that insures privacy and comfort. The space should be quiet and well ventilated. Although the type of test, protocol, and equipment may vary, Table 77.5 describes equipment that should be incorporated into an exercise testing area. A crash cart, an ECG defibrillator and a spine board should be incorporated into the testing area if maximal graded tests are performed. A physician or other legally authorized individual must have authority to use the emergency equipment.

Table 77.5. Fitness Testing Area Equipment*

- Bicycle ergometer or treadmill
- Body composition or other body composition measuring device
- Sit and reach bench or goniometer
- Tensiometer or other device for measuring muscular strength/endurance
- Perceived exertion chart
- Clock
- Metronome
- Sphygmomanometer (blood pressure cuff)
- Stethoscope
- Tape measure
- Scale
- First-aid kit

* Adapted from ACSM. *ACSM Fitness Facility Standards and Guidelines.* Champaign IL: Human Kinetics, 1992.

An air handling system that ensures negative air pressure should be designed and installed to ensure constant circulation in all fitness testing, health promotion, and wellness areas. Appropriate temperature, humidity, and air circulation levels should be maintained in the fitness testing area. The following levels are recommended:

- Air temperature: 68–72°F
- Humidity: 60% or less
- Air circulation: 6–8 exchanges per hour

▶ SUMMARY

Selection, purchase, and maintenance of equipment are all processes critical to the effective operation of a fitness facility. In addition, they contribute to member satisfaction, marketing, and attracting new members. All exercise professionals should be familiar with different types of equipment, maintenance of that equipment, and proper use of the equipment.

Suggested Readings

ACSM. *ACSM Fitness Facility Standards and Guidelines.* Champaign IL: Human Kinetics, 1989.

Patton R, et al. *Developing and Managing Health/Fitness Facilities.* Champaign IL: Human Kinetics, 1989.

226, 270 442, 449

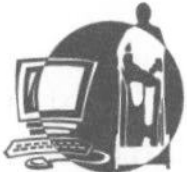 

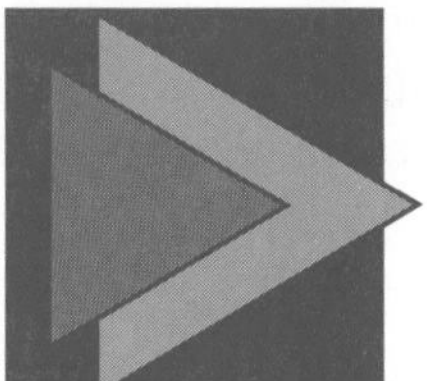

CHAPTER 78
Policies and Procedures

Linda K. Hall

There is no health care organization in existence today that has not undergone the panic-stricken year preceding a visit from the Joint Commission on Accreditation of Healthcare Organization (JCAHO) or another accrediting organization. The JCAHO is an accrediting organization to which any healthcare organization meeting the following definitions may apply to for accreditation to provide services and meet reimbursement criteria from federal agencies (1):

- Hospitals
- Nonhospital-based psychiatric and substance abuse organizations, including community mental health centers, freestanding chemical dependency providers, and organizations that serve persons with mental retardation and other developmental disabilities
- Long term care organizations
- Home care organizations
- Ambulatory care organizations
- Organization-based pathology and clinical laboratory services
- Health care networks

Additionally, a facility may be visited by the American Public Health Association (APHA), the Commission on Accreditation of Rehabilitation Facilities (CARF), the American College of Sports Medicine (ACSM), the American Association of Cardiovascular and Pulmonary Rehabilitation (AACVPR), and state agencies. All of these have or are developing certification procedures for facilities and programs that examine quality control, licensure, appropriateness of care, policies and procedures and, in essence, everything in the performance of business.

These review and accreditation processes require organizations involved in the delivery of rehabilitation, fitness, health enhancement, and preventive programs to establish an operational design that includes individualized policies and procedures for activities, application of therapies, and programming. Policies and procedures should be developed using standards of care promulgated by professional organizations and associations. Additionally, the policies and procedures should be reviewed by appropriate medical and legal persons so that they may serve as the immediate line of defense for a program in the event of legal claim and lawsuit (2).

DESIGN AND STRUCTURE

There are several steps to be taken when developing a program, re-engineering an existing program or actually designing the physical structure of a new fitness or wellness center before writing policies and procedures.

1. Develop a vision and mission statement that defines the philosophy and purpose of the program or center.
2. Find "centers of excellence" that have developed similar programs and centers.
3. Acquire and read published standards and guidelines.
4. Review policy and procedure manuals currently in use within the organization.

Vision and Mission Statement

The development of vision and mission statements is a group effort. Every level of employee should be involved in the process to ensure success. "Ownership" by all levels within the organization is required to carry out the statements. A vision statement is a broad, powerful, and futuristic description of the ideal state that a center may achieve. The mission statement is a broad, powerful, futuristic description of how the vision will be accomplished. If the program or center is a part of a large organization, such as a hospital system or a company (e.g., Procter & Gamble or IBM), the vision and mission statement will reflect a similar philosophical direction.

Sample Vision Statement: "Baptist Memorial Hospital will be THE leader in health care quality, value and service in this region, and one of the leading health care providers in the world" (3).

Sample Mission Statement: "Ford motor company is a world wide leader in automotive and automotive-related products and services as well as in newer industries such as aerospace, communications, and financial services. Our mission is to improve continually our products and services to meet our customers' needs, allowing us to prosper as a business and to provide a reasonable return for our stockholders, the owners of our business" (4).

Vision and mission statements are fluid and should be reviewed regularly and rewritten as required by changing circumstances within or outside the organization. If new programs have been added, the direction of services has changed, or other therapies are included in delivery of services, these statements may be rewritten. Additionally, reviewing them is an important step to help remind staff of the vision and mission and may renew vigor and enthusiasm. The major thrust of the vision and mission should be to provide optimum quality programs, producing positive outcomes that may be benchmarked against local, regional and national programs.

Centers of Excellence

When designing a program, center, or facility it is important to see what others have done. Some programs, deemed "centers of excellence," should be used as models for program development. These can be identified by reading journals from professional organizations such as the ACSM, *Fitness in Business and Industry,* and the American Association of Cardiac and Pulmonary Rehabilitation. These journals have articles written by national leaders about programs or about research that may assist in structuring programs. Additionally, attending regional or national meetings can help identify centers of excellence. Talking with or visiting these experts can help in program or facility design and equipment purchase; in addition they may be willing to share policies and procedures.

Published Standards and Guidelines

Collect and review the most recent publications of standards and guidelines promulgated by national organizations such as the ACSM *Guidelines for Graded Exercise Testing and Exercise Prescription, 5th edition* (American College of Sports Medicine); the *Guidelines for Cardiac Rehabilitation Programs, 2nd edition* (American Association of Cardiovascular and Pulmonary Rehabilitation); *Health/Fitness Facility Standards and Guidelines* (American College of Sports Medicine); and other federal, state, and local agency documents and standards to which a program or facility may be held accountable.

The policies and procedures that are formulated for programs and facilities should not have a standard that requires less or a level below that which is a part of a local, state, regional or national standard. In cases where legal liability may be in question, these "gold" standards have been and continue to be used as the baseline for determination of a "standard of care" against which the alleged liability issue in question will be compared.

Organizational Policies and Procedures

Collect policy and procedural manuals that currently existing within the parent organization. For example, in most hospitals, the following policy and procedural manuals are generally available:

- Infection Control and Hazardous Waste
- Human Resource Management Nursing Practice
- Emergency Management
- Hospital Policy and Procedure Manual

A complete review of these manuals should be completed before attempting to write policies and procedures for programs, facilities, or staff. If a standard or guideline exists in these manuals or in the state, regional, or national guideline and it is exactly what will be followed, do not rewrite it; reference it in the policy. Establish a central location where all staff have access to copies of program (or facility) policy and procedure manuals and state, regional, and national guidelines and standards. This area contains the directional "atlas" for the facility, program(s), and staff.

PREVENTIVE AND REHABILITATIVE EXERCISE PROGRAMS

There are 16 key areas that must be considered when identifying and writing policies for the process of delivering preventive and rehabilitative exercise programs. These key areas contain basic standards of care and program implementation. The policies should not hold staff or facility to a level of practice less than found in any state, regional, or national guideline regarding the same practice. These policies and procedures become standard operating procedure for all staff in operating the facility, dealing with patients, and applying therapy. During orientation, new staff should read the policy and procedure manual and be trained in the application of the policies and procedures. This manual must identify the right thing to do and define how to do it. Leadership must ensure that the staff carries this out (5). Once training is complete, a competency checklist should be completed and placed in the personnel file.

Leadership

Providing excellent services to patients and clients requires effective leadership. Effective leadership is based on planning and designing programs, facility utilization, staff growth and assignments and all other areas of program development. Leadership is responsible for directing, integrating and coordinating services. There are several potential levels of organization, usually including a board of directors (or a president or vice president), a medical director, and/or a board of medical advisors. The leadership is responsible for coordinating meetings, agendas, and carrying out decisions and recommendations from these boards. An organizational chart designating lines of authority should be placed at the beginning of the policies and procedures. Generally, the medical director or board is responsible for establishing guidelines and processes for clinical practice. The medical director or board approves the process of patient/client evaluation and exercise prescription. The board of directors (president/vice president) establish business policies and practices. The manager/director carries out the policies and processes instituted by these governing bodies.

Effective leadership creates a clear vision for the future and defines values that underlie day to day operations. This type of leadership is evaluated by accrediting organizations (JCAHO, CARF, etc.) for being inclusive, not exclusive, and for encouraging staff participation in shaping the vision and values that are the backbone of excellent program delivery. Effective leadership is guided by the principle of leadership development at every level of the organization. This type of leadership is reflected in the development of the chain of command that, in modern management practice, is more horizontal than vertical in structure.

Effective leadership accurately assesses the needs of patients, clients, and future customers to shape and reshape programs to meet these needs. The program should foster a culture in which staff are focused on continuous customer service and quality improvement of processes. The responsibility of the program and facility includes an awareness of issues related to the community in which it resides. Additionally, leadership ensures that all services within the scope of the program/facility are integrated and imbued with the same culture and theme of excellent, safe, and high quality provision of care.

Environmental Concerns

Policies and procedures regarding management of the environment are aimed at providing safe, functional and effective surroundings for program delivery. The components of the policies should include:

- Planning of space utilization
- Acquisition of equipment, dispersal of resources, and maintenance
- Reduction and control of environmental hazards and risks
- Prevention of accidents and injuries
- Maintenance of safe conditions
- Provision for emergency treatment, training and practice programs
- Staff training with regard to emergencies such as disaster, bomb threats, fire, earthquake, hazardous waste, power failures, etc.
- Climate control

These policies should reflect national, state and local regulations and all staff should be aware of them. If they are described in the parent organization policy and procedure manual, then only those which apply specifically need to be developed.

Improving Performance

The success of any program, organization, or company is predicated on the delivery of excellent services, new and innovative techniques, and application of scientifically based information aimed at producing proven outcomes. The mechanism for achieving success is through analysis of performance, continued evaluation and current scientific knowledge. This is managed through designing a process for examination of efficacy, appropriateness and availability of programs. The mechanism for continuous performance improvement should mirror the plan within the parent organization and includes the following:

- Regular review of policy and procedure manuals to assure comprehensiveness and accuracy
- Evaluation of performance dimensions (e.g., timeliness, effectiveness, continuity, safety, and efficiency)
- Evaluation of client satisfaction
- Continued scrutiny of national, regional and local programs for benchmarking outcomes
- Regulating agencies involved in accrediting organizations require that the organization, both as a whole and within individual departments, is able to demonstrate a continuing process of evaluation performance, outcomes and processes

Information Management

This section describes how to manage the storage, transmission, use, and tracking of information related to operation. Included are policies and procedures with regard to:

- Patient records, patient privacy and confidentiality, storage and outcome data
- Financial records, analysis, budget allocation and capital and operational expenses
- Insurance billing, precertification, and reimbursement
- Provision of charity and scaled remunerative services
- Patient/client registration and procedure scheduling

Policies for information management are usually determined by the parent organization. There is usually an information services department that coordinates tracking programs, billing and registration processes, and patient records and is responsible for developing organization-wide policies related to patient records, data collection, clinical outcomes, and reporting channels. Individual services, such as cardiac rehabilitation and preventive services, may write program-specific guidelines unique to the application of those services and consistent with policies of the parent organization.

Human Resources

The program should have a master staffing plan including an evaluation of the complexity of patient and client care and delivery of services, information management, fiscal management (including purchasing, billing, insurance pre-certification and financial resource management), facility maintenance, and other areas involved in facility and program management. Policies and procedures should include the following:

1. Job descriptions for each position with baseline educational requirements and knowledge. The job description should outline primary responsibilities and competencies required and include a description of the physical demands and working conditions (OSHA, blood born pathogen, lifting, carrying, job classification, etc.).
2. A description of the orientation and initial 90-day evaluation to ensure proper job training of new employees.
3. A description of the annual performance appraisal of employees and mechanism of remuneration.
4. A list of required staff certifications and licenses. Current staff should have copies of these on file.
5. Clearly delineated staff rights

Staff Education and Inservices

Continuing education for staff is critical to providing quality programs and facilities. Policies concerning continuing education, inservices, and educational experiences required should be written. A number of national guidelines require a monthly inservice for emergency education and skill training. Surveying agencies may review documentation of department meetings, agendas, inservices, educational programs and certifications. The policy and procedure manual should describe what, when, how, and where these should be delivered, evaluated, and recorded. Included are policies for staff performance review and evaluation and, perhaps, staff advancement and promotion.

Patient and Client Rights

Preventive, rehabilitative, and exercise programs/facilities survive by the volume of patients and clients they serve, either temporarily or through continuing membership. Maintaining patient/client loyalty and satisfaction is an optimum requirement. The patient/client has rights that must be made public within the facility. The patient/client has the right to:

- Considerate care that safeguards personal dignity
- Respect for cultural, psychosocial and spiritual values
- Know the personal responsibility in the care process

There should be policies and procedures establishing guidelines that ensure patient privacy and confidentiality. The delivery of patient/client care should improve outcomes by respecting individual rights and conducting the business of the program/facility ethically. This includes promoting consideration of patient/client values and preferences, recognizing the facility/program responsibility, and comprehensive communication and record keeping. Record keeping includes informing the patient/client of risks and processes involved in the provision of evaluation, exercise prescription, rehabilitation and exercise programs and receiving informed consent to provide these services.

Patient/Client Assessment and Provision of Care

Provision of comprehensive services to the patient/client occurs only when initial and ongoing assessment is the basis for determining and addressing specific care needs. This assessment is accomplished by collecting data specific to physical, psychosocial status and health history, analyzing the data and making care decisions based on the data. In ongoing assessment, there are specific guidelines delineating patient/client participation in goal setting for personal health and lifestyle achievements. The major phases for delivery of services involve assessment, development and application of a care plan, monitoring and determining outcomes and endpoints, modification of the plan, and coordination of follow-up. Included in these policies should be specific guidelines for:

- Assessment of patient/client medications and potential interaction with application of therapy
- Consideration and assessment of medication efficacy and impact on function and side effects
- Communication with referring physicians regarding patient/client compliance to medication regime
- Assessment of nutrition and dietary needs and establishment of a diet plan appropriate to the diagnosis and treatment plan

Rehabilitative Care

This area outlines tasks after completion of the assessment. It includes the following areas:

- A description of the risk stratification process and assignment of risk status
- A decision concerning monitoring and supervision in light of risk status (e.g., continuous ECG, intermittent ECG, blood pressure, heart rate, signs and symptoms, rating of perceived exertion)
- Exercise prescription methodology including mode, time, intensity, frequency, progression
- Risk factor evaluation, goal setting and expected outcomes
- Vocational retraining
- Discharge planning and follow-up

The objective is to establish a protocol in which the patient achieves optimal functioning, self care/responsibility, independence and an acceptable quality of life. Additionally, it is important to recognize that outcomes are projected based on national norms and scientific data with the objective of reducing future clinical events and minimizing development or exacerbation of chronic illness.

Patient/Client and Family Education

Education promotes healthy behavior, thus educational programs are a key function of any wellness, rehabilitative and preventive center. It is important to establish policies regarding development of and referral to educational programs dealing with risk factors that are common across the chronic and acute disease spectrum, such as smoking cessation, stress management, hypertension, dietary programs for diabetes, cholesterol, weight loss, pulmonary disease, sports nutrition, and relaxation, as well as exercise training and behavior management. The goals of the educational programs should be to help people:

- Change lifestyle to effect a positive health status
- Exchange negative for positive health behaviors
- Reduce risk for future chronic and acute disease
- Develop and use skills for coping with chronic disease
- Acquire physical skills
- Optimize health status
- Optimally function in vocational and avocational activities

Policies and procedures establish protocols for the patient/client to become self-directed, participate in the decision making process, and use experience and problem solving skills as a learning resource. The educational policies should be formulated around principles of adult education, evaluation of readiness to learn and principles of lapse and relapse prevention.

The intent of the educational programs is to improve health outcomes by promoting healthy behavior and involving patients in care and life decisions. The basis of this education is founded in encouraging acceptance of personal responsibility for self-teaching. Materials and knowledge that patients are unable to accomplish for themselves should be provided by the educational program.

Continuum of Care/Services

Policies describing the integration of settings for all phases of the care continuum from entry through discharge should be in place. The needs of patients/clients should be matched with appropriate services, appraisals, and programs. Policies in this section include:

- Appointment scheduling
- Parking
- Registration
- Insurance precertification and enrollment
- Informed consent
- Program evaluation
- Referral to other disciplines as needed (e.g., Occupational and Physical Therapy)
- Intermittent progress evaluations
- Discharge planning and follow-up

This section should establish the process by which the patient/client is able to move within the rehabilitative system and facility from parking through registration with a minimum of difficulty or excess time involvement with a clear understanding of the process.

SUMMARY

As with the vision and mission statements, policies and procedures are fluid. They should be reviewed regularly and updated similarly to any new application or process. The rapidly changing nature of health care delivery and reimbursement coupled with the increasing number of preventive and rehabilitation programs makes regular review and revision of the policies and procedure (every 6–12 months) prudent. This should ensure adherence with national standards and guidelines and accrediting organizations.

The baseline of a comprehensive policy and procedure document is the goals and objectives of the program. A written statement describing the process of who, when, where, why, and how delivery of services occurs is the content. Finally, those policies must be aligned with existing national, regional, state, and local standards and guidelines.

References

1. Joint Commission on Accreditation of Healthcare Organizations, 1996. Comprehensive Accreditation Manual for Hospitals. Oakbrook Terrace, Illinois: JCAHO; 1995.
2. Herbert DL, Herbert WG. Medicoleagal aspects of rehabilitation of the coronary patient. In: Wenger NK, Hellerstein HK eds. *Rehabilitation of the Coronary Patient.*

3. Baptist Memorial Hospital. Vision Statement, 1996. Baptist Memorial Hospital, Memphis, Tennessee.
4. Ford Motor Company, Mission Statement, 1988, Detroit, Michigan.
5. Deming WE. Quality Productivity and Competitive Position. Cambridge, MA: Massachusetts Institute of Technology, Center for Advanced Engineering Study.

Suggested Readings

Monthly

Hospitals and Health Networks. American Hospital Publishing, Inc., Chicago, IL.

Circulation. American Heart Association, Dallas, Texas.

Medicine and Science in Sports and Exercise. ACSM, Indianapolis, IN.

Journal of Cardiopulmonary Rehabilitation. Lippincott, Philadelphia, PA.

Books

Froelicher VF. *Manual of Exercise Testing.* 2nd ed. St. Louis: Mosby-Yearbook, 1994.

Pollock ML, Schmidt DH, eds. *Heart Disease and Rehabilitation.* Champaign, IL: Human Kinetics, 1995.

132, 135, 167 136, 141 144, 146

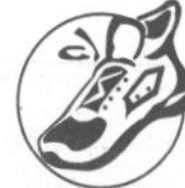
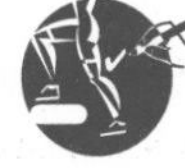
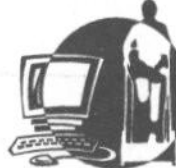

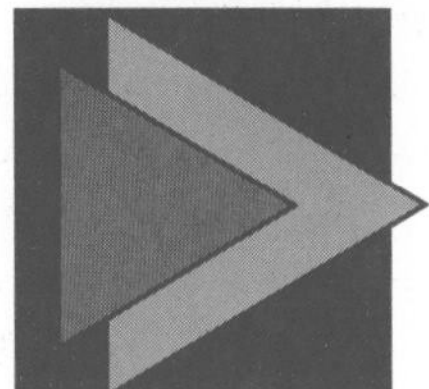

CHAPTER 79

Emergency Procedures and Exercise Safety

Sue Beckman

Although there is always risk with exercise programs, most health and fitness professionals believe that the benefits outweigh the risks. However, vigorous exercise involves a variety of risks, including musculoskeletal injury and cardiovascular complications. The risk of injury and myocardial infarction related to exercise and exercise testing can be reduced through appropriate screening and risk stratification procedures, exercise prescription techniques, and facility safety standards. Furthermore, rehearsing emergency procedures reduces risk of serious complications in the event of emergency. Staff training and client orientation sessions maximize safety and minimize employee and facility liability. The information presented in this chapter is intended as a template for the exercise professional for developing policies and procedures specific to facility, clientele, staff, and community medical resources. Numerous resources are available to assist in the development of safe and effective exercise programs for clientele and staff.

DEATH AND CARDIAC ARREST

The incidence of sudden death and cardiac arrest during exercise has been investigated by many researchers. In cases of sudden cardiac death, under age 30, coronary artery disease is rare; congenital or other abnormalities such as valvular heart disease, myocardial hypertrophy, and cardiomyopathy are often associated with exercise-related deaths. Thompson, et al. showed men between 30 and 64 years of age who jog at least 2 days a week had a yearly sudden death rate of 1 per 7,620. By excluding men with known heart disease, the death rate dropped to 1 per 15,200 joggers per year. The incidence of cardiac arrest during vigorous activity was reported as 1 in 18,000 healthy men per year. The incidence of exercise-related deaths and cardiac events is lower in women due to the lower prevalence of coronary artery disease in young and middle-aged women. These studies emphasize the need for appropriate medical screening, risk factor stratification, and exercise prescription to reduce the risk of exercise-related complications and death.

Exercise-related risk should be examined relative to the risks of physical inactivity. Physical inactivity is a major risk factor for coronary artery disease. The average relative risk of coronary artery disease in inactive individuals is approximately twice the risk of an active person. This is similar to the risk associated with smoking, hypertension and hypercholesterolemia. Based on percentages of U.S. population at increased risk for coronary artery disease, 59% are physically inactive; this exceeds the combined percentages of individuals with risk factors for hypertension, hypercholesterolemia and smoking, suggesting physical activity should be vigorously targeted for intervention. In view of this epidemiological evidence, the benefits of exercise outweigh the risks in most individuals, assuming that ACSM Guidelines for health screening, risk stratification, and exercise prescription are followed.

MUSCULOSKELETAL INJURY

Epidemiological studies investigating the incidence of injury during vigorous activity provide valuable information for the selection of appropriate activities, based on health history and fitness evaluation. More epidemiological data are available regarding running compared to other fitness related activities. Studies investigating the incidence of running injuries report yearly rates of 24–54%; generally, lower rates are reported in recreational runners and higher rates in competitive athletes. Differences in the definition of injury among studies also contribute to variation in the incidence of injury. A higher weekly mileage was associated with an increased incidence of injury.

Injury rates for other weight-bearing activities, such as aerobic dance, are often reported based on exposure or hours spent in aerobic dance classes. A study by Garrick, et al. reported that injuries resulting in an alteration of aerobic dance activity were 0.29 and 0.26 per 100 hours of activity for students and instructors, respectively. In other words, one injury-altering participation occurred for every 344 hours of activity; instructors report one injury per 384 hours. Prior orthopedic problems, lack of alternate fitness activities and minimal weekly participation in aerobic dance classes were associated with increased injury rates. The injury rate for non-weight-bearing activities such as cycling and swimming is lower. The brief discussions below cover simple, concise exercise-related problems. See Chapter 57 for extensive discussion of musculoskeletal injuries related to exercise.

Risk Factors for Musculoskeletal Injury

Risk factors associated with injury in weight-bearing activities can be classified into three broad categories: environmental, program and individual factors. Current research on running suggests that age, gender, body build (large vs. small size), running experience, and speed of running are not independent risk factors for injury. A stronger association has been established for previous history of injury, frequency and duration of training, number of miles run per week, and the incidence of injury. A study by Pollock et al. reports the incidence of injury in 70 men 20–35 years of age increased as the frequency and duration of training increased. The incidence of injury was 22%, 24% and 54% in the 15, 30, and 45 minutes/session groups, respectively; incidence of injury was 0%, 12%, and 39% for the 1, 3, and 5 days/week groups. Training intensity was 85–90% of maximal heart rate for all groups. This study suggests that the incidence of injury in novice runners increases significantly with more than 30 minutes of exercise or more than 3 days/week.

EXERCISE-RELATED INJURIES

Exercise-related injuries can be classified into two categories—acute traumatic and "overuse" injuries. Traumatic injuries usually occur from a single, violent event. Injuries such as strains, sprains, tears, and fractures are considered traumatic injuries. Conversely, overuse injuries are caused by chronic, repetitive, submaximal forces leading to inflammation and pain. Common overuse injuries include tendinitis, strains, shin splints, stress fractures, and blisters. Acute treatments for common injuries are outlined in Table 79.1. Many of the following conditions and injuries are discussed in other chapters in this book. The reader is encouraged to review each of those chapters for in depth information about specific topics of interest.

Skin Wounds

Skin wounds, including blisters, corns, abrasions, lacerations, punctures, sunburn, and infections, are caused by mechanical trauma, environmental factors, or transmission of infectious organisms. Blisters are caused by friction between the surface of the skin and athletic wear or equipment, resulting in fluid accumulation. The blister itself provides a protective dressing and should be covered with a sterile dressing which promotes rapid healing and reduces the risk of infection. Blisters often rupture due to location in areas such as feet, or require drainage for other reasons. To drain a blister, puncture with a sterile needle, treat with antibiotic ointment, and cover with a sterile dressing. Properly fitting socks and shoes and sport-specific gloves help prevent blisters.

Bleeding/open skin wounds such as lacerations may require direct application of pressure and elevation to stop bleeding. Care should be taken to prevent the transfer of blood-borne pathogens during cleaning of the wound. Medical evaluation is indicated for deep or large wounds or if signs of infection such as swelling, redness, and pain are present.

Contusions

Contusions are bruises with intact skin. Common in contact sports, muscle contusions incite an inflammatory response and may involve formation of a hematoma. The treatment of choice is rest, ice, compression, elevation, and stabilization (RICES [Table 79.2]). Severe, painful contusions, especially with hematoma formation, should be evaluated by a physician.

Strains/Sprains

Strains refer to stretching or tearing of the musculotendinous unit and sprains to a ligament. Strains and sprains are classified as Grade I, II, or III, depending upon the severity of tissue tearing. Grade I strains and sprains involve stretching or minor tearing of connective tissue. Grade II strains and sprains result from partial tearing of tissue; Grade III strains and sprains involve extensive tearing or complete rupture of tissue and generally require surgery. The RICES protocol is appropriate for acute strains and sprains.

Following joint injury, proprioception, the ability to perceive position in space and respond, is often affected; mechanoreceptor function and proprioceptive feedback to the brain is decreased. Therefore, proprioceptive exercises should be included in the rehabilitation program to restore kinesthetic awareness, coordination, agility, flexibility, muscular strength, and endurance.

Fractures

Fractures include 3 types: stress, simple and compound. Stress fractures involve microfractures in the bone surface and are caused by repetitive stress. Simple fractures are fractures where the bone remains within the skin. Compound or open fractures involve external exposure of bone, increasing risk of infection. Common in runners, stress fractures are often related to sudden in-

Table 79.1. Acute Responses for Common Injuries/Emergencies

INJURY/EMERGENCY	SIGNS/SYMPTOMS	ACUTE CARE
Closed skin wounds (blisters, corns)	Pain, swelling, infection	Clean with antiseptic soap, apply sterile dressing, antibiotic ointment
Open skin wounds (lacerations, abrasions)	Pain, redness, bleeding, swelling, headache, mild fever	Apply pressure to stop bleeding, clean with soap or sterile saline, apply sterile dressing, refer to physician for stitches/tetanus
Contusions (bruises)	Swelling, localized pain, loss of function if severe	RICES, apply padding if necessary for protection
Strains*		
Grade I	Pain, localized tenderness, tightness	RICES
Grade II	Loss of function, hemorrhage	RICES, refer for physician evaluation if impaired function
Grade III	Palpable defect	Immobilization, RICES, immediate referral to physician
Sprains*		
Grade I	Pain, point tenderness, strength loss, edema	RICES
Grade II	Hemorrhage, measurable laxity	RICES, physician evaluation
Grade III	Palpable or observable defect	Immobilization, RICES, physician evaluation
Fractures		
Stress	Pain, point tenderness	Physician evaluation, rest
Simple	Swelling, disability, pain	Immobilize with splint, physician evaluation, X-rays
Compound	Bleeding, swelling, pain, disability	Immobilize, control bleeding, apply sterile dressing, immediate physician evaluation
Dizziness/Syncope	Disoriented, confused, skin color-pale	Determine responsiveness, place supine with legs elevated, administer fluids if conscious, begin emergency breathing or compressions as needed
Hypoglycemia (Low blood sugar)	Skin color-pale, skin moist and sweaty, tachycardia, hunger, double vision	Administer sugar if conscious, if unconscious, place sugar granules under tongue, if recovery requires more than 1–2 minutes, activate EMS system (12)
Hyperglycemia (high blood sugar)	Confused, nauseous, headache, breathe-sweet, fruity odor, thirsty, abdominal pain and vomiting, hyperventilation	Activate EMS, administer fluids if conscious, turn head to side if vomiting
Hypothermia	Shivering but may stop with extreme drops in core temperature, loss of coordination, muscle stiffness, lethargy	Activate EMS and transport to hospital, remove wet clothing, replace with dry, warm clothing
Hyperthermia		
Heat cramps	Involuntary, isolated muscle spasms	Administer fluids, apply direct pressure to spasm and release, massage cramping area with ice
Heat syncope	Weakness, fatigue, hypotension, pale skin, syncope	Move to cool area, place supine with legs elevated, administer fluids if conscious, check blood pressure
Heat exhaustion	Profuse sweating, cold, clammy skin, multiple muscle spasms, headache, nausea, loss of consciousness, dizziness, tachycardia, low blood pressure	Move to cool area, place supine with feet elevated, administer fluids, monitor body temperature, refer for physician evaluation
Heat stroke	Hot, dry skin, but can be sweating, dyspnea, confusion, often unconscious	Activate EMS and transport to hospital immediately, remove clothing, dowse with cool water, wrap in cool wet sheets, administer fluids if conscious
Angina (Pain, pressure or tingling in the chest, neck, jaw, arm and/or back)	Pain, sweating, denial of medical problem, nausea, shortness of breath	Stop activity, place in seated or supine position (whichever is most comfortable), activate EMS if pain is not relieved, if unresponsive, check breathing and pulse, begin CPR if necessary
Dyspnea, labored breathing	Hyperventilation, dizziness, wheezing, coughing, loss of coordination	Maintain open airway, administer bronchodilator if prescribed, try pursed lip breathing, if no relief, activate EMS and transport

* Signs and symptoms for each grade include those for the Grade below the one listed (i.e., Grade II includes those of Grades I and II; Grade III includes signs and symptoms listed under Grades I, II and III).

Table 79.2. RICES Protocol for Acute Injuries

Treatment	Purpose	Application
Rest	Pain control, prevention of reinjury	Complete rest, immobilization, or reduction in training intensity, duration, frequency or nonweight bearing activities, depending on severity of injury
Ice	Reduction of pain, swelling, inflammation and bleeding	Immediately post injury, 2–4 times daily, 20–30 minutes, plastic bag filled with crushed ice, covered with a warm, moist towel and secured with an elastic bandage; ice massage for small areas, such as tendons and strains for 10–20 minutes
Compression	Reduction of swelling	Elastic wrap/compression sleeve
Elevation	Reduction of swelling	Elevate extremity above heart level
Stabilization	Reduce muscle spasm	Use of braces, splints, wraps to stabilize area around joint injury

creases in running distance and/or intensity. Point tenderness and pain with weight-bearing activity are characteristic of stress fractures which may not appear on x-rays. Nonweight-bearing and partial weight-bearing activities such as swimming and bicycling are recommended for maintenance of cardiovascular fitness until pain-free activity is possible.

Dizziness/Syncope

Dizziness or syncope (temporary loss of consciousness) during exercise may be caused by hyperventilation, cardiac arrhythmias, heat stress, cardiomyopathy (disease of heart muscle resulting in damage and enlargement of the myocardium), aortic stenosis (narrowing of aortic valve) or coronary artery disease. Acute care should always include evaluation of the airway, breathing, and pulse if the individual is unresponsive. Cessation of exercise and physician evaluation is paramount to determine whether an underlying condition is present.

Hypotension can also cause dizziness and fainting. Post-exercise hypotension occurs when blood pools in the lower extremities due to inadequate cool-down. A 5–10 minute, low-intensity cool-down using large muscle groups is effective in preventing post-exercise hypotension. Antihypertensive medications may exacerbate post-exercise hypotension, necessitating a longer cool-down period. **Orthostatic hypotension,** an inability to maintain arterial blood pressure with changes in posture, may occur when moving from the supine to upright position. Gradual movement with momentary sitting is often effective in preventing orthostatic hypotension. Plasma volume depletion is also a causative factor in hypotension. Proper hydration should always be encouraged, especially if dehydration is suspected or diuretic medications are taken.

Hypoglycemia/Hyperglycemia

Hypoglycemic reactions may occur during and after exercise in diabetic and nondiabetic individuals who are taking inadequate quantities of carbohydrate and total calories. Hypoglycemia involves low blood sugar (usually < 50 mg/dl); however, symptoms may occur at higher blood glucose levels in diabetics on insulin.

Hypoglycemia is a medical emergency which must be treated immediately in diabetics. Hypoglycemia may, however, occur in otherwise healthy individuals who are not eating properly. Signs and symptoms of hypoglycemia and hyperglycemia may be similar, however, symptoms of hypoglycemia develop rapidly while signs and symptoms associated with hyperglycemia are slower to manifest. A more detailed discussion of glycemic control during exercise can be found in Chapter 31.

Hypothermia/Hyperthermia

Hypothermia or cold injury involves a decrease in core temperature. Metabolic heat production is inadequate to match the rate of heat lost through evaporation of sweat, radiation, conduction, and convection. Factors such as windchill (wind speed) and moisture increase the risk of hypothermia. Most cases of hypothermia can be prevented if exercise intensity is controlled, adequate clothing made of fabric designed to wick moisture is worn, and alcohol and drugs which impair thermoregulation are avoided. Elderly persons, children, and individuals with ischemic heart disease or poor aerobic capacities should limit physical activity in the cold.

Hyperthermia or heat injury refers to a category of heat-related disorders including heat cramps, syncope, exhaustion and stroke. The combination of high ambient temperatures, humidity and metabolic heat lead to increases in core temperature, increased sweat rate, and dehydration, sometimes resulting in circulatory collapse and death. Therefore, the WBGT Heat Stress Index, an index of temperature and humidity, should be used to determine the risk of heat stress. Prevention of heat-related injuries include heat acclimatization, avoidance of exercise if the heat index is in the high-risk zone, replacement of electrolytes and fluids, monitoring of body weight, and use of light clothing which promotes cooling and evaporation.

Heat cramps, though uncomfortable, represent a benign condition, but exercise should be discontinued and rehydration initiated immediately. Symptoms of heat exhaustion and heat stroke are similar, and heat exhaustion can rapidly deteriorate into life threatening heat stroke. Any mechanisms available to lower core temperature should be attempted immediately. Chapter 24 provides more detailed information concerning environmental considerations during exercise.

Angina

Pain or discomfort in the chest, jaw, neck or arms (or other areas) during exercise that is not altered by movement of the involved areas or extremity may require immediate medical attention. Individuals with anginal-type discomfort should discontinue exercise immediately and rest in a sitting or recumbent position until the discomfort is resolved. Individuals with medication for anginal syndromes should be encouraged to use the medication as directed.

Dyspnea

Dyspnea or labored breathing may occur in response to bronchospasm, which can be triggered by allergens, cold air, airborne irritants, and respiratory infection. Prescription bronchodilators are often used to resolve such episodes.

TREATMENT OF EXERCISE-RELATED INJURIES

The immediate treatment for acute traumatic and overuse injuries follows the RICES protocol. Anti-inflammatory drugs, such as aspirin and ibuprofen, may be useful in treatment of chronic and acute injuries. Acetaminophen may be used for pain relief, but is not considered an anti-inflammatory medication. Anti-inflammatory medications may be most effective if started several days after injury since the inflammatory process plays an important role in healing. For a detailed discussion of RICES, see Chapter 57.

INJURY PREVENTION

Many of injuries occurring in the fitness setting can be prevented with regular maintenance procedures, training of health/fitness personnel, and formal member orientations regarding equipment utilization, weight room etiquette and facility safety policies. Outlined below are precautions which should be taken to insure member and employee safety. The reader is referred to *ACSM's Health/Fitness Facility Standards and Guidelines* for a detailed list of guidelines. The following recommendations for maintenance and safety apply generally to fitness facilities of many different types:

1. Free weight exercises such as squats and bench press should be performed with a spotter. The spotter should, however, be trained as to proper spotting technique. Two spotters are recommended for heavily loaded free weight exercises.
2. The buddy system is ideal for all types of fitness training (resistance, cardiovascular, etc.) One individual monitors form and biomechanics (during resistance training) and provides feedback to the partner. In the event of an emergency, a rapid response is insured.
3. Routine inspection and maintenance of resistance and cardiovascular equipment is necessary to reduce risk of injury related to equipment malfunction.
4. Passageways between equipment should be sufficient (approximately 3 feet) to allow safe movement at all times.
5. Weights and other accessories (pads, attachments, collars, and pins) must be racked or properly stored after use.
6. Members should be oriented to equipment, including proper lifting technique, controlled speed of movement, adjustments required for proper biomechanical alignment, appropriate amount of weight, sets, and repetitions.
7. Weight room etiquette should be shared with members to facilitate courteous flow of members through the weight room. Allowing other members to rotate in during the rest period, racking weights and wiping equipment with towels to decrease the risk of transmitting viral and bacterial infections are examples of such courtesy.
8. All pads should be cleaned by staff daily with antifungal and antibacterial agents.
9. Equipment should be arranged in a manner consistent with the appropriate order of training.

EMERGENCY PROCEDURES

All facilities should have a written emergency plan for medical complications related to fitness testing. The emergency plan should list specific responsibilities of each staff member, required equipment and a predetermined contact for emergency response. Emergency plans including telephone numbers for EMS, police, and fire should be posted adjacent to all telephones. First-aid kits, first responder blood-borne pathogen kits, latex gloves, CPR mouthpieces, and resuscitation bags must be readily available and transportable. The areas where first-aid equipment is stored should be clearly labeled and supplies checked monthly. Regular, periodic review of the emergency plan by a medical professional is recommended to insure that all appropriate steps are outlined. The plan should be practiced with both announced and unannounced drills on a quarterly basis. Potential and common injuries in the exercise and fitness testing setting should be rehearsed. Completion of a written report should follow each emergency drill, including an evaluation of the drill and recommendations for changes, if necessary. Sample emergency reports are provided in *ACSM's Health/Fitness Facility Standards and Guidelines.*

Emergency plans specific to both minor and major medical incidents are required. Minor medical events are not life or limb threatening and can be initially managed within the facility, but may be triaged to a medical resource. Major medical emergencies involve an initial response by the staff followed by immediate transport to a community medical facility. Since a medical emergency may arise at any time and any location, all employees, including secretarial, janitorial and child care staff should be certified in CPR and first-aid. *ACSM's Guidelines for Exercise Testing and Prescription* details emergency plans for nonemergency and life-threatening situations (2). Emergency plans may vary depending on the facility size, staff, and local emergency response.

EVALUATION SKILLS

A crucial responsibility of the exercise professional is evaluation of technique and body position during resistance and cardiovascular training. Early recognition and correction of poor technique may help reduce risk of injury and insure that the client receives the maximum benefit possible. Participants are usually appreciative and respectful if approached in a friendly, knowledgeable manner. The utmost concern for client safety and scientifically based information should be emphasized when correcting form or technique. Additionally, clients should be discouraged from selecting high-risk exercises.

CONTRAINDICATED AND HIGH-RISK EXERCISES

Much controversy surrounds the decision to label specific exercises as contraindicated or inappropriate *for all individuals.* Factors such as age, flexibility, strength, type of exercise performed, history of pre-existing orthopedic problems, and individual ability to perform an exercise properly make it difficult to label exercises as acceptable or unacceptable for all individuals. Therefore, the term high-risk exercises may be more appropriate than contraindicated, since an exercise may be appropriate for an athlete involved in sports requiring high-risk movements, such as gymnastics, but inappropriate for the general fitness setting. See Table 79.3 and Figure 79.1 for a list of commonly performed high-risk exercises and some alternatives.

In a group exercise setting where all individuals are performing the same exercise, caution in selecting appropriate exercises for all ages, disabilities, and skill levels is crucial. Demonstration of a modified form of an exercise is always appropriate in a group since individuals in "advanced" level classes may exhibit high levels of cardiovascular fitness, but poor levels of flexibility, strength and/or muscular endurance. Of additional concern is the ability to perform the exercise correctly to insure safety. Selection of the most effective and safe exercises is crucial as most exercise classes attempt to provide multiple fitness components within a limited (45–60 minute) amount of time. When selecting exercises appropriate for the group exercise setting, the following evaluation is recommended; a yes answer to all questions is required to maximize participant safety:

- Is the exercise safe for all participants based on age and health status?
- If the exercise is safe, are the participants able to perform the exercise properly?
- Is this exercise an effective way to strengthen, tone, increase flexibility or cardiovascular endurance?

Table 79.3. High-Risk Exercises and Alternatives

Contraindicated/High-Risk Exercise	Alternative Exercise
Straight leg/Full sit-ups	Crunches
Risk: Stress on low back due to utilization of hip flexors with origin in the lumbar spine; exercise primarily targets hip flexors	
Double leg raises	Single leg raises-opposite knee flexed
Risk: Hyperextends low back due to utilization of hip flexors with origin in the lumbar spine	
Full squats	Squats to 90° of knee flexion-knee over ankle
Risk: Patellar tendon forces during keep knee bending are 7.6 times body weight (7), increasing the risk of chrondomalacia and meniscal tears; individuals with previous injury to ligamental structures and menisci are at increased risk for injury	
Hurdler's stretch	Seated hamstring stretch
Risk: Knee flexion at end range of motion with rotational forces on hinge joint may stress the medial collateral ligament and menisci	
Plough	Double knee to chest
Risk: Loaded neck flexion can sprain cervical ligaments and increase pressure in cervical discs	
Back hyperextension	Back extension to normal standing lumbar lordosis
Risk: Hyperextension of the back past the anatomical position can strain lumbar musculature	
Full neck rolls	Lateral neck stretches
Risk: Stretches cervical ligaments, increases cervical disc pressure and may impinge arterial flow, resulting in dizziness	
Flexion with rotation	Supine crunches with rotation-flexion followed by rotation
Risk: Flexion with rotation increases pressure and shear forces on spinal discs, common cause of low back injuries	
Standing toe touch	Standing hamstring stretch, back flat
Risk: Increases pressure in lumbar discs and overstretches lumbar ligaments	

Adapted from Corbin B, Lindsey R. Concepts of Physical Fitness with Laboratories. 5th ed. Dubuque, IA: William C. Brown Publishers, 1985.

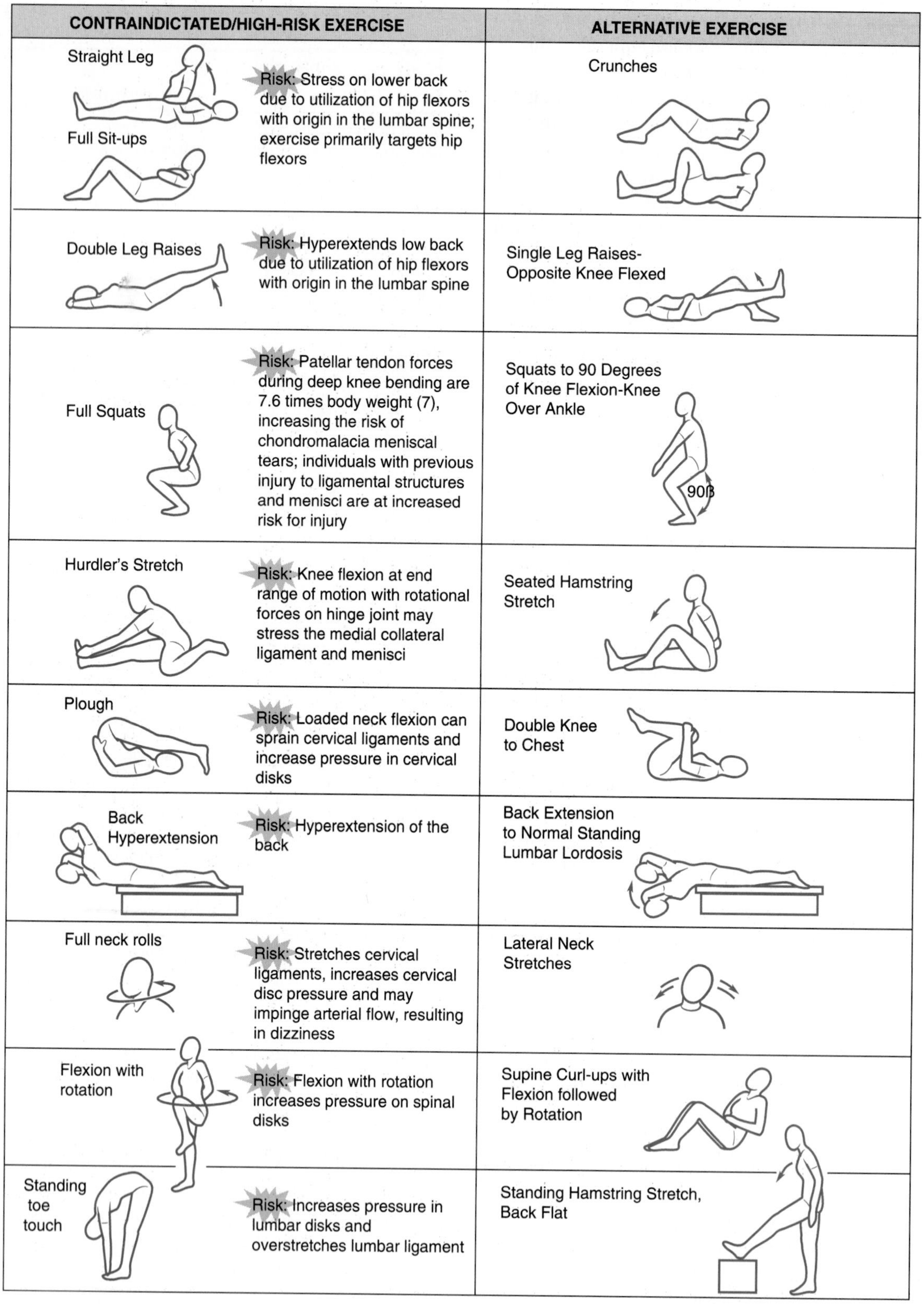

CONTRAINDICTATED/HIGH-RISK EXERCISE		ALTERNATIVE EXERCISE
Straight Leg Full Sit-ups	Risk: Stress on lower back due to utilization of hip flexors with origin in the lumbar spine; exercise primarily targets hip flexors	Crunches
Double Leg Raises	Risk: Hyperextends low back due to utilization of hip flexors with origin in the lumbar spine	Single Leg Raises-Opposite Knee Flexed
Full Squats	Risk: Patellar tendon forces during deep knee bending are 7.6 times body weight (7), increasing the risk of chondromalacia meniscal tears; individuals with previous injury to ligamental structures and menisci are at increased risk for injury	Squats to 90 Degrees of Knee Flexion-Knee Over Ankle 90ß
Hurdler's Stretch	Risk: Knee flexion at end range of motion with rotational forces on hinge joint may stress the medial collateral ligament and menisci	Seated Hamstring Stretch
Plough	Risk: Loaded neck flexion can sprain cervical ligaments and increase pressure in cervical disks	Double Knee to Chest
Back Hyperextension	Risk: Hyperextension of the back	Back Extension to Normal Standing Lumbar Lordosis
Full neck rolls	Risk: Stretches cervical ligaments, increases cervical disc pressure and may impinge arterial flow, resulting in dizziness	Lateral Neck Stretches
Flexion with rotation	Risk: Flexion with rotation increases pressure on spinal disks	Supine Curl-ups with Flexion followed by Rotation
Standing toe touch	Risk: Increases pressure in lumbar disks and overstretches lumbar ligament	Standing Hamstring Stretch, Back Flat

Figure 79.1. Common high-risk exercises and recommendations for alternative exercises.

If any questions are answered with a no response, replace the activity with a safe exercise which is more effective in achieving the ultimate goal.

The personal trainer or fitness instructor working one-on-one has only to make decisions regarding the safety and effectiveness of exercises for one client at a time. This task is easier than evaluating a group exercise class; however, the same procedure should be used. Several of the common high risk exercises and recommendations for alternative exercises are outlined in Figure 79.1.

▶ SUMMARY

First and foremost, the exercise professional should attempt to prevent injury through careful review of the medical history, fitness level, and injury history. Based on this information, an exercise prescription can be developed to prevent exercise-related injuries, improve specific fitness components and assist in meeting goals. Warning signs of overtraining (fatigue, insomnia, and loss of appetite) and injury (pain, stiffness, or a decline in performance) should be monitored by the client and exercise professional. Early recognition and appropriate modification of the exercise program may prevent development of serious overuse injuries. In the event that an injury does occur, prompt recognition and application of acute care treatments will help minimize the time required to return to full activity. If the injury is serious, the exercise professional should refer clients for medical evaluation and diagnosis.

Suggested Readings

American College of Sports Medicine.*ACSM's Health/Fitness Facility Standards and Guidelines.* Champaign: Human Kinetics, 1992.

American College of Sports Medicine. *ACSM's Guidelines for Exercise Testing and Prescription,* 2nd ed. Baltimore: Williams & Wilkins, 1995.

American College of Sports Medicine. *ACSM's Health/Fitness Facility Standards and Guidelines.* Champaign: Human Kinetics, 1992.

American Heart Association. Basic Life Support Heartsaver Guide, 1993.

Blair SE, Kohl HW, Goodyear NN. Rates and risks for runners and exercise injuries: studies in three populations. *Res Q Exerc Sport* 58:221, 1987.

Caspersen CJ. Physical inactivity and coronary heart disease. *Phys Sportsmed* 15:11,43–44, 1987.

Clarke RSJ, Hellon RF, Lind AR. Vascular reactions of the human forearm to cold. *Clin Sci* 14:165, 1958.

Corbin B, Lindsey R. *Concepts of Physical Fitness with Laboratories* 5th ed. Dubuque: Wm.C. Brown Publishers, 1985.

Fahey TD. *Athletic Training: Principles and Practice.* Palo Alto: Mayfield Publishing, 1986.

Frankel VH, Hang YS. Recent advances in the biomechanics of sports injuries. *Acta Orthop Scand* 46:484, 1975.

Garrick JG, Gillien DM, Whiteside P. The epidemiology of aerobic dance injuries. *Am J Sports Med* 14:67, 1986.

Grana WA, Kalenak A, eds. *Clinical Sports Medicine.* Philadelphia: W.B. Saunders, 1991.

Halvorson FA. Therapeutic heat and cold for athletic injuries. *Phys Sportsmed* 18 (5):87–94, 1990.

Hocutt JE, et al. Cryotherapy in ankle sprains. *Am J Sport Med* 10:316, 1982.

Koplan JP, et al. An epidemiologic study of the benefits and risks of running. *JAMA* 248(23):3118, 1982.

Kruse DL, McBeath AA. Bicycle accidents and injuries. *Am J Sport Med* 8:342, 1980.

MacDonald MJ. Postexercise late onset hypoglycemia in insulin-dependent diabetic patients. *Diabetes Care* 10:584, 1987.

McKeag DB, Dolan C. Overuse syndromes of the lower extremity. *Phys Sportsmed* 17:108, 1989.

Mechelen WV. Running injuries: A review of epidemiological literature. *Sports Med* 14:320, 1992.

Meeusen R, Lievens P. The use of cryotherapy in sports injuries. *Sports Med* 3:398, 1986.

Pollock ML, et al. Effects of frequency and duration of training on attrition and incidence of injury. *Med Sci Sport Exerc* 9: 31, 1977.

Powell KE, et al. An epidemiological perspective on the causes of running injuries. *Phys Sportsmed* 14:100, 1986.

Powell KE, et al. Physical activity and the incidence of heart disease. *Ann Rev Publ Health* 8:253, 1987.

Ragosta M, Crabtree J, Sturner WQ, et al. Death during recreational exercise in the State of Rhode Island. *Med Sci Sports Exerc* 16:339, 1984.

Saal JS, Saal JA. Strength training and flexibility. In: White AH, Anderson R, eds. *Conservative Care of Low Back Pain.* Baltimore: Williams & Wilkins, 1991.

Siscovick DS, et al. The incidence of primary cardiac arrest during vigorous exercise. *N Engl J Med* 311, 1984.

Skinner JS. *Exercise Testing and Exercise Prescription for Special Cases.* Philadelphia: Lea & Febiger, 1987.

Thompson PD, et al. Incidence of death during jogging in Rhode Island from 1975 through 1980. *JAMA* 247:2535, 1982.

Thompson PD. The safety of exercise testing and participation. In: Durstine JL, King AC, Painter PL, et al. *Resource Manual for Guidelines for Exercise Testing and Prescription.* 2nd ed. Philadelphia: Lea & Febiger, 1993.

Waylonis GW. The physiologic effects of ice massage. *Arch Phys Med Rehabil* 48:37, 1967.

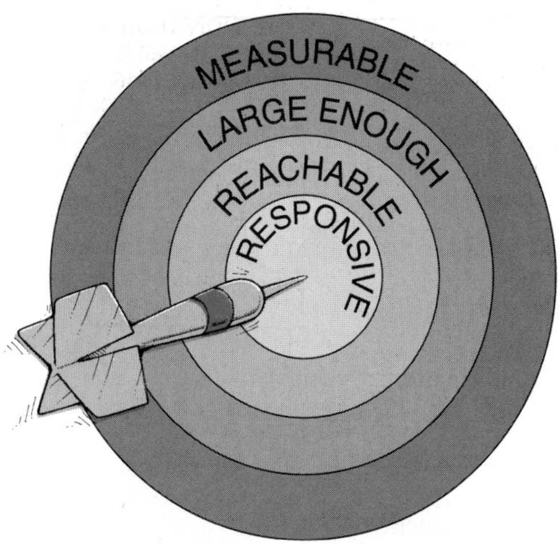

Figure 80.5. Four criteria for a targetable market.

ready has several similar facilities. The key factor is the number of customers an organization can attract to its product and services. All identifiable target segments can potentially be reached. Exercise professionals must be able to answer two basic questions in this regard, however:

1. What is the best method for communication with a specific target segment?
2. How much will it cost?

In the final analysis, the ultimate decision involves the key criterion: profitability.

Are the people in this target segment willing to buy the products and services? Can a marketable product or service and a strategy for selling these products and services be developed that will give an organization a perceived advantage over other organizations with similar products and services? The challenge is to identify consumer needs and wants and then to provide it at a price they are willing to pay. Marketing studies document the fact that people are responsive when needs and wants are satisfied. For example, some individuals question the wide popularity of independent, stairclimbing machines. Several of the reasons advanced including safety, convenience, enjoyment, variety, etc. illustrate the concept of consumer responsiveness in action.

Even with satisfactory answers to questions imposed by the four criteria for market segmentation, the process of identifying appropriate market segments can be a challenging task. At best, markets are complicated, constantly changing entities. To be successful, exercise professionals need to employ the best methods available to identify and define markets. The relatively popular methods of trial and error, intuition, and copying the techniques and focuses of other individuals are often ineffective. Although no single method has been found to work in all situations, the literature suggests at least four effective approaches to market segmentation:

- Demographic
- Geographic
- Psychographic
- Behavioral

Demographic Segmentation

When the market is divided demographically, target groups are identified by variables such as age, gender, income, occupation, education and household. Such variables are relatively accessible and easy to quantify. Demographic variables are often used to shape the size and features of a market segment even when other (non-demographic) factors, such as lifestyle, are also used. In fact, demographic variables often need support from other factors to identify an appropriate segment. For example, a physically active group of individuals with a high degree of disposable income may comprise an excellent target market.

Geographic Segmentation

Where consumers live and work strongly affects needs, wants and behavioral patterns. Subdivision, urban living, commuting distance, county, state, and related variables become the basis for geographic segmentation. If convenience is an important factor in deciding when someone exercises, the location of the fitness center relative to the workplace and the residence becomes a marketing consideration. By the same token, if a fitness center is located in a geographic region where either snow or sunshine is present for most of the year, the organization should (and probably will) gear some products and services to the climate.

Psychographic Segmentation

Psychographic variables include such factors as lifestyle, personality, attitudes, self-concept and other psychological influences on consumer behavior. Although such variables are fairly difficult to obtain and measure, psychographic information is critical to understanding consumer interests, traits they possess that influence behavior, and how they see themselves.

Behavioral Segmentation

In this approach, consumers are grouped behaviorally according to response to specific features of products and services, as well as to benefits they may desire from those products and services. In the fitness and health club arena, several examples illustrate behavioral segmentation including the 30-minute workout, the $99 yearly membership, and exercise programs focused on losing weight.

Identifying Target Markets

Marketing strategies aimed at everyone and all groups in a total market seldom succeed. Results-oriented marketers understand the importance of knowing the characteristics of potential markets. Concurrently, they can successfully implement techniques to identify important target segments within the total market and design a specific marketing mix to appeal to each target segment. The fundamental benefit to the fitness and health club is more aggregate sales and profits from satisfying selected segments, than from unfocused attempts on the total market.

PLANNING A SUCCESSFUL MARKETING PROGRAM

Proper planning and preparation must occur before exercise professionals can act purposefully and effectively to help achieve organizational goals. Planning is deciding in the present what to do in the future. It involves both determining a desired future and taking the necessary steps to bring it about. Collectively, it is a process whereby the decision makers of an organization reconcile resources with goals and opportunities. All organizations carry out some planning. The preparation of an annual budget, for example, represents planning.

Commercial fitness organizations vary considerably in how extensive, thorough, and formally they approach planning marketing. It is indisputable, however, that proper planning for a marketing program can yield positive results. Though planning can be overdone, excessive efforts are usually not a problem in a commercial fitness organization. Rather, the main issue is the development of appropriate planning procedures and systems to enhance organization-wide participation and in finding the competence to carry out these procedures.

If proper procedures are identified and implemented, several distinct benefits from such planning accrue including:

- Encouraging systematic, before-the-fact thinking by management
- Leads to better coordination of organizational efforts
- Facilitates development of performance standards for control
- Causes the organization to sharpen guiding objectives and policies
- Results in better preparation for sudden and unexpected situations
- Brings about a more vivid sense of interacting responsibilities in staff members who participate in planning

The "Truths" of Human Behavior

A successful marketing plan focuses on several fundamental truths concerning business behavior, including the following:

- Most purchase decisions are made unconsciously. Individuals do not react as quickly to promotional efforts as an organization might prefer. Even when individuals finally act, the reason may be unknown.
- Marketing efforts can be almost twice as effective if they are directed at both right-brained and left-brained individuals. Marketing efforts that do not take into account brain orientation of the audience are irresponsible, outdated, wasteful, and ill-advised. Forty-five percent of people are right-brained (influenced by emotional, aesthetic appeals). A comparable number are left-brained individuals who respond to logical, sequential reasoning. The remainder (10%) are "balanced-brained."
- Documented data on individual attitudes and values exists—information that can provide substantial assistance to marketing efforts. Fitness organizations should address marketing efforts to the value structure of the customer base. Health-fitness organizations must recognize that these values may change periodically.
- Sales can be influenced by two bonds—the human bond and the business bond. Positive relationships, as well as basic business considerations affect sales. If all other factors are equal, people prefer to do business with someone with whom they have a human bond, rather than with someone with whom they do not. A human bond involves any act on the part of the organization that reinforces a caring attitude about the customer and meets individual, specific needs.
- One of the most basic human needs is identity. An organization should recognize that each of its customers is a unique person with special qualities and avoid treating individuals as prospects. Potential clients are more than simply members of a particular demographic group, they are people.
- People have a basic need to belong. Steps should be undertaken to intensify that feeling for members of a health-fitness club (e.g., frequent mailings, personal service, first name greetings).
- Customers buy more than merely an organizational product or service. The organization is selling the total of the organization and its employees. In addition to a specific product, the decision to purchase is often influenced by other factors, including reputation, service policies, status of the offerings, personalities and appearance of employees, and the physical plant/facility.
- People tend to remember the most fascinating element of a marketing effort, not necessarily the product or service being marketed. The organization needs a "share of mind" before it can earn a "share of market." In order to interest prospective customers, relate offerings directly to them so that the product or service is the most interesting part of the message.

The "Truths" of Marketing

Understanding the disparity between a marketing myth and a marketing reality may mean the difference between success and failure in efforts to be competitive.

Appendix A.1 *(continued)*

Activity Coding	METs Used	Major Heading	Specific Activity
05030	3.5	Home activities	Cleaning, house or cabin, general
05040	2.5	Home activities	Cleaning, light (dusting, straightening up, vacuuming, changing linen, carrying out trash), moderate effort
05041	2.3	Home activities	Wash dishes-standing or in general (not broken into stand/walk components)
	2.3	Home activities	Wash dishes: cleaning dishes from table-walking
05050	2.5	Home activities	Cooking or food preparation-standing or sitting or in general (not broken into stand/walk components)
05051	2.5	Home activities	Serving food, setting table-implied walking or standing
05052	2.5	Home activities	Cooking or food preparation-walking
05055	2.5	Home activities	Putting away groceries (e.g., carrying groceries, shopping without a grocery cart)
05056	8.0	Home activities	Carrying groceries upstairs
05060	3.5	Home activities	Food shopping, with grocery cart
05065	2.0	Home activities	Standing-shopping (non-grocery shopping)
05066	2.3	Home activities	Walking-shopping (non-grocery shopping)
05070	2.3	Home activities	Ironing
05080	1.5	Home activities	Sitting, knitting, sewing, light wrapping (presents)
05090	2.0	Home activities	Implied standing-laundry, fold or hang clothes, put clothes in washer or dryer, packing suitcase
05095	2.3	Home activities	Implied walking-putting away clothes, gathering clothes to pack, putting away laundry
05100	2.0	Home activities	Making bed
05110	5.0	Home activities	Maple syruping/sugar bushing (including carrying buckets, carrying wood)
05120	6.0	Home activities	Moving furniture, household
05130	5.5	Home activities	Scrubbing floors, on hands and knees
05140	4.0	Home activities	Sweeping garage, sidewalk or outside of house
05145	7.0	Home activities	Moving household items, carrying boxes
05146	3.5	Home activities	Standing-packing/unpacking boxes, occasional lifting of household items light-moderate effort
05147	3.0	Home activities	Implied walking-putting away household items-moderate effort
05150	9.0	Home activities	Move household items upstairs, carrying boxes or furniture
05160	2.5	Home activities	Standing-light (pump gas, change light bulb, etc.)
05165	3.0	Home activities	Walking-light, noncleaning (ready to leave, shut/lock doors, close windows, etc.)
05170	2.5	Home activities	Sitting-playing with children-light
05171	2.8	Home activities	Standing-playing with children-light
05175	4.0	Home activities	Walk/run-playing with children-moderate
05180	5.0	Home activities	Walk/run-playing with children-vigorous
05185	3.0	Home activities	Child care: sitting/kneeling-dressing, bathing, grooming, feeding, occasional lifting of child-light effort
05186	3.5	Home activities	Child care: standing-dressing, bathing, grooming, feeding, occasional lifting of child-light effort
06010	3.0	Home repair	Airplane repair
06020	4.5	Home repair	Automobile body work
06030	3.0	Home repair	Automobile repair
06040	3.0	Home repair	Carpentry, general, workshop (T 620)
06050	6.0	Home repair	Carpentry, outside house (T 640), installing rain gutters
06060	4.5	Home repair	Carpentry, finishing or refinishing cabinets or furniture
06070	7.5	Home repair	Carpentry, sawing hardwood
06080	5.0	Home repair	Caulking, chinking log cabin
06090	4.5	Home repair	Caulking, except log cabin
06100	5.0	Home repair	Cleaning gutters
06110	5.0	Home repair	Excavating garage
06120	5.0	Home repair	Hanging storm windows
06130	4.5	Home repair	Laying or removing carpet
06140	4.5	Home repair	Laying tile or linoleum
06150	5.0	Home repair	Painting, outside house (T 650)
06160	4.5	Home repair	Painting, papering, plastering, scraping, inside house, hanging sheet rock, remodeling (T 630)

Appendix A.1 *(continued)*

Activity Coding	METs Used	Major Heading	Specific Activity
06170	3.0	Home repair	Put on and removal of tarp-sailboat
06180	6.0	Home repair	Roofing
06190	4.5	Home repair	Sanding floors with a power sander
06200	4.5	Home repair	Scrape and paint sailboat or powerboat
06210	5.0	Home repair	Spreading dirt with a shovel
06220	4.5	Home repair	Wash and wax hull of sailboat, car, powerboat, airplane
06230	4.5	Home repair	Washing fence
06240	3.0	Home repair	Wiring, plumbing
07010	0.9	Inactivity, quiet	Lying quietly, reclining (watch television), lying quietly in bed-awake
07020	1.0	Inactivity, quiet	Sitting quietly (riding in a car, listening to a lecture or music, watch television or a movie)
07030	0.9	Inactivity, quiet	Sleeping
07040	1.2	Inactivity, quiet	Standing quietly (standing in a line)
07050	1.0	Inactivity, light	Recline-writing
07060	1.0	Inactivity, light	Recline-talking or talking on phone
07070	1.0	Inactivity, light	Recline-reading
08010	5.0	Lawn and garden	Carrying, loading or stacking wood, loading/unloading or carrying lumber
08020	6.0	Lawn and garden	Chopping wood, splitting logs
08030	5.0	Lawn and garden	Clearing land, hauling branches
08040	5.0	Lawn and garden	Digging sandbox
08050	5.0	Lawn and garden	Digging, spading, filling garden (T 590)
08060	6.0	Lawn and garden	Gardening with heavy power tools, tilling a garden (see occupation, shoveling)
08080	5.0	Lawn and garden	Laying crushed rock
08090	5.0	Lawn and garden	Laying sod
08095	5.5	Lawn and garden	Mowing lawn, general
08100	2.5	Lawn and garden	Mowing lawn, riding mower (T 550)
08110	6.0	Lawn and garden	Mowing lawn, walk, hand mower (T 570)
08120	4.5	Lawn and garden	Mowing lawn, walk, power mower (T 590)
08130	4.5	Lawn and garden	Operating snow blower, walking
08140	4.0	Lawn and garden	Planting seedlings, shrubs
08150	4.5	Lawn and garden	Planting trees
08160	4.0	Lawn and garden	Raking lawn (T 600)
08170	4.0	Lawn and garden	Raking roof with snow rake
08180	3.0	Lawn and garden	Riding snow blower
08190	4.0	Lawn and garden	Sacking grass, leaves
08200	6.0	Lawn and garden	Shoveling, snow, by hand (T 610)
08210	4.5	Lawn and garden	Trimming shrubs or trees, manual cutter
08215	3.5	Lawn and garden	Trimming shrubs or trees, power cutter
08220	2.5	Lawn and garden	Walking, applying fertilizer or seeding a lawn
08230	1.5	Lawn and garden	Watering lawn or garden, standing or walking
08240	4.5	Lawn and garden	Weeding, cultivating garden (T 580)
08245	5.0	Lawn and garden	Gardening, general
08250	3.0	Lawn and garden	Implied walking/standing-picking up yard, light
09010	1.5	Miscellaneous	Sitting, card playing, playing board games
09020	2.0	Miscellaneous	Standing-drawing (writing), casino gambling
09030	1.3	Miscellaneous	Sitting-reading, book, newspaper, etc.
09040	1.8	Miscellaneous	Sitting-writing, desk work
09050	1.8	Miscellaneous	Standing-talking or talking on the phone
09055	1.5	Miscellaneous	Sitting-talking or talking on the phone
09060	1.8	Miscellaneous	Sitting-studying, general, including reading and/or writing
09065	1.8	Miscellaneous	Sitting-in class, general, including note-taking or class discussion
09070	1.8	Miscellaneous	Standing-reading
10010	1.8	Music playing	Accordion
10020	2.0	Music playing	Cello
10030	2.5	Music playing	Conducting
10040	4.0	Music playing	Drums
10050	2.0	Music playing	Flute (sitting)
10060	2.0	Music playing	Horn
10070	2.5	Music playing	Piano or organ

(continued)

Appendix A.1 *(continued)*

Activity Coding	METs Used	Major Heading	Specific Activity
10080	3.5	Music playing	Trombone
10090	2.5	Music playing	Trumpet
10100	2.5	Music playing	Violin
10110	2.0	Music playing	Woodwind
10120	2.0	Music playing	Guitar, classical, folk (sitting)
10125	3.0	Music playing	Guitar, rock and roll band (standing)
10130	4.0	Music playing	Marching band, playing an instrument, baton twirling, walking)
10135	3.5	Music playing	Marching band, drum major (walking)
11010	4.0	Occupation	Bakery, general
11020	2.3	Occupation	Bookbinding
11030	6.0	Occupation	Building road (including hauling debris, driving heavy machinery)
11035	2.0	Occupation	Building road, directing traffic (standing)
11040	3.5	Occupation	Carpentry, general
11050	8.0	Occupation	Carrying heavy loads, such as bricks
11060	8.0	Occupation	Carrying moderate loads up stairs, moving boxes (16–40 pounds)
11070	2.5	Occupation	Chambermaid
11080	6.5	Occupation	Coal mining, drilling coal, rock
11090	6.5	Occupation	Coal mining, erecting supports
11100	6.0	Occupation	Coal mining, general
11110	7.0	Occupation	Coal mining, shoveling coal
11120	5.5	Occupation	Construction, outside, remodeling
11130	3.5	Occupation	Electrical work, plumbing
11140	8.0	Occupation	Farming, bailng hay, cleaning barn, poultry work
11150	3.5	Occupation	Farming, chasing cattle, nonstrenuous
11160	2.5	Occupation	Farming, driving harvester
11170	2.5	Occupation	Farming, driving tractor
11180	4.0	Occupation	Farming, feeding small animals
11190	4.5	Occupation	Farming, feeding cattle
11200	8.0	Occupation	Farming, forking straw bales
11210	3.0	Occupation	Farming, milking by hand
11220	1.5	Occupation	Farming, milking by machine
11230	5.5	Occupation	Farming, shoveling grain
11240	12.0	Occupation	Fire fighter, general
11245	11.0	Occupation	Fire fighter, climbing ladder with full gear
11246	8.0	Occupation	Fire fighter, hauling hoses on ground
11250	17.0	Occupation	Forestry, ax chopping, fast
11260	5.0	Occupation	Forestry, ax chopping, slow
11270	7.0	Occupation	Forestry, barking trees
11280	11.0	Occupation	Forestry, carrying logs
11290	8.0	Occupation	Forestry, felling trees
11300	8.0	Occupation	Forestry, general
11310	5.0	Occupation	Forestry, hoeing
11320	6.0	Occupation	Forestry, planting by hand
11330	7.0	Occupation	Forestry, sawing by hand
11340	4.5	Occupation	Forestry, sawing, power
11350	9.0	Occupation	Forestry, trimming trees
11360	4.0	Occupation	Forestry, weeding
11370	4.5	Occupation	Furriery
11380	6.0	Occupation	Horse grooming
11390	8.0	Occupation	Horse racing, galloping
11400	6.5	Occupation	Horse racing, trotting
11410	2.6	Occupation	Horse racing, walking
11420	3.5	Occupation	Locksmith
11430	2.5	Occupation	Machine tooling, machining, working sheet metal
11440	3.0	Occupation	Machine tooling, operating lathe
11450	5.0	Occupation	Machine tooling, operating punch press
11460	4.0	Occupation	Machine tooling, tapping and drilling
11470	3.0	Occupation	Machine tooling, welding
11480	7.0	Occupation	Masonry, concrete

Appendix A.1 *(continued)*

Activity Coding	METs Used	Major Heading	Specific Activity
11485	4.0	Occupation	Masseur, masseuse (standing)
11490	7.0	Occupation	Moving, pushing heavy objects, 75 lbs or more (desks, moving van work)
11500	2.5	Occupation	Operating heavy duty equipment/automated, not driving
11510	4.5	Occupation	Orange grove work
11520	2.3	Occupation	Printing (standing)
11525	2.5	Occupation	Police, directing traffic (standing)
11526	2.0	Occupation	Police, driving a squad car (sitting)
11527	1.3	Occupation	Police, riding in a squad car (sitting)
11528	8.0	Occupation	Police, making an arrest (standing)
11530	2.5	Occupation	Shoe repair, general
11540	8.5	Occupation	Shoveling, digging ditches
11550	9.0	Occupation	Shoveling, heavy (more than 16 lbs. min^{-1})
11560	6.0	Occupation	Shoveling, light (less than 10 lbs. min^{-1})
11570	7.0	Occupation	Shoveling, moderate (10–15 lbs. min^{-1})
11580	1.5	Occupation	Sitting-light office work, in general (chemistry lab work, light use of handtools, watch repair or micro-assembly, light assembly/repair)
11585	1.5	Occupation	Sitting-meetings, general, and/or with talking involved
11590	2.5	Occupation	Sitting; moderate (heavy levers, riding mower/forklift, crane operation)
11600	2.5	Occupation	Standing; light (bartending, store clerk, assembling, filing, xeroxing, put up Christmas tree)
11610	3.0	Occupation	Standing; light/moderate (assemble/repair heavy parts, welding, stocking, auto repair, pack boxes for moving, etc.), patient care (as in nursing)
11620	3.5	Occupation	Standing; moderate (assembling at fast rate, lifting 50 lbs, hitch/twisting ropes)
11630	4.0	Occupation	Standing; moderate/heavy (lifting more than 50 lb, masonry, painting, paper hanging)
11640	5.0	Occupation	Steel mill, fettling
11650	5.5	Occupation	Steel mill, forging
11660	8.0	Occupation	Steel mill, hand rolling
11670	8.0	Occupation	Steel mill, merchant mill rolling
11680	11.0	Occupation	Steel mill, removing stag
11690	7.5	Occupation	Steel mill, tending furnace
11700	5.5	Occupation	Steel mill, tipping molds
11710	8.0	Occupation	Steel mill, working in general
11720	2.5	Occupation	Tailoring, cutting
11730	2.5	Occupation	Tailoring, general
11740	2.0	Occupation	Tailoring, hand sewing
11750	2.5	Occupation	Tailoring, machine sewing
11760	4.0	Occupation	Tailoring, pressing
11766	6.5	Occupation	Truck driving, loading and unloading truck (standing)
11770	1.5	Occupation	Typing, electric, manual or computer
11780	6.0	Occupation	Using heavy power tools such pneumatic tools (jackhammers, drills, etc.)
11790	8.0	Occupation	Using heavy tools (not power) such as shovel, pick, tunnel bar, spade
11791	2.0	Occupation	Walking on job, less than 2.0 mph (in office or lab area), very slow
11792	3.5	Occupation	Walking on job, 3.0 mph, in office, moderate speed, not carrying anything
11793	4.0	Occupation	Walking on job, 3.5 mph, in office, brisk speed, not carrying anything
11795	3.0	Occupation	Walking, 2.5 mph, slowly and carrying light objects less than 25 lbs
11800	4.0	Occupation	Walking, 3.0 mph, moderately and carrying light objects less than 25 lbs
11810	4.5	Occupation	Walking, 3.5 mph, briskly and carrying objects less than 25 lbs
11820	5.0	Occupation	Walking or walk downstairs or standing, carrying objects about 25–49 lbs
11830	6.5	Occupation	Walking or walk downstairs or standing, carrying objects about 50–74 lbs
11840	7.5	Occupation	Walking or walk downstairs or standing, carrying objects about 75–99 lbs
11850	8.5	Occupation	Walking or walk downstairs or standing, carrying objects about 100 lbs and over
11870	3.0	Occupation	Working in scene shop, theater actor, backstage, employee
12010	6.0	Running	Job/walk combination (jobbing component of less than 10 min) (T 180)
12020	7.0	Running	Jogging, general
12030	8.0	Running	Running, 5 mph (12 min. $mile^{-1}$)
12040	9.0	Running	Running, 5.2 mph (11.5 min. $mile^{-1}$)
12050	10.0	Running	Running, 6 mph (10 min. $mile^{-1}$)

(continued)

Appendix A.1 *(continued)*

Activity Coding	METs Used	Major Heading	Specific Activity
12060	11.0	Running	Running, 6.7 mph (9 min. mile^{-1})
12070	11.5	Running	Running, 7 mph (8.5 min. mile^{-1})
12080	12.5	Running	Running, 7.5 mph (8 min. mile^{-1})
12090	13.5	Running	Running, 8 mph (7.5 min. mile^{-1})
12100	14.0	Running	Running 8.6 mph (7 min. mile^{-1})
12110	15.0	Running	Running, 9 mph (6.5 min. mile^{-1})
12120	16.0	Running	Running, 10 mph (6 min. mile^{-1})
12130	18.0	Running	Running, 10.9 mph (5.5 min. mile^{-1})
12140	9.0	Running	Running, cross-country
12150	8.0	Running	Running, general (T 200)
12160	8.0	Running	Running, in place
12170	15.0	Running	Running, stairs, up
12180	10.0	Running	Running, on a track, team practice
12190	8.0	Running	Running, training, pushing wheelchair, marathon wheeling
12195	3.0	Running	Running, wheeling, general
13000	2.5	Self-care	Standing-getting ready for bed, in general
13009	1.0	Self-care	Sitting on toilet
13010	2.0	Self-care	Bathing (sitting)
13020	2.5	Self-care	Dressing, undressing (standing or sitting)
13030	1.5	Self-care	Eating (sitting)
13035	2.0	Self-care	Talking and eating or eating only (standing)
13040	2.5	Self-care	Sitting or standing-grooming (washing, shaving, brushing teeth, urinating, washing hands, put on make-up)
13050	4.0	Self-care	Showering, toweling off (standing)
14010	1.5	Sexual activity	Active, vigorous effort
14020	1.3	Sexual activity	General, moderate effort
14030	1.0	Sexual activity	Passive, light effort, kissing, hugging
15010	3.5	Sports	Archery (nonhunting)
15020	7.0	Sports	Badminton, competitive (T 450)
15030	4.5	Sports	Badminton, social singles and doubles, general
15040	8.0	Sports	Basketball, game (T 490)
15050	6.0	Sports	Basketball, nongame, general (T 480)
15060	7.0	Sports	Basketball, officiating (T 500)
15070	4.5	Sports	Basketball, shooting baskets
15075	6.5	Sports	Basketball, wheelchair
15080	2.5	Sports	Billiards
15090	3.0	Sports	Bowling (T 390)
15100	12.0	Sports	Boxing, in ring, general
15110	6.0	Sports	Boxing, bunching bag
15120	9.0	Sports	Boxing, sparring
15130	7.0	Sports	Broomball
15135	5.0	Sports	Children's games (hopscotch, 4-square, dodgeball, playground apparatus, t-ball, tetherball, marbles, jacks, arcade games)
15140	4.0	Sports	Coaching: football, soccer, basketball, baseball, swimming, etc.
15150	5.0	Sports	Cricket (batting, bowling)
15160	2.5	Sports	Croquet
15170	4.0	Sports	Curling
15180	2.5	Sports	Darts, wall or lawn
15190	6.0	Sports	Drag racing, pushing or driving a car
15200	6.0	Sports	Fencing
15210	9.0	Sports	Football, competitive
15230	8.0	Sports	Football, touch, flag, general (T 510)
15235	2.5	Sports	Football or baseball, playing catch
15240	3.0	Sports	Frisbee playing, general
15250	3.5	Sports	Frisbee, ultimate
15255	4.5	Sports	Golf, general
15260	5.5	Sports	Golf, carrying clubs (T 090)
15270	3.0	Sports	Golf, miniature, driving range
15280	5.0	Sports	Golf, pulling clubs (T 080)

Appendix A.1 *(continued)*

Activity Coding	METs Used	Major Heading	Specific Activity
15290	3.5	Sports	Golf, using power cart (T 070)
15300	4.0	Sports	Gymnastics, general
15310	4.0	Sports	Hacky sack
15320	12.0	Sports	Handball, general (T 520)
15330	8.0	Sports	Handball, team
15340	3.5	Sports	Hang gliding
15350	8.0	Sports	Hockey, field
15360	8.0	Sports	Hockey, ice
15370	4.0	Sports	Horseback riding, general
15380	3.5	Sports	Horseback riding, saddling horse
15390	6.5	Sports	Horseback riding, trotting
15400	2.5	Sports	Horseback riding, walking
15410	3.0	Sports	Horseshoe pitching, quoits
15420	12.0	Sports	Jai alai
15430	10.0	Sports	Judo, jujitsu, karate, kick boxing, tae kwon do
15440	4.0	Sports	Juggling
15450	7.0	Sports	Kickball
15460	8.0	Sports	Lacrosse
15470	4.0	Sports	Moto-cross
15480	9.0	Sports	Orienteering
15490	10.0	Sports	Paddleball, competitive
15500	6.0	Sports	Paddleball, casual, general (T 460)
15510	8.0	Sports	Polo
15520	10.0	Sports	Racquetball, competitive
15530	7.0	Sports	Racketball, casual, general (T 470)
15535	11.0	Sports	Rock climbing, ascending rock
15540	8.0	Sports	Rock climbing, rapelling
15550	12.0	Sports	Rope jumping, fast
15551	10.0	Sports	Rope jumping, moderate, general
15552	8.0	Sports	Rope jumping, slow
15560	10.0	Sports	Rugby
15570	3.0	Sports	Shuffleboard, lawn bowling
15580	5.0	Sports	Skateboarding
15590	7.0	Sports	Skating, roller (T 360)
15600	3.5	Sports	Sky diving
15605	10.0	Sports	Soccer, competitive
15610	7.0	Sports	Soccer, casual, general (T 540)
15620	5.0	Sports	Softball or baseball, fast or slow pitch, general (T 440)
15630	4.0	Sports	Softball, officiating
15640	6.0	Sports	Softball, pitching
15650	12.0	Sports	Squash (T 530)
15660	4.0	Sports	Table tennis, ping pong (T 410)
15670	4.0	Sports	Tai chi
15675	7.0	Sports	Tennis, general
15680	6.0	Sports	Tennis, doubles (T 430)
15690	8.0	Sports	Tennis, singles (T 420)
15700	3.5	Sports	Trampoline
15710	4.0	Sports	Volleyball, competitive, in gymnasium (T 400)
15720	3.0	Sports	Volleyball, noncompetitive; 6–9 member team, general
15725	8.0	Sports	Volleyball, beach
15730	6.0	Sports	Wrestling (one match = 5 min)
15731	7.0	Sports	Wallyball, general
16010	2.0	Transportation	Automobile or light truck (not a semi) driving
16020	2.0	Transportation	Flying airplane
16030	2.5	Transportation	Motor scooter, motor cycle
16040	6.0	Transportation	Pushing plane in and out of hangar
16050	3.0	Transportation	Driving heavy truck, tractor, bus
17010	7.0	Walking	Backpacking, general (T 050)
17020	3.5	Walking	Carrying infant or 15-lb load (e.g., suitcase), level ground or downstairs

(continued)

Appendix A.1 *(continued)*

Activity Coding	METs Used	Major Heading	Specific Activity
17025	9.0	Walking	Carrying load upstairs, general
17026	5.0	Walking	Carrying 1- to 15-lb load, upstairs
17027	6.0	Walking	Carrying 16- to 24-lb load, upstairs
17028	8.0	Walking	Carrying 25- to 49-lb load, upstairs
17029	10.0	Walking	Carrying 50- to 74-lb load, upstairs
17030	12.0	Walking	Carrying 74 + lb load, upstairs
17035	7.0	Walking	Climbing hills with 0- to 9-lb load
17040	7.5	Walking	Climbing hills with 10- to 20-lb load
17050	8.0	Walking	Climbing hills with 21- to 42-lb load
17060	9.0	Walking	Climbing hills with 42 + lb load
17070	3.0	Walking	Downstairs
17080	6.0	Walking	Hiking, cross country (T 040)
17090	6.5	Walking	Marching, rapidly, military
17100	2.5	Walking	Pushing or pulling stroller with child
17110	6.5	Walking	Race walking
17120	8.0	Walking	Rock or mountain climbing (T 060)
17130	8.0	Walking	Up stairs, using or climbing up ladder (T 030)
17140	4.0	Walking	Using crutches
17150	2.0	Walking	Walking, less than 2.0 mph, level ground, strolling, household walking, very slow
17160	2.5	Walking	Walking, 2.0 mph, level, slow pace, firm surface
17170	3.0	Walking	Walking, 2.5 mph, firm surface
17180	3.0	Walking	Walking, 2.5 mph, downhill
17190	3.5	Walking	Walking, 3.0 mph, level, moderate pace, firm surface
17200	4.0	Walking	Walking, 3.5 mph, level, brisk, firm surface
17210	6.0	Walking	Walking, 3.5 mph, uphill
17220	4.0	Walking	Walking, 4.0 mph, level, firm surface, very brisk pace
17230	4.5	Walking	Walking, 4.5 mph, level, firm surface, very, very brisk
17250	3.5	Walking	Walking, for pleasure, work break, walking the dog
17260	5.0	Walking	Walking, grass track
17270	4.0	Walking	Walking, to work or class (T 015)
18010	2.5	Water activities	Boating, power
18020	4.0	Water activities	Canoeing, on camping trip (T 270)
18030	7.0	Water activities	Canoeing, portaging
18040	3.0	Water activities	Canoeing, rowing, 2.0–3.9 mph, light effort
18050	7.0	Water activities	Canoeing, rowing, 4.0–5.9 mph, moderate effort
18060	12.0	Water activities	Canoeing, rowing, > 6 mph, vigorous effort
18070	3.5	Water activities	Canoeing, rowing, for pleasure, general (T 250)
18080	12.0	Water activities	Canoeing, rowing, in competition, or crew or sculling (T 260)
18090	3.0	Water activities	Diving, springboard or platform
18100	5.0	Water activities	Kayaking
18110	4.0	Water activities	Paddleboat
18120	3.0	Water activities	Sailing, boat and board sailing, windsurfing, ice sailing, general (T 235)
18130	5.0	Water activities	Sailing, in competition
18140	3.0	Water activities	Sailing, Sunfish/Laser/Hobby Cat, keel boats, ocean sailing, yachting
18150	6.0	Water activities	Skiing, water (T 220)
18160	7.0	Water activities	Skimobiling
18170	12.0	Water activities	Skindiving or scuba diving as frogman
18180	16.0	Water activities	Skindiving, fast
18190	12.5	Water activities	Skindiving, moderate
18200	7.0	Water activities	Skindiving, scuba diving, general (T 310)
18210	5.0	Water activities	Snorkeling (T 320)
18220	3.0	Water activities	Surfing, body or board
18230	10.0	Water activities	Swimming laps, freestyle, fast, vigorous effort
18240	8.0	Water activities	Swimming laps, freestyle, slow, moderate or light effort
18250	8.0	Water activities	Swimming, backstroke, general
18260	10.0	Water activities	Swimming, breaststroke, general
18270	11.0	Water activities	Swimming, butterfly, general
18280	11.0	Water activities	Swimming, crawl, fast (75 yards-min^{-1}), vigorous effort

Appendix A.1 *(continued)*

Activity Coding	METs Used	Major Heading	Specific Activity
18290	8.0	Water activities	Swimming, crawl, slow (50 yards-min/mile^{-1}), moderate or light effort
18300	6.0	Water activities	Swimming, lake, ocean, river (T 280, T 295)
18310	6.0	Water activities	Swimming, leisurely, not lap swimming, general
18320	8.0	Water activities	Swimming, sidestroke, general
18330	8.0	Water activities	Swimming, synchronized
18340	10.0	Water activities	Swimming, treading water, fast vigorous effort
18350	4.0	Water activities	Swimming, treading water, moderate effort, general
18360	10.0	Water activities	Water polo
18365	3.0	Water activities	Water volleyball
18370	5.0	Water activities	Whitewater rafting, kayaking, or canoeing
19010	6.0	Winter activities	Moving ice house (set up/drill holes, etc.)
19020	5.5	Winter activities	Skating, ice, 9 mph or less
19030	7.0	Winter activities	Skating, ice, general (T 360)
19040	9.0	Winter activities	Skating, ice, rapidly, more than 9 mph
19050	15.0	Winter activities	Skating, speed, competitive
19060	7.0	Winter activities	Ski jumping (climb up carrying skis)
19075	7.0	Winter activities	Skiing, general
19080	7.0	Winter activities	Skiing, cross-country, 2.5 mph, slow or light effort, ski walking
19090	8.0	Winter activities	Skiing, cross-country, 4.0–4.9 mph, moderate speed and effort, general
19100	9.0	Winter activities	Skiing, cross-country, 5.0–7.9 mph, brisk speed, vigorous effort
19110	14.0	Winter activities	Skiing, cross-country, > 8.0 mph, racing
19130	16.5	Winter activities	Skiing, cross-country, hard snow, uphill, maximum
19150	5.0	Winter activities	Skiing, downhill, light effort
19160	6.0	Winter activities	Skiing, downhill, moderate effort, general
19170	8.0	Winter activities	Skiing, downhill, vigorous effort, racing
19180	7.0	Winter activities	Sledding, tobogganing, bobsledding, luge (T 370)
19190	8.0	Winter activities	Snow shoeing
19200	3.5	Winter activities	Snowmobiling

coding physical data on physical activity by purpose and energy cost. The energy cost of specific activities listed in this Compendium were obtained primarily from the following previously published physical activity energy expenditure lists: Tecumseh Occupational Questionnaire (13, 14), Minnesota Leisure Time Physical Activity Questionnaire (LTPA) (5, 10), McArdle, Katch, and Katch's physical activity list (7, 9), the 7-Day Recall Physical Activity Questionnaire (2), and the American Health Foundation's physical activity list (8). Activities from the LTPA were identified by a T followed by a number (e.g., T115). By retaining the LTPA designator codes, the new list may be used to score the LTPA with its original physical activity intensity codes.

As would be expected, there was considerable overlap in energy expenditure values among the supplied lists. For example, the Minnesota LTPA, which was developed from the Tecumseh Leisure Time Questionnaire, identifies similar activities; while the list of activities from the 7-Day Physical Activity Recall questionnaire is nearly identical to that of McArdle, Katch, and Katch (9). In general, the majority of the energy expenditure lists were generated from Passmore and Durnin (11); while McArdle, Katch, and Katch (9) also used data derived from Bannister and Brown (1) and Howley and Glover (6). The intensity assigned to activities in this publication were determined by selecting a mean energy expenditure value from the eight sources mentioned previously. The representative intensity levels were determined by consensus of the authors.

Organization

The Compendium of Physical Activities is organized to maximize flexibility in coding, data entry, and interpretation of energy cost for each class and type of activity.

The coding scheme for the Compendium of Activities employs a five-digit code in order to categorize activities by their major heading (first two digits on the left), specific activity (last three digits on the right), and intensity (3-digit column). The coding scheme is organized in the following way:

00	000	0.0
major headings	specific activity	intensity

For example:

01	009	08.5
bicycling	bmx	METs

The Compendium is organized by activity types or purpose and includes activities of daily living or self care, leisure and recreation, occupation, and rest (Table A.1). The major head-

Table A.1. Major Types of Activities

Bicycling	Lawn and garden	Sexual activity
Conditioning exercises	Miscellaneous	Sports
Dancing	Music playing	Transportation
Fishing and hunting	Occupation	Walking
Home activities	Running	Water activities
Home repair	Self-Care	Winter activities
Inactivity		

ings explain the reason a person is engaging in a specific activity and is useful in categorizing activity types.

Identification of the proper major heading is the initial step in classifying an activity. However, it is possible that there may be more than one reason for performing an activity; thus, a specific activity may be listed under more than one major heading. For example, an individual may sit and read a book for pleasure in one situation and at another time read a document as a job requirement. These may be classified under the major headings of rest or inactivity and occupation depending on their purpose. Assumptions made for the placement of activities into major headings are listed in Appendix A.2.

The specific activity descriptions range from a general classification of an activity (e.g., tennis, general) to a detailed description that includes the form and intensity of the activity (e.g., tennis, singles, vigorous effort) depending on the information gathered by the survey method. Activities without a specified intensity are classified as "general." More detailed descriptions of activities are preferred since an appropriate intensity can be assigned. Guidelines for coding specific activities within major headings are listed in Appendix A.3.

All activities are assigned an intensity unit based on their rate of energy expenditure expressed as METs. The intensity of activities in the Compendium are classified as multiples of one MET or the ratio of the associated metabolic rate for the specific activity divided by the resting metabolic rate (RMR). For example, a 2-MET activity requires two times the metabolic energy expenditure of sitting quietly. One MET is also defined as the energy expenditure for sitting quietly, which for the average adult is approximately 3.5 ml of oxygen/kg body weight^{-1}/min^{-1} or 1 kcal/kg^{-1} body weight/h^{-1}.

A MET value was assigned to each activity in the Compendium and was based on the "best representation" from published lists and selected unpublished data as was previously mentioned. For activities not in the original lists, intensity was obtained from published literature, if possible, and assigned a MET value or estimated from similar known activities (3, 4, 11, 16).

Only data for adults were included in this Compendium. When children's games are listed in the Compendium, the intensity level is for adults participating in children's activities. Further, the Compendium is not intended to be used for adults with major neuromuscular handicaps or other conditions that would significantly alter their mechanical or metabolic efficiency.

Appendix A.2. Guidelines for Assigning Activities by Major Purpose or Intent

1. Conditioning exercises include activities with the intent of improving physical condition. This includes stationary ergometers (bicycling, rowing machines, treadmills, etc.) health club exercise, calisthenics, and aerobics.
2. Home repair includes all activity associated with the repair of a house and does not include housework. This is not an occupational task.
3. Sleeping, lying, sitting, and standing are classified as inactivity.
4. Home activities include all activities associated with maintaining the inside of a house and includes house cleaning, laundry, grocery shopping, and cooking.
5. Lawn and garden includes all activity associated with maintaining the yard and includes yard work, gardening, and snow removal.
6. Occupation includes all job-related physical activity where one is paid (gainful employment). Specific activities may be cross-referenced in other categories (such as reading, writing, driving a car, walking) and should be coded in this major heading if related to employment. Housework is occupational only if the person is earning money for the task.
7. Self-care includes all activity related to grooming, eating, bathing, etc.
8. Transportation includes energy expended for the primary purpose of going somewhere in a motorized vehicle.

Calculation of Energy Cost

Energy expenditure values can be expressed in kcal/kg^{-1} body weight/h^{-1}, kcal/min^{-1}, kcal/h^{-1} or kcal/24 h^{-1}. The most accurate way to determine the kilocalorie energy cost of an activity is to measure the kcal expended during rest (i.e., the RMR) and multiply that value by the MET values listed in the Compendium. Because RMR is fairly close to 1 kcal/kg body weight^{-1}/h^{-1}, the energy cost of activities may be expressed as multiples of the RMR (15). By multiplying the body weight in kg by the MET value and duration of activity, it is possible to estimate a kcal energy expenditure that is specific to a person's body weight. For example, bicycling at a 4 MET value expends 4 kcal/kg^{-1} body weight/h^{-1}. A 60 kg individual bicycling for 40 min expends the following: (4 METs $\times$ 60 kg body weight) $\times$ (40 min/60 min) $=$ 160 kcal. Dividing 160 kcal by 40 min equals 4 kcal/min^{-1}. Using the same formula for an 80 kg person would yield an energy expenditure of 213 kcal or 5.3 kcal/min^{-1}. However, it is important to note that to the extent the RMR is not equal to 1 kcal/kg body weight^{-1}/h^{-1} for individuals, then estimates of energy expenditure that include weight will more closely reflect body weight than the metabolic rate (2).

Use of the Compendium for PA Records or Diaries

For records or diaries the data collection forms should be organized in a way to identify each activity's major heading,

Appendix A.3. Guidelines for Coding Specific Activities

A. General guidelines: All activities should be coded as "general" if no other information about the activity is given. This applies primarily to intensity ratings. If any additional information is given, activities should be coded accordingly.

B. Specific guidelines

1. Bicycling
   a. Stationary cycling using cycle ergometers (all types), wind trainers, or other conditioning devices should be classified under the major heading of Conditioning Exercise, stationary cycling specific activities (codes 02010 to 02015).
   b. The list does not account for differences in wind conditions.
   c. If bicycling is performed in a race, classify it as general racing if no descriptions are given about drafting (code 01050). If information is given about the speed or drafting code as 01050 (bicycling, 16–19 mph, racing/not drafting or > 19 mph drafting, very fast) or 01060 (bicycling, ≤ 20 mph, racing, not drafting).
   d. Using a mountain bike in the city should be classified as bicycling, general (code 01010). Cycling on mountain trails or on a BMX course is coded 01009.
2. Conditioning Exercises.
   a. If a calisthenics program is described as a light or moderate type of activity (e.g., performing back exercises) but indicates a vigorous effort on the part of the participant, code the activity as calisthenics, general (code 02030).
   b. Exercise performed at a health club that is not described should be classified as health club, general (code 02060). Other activities performed at a health club (e.g., weight lifting, aerobic dance, circuit training, treadmill running, etc. at a health club) should be classified under separate major headings.
   c. Regardless of whether aerobic dance, conditioning, circuit training, or water calisthenics programs are described by their component parts (i.e., 10 min jogging in place, 10 min sit-ups, 10 min stretching, etc.), code the activity as one activity (e.g., water aerobics, code 02120).
   d. Effort, speed, or intensity breakdowns for the specific activities of stair-treadmill ergometer (code 02065), ski machine (code 02080), water aerobics or water calisthenics (code 02120), circuit training (code 02040), and slimnastics (code 02090) are not given. Code these as general, even though effort or intensities may vary in the descriptions of the activity.
3. Dancing
   a. If the type of dancing performed is not described, code it as dancing, general (code 03025).
4. Home Activities
   a. House cleaning should be coded as light (code 05040) or heavy (code 05020). Examples for each are given in the description of the specific activities.
   b. Making the bed on a daily basis is coded 05100. Changing the bed sheets is coded as cleaning, light (code 05040).
5. Home Repair
   a. Any painting outside of the house (i.e., fence, the house, barn) is coded, painting, outside house (code 60150).
6. Inactivity
   a. Sitting and reading a book or newspaper is listed under the major heading of Miscellaneous, reading, book, newspaper, etc. (code 09030).
   b. Sitting and writing is listed under the major heading of Miscellaneous, writing (code 09040).
7. Lawn and Garden
   a. Working in the garden with a specific type of tool (e.g., hoe, spade) is coded as digging, spading, filling garden (code 08050).
   b. Removing snow may be done by one of three methods: shoveling snow by hand (code 08200), walking and operating a snow blower (code 08130), or riding a snow blower (code 08180).
8. Music Playing
   a. Most variation in music playing will be according to the setting (i.e., rock and roll band, orchestra, marching band, concert band, standing on the stage, performance, practice, in a church etc.). The compendium does not consider differences in the setting (except for marching band and guitar playing).
9. Occupation
   a. Types of occupational activities not listed separately under specific activities (e.g., chemistry laboratory experiments), should be placed into the types of energy expenditure classifications best describing the activity. See sitting: light (code 11580), sitting: moderate (code 11590), standing: light (code 11600), standing: light to moderate (code 11610), standing: moderate (code 11620), standing: moderate to heavy code 11630).
   b. Driving an automobile or a light truck for employment (taxi cab, salesman, contractor, ambulance driver, bus driver), should be listed under the major heading of Transportation, automobile or light truck (not a semi) driving (code 06010).
   c. Performing skin or SCUBA diving as an occupation is listed under the major heading of Water Activities, and the specific activity of skindiving or SCUBA diving as a frogman (code 18170).
10. Running
   a. Running is not classified as treadmill or outdoor running. Running on a treadmill or outdoors should be coded by the speed of the run (codes 12030 to 12130). If speed is not given, code it as running, general (code 12150).
11. Self-care
   a. The compendium does not account for effort ratings. All items are considered to be general.
12. Transportation
   a. Being a passenger in an automobile is coded under the major heading of inactivity, sitting quietly (code 07020).

(continued)

Appendix A.3. *(continued)*

13. Walking
    a. Household walking is coded 17150, regardless if the subject identified a walking speed.
    b. If the walking speed is unidentified, use 3.0 mph, level, moderate, firm surface as the standard speed (code 17190). This should not be used for household walking.
    c. Walking during a household move, shopping, or for household work is coded under the major heading of Home Activities. Walking for job-related activities is coded under Occupational Activities.
    d. If a subject is backpacking, regardless of descriptors attached, the code is backpacking, general (code 17010).
    e. The compendium does not account for variations in speed or effort while carrying luggage or a child.
    f. Mountain climbing should be classified as general (rock or mountain climbing, code 17120) if no descriptors are given. If the weight of the load is described, code the activity as climbing hills with the appropriate load (codes 17030 to 17060).
    g. Walking on a grassy area (golf course, in a park, etc.) should be coded as walking, grass track (code 17260). The compendium does not account for variations in walking speed on a grassy area, so ignore recording walking speed or effort. If the walking is not on a grassy area, code activity according to the walking speed (codes 17150 to 17230).
    h. Walking to work or to class should be coded as 17270. The compendium does not account for walking speed or effort in this activity.
    i. Hiking and cross-country walking (code 17080) should be used when the walking activity lasted 3 h or more. Do not use this category backpacking, but for day hikes.

14. Water Activities
    a. Swimming should be coded as leisurely, not lap swimming, general (code 18310) if descriptors about stroke, speed, or swimming location are not given.
    b. Lap swimming should be coded as swimming laps, freestyle, slow (code 18240) if the activity is described as lap swimming, light or moderate effort, but stroke or speed are not indicated. Swimming laps should be coded as swimming, laps, freestyle, fast (code 18230) if the activity described as lap swimming, vigorous effort, but stroke or speed are not given.
    c. Swimming crawl should be coded as swimming, crawl, slow (50 yards/min^{-1}) if speed is not given and the effort is rated light or moderate (code 18290). Swimming crawl should be coded as swimming, crawl, fast (yards/min^{-1}) if speed is not given, but the effort is rated as vigorous (code 18280).
    d. The swimming strokes of backstroke (code 18250), breaststroke (code 18260), butterfly (code 18270), and sidestroke (code 18230) are code as general for speed and intensity.
    e. If a swimming activity is not identified as lake, ocean, or river swimming (code 18300), assume that the swimming was performed in a swimming pool.
    f. If canoeing is related to a canoe trip, code as canoeing, on a camping trip (code 18020). Otherwise, code it according to the speed and effort listed.

classify the intensity level, and the record the duration to ensure accurate data entry.

It is important the participant complete all questions except the space labeled "for clinic use only." The clinic staff will use this space to record the activity code or MET value for data analysis. The space labeled "reason for activity" is to help the coder decide under which major heading to place the activity. The intensity rating is designed to help the coder in assigning the appropriate MET value. Intensity terms of light, moderate, heavy or vigorous, and very heavy or very vigorous should be used in classifying intensity. In the case of walking, the corresponding intensity terms are very slow, slow, moderate, brisk, and very brisk. If a coder does not plan to use the five digit code for data analysis, a space can be provided on the questionnaire to record the MET values to calculate kcal scores.

Discussion and Limitations

The Compendium of Activities is a classification system that groups physical activities by purpose and provides flexibility in determining energy cost. However, there are several factors that may limit the use of the Compendium for determining the precise energy cost of PA. The activity classification system was primarily based on previously published data and as such may not reflect the exact energy cost of all physical activities. Since often the values are merely averages, they do not take into account that some people perform activities more vigorously than others. In addition, the MET values of some activities were not derived from actual measurements of oxygen consumption; instead they were estimated from the energy cost of activities having similar movement patterns. Therefore, the estimates may have ill-defined confidence limits around the mean MET values. For activities in which the parameters are undefined, individual differences in energy expenditure can be large and the true energy cost for a person may or may not be close to the stated mean. This does not reduce the value of the standard intensity codes, but it is an important perspective from which to view the Compendium. Calculation of kcal energy expenditure from body weight and MET values may also affect the energy cost of activities. Therefore, the kcal scores should be used with caution in correlation analyses since coefficients may reflect body weight rather than the actual energy cost of activities. Expression of energy expenditure scores as kcal/kg^{-1} body weight/h^{-1} or kcal/kg^{-1} body weight/day^{-1} will eliminate this effect. Individual variation in movement patterns and differences in the way activity is reported (i.e., effort, pace, age, and gender differences) may influence the energy cost of activities also. For example, one person may rate his or her walking pace as "brisk" while another classifies the same pace as "slow." The Compendium cannot account for individual differences in movement efficiency; however, variation in how physical activities are recorded can be reduced by providing instruction to participants on how to classify energy expenditure (i.e., 3 mph is moderate walking), standardizing data recording techniques, and having trained interviewers review the data with participants for clarity before energy costs are calculated.

▶ SUMMARY

The Compendium of Physical Activities is a unique coding system that classifies the energy cost of physical activities. Based on previously published data, it groups activities by purpose and intensity expressed as METs. The Compendium is easy to use and provides flexibility in calculating the energy cost of various types of physical activities. Despite its possible limitations, the Compendium of Physical Activities is useful for coding physical activity questionnaires or records used in physical activity research, education, and clinic settings.

We wish to thank M. Carl McNally, Mark Richardson, Terri Hartman, and Yvonne Guptill (University of Minnesota) and Martin Yee (Stanford University) for their contributions in creating and organizing the Compendium of Physical Activities. We offer a special thank you to Carl McNally for writing the SAS data analysis program to score the Compendium of Physical Activities.

This work was supported by grants NHLBI (RFA-86-90-P) to Drs. Leon and Jacobs: NHLBI (5-R01-HL-37561) to Dr. Montoye; NHLBI (HL-362-72) to Dr. Haskell; and NHLBI (RFA-86-HL-9-P) to Dr. Sallis.

Dr. Barbara Ainsworth was a post-doctoral associate in the Division of Epidemiology, School of Public Health, University of Minnesota at the time of this project. Dr. Ainsworth is currently with the Applied Physiology Laboratory, Department of Physical Education, Exercise and Sport Science, University of North Carolina at Chapel Hill.

References

1. Bannister EW, Brown SR. The relative energy requirements of physical activity. In: Falls HB, ed. *Exercise Physiology.* New York: Academic Press, 1968.
2. Blair SN, Haskell WL, Ho P, et al. Assessment of habitual physical activity by a 7-day recall in a community survey and controlled experiment. *Am J Epidemiol* 1985;122:794–804,1985.
3. Burke EJ, Auchinachie JA, Hayden R, et al. Energy cost of wheelchair basketball. *Physician Sportsmed;*13:99–105.
4. Fisher SV, Patterson RP. Energy cost of ambulation with crutches. *Arch Phys Med Rehabil* 1981;62:250–256.
5. Folsom AR, Caspersen CJ, Taylor HL, et al. Leisure time physical activity and its relationship to coronary risk factors in a population-based sample: the Minnesota Heart Survey. *Am J Epidemiol* 1985;121:570–579.
6. Howley ET, Glover ME. The caloric costs of running and walking one mile for men and women. *Med Sci Sports Exerc* 1974;6:235.
7. Katch FI, McArdle WD. *Nutrition, Weight Control, and Exercise.* 3rd Ed. Philadelphia: Lea & Febiger, 1988.
8. Leon AS. Approximate energy expenditures and fitness values of sports and recreational and household activities. In: Wynder EL, ed. *The Book of Health Physical Fitness.* 1981;283–341.
9. McArdle WD, Katch FI, Katch VL. *Exercise physiology: Energy, Nutrition, and Human Performance.* 2nd Ed. Philadelphia: Lea & Feriger, 1988;642–649.
10. Minnesota Leisure Time Physical Activity Questionnaire Manual. Division of Epidemiology. School of Public Health. University of Minnesota, Minneapolis, MN 55455.
11. O'Connell ER, Thomas PC, Cady LD, et al. Energy costs of simulated stair climbing as a job-related task in fire fighting. *J Occup Med* 1986;28:282–284.
12. Passmore R, Durnin JVGA. Human energy expenditure. *Physiol Rev* 1955;35:801–840.
13. Reiff GG, Montoye HJ, Remington RD, et al. Assessment of physical activity by questionnaire and interview. In: Karvonen MJ, Barry AJ, eds. *Physical Activity and the Heart.* Springfield, IL: Charles C Thomas, 1967;336–371.
14. Reiff GG, Montoye HJ, Remington RD, et al. Assessment of physical activity by questionnaire and interview. *J Sports Med Phys Fitness* 1967;7:1-32.
15. Taylor H, Jacobins DR Jr., Schucker B, et al. A questionnaire for the assessment of leisure time physical activities. *J Chronic Dis* 1978;31:741–755.
16. Town GP, Sol N, Sinning WE. The effect of rope skipping rate on energy expenditure of males and females. *Med Sci Sport Exerc* 1980;12:295–298.

APPENDIX **B**

IHRSA Briefing Paper: OSHA Blood-borne Pathogen Standard HIV and Hepatitis B Regulatory Alert

WHAT IS THE PURPOSE OF THE BLOOD-BORNE PATHOGENS STANDARD?

The Occupational Safety and Health Administration (OSHA) has issued standards to reduce occupational exposure to blood and other potentially infectious materials that could lead to disease or death in the workplace.

Blood-borne pathogens are microorganisms in human blood that can cause disease in humans, which include the hepatitis B virus (HBV) and the human immunodeficiency virus (HIV).

WHO IS COVERED BY THE STANDARDS?

The standards apply to employers with employees who may be "reasonably anticipated" to come in contact with human blood and other potentially infectious materials to perform their job.

ARE HEALTH CLUBS COVERED BY THE STANDARDS?

Yes, since it is likely clubs have employees that may be "reasonably anticipated" to come in contact with human blood or other infectious fluids, such as:

- Any club personnel responsible for first aid
- Housekeeping/laundry staff that could handle bloody towels, razors, or other potentially infectious waste
- Fitness staff with close contact with members or sharp objects or equipment that could be bloody
- Personal service workers whose jobs involve close personal contact with clients/members such as hairdressers, barbers and massage therapists

WHAT ARE THE OTHER POTENTIALLY INFECTIOUS MATERIALS BESIDES BLOOD?

Potential infectious materials include semen, vaginal secretions, cerebrospinal fluid, synovial fluid, pleural fluid, pericardial fluid, peritoneal fluid, amniotic fluid, saliva in dental procedures, and any body fluid visibly contaminated with blood.

WHAT DOES THE STANDARD REQUIRE EMPLOYERS TO DO?

The standard requires an employer to establish a written exposure control plan and other procedures for reducing the risk of disease or death from blood-borne pathogens. The written plan must:

1. Identify the tasks, procedures, and job classifications where occupational exposure to blood occurs.
2. Set forth a schedule for implementing the provisions of the plan.
3. Specify the means to protect and train those employees.

Procedures that employers are required to perform include:

1. Using engineering controls where appropriate, i.e., controls that isolate or remove the blood-borne pathogens from the workplace, such as puncture-resistant containers for used needles.
2. Introducing work practices to reduce contamination, such as providing hand-washing facilities which are readily accessible to employees.
3. Providing, at no cost to the employee, appropriate personal protective equipment such as gowns and gloves.
4. Introducing requirements for housekeeping-covered decontamination procedures, a written schedule for cleaning, and handling of regulated waste and specific procedures for handling contaminated laundry.
5. Offering, at the employer's expense, voluntary hepatitis B vaccinations to all employees with occupational exposure and prescribing appropriate medical follow-up and counseling after an exposure incident.

6. Training workers initially and then annually thereafter to alert them to the risks posed by blood-borne pathogens.
7. Providing appropriate labels and maintaining records of exposure incidents, post exposure follow-ups, hepatitis B vaccinations and employee training.

WHEN DOES THIS REGULATION BECOME EFFECTIVE?

In most states, covered employees are required to have an Exposure Control Plan by May 5, 1992. Information, training requirements, and record keeping are required by June 4, 1992. All other provisions take effect on July 6, 1992.

While it is important to take steps to comply with this standard immediately, OSHA is currently focusing its enforcement on the medical and dental community.

If your club is in Alaska, Arizona, California, Connecticut, Hawaii, Indiana, Iowa, Kentucky, Maryland, Michigan, Minnesota, Nevada, New Mexico, New York, North Carolina, Oregon, South Carolina, Tennessee, Utah, Vermont, Virginia, Washington, and Wyoming, you may have up to an additional 6 months before the regulation becomes effective. Call your state department of occupational safety and health to determine the effective date of the new standards for your state.

WHAT IS THE PENALTY FOR FAILURE TO COMPLY WITH BLOOD-BORNE PATHOGENS STANDARD?

The violation of an OSHA standard can involve potential criminal liability or civil liability and fines. The severity of the penalty is directly related to the seriousness and willfulness of the violation.

WHERE CAN WE GET MORE INFORMATION ON THE BLOOD-BORNE PATHOGENS STANDARD?

Check your phone book under the US Government: Department of Labor, Occupational Safety and Health Administration (OSHA). Ask you local OSHA office to send you the "Prototype Blood-borne Exposure Control Plan."

You may also want to contact local medical providers or local medical societies to see if they will share their plan with you. In addition, there are some private companies that will assist you in meeting the requirements of the regulations.

APPENDIX **C**

Common Medications

Table C.1. **Generic and Brand Names of Common Drugs by Class**

Generic Name	Brand Name
Beta Blockers	
Acebutolol	Sectral
Atenolol	Tenormin
Bisopropolol	Zebeta
Esmolol	Brevibloc (IV)
Metoprolol	Lopressor, Toprol
Nadolol	Corgard
Pindolol	Visken
Propranolol	Inderal
Sotalol	Betapace
Timolol	Blocadren
Carteolol	Cartrol
Betaxolal	Kerlone
Bisoprolol	Zebeta
Penbutolol	Levatol
Alpha$_1$ Blockers	
Prazosin	Minipress
Terazosin	Hytrin
Doxazosin	Cardura
Alpha and Beta Blockers	
Carvedilol	Coreg
Labetalol	Trandate, Normodyne
Antiadrenergic Agents Without Selective Receptor Blockade	
Clonidine	Catapres
Guanabenz	Wyntensin
Guanethidine	Ismelin
Guanfacine	Tenex
Methyldopa	Aldomet
Reserpine	Serapasil
Guanadrel	Hylorel
Nitrates and Nitoglycerin	
Isosorbide dinitrate	Isordil, Diltrate
Nitroglycerin	Nitrostat, Nitrolingual spray
Nitroglycerin ointment	Nitrol ointment
Nitroglycerin patches	Transderm Nitro, Nitro-Dur II, Nitrodisc
Isosorbide mononitrate	Ismo, Monoket, Imdur
Calcium Channel Blockers	
Diltiazem	Cardizem, Dilacor, Tiazac
Meberfradil	Posicard
Nifedipine	Procardia, Adalat
Nisoldipine	Sular
Verapamil	Calan, Isoptin
Nicardipine	Cardene
Amlodipine	Norvasc
Felodipine	Plendil
Isradipine	DynaCirc
Nimodipine	Nimotop
Bepridil	Vascor
Cardiac Glycosides	
Digitalis	Digoxin, Lanoxin
Diuretics	
Thiazides	
Chlorthiazide	Diuril
Hydrochlorothiazide (HCTZ)	Esidrix, Hydrodiuril
Indapamide	Lozol
"Loops"	
Furosemide	Lasix
Bumetanidine	Bumex
Ethacrynic acid	Edecrin
Torsemide	Demadex
Potassium-Sparing	
Spironolactone	Aldactone
Triamterene	Dyrenium
Amiloride	Midamor
Combinations	
Trimterine and hydrochlorothiazide	Dyazide, Maxzide
Amiloride and hydrochlorothiazide	Moduretic
Others	
Metolazone	Zaroxolyn
Peripheral Vasodilators (Nonadrenergic)	
Hydralazine	Apresoline
Minoxidil	Loniten
Angiotensin-Converting Enzyme (ACE) Inhibitors	
Captopril	Capoten
Enalapril	Vasotec
Lisinopril	Prinivil, Zestril, Prinzide
Moexipril	Univasc

Table C.1. *(continued)*

GENERIC NAME	BRAND NAME
Ramipril	Altace
Benazepril	Lotensin
Fosinopril	Monopril
Quinapril	Accupril
Trandolapril	Mavik
Angiotensin II Receptor Antagonist	
Losartan	Cozaar
Valsartan	Diovan
Antiarrhythmic Agents	
Class I	
IA	
Quinidine	Quinidex, Quinaglute
Procainamide	Pronestyl, Procan SR
Disopyramide	Norpace
IB	
Tocainide*	Tonocard*
Mexiletine	Mexitil
Phenytoin	Dilantin
Lidocaine	Xylocaine, Xylocard
IC	
Encainidine	Enkaid
Flecainide	Tambocor
Propafenone	Rythmol
Multiclass	
Moricizine	Ethmozine
Class II	
β-Blockers	
Propranolol	Inderal
Acebutolol	Sectral
Esmolol	Brevibloc
Class III	
Amiodarone	Cordarone
Bretylium	Bretylol
Ibutilide	Corvet
Sotalol	Betapace
Class IV	
Calcium channel blockers	
Verapamil	Procardia
Diltiazem	Cardizem
Other	
Digoxin	Digitalis
Adenosine	Adenocard (IV), Adenoscan (IV)
Sympathomimetic Agents	
Ephedrine	Adrenalin
Epinephrine	Alupent
Metaproterenol	Proventil, Ventolin
Albuterol	Bronkosol
Isoetharine	Brethine
Cromolyn sodium	Intal
Antihyperlipidemic Agents	
Atorvastatin	Lipitor
Cerivastatin	Baycol
Cholestyramine	Questran
Clofibrate	Atromid-S
Colestipol	Colestid
Gemfibrozil	Lopid
Lovastatin	Mevacor
Nicotinic acid (niacin)	Nicobid, Nicolar, Slo-Niacin
Pravastatin	Pravachol
Simvastatin	Zocor
Fluvastatin	Lescol
Anticoagulants	
Ticlopidine Hydrocloride	Ticlid
Warfarin	Coumadin
Pentoxifylline	Trental
Dypridamole	Persantine
Abcixamab	ReoPro
Oral-antihyperglycemics	
Glyburide	DiaBeta, Glynase, Micronase
Metformin hydrochloride	Glucophage
Troglitazone	Rezulin

* limited clinical use

Index

Page numbers in *italics* denote figures; those followed by "t" denote tables

I

Q

R